The American Psychiatric Publishing
Textbook of
Personality Disorders

The American Psychiatric Publishing

Textbook of
Personality Disorders

Edited by

John M. Oldham, M.D., M.S.

Andrew E. Skodol, M.D.

Donna S. Bender, Ph.D.

Associate Editors

Glen O. Gabbard, M.D.

Joel Paris, M.D.

M. Tracie Shea, Ph.D.

Thomas A. Widiger, Ph.D.

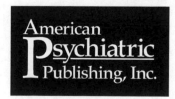

Washington, DC
London, England

Copyright © 2005 American Psychiatric Publishing, Inc.
ALL RIGHTS RESERVED

Manufactured in the United States of America on acid-free paper
09 08 07 06 05   5 4 3 2 1
First Edition

Typeset in Adobe's Palatino and Optima.

American Psychiatric Publishing, Inc.
1000 Wilson Boulevard
Arlington, VA 22209-3901
www.appi.org

Library of Congress Cataloging-in-Publication Data
The American Psychiatric Publishing textbook of personality disorders / edited by John M. Oldham, Andrew E. Skodol, Donna S. Bender.—1st ed.
     p. ; cm.
   Includes bibliographical references and index.
   ISBN 1-58562-159-5 (hardcover : alk. paper)
  1. Personality disorders. 2. Personality disorders—Treatment.
   [DNLM: 1. Personality Disorders—therapy. 2. Personality Disorders—diagnosis. 3. Personality Disorders—etiology. WM 190 A5125 2005] I. Title: Textbook of personality disorders. II. Oldham, John M. III. Skodol, Andrew E. IV. Bender, Donna S., 1960– V. American Psychiatric Publishing.
   RC554.A247 2005
   616.85'81–dc22
                                                                                                                    2004023812

British Library Cataloguing in Publication Data
A CIP record is available from the British Library.

To our families, who have supported us:

Karen, Madeleine, and Michael Oldham;
Laura, Dan, and Ali Skodol; and
John and Joseph Rosegrant.

To our colleagues, who have helped us.

To our patients, who have taught us.

And to each other, for the friendship that has enriched our work together.

Contents

Part I
Basic Concepts

Part II
Clinical Evaluation

Part III
Etiology

Part IV
Treatment

Part VI
New Developments and
Future Directions

Contributors

Renato D. Alarcón, M.D., M.P.H.
Professor of Psychiatry, Mayo Clinic College of Medicine; Chair, Inpatient Psychiatry and Psychology Division, and Medical Director, Mayo Psychiatry and Psychology Treatment Center, Rochester, Minnesota

Gerianne M. Alexander, Ph.D.
Assistant Professor of Psychology, Department of Psychology, Texas A&M University, College Station, Texas

Ann H. Appelbaum, M.D.
Clinical Professor of Psychiatry, Department of Psychiatry, Columbia University College of Physicians and Surgeons, New York, New York

Samuel A. Ball, Ph.D.
Associate Professor of Psychiatry, Department of Psychiatry, Yale University School of Medicine, West Haven, Connecticut

Anthony W. Bateman, M.A., F.R.C.Psych.
Visiting Professor, Sub-Department of Clinical Health Psychology, University College London; Consultant Psychotherapist, Barnet, Enfield, and Haringey Mental Health Trust, London, England

Donna S. Bender, Ph.D.
Assistant Clinical Professor of Medical Psychology in Psychiatry, Columbia University College of Physicians and Surgeons; Research Scientist, Department of Personality Studies, New York State Psychiatric Institute, New York, New York

Christina Boggs, M.S.
Graduate Student, Department of Psychology, Texas A&M University, College Station, Texas

Martin Bohus, M.D.
Chair in Psychosomatic Medicine, University of Heidelberg; Director, Department of Psychosomatic Medicine and Psychotherapy, Central Institute of Mental Health, Mannheim, Germany

Michael Bond, M.D.
Psychiatrist-in-Chief, Sir Mortimer B. Davis Jewish General Hospital; Associate Professor, Department of Psychiatry, McGill University, Montréal, Québec, Canada

Beth S. Brodsky, Ph.D.
Assistant Clinical Professor of Medical Psychology, Department of Psychiatry, Columbia University College of Physicians and Surgeons; Research Scientist, Department of Neuroscience, New York State Psychiatric Institute, New York, New York

Elizabeth Bromley, M.D.
Robert Wood Johnson Clinical Scholar, West Los Angeles VA Mental Illness Research, Education, and Clinical Center (MIRECC) and Department of Psychiatry and Biobehavioral Sciences, University of California, Los Angeles, California

John F. Clarkin, Ph.D.
Professor of Clinical Psychology in Psychiatry, Department of Psychiatry, Weill Medical College of Cornell University, New York, New York

C. Robert Cloninger, M.D.
Wallace Renard Professor of Psychiatry, Genetics, and Psychology, Washington University School of Medicine, St. Louis, Missouri

Emil F. Coccaro, M.D.
Ellen C. Manning Professor and Chairman, Department of Psychiatry, University of Chicago, Chicago, Illinois

Patricia Cohen, Ph.D.
Professor of Psychiatry, Columbia University College of Physicians and Surgeons, New York, New York

Jeremy Coid, M.D.
Professor of Forensic Psychiatry, Forensic Psychiatry Research Unit, St. Bartholomew's Hospital, London, England

Thomas Crawford, Ph.D.
Assistant Clinical Professor of Medical Psychology, Columbia University College of Physicians and Surgeons, New York, New York

Amit Etkin, M.Phil.
Center for Neurobiology and Behavior, Kavli Institute for Brain Sciences, Columbia University, New York, New York

Peter Fonagy, Ph.D., F.B.A.
Freud Memorial Professor of Psychoanalysis and Director of the Sub-Department of Clinical Health Psychology, University College London; Chief Executive of the Anna Freud Centre, London, England; and Consultant to the Child and Family Program, Menninger Department of Psychiatry, Baylor College of Medicine, Houston, Texas

Alan E. Fruzzetti, Ph.D.
Associate Professor and Director, Dialectical Behavior Therapy Program, University of Nevada, Reno, Nevada

Glen O. Gabbard, M.D.
Brown Foundation Chair of Psychoanalysis and Professor, Department of Psychiatry, Baylor College of Medicine; Training and Supervising Analyst, Houston-Galveston Psychoanalytic Institute; Joint Editor-in-Chief, International Journal of Psychoanalysis, Houston, Texas

Mark S. George, M.D.
Distinguished Professor of Psychiatry, Neurology, and Radiology, Brain Stimulation Laboratory, Center for Advanced Imaging Research, Medical University of South Carolina, Charleston, South Carolina

Kim L. Gratz, Ph.D.
Clinical and Research Fellow, Center for the Treatment of Borderline Personality Disorder, McLean Hospital, Harvard Medical School, Boston, Massachusetts

Carlos M. Grilo, Ph.D.
Professor of Psychiatry, Department of Psychiatry, Yale University School of Medicine, New Haven, Connecticut

Seth D. Grossman, Psych.D.
Research Associate, Institute for Advanced Studies in Personology and Psychopathology, Coral Gables, Florida

John G. Gunderson, M.D.
Professor of Psychiatry, Harvard Medical School; Director, Psychosocial and Personality Research, McLean Hospital, Boston, Massachusetts

Thomas G. Gutheil, M.D.
Professor of Psychiatry, Harvard Medical School, and Co-Director, Program in Psychiatry and the Law, Massachusetts Mental Health Center, Boston, Massachusetts

Amy Heim, Ph.D.
Private practice, Hoover & Associates, Chicago, IL

Perry D. Hoffman, Ph.D.
President, National Education Alliance for Borderline Personality Disorder (NEA-BPD), Rye, New York; Research Associate, Department of Psychiatry, White Plains, New York, and Weill Medical College of Cornell University, New York, New York

Jeffrey G. Johnson, Ph.D.
Associate Professor of Clinical Psychology, Department of Psychiatry, College of Physicians and Surgeons, Columbia University; and Research Scientist IV, Epidemiology of Mental Disorders Department, New York State Psychiatric Institute, New York, New York

Eric R. Kandel, M.D.
Center for Neurobiology and Behavior, Kavli Institute for Brain Sciences, Howard Hughes Medical Institute, Columbia University, New York, New York

Janet Klosko, Ph.D.
Codirector, Cognitive Therapy Center of Long Island, Great Neck, New York; Senior Therapist, Cognitive Therapy Center of New York, New York, New York; and Clinical Psychologist, Woodstock Woman's Health, Woodstock, New York

Nathan Kolla
Undergraduate Research Program, Suicide Studies Unit, Department of Psychiatry, St. Michael's Hospital, University of Toronto, Toronto, Ontario, Canada

Kenneth N. Levy, Ph.D.
Assistant Professor, Department of Psychology, Pennsylvania State University, University Park, Pennsylvania; Adjunct Assistant Professor of Psychology, Department of Psychiatry, Joan and Sanford I. Weill Medical College of Cornell University, New York, New York

Paul S. Links, M.D., F.R.C.P.C.
Arthur Sommer Rotenberg Chair in Suicide Studies, Professor of Psychiatry, Department of Psychiatry, St. Michael's Hospital, University of Toronto, Toronto, Ontario, Canada

José R. Maldonado, M.D.
Associate Professor and Chief, Medical and Forensic Psychiatry Section; Chief, Medical Psychotherapy Clinic, Department of Psychiatry and Behavioral Sciences, Stanford University School of Medicine; Medical Director, Psychiatry Consultation/Liaison Service, Stanford University Medical Center; Faculty, Center for Biomedical Ethics and Chair, Ethics Committee, Stanford University Medical Center, Stanford, California

John C. Markowitz, M.D.
Research Psychiatrist 2, New York State Psychiatric Institute; Clinical Associate Professor of Psychiatry, Weill Medical College of Cornell University; Adjunct Clinical Associate Professor of Psychiatry, Columbia University College of Physicians and Surgeons, New York, New York

Wilson McDermut, Ph.D.
Assistant Professor, Department of Psychology, St. John's University, Jamaica, New York, and Staff Psychologist, Albert Ellis Institute, New York

Pamela G. McGeoch, M.A.
Graduate Faculty, Department of Psychology, The New School University, New York, New York; Psychology Intern, Creedmoor Psychiatric Center, Queens Village, New York

Thomas H. McGlashan, M.D.
Professor of Psychiatry, Department of Psychiatry, Yale University School of Medicine, New Haven, Connecticut

Michael J. Meaney, Ph.D.
James McGill Professor of Medicine and Director, McGill Program for the Study of Behavior, Genes, and Environment, Douglas Hospital Research Center, McGill University, Montréal, Québec, Canada

Theodore Millon, Ph.D., D.Sc.
Dean and Scientific Director, Institute for Advanced Studies in Personology and Psychopathology, Coral Gables, Florida; Postdoctoral Fellow, Florida International University, Miami, Florida

Chris Molnar, Ph.D.
Postdoctoral Fellow, Brain Stimulation Laboratory, Center for Advanced Imaging Research, Medical University of South Carolina, Charleston, South Carolina

Leslie C. Morey, Ph.D.
Professor of Psychology, Department of Psychology, Texas A&M University, College Station, Texas

Stephanie N. Mullins-Sweatt, M.A.
Graduate Student, Department of Psychology, University of Kentucky, Lexington, Kentucky

Ziad Nahas, M.D.
Assistant Professor, Department of Psychiatry; Medical Director, Brain Stimulation Laboratory, Center for Advanced Imaging Research, Medical University of South Carolina, Charleston, South Carolina

Edmund C. Neuhaus, Ph.D.
Director, Behavioral Health Partial Hospital, McLean Hospital, Boston, Massachusetts

John S. Ogrodniczuk, Ph.D.
Assistant Professor, Department of Psychiatry, University of British Columbia, Vancouver, British Columbia, Canada

John M. Oldham, M.D., M.S.
Professor and Chairman, Department of Psychiatry and Behavioral Sciences, Medical University of South Carolina, Charleston, South Carolina

Joel Paris, M.D.
Professor of Psychiatry, McGill University, Montréal, Québec, Canada

J. Christopher Perry, M.P.H., M.D.
Professor of Psychiatry, McGill University; Director of Psychotherapy Research, Institute of Community and Family Psychiatry, Sir Mortimer B. Davis Jewish General Hospital, Montréal, Québec, Canada; Research Affiliate, The Austen Riggs Center, Stockbridge, Massachusetts

William E. Piper, Ph.D.
Professor and Head, Division of Behavioural Science; Director, Psychotherapy Program, Department of Psychiatry, University of British Columbia, Vancouver, British Columbia, Canada

Christopher J. Pittenger, M.D., Ph.D.
Neuroscience Research Training Program, Department of Psychiatry, Yale University, New Haven, Connecticut

Christian Schmahl, M.D.
Assistant Medical Director, Department of Psychosomatic Medicine and Psychotherapy, Central Institute of Mental Health, Mannheim, Germany

Abigail Schlesinger, M.D.
Child Fellow, Western Psychiatric Institute and Clinic, University of Pittsburgh School of Medicine, Pittsburgh, Pennsylvania

M. Tracie Shea, Ph.D.
Associate Professor, Department of Psychiatry and Human Behavior, Brown University Medical School, Providence, Rhode Island

G. Pirooz Sholevar, M.D.
Clinical Professor of Psychiatry, Jefferson Medical College, Thomas Jefferson University, Philadelphia, Pennsylvania

Larry J. Siever, M.D.
Executive Director, Mental Illness Research, Education and Clinical Center, Bronx Veterans Administration Medical Center, Bronx, New York; Professor of Psychiatry, Department of Psychiatry, The Mount Sinai School of Medicine, New York, New York

Kenneth R. Silk, M.D.
Professor and Associate Chair, Clinical and Administrative Affairs, University of Michigan Health System, Ann Arbor, Michigan

Andrew E. Skodol, M.D.
Professor of Clinical Psychiatry, Columbia University College of Physicians and Surgeons, and Director, Department of Personality Studies, New York State Psychiatric Institute, New York, New York

George W. Smith, M.S.W.
Director, Outpatient Personality Disorder Services, McLean Hospital, Boston, Massachusetts

Paul H. Soloff, M.D.
Professor of Psychiatry, Western Psychiatric Institute and Clinic, Pittsburgh, Pennsylvania

David Spiegel, M.D.
Willson Professor and Associate Chair of Psychiatry and Behavioral Sciences, Department of Psychiatry and Behavioral Sciences, Stanford University School of Medicine, Stanford, California; Director, Center for Integrative Medicine, Stanford Hospital and Clinics

Barbara Stanley, Ph.D.
Lecturer, Department of Psychiatry, Columbia University College of Physicians and Surgeons; Research Scientist, Department of Neuroscience, New York State Psychiatric Institute; and Professor, Department of Psychology, City University of New York–John Jay College, New York, New York

Michael H. Stone, M.D.
Professor of Clinical Psychiatry, Columbia College of Physicians and Surgeons, New York, New York

Svenn Torgersen, Ph.D.
Professor, Department of Psychology, University of Oslo, Blindern, Norway

Peter Tyrer, M.D.
Professor of Community Psychiatry and Head of Department, Department of Psychological Medicine, Imperial College, London, United Kingdom

Louisa M.C. van den Bosch, Ph.D.
Clinical Psychologist and Administrative Executive, Forensic Psychiatric Hospital, Oldenkotte, Eibergen, The Netherlands

Roel Verheul, Ph.D.
Professor of Personality Disorders, Viersprong Institute for Studies on Personality Disorders (VISPD), Center of Psychotherapy De Viersprong, Halsteren, University of Amsterdam, Department of Clinical Psychology, Amsterdam, The Netherlands

Drew Westen, Ph.D.
Professor, Department of Psychiatry and Behavioral Sciences and Department of Psychology, Emory University, Atlanta, Georgia

Thomas A. Widiger, Ph.D.
Professor, Department of Psychology, University of Kentucky, Lexington, Kentucky

Frank E. Yeomans, M.D.
Clinical Associate Professor of Psychiatry, Department of Psychiatry, Weill Medical College of Cornell University, New York, New York

Jeffrey Young, Ph.D.
Assistant Professor of Clinical Psychology in Psychiatry, Department of Psychiatry, Columbia University; Director, Cognitive Therapy Centers of New York & Connecticut; Director, Schema Therapy Institute, New York, New York

Mark Zimmerman, M.D.
Associate Professor, Department of Psychiatry and Human Behavior, Brown University School of Medicine, and Director of Outpatient Psychiatry, Department of Psychiatry, Rhode Island Hospital, Providence, Rhode Island

Introduction

From as early as the fifth century B.C., it has been recognized that every human being develops an individualized signature pattern of behavior that is reasonably persistent and predictable throughout life. Hippocrates proposed that the varieties of human behavior could be organized into what we might now call prototypes—broad descriptive patterns of behavior characterized by typical, predominant, easily recognizable features—and that most individuals could be sorted into these broad categories. Sanguine, melancholic, choleric, and phlegmatic types of behavior were, in turn, thought to derive from "body humors," such as blood, black bile, yellow bile, and phlegm, and the predominance of a given body humor in an individual was thought to correlate with a particular behavior pattern. Although we now call body humors by different names (neurotransmitters, transcription factors, second messengers), the ancient principle that fundamental differences in biology correlate with relatively predictable patterns of behavior is strikingly familiar.

In spite of long-standing worldwide interest in personality types, however, remarkably little progress has been made, until recently, in our understanding of those severe and persistent patterns of inner experience and behavior that result in enduring emotional distress and impairment in occupational functioning and interpersonal relationships—the conditions we now refer to as personality disorders. For decades, it was widely recognized that some severely disturbed individuals just seemed to have been "born that way," a view we now know to be true in some cases involving significant genetic loading or risk. In the twentieth century, however, we became more interested in the role of the environment during early development in determining the shape of lasting adult behavior—a view that for a while extended well beyond the realm of the personality disorders to include most major mental disorders. We know, of course, that the early life environment is indeed critically important—from health-promoting, highly nurturing environments to stressful and neglectful environments from which only the most resilient emerge unscathed. But we also know that variable degrees of genetic risk predispose many of us to become ill in very specific ways, should we unluckily encounter more stress than we can tolerate.

In recent years, we have begun to see an upsurge of empirical and clinical interest in personality disorders. Improved standardized diagnostic systems have led to semistructured research interviews that are being used not only in studies of clinical populations but also in community-based studies, to give us, for the first time, good data about the epidemiology of these disorders. Personality disorders represent about 12% of the general population, and their public health significance has been documented by studies showing their extreme social dysfunction and high health care utilization. As clinical populations are becoming better defined, new and more rigorous treatment studies are being carried out, with increasingly promising results. No longer are personality disorders swept into the "hopeless cases" bin. An explosion of knowledge and technology in the neurosciences has made the formerly black box, the brain, more and more transparent. Mapping the human genome paved the way for new gene-finding technologies that are being put to work to tackle complex psychiatric disorders, including the personality disorders. New transgenic animal models are providing important hints about the genetic loci driving certain behavior types, such as attachment and bonding behavior. Brain imaging studies are allowing researchers to zero in on malfunctioning areas of the brain in specific personality disorders.

A great deal of work must still be done. Fundamental questions remain, such as what is the relationship between traits of general, or normal, personality functioning and personality psychopathology. Directly related to this issue is the ongoing debate about whether dimensional or categorical systems best capture the full scope of personality differences and personality pathology. The extent of impairment associated with personality disorders highlights the significance of gaining knowledge regarding their longer-term course and increased understanding of factors contributing to variations in course. But there is a strong momentum of interest internationally in these issues, as new research findings emerge daily to inform the process.

In light of the acceleration of interest and progress in the field of personality studies and personality disorders, we judged the time to be right to develop a comprehensive textbook of personality disorders, recognizing that "comprehensive" coverage of the field would be a daunting goal and that even newer findings would likely appear by the time the book was published. However, our attempt has been to assemble as many of the best experts in the field as we could, to present a thorough and informative survey of what we now know about the personality disorders. Thus, this book is organized into several parts: 1) Basic Concepts, 2) Clinical Evaluation, 3) Etiology, 4) Treatment, 5) Special Problems and Populations, and 6) New Developments and Future Directions.

PART I: BASIC CONCEPTS

Basic Concepts, the first part of _The American Psychiatric Publishing Textbook of Personality Disorders_, might be thought of as setting the stage for the parts that follow. In Chapter 1, Oldham presents a brief overview of the recent history of the personality disorders, along with a summary look at current controversies and possible future developments in the field. Heim and Westen, in the next chapter, review the major theories that have influenced our thinking about the nature of personality and personality disorders. In Chapter 3, Widiger and Mullins-Sweatt discuss in depth the arguments and evidence supporting either categorical models of personality pathology or dimensional, continuous models of personality styles and disorders.

PART II: CLINICAL EVALUATION

In the section on clinical evaluation beginning with Chapter 4, Skodol reviews the defining features of DSM-IV-TR personality disorders, discusses comple-

mentary approaches to the clinical assessment of a patient with a possible personality disorder, provides guidance on general problems encountered in the routine clinical evaluation, and describes patterns of Axis I and Axis II disorder comorbidity. The chapter concludes with a disorder-by-disorder discussion of specific problems in the differential diagnosis of the personality disorders and how the clinician might resolve them. In Chapter 5, McDermut and Zimmerman review the assessment instruments available for conducting standardized evaluations of personality disorders, including semistructured interviews, other clinician-administered instruments, and self-report questionnaires. The instruments covered are those that measure personality psychopathology according to the DSM-IV-TR taxonomy, as well as those that measure alternative concepts of personality and its pathology, such as the Five-Factor Model. Part II concludes with Chapter 6, in which Grilo and McGlashan provide an overview of the clinical course and outcome of personality disorders, synthesizing the empirical literature on the stability of personality disorder psychopathology.

PART III: ETIOLOGY

The section on etiology of the personality disorders begins with Chapter 7, a presentation by Paris of an integrative perspective on the personality disorders. Paris reviews the increasingly useful bidirectional stress-diathesis framework, along with its relevance to our understanding of the dual roles of genes and environment in the etiology of the personality disorders. Torgersen then presents, in Chapter 8, the best data we have to date on the population-based epidemiology of the personality disorders. Although there are relatively few well-designed population-based studies, Torgersen selects eight studies, including his own Norwegian study, and tabulates prevalence ranges and averages for individual DSM-defined personality disorders as well as for all personality disorders taken together (showing an overall average prevalence rate for the personality disorders of over 12%). Of particular interest in these data are cross-cultural comparisons, suggesting significant cultural differences in the prevalence of selected personality disorders. The genetic role in the etiology of personality disorders is summarized by Cloninger in Chapter 9, who argues that personality styles and disorders are comprised of multiple heritable dimensions, variably expressed, in combination with environmental factors. Substantial progress has been made in our understanding of these genetic influences, and new findings are emerging steadily on the neurobiology of the personality disorders, as reviewed in Chapter 10 by Coccaro and Siever. Although a great deal more is known about the neurobiology of some personality disorders (e.g., schizotypal personality disorder and borderline personality disorder) than others (e.g., Cluster C personality disorders), the underlying neurobiological dysfunction involved in personality disorders characterized by cognitive symptomatology, impulsivity, and mood dysregulation is becoming increasingly clear.

Understanding the etiology of the personality disorders involves not just cross-sectional genetic and neurobiological analysis; environmental influences shaping personality must be understood as well. In Chapter 11, Cohen and Crawford provide a developmental perspective. Although by convention DSM-IV-TR personality disorders are generally not diagnosed until late adolescence, there is increasing recognition of early patterns of behavior that are thought to be precursors to certain personality disorders. The challenge to identify true early precursors of personality disorders, versus the risk of inaccurate labeling of transient symptoms, is central to the work ahead of us as we focus more and more on prevention strategies. Developmental issues are central to an increasingly persuasive "mentalization model" of understanding borderline personality disorder, deriving from basic concepts of attachment theory—reviewed in Chapter 12 by Fonagy and Bateman. In this model, borderline personality disorder is seen as dysfunction in self-regulation, critically related to interpersonal dynamics. Complementing this model specific to borderline personality disorder, the authors of Chapter 13, Johnson, Bromley, and McGeoch, review the relevance of childhood experiences in the development of maladaptive personality traits. Consistent with the stress-diathesis model presented earlier by Paris in Chapter 7, Johnson and colleagues emphasize not just the importance of stress, but also the role of protective factors that can offset and even prevent the development of maladaptive traits in vulnerable individuals. Finally, the section on etiology closes with Chapter 14, a thoughtful review by Millon and Grossman of the many sociocultural factors that shape our behavior, both ordered and disordered.

PART IV: TREATMENT

The treatment section begins with Chapter 15, a discussion of the levels of care available for patients with personality disorders. Gunderson, Gratz, Neuhaus, and Smith offer guidelines for determining the appropriate intensity of treatment services for individual patients. Four levels of care are addressed: hospital, partial hospitalization/day treatment, intensive outpatient, and outpatient.

Chapters 16 through 21 offer a range of outpatient treatment options that are, for the most part, centered on interventions within a patient-therapist dyad. Gabbard (Chapter 16) summarizes the salient features of psychoanalysis as applied to patients with character pathology, while Yeomans, Clarkin, and Levy offer a review of various psychodynamic psychotherapy approaches in Chapter 17. In the cognitive-behavioral realm, Chapter 18 by Young and Klosko describes the latest schema-therapy developments for personality disorders, and in Chapter 19, Stanley and Brodsky outline the core elements of dialectical behavior therapy, which includes individual and group interventions, and is chiefly used to treat parasuicidal behaviors in patients with borderline personality disorder. Patients with borderline pathology are also the focus of a new treatment approach based on interpersonal principles, presented by Markowitz in Chapter 20. Appelbaum's (Chapter 21) synthesis of theories and techniques underpinning supportive psychotherapy provides a fundamental backdrop for many clinicians engaged in the treatment of personality disorders.

Apart from the realm of individual treatments, there are other venues for therapeutic interventions. In Chapter 22, Piper and Ogrodniczuk demonstrate the application of group therapy to personality disorders, and the family is the context for Sholevar's work, detailed in Chapter 23. In addition, Hoffman and Fruzzetti (Chapter 24) suggest various psychoeducational programs that might benefit personality disorder patients and their families. Further, Soloff (Chapter 25) takes up the issue of pharmacotherapy and other somatic treatments, because many patients with personality disorders may benefit by complementing their psychosocial treatments with medication.

The final three chapters of this section address issues of great importance pertaining to most, if not all, treatments. Bender (Chapter 26) underscores the necessity of explicitly considering alliance-building across all treatment modalities, while Gutheil (Chapter 27) cautions practitioners about dynamics that can lead treaters to boundary violations when working with certain patients with personality disorders. Finally, as many of these patients with personality disorders are engaged in several modalities with several clinicians at the same time, Schlesinger and Silk, in Chapter 28, provide recommendations about the best way of negotiating collaborative treatments.

PART V: SPECIAL PROBLEMS AND POPULATIONS

In recognition of the fact that patients with personality disorders can be particularly challenging, we have devoted a section of the Textbook to special problems and populations. Of prime importance is the risk for suicide. In Chapter 29, Links and Kolla provide evidence on the association of suicidal behavior and personality disorders, examine modifiable risk factors, and discuss clinical approaches to the assessment and management of suicide risk. In Chapter 30, Verheul, van den Bosch, and Ball focus on pathways to substance abuse in patients with personality disorders, and discuss issues of differential diagnosis and treatment.

Patients with personality disorders may be not only a danger to themselves, but also sometimes a danger to others. Stone, in Chapter 31, discusses aggression and violence associated with specific personality disorder types and factors predisposing to violent behavior. The chapter is illustrated by many clinical vignettes from literature and Stone's personal clinical experience. Chapter 32, by Maldonado and Spiegel, is a review of the literature on dissociative states and their relationship to personality disorder psychopathology. Chapter 33, by Perry and Bond, presents the theory and measurement of defense mechanisms relevant to personality disorders, with a discussion of how the management and interpretation of defenses can further psychotherapy. This chapter also includes many clinical examples of defenses observed in specific therapeutic interactions.

Gender and culture play important roles in the evaluation and treatment of personality disorders. These issues are dissected in Chapters 34 and 35. In Chapter 34, Morey, Alexander, and Boggs look at gender differences in the prevalence of personality disorders, discuss research bearing on the issue of gender bias in the diagnosis of personality disorders that may or may not account for gender distributions, and, finally, describe the interaction of biological and social factors in determining gender differences in personality traits and behaviors. In Chapter 35, Alarcón discusses the role of culture in the etiology, diagnosis, and treatment of personality disorders.

As personality disorders have received greater attention from the mental health fields, it has become increasingly apparent that they may be encountered outside of traditional mental health treatment settings, where they can present special problems in detection and management. In Chapter 36, Coid describes personality disorders as they are found in prison popula-tions and the role of personality disorders in determining the risks for the development of "career criminals." Tyrer's Chapter 37 on the significance of personality disorders occurring in the medically ill concludes the section on special problems and populations.

PART VI: NEW DEVELOPMENTS AND FUTURE DIRECTIONS

In the final section of *The American Psychiatric Publishing Textbook of Personality Disorders*, we have selected a few areas in which research is intensifying and key findings are anticipated that will increase our understanding of the personality disorders. In Chapter 38, Nahas, Molnar, and George review brain imaging studies of patients with personality disorders. Both structural and functional imaging studies are beginning to shed light on dysfunctions in the brain in a number of the personality disorders, particularly in schizotypal personality disorder, borderline personality disorder, and antisocial personality disorder. The very application of basic research methods to the study of personality disorders is illustrated not only by brain imaging research but by the utility of the principles of translational research, illustrated in Chapter 39 by Bohus and Schmahl, and by the relevance of animal models for the study of personality disorders, reviewed in Chapter 40 by Meaney. Finally, in Chapter 41, Etkin, Pittenger, and Kandel present what is currently known about biological changes in the brain produced by psychotherapy, from the vantage point of psychotherapy as a form of learning. Of particular relevance, they suggest that neuroimaging techniques may enable us to identify brain substrates that are particularly relevant to patients with personality disorders, in order to guide prediction of treatment outcome.

We are grateful to all of the authors of each chapter for their careful and thoughtful contributions, and we hope that we have succeeded in providing a current, definitive review of the field. We would particularly like to thank Liz Bednarowicz for her organized and steadfast administrative support, without which this volume would not have been possible.

John M. Oldham, M.D., M.S.
Charleston, South Carolina

Andrew E. Skodol, M.D.
New York, New York

Donna S. Bender, Ph.D.
New York, New York

Part I

Basic Concepts

1

Personality Disorders

Recent History and Future Directions

John M. Oldham, M.D., M.S.

PERSONALITY TYPES AND PERSONALITY DISORDERS

Charting a historical review of efforts to understand personality types and the differences among them would involve exploring centuries of scholarly archives, worldwide, on the varieties of human behavior. For it is human behavior, in the end, that serves as the most valid measurable and observable benchmark of personality. In many important ways, we are what we do. The "what" of personality is easier to come by than the "why," and each of us has a personality style that is unique, almost like a fingerprint. At a school reunion, recognition of classmates not seen for decades derives as much from familiar behavior as from physical appearance.

As to why we behave the way we do, we know now that a fair amount of the reason relates to our "hardwiring." To varying degrees, heritable temperaments that vary widely from one individual to another determine the amazing range of behavior in the newborn nursery, from cranky to placid. Each individual's temperament remains a key component of that person's developing personality, to which is added the shaping and molding influences of family, caretakers, and environmental experiences. This process is, we now know, bidirectional, so that the "in-born" behavior of the infant can elicit behavior in parents or caretakers that can, in turn, reinforce infant behavior: placid, happy babies may elicit warm and nurturing behaviors; irritable babies may elicit impatient and neglectful behaviors.

However, even-tempered, easy-to-care-for babies can have bad luck and land in a nonsupportive or even abusive environment that may set the stage for a personality disorder, and difficult-to-care-for babies can have good luck and be protected from future personality pathology by specially talented and attentive caretakers. Once these highly individualized dynamics have had their main effects and an individual has reached late adolescence or young adulthood, his or her personality will usually have been pretty well established. We know that this is not an ironclad rule;

Sections of this chapter have been modified with permission from Oldham JM, Skodol AE: "Charting the Future of Axis II." *Journal of Personality Disorders* 14:17–29 2000.

there are "late bloomers," and high-impact life events can derail or reroute any of us. How much we can change if we need and want to is variable, but change is possible. How we define the differences between personality styles and personality disorders, how the two relate to each other, what systems best capture the magnificent variety of nonpathological human behavior, and how we think about and deal with extremes of behavior that we call personality disorders are all spelled out in great detail in the chapters of this textbook. In this first chapter, I briefly describe how psychiatrists in the United States have approached the definition and classification of the personality disorders, building on broader international concepts and theories of psychopathology.

TWENTIETH-CENTURY CONCEPTS OF PERSONALITY PSYCHOPATHOLOGY

Personality pathology has been recognized in most influential systems of classifying psychopathology. The well-known contributions by European pioneers of descriptive psychiatry, such as Kraepelin (1904), Bleuler (1924), Kretschmer (1926), and Schneider (1923) had an important impact on early twentieth-century American psychiatry. For the most part, Kraepelin, Bleuler, and Kretschmer described personality types or temperaments, such as aesthenic, autistic, schizoid, cyclothymic, or cycloid, that were thought to be precursors or less extreme forms of psychotic conditions, such as schizophrenia or manic-depressive illness—systems that can clearly be seen as forerunners of current Axis I/Axis II "spectrum" models. Schneider, on the other hand, described a set of "psychopathic personalities" that he viewed as separate disorders co-occurring with other psychiatric disorders. Although these classical systems of descriptive psychopathology resonate strongly with the framework eventually adopted by the American Psychiatric Association (APA) and published in its *Diagnostic and Statistical Manual of Mental Disorders* (DSM), they were widely overshadowed in American psychiatry during the mid-twentieth century by theory-based psychoanalytic concepts stimulated by the work of Sigmund Freud and his followers.

Freud emphasized the presence of a dynamic unconscious, a realm that, by definition, is mostly unavailable to conscious thought but is a powerful motivator of human behavior (key ingredients of his topographical model). His emphasis on a dynamic unconscious was augmented by his well-known tripartite structural theory, a conflict model serving as the bedrock of his psychosexual theory of pathology (Freud 1926). Freud theorized that certain unconscious sexual wishes or impulses (id) could threaten to emerge into consciousness (ego), thus colliding wholesale with strict conscience-driven prohibitions (superego) and producing "signal" anxiety, precipitating unconscious defense mechanisms and, when these coping strategies prove insufficient, leading to frank symptom formation. For the most part, this system was proposed as an explanation for what were called at the time the *symptom neuroses,* such as hysterical neurosis or obsessive-compulsive neurosis. During the 1940s, 1950s, and 1960s, these ideas became dominant in American psychiatry, followed later by interest in other psychoanalytic principles, such as object relations theory.

Freud's concentration on the symptom neuroses involved the central notion of anxiety as the engine that led to defense mechanisms and to symptom formation, and as a critical factor in motivating patients to work hard in psychoanalysis to face painful realizations and to tolerate stress within the treatment itself (such as that involved in the "transference neurosis"). Less prominently articulated were Freud's notions of character pathology, but generally character disorders were seen to represent "pre-oedipal" pathology. As such, patients with these conditions were judged less likely to be motivated to change. Instead of experiencing anxiety related to the potential gratification of an unacceptable sexual impulse, patients with "fixations" at the oral-dependent stage, for example, experienced anxiety when *not* gratifying the impulse—in this case, the need to be fed. Relief of anxiety thus could be accomplished by some combination of real and symbolic feeding—attention from a parent or parent figure or consumption of alcohol or drugs. Deprivations within the psychoanalytic situation, then—inevitable by its very nature—could lead to patient flight and interrupted treatment.

In a way, social attitudes mirrored and extended these beliefs such that although personality pathology was well known, it was often thought to reflect weakness of character or willfully offensive or socially deviant behavior produced by faulty upbringing, rather than understood as "legitimate" psychopathology. A good example of this view could be seen in military psychiatry in the mid-1900s, where those discharged from active duty for mental illness, with eligibility for disability and medical benefits, did not include individuals with "character disorders" (or alcoholism and substance abuse) because these conditions were seen as "bad behavior" and led to administrative, nonmedical separation from the military.

In spite of these common attitudes, clinicians recognized that many patients with significant impairment in social or occupational functioning, or with significant emotional distress, needed treatment for psychopathology that did not involve frank psychosis or other syndromes characterized by discrete, persistent symptom patterns such as major depressive episodes, persistent anxiety, or dementia. General clinical experience and wisdom guided treatment recommendations for these patients, at least for those who sought treatment. Patients with paranoid, schizoid, or antisocial patterns of thinking and behaving often did not seek treatment. Others, however, often resembled patients with symptom neuroses and did seek help for problems ranging from self-destructive behavior to chronic misery. The most severely and persistently disabled of these patients were often referred for intensive, psychoanalytically oriented long-term inpatient treatment at treatment centers such as Austen Riggs, Chestnut Lodge, Menninger Clinic, McLean Hospital, New York Hospital Westchester Division, New York State Psychiatric Institute, Sheppard Pratt, and other long-term inpatient facilities available at the time. Other patients, able to function outside of a hospital setting and often hard to distinguish from patients with neuroses, were referred for outpatient psychoanalysis or intensive psychoanalytically oriented psychotherapy. As Gunderson (2001) described, the fact that many such patients in psychoanalysis regressed and seemed to get worse, rather than showing improvement in treatment, was one factor that contributed to the emerging concept of borderline personality disorder (BPD), thought initially to be in the border zone between the psychoses and the neuroses. Patients in this general category included some who had previously been labeled as having latent schizophrenia (Bleuler 1924), ambulatory schizophrenia (Zillborg 1941), pseudoneurotic schizophrenia (Hoch and Polatin 1949), psychotic character (Frosch 1964), or "as-if" personality (Deutsch 1942).

These developments coincided with new approaches based on alternative theoretical models that were emerging within the psychoanalytic framework, such as the British object relations school. New conceptual frameworks, such as Kernberg's (1975) model of borderline personality organization or Kohut's (1971) concept of the central importance of empathic failure in the histories of narcissistic patients, served as the basis for an intensive psychodynamic treatment approach for selected patients with personality disorders. These strategies and others are reviewed in detail in Chapter 16, "Psychoanalysis."

The DSM System

Contrary to assumptions commonly encountered, personality disorders have been included in every edition of the APA's *Diagnostic and Statistical Manual of Mental Disorders*. Largely driven by the need for standardized psychiatric diagnosis in the context of World War II, the United States War Department in 1943 developed a document labeled "Technical Bulletin 203," representing a psychoanalytically oriented system of terminology for classifying mental illness precipitated by stress (Barton 1987). The APA charged its Committee on Nomenclature and Statistics to solicit expert opinion and to develop a diagnostic manual that would codify and standardize psychiatric diagnoses. This diagnostic system became the framework for the first edition of DSM (DSM-I; American Psychiatric Association 1952). This manual was widely utilized, and it was subsequently revised on several occasions, leading to DSM-II (American Psychiatric Association 1968), DSM-III (American Psychiatric Association 1980), DSM-III-R (American Psychiatric Association 1987), DSM-IV (American Psychiatric Association 1994), and DSM-IV-TR (American Psychiatric Association 2000). Figure 1–1 (Skodol 1997) portrays the ontogeny of diagnostic terms relevant to the personality disorders from DSM-I through DSM-IV (DSM-IV-TR involved only text revisions; it used the same diagnostic terms as DSM-IV).

Although not explicit in the narrative text, DSM-I reflected the general view of personality disorders at the time, elements of which persist to the present. Generally, personality disorders were viewed as more or less permanent patterns of behavior and human interaction that were established by early adulthood and were unlikely to change throughout the life cycle. Thorny issues such as how to differentiate personality disorders from personality styles or traits, which remain actively debated today, were clearly identified at the time. Personality disorders were contrasted with the symptom neuroses in a number of ways, particularly that the neuroses were characterized by anxiety and distress, whereas the personality disorders were often ego-syntonic and thus not recognized by those who had them. Even today, we hear descriptions of some personality disorders as "externalizing"—that is, disorders in which the patient disavows any problem but blames all discomfort on the real or perceived unreasonableness of others. Notions of personality

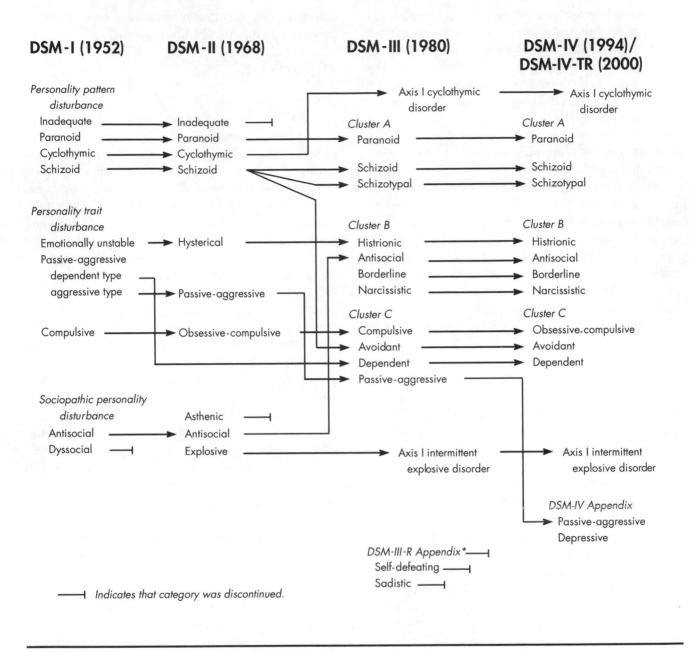

Figure 1–1.   Ontogeny of personality disorder classification.

*No changes were made to the personality disorder classification in DSM-III-R except for the inclusion of self-defeating and sadistic personality disorders in Appendix A: Proposed Diagnostic Categories Needing Further Study. These two categories were not included in DSM-IV or in DSM-IV-TR.

Source.   Reprinted with permission from Skodol AE: "Classification, Assessment, and Differential Diagnosis of Personality Disorders." *Journal of Practical Psychiatry and Behavioral Health* 3:261–274, 1997.

psychopathology still resonate with concepts such as those of Reich (1933/1945), who described defensive "character armor" as a lifetime protective shield.

In DSM-I, personality disorders were generally viewed as deficit conditions reflecting partial developmental arrests or distortions in development secondary to inadequate or pathological early caretaking. The personality disorders were grouped primarily into "personality pattern disturbances," "personality trait disturbances," and "sociopathic personality disturbances." *Personality pattern disturbances* were viewed as the most entrenched conditions and likely to be recalcitrant to change, even with treatment; these included inadequate personality, schizoid personality, cyclothymic personality, and paranoid personality. *Personality trait disturbances* were thought to be less pervasive and disabling, so that in the absence of stress these patients could function relatively well. If under significant stress, however, patients with emotionally unstable, passive-aggressive, or compulsive personalities were thought to show emotional distress and deterioration in functioning, and they were variably motivated for and amenable to treatment. The category of *sociopathic personality disturbances* reflected what were generally seen as types of social deviance at the time, including antisocial reaction, dyssocial reaction, sexual deviation, and addiction (subcategorized into alcoholism and drug addiction).

The primary stimulus leading to the development of a new, second edition of DSM was the publication of the eighth edition of the International Classification of Diseases (World Health Organization 1968) and the wish of the APA to reconcile its diagnostic terminology with this international system. In the DSM revision process, an effort was made to move away from theory-derived diagnoses and to attempt to reach consensus on the main constellations of personality that were observable, measurable, enduring, and consistent over time. The earlier view that patients with personality disorders did not experience emotional distress was discarded, as were the DSM-I subcategories of personality pattern, personality trait, and sociopathic personality disturbances. One new personality disorder was added, called asthenic personality disorder, only to be deleted in the next edition of the DSM.

By the mid 1970s, greater emphasis was placed on increasing the reliability of all diagnoses; whenever possible, diagnostic criteria that were observable and measurable were developed to define each diagnosis. DSM-III, the third edition of the diagnostic manual, was developed and introduced a multiaxial system. Disorders classified on Axis I included those generally seen as episodic, characterized by exacerbations and remissions, such as psychoses, mood disorders, and anxiety disorders. Axis II was established to include the personality disorders as well as mental retardation; both groups were seen as composed of early onset, persistent conditions, but mental retardation was understood to be "biological" in origin, in contrast to the personality disorders, which were generally regarded as "psychological" in origin. The stated reason for placing the personality disorders on Axis II was to ensure that "consideration is given to the possible presence of disorders that are frequently overlooked when attention is directed to the usually more florid Axis I disorders" (American Psychiatric Association 1980, p. 23). It is generally agreed that the decision to place the personality disorders on Axis II led to greater recognition of the personality disorders and

stimulated extensive research and progress in our understanding of these conditions.

As shown in Figure 1–1, the DSM-II diagnoses of inadequate personality disorder and asthenic personality disorder were discontinued in DSM-III. The diagnosis of explosive personality disorder was changed to intermittent explosive disorder, cyclothymic personality disorder was renamed cyclothymic disorder, and both of these diagnoses were moved to Axis I. Schizoid personality disorder was felt to be too broad a category in DSM-II, and it was recrafted into three personality disorders: *schizoid personality disorder*, reflecting "loners" who are uninterested in close personal relationships; *schizotypal personality disorder*, understood to be on the schizophrenia spectrum of disorders and characterized by eccentric beliefs and nontraditional behavior; and *avoidant personality disorder*, typified by self-imposed interpersonal isolation driven by self-consciousness and anxiety. Two new personality disorder diagnoses were added in DSM-III: BPD and narcissistic personality disorder. In contrast to initial notions that patients called "borderline" were on the border between the psychoses and the neuroses, the criteria defining BPD in DSM-III emphasized emotional dysregulation, unstable interpersonal relationships, and loss of impulse control more than cognitive distortions and marginal reality testing, which were more characteristic of schizotypal personality disorder. Among many scholars whose work greatly influenced and shaped our understanding of borderline pathology were Kernberg (1975) and Gunderson (1984, 2001). Although concepts of narcissism had been described by Freud, Reich, and others, the essence of the current views of narcissistic personality disorder emerged from the work of Millon (1969), Kohut (1971), and Kernberg (1975).

DSM-III-R was published in 1987 after an intensive process to revise DSM-III involving widely solicited input from researchers and clinicians and following similar principles to those articulated in DSM-III, such as assuring reliable diagnostic categories that were clinically useful and consistent with research findings and thus minimizing reliance on theory. Efforts were made for diagnoses to be "descriptive" and to require a minimum of inference, although the introductory text of DSM-III-R acknowledged that for some disorders, "particularly the Personality Disorders, the criteria require much more inference on the part of the observer" (American Psychiatric Association 1987, p. xxiii). No changes were made in DSM-III-R diagnostic categories of personality disorders, although some adjustments were made in certain criteria sets, for example, making them uniformly polythetic instead of defining some personality disorders with monothetic criteria sets (e.g., dependent personality disorder) and others with polythetic criteria sets (e.g., borderline personality disorder). In addition, two personality disorders were included in DSM-III-R in Appendix A ("Proposed Diagnostic Categories Needing Further Study")—self-defeating personality disorder and sadistic personality disorder—based on prior clinical recommendations to the DSM-III-R personality disorder subcommittee. These diagnoses were considered provisional, pending further review and research.

DSM-IV was derived after an extensive process of literature review, data analysis, field trials, and feedback from the profession. Because of the increase in research stimulated by the criteria-based multiaxial system of DSM-III, a substantial body of evidence existed to guide the DSM-IV process. As a result, the threshold for approval of revisions for DSM-IV was higher than that used in DSM-III or DSM-III-R. DSM-IV introduced, for the first time, a set of general diagnostic criteria for any personality disorder (Table 1–1), underscoring qualities such as early onset, long duration, inflexibility, and pervasiveness. Diagnostic categories and dimensional organization of the personality disorders into clusters remained the same in DSM-IV as in DSM-III-R, with the exception of the relocation of passive-aggressive personality disorder from the "official" diagnostic list to Appendix B ("Criteria Sets and Axes Provided for Further Study"). Passive-aggressive personality disorder, as defined by DSM-III and DSM-III-R, was thought to be too unidimensional and generic; it was tentatively retitled "negativistic personality disorder," and the criteria were revised. In addition, the two provisional Axis II diagnoses in DSM-III-R, self-defeating personality disorder and sadistic personality disorder, were dropped because of insufficient research data and clinical consensus to support their retention. One other personality disorder was proposed and added to Appendix B: depressive personality disorder. Although substantially controversial, this provisional diagnosis was proposed as a pessimistic cognitive style; its validity and its distinction from passive-aggressive personality disorder on Axis II or dysthymic disorder on Axis I, however, remain to be established.

DSM-IV-TR, published in 2000, did not change the diagnostic terms or criteria of DSM-IV. The intent of DSM-IV-TR was to revise the descriptive, narrative text accompanying each diagnosis where it seemed indicated and to update the information provided. Only

Table 1–1.   General diagnostic criteria for a personality disorder

A. An enduring pattern of inner experience and behavior that deviates markedly from the expectations of the individual's culture. This pattern is manifested in two (or more) of the following areas:

    (1) cognition (i.e., ways of perceiving and interpreting self, other people, and events)

    (2) affectivity (i.e., the range, intensity, lability, and appropriateness of emotional response)

    (3) interpersonal functioning

    (4) impulse control

B. The enduring pattern is inflexible and pervasive across a broad range of personal and social situations.

C. The enduring pattern leads to clinically significant distress or impairment in social, occupational, or other important areas of functioning.

D. The pattern is stable and of long duration, and its onset can be traced back at least to adolescence or early adulthood.

E. The enduring pattern is not better accounted for as a manifestation or consequence of another mental disorder.

F. The enduring pattern is not due to the direct physiological effects of a substance (e.g., a drug of abuse, a medication) or a general medical condition (e.g., head trauma).

Source.   Reprinted with permission from American Psychiatric Association: *Diagnostic and Statistical Manual of Mental Disorders*, 4th Edition, Text Revision. Washington, DC, American Psychiatric Association, 2000.

minimal revisions were made in the text material accompanying the personality disorders.

Current Controversies and Future Directions

There is a general consensus, at least in the United States, that the placement of the personality disorders on Axis II has stimulated research and focused clinical and educational attention on these disabling conditions. However, there is growing debate about the continued appropriateness of maintaining the personality disorders on a separate axis in future editions of the diagnostic manual and about whether a dimensional or a categorical system of classification is preferable. As new knowledge has rapidly accumulated about the personality disorders, these controversies take their places among many ongoing constructive dialogues, such as the relationship of normal personality to personality disorder, the pros and cons of polythetic criteria sets, how to determine the appropriate number of criteria (i.e., threshold) required for each diagnosis, which personality disorder categories have construct validity, which dimensions best cover the scope of normal and abnormal personality, and others. Many of these discussions overlap with and inform each other, yet a central issue under scrutiny is whether or not to maintain a separate diagnostic axis for the personality disorders. I briefly review some ongoing challenges and debates in the following sections, all of which are examined in greater detail in the subsequent chapters in this volume.

Dimensional or Categorical?

Much of the literature poses the question of a dimensional or categorical system as a debate or competition, as though one must choose sides in a "dimensional versus categorical" Super Bowl. Blashfield and McElroy (1995) provided helpful clarification about our terminology, pointing out that a "categorical model is a more complex, elaborated version of a dimensional model" (p. 409). They noted that the DSM-IV system includes 10 categories grouped into three dimensions (called clusters), and they clarified, as did Livesley et al. (1994), Clark (1995), Widiger (1993) and others (Gunderson et al. 1991; Livesley 1998), that dimensional structure implies continuity whereas categorical structure implies discontinuity. For example, being pregnant is a categorical concept (either one is pregnant or one is not, even though we speak of how "far along" one is), whereas being tall or short might better be conceptualized dimensionally, because there is no exact definition of either, notions of tallness or shortness may vary among different cultures, and all gradations of height exist along a continuum.

We know, of course, that the DSM system is referred to as categorical and is contrasted to any number of systems referred to as dimensional, such as the interpersonal circumplex (Benjamin 1993; Kiesler 1983; Wiggins 1982), the three-factor model (Eysenck and Eysenck 1975), several four-factor models (Clark et al. 1996; Livesley et al. 1993, 1998; Watson et al. 1994; Widiger 1998), the five-factor model (Costa and McCrae 1992), and the seven-factor model (Cloninger et al. 1993). How fundamental is the difference between the two types of systems? Livesley et al. (1994) went so far as to say that "DSM-III-R categorical diagnoses are based on cutting scores. Individuals who meet more than a threshold number of criteria are believed to be qualitatively different from those who meet fewer criteria" (p. 8). They added that "[a]lthough many of the features of the DSM-III-R and DSM-IV...personality disorder diagnoses are not substantively different from features of normal personality, they are used to define discontinuous categories" (p. 8). Although this

concept of discontinuity is implied by a categorical system, clinicians do not necessarily think in such dichotomous terms. Thresholds defining disease categories, such as hypertension, are in fact somewhat arbitrary, as is certainly the case with the personality disorders. In addition, the polythetic criteria sets for the DSM-IV personality disorders contain an element of dimensionality, because one can just meet the threshold or can have all of the criteria (and thus presumably a more extreme version of the disorder). Widiger (1991a, 1993) and Widiger and Sanderson (1995) suggested that this inherent dimensionality in our existing system could be usefully operationalized by stratifying each personality disorder into subcategories of "absent, traits, subthreshold, threshold, moderate, and extreme" according to the number of criteria met. Certainly if an individual is one criterion short of being diagnosed with a personality disorder, clinicians do not necessarily assume that there is no element of the disorder present; instead, prudent clinicians would understand that features of the disorder need to be recognized if present and may need attention. Nonetheless, a prudent, thoughtful clinician is one thing, and a busy, pressured clinician hustling to get paperwork finished may be another; there would be a natural tendency to think categorically—that is, to decide what disorders the patient "officially" has and to disregard all else. In fact, studies of clinical practice patterns reveal that clinicians generally assign only one Axis II diagnosis (Westen 1997), whereas systematic studies of clinical populations utilizing semistructured interviews generally reveal multiple Axis II diagnoses and significant traits in individuals who have pathology on Axis II (Oldham et al. 1992; Shedler and Westen 2004; Skodol et al. 1988; Widiger et al. 1991).

Definition of a Personality Disorder

As mentioned previously, DSM-IV introduced general criteria defining personality disorders that emphasize the early onset; the primary, enduring and cross-situational nature of the pathology; and the presence of emotional distress or impairment in social or occupational functioning. Although this effort to specify the generic components of all personality disorders has been helpful, the definition is relatively nonspecific and could apply to many Axis I disorders as well, such as dysthymia or even schizophrenia. In fact, DSM-IV-TR states that it

> may be particularly difficult (and not particularly useful) to distinguish Personality Disorders from those Axis I disorders (e.g., Dysthymic Disorder) that have an early onset and a chronic, relatively sta-

ble course. Some Personality Disorders may have a 'spectrum' relationship to particular Axis I conditions (e.g., Schizotypal Personality Disorder with Schizophrenia; Avoidant Personality Disorder with Social Phobia) based on phenomenological or biological similarities or familial aggregation. (American Psychiatric Association 2000, p. 688)

Livesley (1998) and Livesley and Jang (2000) proposed that the two key ingredients of a revised definition for personality disorder might be chronic interpersonal difficulties and problems with a sense of self, notions consistent with Kernberg's umbrella concept of borderline personality organization (Kernberg 1975) that encompasses many of the DSM-IV personality disorder categories and also consistent with earlier concepts of personality pathology (Schneider 1923). Livesley (1998) proposed a working definition for *personality disorder* as a "tripartite failure involving 3 separate but interrelated realms of functioning: self-system, familial or kinship relationships, and societal or group relationships" (p. 141). This proposed revision was suggested as one that could more readily be translated into reliable measures and as one that derives from an understanding of the "functions of normal personality." Although this definition conceptually links personality pathology with normal personality traits and emphasizes dimensional continuity, how readily measurable a "failure in a self-system" would be seems unclear. More importantly, this proposed definition could be applied to major Axis I conditions such as schizophrenia, unless one added the third criterion for borderline personality organization described by Kernberg (1975): maintenance of reality testing.

Whether the current generic personality disorder definition is retained or a new one such as that just described were to be adopted, there would still be a need for specified types of personality disorders—retaining or modifying the existing categories or replacing them with selected dimensions. In either case, criteria defining the types would be needed. Problems with the current criteria include the hodgepodge mixture of traits and behavioral measures, a confusion that has been criticized (Livesley and Jackson 1992; Widiger 1991a). Widiger (1991a) described the problems in the DSM system that resulted from the unsuccessful efforts of the DSM authors to devise criteria sets that *define* each personality disorder and that provide measures with which to *diagnose* each disorder at the same time. Initial attempts by the DSM-III committee to include only measurable and observable (i.e., behavioral) criteria were most evident in the much-criticized criteria set for antisocial personality disorder (seen as a checklist

for criminal behavior that omitted "lack of remorse" [later added in DSM-III-R], a fundamental defining feature of psychopathy), yet not so evident in other cases such as narcissistic personality disorder (which *did* include "lack of empathy" as one type of disturbance in interpersonal relationships—a defining feature of the concept of narcissism rather than a readily assessed or measured behavior).

Widiger (1991a) suggested that two criteria sets might be devised, one to define a disorder and a different one to diagnose it, but he admitted that sufficiently comprehensive behavioral criteria sets would be too lengthy to be practical. Livesley and Jackson (1992) also suggested developing a definitional system based on expert opinion and complemented by a set of diagnostic "exemplars," each of which should be direct, noncomplex, and relevant to only one trait of a diagnosis and only one diagnosis. Although perhaps this model represents a laudable goal, it would be a daunting challenge to identify such specific behavioral criteria (exemplars). For example, a simple, direct, measurable behavior such as spending most of one's time alone could reflect anxiety, depression, low self-esteem, lack of self-confidence, schizoid disconnectedness, or paranoid suspiciousness. Finally, even if one succeeded in developing a reasonably representative set of behavioral criteria considered diagnostic of a personality disorder, it is unlikely, as a number of authors have pointed out (Gunderson 1987; Widiger 1991a), that such a set would be optimal in all situations, because personality pathology is often activated or intensified by circumstance, such as loss of a job or of a meaningful relationship. In the ongoing findings of the Collaborative Longitudinal Study of Personality Disorders (Grilo et al. 2004; Shea et al. 2002), this problem has become evident, because stability of diagnosis must rely on sustained pathology above the DSM-IV-TR diagnostic threshold, and substantial percentages of patients show fluctuation over time, sometimes being above and sometimes below the diagnostic threshold. These data support an argument for a more flexible dimensional component to our diagnostic system, perhaps along the lines of Widiger's stratification scheme (Widiger 1991a, 1993; Widiger and Sanderson 1995).

One suggested way to better capture the essence of each personality disorder is to define the "classic" case—that is, the prototype. Livesley (1986, 1987) utilized DSM-III categories and reported that clinicians could reliably agree on prototypical traits and behaviors of the personality disorders. Widiger (1991a) cautioned, however, that such prototypes might not apply to most cases seen in clinical practice and thus might be of little utility. Although it does seem clear that clinicians can prioritize the criteria of each Axis II diagnosis when asked to list, in order of importance, the criteria they believe to be most representative of the disorder, different information may be obtained when clinicians are asked different questions. Westen and Arkowitz-Westen (1998) reported the results of a survey of clinicians who were asked if they were treating patients with personality pathology who could not be diagnosed on Axis II. They found, in a survey of clinicians, that over 60% of patients reported to have personality pathology for which treatment was indicated were "currently undiagnosable on Axis II." The results suggested that "much of the personality pathology clinicians see and treat in practice may not be captured by Axis II of DSM-IV" (p. 1767). Westen and Shedler (1999a, 1999b) devised a method based on a Q-score system to develop clinician-derived prototypes. They presented seven Q-factors (dysphoric, antisocial-psychopathic, schizoid, paranoid, obsessional, histrionic, and narcissistic), the psychological features of which, they proposed, represent coherent, meaningful clinical syndromes. In later work, Shedler and Westen (2004) again proposed a prototype matching model for diagnosing personality disorders in the context of concerns about the narrowness of the DSM criteria sets and the resulting extensive overlap among some diagnostic categories.

Reliability and Validity

Many authors have discussed the continuing questions of reliability and validity, which inevitably must be considered together (Clark et al. 1997; Lenzenweger and Clarkin 1996; Livesley 1998; Perry 1990). Debates continue regarding the most reliable ways to assess the Axis II categories. In clinical research, semistructured interviews have been developed, such as the International Personality Disorder Examination (Loranger 1999), the Structured Interview for DSM-IV Personality Disorders (Pfohl et al. 1997), and the Structured Clinical Interview for DSM-IV (First et al. 1997; see Chapter 4, "Manifestations, Clinical Diagnosis, and Comorbidity," and Chapter 5, "Assessment Instruments and Standardized Evaluation"). These interviews are called semistructured because they are administered by a clinician rather than an untrained technician so that the clinician can probe and explore areas of confusion or inconsistency and can employ clinical judgment in making ratings. These methods involve at least two data sources, the clinician and the patient, and some require input from collateral informants.

Studies have repeatedly shown that good interrater reliability can be achieved for most Axis II semistructured interviews, but inter-interview agreement is consistently poor (Oldham et al. 1992; Perry 1992; Pilkonis et al. 1991; Skodol et al. 1988). This inability to obtain the same data from the same patient with different interview instruments may indeed relate to differences in interview construction, but it may also reflect underlying questions about the construct validity of the diagnostic categories themselves (Livesley 1998; Perry 1990). Overlapping criteria in many of the categories diminish the "points of rarity" (Kendell 1975; Livesley et al. 1994) or discontinuity between categories. Systematic studies reveal high levels of comorbidity within Axis II itself, suggesting that the various categories may not be independent, valid constructs. Spitzer (1983) proposed a LEAD ("longitudinal expert evaluation using all data") standard, but operationalization of this standard in clinical research or in efficient clinical care is formidable.

Future Directions

Where do we go from here? Livesley (1998) contended that "[w]hatever advantages accrued from forcing clinicians to consider personality during the diagnostic process by placing personality disorders on a separate axis have been realized" (p. 139). The problems and concerns about the justification of maintaining the personality disorders on Axis II have been discussed at length (Krueger and Tackett 2003; Millon 2000; Shea and Yen 2003; Widiger 2003), particularly as potential changes that might be incorporated into DSM-V are anticipated. What are the suggestions for change and how feasible are they?

Move Personality Disorders to Axis I

In the context of addressing the lack of clear differentiation between Axis I and Axis II (Pfohl 1999), Widiger and Shea (1991) suggested that some Axis II disorders could be shifted to Axis I, and vice versa. A variation of this suggestion would be "to move some of the personality disorders to Axis I but to retain each's label as a personality disorder (or code them on both Axes I and II). This acknowledges that the Axes I and II boundary is fluid, at times with no real distinction" (p. 402). Livesley et al. (1994) broadened this suggestion, stating that "[b]ecause personality disorder does not appear to be substantially different in kind from other mental disorders, we would prefer to classify personality disorder on Axis I and to use a separate axis (perhaps Axis II) to code personality traits" (p. 14). Arguments are increasingly persuasive that Axis II disorders, as currently defined in DSM-IV-TR, are not fundamentally distinct from Axis I disorders. Nonetheless, there might still be plausible reasons to maintain the personality disorders on Axis II, in the context of significant revisions.

Replace the Current Axis II Categorical System With a Dimensional System

Frances (1993) stated that "[s]omeday (perhaps in time for the fifth edition of [DSM]), we will almost certainly be applying a dimensional model of personality diagnosis" (p. 110). The overwhelming majority of opinion in the literature on this subject favors the adoption of some type of dimensional approach (Clark et al. 1996; Cloninger et al. 1993; Costa and Widiger 1994; First et al. 2002; Frances 1993; Livesley 1998; Livesley and Jackson 1992; Livesley et al. 1993, 1998; Tellegen 1993; Watson et al. 1994; Westen and Shedler 1999a, 1999b; Widiger 1991a, 1991b, 1992, 1993, 1998; Widiger and Shea 1991). There is evidence supporting the dimensional view that personality psychopathology represents a crescendo on the end of a continuous scale defining personality traits (the "hypertension model") (Livesley et al. 1993, 1998). Conceptualized, then, as exaggerations of normal functioning (intense, extreme, hence maladaptive personality traits), the challenge to those creating the diagnostic manual is to develop a scheme that portrays this dimensional continuity and includes normal personality types or traits. Advocates of the categorical system contend that such a change would be too discrepant from traditional medical and clinical tradition and that the categorical system, admittedly a somewhat artificial convention, should be maintained.

Emphasize Level of Functioning

A number of authors emphasize the importance of level of functioning in the classification of personality and personality disorders (Gunderson et al. 1991; Kernberg 1975; Livesley et al. 1994; Skodol et al. 2002; Tyrer 1995; Westen and Arkowitz-Westen 1998). Kernberg's (1975) concept of borderline personality organization implies such a hierarchy, distinguishing three broad categories of intrapsychic structure (neurotic, borderline, and psychotic) that roughly correlate with decreasingly successful functioning. Gunderson et al. (1991) broadened this concept, portraying individuals with all personality disorders in an intermediate level between higher-functioning neurotic patients and lower-functioning psychotic patients. Such schemes

represent, in effect, dimensions of severity (e.g., mild, moderate, and severe) into which all mental illnesses could, theoretically, be sorted. In contrast, DSM-IV included impairment in social or occupational functioning as one of the defining criteria for personality disorders, which could then be evaluated utilizing Axis V, the Global Assessment of Functioning (GAF) Scale. Skodol et al. (1988) and Goldman et al. (1992) criticized the use of the GAF Scale because it confounds impairment in social and occupational functioning with symptom levels. Westen and Arkowitz-Westen (1998) argued in favor of a "functional assessment of personality," representing a case-formulation approach. They argued that instead of asking diagnostic questions such as "Does the patient cross the threshold for a personality disorder?" or "How low is the patient on the trait of agreeableness?" a functional assessment would ask, "Under what circumstances are which dysfunctional cognitive, affective, motivational, and behavioral patterns likely to occur?" Although approaches such as these are appealing, they represent a plea to return to the time-honored tradition of careful clinical assessment and formulation; how effectively such systems could be standardized for research purposes or for clinical use is not clear.

Retain Personality Disorders on Axis II but Collapse and Stratify the Current Categories

One possible modification of the current system would be to retain the categorical system but specify that no patient should be given more than two comorbid personality disorder diagnoses using the existing categories (Oldham and Skodol 2000; Oldham et al. 1992). In such a model, when three or more personality disorders are determined to be present (above threshold) in any given patient, a single diagnosis could be utilized (e.g., "extensive personality disorder"). Widiger and Sanderson (1995) noted that this suggestion "would eliminate the conceptual and clinical oddity of diagnosing a patient with three, four, or more purportedly comorbid and distinct personality disorders" (p. 445). They also noted, however, that it would fail to address the presence of clinically significant traits that are below the diagnostic threshold. This concern could be addressed in the following way: for patients with more than two comorbid personality disorder diagnoses, one could diagnose "extensive personality disorder," characterized by (a, b, c) components (above-threshold categories) and (x, y, z) features (clinically significant traits). The determination of which below-threshold traits are clinically significant could be either a matter of judgment by the clinician or based on a designated number of criteria met, as proposed by Widiger (1991a, 1993) and Widiger and Sanderson (1995).

Although the nature of personality disorders is not, after all, fundamentally distinct from that of many disorders on Axis I—hence conceptual consistency might better be approached by relocating them on Axis I—a preferable model for DSM-V might be to reconfigure and retain the personality disorders on Axis II. The primary justification for maintaining the personality disorders on a separate axis would be to allow the inclusion of trait assessment in DSM, a manual dedicated to the diagnosis of psychopathology. Eventually (perhaps beyond DSM-V), continuous concepts could be developed that encompass normal personality styles, personality disorder traits, and personality disorders themselves. Clinicians could evaluate potentially clinically significant traits within a dimensional *and* categorical system. (As Tellegen [1993] stated, "[t]he terms *dimensional* and *categorical* are sometimes contrasted as if standing for mutually exclusive alternatives. In reality, valid dimensional and categorical distinctions exist side by side, both among indicators and among latent variables" [p. 123].) It would then be possible, by retaining existing or revised personality disorder categories, to stratify them in a more systematic way, such as that described by Widiger (1991a, 1993) and Widiger and Sanderson (1995).

Such a scheme could be readily charted and displayed on a graph like that of the Minnesota Multiphasic Personality Inventory, further conveying the integration of its categorical and dimensional aspects. In this proposal, dimensional traits are pathology-defined because they represent the presence of some of the criteria of the disorders. A more ambitious proposal would be to develop criteria for normal personality types that correspond to their extreme forms—that is, the disorders. Such a DSM-IV–based system has been described (Oldham and Morris 1995), but the criteria for normal personality types (or others that could be developed) would need to be validated.

Finally, a decision to maintain the personality disorders on Axis II—but to introduce a stratification system such as that described above—would not require retention of the exact categories presently included in DSM-IV. An empirically based set of diagnoses such as the prototypes described by Westen and Shedler (1999a, 1999b) could be adopted. This set of categories was developed based on clinician opinion and is based on prototypes derived from clinical constructs closely related

to DSM-IV. As a result, these categories would be quite familiar to the clinical world and could be readily accepted. Although a broader revision could be attempted that could include normal personality types and that might incorporate a well-researched dimensional approach such as the five-factor model, such an undertaking might still be premature for DSM-V.

CONCLUSIONS

This brief review of recent notions of personality pathology serves as a window on the rapid progress in our field and in our understanding of psychiatric disorders. Increasingly, a stress/diathesis framework seems applicable in medicine in general as a unifying model of illness—a model that can easily encompass the personality disorders (Paris 1999). Variable genetic vulnerabilities predispose us all to potential future illness that may or may not develop depending on the balance of specific stressors and protective factors.

The personality disorders represent maladaptive exaggerations of nonpathological personality styles resulting from predisposing temperaments combined with stressful circumstances. Neurobiology can be altered in at least some Axis II disorders, as it can be in Axis I disorders. Our challenge for the future is to recognize that not all personality disorders are alike, nor are personality disorders fundamentally different from many other psychiatric disorders. What may be somewhat unique to the personality disorders is their correlation and continuity with normal functioning, which could be an important consideration in future revisions of our diagnostic system. As we learn more about the etiologies and pathology of the personality disorders, it will no longer be necessary, or even desirable, to limit our diagnostic schemes to atheoretical, descriptive phenomena, and we can look forward to an enriched understanding of these disorders.

REFERENCES

American Psychiatric Association: Diagnostic and Statistical Manual of Mental Disorders. Washington, DC, American Psychiatric Association, 1952

American Psychiatric Association: Diagnostic and Statistical Manual of Mental Disorders, 2nd Edition. Washington, DC, American Psychiatric Association, 1968

American Psychiatric Association: Diagnostic and Statistical Manual of Mental Disorders, 3rd Edition. Washington, DC, American Psychiatric Association, 1980

American Psychiatric Association: Diagnostic and Statistical Manual of Mental Disorders, 3rd Edition, Revised. Washington, DC, American Psychiatric Association, 1987

American Psychiatric Association: Diagnostic and Statistical Manual of Mental Disorders, 4th Edition. Washington, DC, American Psychiatric Association, 1994

American Psychiatric Association: Diagnostic and Statistical Manual of Mental Disorders, 4th Edition, Text Revision. Washington, DC, American Psychiatric Association, 2000

Barton WE: The History and Influence of the American Psychiatric Association. Washington, DC, American Psychiatric Press, 1987

Benjamin LS: Interpersonal Diagnosis and Treatment of Personality Disorders. New York, Guilford, 1993

Blashfield RK, McElroy RA: Confusions in the terminology used for classificatory models, in The DSM-IV Personality Disorders. Edited by Livesley WJ. New York, Guilford, 1995, pp 407–416

Bleuler E: Textbook of Psychiatry (English translation). New York, Macmillan, 1924

Clark LA: The challenge of alternative perspectives in classification: a discussion of basic issues, in The DSM-IV Personality Disorders. Edited by Livesley WJ. New York, Guilford, 1995, pp 482–496

Clark LA, Livesley WJ, Schroeder ML, et al: Convergence of two systems for assessing specific traits of personality disorder. Psychol Assess 8:294–303, 1996

Clark LA, Livesley WJ, Morey L: Special feature: personality disorder assessment: the challenge of construct validity. J Personal Disord 11:205–231, 1997

Cloninger CR, Svrakic DM, Przybeck TR: A psychobiological model of temperament and character. Arch Gen Psychiatry 50:975–990, 1993

Costa PT, McCrae RR: The five-factor model of personality and its relevance to personality disorders. J Personal Disord 6:343–359, 1992

Costa PT, Widiger TA: Personality Disorders and the Five-Factor Model of Personality. Washington, DC, American Psychological Association, 1994

Deutsch H: Some forms of emotional disturbance and their relationship to schizophrenia. Psychoanal Q 11:301–321, 1942

Eysenck HJ, Eysenck SBG: Manual of the Eysenck Personality Questionnaire. San Diego, CA, Educational and Industrial Testing Service, 1975

First M, Gibbon M, Spitzer RL, et al: User's Guide for the Structured Clinical Interview for DSM-IV Axis II Personality Disorders. Washington, DC, American Psychiatric Press, 1997

First MB, Bell CC, Cuthbert B, et al: Personality disorders and relational disorders: a research agenda for addressing crucial gaps in DSM, in A Research Agenda for DSM-V. Edited by Kupfer DJ, First MB, Regier DA. Washington, DC, American Psychiatric Association, 2002, pp 123–199

Frances A: Dimensional diagnosis of personality: not whether, but when and which (commentary). Psychological Inquiry 4:110–111, 1993

Freud S: Inhibitions, Symptoms and Anxiety, Standard Edition, London, Hogarth Press, 1926

Frosch J: The psychotic character: clinical psychiatric considerations. Psychiatr Q 38:81–96, 1964

Goldman HH, Skodol AE, Lave TR: Revising axis V for DSM-IV: a review of measures of social functioning. Am J Psychiatry 149:1148–1156, 1992

Grilo CM, Shea MT, Sanislow CA et al: Two-year stability and change in schizotypal, borderline, avoidant, and obsessive-compulsive personality disorders. J Consult Clin Psychol 72:767–775, 2004

Gunderson JG: Borderline Personality Disorder. Washington, DC, American Psychiatric Press, 1984

Gunderson JG: Interfaces between psychoanalytic and empirical studies of borderline personality, in The Borderline Patient, Vol 1. Edited by Grotstein J, Solomon M, Lang J. Hillsdale, NJ, The Analytic Press, 1987

Gunderson JG: Borderline Personality Disorder: A Clinical Guide. Washington, DC, American Psychiatric Publishing, 2001

Gunderson JG, Links PS, Reich JH: Competing models of personality disorders. J Personal Disord 5:60–68, 1991

Hoch PH, Polatin P: Pseudoneurotic forms of schizophrenia. Psychiatr Q 23:248–276, 1949

Kendell RE: The Role of Diagnosis in Psychiatry. Oxford, England, Basil Blackwell, 1975

Kernberg O: Borderline Conditions and Pathological Narcissism. New York, Jason Aronson, 1975

Kiesler DJ: The 1982 interpersonal circle: a taxonomy for complementarity in human transactions. Psychol Rev 90:185–214, 1983

Kohut H: The Analysis of the Self. New York, International Universities Press, 1971

Kraepelin E: Lectures on Clinical Psychiatry (English translation). New York, Wood Press, 1904

Kretschmer E: Hysteria (English translation). New York, Nervous and Mental Disease Publishers, 1926

Krueger RF, Tackett MA: Personality and psychopathology: working toward the bigger picture. J Personal Disord 17:109–128, 2003

Lenzenweger MF, Clarkin JF: The personality disorders: history, classification, and research issues, in Major Theories of Personality Disorder. Edited by Clarkin JF, Lenzenweger MF. New York, Guilford, 1996

Livesley WJ: Trait and behavioral prototypes of personality disorder. Am J Psychiatry 143:728–732, 1986

Livesley WJ: A systematic approach to the delineation of personality disorders. Am J Psychiatry 144:772–777, 1987

Livesley WJ: Suggestions for a framework for an empirically based classification of personality disorder. Can J Psychiatry 43:137–147, 1998

Livesley WJ, Jackson DN: Guidelines for developing, evaluating, and revising the classification of personality disorders. J Nerv Ment Disease 180:609–618, 1992

Livesley WJ, Jang KL: Toward an empirically based classification of personality disorder. J Personal Disord 14:137–151, 2000

Livesley WJ, Jang KL, Jackson DN, et al: Genetic and environmental contributions to dimensions of personality disorder. Am J Psychiatry 150:1826–1831, 1993

Livesley WJ, Schroeder ML, Jackson DN, et al: Categorical distinctions in the study of personality disorder: implications for classification. J Abnorm Psychol 103:6–17, 1994

Livesley WJ, Jang KL, Vernon PA: Phenotypic and genetic structure of traits delineating personality disorder. Arch Gen Psychiatry 55:941–948, 1998

Loranger AW: International Personality Disorder Examination (IPDE). Odessa, FL, Psychological Assessment Resources, 1999

Millon T: Modern Psychopathology. Philadelphia, PA, WB Saunders, 1969

Millon T: Reflections on the future of DSM Axis II. J Personal Disord 14:30–41, 2000

Oldham JM, Morris LB: The New Personality Self-Portrait, New York, Bantam, 1995

Oldham JM, Skodol AE: Charting the future of Axis II. J Personal Disord 14:17–29, 2000

Oldham JM, Skodol AE, Kellman HD, et al: Diagnosis of DSM-III-R personality disorders by two structured interviews: patterns of comorbidity. Am J Psychiatry 149:213–220, 1992

Paris J: Nature and Nurture in Psychiatry: A Predisposition-Stress Model of Mental Disorders. Washington, DC, American Psychiatric Press, 1999

Perry JC: Challenges in validating personality disorders: beyond description. J Personal Disord 4:273–289, 1990

Perry JC: Problems and considerations in the valid assessment of personality disorders. Am J Psychiatry 149:1645–1653, 1992

Pfohl B: Axis I and Axis II: comorbidity or confusion? in Personality and Pathology. Edited by Cloninger CR. Washington, DC, American Psychiatric Press, 1999, pp 83–98

Pfohl B, Blum N, Zimmerman M: Structured Interview for DSM-IV Personality. Washington, DC, American Psychiatric Press, 1997

Pilkonis PA, Heape CL, Ruddy J, et al: Validity in the diagnosis of personality disorders: the use of the LEAD standard. Psychol Assess 3:46–54, 1991

Reich W: Character Analysis (1933). New York, Simon and Schuster, 1945

Schneider K: Psychopathic Personalities (1923). London, Cassell, 1950

Shea MT, Yen S: Stability as a distinction between Axis I and Axis II disorders. J Personal Disord 17:373–386, 2003

Shea MT, Stout R, Gunderson J, et al: Short-term diagnostic stability of schizotypal, borderline, avoidant, and obsessive-compulsive personality disorders. Am J Psychiatry 159:2036–2041, 2002

Shedler J, Westen D: Refining personality disorder diagnosis: integrating science and practice. Am J Psychiatry 161:1350–1365, 2004

Skodol AE: Classification, assessment, and differential diagnosis of personality disorders. Journal of Practical Psychology, Behavior and Health 3:261–274, 1997

Skodol AE, Link BG, Shrout PE, et al: The revision of Axis V in DSM-III-R: should symptoms have been included? Am J Psychiatry 145:825–829, 1988

Skodol AE, Gunderson JG, McGlashan TH, et al: Functional impairment in patients with schizotypal, borderline, avoidant, or obsessive-compulsive personality disorder. Am J Psychiatry 159:276–283, 2002

Spitzer RL: Psychiatric diagnosis: are clinicians still necessary? Compr Psychiatry 24:399–411, 1983

Tellegen A: Folk concepts and psychological concepts of personality and personality disorder (commentary). Psychological Inquiry 4:122–130, 1993

Tyrer P: Are personality disorders well classified in DSM-IV? in The DSM-IV Personality Disorders. Edited by Livesley WJ. New York, Guilford, 1995, pp 29–42

Watson D, Clark LA, Harkness AR: Structures of personality and their relevance to psychopathology. J Abnorm Psychol 103:18–31, 1994

Westen D: Divergences between clinical and research methods for assessing personality disorders: implications for research and the evolution of Axis II. Am J Psychiatry 154:895–903, 1997

Westen D, Arkowitz-Westen L: Limitations of Axis II in diagnosing personality pathology in clinical practice. Am J Psychiatry 155:1767–1771, 1998

Westen D, Shedler J: Revising and assessing Axis II, part I: developing a clinically and empirically valid assessment method. Am J Psychiatry 156:258–272, 1999a

Westen D, Shedler J: Revising and assessing Axis II, part II: toward an empirically based and clinically useful classification of personality disorders. Am J Psychiatry 156:273–285, 1999b

Widiger TA: Definition, diagnosis, and differentiation. J Personal Disord 5:42–51, 1991a

Widiger TA: Personality disorder dimensional models proposed for DSM-IV. J Personal Disord 5:386–398, 1991b

Widiger TA: Categorical versus dimensional classification: implications from and for research. J Personal Disord 6:287–300, 1992

Widiger TA: The DSM-III-R categorical personality disorder diagnoses: a critique and an alternative. Psychological Inquiry 4:75–90, 1993

Widiger TA: Four out of five ain't bad (commentary). Arch Gen Psychiatry 55:865–866, 1998

Widiger TA: Personality disorder and Axis I psychopathology: the problematic boundary of Axis I and Axis II. J Personal Disord 17:90–108, 2003

Widiger TA, Sanderson CJ: Toward a dimensional model of personality disorders, in The DSM-IV Personality Disorders. Edited by Livesley WJ. New York, Guilford, 1995, pp 433–458

Widiger TA, Shea T: Differentiation of Axis I and Axis II disorders. J Abnorm Psychol 100:399–406, 1991

Widiger TA, Frances AJ, Harris M, et al: Comorbidity among Axis II disorders, in Personality Disorders: New Perspectives on Diagnostic Validity. Edited by Oldham JM. Washington, DC, American Psychiatric Press, 1991

Wiggins J: Circumplex models of interpersonal behavior in clinical psychology, in Handbook of Research Methods in Clinical Psychology. Edited by Kendall P, Butcher J. New York, Wiley, 1982

World Health Organization: International Classification of Diseases, 8th Revision. Geneva, Switzerland, World Health Organization, 1968

Zillborg G: Ambulatory schizophrenia. Psychiatry 4:149–155, 1941

2

Theories of Personality and Personality Disorders

Amy Heim, Ph.D.
Drew Westen, Ph.D.

Personality refers to enduring patterns of cognition, emotion, motivation, and behavior that are activated in particular circumstances (see Mischel and Shoda 1995; Westen 1995). This minimalist definition (i.e., one that most personality psychologists would accept, despite widely differing theories) underscores two important aspects of personality. First, personality is dynamic, characterized by an ongoing interaction of mental, behavioral, and environmental events). Second, inherent in personality is the potential for variation and flexibility of responding (activation of specific processes under particular circumstances). Enduring ways of responding need not be broadly generalized to be considered aspects of personality (or to lead to dysfunction), because many aspects of personality are triggered by specific situations, thoughts, or feelings. For example, a tendency to bristle and respond with opposition, anger, or passive resistance to perceived demands of male authority figures may or may not occur with female authorities, peers, lovers, or subordinates. Nevertheless,

this response tendency represents an enduring way of thinking, attending to information, feeling, and responding that is clearly an aspect of personality (and one that can substantially affect adaptation).

Among the dozens of approaches to personality advanced over the past century, two are of the most widespread use in clinical practice: the psychodynamic and the cognitive-social or cognitive-behavioral. Two other approaches have gained increased interest among personality disorder researchers: trait psychology, one of the oldest and most enduring empirical approaches to the study of normal personality; and biological approaches, which reflect a long-standing tradition in descriptive psychiatry as well as more recent developments in behavior genetics and neuroscience. Although most theories have traditionally fallen into a single "camp," several other approaches are best viewed as integrative. These include Benjamin's (1996a, 1996b) interpersonal approach, which integrates interpersonal, psychodynamic, and social

Preparation of this manuscript was supported in part by NIMH MH62377 and MH62378 to the second author.

learning theories; Millon's (1990) evolutionary–social learning approach, which has assimilated broadly from multiple traditions (e.g., psychoanalytic object relations theory); and Westen's (1995, 1998) functional domains model, which draws on psychodynamic, evolutionary, behavioral, cognitive, and developmental research. In this chapter we briefly consider how each approach conceptualizes personality disorders.

PSYCHODYNAMIC THEORIES

Psychoanalytic theorists were the first to generate a concept of personality disorder (also called *character disorder*, reflecting the idea that personality disorders involve character problems not isolated to a specific symptom or set of independent symptoms). Personality disorders began to draw considerable theoretical attention in psychoanalysis by the middle of the twentieth century (e.g., Fairbairn 1952; Reich 1933/1978), in part because they were common and difficult to treat, and in part because they defied understanding using the psychoanalytic models prevalent at the time. For years, analysts had understood psychological problems in terms of conflict and defense using Freud's topographic model (conscious, preconscious, unconscious) or his structural model (id, ego, superego). In classical psychoanalytic terms, most symptoms reflect maladaptive compromises, forged outside of awareness, among conflicting wishes, fears, and moral standards. For example, a patient with anorexia nervosa who is uncomfortable with her impulses and who fears losing control over them may begin to starve herself as a way of demonstrating that she can control even the most persistent of desires, hunger. Some of the personality disorders currently identified in DSM-IV (American Psychiatric Association 1994) and its update, DSM-IV-TR (American Psychiatric Association 2000), have their roots in early psychoanalytic theorizing about conflict—notably dependent, obsessive-compulsive, and to some extent histrionic personality disorders (presumed to reflect fixations at the oral, anal, and phallic stages, respectively).

Although some psychoanalysts have argued that a conflict model can account for severe personality pathology (e.g., Abend et al. 1983), most analytic theorists have turned to ego psychology, object relations theory, self psychology, and relational theories to help understand patients with personality disorders. According to these approaches, the problems seen in patients with character disorders run deeper than maladaptive compromises among conflicting motives,

and reflect derailments in personality development reflecting temperament, early attachment experiences, and their interaction (e.g., Balint 1969; Kernberg 1975b). Many of the DSM-IV personality disorders have roots in these later approaches, notably schizoid, borderline, and narcissistic personality disorders.

Psychoanalytic ego psychology focuses on the psychological functions (in contemporary cognitive terms, the skills, procedures, and processes involved in self-regulation) that must be in place for people to behave adaptively, attain their goals, and meet external demands (see Bellak et al. 1973; Blanck and Blanck 1974; Redl and Wineman 1951). From this perspective, patients with personality disorders may have various deficits in functioning, such as poor impulse control, difficulty regulating affects, and deficits in the capacity for self-reflection. These deficits may render them incapable of behaving consistently in their own best interest or of taking the interests of others appropriately into account (e.g., they lash out aggressively without forethought or cut themselves when they become upset).

Object relations, relational, and self psychological theories focus on the cognitive, affective, and motivational processes presumed to underlie functioning in close relationships (Aron 1996; Greenberg and Mitchell 1983; Mitchell 1988; Westen 1991b). From this point of view, personality disorders reflect a number of processes. Internalization of attitudes of hostile, abusive, critical, inconsistent, or neglectful parents may leave patients with personality disorder vulnerable to fears of abandonment, self-hatred, a tendency to treat themselves as their parents treated them, and so forth (Benjamin 1996a, 1996b; Masterson 1976; McWilliams 1998). Patients with personality disorder often fail to develop mature, constant, multifaceted representations of the self and others. As a result, they may be vulnerable to emotional swings when significant others are momentarily disappointing, and they may have difficulty understanding or imagining what might be in the minds of the people with whom they interact (Fonagy and Target 1997; Fonagy et al. 1991, 2003). Those with personality disorder often appear to have difficulty forming a realistic, balanced view of themselves that can weather momentary failures or criticisms and may have a corresponding inability to activate procedures (hypothesized to be based on loving, soothing experiences with early caregivers) that would be useful for self-soothing in the face of loss, failure, or threats to safety or self-esteem (e.g., Adler and Buie 1979). A substantial body of research supports many of these propositions, particularly vis-à-vis borderline personality disorder (BPD), the most extensively studied personality disorder (e.g., Baker et al. 1992; Gunderson 2001; Westen 1990a, 1991a).

From a psychodynamic point of view, perhaps the most important features of personality disorders are the following: a) they represent constellations of psychological processes, not distinct symptoms that can be understood in isolation; b) they can be located on a continuum of personality pathology from relative health to relative sickness; c) they can be characterized in terms of character style, which is orthogonal to level of disturbance (e.g., a patient can have an obsessional style but be relatively sick or relatively healthy); d) they involve both implicit and explicit personality processes, only some of which are available to introspection (and thus amenable to self-report); and e) they reflect processes that are deeply entrenched, often serve multiple functions, and/or have become associated with regulation of affects and are hence resistant to change.

The most comprehensive theory that embodies these principles is the theory of personality structure or organization developed by Otto Kernberg (1975a, 1984, 1996). In his theory, Kernberg proposed a continuum of pathology, from chronically psychotic levels of functioning, through borderline functioning (severe personality disorders), through neurotic to normal functioning. In Kernberg's view, people with severe personality pathology are distinguished from people whose personality is organized at a psychotic level by their relatively intact capacity for reality testing (the absence of hallucinations or psychotic delusions) and their relative ability to distinguish between their own thoughts and feelings and those of others (the absence of beliefs that their thoughts are being broadcast on the radio; their recognition, although sometimes less than complete, that the persecutory thoughts in their heads are voices from the past rather than true hallucinations, etc.). What distinguishes individuals with severe personality pathology from people with "neurotic" (that is, healthier) character structures includes 1) their more maladaptive modes of regulating their emotions through immature, reality-distorting defenses such as denial and projection (e.g., refusing to recognize the part they play in generating some of the hostility they engender from others); and 2) their difficulty in forming mature, multifaceted representations of themselves and significant others (e.g., believing that a person they once loved is really all bad, with no redeeming features, and is motivated only by the desire to hurt them). Kernberg refers to these two aspects of borderline personality organization as "primitive defenses" and "identity diffusion." This level of severe personality disturbance, which

Kernberg calls "borderline personality organization," shares some features with the DSM-IV's BPD diagnosis. However, borderline personality organization is a broader construct, encompassing patients with paranoid, schizoid, schizotypal, and antisocial personality disorders as well as some patients who would receive a DSM-IV diagnosis of narcissistic, histrionic, or dependent personality disorder. (Some schizotypal and borderline patients may at times fall "south of the border" into the psychotic range.) Recent research supports the notion that patients fall on a continuum of severity of personality pathology (see Millon and Davis 1995; Tyrer and Johnson 1996), with disorders such as paranoid and borderline personality disorder representing more severe forms, and disorders such as obsessive-compulsive personality disorder less severe (Westen and Shedler 1999a).

Although many of Kernberg's major contributions have been in the understanding of borderline phenomena, his theory of narcissistic disturbance contributed substantially to the development of the diagnosis of narcissistic personality disorder in DSM-III (American Psychiatric Association 1980), just as his understanding of borderline phenomena contributed to the borderline diagnosis. According to Kernberg, whereas borderline patients lack an integrated identity, narcissistic patients are typically developmentally more advanced, in that they have been able to develop a coherent (if distorted) view of themselves. Narcissistic phenomena, in Kernberg's view, lie on a continuum from normal (characterized by adequate self-esteem regulation) to pathological (narcissistic personality disorder) (Kernberg 1984, 1998). Individuals with narcissistic personality disorder need to construct a grossly inflated view of themselves to maintain self-esteem and may appear grandiose, sensitive to the slightest attacks on their self-esteem (and hence vulnerable to rage or depression), or both. Not only are the conscious self-representations of narcissistic patients inflated but so too are the representations that constitute their ideal selves. Actual and ideal self-representations stand in dynamic relation to one another. Thus, one reason narcissistic patients must maintain an idealized view of self is that they have a correspondingly grandiose view of who they should be, a divergence that leads to tremendous feelings of shame, failure, and humiliation.

The concept of a grandiose self is central to the self psychology of Heinz Kohut, a major theorist of narcissistic personality pathology whose ideas, like those of Kernberg, contributed to the DSM-III diagnosis of narcissistic personality disorder (Goldstein 1985). Kohut's theory grew out of his own and others' clinical experiences with patients whose problems (such as feelings of emptiness or unstable self-esteem) did not respond well to existing (psychoanalytic) models. Narcissistic pathology, according to Kohut, results from faulty self-development. Kohut's concept of the *self* refers to the nucleus of a person's central ambitions and ideals and the talents and skills used to actualize them (Kohut 1971, 1977; Wolf 1988). It develops through two pathways ("poles") that provide the basis for self-esteem. The first is the *grandiose self*—an idealized representation of self that emerges in children through empathic mirroring by their parents ("Mommy, watch!") and provides the nucleus for later ambitions and strivings. The second is the *idealized parent imago*—an idealized representation of the parents that provides the foundation for ideals and standards for the self. Parental mirroring allows the child to see his reflection in the eyes of a loving and admiring parent; idealizing a parent or parents allows the child to identify with and become like them. In the absence of adequate experiences with parents who can mirror the child or serve as appropriate targets of idealization (for example, when the parents are self-involved or abusive), the child's self-structure cannot develop, preventing the achievement of cohesion, vigor, and normal self-esteem (described by Kohut as "healthy narcissism"). As a result, the child develops a disorder of the self, of which pathological narcissism is a prototypic example.

COGNITIVE-SOCIAL THEORIES

Cognitive-social theories (Bandura 1986; Mischel 1973, 1979) offered the first comprehensive alternative to psychodynamic approaches to personality. First developed in the 1960s, these approaches are sometimes called social learning theory, cognitive-social learning theory, social cognitive theory, and cognitive-behavioral theories. Cognitive-social theories developed from behaviorist and cognitive roots. From a behaviorist perspective, personality consists of learned behaviors and emotional reactions that tend to be relatively specific (rather than highly generalized) and tied to particular environmental contingencies. Cognitive-social theories share the behaviorist belief that learning is the basis of personality and that personality dispositions tend to be relatively specific and shaped by their consequences. They share the cognitive view that the way people encode, transform, and retrieve information, particularly about themselves and others, is central to personality. From a cognitive-social perspective, personality reflects a constant interplay between environmental demands and the way

the individual processes information about the self and the world (Bandura 1986).

Cognitive-social theorists have only recently begun to write about personality disorders (e.g., Beck et al. 2003; Linehan 1993a; Pretzer and Beck 1996; Young 1990). In large part this late entrance into the study of personality disorders reflects the assumption, initially inherited from behaviorism, that personality is composed of relatively discrete, learned processes that are more malleable and situation specific than implied by the concept of personality disorder. Cognitive-social theories focus on a number of variables presumed to be most important in understanding personality disorders, including schemas, expectancies, goals, skills and competencies, and self-regulation (Bandura 1986, 1999; Cantor and Kihlstrom 1987; Mischel 1973, 1979; Mischel and Shoda 1995). Although particular theorists have tended to emphasize one or two of these variables in explaining personality disorders, such as the schemas involved in encoding and processing information about the self and others (Beck et al. 2003) or the deficits in affect regulation seen in borderline patients (Linehan 1993a), a comprehensive cognitive-social account of personality disorders would likely address all of them.

For example, patients with personality disorders have dysfunctional schemas that lead them to misinterpret information (as when patients with BPD misread and misattribute people's intentions); attend to and encode information in biased ways (as when patients with paranoid personality disorder maintain vigilance for perceived slights or attacks); or view themselves as bad or incompetent (pathological self-schemas). Related to these schemas are problematic expectancies, such as pessimistic expectations about the world, beliefs about the malevolence of others, and fears of being mocked. Patients with personality disorders may have pathological self-efficacy expectancies, such as the dependent patient's belief that he cannot survive on his own; the avoidant patient's belief that she is likely to fail in social circumstances, or the narcissistic patient's grandiose expectations about what he can accomplish. Equally important are competencies—that is, skills and abilities used for solving problems. In social-cognitive terms, social intelligence includes a variety of competencies that help people navigate interpersonal waters (Cantor and Harlow 1994; Cantor and Kihlstrom 1987), and patients with personality disorders tend to be notoriously poor interpersonal problem solvers.

Of particular relevance to severe personality disorders is self-regulation, which refers to the process of setting goals and subgoals, evaluating one's performance in meeting these goals, and adjusting one's behavior to achieve these goals in the context of ongoing feedback (Bandura 1986; Mischel 1990). Problems in self-regulation, including a deficit in specific skills, form a central aspect of Linehan's (1993a, 1993b) work on BPD. Linehan regards emotion dysregulation as the essential feature of BPD. The key characteristics of emotion dysregulation include difficulty 1) inhibiting inappropriate behavior related to intense affect, 2) organizing oneself to meet behavioral goals, 3) regulating physiological arousal associated with intense emotional arousal, and 4) refocusing attention when emotionally stimulated (Linehan 1993b). Many of the behavioral manifestations of BPD (e.g., cutting) can be viewed as consequences of emotional dysregulation. Deficits in emotion regulation lead to other problems, such as difficulties with interpersonal functioning and with the development of a stable sense of self.

According to another cognitive-behavioral approach, Beck's cognitive theory (Beck 1999; Beck et al. 2003; Pretzer and Beck 1996), dysfunctional beliefs constitute the primary pathology involved in the personality disorders (Beck et al. 2001), which are viewed as "pervasive, self-perpetuating cognitive-interpersonal cycles" (Pretzer and Beck 1996, p. 55). Beck's theory highlights three aspects of cognition: 1) automatic thoughts (beliefs and assumptions about the world, the self, and others); 2) interpersonal strategies; and 3) cognitive distortions (systematic errors in rational thinking). Beck and colleagues have described a unique cognitive profile characteristic of each of the DSM-IV personality disorders. For example, an individual diagnosed with schizoid personality disorder would have a view of himself as a self-sufficient loner, a view of others as unrewarding and intrusive, and a view of relationships as messy and undesirable, and his primary interpersonal strategy would involve keeping his distance from other people (Pretzer and Beck 1996). He would use cognitive distortions that minimize his recognition of how relationships with others can be sources of pleasure. A recent study of dysfunctional beliefs (as assessed by the Personal Beliefs Questionnaire [A.T. Beck, J.S. Beck, unpublished assessment instrument, The Beck Institute for Cognitive Therapy and Research, Bala Cynwyd, Pennsylvania, 1991]) provides some initial support for the link between particular beliefs and the DSM-IV personality disorders (Beck et al. 2001).

Building on Beck's cognitive theory, Young and colleagues (Young and Gluhoski 1996; Young and Lindemann 2002; Young et al. 2003) have added a fourth level of cognition: early maladaptive schemas, which they have defined as "broad and pervasive themes regarding oneself and one's relationships with others, developed during childhood and elaborated throughout one's life" (Young and Lindemann 2002, p. 95). The authors distinguish these schemas from automatic thoughts and underlying assumptions, noting that the schemas are associated with greater levels of affect, are more pervasive, and involve a strong interpersonal aspect. Young and colleagues have identified 16 early maladaptive schemas, each of which comprises cognitive, affective, and behavioral components. They have also identified three cognitive processes involving schemas that define key features of personality disorders: *schema maintenance*, which refers to the processes by which maladaptive schemas are rigidly upheld (e.g., cognitive distortions, self-defeating behaviors); *schema avoidance*, which refers to the cognitive, affective, and behavioral ways individuals avoid the negative affect associated with the schema; and *schema compensation*, which refers to ways of overcompensating for the schema (e.g., becoming a workaholic in response to a schema of self as failure).

Mischel and Shoda (1995) have offered a compelling social-cognitive account of personality that focuses on if–then contingencies—that is, conditions that activate particular thoughts, feelings, and behaviors. Although they have not linked this model to personality disorders, one could view personality disorders as involving a host of rigid, maladaptive if–then contingencies. For example, for some patients, the first hints of trouble in a relationship may activate concerns about abandonment. These in turn may elicit anxiety or rage, to which the patient responds with desperate attempts to lure the person back that often backfire (such as manipulative statements and suicidal gestures). From an integrative psychodynamic-cognitive viewpoint, Horowitz (1988, 1998) offered a model that similarly focused on the conditions under which certain states of mind become active, which he has tied more directly to a model of personality disorders; and Wachtel (1977, 1997) has similarly described cyclical psychodynamics, in which people manage to elicit from others precisely the kind of reactions of which they are the most vigilant and afraid.

TRAIT THEORIES

Trait psychology focuses less on personality processes or functions than do psychodynamic or cognitive-social approaches, and hence has not generated an approach to treatment, although it has generated highly productive empirical research programs. *Traits* are emotional, cognitive, and behavioral tendencies on which individuals vary (e.g., the tendency to experience negative emotions). According to Gordon Allport (1937), who pioneered the trait approach to personality, the concept of *trait* has two separate but complementary meanings: it is both an observed tendency to behave in a particular way and an inferred underlying personality disposition that generates this behavioral tendency. In the empirical literature, traits have largely been defined operationally, as the average of a set of self-report items designed to assess a given trait (e.g., items indicating a tendency to feel anxious, sad, ashamed, guilty, self-doubting, and angry that all share a common core of negative affectivity or neuroticism).

Researchers have recently begun recasting personality disorders in terms of the most prominent contemporary trait theory, the Five-Factor Model of personality (FFM; McCrae and Costa 1997; Widiger 2000; Widiger and Costa 1994). (We address other trait models that have been more closely associated with biological theories later.) The FFM is a description of the way personality descriptors tend to covary and hence can be understood in terms of latent factors (traits) identified via factor analysis. Based on the lexical hypothesis of personality—that important personality attributes will naturally find expression in words used in everyday language—the FFM emerged from factor analysis of adjectival descriptions of personality originally selected from *Webster's Unabridged Dictionary* (Allport and Odbert 1936). Numerous studies, including cross-cultural investigations, have found that when participants in nonclinical (normal) samples are asked to rate themselves on dozens or hundreds of adjectives or brief sentences, the pattern of self-descriptions can often be reduced to five overarching constructs (Costa and McCrae 1997; Goldberg 1993): 1) neuroticism or negative affect (how much they tend to be distressed); 2) extraversion or positive affect (the extent to which they tend to be gregarious, high-energy, and happy); 3) conscientiousness; 4) agreeableness; and 5) openness to experience (the extent to which they are open to emotional, aesthetic, and intellectual experiences).

McCrae and Costa (1990, 1997) proposed a set of lower-order traits, or facets, within each of these broadband traits that can allow a more discriminating portrait of personality. Thus, an individual's personality profile is represented by a score on each of the five factors plus scores on six lower-order facets or subfactors within each of these broader constructs (e.g., anxiety and depression as facets of neuroticism). Advo-

cates of the FFM argue that personality disorders reflect extreme versions of normal personality traits, so that the same system can be used for diagnosing normal and pathological personality. From the perspective of the FFM, personality disorders are not discrete entities separate and distinct from normal personality. Rather, they represent extreme variants of normal personality traits or blends thereof.

In principle, one could classify personality disorders in one of two ways using the FFM. The first, and that more consistent with the theoretical and psychometric tradition within which the FFM developed, is simply to identify personality pathology by extreme values on each of the five factors (and perhaps on their facets). For example, extremely high scores on the neuroticism factor and its facets (anxiety, hostility, depression, self-consciousness, impulsivity, and vulnerability) all represent aspects of personality pathology. Whether this strategy is appropriate for all factors and facets, and when to consider extreme responses on one or both poles of a dimension pathological, are matters of debate. Extreme extraversion, for example, may or may not be pathological, depending on the social milieu and the person's other traits. Similarly, extreme openness to experience could imply a genuinely open attitude toward emotions, art, and so forth or an uncritical, "flaky," or schizotypal cognitive style. The advantages of this approach, however, are that it integrates the understanding and assessment of normal and pathological personality and that it establishes dimensions of personality pathology using well-understood empirical procedures (factor analysis).

Another way to proceed using the FFM is to translate clinically derived categories into five-factor language (Coker et al. 2002; Lynam and Widiger 2001; Widiger and Costa 1994). For example, Widiger and colleagues (2002) described antisocial personality disorder (ASPD) as combining low agreeableness with low conscientiousness. Because analysis at the level of five factors often lacks the specificity to characterize complex disorders such as BPD (high neuroticism plus high extraversion), proponents of the FFM have often moved to the facet level. Thus, whereas all six neuroticism facets (anxiety, hostility, depression, self-consciousness, impulsivity, and vulnerability) are characteristic of patients with BPD, patients with avoidant personality disorder are characterized by only four of these facets (anxiety, depression, self-consciousness, and vulnerability). Similarly, Widiger and colleagues (1994, 2002) described obsessive-compulsive personality disorder as primarily an extreme, maladaptive variant of conscientiousness. They add, however, that obsessive-compulsive patients tend to be low on the compliance and altruism facets of agreeableness (i.e., they are oppositional and stingy) and low on some of the facets of openness to experience as reflected in being closed to feelings and closed to values (i.e., morally inflexible). Numerous studies have shown predicted links between DSM-IV Axis II disorders and FFM factors and facets (Axelrod et al. 1997; Ross et al. 2002; Trull et al. 2001), although other studies have found substantial overlap among the FFM profiles of patients with very different disorders (e.g., borderline and obsessive-compulsive) using major FFM self-report inventories (Morey et al. 2002).

BIOLOGICAL PERSPECTIVES

The first biological perspectives on personality disorders, which influenced the current Axis II classification, stemmed from the observations of the pioneering psychiatric taxonomists in the early twentieth century, notably Bleuler (1911/1950) and Kraepelin (1896/1919). These authors and others noticed, for example, that the relatives of schizophrenic patients sometimes appeared to have attenuated symptoms of the disorder that endured as personality traits, such as interpersonal and cognitive peculiarity. More recently, researchers have used the methods of trait psychology (particularly the reliance on self-report questionnaires and factor analysis) to study personality disorders from a biological viewpoint. In some cases, they have developed item sets with biological variables in mind (e.g., neurotransmitters and their functions) or have reconsidered patterns of covariation among different traits in light of hypothesized neurobiological systems or circuits. In other cases, they have applied behavior-genetic approaches to study personality traits (as well as DSM-IV disorders). We explore each of these approaches in turn. (Researchers are just beginning to use neuroimaging to study personality disorders, particularly BPD [e.g., Herpertz et al. 2001], but the results at this point are preliminary, and hence we do not address them further here.)

Traits and Neural Systems

Siever and Davis (1991) provided one of the first attempts to reconsider the personality disorders from a neurobiology perspective. They proposed a model based on core characteristics of Axis I disorders relevant to personality disorders and related these characteristics to emerging knowledge of their underlying neurobiology. They focused on cognitive/perceptual organization (schizophrenia and other psychotic disorders); impulsivity/aggression (impulse control disorders); affective instability (mood disorders); and anxiety/inhibition (anxiety disorders). Conceptualized in dimensional terms, Axis I disorders such as schizophrenia represent the extreme end of a continuum. Milder abnormalities can be seen in patients with personality disorder, either directly (as subthreshold variants) or through their influence on adaptive strategies (coping and defense).

Siever and Davis linked each dimension to biological correlates and indicators, some presumed to be causal and others to provide markers of underlying biological dysfunction (e.g., eye movement dysfunction in schizophrenia, which is also seen in individuals with schizotypal personality disorder and in nonpsychotic relatives of schizophrenic probands). They also pointed to suggestive data on neurotransmitter functioning that might link Axis II disorders with Axis I syndromes such as depression. More recently, Siever and colleagues (New and Siever 2002; Siever et al. 2003) proposed an approach to BPD that tries to circumvent the problems created by the heterogeneity of the diagnosis by examining the neurobiology of specific dimensions thought to underlie the disorder (endophenotypes), especially impulsive aggression and affective instability.

The major attempt thus far to develop a trait model of personality disorders based on a neurobiological model is Cloninger's seven-factor model of personality (Cloninger 1998; Cloninger et al. 1993). In his model, Cloninger divided personality structure into two domains: *temperament* ("automatic associative responses to basic emotional stimuli that determine habits and skills") and *character* ("self-aware concepts that influence voluntary intentions and attitudes") (Cloninger 1998, p. 64). According to Cloninger, each of these domains is defined by a mode of learning and the underlying neural systems involved in that learning: temperament is associated with associative/procedural learning, and character is associated with insight learning. The temperament domain includes four dimensions, each theoretically linked to particular neurotransmitter systems: 1) novelty seeking (exploration, extravagance, impulsivity), associated with dopamine; 2) harm avoidance (characterized by pessimism, fear, timidity), associated with serotonin and GABA (γ-aminobutyric acid); 3) reward dependence (sentimentality, social attachment, openness), associated with norepinephrine and serotonin; and 4) persistence (industriousness, determination, ambitiousness, perfectionism), associated with glutamate and seroto-nin (Cloninger 1998, p. 70). The character domain in-cludes three dimensions: 1) self-directedness (respon-sibility, purposefulness, self-acceptance), considered the "major determinant of the presence or absence of personality disorder" (Cloninger et al. 1993, p. 979); 2) cooperativeness (empathy, compassion, helpfulness); and 3) self-transcendence (spirituality, idealism, en-lightenment).

Cloninger (1998) proposed that all personality dis-orders are low on the character dimensions of self-directedness and cooperativeness. What distinguishes patients with different disorders are their more spe-cific profiles. In broad strokes, the Cluster A personal-ity disorders (schizotypal, schizoid, paranoid) are as-sociated with low reward dependence; the Cluster B personality disorders (borderline, antisocial, narcissis-tic, histrionic) are associated with high novelty seek-ing; and the Cluster C personality disorders (depen-dent, avoidant, obsessive-compulsive) are associated with high harm avoidance. Individual personality dis-orders may be described more fully by profiles ob-tained from Cloninger's self-report Temperament and Character Inventory (Cloninger and Svrakic 1994). For example, BPD would consist of high harm avoidance, high novelty seeking, and low reward dependence as well as low scores on the character dimensions.

More recently, a dimensional neurobehavioral model was offered by Depue, Lenzenweger, and col-leagues (e.g., Depue and Collins 1999; Depue and Lenzenweger 2001). Their model regards personality disorders as emergent phenotypes arising from the in-teraction of basic neurobehavioral systems that under-lie major personality traits (Depue and Lenzenweger 2001, p. 165). Through an extensive examination of the psychometric literature on the structure of personality traits as well as a theoretical analysis of the neurobe-havioral systems likely to be relevant to personality and personality dysfunction, they identified five trait dimensions that may account for the range of person-ality disorder phenotypes. They labeled these five traits 1) agentic extraversion (reflecting both the activ-ity and gregariousness components of extraversion); 2) neuroticism; 3) affiliation; 4) nonaffective constraint (the opposite pole of which is impulsivity); and 5) fear. For example, the neurobehavioral system underlying the trait of agentic extraversion is positive incentive motivation, which is common to all mammalian spe-cies and involves positive affect and approach motiva-tion. The dopaminergic system has been strongly im-plicated in incentive-motivated behavior, such that individual differences in the former predict differ-ences in the latter. Research on this model is just begin-ning, but the model is promising in its integration of research on neural systems involved in fundamental functions common to many animal species (such as approach, avoidance, affiliation with conspecifics, and inhibition of punished behavior) with individual dif-ferences research in personality psychology.

Behavior-Genetic Approaches

The vast majority of behavior-genetic studies of per-sonality have focused on normal personality traits, such as those that compose the FFM and Eysenck's (1967, 1981) three-factor model (extraversion, neuroti-cism, and psychoticism). These studies have generally shown moderate to high heritability (30%–60%) for a range of personality traits (Livesley et al. 1993; Plomin and Caspi 1999) relevant to personality disorders. The most frequently studied traits, extraversion and neu-roticism, have produced heritability estimates of 54%–74% and 42%–64%, respectively (Eysenck 1990).

Behavior-genetic data are proving increasingly useful in both etiological and taxonomic work (e.g., Krueger 1999; Livesley et al. 1998). Livesley and col-leagues (2003) noted that behavior-genetic data can help address the persistent lack of consensus among trait psychologists regarding which traits to study by helping them study the causes of trait covariation (as opposed to simply describing it). Establishing con-gruence between a proposed phenotypic model of personality traits and the genetic structure underlying it would support the validity of a proposed factor model. The same holds true for models of personality disorders. To test this approach, Livesley et al. (1998) administered the Dimensional Assessment of Person-ality Pathology—Basic Questionnaire to a large sam-ple of individuals with and without personality disor-ders, including twin pairs. This self-report measure consists of 18 traits considered to underlie personality disorder diagnoses (e.g., identity problems, opposi-tionality, social avoidance). Factor analysis indicated a four-factor solution: emotional dysregulation, disso-cial behavior, inhibition, and compulsivity. Results showed high congruence for all four factors between the phenotypic and behavior-genetic analyses, indi-cating strong support for the proposed factor solution. In addition, the data showed substantial residual her-itability for many lower-order traits, suggesting that these traits likely are not simply components of the higher-order factors but include unique components (specific factors) as well. Krueger and colleagues (e.g., Krueger 1999) have similarly found, using structural equation modeling with a large twin sample, that broadband internalizing and externalizing personality factors account for much of the variance in many common Axis I disorders (e.g., mood, anxiety, and substance use) and that genetic and environmental sources of variance are associated with many of both the higher- and lower-order factors they identified.

Compared with research on normal personality traits (as well as many Axis I disorders), behavior-genetic studies of personality disorders are relatively rare. The most common designs have been family studies in which researchers begin with the personality disorder proband and then assess other family members. The major limitation of this method is that familial aggregation of disorders can support either genetic or environmental causes. As in all behavior-genetic research, twin and adoption studies provide more definitive data. Most of these studies have examined only a subset of the DSM personality disorders, particularly schizotypal, antisocial, and borderline personality disorders. These disorders appear to reflect a continuum of heritability, with schizotypal most strongly linked to genetic influences, antisocial linked both to environmental and genetic variables, and borderline showing the smallest estimates of heritability in the majority of studies (see Nigg and Goldsmith 1994).

Research on the heritability of schizotypal personality disorder provides the clearest evidence of a genetic component to a personality disorder. (Schizotypal personality disorder is defined by criteria such as odd beliefs or magical thinking, unusual perceptual experiences, odd thinking and speech, suspiciousness, inappropriate or constricted affect, and behavior or appearance that is odd or eccentric.) As mentioned earlier, Bleuler and Kraepelin noted peculiarities in language and behavior among some relatives of their schizophrenic patients. Bleuler called this presentation "latent schizophrenia" and considered it to be a less severe and more widespread form of schizophrenia. Further research into the constellation of symptoms characteristic of relatives of schizophrenic patients ultimately resulted in the creation of the DSM diagnosis of schizotypal personality disorder (Spitzer et al. 1979). A genetic relationship between schizophrenia and schizotypal personality disorder is now well established (Kendler and Walsh 1995; Lenzenweger 1998). In one study, Torgersen (1984) found that 33% (7 of 21) of identical co-twins had schizotypal personality disorder, whereas only 4% (1 of 23) of fraternal co-twins shared the diagnosis. Data from a later twin study (Torgersen et al. 2000), which used structural equation modeling, estimated heritability at 0.61.

ASPD, in contrast, appears to have both genetic and environmental roots, as documented in adoption studies (Cadoret et al. 1995). An adult adoptee whose biological parent has an arrest record for antisocial behavior is four times more likely to have problems with aggressive behavior than a person without a biological vulnerability. At the same time, a person whose adoptive parent has ASPD is more than three times more likely to develop the disorder, regardless of biological history. As is the case with other behavior-genetic findings, twin studies suggest that environmental genetic factors grow more predictive as individuals get older (Lyons et al. 1995). In considering the data on ASPD and other personality disorders, however, it is important to remember that all estimates of heritability are sample dependent. Turkheimer et al. (2003) recently found, for example, that genes account for most of the variability in IQ among middle-class children but that over 60% of the variance in IQ in samples from low socioeconomic backgrounds reflects shared environment. Socioeconomic status may similarly moderate the relation between genes and environment and antisocial behavior.

Data on the behavioral genetics of BPD are mixed. Several studies have found only modest evidence of heritability (e.g., Dahl 1993; Nigg and Goldsmith 1994; Reich 1989). A rare twin study conducted by Torgersen (1984) failed to find evidence for the genetic transmission of the disorder, although the sample was relatively small. A more recent twin study by Torgersen et al. (2000) focused on the heritability of several personality disorders, finding a substantial genetic component to several personality disorders, with most heritability estimates between 0.50 and 0.60, including BPD. Increasingly, researchers are suggesting that specific components of BPD may have higher heritability than the BPD diagnosis taken as a whole. For example, several authors (Nigg and Goldsmith 1994; Widiger and Frances 1994) suggest that neuroticism, which is highly heritable, is at the core of many borderline features (e.g., negative affect and stress sensitivity). Other components of BPD have shown substantial heritability as well (e.g., problems with identity, impulsivity, affective lability) (Livesley et al. 1993; Skodol et al. 2002).

A caveat worth mentioning, however, is that behavior-genetic studies that systematically measure environmental influences directly (e.g., measuring developmental toxins such as sexual abuse), rather than deriving estimates of shared and nonshared environment statistically from residual terms, often obtain very different estimates of environmental effects, and this may well be the case with many personality disorders. For example, if one child in a family responds to sexual abuse by becoming avoidant and constricted and another responds to the same experience by becoming borderline and impulsive, researchers will mistakenly conclude—unless they actually measured developmental variables—that shared environment has no effect, because a shared environmental event led to nonshared responses (see Turkheimer and Waldron 2000; Westen 1998). Recent work by Caspi, Moffitt, and colleagues (2002) showing genes and environmental events (e.g., sexual abuse) interacting in predicting subsequent personality and psychopathology emphasize the same point.

INTEGRATIVE THEORIES

Of all the disorders identified in DSM-IV-TR, the personality disorders are likely to be among those that most require biopsychosocial perspectives. They are also disorders for which we may gain substantially by integrating data from both clinical observation and research, from classical theories of personality that delineate personality functions, and from more contemporary research that emphasizes traits. The emergence of several integrative models is thus perhaps not surprising. We briefly describe three such models in the following discussion: Millon's evolutionary–social learning model, Benjamin's interpersonal model, and Westen's functional-domains model.

Millon's Evolutionary–Social Learning Model

Millon developed a comprehensive model of personality and personality disorders that he initially framed in social learning terms (Millon 1969), describing personality in terms of three polarities: pleasure/pain, self/other, and passive/active. These polarities reflect the nature of reinforcement that controls the person's behavior (rewarding or aversive), the source or sources that provide reinforcement (oneself or others), and the instrumental behaviors and coping strategies used to pursue reinforcement (active or passive). Millon (Davis and Millon 1999; Millon 1990; Millon and Davis 1996; Millon's Chapter 14, "Sociocultural Factors," this volume) eventually reconceptualized his original theory in evolutionary terms. In doing so, he added a fourth polarity, thinking/feeling, which reflects the extent to which people rely on abstract thinking or intuition.

Millon's reconceptualized theory outlined four basic evolutionary principles consistent with the polarities described by his earlier theory: 1) aims of existence, which refer to life enhancement and life preservation, and which are reflected in the pleasure/pain polarity; 2) modes of adaptation, which he described in terms of accommodation to, versus modification of, the environment (whether one adjusts or tries to adjust the world, particularly other people) and which are reflected in the passive/active polarity; 3) strategies of replication or reproduction, which refer to the extent to which the person focuses on individuation or nurturance of others and which are reflected in the self/other polarity; and 4) processes of abstraction, which refer to the ability for symbolic thought and which are represented by the thinking/feeling polarity.

Millon identified 14 personality prototypes that can be understood in terms of the basic polarities. For example, patients with schizoid personality disorder tend to have little pleasure, to have little involvement with others, to be relatively passive in their stance to the world, and to rely on abstract thinking over intuition. In contrast, patients with histrionic personality disorder are pleasure seeking, interpersonally focused (although in a self-centered way), highly active, and short on abstract thinking. Millon's theory led to the distinction between avoidant and schizoid personality disorder in DSM-III. Whereas schizoid personality disorder represents a passive-detached personality style, avoidant personality disorder represents an active-detached style characterized by active avoidance motivated by avoidance of anxiety. Millon also developed both a comprehensive measure to assess the DSM personality disorders and his own theory-driven personality disorder classification, the Millon Clinical Multiaxial Inventory (Millon and Davis 1997). The instrument, now in its third edition, has been used in hundreds of studies and is widely used as an assessment tool in clinical practice (e.g., Espelage et al. 2002; Kristensen and Torgersen 2001).

Benjamin's Interpersonal Model

Benjamin's (1993, 1996a, 1996b) interpersonal theory, called Structural Analysis of Social Behavior (SASB), focuses on interpersonal processes in personality and psychopathology and their intrapsychic causes, correlates, and sequelae. Influenced by Sullivan's (1953) interpersonal theory of psychiatry, by object relations approaches, and by research using the interpersonal circumplex (e.g., Kiesler 1983; Leary 1957; Schaefer 1965), the SASB is a three-dimensional circumplex model with three "surfaces," each of which represents a specific focus. The first surface focuses on actions directed at a person (e.g., abuse by a parent toward the patient). A second surface focuses on the person's response to real or perceived actions by the other (e.g., recoiling from the abusive parent). The third focus is on the person's actions toward him- or herself, or what Benjamin calls the "introject" (e.g., self-abuse). The notion behind the surfaces is that the first two are interpersonal and describe the kinds of interaction patterns (self with other) in which the patient engages with significant others (e.g., parents, attachment figures, therapists). The third surface represents internalized attitudes and actions toward the self (e.g., self-criticism that began as criticism from parents). According to Benjamin, children learn to respond to themselves and others by identifying with significant others (acting like them), recapitulating what they experienced with significant others (e.g., eliciting from others what they experienced before), and introjecting others (treating themselves as others have treated them).

As with all circumplex models, each surface has two axes that define its quadrants. In the SASB (as in other interpersonal circumplex models), love and hate represent the two poles of the horizontal axis. Enmeshment and differentiation are the endpoints of the vertical axis. The SASB offers a translation of each of the DSM Axis II criteria (and disorders) into interpersonal terms (Benjamin 1993, 1996b). In this respect, it has two advantages. First, it reduces comorbidity among disorders by specifying the interpersonal antecedents that elicit the patient's responses. For example, maladaptive anger is characteristic of many of the DSM-IV personality disorders but has different interpersonal triggers and meanings (Benjamin 1993). Anger in patients with BPD often reflects perceived neglect or abandonment. Anger in narcissistic personality disorder tends to follow from perceived slights or failures of other people to give the patient everything he or she wants (entitlement). Anger in patients with ASPD is often cold, detached, and aimed at controlling the other person. Second, the SASB model is able to represent multiple, often conflicting aspects of the way patients with a given disorder behave (or complex, multifaceted aspects of a single interpersonal interaction) simultaneously. Thus, a single angry outburst by a borderline patient could reflect an effort to get distance from the other, to hurt the other, and to get the other to respond and hence be drawn back into the relationship. Benjamin has devised several ways of operationalizing a person's dynamics or an interpersonal interaction (e.g., in a therapy hour), ranging from direct observation and coding of behavior to self-report questionnaires, all of which yield descriptions using the same circumplex model.

Westen's Functional-Domains Model

Westen (1995, 1996, 1998) described a model of domains of personality functioning that draws substantially on psychoanalytic clinical theory and observation as well as on empirical research in personality, cognitive, developmental, and clinical psychology. Although some aspects of the model are linked to research on etiology, the model is less a theory of personality disorders than an attempt to delineate and systematize the major elements of personality that define a patient's personality, whether or not the patient has a personality disorder. The model differs from trait approaches in its focus on personality processes and functions (e.g., the kinds of affect regulation strategies the person uses, the ways she represents the self and others mentally, as well as more behavioral dispositions, such as whether she engages in impulsive or self-destructive behavior). However, it shares with trait approaches the view that a single model should be able to accommodate relatively healthy as well as relatively disturbed personality styles and dynamics.

The model suggests that a systematic personality case formulation must answer three questions, each composed of a series of subquestions or variables that require assessment: 1) What does the person wish for, fear, and value, and to what extent are these motives conscious or unconscious, collaborating or conflicting? 2) What psychological resources—including cognitive processes (e.g., intelligence, memory, intactness of thinking processes), affects, affect regulation strategies (conscious coping strategies and unconscious defenses), and behavioral skills—does the person have at his or her disposal to meet internal and external demands? 3) What is the person's experience of the self and others, and how able is the individual—cognitively, emotionally, motivationally, and behaviorally—to sustain meaningful and pleasurable relationships?

From a psychodynamic perspective, these questions correspond roughly to the issues raised by classical psychoanalytic theories of motivation and conflict (Brenner 1982); ego-psychological approaches to adaptive functioning; and object-relational, self-psychological, attachment, and contemporary relational (Aron 1996; Mitchell 1988) approaches to understanding people's experience of self with others. Each of these questions and subdimensions, however, is also associated with a number of research traditions in personality, clinical, cognitive, and developmental psychology (e.g., on the development of children's representations of self, representations of others, moral judgment, attachment styles, ability to tell coherent narratives) (see Damon and Hart 1988; Fonagy et al. 2002; Harter 1999; Livesley and Bromley 1973; Main 1995; Westen 1990a, 1990b, 1991b, 1994). Westen and Shedler (1999a) used this model as a rough theoretical guide to ensure comprehensive coverage of personality domains in developing items for the Shedler-Westen Assessment Procedure Q-Sort, a personality pathology measure for use by expert informants, although the model and the measure are not closely linked (i.e., one does not require the other).

From this point of view, individuals with particular personality disorders are likely to be characterized by a) distinct constellations of motives and conflicts, such as chronic worries about abandonment in BPD or a conflict between the wish for and fear of connectedness to others in avoidant personality disorder; b) deficits in adaptive functioning, such as poor impulse control, lack of self-reflective capacities (see Fonagy and Target 1997), and difficulty regulating affect (Linehan 1993a; Westen 1991a) in BPD or subclinical cognitive disturbances in schizotypal personality disorder; and c) problematic ways of thinking, feeling, and behaving toward themselves and significant others, such as a tendency to form simplistic, one-dimensional representations of the self and others, to misunderstand why people (including the self) behave as they do, and to expect malevolence from other people (characteristics seen in patients with many personality disorders, such as paranoid, schizoid, and borderline) (Kernberg 1975a, 1984; Westen 1991a). In this model, a person's level of personality health–sickness (from severe personality disorder to relatively healthy functioning), which can be assessed reliably using a personality health prototype or a simple rating of level of personality organization derived from Kernberg's work (Westen and Muderrisoglu 2003; Westen and Shedler 1999b), reflects his or her functioning in each of these three domains.

People who do not have severe enough pathology to receive a personality disorder diagnosis can similarly be described using this approach. For example, a successful male executive presented for treatment with troubles in his marriage and his relationships at work, as well as low-level feelings of anxiety and depression. None of these characteristics approached criteria for a personality disorder (or any Axis I disorders, except the relatively nondescript diagnosis of adjustment disorder with mixed anxious and depressed mood). Using this model, one would note that

he was competitive with other people, a fact of which he was unaware (Question 1); had impressive capacities for self-regulation but was intellectualized and afraid of feelings and often used his enjoyment of his work as a way of retreating from his family (Question 2); and had surprisingly noncomplex representations of others' minds (for a person who could solve noninterpersonal problems in complex ways) and consequently would often became angry and attack at work without stopping to empathize with the other person's perspective (Question 3). This description is, of course, highly oversimplified, but it gives a sense of how the model can be used to describe personality dynamics in patients without a diagnosable personality disorder (Westen 1998; Westen and Shedler 1999b).

CASE EXAMPLE

To see how some of the models discussed here operate in practice, consider the following brief case description:

Mr. A was a man in his early 20s who came to treatment for lifelong problems with depression, anxiety, and feelings of inadequacy. He was a kind, introspective, sensitive man who nevertheless had tremendous difficulty making friends and interacting comfortably with people. He was constantly worried that he would misspeak, he would ruminate after conversations about what he had said and the way he was perceived, and he had only one or two friends with whom he felt comfortable. He wanted to be closer to people, but he was frightened that he would be rejected and was afraid of his own anger in relationships. While interacting with people (including his therapist), he would often have a running commentary with them in his mind, typically filled with aggressive content. He was in a 2-year relationship with a woman who was emotionally and physically very distant, whom he saw twice a month and with whom he rarely had sex. Prior to her, his sexual experiences had all been anxiety provoking and short lived, in every sense.

Mr. A tended to be inhibited in many areas of his life. He was emotionally constricted and seemed particularly uncomfortable with pleasurable feelings. He tended to speak in intellectualized terms about his life and history and seemed afraid of affect. He felt stifled in his chosen profession, which did not allow him to express many of his intellectual abilities or creative impulses. He alternated between overcontrol of his impulses, which was his modal stance in life, and occasional breakthroughs of poorly thought-out, impulsive actions (as when he bought an expensive piece of equipment with little forethought about how he would pay for it).

Mr. A came from a working class family in Boston and had lost his father, a policeman, as a young boy. He was reared by his mother and later by a stepfather with whom he had a positive relationship. He also described a good relationship with his mother, although she, like several members of her extended family, struggled with depression, and she apparently suffered a lengthy major depressive episode after her husband's death.

For purposes of brevity, we briefly explicate this case from two theoretical standpoints that provide very different approaches to case formulation: the FFM and the functional-domains viewpoint. (In clinical practice, a functional-domains account and a psychodynamic account are similar, because the former reflects an attempt to systematize and integrate with empirical research [and minimal jargon] the major domains emphasized by classical psychoanalytic, ego-psychological, and object-relational/self-psychological/relational approaches.)

From a five-factor perspective, the most salient features of Mr. A's personality profile were his strong elevations in neuroticism and introversion (low extraversion). He was high on most of the facets of neuroticism, notably anxiety, depression, anger, self-consciousness, and vulnerability. He was low on most facets of extraversion as well, particularly gregariousness, assertiveness, activity, and happiness. This combination of high negative affectivity and low positive affectivity, which left him vulnerable to feelings of depression, captures his anxious, self-conscious social avoidance.

No other broadband factors describe Mr. A adequately, although specific FFM facets provide insight into his personality. He was moderately high in agreeableness, being compliant, modest, and tender-minded; however, he was not particularly high on trust, altruism, or straightforwardness (reflecting his tendency to behave passive-aggressively). He was moderately conscientious, showing moderate scores on the facets of orderliness and discipline. He similarly showed moderate openness to experience, being artistically oriented but low on comfort with feelings. His scores on facets such as intellectual curiosity would likely be moderate, reflecting both an interest and an inhibition. Indeed, a tendency to receive moderate scores because of opposing dynamics would be true of his facet scores on several traits, such as achievement orientation.

A functional domains perspective would offer a similar summary diagnosis to that of a psychodynamic approach, along with a description of his functioning on the three major domains outlined in the model. In broadest outline, from this point of view Mr. A had a depressive, avoidant, and obsessional

personality style organized at a low-functioning neurotic level. In other words, he did not have a personality disorder, as evidenced by his ability to maintain friendships and stable employment, but he had considerable psychological impediments to love, work, and life satisfaction, with a predominance of depressive, avoidant, and obsessional dynamics.

With respect to motives and conflicts (and interpersonal issues, around which many of his conflicts centered), Mr. A had a number of conflicts that impinged on his capacity to lead a fulfilling life. He wanted to connect with people, but he was inhibited by social anxiety, feelings of inadequacy, and an undercurrent of anger toward people that he could not directly express (which emerged in his "running commentaries" in his mind). Although he worried that he would fail others, he always felt somehow unfulfilled in his relationships with them and could be subtly critical. He likely had high standards with which he compared himself and others and against which both frequently fell short. He also had trouble handling his anger, aggressive impulses, and desires for self-assertion. He would frequently behave in passive or self-punitive ways rather than appropriately asserting his desires or expressing his anger. This pattern contributed in turn to a lingering hostile fantasy life and a tendency at times to behave passive-aggressively.

Sex was particularly conflictual for Mr. A, not only because it forced him into an intimate relationship with another person but because of his feelings of inadequacy, his discomfort in looking directly at a woman's body (because of his associations to sex and women's bodies), and his worries that he was homosexual. When with a woman, he frequently worried that he would "accidentally" touch her anus and be repulsed, although interestingly, his sexual fantasies (and humor) had a decidedly anal tone. Homosexual images would also jump into his mind in the middle of sexual activity, which led to considerable anxiety.

With respect to adaptive resources, Mr. A had a number of strengths, notably his impressive intellect, a dry sense of humor, a capacity to introspect, and an ability to persevere. Nevertheless, his overregulation of his feelings and impulses left him vulnerable to breakthroughs of anger, anxiety, and impulsive action. He distanced himself from emotion, in an effort both to regulate anxiety and depression and to regulate excitement and pleasure, which seemed to him both undeserved and threatening.

With respect to his experience of self and relationships, Mr. A's dominant interpersonal concerns centered around rejection, shame, and aloneness. He was able to think about himself and others in complex ways and to show genuine care and concern toward other people, although these strengths were often not manifest because of his interpersonal avoidance. He had low self-esteem, although he had some intellectual awareness that his feelings toward himself were unrealistically negative. He often voiced identity concerns, wondering what he was going to do with his life and where he would fit in and feeling adrift without either meaningful work or love relationships that were sustaining. (This is, of course, a very skeletal description of functional domains in Mr. A; for a more thorough description, and an empirical description using the Shedler-Westen Assessment Procedure Q-Sort, see Westen 1998.)

Conclusions

These observations are highly schematic versions of what an FFM or functional-domains (or psychodynamic) account might offer in describing this case. Nevertheless, they provide some sense of how one might conceptualize a case from two very different theoretical perspectives—notably a case on which Axis II would be silent because the patient's pathology is not severe enough for an Axis II diagnosis. Theory, research, and this brief case example all suggest that including a broader range of personality pathology should be one of the primary goals guiding the revision of Axis II in DSM-V.

REFERENCES

Abend S, Porder MS, Willick MS: Borderline Patients: Psychoanalytic Perspectives. Madison, CT, International Universities Press, 1983

Adler G, Buie D: Aloneness and borderline psychopathology: the possible relevance of child development issues. Int J Psychoanal 60:83–96, 1979

Allport G: Personality: A Psychological Interpretation. New York, Henry Holt, 1937

Allport G, Odbert H: Trait-names: a psycho-lexical study, in Psychological Monographs, Vol 47. Princeton, NJ, Psychological Review Co, 1936

American Psychiatric Association: Diagnostic and Statistical Manual of Mental Disorders, 3rd Edition. Washington, DC, American Psychiatric Association, 1980

American Psychiatric Association: Diagnostic and Statistical Manual of Mental Disorders, 4th Edition. Washington, DC, American Psychiatric Association, 1994

American Psychiatric Association: Diagnostic and Statistical Manual of Mental Disorders, 4th Edition, Text Revision. Washington, DC, American Psychiatric Association, 2000

Aron L: A Meeting of Minds: Mutuality in Psychoanalysis, Vol 4. New York, The Analytic Press, 1996

Axelrod S, Widiger T, Trull T, et al: Relations of five-factor model antagonism facets with personality disorder symptomatology. J Pers Assess 69:297–313, 1997

Baker L, Silk KR, Westen D, et al: Malevolence, splitting, and parental ratings by borderlines. J Nerv Ment Dis 180:258–264, 1992

Balint M: The Basic Fault: Therapeutic Aspects of Regression. Evanston, IL, Northwestern University Press, 1969

Bandura A: Social Foundations of Thought and Action. Englewood Cliffs, NJ, Prentice-Hall, 1986

Bandura A: Social cognitive theory of personality, in Handbook of Personality: Theory and Research, 2nd Edition. Edited by Pervin L, John O. New York, Guilford, 1999, pp 154–196

Beck A: Cognitive aspects of personality disorders and their relation to syndromal disorders: a psychoevolutionary approach, in Personality and Psychopathology. Edited by Cloninger CR. Washington, DC, American Psychiatric Association, 1999, pp 411–429

Beck A, Butler A, Brown G, et al: Dysfunctional beliefs discriminate personality disorders. Behav Res Ther 39:1213–1225, 2001

Beck A, Freeman A, Davis DD: Cognitive Therapy of Personality Disorders, 2nd Edition. New York, Guilford, 2003

Bellak L, Chassan JB, Gediman HK, et al: Ego function assessment of analytic psychotherapy combined with drug therapy. J Nerv Ment Dis 157:465–469, 1973

Benjamin L[S]: Interpersonal Diagnosis and Treatment of Personality Disorders. New York, Guilford, 1993

Benjamin LS: Interpersonal Diagnosis and Treatment of Personality Disorders, 2nd Edition. New York, Guilford, 1996a

Benjamin LS: An interpersonal theory of personality disorders, in Major Theories of Personality Disorder. Edited by Clarkin JF, Lenzenweger MF. New York, Guilford, 1996b, pp 141–220

Blanck G, Blanck R: Ego Psychology: Theory and Practice. New York, Columbia University Press, 1974

Bleuler E: Dementia Praecox or the Group of Schizophrenias (1911). New York, International Universities Press, 1950

Brenner C: The Mind in Conflict. New York, International Universities Press, 1982

Cadoret RJ, Yates WR, Troughton E, et al: Genetic–environmental interaction in the genesis of aggressivity and conduct disorders. Arch Gen Psychiatry 52:916–924, 1995

Cantor N, Harlow RE: Personality, strategic behavior, and daily life problem solving. Current Directions in Psychological Science 3:169–172, 1994

Cantor N, Kihlstrom JF: Personality and Social Intelligence. Englewood Cliffs, NJ, Prentice-Hall, 1987

Caspi A, McClay J, Moffitt T, et al: Role of genotype in the cycle of violence in maltreated children. Science 297:851–853, 2002

Cloninger CR: The genetics and psychobiology of the seven-factor model of personality, in Biology of Personality Disorders. Edited by Silk KR (Review of Psychiatry Series, Vol 17; Oldham JM, Riba MB, series eds). Washington, DC, American Psychiatric Press, 1998, pp 63–92

Cloninger RC, Svrakic D: Differentiating normal and deviant personality by the seven-factor personality model, in Differentiating Normal and Abnormal Personality. Edited by Strack S, Lorr M. New York, Springer, 1994, pp 40–64

Cloninger RC, Svrakic D, Przybeck T: A psychobiological model of temperament and character. Arch Gen Psychiatry 50:975–990, 1993

Coker L, Samuel D, Widiger T: Maladaptive personality functioning within the Big Five and the five-factor model. J Personal Disord 16:385–401, 2002

Costa P, McCrae R: Longitudinal stability of adult personality, in Handbook of Personality Psychology. Edited by Hogan R, Johnson J. San Diego, CA, Academic Press, 1997, pp 269–290

Dahl A: The personality disorders: a critical review of family, twin, and adoption studies. J Personal Disord 7 (suppl):86–99, 1993

Damon W, Hart D: Self-Understanding in Childhood and Adolescence. New York, Cambridge University Press, 1988

Davis R: Millon: Essentials of his science, theory, classification, assessment, and therapy. J Pers Assess 72:330–352, 1999

Depue R, Collins P: Neurobiology of the structure of personality: dopamine, facilitation of incentive motivation, and extraversion. Behav Brain Sci 22:491–569, 1999

Depue R, Lenzenweger M: A neurobehavioral dimensional model, in Handbook of Personality Disorders: Theory, Research, and Treatment. Edited by Livesley J. New York, Guilford, 2001, pp 136–176

Espelage DL, Mazzeo SE, Sherman R, et al: MCMI-II profiles of women with eating disorders: a cluster analytic investigation. J Personal Disord 16:453–463, 2002

Eysenck H: The Biological Basis of Personality. Springfield, IL, Charles C Thomas, 1967

Eysenck H: A Model for Personality. New York, Springer-Verlag, 1981

Eysenck HJ: Biological dimensions of personality, in Handbook of Personality: Theory and Research. Edited by Pervin LA. New York, Guilford, 1990, pp 244–276

Fairbairn WR: Psychoanalytic Studies of the Personality. London, England, Tavistock, 1952

Fonagy P, Target M: Attachment and reflective function: their role in self-organization. Dev Psychopathol 9:679–700, 1997

Fonagy P, Steele H, Steele M: Maternal representations of attachment during pregnancy predict the organization of infant–mother attachment at one year of age. Child Dev 62:891–905, 1991

Fonagy P, Gergely G, Jurist EL, et al: Affect Regulation, Mentalization, and the Development of the Self. New York, Other Press, 2002

Fonagy P, Target M, Gergely G, et al: The developmental roots of borderline personality disorder in early attachment relationships: a theory and some evidence. Psychoanalytic Inquiry 23:412–459, 2003

Goldberg L: The structure of phenotypic personality traits. Am Psychol 48:26–34, 1993

Goldstein W: DSM-III and the narcissistic personality. Am J Psychother 39:4–16, 1985

Greenberg JR, Mitchell S: Object Relations in Psychoanalytic Theory. Cambridge, MA, Harvard University Press, 1983

Gunderson JG: Borderline Personality Disorder: A Clinical Guide. Washington, DC, American Psychiatric Publishing, 2001

Harter S: The Construction of the Self: A Developmental Perspective. New York, Guilford, 1999

Herpertz SC, Dietrich TM, Wenning B, et al: Evidence of abnormal amygdala functioning in borderline personality disorder: a functional MRI study. Biol Psychiatry 50:292–298, 2001

Horowitz M: Introduction to Psychodynamics: A Synthesis. New York, Basic Books, 1988

Horowitz M: Cognitive Psychodynamics: From Conflict to Character. New York, Wiley, 1998

Kendler K, Walsh D: Schizotypal personality disorder in parents and the risk for schizophrenia in siblings. Schizophr Bull 21:47–52, 1995

Kernberg O: Borderline Conditions and Pathological Narcissism. Northvale, NJ, Jason Aronson, 1975a

Kernberg O: Transference and countertransference in the treatment of borderline patients. J Natl Assoc Priv Psychiatr Hosp 7:14–24, 1975b

Kernberg O: Severe Personality Disorders. New Haven, CT, Yale University Press, 1984

Kernberg O: A psychoanalytic theory of personality disorders, in Major Theories of Personality Disorder. Edited by Clarkin J, Lenzenweger M. New York, Guilford, 1996, pp 106–140

Kernberg O: Pathological narcissism and narcissistic personality disorder: theoretical background and diagnostic classification, in Disorders of Narcissism: Diagnostic, Clinical, and Empirical Implications. Edited by Ronningstam E. Washington, DC, American Psychiatric Association, 1998, pp 29–51

Kiesler D: The 1982 interpersonal circle: a taxonomy for complementarity in human transactions. Psychol Rev 90:185–214, 1983

Kohut H: The Analysis of the Self: A Systematic Approach to the Treatment of Narcissistic Personality Disorders. New York, International Universities Press, 1971

Kohut H: The Restoration of the Self. Madison, WI, International Universities Press, 1977

Kraepelin E: Dementia Praecox and Paraphrenia (1896). Chicago, IL, Chicago Medical Book Co, 1919

Kristensen H, Torgersen S: MCMI-II personality traits and symptom traits in parents of children with selective mutism: a case-control study. J Abnorm Psychol 110:648–652, 2001

Krueger RF: The structure of common mental disorders. Arch Gen Psychiatry 56:921–926, 1999

Leary T: Interpersonal Diagnosis of Personality: A Functional Theory and Methodology for Personality Evaluation. Oxford, England, Ronald Press, 1957

Lenzenweger M: Schizotypy and schizotypic psychopathology, in Origins and Development of Schizophrenia: Advances in Experimental Psychopathology. Edited by Lenzenweger M, Dworkin R. Washington, DC, American Psychological Association, 1998, pp 93–122

Linehan M: Cognitive-Behavioral Treatment of Borderline Personality Disorder. New York, Guilford, 1993a

Linehan M: Skills-Training Manual for Treatment of Borderline Personality Disorder. New York, Guilford, 1993b

Livesley WJ, Bromley DB: Person Perception in Childhood and Adolescence. London, England, Wiley, 1973

Livesley WJ, Jang K, Jackson D, et al: Genetic and environmental contributions to dimensions of personality disorder. Am J Psychiatry 150:1826–1831, 1993

Livesley WJ, Jang KL, Vernon PA: Phenotypic and genetic structure of traits delineating personality disorder. Arch Gen Psychiatry 55:941–948, 1998

Livesley WJ, Jang K, Vernon P: Genetic basis of personality structure, in Handbook of Psychology: Personality and Social Psychology, Vol 5. Edited by Millon T, Lerner M. New York, Wiley, 2003, pp 59–83

Lynam DR, Widiger TA: Using the five-factor model to represent the DSM-IV personality disorders: an expert consensus approach. J Abnorm Psychol 110:401–412, 2001

Lyons M, Toomey R, Faraone S, et al: Correlates of psychosis proneness in relatives of schizophrenic patients. Journal of Abnormal Psychology and Psychotherapy: Theory, Research and Practice 104:390–394, 1995

Main M: Recent studies in attachment: overview, with selected implications for clinical work, in Attachment Theory: Social, Developmental, and Clinical Perspectives. Edited by Goldberg S, Muir R, Kerr J. Hillsdale, NJ, Analytic Press, 1995, pp 407–474

Masterson J: Psychotherapy of the Borderline Adult: A Developmental Approach. New York, Brunner/Mazel, 1976

McCrae R, Costa P: Personality in Adulthood. New York, Guilford, 1990

McCrae R, Costa PL: Personality trait structure as a human universal. Am Psychol 52:509–516, 1997

McWilliams N: Relationship, subjectivity, and inference in diagnosis, in Making Diagnosis Meaningful: Enhancing Evaluation and Treatment of Psychological Disorders. Edited by Barron JW. Washington, DC, American Psychological Association, 1998, pp 197–226

Millon T: Modern Psychopathology: A Biosocial Approach to Maladaptive Learning and Functioning. Philadelphia, PA, WB Saunders, 1969

Millon T: Toward a New Psychology. New York, Wiley, 1990

Millon T, Davis R: Conceptions of personality disorders: historical perspectives, the DSMs, and future directions, in The DSM-IV Personality Disorders: Diagnosis and Treatment of Mental Disorders. Edited by Livesley WJ. New York, Guilford, 1995, pp 3–28

Millon T, Davis R: An evolutionary theory of personality disorders, in Major Theories of Personality Disorder. Edited by Clarkin J, Lenzenweger M. New York, Guilford, 1996, pp 221–346

Millon T, Davis R: The MCMI-III: present and future directions. J Pers Assess 68:69–85, 1997

Mischel W: Toward a cognitive social learning reconceptualization of personality. Psychol Rev 39:351–364, 1973

Mischel W: On the interface of cognition and personality: beyond the person-situation debate. Am Psychol 34:740–754, 1979

Mischel W: Personality dispositions revisited and revised: a view after three decades, in Handbook of Personality: Theory and Research. Edited by Pervin L. New York, Guilford, 1990, pp 111–134

Mischel W, Shoda Y: A cognitive-affective system theory of personality: reconceptualizing situations, dispositions, dynamics, and invariance in personality structure. Psychol Rev 102:246–268, 1995

Mitchell SA: Relational Concepts in Psychoanalysis: An Integration. Cambridge, MA, Harvard University Press, 1988

Morey L, Gunderson J, Quigley B, et al: The representation of borderline, avoidant, obsessive-compulsive, and schizotypal personality disorders by the five-factor model. J Personal Disord 16:215–234, 2002

New A, Siever L: Neurobiology and genetics of borderline personality disorder. Psychiatric Annals of Clinical Psychiatry 32:329–336, 2002

Nigg JT, Goldsmith H: Genetics of personality disorders: perspectives from personality and psychopathology research. Psychol Bull 115:346–380, 1994

Plomin R, Caspi A: Behavioral Genetics and Personality. New York, Guilford, 1999

Pretzer JL, Beck AT: A cognitive theory of personality disorders, in Major Theories of Personality Disorder. Edited by Clarkin J, Lenzenweger M. New York, Guilford, 1996, pp 36–105

Redl F, Wineman D: Children Who Hate: The Disorganization and Breakdown of Behavior Controls. Glencoe, IL, Free Press, 1951

Reich J: Familiality of DSM-III dramatic and anxious personality clusters. J Nerv Ment Dis 177:96–100, 1989

Reich W: Character Analysis, 3rd Edition (1933). New York, Simon and Schuster, 1978

Ross S, Lutz C, Bailley S: Positive and negative symptoms of schizotypy and the five-factor model: a domain and facet level analysis. J Pers Assess 79:53–72, 2002

Schaefer E: Configurational analysis of children's reports of parent behavior. J Consult Psychol 29:552–557, 1965

Siever L, Davis K: A psychobiological perspective on the personality disorders. Am J Psychiatry 148:1647–1658, 1991

Siever L, Torgersen S, Gunderson J, et al: The borderline diagnosis III: identifying endophenotypes for genetic studies. Biol Psychiatry 51:964–968, 2003

Skodol A, Siever L, Livesley W, et al: The borderline diagnosis II: biology, genetics, and clinical course. Biol Psychiatry 51:951–963, 2002

Spitzer RL, Endicott J, Gibbon M: Crossing the border into borderline personality and borderline schizophrenia. Arch Gen Psychiatry 36:17–24, 1979

Sullivan HS: The Interpersonal Theory of Psychiatry. New York, Norton, 1953

Torgersen S: Genetic and nosological aspects of schizotypal and borderline personality disorders. Arch Gen Psychiatry 41:546–554, 1984

Torgersen S, Lygren S, Oien PA, et al: A twin study of personality disorders. Compr Psychiatry 41:416–425, 2000

Trull T, Widiger T, Burr R: A structured interview for the assessment of the Five-Factor Model of personality: facet-level relations to the axis II personality disorders. J Pers 69:175–198, 2001

Turkheimer E, Waldron M: Nonshared environment: a theoretical, methodological, and quantitative review. Psychol Bull 126:78–108, 2000

Turkheimer E, Haley A, Waldron M, et al: Socioeconomic status modifies heritability of IQ in young children. Psychol Sci 14:623–628, 2003

Tyrer P, Johnson T: Establishing the severity of personality disorder. Am J Psychiatry 153:1593–1597, 1996

Wachtel P: Psychoanalysis and Behavior Therapy. New York, Basic Books, 1977

Wachtel P: Psychoanalysis, Behavior Therapy, and the Relational World. Washington, DC, American Psychological Association, 1997

Westen D: The relations among narcissism, egocentrism, self-concept, and self-esteem: experimental, clinical and theoretical considerations. Psychoanalysis and Contemporary Thought 13:183–239, 1990a

Westen D: Towards a revised theory of borderline object relations: contributions of empirical research. Int J Psychoanal 71:661–693, 1990b

Westen D: Cognitive-behavioral interventions in the psychoanalytic psychotherapy of borderline personality disorders. Clin Psychol Rev 11:211–230, 1991a

Westen D: Social cognition and object relations. Psychol Bull 109:429–455, 1991b

Westen D: Toward an integrative model of affect regulation: applications to social-psychological research. J Pers 62:641–667, 1994

Westen D: A clinical-empirical model of personality: life after the Mischelian ice age and the NEO-lithic era. J Pers 63:495–524, 1995

Westen D: A model and a method for uncovering the nomothetic from the idiographic: an alternative to the five-factor model? J Res Pers 30:400–413, 1996

Westen D: Case formulation and personality diagnosis: two processes or one? In Making Diagnosis Meaningful: Enhancing Evaluation and Treatment of Psychological Disorders. Edited by Barron JW. Washington, DC, American Psychological Association, 1998, pp 111–138

Westen D, Muderrisoglu S: Assessing personality disorders using a systematic clinical interview: evaluation of an alternative to structured interviews. J Personal Disord 17:351–369, 2003

Westen D, Shedler J: Revising and assessing Axis II, part 1: developing a clinically and empirically valid assessment method. Am J Psychiatry 156:258–272, 1999a

Westen D, Shedler J: Revising and assessing Axis II, part 2: toward an empirically based and clinically useful classification of personality disorders. Am J Psychiatry 156:273–285, 1999b

Widiger T: Personality disorders in the 21st century. J Personal Disord 14:3–16, 2000

Widiger T, Costa P: Personality and personality disorders. Journal of Abnormal Psychology and Psychotherapy: Theory, Research, and Practice 103:78–91, 1994

Widiger T, Frances A: Towards a dimensional model for the personality disorders, in Personality Disorders and the Five-Factor Model of Personality. Edited by Costa P, Widiger T. Washington, DC, American Psychological Association, 1994, pp 19–39

Widiger T, Trull TJ, Clarkin JF, et al: A description of the DSM-IV personality disorders with the five-factor model of personality, in Personality Disorders and the Five-Factor Model of Personality, 2nd Edition. Washington, DC, American Psychological Association, 2002, pp 89–99

Wolf E: Treating the Self: Elements of Clinical Self-Psychology. New York, Guilford, 1988

Young J: Cognitive Therapy for Personality Disorders: A Schema-Focused Approach. Sarasota, FL, Professional Resource Exchange, 1990

Young J, Gluhoski V: Schema-focused diagnosis for personality disorders, in Handbook of Relational Diagnosis and Dysfunctional Family Patterns. Edited by Kaslow F. Oxford, England, Wiley, 1996, pp 300–321

Young J, Lindemann M: An integrative schema-focused model for personality disorders, in Clinical Advances in Cognitive Psychotherapy: Theory and Application. Edited by Leahy R, Dowd T. New York, Springer, 2002, pp 93–109

Young J, Klosko J, Weishaar M: Schema therapy for borderline personality disorder, in Schema Therapy: A Practitioner's Guide. New York, Guilford, 2003

3

Categorical and Dimensional Models of Personality Disorders

Thomas A. Widiger, Ph.D.
Stephanie N. Mullins-Sweatt, M.A.

CATEGORICAL AND DIMENSIONAL MODELS OF PERSONALITY DISORDERS

The conceptualization of personality disorders in the American Psychiatric Association's *Diagnostic and Statistical Manual of Mental Disorders* (DSM-IV-TR; American Psychiatric Association 2000) "represents the categorical perspective that [p]ersonality [d]isorders are qualitatively distinct clinical syndromes" (p. 689). Nevertheless, it is also acknowledged that "an alternative to the categorical approach is the dimensional perspective that [p]ersonality [d]isorders represent maladaptive variants of personality traits that merge imperceptibly into normality and into one another" (p. 689). As concluded by a joint committee of the American Psychiatric Association and the National Institute of Mental Health addressing issues and proposals for DSM-V, "there is a clear need for dimensional models to be developed and for their utility to be compared with that of existing typologies" (Rounsaville et al. 2002, p. 12). The committee emphasized in particular the development of a dimensional model of

personality disorder. The purpose of this chapter is to provide the rationale and empirical support for this perspective and to indicate how personality disorders could be conceptualized as maladaptive variants of continuously distributed personality traits.

LIMITATIONS OF THE CATEGORICAL MODEL

Four concerns commonly cited with respect to the categorical model of personality disorder diagnosis are excessive diagnostic co-occurrence, heterogeneity among persons with the same diagnosis, absence of a nonarbitrary boundary with normal functioning, and inadequate coverage of maladaptive personality functioning. Each of these concerns is discussed briefly in turn.

Excessive Diagnostic Co-Occurrence

DSM-IV-TR provides diagnostic criteria sets to help guide the clinician toward the correct diagnosis and a section devoted to differential diagnosis that indicates "how to differentiate [the] disorder from other disorders that have similar presenting characteristics" (American Psychiatric Association 2000, p. 10). The intention of this information is to help the clinician determine which particular disorder is present, the selection of which would ideally indicate the presence of a specific pathology that will explain the occurrence of the symptoms and suggest a specific treatment to ameliorate the patient's suffering (Frances et al. 1995).

It is evident, however, that DSM-IV-TR routinely fails in the goal of guiding the clinician to the presence of one specific personality disorder. A number of reviews have indicated that many patients meet diagnostic criteria for an excessive number of personality disorder diagnoses (Bornstein 1998; Lilienfeld et al. 1994; Livesley 2003; Oldham et al. 1992; Widiger and Trull 1998). Thus, the maladaptive personality functioning of patients does not appear to be adequately described by a single diagnostic category. No person is generally well described by just one word. Each person is more accurately described by a constellation of personality traits (John and Srivastava 1999).

One approach to diagnostic co-occurrence is to implement hierarchical decision rules. Hierarchical decision rules would eliminate the occurrence of multiple diagnoses, and they may be consistent with how personality disorders are diagnosed in clinical practice (Gunderson 1992). Clinicians generally provide only one personality disorder diagnosis per patient, possibly using their own decision rules for which diagnosis takes precedence (Herkov and Blashfield 1995; Zimmerman and Mattia 1999). However, one limitation of a hierarchical decision rule is the difficulty of establishing a compelling rationale for which diagnosis should take precedence (Gunderson 1992). In addition, any such rule would not actually make the comorbidity go away. For example, borderline patients with obsessive-compulsive personality traits will still have obsessive-compulsive personality traits even if those traits are not included in the diagnosis (Zimmerman and Mattia 1999).

Heterogeneity Among Persons With the Same Diagnosis

There are also important differences among the persons who share the same personality disorder diagnosis. For example, patients with the same diagnosis will vary substantially with respect to which diagnostic criteria were used to make the diagnosis (Clark 1992; Shea 1992), and the differences are not trivial (Millon et al. 1996). For example, only a subset of persons who

meet the DSM-IV-TR criteria for antisocial personality disorder will have the prototypic features of the callous, ruthless, arrogant, charming, and scheming psychopath (Hare et al. 1991), and there are even important differences among the persons who would be diagnosed as psychopathic (Brinkley et al. 2004). One common distinction is between the successful and unsuccessful psychopath, with the former having high levels of diligence, competence, and achievement-striving, whereas the latter is characterized by a laxness, irresponsibility, and negligence (Lynam 2002). Similar distinctions are made for other personality disorders (Millon et al. 1996), such as the differentiation of borderline psychopathology with respect to the dimensions of affective dysregulation, impulsivity, and behavioral disturbance (Sanislow et al. 2002), and the differentiation of dependent personality disorder into submissive, exploitable, and affectionate variants (Pincus and Wilson 2001).

Inconsistent, Unstable, and Arbitrary Diagnostic Boundaries

An additional limitation of the categorical model is the difficulty of establishing a nonarbitrary boundary between disordered and normal personality functioning. One of the innovations of DSM-III (American Psychiatric Association 1980) was the provision of explicit diagnostic criteria, including a specified threshold for a disorder's diagnosis. However, the diagnostic thresholds lack a compelling rationale (Tyrer and Johnson 1996). In fact, no explanation or justification has ever been provided for most of them (Widiger and Corbitt 1994).

The thresholds for the DSM-III schizotypal and borderline diagnoses are the only two for which a rationale has been provided. The DSM-III requirements that the patient have four of eight features for the schizotypal and five of eight for the borderline diagnosis were determined on the basis of maximizing agreement with similar diagnoses provided by clinicians (Spitzer et al. 1979). However, the current diagnostic thresholds for these personality disorders bear little resemblance to the original thresholds established for DSM-III. Blashfield et al. (1992) reported a kappa of only -0.025 for the DSM-III and DSM-III-R (American Psychiatric Association 1987) schizotypal personality disorders, with a reduction in prevalence from 11% to 1%. Seemingly minor changes to diagnostic criteria sets have resulted in unexpected and substantial shifts in prevalence rates that profoundly complicate scientific theory and public health decisions (Blashfield et al. 1992; Narrow et al. 2002).

Inadequate Coverage

In addition to the problem of excessive diagnostic co-occurrence, there is the opposite problem of inadequate coverage. Clinicians provide a diagnosis of personality disorder not otherwise specified (NOS) when they determine that a person has a personality disorder that is not adequately represented by any one of the 10 officially recognized diagnoses (American Psychiatric Association 2000). Personality disorder NOS is often the single most frequently used diagnosis in clinical practice; one explanation for this is that the existing categories are not providing adequate coverage (Verheul and Widiger 2004). Westen and Arkowitz-Westen (1998) surveyed 238 psychiatrists and psychologists with respect to their clinical practice and reported that "the majority of patients with personality pathology significant enough to warrant clinical psychotherapeutic attention (60.6%) are currently undiagnosable on Axis II" (p. 1769). The clinicians reported personality traits concerning commitment, intimacy, shyness, work inhibition, perfectionism, and devaluation of others that were not well described by any of the existing diagnostic categories.

One approach to this problem is to add more diagnostic categories, but there is considerable reluctance to do so, in part because adding categories would increase further the difficulties with excessive diagnostic co-occurrence and differential diagnosis (Pincus et al. 2003). A dimensional model that is reasonably comprehensive would be able to cover a greater range of maladaptive personality functioning without requiring additional diagnostic categories: by avoiding the inclusion of redundant, overlapping diagnoses; by organizing the traits within a hierarchical structure; by representing a broader range of maladaptive personality functioning along a single dimension; and by allowing for the representation of relatively unique or atypical personality profiles (Samuel and Widiger 2004).

VALIDITY OF DIMENSIONAL AND CATEGORICAL MODELS

A variety of statistical and methodological approaches for addressing the validity of categorical and dimensional models of classification have been used, including (but not limited to) the search for evidence of incremental validity, bimodality, discrete breaks within distributions, and reproducibility of factor analytic solutions across groups; as well as latent class, item response, taxometric, and admixture analyses (Haslam 2003; Klein and Riso 1993).

Support for a dimensional model is provided in part by the finding that the maladaptive personality traits included within the diagnostic criteria for the DSM-IV-TR personality disorders are present within members of the general population who would not be diagnosed with a DSM-IV-TR personality disorder. For example, much (if not all) of the fundamental symptomatology of the DSM-IV-TR personality disorders can be understood as maladaptive variants of personality traits included within general models of personality functioning (Saulsman and Page 2004; Widiger and Costa 2002). The symptoms of borderline personality disorder (BPD) can be understood as extreme variants of the angry hostility, vulnerability, anxiousness, depressiveness, and impulsivity included within the broad domain of neuroticism (identified by others as negative affectivity or emotional instability) that is evident within the general population (Clarkin et al. 1993; Morey and Zanarini 2000; Trull et al. 2003). Similarly, much of the symptomatology of antisocial personality disorder appears to be an extreme variant of low conscientiousness (rashness, negligence, hedonism, immorality, undependability, and irresponsibility) and high antagonism (manipulativeness, deceptiveness, exploitativeness, aggressiveness, callousness, and ruthlessness) that have long been evident within the general population (Miller and Lynam 2003; Miller et al. 2001).

Over 50 published studies have suggested that the personality disorders included within DSM-IV appear to be maladaptive variants of common personality traits identified within the general population (Widiger and Costa 2002). Trull et al. (2003) demonstrated that the extent to which a person's personality trait profile matched the profile of a prototypic case of BPD correlated as highly with measures of BPD as measures of BPD correlated with one another, and that this general personality trait index of BPD replicated the relationship of the clinical measures with external validators. Miller and Lynam (2003) demonstrated similarly that a general personality measure of psychopathy predicted drug usage, delinquency, risky sexual behavior, and aggression; as well as several laboratory assessments of pathologies hypothesized to underlie the personality disorder of psychopathy, including willingness to delay gratification in a time-discounting task and a preference for aggressive responses in a social-information processing paradigm.

The structure and heritability of personality disorder symptomatology within general community samples of persons without DSM-IV-TR personality disorders is convergent with the structure and heritability observed among persons who have been diagnosed with these disorders (Tyrer and Alexander 1979). Livesley et al. (1998) compared the phenotypic and genetic structure of a comprehensive set of personality disorder symptoms in samples of 656 patients with personality disorder, 939 general community participants, and 686 twin pairs. Principal components analysis yielded four broad dimensions (emotional dysregulation, dissocial behavior, inhibitedness, and compulsivity) that were replicated across all three samples. Multivariate genetic analyses also yielded the same four factors. "The stable structure of traits across clinical and nonclinical samples is consistent with dimensional representations of personality disorders" (Livesley et al. 1998, p. 941). Livesley and colleagues also noted the remarkable consistency of the four broad domains of personality disorder with four of the five broad domains consistently identified in studies of general personality functioning. They concluded that "the higher-order traits of personality disorder strongly resemble dimensions of normal personality" (p. 941).

Joint factor analyses of measures of the general personality functioning and comprehensive representations of personality disorder symptomatology have consistently confirmed a common underlying structure (Cannon et al. 2003; Clark and Livesley 2002). In sum, it is "striking that an extensive history of research to develop a dimensional model of normal personality functioning that has been confined to community populations is so closely congruent with a model that was derived from an analysis confined to personality disorder symptoms" (Widiger 1998, p. 865). O'Connor (2002) submitted the correlation and factor loading matrices for 37 psychopathology and personality inventories obtained from multiple data sets to round-robin confirmatory factor analyses to determine whether there are differences in the dimensional structure between clinical and nonclinical respondents. He reported quite consistent evidence for high levels of similarity between the normal and abnormal populations with respect both to the number of factors and the factor patterns. O'Connor concluded that "the dimensional universes of normality and abnormality are apparently the same, at least according to data derived from contemporary assessment instruments" (p. 962).

ALTERNATIVE MODELS

The limitations of the categorical model are becoming increasingly recognized by theorists, researchers, and clinicians (Oldham and Skodol 2000; Rounsaville et al. 2002). An expected response to this recognition is the development of proposals for alternative dimensional models. Quite a few dimensional models of personality disorder have been developed; however, space limitations prohibit a comprehensive summary of all of them. We describe in this section several alternative strategies for developing a dimensional model of personality disorder. Additional models beyond those described herein are 1) Eysenck's (1987) three dimensions of neuroticism, extraversion, and psychoticism; 2) the Personality Psychopathology–Five (PSY-5), consisting of positive emotionality/extraversion, aggressiveness, constraint, negative emotionality/neuroticism, and psychoticism (Harkness et al. 1995); 3) the three self-other, pleasure-pain, and active-passive polarities hypothesized by Millon et al. (1996) and assessed by the Millon Index of Personality Styles (MIPS, Millon 1994); 4) Tyrer's (1988) four antisocial, dependent, inhibited, and withdrawn dimensions of personality disorder; and 5) Zuckerman's (2002) five dimensions of sociability, activity, aggression-hostility, impulsive sensation-seeking, and neuroticism-anxiety.

Dimensional Profile of Personality Disorder Diagnostic Categories

A straightforward approach that would involve the least amount of disruption to the existing nomenclature is to provide a dimensional profile of maladaptive personality functioning in terms of the existing (or somewhat revised) diagnostic categories (Oldham and Skodol 2000; Tyrer and Johnson 1996; Widiger and Sanderson 1995). A personality disorder could be characterized as prototypic if all of the diagnostic criteria are met, moderately present if one or two criteria beyond the threshold for a categorical diagnosis are present, threshold if the patient just barely meets diagnostic threshold, subthreshold if symptoms are present but are just below diagnostic threshold, traits if one to three symptoms are present, and absent if no diagnostic criteria are present (Oldham and Skodol 2000). Oldham and Skodol (2000) proposed further that if a patient meets diagnostic criteria for three or more personality disorders, then a diagnosis of "extensive personality disorder" could be provided, along with an indication of the extent to which each personality disorder is present.

Westen and Shedler's (2000) prototypal matching proposal is similar to the proposal of Oldham and Skodol (2000) in that it retains the existing or at least somewhat revised diagnostic categories, each of which would be rated on a five-point scale. However, an important difference is that this five-point rating would not be based on the number of diagnostic criteria. Shedler and Westen (2004) suggested that specific and explicit diagnostic criteria sets are impractical and unnecessary in clinical practice. They proposed instead that the diagnostic manual provide a narrative description of a prototypic case of each personality disorder, with the clinician indicating on a five-point scale the extent to which the actual case matches this description (i.e., 1=description does not apply; 2=only minor features; 3=significant features; 4=strong match, patient has the disorder; and 5=exemplifies the disorder, prototypic case). An additional distinction is that the narrative descriptions would not be confined to the eight or nine diagnostic criteria currently provided but could instead be expanded to provide more extensive descriptions of prototypic cases. Shedler and Westen (2004) provide descriptions of each personality disorder using the Shedler-Westen Assessment Procedure-200 (SWAP-200). The SWAP-200 includes 200 diagnostic criteria (approximately half of which are taken from DSM-IV-TR), drawn from the psychoanalytic and wider personality disorder literature (Shedler 2002).

Dimensional Reorganization of Personality Disorder Symptoms

The proposals of Oldham and Skodol (2000), Tyrer and Johnson (1996), and Westen and Shedler (2000) would largely retain the existing personality disorder categories but provide a means for how each could be described in a more quantitative manner. A potential limitation of these proposals is that there might be underlying dimensions of maladaptive personality functioning that cut across the existing diagnostic constructs, contributing to their diagnostic co-occurrence. The proposals of Livesley (2003) and Clark (1993) are efforts to identify these underlying dimensions of maladaptive personality functioning.

Livesley (2003) approached the development of a dimensional model of personality disorders empirically. He obtained personality disorder symptoms and features from a thorough content analysis of the personality disorder literature. An initial list of criteria was then coded by clinicians with respect to their prototypicality for respective personality disorders. One hundred scales (each with 16 items) were submitted to a series of factor analyses to derive a set of 18 fundamental dimensions of personality disorder that cut across the existing diagnostic categories (e.g., anxiousness, self-harm, intimacy problems, social avoidance,

passive opposition, and interpersonal disesteem). Additional analyses indicate that these 18 dimensions can be subsumed within four higher-order dimensions: emotional dysregulation, dissocial behavior, inhibitedness, and compulsivity. Assessment of the 18-factor model has been provided by the self-report Dimensional Assessment of Personality Pathology–Basic Questionnaire (DAPP-BQ; Livesley 2003).

Clark's (1993) approach was quite similar to that of Livesley (2003). The DSM-III-R personality disorder criteria, along with items obtained from the broader personality disorder literature and selected Axis I disorders (i.e., traitlike manifestations of anxiety and mood disorders), were sorted by clinicians into 22 conceptually similar symptom clusters. Factor analyses of these 22 symptom clusters yielded 12 dimensions of maladaptive personality functioning (e.g., self-harm, entitlement, eccentric perceptions, workaholism, detachment, and manipulation). These 12 dimensions of abnormal personality functioning are related conceptually to three higher-order factors of general personality hypothesized by Watson and colleagues (1999): negative affectivity, positive affectivity, and constraint. Assessment of the 12-factor model has been provided by the self-report Schedule for Nonadaptive and Adaptive Personality (SNAP; Clark 1993). However, support for the three-factor structure of the SNAP has been provided by other instruments, particularly the Multidimensional Personality Questionnaire (MPQ; Tellegen in press). The MPQ has alternative subscales for the three broad domains, including stress reaction, alienation, and aggression within negative emotionality; control, traditionalism, and harm avoidance within constraint; and achievement, social closeness, social potency, and well-being within positive emotionality, and it also has an additional scale of absorption.

Clinical Spectra Models

Clark (1993) included within her factor analyses of personality disorder symptoms traitlike manifestations of anxiety and mood disorders because the diagnostic co-occurrence of personality and Axis I disorders could be due to the presence of common underlying dimensions of maladaptive personality functioning (i.e., temperaments of negative affectivity, positive affectivity, and constraint; Clark and Watson 1999). A proposal by Siever and Davis (1991) was concerned specifically with the diagnostic co-occurrence of the personality and Axis I disorders. The authors suggested that there is no meaningful boundary between the personality and Axis I disorders and proposed that personality and other mental disorders be collapsed into four broad clinical spectra consisting of cognitive/perceptual organization, impulsivity/aggression, affective instability, and anxiety/inhibition.

A suggestion of the clinical spectra model is to reformulate most of the existing personality disorders as early onset, chronic variants of an existing Axis I disorder (First et al. 2002; Siever and Davis 1991). Avoidant personality disorder could be replaced by generalized social phobia; depressive personality disorder by early onset dysthymia; BPD by an affective dysregulation disorder; schizotypal and schizoid personality disorders by an early onset and chronic variant of schizophrenic pathology (as schizotypal is already classified in ICD-10; World Health Organization 1992); paranoid personality disorder by an early onset, chronic, and milder variant of a delusional disorder; obsessive-compulsive personality disorder by a generalized and chronic variant of obsessive-compulsive anxiety disorder; and antisocial personality disorder by an adult variant of conduct (disruptive behavior) disorder. This reformulation would leave just four personality disorders unaccounted for (i.e., histrionic, narcissistic, dependent, and passive-aggressive) that could then be deleted from the manual as falling outside of the existing clinical spectra.

There is little direct empirical support for the four clinical spectra proposal of Siever and Davis (1991), due in part to the absence of an instrument for its assessment. Nevertheless, there is substantial empirical support for the existence of two fundamental dimensions of internalization and externalization that cut across the Axes I and II division (Krueger 1999; Krueger and Tackett 2003). The internalization and externalization dimensions identified by Krueger and colleagues do not map perfectly onto the four clinical spectra of Siever and Davis, but it is apparent that the spectra of affective instability and anxiety/inhibition could be folded into the domain of internalization, and that of impulsivity/aggression into the domain of externalization.

Dimensional Models of General Personality Functioning

Personality disorders may not only be on a continuum with Axis I disorders, they may also be on a continuum with general personality functioning, contributing to the absence of a clear boundary between normal and abnormal personality functioning and to the presence of a considerable amount of personality disorder symp-

tomatology within the general population (Livesley 2003; Widiger and Sanderson 1995). As indicated earlier, the 12 personality disorder scales of the SNAP are related conceptually to the three-factor model of general personality functioning proposed by Watson et al. (1999).

Five-Factor Model

An additional model of general personality functioning is the five-factor model (FFM), derived originally from factor analytic studies of extensive samples of trait terms within the English language (John and Srivastava 1999). In the FFM, the relative importance of a trait is indicated by the number of terms that have been developed within a language to describe the various degrees and nuances of that trait, and the structure of the trait is evident by the relationship among the trait terms (Goldberg 1993). This lexical approach to personality description has emphasized five broad domains of personality, presented in their order of importance as extraversion (or surgency) versus introversion; agreeableness versus antagonism; conscientiousness; emotional instability (or neuroticism); and unconventionality (or openness). The five broad domains have been replicated in lexical studies of the trait terms in a wide variety of other languages, including Czech, Dutch, French, German, Hungarian, Italian, Korean, and Polish, although this research has also suggested that an additional, smaller factor may also emerge—honesty-humility—that is currently included largely as a component of agreeableness (Ashton et al. 2004). Each of the five broad domains has been further differentiated by Costa and McCrae (1992) into more specific facets. For example, the facets of agreeableness versus antagonism are trust versus mistrust, straightforwardness versus deception, altruism versus exploitation, compliance versus opposition, modesty versus arrogance, and tender-mindedness versus tough-mindedness.

The FFM is the predominant model in general personality research, with extensive applications in the fields of health psychology, aging, and developmental psychology (McCrae and Costa 1999). Empirical support for the FFM is extensive, including convergent and discriminant validity at both the domain and facet levels across self, peer, and spouse ratings; temporal stability across 7–10 years; and heritability (McCrae and Costa 1999; Plomin and Caspi 1999); as well as links to a wide variety of important life outcomes, such as mental health (Basic Behavioral Science Task Force of the National Advisory Mental Health Council 1996), career success (Judge et al. 1999), and mortality

(Friedman et al. 1995). Adaptive and maladaptive variants of each of the two poles of the 30 facets have been described (Widiger et al. 2002), and descriptions by researchers (Lynam and Widiger 2001) and by clinicians (Samuel and Widiger 2004) of each of the DSM-IV-TR personality disorders in terms of the FFM have been provided. A number of alternative measures of the FFM have been developed. The most commonly used self-report measure is the NEO Personality Inventory–Revised (NEO-PI-R, Costa and McCrae 1992); a semistructured interview that includes the maladaptive variants of each pole of each facet was developed by Trull et al. (1998).

Interpersonal Circumplex

Some theoretical models of personality disorders suggest that they are essentially, if not entirely, disorders of interpersonal relatedness (Benjamin 1996; Kiesler 1996). All forms of normal and abnormal interpersonal relatedness can be well described as some combination of two fundamental dimensions, identified by Wiggins (2003) as agency (dominance versus submission) and communion (affiliation, or love versus hate). Dependent personality disorder, for example, would represent maladaptively extreme levels of submissiveness and affiliation (Pincus and Wilson 2001).

There are a number of different self-report measures of this interpersonal circumplex (IPC) (Wiggins 2003), with the most popular being perhaps the Interpersonal Adjective Scale–Big Five Version (which includes three additional scales to provide a joint assessment of the FFM and the IPC; Wiggins 2003). The Wisconsin Personality Disorders Inventory (Klein et al. 1993) is a self-report inventory for the assessment of the DSM-IV personality disorders from the perspective of the IPC. Compelling empirical support has been obtained for an IPC understanding of many of the personality disorders (Kiesler 1996), particularly dependent, schizoid, avoidant, histrionic, and passive-aggressive, although this research has also suggested that some aspects of other personality disorders are not well accounted for by the IPC, such as the affective dysregulation of BPD, the impulsivity of antisocial personality, and the workaholism of obsessive-compulsive disorder (Widiger and Hagemoser 1997).

Seven-Factor Model of Cloninger

Cloninger (2000) also developed a dimensional model of general personality functioning that would include both normal and abnormal personality traits. He originally hypothesized the existence of three fundamental dimensions of personality "based on a synthesis of information from family studies, studies of longitudinal development, and psychometric studies of personality structure, as well as neuropharmacologic and neuroanatomical studies of behavioral conditioning and learning in man and other animals" (p. 574). The three dimensions were novelty seeking (behavioral activation: exhilaration or excitement in response to novel stimuli or cues for potential rewards or potential relief from punishment); harm avoidance (behavioral inhibition: intense response to signals of aversive stimuli); and reward dependence (behavioral maintenance: response to signals of reward or to resist extinction of behavior that has been previously reinforced). Each was hypothesized to be associated with a particular monoamine neuromodulator (i.e., dopamine, serotonin, and norepinephrine, respectively). The theory was revised subsequently to include four rather than three temperaments (persistence was separated from reward dependence), along with three additional character dimensions.

The four temperaments reflect innate dispositions to respond to stimuli in a consistent manner; the character dimensions are considered to be individual differences that develop through a nonlinear interaction of temperament, family environment, and life experiences (Svrakic et al. 2002). The three character dimensions are self-directedness (responsible, goal-directed vs. insecure, inept); cooperativeness (helpful, empathic vs. hostile, aggressive); and self-transcendence (imaginative, unconventional vs. controlling, materialistic). The presence of a personality disorder is indicated by low levels of cooperativeness, self-transcendence, and, most importantly, self-directedness (the ability to control, regulate, and adapt behavior); and the specific variants of personality disorder are governed by the four temperaments (Cloninger 2000). The seven factors (four temperament and three character dimensions) are assessed by the self-report Temperament and Character Inventory (TCI; Cloninger 2000). Extensive research concerning Cloninger's seven-factor model is detailed within his chapter in this text (Chapter 9, "Genetics") and elsewhere (Cloninger 1998; Cloninger and Svrakic 1999).

INTEGRATION OF ALTERNATIVE MODELS

There are notable differences among the many alternative proposals. Some of the proposed models have been developed largely on the basis of theoretical reasoning informed by research (e.g., the TCI, MIPS, and four clinical spectra), whereas others were developed empirically through analyses of systematically sampled sets of personality traits or symptoms (e.g., DAPP-BQ, FFM, IPC, SNAP, SWAP-200, and PSY-5). The models can also be differentiated with respect to whether they are confined largely to personality disorder symptoms (e.g., DAPP-BQ, SNAP, and SWAP-200); whether they include a full range of normal and abnormal personality functioning (e.g., FFM, IPC, TCI, and MIPS); and whether they also include Axis I symptoms, e.g., the four clinical spectra and SNAP). The models also differ with respect to their hierarchical level of description. Some of the models are confined to broad domains of personality functioning (e.g., the four clinical spectra, the three MIPS polarities, the Zuckerman five dimensions, and the PSY-5), whereas others include lower-order traits within a hierarchical structure (e.g., the DAPP-BQ, SNAP, FFM, and TCI).

Common Higher-Order Domains

Fortunately, most of the alternative models do appear to be readily integrated within a common hierarchical structure (Bouchard and Loehlin 2001; John and Srivastava 1999; Krueger and Tackett 2003; Larstone et al. 2002; Livesley 2003; Zuckerman 2002). This common structure is hardly surprising, because most of them are attempting to do largely the same thing (i.e., identify the fundamental dimensions of maladaptive personality functioning that underlie and cut across the existing diagnostic categories). Table 3–1 lists how the broad domains of the DAPP-BQ, FFM, SNAP, MPQ, PSY-5, IPC, Eysenck (1987), Zuckerman (2002), Siever and Davis (1991), Tyrer (1988), and Cloninger (2000) models might be aligned with one another. The self-other, pleasure-pain, and active-passive polarity model of Millon et al. (1996) is not included in the table because its alignment with the other models is ambiguous and because only one study has empirically related these polarities to the other models (Millon 1994). The placement of Cloninger's (2000) model is also perhaps relatively more difficult than the others (De Fruyt et al. 2000; Zuckerman 2002).

It is evident from Table 3–1 that all of the models include a domain that concerns extraversion, otherwise described as sociability, activity, positive emotionality, or inhibition (when keyed in the negative direction). This domain contrasts being gregarious, talkative, assertive, and active with being withdrawn, isolated, introverted, and anhedonic. The terms *extraversion* and *positive emotionality* might appear to suggest different domains of personality functioning. However, many studies have confirmed that these are in fact the same domains (Bouchard and Loehlin 2001; Harkness et al. 1995; John and Srivastava 1999; Watson et al. 1994). The title *positive affectivity* is preferred by some authors because it is believed that positive affectivity might be providing the motivating force for extraversion, reflecting individual differences in a behavioral activation (or reward sensitivity) system (Depue and Collins 1999; Pickering and Gray 1999; Watson and Clark 1997). The Zuckerman domains of sociability and activity and the Siever and Davis domain of inhibition are italicized in Table 3–1 because they are relatively more narrow in their scope and coverage. Neither agency nor communion from the IPC are aligned directly under this domain because they are 45°-rotated versions of extraversion and agreeableness (Wiggins 2003).

All of the dimensional models also include traits referring to aggressive, dissocial, or antagonistic interpersonal relatedness. This domain contrasts being suspicious, rejecting, exploitative, antagonistic, callous, deceptive, and manipulative with being trusting, compliant, agreeable, modest, dependent, diffident, and empathic. This domain is represented more narrowly by the PSY-5 and by Zuckerman because their versions of this domain are confined largely to interpersonal aggressiveness, whereas the other models include such additional components as mistrust, exploitation, suspiciousness, deception, and arrogance. Psychoticism from Eysenck's dimensional model is not aligned perfectly with this domain because he includes within "psychoticism" both interpersonal antagonism and impulsive disinhibition (Bouchard and Loehlin 2001; Eysenck 1987; John and Srivastava 1999), comparable with the conceptualization of this domain by Siever and Davis. It should also be noted that the title *psychoticism* is perhaps somewhat unusual, because this term is more typically understood to refer to cognitive-perceptual aberrations (as it is understood within the PSY-5).

The three-dimensional models of the MPQ and SNAP do not include an antagonistic, aggressive domain of personality functioning at this higher-order level. The SNAP does include scales for mistrust, manipulativeness, and aggression but these are placed within the domain of negative affectivity, and the MPQ includes an aggression scale within the domain of negative emotionality. However, joint factor analyses of the DAPP-BQ and SNAP subscales have yielded consistently a four-factor solution (Clark and Livesley 2002; Clark et al. 1996) that corresponds to the first

Table 3–1. Alignment of alternative dimensional models: broad domains

	First	Second	Third	Fourth	Fifth
DAPP-BQ	–Inhibition	Dissocial	Compulsivity	Emotional dysregulation	
Five-factor model	Extraversion	Antagonism	Conscientiousness	Neuroticism	Openness
SNAP and MPQ	*Positive affectivity*	*(Negative affectivity)*	*Constraint*	Negative affectivity	
PSY-5	*Positive emotionality*	*Aggressiveness*	*Constraint*	Negative emotionality	*Psychoticism*
IPC		Agency / Communion			
Eysenck	Extraversion		Psychoticism	Neuroticism	
Zuckerman	*Sociability / Activity*	*Aggression-Hostility*	*–Impulsive*	*Neuroticism*	
Tyrer	*–Withdrawn*	*Antisocial-Dependent*		*Inhibited*	
Siever and Davis	(–Inhibition)		*Aggression/Impulsivity*	*Affective instability / Anxiety/Inhibition*	*Cognitive/Perceptual*
TCI	*Reward dependence*	*–Cooperativeness*	*Persistence / Novelty seeking*	*Harm avoidance / Self-directedness*	*Self-transcendence*

Note. Selected scales from the IPC, Eysenck, Siever and Davis, and Cloninger models are off-center because they lie between the domains defined by the adjoining columns. Selected scales from the SNAP, PSY-5, Zuckerman, Siever and Davis, and TCI models are italicized because they describe domains that are somewhat narrower in scope. Selected scales from the SNAP, Siever and Davis, and TCI models are noted parenthetically because they are more strongly related to another domain. Selected scales from the DAPP-BQ, Zuckerman, Tyrer, and Siever and Davis include the symbol – because they are keyed in the opposite direction of the other scales. DAPP-BQ=Dimensional Assessment of Personality Pathology–Basic Questionnaire; IPC=interpersonal circumplex; MPQ=Multidimensional Personality Questionnaire; PSY-5=Personality Psychopathology–Five; SNAP=Schedule for Nonadaptive and Adaptive Personality; TCI=Temperament and Character Inventory.

four domains of Table 3–1. As indicated by Watson et al. (1994), "extensive data indicate that...the Big Three and Big Five models define a common 'Big Four' space" (p. 24), consisting of negative affectivity (neuroticism), positive affectivity (extraversion), antagonism, and constraint.

All but two of the models also include a domain concerned with the control and regulation of behavior, referred to as constraint, compulsivity, and conscientiousness or, when keyed in the opposite direction, impulsivity and disinhibition. This domain contrasts being disciplined, compulsive, dutiful, conscientious, deliberate, workaholic, and achievement-oriented with being irresponsible, lax, impulsive, negligent, and hedonistic. The only models not to include this domain of personality functioning are the IPC and Tyrer's (1988) four-domain model. Tyrer placed the symptoms of the obsessive-compulsive (anankastic) personality disorder within his inhibited domain, which is defined largely by traits of anxiousness and dysphoria (i.e., a different meaning for the term *inhibition* than is used by the DAPP-BQ). The IPC does not include constraint versus disinhibition because it is a two-dimensional model confined to interpersonal relatedness.

Finally, it is also evident from Table 3–1 that all but one of the models includes a broad domain of emotional dysregulation, otherwise described as negative affectivity or neuroticism. The domain of emotional dysregulation contrasts feeling anxious, depressed, despondent, labile, helpless, self-conscious, and vulnerable (and within some models, feeling angry) with feeling invulnerable, self-assured, and perhaps even glib, shameless, and fearless. The only model not to include this domain of personality functioning is again the IPC. This fourth domain is also somewhat more narrowly defined by Siever and Davis (1991) because they separate anxiousness from affective instability.

In summary, the predominant models of normal and abnormal personality functioning do appear to converge onto four broad domains of personality functioning that can be described as extraversion versus introversion, antagonism versus agreeableness, constraint versus impulsivity, and emotional dysregulation versus emotional stability. The authors of these various models would not all agree on the best names for each dimension, due in part to the fact that no single name is likely to optimally describe an entire domain. Some models place more emphasis on the normal variants (e.g., NEO-PI-R and TCI), whereas other models place more emphasis on the abnormal variants (e.g., DAPP-BQ and SNAP). Finally, the models vary in how broadly

or narrowly they define each domain. Nevertheless, the convergence among them is quite evident with respect to the existence of the four domains. Empirical support for the convergence of these models within a four-factor structure has been provided in a number of studies (e.g., Austin and Deary 2000; Clark et al. 1996; Deary et al. 1998; Livesley et al. 1998; Mulder and Joyce 1997), and perhaps even within some of the earliest, original efforts to develop dimensional models of personality disorder by Presly and Walton (1973) and Tyrer and Alexander (1979).

Only three of the models include a fifth broad domain, characterized within the FFM as openness to experience (or as unconventionality), within the PSY-5 as psychoticism (i.e., illusions, misperceptions, perceptual aberrations, and magical ideation), and by Siever and Davis (1991) as cognitive-perceptual aberrations. Subscales within the SNAP (e.g., schizotypal thought), DAPP-BQ (perceptual cognitive distortion), and the MPQ (absorption) relate empirically to FFM unconventionality (Bouchard and Loehlin 2001; Clark and Livesley 2002). A domain of openness is obtained in joint factor analytic studies that provide sufficient representation of the domain (e.g., Clark and Livesley 2002). However, it appears to be the case that when this domain of openness or unconventionality is narrowly defined as simply cognitive-perceptual aberrations, scales to assess the domain either load on other factors (typically negative affectivity) or they define a factor that is so small that it might not appear to be worth identifying (Austin and Deary 2000; Clark et al. 1996; Larstone et al. 2002). Openness to experience is itself the fifth and smallest domain of the FFM (Goldberg 1993). It is also possible that cognitive-perceptual aberrations do not belong within a dimensional model of normal and abnormal personality functioning, consistent with the ICD-10 inclusion of schizotypal as a variant of schizophrenia rather than a personality disorder.

Note that Table 3–1 does not include the proposals of Oldham and Skodol (2000), Tyrer and Johnson (1996), or Westen and Shedler (2000), because the models provided in the table concern dimensions of maladaptive (and at times also adaptive) personality functioning that, for the most part, cut across the existing diagnostic categories. Some personality disorders might be confined largely to one broad domain (e.g., schizoid within the introversion domain and obsessive-compulsive within the compulsivity domain), but most are more aptly described in terms of more than one domain (e.g., antisocial personality disorder would be represented by antagonism and disinhibi-

Table 3–2.   Lower-order facets and diagnostic criteria within the domain of antagonism versus agreeableness

Abnormal high traits

DAPP-BQ: Suspiciousness, interpersonal disesteem, conduct problems, passive oppositionality, rejection, narcissism

SNAP: Mistrust, manipulativeness, aggression, entitlement

DSM-IV-TR diagnostic criteria

Antisocial: Unlawful behaviors, lying, aliases, physical fights, lacks remorse, deceitfulness

Paranoid: Recurrent suspicions, preoccupation with doubts about loyalty or trustworthiness, reluctance to confide in others, reading hidden demeaning or threatening messages, persistent bearing of grudges, perceptions of attacks on character that are not apparent to others

Narcissistic: Arrogant attitudes, sense of entitlement, interpersonally exploitative, preoccupation with fantasies of unlimited success, grandiose sense of self-importance, lack of empathy

Schizotypal: Suspicious or paranoid ideation

Normal high traits

NEO-PI-R: Skepticism, self-confidence, tough-mindedness, cunning, shrewd, competitive

Normal low traits

NEO-PI-R: Trust, straightforwardness, altruism, compliance, modesty, tender-mindedness, agreeableness

TCI: Helpfulness, compassion, pure-heartedness, sentimentality, empathy

Abnormal low traits

DAPP-BQ: Diffidence

SNAP: Dependency

TCI: Dependence

DSM-IV-TR diagnostic criteria

Dependent: Difficulty expressing disagreement, difficulty making everyday decisions without excessive amount of advice

Histrionic: Suggestible, easily influenced by others

Note.   DAPP-BQ=Dimensional Assessment of Personality Pathology–Basic Questionnaire; NEO-PI-R=NEO Personality Inventory–Revised; SNAP=Schedule for Nonadaptive and Adaptive Personality; TCI=Temperament and Character Inventory.

tion, avoidant by neuroticism and introversion, and dependent by agreeableness and neuroticism). The representation of the DSM-IV-TR personality disorders becomes more evident when the lower-order facets of each domain are articulated.

Lower-Order Traits and Symptoms

Some of the dimensional models include lower-order scales beneath the four (or five) broad domains of personality functioning. Table 3–2 provides a description of how the respective personality trait scales from the DAPP-BQ, SNAP, TCI, and FFM within the domain of agreeableness versus antagonism are aligned with one another, along with the respective personality disorder diagnostic criteria that correspond to these personality traits.

The alignment of the lower-order scales is helpful in illustrating the hierarchical relationship among the domains, traits, and behavioral diagnostic criteria. All of the lower-order scales included within Table 3–2 (i.e., DAPP-BQ, SNAP, NEO-PI-R, and TCI scales) have been shown empirically to be organized within a higher-order domain of antagonism versus agreeableness (De Fruyt et al. 2000; Reynolds and Clark 2001), but one can also proceed even lower in the hierarchy to the level of the behavioral symptoms or expressions of these traits, as illustrated by diagnostic criteria from the antisocial, paranoid, narcissistic, schizotypal, dependent, and histrionic personality disorders. For example, it is evident that antisocial lying is a behavioral example of the broader trait of manipulation, and reading hidden or demeaning messages in statements by others is a more specific expression of the general trait of mistrust or suspiciousness. Some DSM-IV-TR diagnostic criteria, however, are also at the level of the personality traits (e.g., sense of entitlement) rather than being specific behavioral acts (Clark 1992; Shea 1992).

Table 3–2 is also useful in illustrating the close relationship of the normal and abnormal variants of these traits. Scales from the NEO-PI-R and TCI refer largely to normal variants of agreeableness (i.e., being trusting, compliant, straightforward, altruistic, modest, helpful, compassionate, sentimental, and empathic), whereas the scales from the DAPP-BQ and SNAP refer largely to abnormal, maladaptive variants of these same traits (i.e., being dependent, diffident, gullible, sacrificial, meek, docile, submissive, or self-denigrating).

Finally, Table 3–2 also illustrates normal and abnormal variants at both of the antagonism and agreeableness poles of this domain of personality functioning. There are abnormal variants of being excessively high in antagonism (e.g., suspicious, aggressive, or callous) and abnormal variants for the opposite pole, being excessively high in agreeableness (e.g., diffidence, dependency, gullibility, and meekness). There are maladaptive variants for both poles of all of the domains of general personality functioning (Coker et al. 2002; Trull et al. 1998).

Table 3–3 provides a comparable illustration for the domain of emotional dysregulation versus emotional stability. In this instance, the lack of a clear boundary between the normal and abnormal variants is even more apparent, particularly for the low levels of emotional dysregulation. For example, the neuroticism scales of the NEO-PI-R assess levels of anxiousness, depressiveness, self-consciousness, and vulnerability that are present within persons of the general population who would not typically be diagnosed as having a personality disorder, whereas the anxiousness scale from the DAPP-BQ was derived from studies of maladaptive personality functioning. The maladaptivity of the most extreme expressions of normal anxiousness, depressiveness, helplessness, and vulnerability, however, are self-evident, as in the suicidal behavior and self-mutilation evident within persons diagnosed with BPD.

Table 3–3 also illustrates that one can even identify maladaptive variants of extremely high emotional regulation (i.e., the lower half of Table 3–3), evident in psychopathic persons who may lack the ability to experience normal adaptive feelings of vulnerability, anxiousness, or self-consciousness (Hare 1991; Hare et al. 1991). Cleckley (1976) had included in his original description of psychopathy an "absence of 'nervousness' or psychoneurotic manifestations" (p. 206). "The psychopath is nearly always free from minor reactions popularly regarded as 'neurotic' or as constituting 'nervousness'" (p. 54), contributing perhaps to the (unself-conscious) glib charm of the psychopath and to the failure to adequately experience signs of threat or to respond effectively to punishment, and to feelings of invulnerability and invincibility (Lykken 1995; Lynam 2002).

Table 3–4 provides trait terms and diagnostic criteria from the domain of constraint versus disinhibition. Normal and abnormal variants of constraint are again readily identified, with a number of scales from the TCI and the NEO-PI-R that refer to normal, adaptive levels of constraint (or conscientiousness)—such as dutifulness, responsibility, ambitiousness, resourcefulness, deliberation, and self-discipline—with maladaptive variants of these traits emphasized by the DAPP-BQ and the SNAP (i.e., compulsivity, workaholism, and propriety) that are in turn evident within the more behavioral diagnostic criteria for the obsessive-compulsive personality disorder (e.g., excessive devotion to work and preoccupation with details, rules, and organization). At the opposite pole of the constraint domain are the impulsivity and disorderliness scales from the SNAP and TCI and the disinhibited, lax, negligent, disorderly, and irresponsible behaviors of the antisocial and passive-aggressive personality disorders.

CLINICAL UTILITY

Categorical models of classification are often preferred because they appear to be easier to use (Frances et al. 1995). One diagnostic label can convey a considerable amount of useful information in a vivid and succinct manner. Dimensional models of classification are, in one respect, inherently more complex than diagnostic categories because they generally provide more specific and precise information. For example, it is simpler to inform a colleague that a patient has BPD than to describe the patient in terms of the 30 facets of the FFM.

However, the existing diagnostic categories are frustrating and troublesome to clinicians in part because the simplicity of the categorical model provides inaccurate and misleading descriptions (Kass et al. 1985; Maser et al. 1991). Clinicians could find a dimensional model of classification to be easier to use because it provides a more valid and internally consistent means with which to describe a particular patient's psychopathology (Kass et al. 1985). A dimensional classification could be less cumbersome because it would not require the assessment of numerous diagnostic criteria from overlapping categories in

Table 3–3. Lower-order traits, facets, and diagnostic criteria within the domain of emotional dysregulation versus emotional stability

Abnormal high traits

DAPP-BQ: Affective lability, self-harm, anxiousness, identity problems, (insecure attachment), (intimacy problems), (social avoidance)

SNAP: Suicide potential, (dependency)

DSM-IV diagnostic criteria

Borderline: Affective instability, recurring suicidal behavior, unstable and intense relationships, frantic efforts to avoid abandonment, inappropriate and intense anger

Avoidant: Fear of being shamed or ridiculed, feelings of inadequacy, view of self as inept or inadequate

Dependent: Preoccupation with fears of being alone, losing support, or being left to care of self

Schizotypal: Social anxiety

Normal high traits

NEO-PI-R: Self-consciousness, anxiousness, depressiveness, vulnerability, responsive

TCI: Shyness, worry/pessimism, fear of uncertainty

Normal low traits

NEO-PI-R: Calm, low self-consciousness, self-assured, relaxed, resilient

TCI: Self-acceptance

Abnormal low traits

DAPP-BQ: (Narcissism)

PCL-R: Glib and superficial charm

Personality disorder diagnostic criteria

Psychopathic: Shamelessness, fearlessness, feelings of invulnerability or invincibility, inability to feel anxious

Note. Some scales from the DAPP-BQ and SNAP are noted parenthetically because they include aspects of personality function from another domain. DAPP-BQ=Dimensional Assessment of Personality Pathology–Basic Questionnaire; NEO-PI-R=NEO Personality Inventory–Revised; PCL-R=Hare Psychopathy Checklist—Revised; SNAP=Schedule for Nonadaptive and Adaptive Personality; TCI=Temperament and Character Inventory.

a frustratingly unsuccessful effort to make illusory distinctions. Semistructured interviews for the DSM-IV-TR personality disorders must evaluate approximately 100 diagnostic criteria, whereas a semistructured interview for the FFM that covers both normal and maladaptive personality functioning requires the assessment of only 30 facets of personality functioning (Trull et al. 1998). A dimensional model of classification would have an immediate benefit to clinical practice through its resolution of the problems of diagnostic co-occurrence, heterogeneity of membership, inconsistent and ill-defined diagnostic boundaries, inadequate coverage, and illusory diagnostic distinctions.

A potential limitation of some of the dimensional models is the absence of much literature on the treatment implications for elevations on some of the respective scales, or at least an absence of familiarity among clinicians with respect to this literature (Sprock 2003). For example, many clinicians might feel lost when informed that their client has maladaptively low

or high levels of TCI persistence, FFM altruism, or MIPS active instrumental behavior. On the other hand, the dimensional models of personality disorder that are closest to the existing diagnostic categories (e.g., DAPP-BQ and SNAP) are readily able to draw upon the extensive clinical literature concerning the treatment implications of each personality disorder. Very little additional training would be necessary for the clinician to apply the profile descriptions proposal of Oldham and Skodol (2000), Tyrer and Johnson (1996), or Westen and Shedler (2000).

In addition, it is also apparent from Tables 3–2 through 3–4 that a dimensional model could retain the existing personality disorder symptoms as lower-order (behavioral) manifestations of a respective personality trait. Clinicians familiar with the treatment of borderline suicidal behavior, avoidant social anxiety, dependent feelings of inadequacy, or paranoid recurrent suspiciousness would still be treating these symptoms, and a dimensional model of personality disorder could still refer explicitly to them. The major difference

Table 3–4.   Lower-order traits, facets, and diagnostic criteria within the domain of constraint versus disinhibition

Abnormal high traits

DAPP-BQ:	Compulsivity
SNAP:	Workaholism, propriety
TCI:	Perfectionism, work-hardened

     DSM-IV diagnostic criteria

     Obsessive-compulsive: Preoccupation with details, rules, lists, order and organization; perfectionism; excessive devotion to work; overly conscientious; scrupulous; unable to discard worn-out or worthless objects

Normal high traits

NEO-PI-R:	Dutifulness, order, achievement striving, self-discipline, deliberation, competence
TCI:	Resourcefulness, eagerness of effort, responsibility, ambitiousness, purposefulness

Normal low traits

NEO-PI-R:	Casual, easygoing, intuitive, playful

Abnormal low traits

DAPP-BQ:	(Conduct problems), (stimulus-seeking), (passive-oppositionality)
SNAP:	Impulsivity
TCI:	Disorderliness

     DSM-IV diagnostic criteria

Passive-aggressive:	Passive resistance to fulfilling routine social and occupational tasks
Antisocial:	Impulsivity, failure to plan ahead, consistent irresponsibility, recklessness

Note. Some scales from the DAPP-BQ are noted parenthetically because they include aspects of personality function from another domain. DAPP-BQ=Dimensional Assessment of Personality Pathology–Basic Questionnaire; NEO-PI-R=NEO Personality Inventory–Revised; SNAP=Schedule for Nonadaptive and Adaptive Personality; TCI=Temperament and Character Inventory.

would just be that the dimensional models would provide these symptoms within dimensions that would be appreciably less overlapping than the existing diagnostic categories.

The personality domain organization provided in Table 3–1 could in fact facilitate treatment recommendations, as each domain would have more differentiated implications for functioning and treatment planning than the existing diagnostic categories. For example, the first two domains concern disorders of interpersonal relatedness that would be of particular interest and concern to clinicians specializing in marital or family therapy. The third domain involves, at one pole, disorders of impulse dysregulation and disinhibition for which there is again a considerable amount of treatment literature (Coccaro 1998). Disorders within this realm would be particularly evident in behavior that affects work, career, and parenting, with laxness, irresponsibility, and negligence at one pole and a maladaptively excessive perfectionism and workaholism at the other pole. The fourth domain would be most suggestive of pharmacotherapy (as well as psychotherapeutic) interventions for the treat-

ment of various forms of affective dysregulation that are currently spread across the diagnostic categories, including anxiousness, depressiveness, anger, and instability of mood. If the fifth domain of unconventionality was included, it would have specific implications for impaired reality testing, magical thinking, and perceptual aberrations at one pole (Siever and Davis 1991) and perhaps alexithymia, closed-mindedness, and a sterile absence of imagination at the other.

A dimensional model of classification would also have the potentially useful advantage of providing both adaptive and maladaptive personality traits. One can indicate whether a patient is trusting, gregarious, agreeable, and achievement striving, as well as whether the patient shows the maladaptive variants of these traits (i.e., gullibility, intolerance of being alone, docile acquiescence, and workaholism, respectively). Clinicians can then not only describe their patients in a more accurate and specific manner by indicating their precise location along the various dimensions of personality functioning, but also provide a more thorough and comprehensive description by including traits that contribute to adaptive functioning and treatment responsivity. This comprehensive profile description would then draw not only on the existing clinical literature concerning affective dysregulation, impulsivity, workaholism, and interpersonal relatedness but also on the basic science literature concerning the etiology and development of general personality functioning.

Case Example

This case is a summary of a woman, Ms. B, who participated in a dialectical behavior therapy (DBT) program, described by Sanderson and Clarkin (2002). Ms. B was a 37-year-old, married Hispanic woman with three children. She had a bachelor's degree in nursing but had been on psychiatric disability leave for the past 2 years.

Ms. B had done well in school as a child, although she was at times a problem for her teachers because she would occasionally seem to explode in an inexplicable anger and tirade. She was the second of eight children in a family in which there was quite severe corporal punishment. Whenever her parents discovered that she had been reprimanded at school, she would be severely punished at home, at times reaching the level of bruises, wounds, and scars. At the age of 14, she began to be repeatedly sexually abused by a "friend" of the family. The abuse ended when it became known to her parents, but Ms. B felt that they also considered her to be at least partly responsible. Her mother often prayed for her lost soul, and her father often referred to her as "the lost one." As the second oldest child, she had considerable household responsibilities, and she would often be punished severely for failing to meet them. She described having very mixed feelings toward her mother, feeling that she let her mother down yet also feeling bitter and angry in not being adequately protected from the sexual abuser or her physically abusive father.

Ms. B had been hospitalized seven times prior to her entry into the DBT program. Her previous diagnoses included major depressive disorder, posttraumatic stress disorder, generalized anxiety disorder, and BPD. She was given a diagnosis of BPD upon entry into the DBT program, but it did not appear to her therapist that this diagnosis adequately described her difficulties or her strengths. From the perspective of the dimensional model of description of Table 3–1, she clearly had difficulty with affective regulation. She would be expected to have elevations on the DAPP-BQ scales for affective lability and self-harm, the SNAP scale for suicide potential, and perhaps the DAPP-BQ scales for identity problems and insecure attachment as well (see Table 3–3). She completed the self-report NEO-PI-R inventory (Costa and McCrae 1992), which indicated substantial elevations on anxiousness, depressiveness, angry hostility, and vulnerability. She also obtained markedly low elevations on facets of agreeableness (compliance and straightforwardness) that are commonly seen in persons diagnosed with BPD (Clarkin

et al. 1993), indicating defiance and manipulative deception. However, inconsistent with these expressions of antagonism were adaptive elevations on the agreeableness facets of modesty and altruism and the extraversion facet of warmth. "Ms. B was often defiant, oppositional, and angry, particularly toward people in authority, but she was also very self-sacrificial, self-denying, and self-deprecating" (Sanderson and Clarkin 2002, p. 367). The borderline diagnosis did not do justice to these specific aspects of her personality. "She would often get into verbal fights and arguments, but these arguments were also coupled with sincere feelings of warmth and concern toward others" (p. 367).

Of particular importance to her entry into the DBT program were her adaptive elevations within the domain of constraint (conscientiousness; see Table 3–4). "Elevations on facets of conscientiousness are not usually seen in patients with BPD, but they bode well for a potential responsivity to the rigors and demands of the DBT program" (Sanderson and Clarkin 2002, p. 367). On the one hand, Ms. B had a very dysfunctional life, with seven hospitalizations and loss of employment due to a psychiatric disability. On the other hand, she had also accomplished a great deal despite her abusive past and negative emotionality, including good grades in school, a bachelor's degree, a (temporarily suspended) nursing career, and a successful marriage. "She clearly did aspire to be successful and competent in all that she did" (p. 367), including the DBT program. Ms. B responded well to the DBT social skills group and eventually even became a mentor to the younger patients within the group.

Complicating her involvement in the DBT program, however, were her relatively low scores on the NEO-PI-R scales for openness to values and ideas. Ms. B came from a relatively conservative background, and she had an unwavering attitude regarding many matters of life. Fundamental to her depressiveness was her self-deprecation and self-blame, but she was also highly resistant to questioning this self-criticism. Her therapist eventually abandoned her effort to confront Ms. B's strong moral attitudes, focusing instead on developing a forgiveness of others for the pain she had suffered at their hands.

CONCLUSIONS AND RECOMMENDATIONS

The description and classification of personality disorders currently use a categorical model, wherein a person is provided with a single diagnostic label to describe his or her maladaptive personality traits. However, it appears that personality disorders, like general personality functioning, are not summarized well by one single diagnostic label. Persons appear instead to have constellations of maladaptive (and adaptive) personality traits that might be better described in terms of dimensional models. A number of alternative dimensional models of personality disorder have now been developed, and it appears that most of them can be readily integrated into a common hierarchical structure.

REFERENCES

American Psychiatric Association: Diagnostic and Statistical Manual of Mental Disorders, 3rd Edition. Washington, DC, American Psychiatric Association, 1980

American Psychiatric Association: Diagnostic and Statistical Manual of Mental Disorders, 3rd Edition, Revised. Washington, DC, American Psychiatric Association, 1987

American Psychiatric Association: Diagnostic and Statistical Manual of Mental Disorders, 4th Edition, Text Revision. Washington, DC, American Psychiatric Association, 2000

Ashton MC, Lee K, Goldberg LR: A hierarchical analysis of 1,710 English personality-descriptive adjectives. J Pers Soc Psychol 87:707–721, 2004

Austin EJ, Deary IJ: The 'four As': a common framework for normal and abnormal personality? Pers Individ Dif 28:977–995, 2000

Basic Behavioral Science Task Force of the National Advisory Mental Health Council: Basic behavioral science research for mental health: vulnerability and resilience. Am Psychol 51:22–28, 1996

Benjamin LS: Interpersonal Diagnosis and Treatment of Personality Disorders, 2nd Edition. New York, Guilford, 1996

Blashfield RK, Blum N, Pfohl B: The effects of changing Axis II diagnostic criteria. Compr Psychiatry 33:245–252, 1992

Bornstein RF: Reconceptualizing personality disorder diagnosis in the DSM-V: the discriminant validity challenge. Clin Psychol 5:333–343, 1998

Bouchard TJ, Loehlin JC: Genes, evolution, and personality. Behav Genet 31:243–273, 2001

Brinkley CA, Newman JP, Widiger TA, et al: Two approaches to parsing the heterogeneity of psychopathy. Clin Psychol 11:69–94, 2004

Cannon T, Turkheimer E, Oltmanns TF: Factorial structure of pathological personality as evaluated by peers. J Abnorm Psychol 112:81–91, 2003

Clark LA: Resolving taxonomic issues in personality disorders. J Personal Disord 6:360–378, 1992

Clark LA: Manual for the Schedule for Nonadaptive and Adaptive Personality. Minneapolis, MN, University of Minnesota Press, 1993

Clark LA, Livesley WJ: Two approaches to identifying the dimensions of personality disorder: convergence on the five-factor model, in Personality Disorders and the Five-Factor Model of Personality, 2nd Edition. Edited by Costa PT, Widiger TA. Washington, DC, American Psychological Association, 2002, pp 161–176

Clark LA, Watson D: Temperament: a new paradigm for trait psychology, in Handbook of Personality: Theory and Research, 2nd Edition. Edited by Pervin L, John O. New York, Guilford, 1999, pp 399–423

Clark LA, Livesley WJ, Schroeder ML, et al: Convergence of two systems for assessing personality disorder. Psychol Assess 8:294–303, 1996

Clarkin JF, Hull JW, Cantor J, et al: Borderline personality disorder and personality traits: a comparison of SCID-II BPD and NEO-PI. Psychol Assess 5:472–476, 1993

Cleckley H: The Mask of Sanity, 5th Edition. St Louis, MO, Mosby, 1976

Cloninger CR: The genetics and psychobiology of the seven-factor model of personality, in Biology of Personality Disorders. Edited by Silk KR. Washington, DC, American Psychiatric Press, 1998, pp 63–92

Cloninger CR: A practical way to diagnosis personality disorders: a proposal. J Personal Disord 14:99–108, 2000

Cloninger CR, Svrakic D: Personality disorder, in Comprehensive Textbook of Psychiatry, 7th Edition. Edited by Sadock B, Kaplan H. Baltimore, MD, Williams and Wilkins, 1999, pp 1567–1588

Coccaro EF: Neurotransmitter function in personality disorders, in Biology of Personality Disorders. Edited by Silk KR. Washington, DC, American Psychiatric Press, 1998, pp 1–25

Coker LA, Samuel DB, Widiger TA: Maladaptive personality functioning within the Big Five and the FFM. J Personal Disord 16:385–401, 2002

Costa PT, McCrae RR: Revised NEO Personality Inventory (NEO PI-R) and NEO Five-Factor Inventory (NEO-FFI) Professional Manual. Odessa, FL, Psychological Assessment Resources, 1992

Deary IJ, Peter A, Austin E, et al: Personality traits and personality disorders. Br J Psychol 89:647–661, 1998

De Fruyt F, van De Wiele L, van Heeringen C: Cloninger's psychobiological model of temperament and character and the five-factor model of personality. Pers Individ Dif 29:441–452, 2000

Depue RA, Collins PF: Neurobiology of the structure of personality: dopamine facilitation of incentive motivation and extraversion. Behav Brain Sci 22:491–569, 1999

Eysenck HJ: The definition of personality disorders and the criteria appropriate for their description. J Personal Disord 1:211–219, 1987

First MB, Bell CB, Cuthbert B, et al: Personality disorders and relational disorders: a research agenda for addressing crucial gaps in DSM, in A Research Agenda for DSM-V. Edited by Kupfer DJ, First MB, Regier DA. Washington, DC, American Psychiatric Association, 2002, pp 123–199

Frances AJ, First MB, Pincus HA: DSM-IV Guidebook. Washington, DC, American Psychiatric Press, 1995

Friedman HS, Tucker JS, Schwartz JE, et al: Childhood conscientiousness and longevity: health behaviors and cause of death. J Pers Soc Psychol 68:696–703, 1995

Goldberg LR: The structure of phenotypic personality traits. Am Psychol 48:26–34, 1993

Gunderson JG: Diagnostic controversies, in American Psychiatric Press Review of Psychiatry, Vol 11. Edited by Tasman A, Riba MB. Washington, DC, American Psychiatric Press, 1992, pp 9–24

Hare RD: The Hare Psychopathy Checklist–Revised Manual. North Tonawanda, NY, Multi-Health Systems, 1991

Hare RD, Hart SD, Harpur TJ: Psychopathy and the DSM-IV criteria for antisocial personality disorder. J Abnorm Psychol 100:391–398, 1991

Harkness AR, McNulty JL, Ben Porath YS: The Personality Psychopathology Five (PSY-5): constructs and MMPI-2 scales. Psychol Assess 7:104–114, 1995

Haslam N: The dimensional view of personality disorders: a review of the taxometric evidence. Clin Psychol Rev 23:75–93, 2003

Herkov MJ, Blashfield RK: Clinicians' diagnoses of personality disorder: evidence of a hierarchical structure. J Pers Assess 65:313–321, 1995

John OP, Srivastava S: The big five trait taxonomy: history, measurement, and theoretical perspectives, in Handbook of Personality: Theory and Research, 2nd Edition. Edited by Pervin LA, John OP. New York, Guilford, 1999, pp 102–138

Judge TA, Higgins CA, Thoresen CJ, et al: The big five personality traits, general mental ability, and career success across the life span. Personnel Psychology 52:621–652, 1999

Kass F, Skodol A, Charles E, et al: Scaled ratings of DSM-III personality disorders. Am J Psychiatry 142:627–630, 1985

Kiesler DJ: Contemporary Interpersonal Theory and Research: Personality, Psychopathology, and Psychotherapy. New York, Wiley, 1996

Klein DN, Riso LP: Psychiatric disorders: problems of boundaries and comorbidity, in Basic Issues in Psychopathology. Edited by Costello CG. New York, Guilford, 1993, pp 19–66

Klein MH, Benjamin LS, Rosenfeld R, et al: The Wisconsin Personality Disorders Inventory, I: development, reliability, and validity. J Personal Disord 7:285–303, 1993

Krueger RF: The structure of common mental disorders. Arch Gen Psychiatry 56:921–926, 1999

Krueger RF, Tackett JL: Personality and psychopathology: working toward the bigger picture. J Personal Disord 17:109–128, 2003

Larstone RM, Jang KL, Livesley WJ, et al: The relationship between Eysenck's P-E-N model of personality, the five factor model of personality, and traits delineating personality dysfunction. Pers Individ Dif 33:25–37, 2002

Lilienfeld SO, Waldman ID, Israel AC: A critical examination of the use of the term "comorbidity" in psychopathology research. Clin Psychol 1:71–83, 1994

Livesley WJ: Diagnostic dilemmas in classifying personality disorder, in Advancing DSM: Dilemmas in Psychiatric Diagnosis. Edited by Phillips KA, First MB, Pincus HA. Washington, DC, American Psychiatric Association, 2003, pp 153–190

Livesley WJ, Jang KL, Vernon PA: Phenotypic and genetic structure of traits delineating personality disorder. Arch Gen Psychiatry 55:941–948, 1998

Lykken DT: The Antisocial Personalities. Hillsdale, NJ, Erlbaum, 1995

Lynam DR: Psychopathy from the perspective of the five factor model, in Personality Disorders and the Five Factor Model, 2nd Edition. Edited by Costa PT, Widiger TA. Washington DC, American Psychological Association, 2002, pp 325–348

Lynam DR, Widiger TA: Using the five-factor model to represent the DSM-IV personality disorders: an expert consensus approach. J Abnorm Psychol 110:401–412, 2001

Maser JD, Kaelber C, Weise RF: International use and attitudes toward DSM-III and DSM-III-R: growing consensus in psychiatric classification. J Abnorm Psychol 100:271–279, 1991

McCrae RR, Costa PT: A five-factor theory of personality, in Handbook of Personality: Theory and Research, 2nd Edition. Edited by Pervin LA, John OP. New York, Guilford, 1999, pp 139–153

Miller JD, Lynam DR: Psychopathy and the five-factor model of personality: a replication. J Pers Assess 81:168–178, 2003

Miller JD, Lynam DR, Widiger TA, et al: Personality disorders as extreme variants of common personality dimensions: can the five-factor model adequately represent psychopathy? J Pers 69:253–276, 2001

Millon T: Millon Index of Personality Styles Manual. San Antonio, TX, The Psychological Corporation, 1994

Millon T, Davis RD, Millon CM, et al: Disorders of Personality: DSM-IV and Beyond. New York, Wiley, 1996

Morey LC, Zanarini MC: Borderline personality: traits and disorder. J Abnorm Psychol 109:733–737, 2000

Mulder RT, Joyce PR: Temperament and the structure of personality disorder symptoms. Psychol Med 27:99–106, 1997

Narrow WE, Rae DS, Robins LN, et al: Revised prevalence estimates of mental disorders in the United States: using a clinical significance criterion to reconcile 2 surveys' estimates. Arch Gen Psychiatry 59:115–123, 2002

O'Connor BP: The search for dimensional structure differences between normality and abnormality: a statistical review of published data on personality and psychopathology. J Pers Soc Psychol 83:962–982, 2002

Oldham JM, Skodol AE: Charting the future of Axis II. J Personal Disord 14:17–29, 2000

Oldham JM, Skodol AE, Kellman HD, et al: Diagnosis of DSM-III-R personality disorders by two semistructured interviews: patterns of comorbidity. Am J Psychiatry 149:213–220, 1992

Pickering AD, Gray JA: The neuroscience of personality, in Handbook of Personality: Theory and Research, 2nd Edition. Edited by Pervin LA, John OP. New York, Guilford, 1999, pp 277–299

Pincus AL, Wilson KR: Interpersonal variability in dependent personality. J Pers 69:223–251, 2001

Pincus HA, McQueen LE, Elinson L: Subthreshold mental disorders: nosological and research recommendations, in Advancing DSM: Dilemmas in Psychiatric Diagnosis. Edited by Phillips KA, First MB, Pincus HA. Washington, DC, American Psychiatric Association, 2003, pp 129–144

Plomin R, Caspi A: Behavioral genetics and personality, in Handbook of Personality: Theory and Research, 2nd Edition. Edited by Pervin LA, John OP. New York, Guilford, 1999, pp 251–276

Presly AS, Walton HJ: Dimensions of abnormal personality. Br J Psychiatry 122:269–276, 1973

Reynolds SK, Clark LA: Predicting dimensions of personality disorder from domains and facets of the Five-Factor Model. J Pers 69:199–222, 2001

Rounsaville BJ, Alarcón RD, Andrews G, et al: Basic nomenclature issues for DSM-V, in A Research Agenda for DSM-V. Edited by Kupfer DJ, First MB, Regier DE. Washington, DC, American Psychiatric Association, 2002, pp 1–29

Samuel DB, Widiger TA: Clinicians' personality descriptions of prototypic personality disorders. J Personal Disord 18:286–308, 2004

Sanderson C, Clarkin JF: Further use of the NEO PI-R personality dimensions in differential treatment planning, in Personality Disorders and the Five Factor Model of Personality, 2nd Edition. Edited by Costa PT, Widiger TA. Washington, DC, American Psychological Association, 2002, pp 351–375

Sanislow CA, Morey LC, Grilo CM, et al: Confirmatory factor analysis of DSM-IV borderline, schizotypal, avoidant and obsessive-compulsive personality disorders: findings from the Collaborative Longitudinal Personality Disorders Study. Acta Psychiatr Scand 105:28–36, 2002

Saulsman LM, Page AC: The five-factor model and personality disorder empirical literature: a meta-analytic review. Clin Psychol Rev 23:1055–1085, 2004

Shea MT: Some characteristics of the Axis II criteria sets and their implications for assessment of personality disorders. J Personal Disord 6:377–381, 1992

Shedler J: A new language for psychoanalytic diagnosis. J Am Psychoanal Assoc 50:429–456, 2002

Shedler J, Westen D: Refining DSM-IV personality disorder diagnosis: integrating science and practice. Am J Psychiatry 161:1350–1365, 2004

Siever LJ, Davis KL: A psychobiological perspective on the personality disorders. Am J Psychiatry 148:1647–1658, 1991

Spitzer R, Endicott J, Gibbon M: Crossing the border into borderline personality and borderline schizophrenia. Arch Gen Psychiatry 36:17–24, 1979

Sprock J: Dimensional versus categorical classification of prototypic and nonprototypic cases of personality disorder. J Clin Psychol 59:991–1014, 2003

Svrakic DM, Draganic S, Hill K, et al: Temperament, character, and personality disorders: etiologic, diagnostic, and treatment issues. Acta Psychiatr Scand 106:189–195, 2002

Tellegen A: Multidimensional Personality Questionnaire: Manual for Administration, Scoring, and Interpretation. Minneapolis, MN, University of Minnesota Press (in press)

Trull TJ, Widiger TA, Useda JD, et al: A structured interview for the assessment of the five-factor model of personality. Psychol Assess 10:229–240, 1998

Trull TJ, Widiger TA, Lynam DR, et al: Borderline personality disorder from the perspective of general personality functioning. J Abnorm Psychol 112:193–202, 2003

Tyrer P: Personality Disorders: Diagnosis, Management, and Course. London, Wright, Butterworth and Co, 1988

Tyrer P, Alexander J: Classification of personality disorder. Br J Psychiatry 135:163–167, 1979

Tyrer P, Johnson T: Establishing the severity of personality disorder. Am J Psychiatry 153:1593–1597, 1996

Verheul R, Widiger TA: A meta-analysis of the prevalence and usage of the personality disorder not otherwise specified (PDNOS) diagnosis. J Personal Disord 18:309–319, 2004

Watson D, Clark LA: Extraversion and its positive emotional core, in Handbook of Personality Psychology. Edited by Hogan R, Johnson J, Briggs S. New York, Academic Press, 1997, pp 767–793

Watson D, Clark LA, Harkness AR: Structures of personality and their relevance to psychopathology. J Abnorm Psychol 103:18–31, 1994

Watson D, Wiese D, Vaidya J, et al: The two general activation systems of affect: structural findings, evolutionary considerations, and psychobiological evidence. J Pers Soc Psychol 76:820–838, 1999

Westen D, Arkowitz-Westen L: Limitations of Axis II in diagnosing personality pathology in clinical practice. Am J Psychiatry 155:1767–1771, 1998

Westen D, Shedler J: A prototype matching approach to diagnosing personality disorders: toward DSM-V. J Personal Disord 14:109–126, 2000

Widiger TA: Four out of five ain't bad. Arch Gen Psychiatry 55:865–866, 1998

Widiger TA, Corbitt E: Normal versus abnormal personality from the perspective of the DSM, in Differentiating Normal and Abnormal Personality. Edited by Strack S, Lorr M. New York, Springer, 1994, pp 158–175

Widiger TA, Costa PT: Five factor model personality disorder research, in Personality Disorders and the Five Factor Model of Personality, 2nd Edition. Edited by Costa PT, Widiger TA. Washington, DC, American Psychological Association, 2002, pp 59–87

Widiger TA, Hagemoser S: Personality disorders and the interpersonal circumplex, in Circumplex Models of Personality and Emotions. Edited by Plutchik R, Conte HR. Washington, DC, American Psychological Association, 1997, pp 299–325

Widiger TA, Sanderson CJ: Towards a dimensional model of personality disorders in DSM-IV and DSM-V, in The DSM-IV Personality Disorders. Edited by Livesley WJ. New York, Guilford, 1995, pp 433–458

Widiger TA, Trull TJ: Performance characteristics of the DSM-III-R personality disorder criteria sets, in DSM-IV Sourcebook, Vol 4. Edited by Widiger TA, Frances AJ, Pincus HA, et al. Washington, DC, American Psychiatric Association, 1998, pp 357–373

Widiger TA, Costa PT, McCrae RR: A proposal for Axis II: diagnosing personality disorders using the five factor model, in Personality Disorders and the Five Factor Model of Personality, 2nd Edition. Edited by Costa PT, Widiger TA. Washington, DC, American Psychological Association, 2002, pp 431–456

Wiggins JS: Paradigms of Personality Assessment. New York, Guilford, 2003

World Health Organization: The ICD-10 Classification of Mental and Behavioural Disorders: Clinical Descriptions and Diagnostic Guidelines. Geneva, Switzerland, World Health Organization, 1992

Zimmerman M, Mattia JI: Psychiatric diagnosis in clinical practice: is comorbidity being missed? Compr Psychiatry 40:182–191, 1999

Zuckerman M: Zuckerman-Kuhlman Personality Questionnaire (ZKPQ): an alternative five-factorial model, in Big Five Assessment. Edited by de Raad B, Perugini M. Kirkland, WA, Hogrefe and Huber, 2002, pp 377–397

Part II

Clinical Evaluation

4

Manifestations, Clinical Diagnosis, and Comorbidity

Andrew E. Skodol, M.D.

A *personality disorder* is defined in DSM-IV-TR as an "enduring pattern of inner experience and behavior that deviates markedly from the expectations of the individual's culture, is pervasive and inflexible, has an onset in adolescence or early adulthood, is stable over time, and leads to distress or impairment" (American Psychiatric Association 2000, p. 685). Personality disorders are reported on Axis II of the DSM-IV-TR multiaxial system to ensure that consideration is given to their presence in all patient evaluations, even when Axis I disorder psychopathology is present and prominent.

DSM-IV-TR includes criteria for the diagnosis of 10 specific personality disorders, arranged into three clusters based on descriptive similarities. Cluster A is commonly referred to as the "odd or eccentric" cluster and includes paranoid, schizoid, and schizotypal personality disorders. Cluster B, the "dramatic, emotional, or erratic" cluster, includes antisocial, borderline, histrionic, and narcissistic personality disorders. Cluster C, the "anxious and fearful" cluster, includes avoidant, dependent, and obsessive-compulsive personality disorders. DSM-IV-TR also provides for a residual category of personality disorder not otherwise specified (PDNOS). This category is to be used when a patient meets the general criteria for a personality disorder and has features of several different types but does not meet criteria for any specific personality disorder (i.e., "mixed" personality disorder) or is considered to have a personality disorder not included in the official classification (e.g., self-defeating or depressive personality disorders).

DEFINING FEATURES OF PERSONALITY DISORDERS

Patterns of Inner Experience and Behavior

The general diagnostic criteria for a personality disorder in DSM-IV-TR (see Table 4–1) indicate that a pattern

---

Sections of this chapter have been modified with permission from Skodol AE: *Problems in Differential Diagnosis: From DSM-III to DSM-III-R in Clinical Practice*. Washington, DC, American Psychiatric Press, 1989

Table 4–1.   General diagnostic criteria for a personality disorder

A.   An enduring pattern of inner experience and behavior that deviates markedly from the expectations of the individual's culture. This pattern is manifested in two (or more) of the following areas:

    (1)   cognition (i.e., ways of perceiving and interpreting self, other people, and events)

    (2)   affectivity (i.e., the range, intensity, lability, and appropriateness of emotional response)

    (3)   interpersonal functioning

    (4)   impulse control

B.   The enduring pattern is inflexible and pervasive across a broad range of personal and social situations.

C.   The enduring pattern leads to clinically significant distress or impairment in social, occupational, or other important areas of functioning.

D.   The pattern is stable and of long duration, and its onset can be traced back at least to adolescence or early adulthood.

E.   The enduring pattern is not better accounted for as a manifestation or consequence of another mental disorder.

F.   The enduring pattern is not due to the direct physiological effects of a substance (e.g., a drug of abuse, a medication) or a general medical condition (e.g., head trauma).

Source.   Reprinted from American Psychiatric Association: *Diagnostic and Statistical Manual of Mental Disorders*, 4th Edition, Text Revision. Washington, DC, American Psychiatric Association, 2000. Used with permission. Copyright 2000 American Psychiatric Association.

of inner experience and behavior is manifest by characteristic patterns of 1) cognition (i.e., ways of perceiving and interpreting self, other people, and events); 2) affectivity (i.e., the range, intensity, lability, and appropriateness of emotional response); 3) interpersonal functioning; and 4) impulse control. Patients with personality disorders are expected to have manifestations in at least two of these areas.

Cognitive Features

Personality disorders commonly affect the ways patients think about their relationships with other people and about themselves. Most of the DSM-IV-TR diagnostic criteria for paranoid personality disorder reflect a disturbance in cognition, characterized by pervasive distrust and suspiciousness of others. Patients with paranoid personality disorder suspect that others are exploiting, harming, or deceiving them; doubt the loyalty or trustworthiness of others; read hidden, demeaning, or threatening meanings into benign remarks or events; and perceive attacks on their character or reputation. Among the major symptoms of schizotypal personality disorder are characteristic cognitive and perceptual distortions, such as ideas of reference; odd beliefs and magical thinking (e.g., superstitiousness, belief in clairvoyance or telepathy); bodily illusions; and suspiciousness and paranoia similar to that observed in patients with paranoid personality disorder.

Patients with borderline personality disorder (BPD) may also experience transient paranoid ideation when under stress, but the characteristic cognitive manifestations of borderline patients are dramatic shifts in their

views toward people with whom they are intensely emotionally involved. These shifts result in their over-idealizing others at one point and then devaluating them at another point, when they feel disappointed, neglected, or uncared for. This phenomenon is commonly referred to as "splitting." Patients with narcissistic personality disorder exhibit a grandiose sense of self; have fantasies of unlimited success, power, brilliance, beauty, or ideal love; and believe that they are special or unique.

Patients with avoidant personality disorder have excessively negative opinions of themselves, in contrast to patients with narcissistic personality disorder. They see themselves as inept, unappealing, and inferior, and they constantly perceive that they are being criticized or rejected. Patients with dependent personality disorder also lack self-confidence and believe that they are unable to make decisions or to take care of themselves. Patients with obsessive-compulsive personality disorder (OCPD) are perfectionistic and rigid in their thinking and are often preoccupied with details, rules, lists, and order.

Affective Features

Some patients with personality disorders are emotionally constricted, whereas others are excessively emotional. Among the constricted types are patients with schizoid personality disorder, who experience little pleasure in life, appear indifferent to praise or criticism, and are generally emotionally cold, detached, and unexpressive. Patients with schizotypal personality disorder also often have constricted or inappropriate affect, although they can exhibit anxiety in relation to their paranoid fears. Patients with OCPD have considerable difficulty expressing loving feelings toward others, and when they do express affection, they do so in a highly controlled or stilted manner.

Among the most emotionally expressive patients with personality disorders are those with borderline and histrionic personality disorders. Patients with BPD are emotionally labile and react very strongly, particularly in interpersonal contexts, with a variety of intensely dysphoric emotions, such as depression, anxiety, or irritability. They are also prone to inappropriate, intense outbursts of anger and are often preoccupied with fears of being abandoned by those they are attached to and reliant upon. Patients with histrionic personality disorder often display rapidly shifting emotions that seem to be dramatic and exaggerated but are shallow in comparison to the intense emotional expression seen in BPD. Patients with antisocial personality disorder (ASPD) characteristically have problems with irritability and aggressive feelings toward others, which are expressed in the context of threat or intimidation. Patients with narcissistic personality disorder display arrogant, haughty attitudes and have no empathy for other people. Patients with avoidant personality disorder are dominated by anxiety in social situations; those with dependent personality disorder are preoccupied by anxiety over the prospects of separation from caregivers and the need to be independent.

Interpersonal Features

Interpersonal problems are probably the most typical of personality disorders (Benjamin 1996; Kiesler 1996). Other mental disorders are characterized by prominent cognitive or affective features or by problems with impulse control. All personality disorders, however, also have interpersonal manifestations that can be described along the two orthogonal poles of the so-called interpersonal circumplex: dominance versus submission and affiliation versus detachment (Wiggins 2003; see also Chapter 3, "Categorical and Dimensional Models of Personality Disorders," and Chapter 20, "Interpersonal Therapy").

Personality disorders characterized by a need for or a tendency toward dominance in interpersonal relationships include antisocial, histrionic, narcissistic, and obsessive-compulsive. Patients with ASPD deceive and intimidate others for personal gain. Patients with histrionic and narcissistic personality disorders need to be the center of attention and require excessive admiration, respectively. Patients with OCPD need to control others and have them submit to their ways of

doing things. On the submissive side are patients with avoidant and dependent personality disorders. Patients with avoidant personality disorder are inhibited in interpersonal relationships because they are afraid of being shamed or ridiculed. Patients with dependent personality disorder will not disagree with important others for fear of losing their support or approval and will actually do things that are unpleasant, demeaning, or self-defeating in order to receive nurturance from them. Patients with BPD may alternate between submissiveness and dominance, seeming to become deeply involved and dependent only to turn manipulative and demanding when their needs are not met.

In the domain of affiliation versus detachment, patients with histrionic, narcissistic, and dependent personality disorders have the greatest degrees of affiliative behavior, whereas patients with paranoid, schizoid, schizotypal, avoidant, and obsessive-compulsive personality disorders are the most detached. Patients with histrionic, narcissistic, and dependent personality disorders are pro-social because of their needs for attention, admiration, and support, respectively. Patients with paranoid personality disorder do not trust others enough to become deeply involved; patients with schizotypal personality disorder have few friends or confidants, in part from a lack of trust and in part as a result of poor communication and inadequate relatedness. Patients with avoidant personality disorder are socially isolated because of their feelings of inadequacy and their fears of rejection, whereas those with schizoid personality disorder neither desire nor enjoy relationships. Patients with OCPD opt for work and productivity over friendships and interpersonal activity because they feel more in control in the former than the latter. Patients with BPD again can vacillate between being overly attached and dependent on someone (often one who is not the best match) and being isolated, distant, and aloof.

Problems With Impulse Control

Problems with impulse control can also be viewed as extremes on a continuum. Personality disorders characterized by a lack of impulse control include ASPD and BPD. Disorders involving problems with overcontrol include avoidant, dependent, and obsessive-compulsive personality disorders. ASPD is a prototype of a personality disorder characterized by impulsivity. Patients with ASPD break laws, exploit others, fail to plan ahead, get into fights, ignore commitments and obligations, and exhibit generally reckless behaviors without regard to consequences, such as speeding, driving while intoxicated, having impulsive sex, or abusing drugs. Patients with BPD also show many problems with impulse con-

Table 4–2. DSM-IV-TR personality clusters, specific types, and their defining clinical features

Cluster	Type	Characteristic Features
A		**Odd or eccentric**
	Paranoid	Pervasive distrust and suspiciousness of others such that their motives are interpreted as malevolent
	Schizoid	Pervasive pattern of detachment from social relationships and restricted range of expression of emotions in interpersonal settings
	Schizotypal	Pervasive pattern of social and interpersonal deficits marked by acute discomfort with, and reduced capacity for, close relationships as well as by cognitive or perceptual distortions and eccentricities of behavior
B		**Dramatic, emotional, or erratic**
	Antisocial	History of conduct disorder before age 15; pervasive pattern of disregard for and violation of the rights of others; current age at least 18
	Borderline	Pervasive pattern of instability of interpersonal relationships, self-image, and affects, and marked impulsivity
	Histrionic	Pervasive pattern of excessive emotionality and attention seeking
	Narcissistic	Pervasive pattern of grandiosity (in fantasy or behavior), need for admiration, and lack of empathy
C		**Anxious or fearful**
	Avoidant	Pervasive pattern of social inhibition, feelings of inadequacy, and hypersensitivity to negative evaluation
	Dependent	Pervasive and excessive need to be taken care of that leads to submissive and clinging behavior and fears of separation
	Obsessive-compulsive	Pervasive pattern of preoccupation with orderliness, perfectionism, and mental and interpersonal control at the expense of flexibility, openness, and efficiency

Source. Adapted from American Psychiatric Association: *Diagnostic and Statistical Manual of Mental Disorders,* Fourth Edition, Text Revision. Washington, DC, American Psychiatric Association, 2000, p. 685. Used with permission. Copyright 2000 American Psychiatric Association.

trol, including impulsive spending, indiscriminate sex, substance abuse, reckless driving, and binge eating. In addition, patients with BPD engage in recurrent suicidal threats, gestures, or attempts and in self-mutilating behavior such as cutting or burning. Finally, patients with BPD have problems with anger management, have frequent temper outbursts, and at times may even engage in physical fights.

In contrast, patients with avoidant personality disorder are generally inhibited, especially in relation to people, and are reluctant to take risks or to undertake new activities. Patients with dependent personality disorder cannot even make decisions and do not take initiative to start things. Patients with OCPD are overly conscientious and scrupulous about morality, ethics, and values; they cannot bring themselves to throw away even worthless objects and are miserly.

The DSM-IV-TR personality disorder clusters, specific personality disorder types, and their principal defining clinical features are presented in Table 4–2.

Pervasiveness and Inflexibility

For a personality disorder to be present, the disturbances reviewed earlier have to be manifest frequently over a wide range of behaviors, feelings, and perceptions and in many different contexts. In DSM-IV-TR, attempts are made to stress the pervasiveness of the behaviors caused by personality disorders. Added to the basic definition of each personality disorder, serving as the "stem" to which individual features apply, is the phrase "present in a variety of contexts." For example, the essential features of paranoid personality disorder in DSM-IV-TR, preceding the specific criteria, begin: "A pervasive distrust and suspiciousness of others such that their motives are interpreted as malevolent, beginning by early adulthood and present in a variety of contexts, as indicated by four (or more) of the following" (American Psychiatric Association 2000, p. 694). Similarly, for dependent personality disorder, the criteria are preceded by the description: "A pervasive and excessive need to be taken care of that leads to submissive and clinging behavior and fears of separation, beginning by early adulthood and present in a variety of contexts, as indicated by five (or more) of the following" (American Psychiatric Association 2000, p. 725).

Inflexibility is a feature that helps to distinguish personality traits or styles and personality disorders. Inflexibility is indicated by a narrow repertoire of responses that are repeated even when the situation calls for an alternative behavior or in the face of clear evidence that a behavior is inappropriate or not working. For example, an obsessive-compulsive person rigidly adheres to rules and organization even in recreation and loses enjoyment as a consequence. An avoidant person is so fearful of being scrutinized or criticized, even in group situations in which he or she could hardly be the focus of such attention, that life becomes painfully lonely.

Onset and Clinical Course

Personality and personality disorders have traditionally been assumed to reflect stable descriptions of a person, at least after a certain age. Thus, the patterns of inner experience and behaviors described earlier are called "enduring." Personality disorder is also described as "of long duration," with an onset that "can be traced back to at least adolescence or early adulthood" (American Psychiatric Association 2000, p. 686). These concepts persist as integral to the definition of personality disorder despite a large body of empirical evidence that suggests that personality disorder psychopathology is not as stable as the DSM definition would indicate. Longitudinal studies indicate that personality disorders tend to improve over time, at least from the point of view of their overt clinical signs and symptoms (Grilo et al. 2004b; Johnson et al. 2000; Lenzenweger 1999; Shea et al. 2001). Furthermore, personality disorder criteria sets consist of combinations of pathological personality traits and symptomatic behaviors (McGlashan et al. in press). Some behaviors, such as self-mutilating behavior (BPD), may be evidenced much less frequently than traits such as "views self as socially inept, personally unappealing or inferior to others" (avoidant personality disorder). How stable individual manifestations of personality disorders actually are and what the stable components of personality disorders are have become areas of active empirical research. It may be that personality psychopathology waxes and wanes depending on the circumstances of a person's life (see Chapter 6, "Course and Outcome of Personality Disorders").

Distress or Impairment in Functioning

Another important aspect of personality disorders that distinguishes them from traits or styles is that personality disorders lead to distress or impairment in functioning. By their nature, some personality disorders may not be accompanied by obvious subjective distress on the part of the patient. Examples would include schizoid personality disorder, in which a patient is ostensibly satisfied with his or her social isolation and does not seem to need or desire the companionship of others, and ASPD, in which the patient has utter disdain and disregard for social norms and will not experience distress unless his activities are thwarted. On the other side of the coin are patients with BPD, who are likely to experience and express considerable distress, especially when disappointed in a significant other, or patients with avoidant personality disorder, who, in contrast with schizoid patients, are usually very uncomfortable and unhappy with their lack of close friends and companions.

All personality disorders are maladaptive, however, and are accompanied by functional problems in school or at work, in social relationships, or at leisure. The requirement for impairment in psychosocial functioning is codified in DSM-IV-TR in its criterion C of the general diagnostic criteria for a personality disorder, which states that "the enduring pattern [of inner experience and behavior, i.e., personality] leads to clinically significant distress or impairment in social, occupational, or other important areas of functioning" (American Psychiatric Association 2000, p. 689).

A number of studies have compared patients with personality disorders to patients with no personality disorder or with Axis I disorders and have found that patients with personality disorders were more likely to be separated, divorced, or never married (Drake and Vaillant 1985; Pfohl et al. 1984; Zimmerman and Coryell 1989) and to have had more unemployment, frequent job changes, or periods of disability (McGlashan 1986; Modestin and Villiger 1989; Paris et al. 1987; Swartz et al. 1990). It is interesting that only rarely have patients with personality disorders been found to be less well educated (Reich et al. 1989; Soloff and Ulrich 1981). Fewer studies have examined quality of functioning, but in those that have, poorer social functioning or interpersonal relationships (Noyes et al. 1990; Torgersen 1984; Turner et al. 1991) and poorer work functioning or occupational achievement and satisfaction have been found among patients with personality disorders than with others (Andreoli et al. 1989; Casey and Tyrer 1990; Pope et al. 1983; Shea et al.

1990). When patients with different personality disorders have been compared with each other on levels of functional impairment, those with severe personality disorders such as schizotypal and borderline have been found to have significantly more impairment at work, in social relationships, and at leisure than patients with less severe personality disorders, such as OCPD, or with an impairing Axis I disorder, such as major depressive disorder (MDD) without personality disorder. Patients with avoidant personality disorder had intermediate levels of impairment. Even the less impaired patients with personality disorders (i.e., OCPD), however, had moderate to severe impairment in at least one area of functioning (or a Global Assessment of Functioning rating of 60 or less) (Skodol et al. 2002). The finding that significant impairment may be in only one area suggests that patients with personality disorders differ not only in the degree of associated functional impairment but also in the breadth of impairment across functional domains.

Another important aspect of the impairment in functioning in patients with personality disorders is that it tends to be persistent even beyond apparent improvement in personality disorder psychopathology itself (Seivewright et al. 2004; Skodol et al. in press). The persistence of impairment is understandable if one considers that personality disorder psychopathology has usually been long-standing and, therefore, has disrupted a person's work and social development over a period of time (Roberts et al. 2003). The "scars" or residua of personality disorder pathology take time to heal or be overcome. With time (and treatment), however, improvements in functioning can occur.

APPROACHES TO CLINICAL INTERVIEWING

Interviewing a patient to assess for a possible personality disorder presents certain challenges that are somewhat unique. Thus, the interviewer is likely to need to rely on a variety of techniques for gathering information to arrive at a clinical diagnosis, including observation and interaction with the patient, direct questioning, and interviewing informants.

Observation and Interaction

One problem in evaluating a patient for a personality disorder arises from the fact that most people are not able to view their own personality objectively (Zimmerman 1994). Because personality is, by definition, the way a person sees, relates to, and thinks about

himself or herself and the environment, a person's assessment of his or her own personality must be colored by it. The expression of Axis I psychopathology may also be colored by Axis II personality style—for example, symptoms exaggerated by the histrionic or minimized by the compulsive personality—but the symptoms of Axis I disorders are usually more clearly alien to the patient and more easily identified as problematic. People usually learn about their own problem behavior and their patterns of interaction with others through the reactions or observations of other people in their environments.

Traditionally, clinicians have not conducted the same kind of interview in assessing patients suspected of having a personality disturbance as they do with persons suspected of having, for example, a mood or an anxiety disorder. Rather than directly questioning the patient about characteristics of his or her personality, the clinician, assuming that the patient cannot accurately describe these traits, looks for patterns in the way the patient describes social relations and work functioning. These two areas usually give the clearest picture of personality style in general and personality problems specifically. Clinicians have also relied heavily on their observations of how patients interact with them during an evaluation interview or in treatment as manifestations of their patients' personalities (Westen 1997).

These approaches have the advantage of circumventing the lack of objectivity patients might have about their personalities, but they also create problems. The clinician usually comes away with a global impression of the patient's personality but frequently is not aware of many of that patient's specific personality characteristics because he or she has not made a systematic assessment of the signs and symptoms of the wide range of personality disorders (Blashfield and Herkov 1996; Morey and Ochoa 1989; Zimmerman and Mattia 1999b). In routine clinical practice, clinicians tend to use the nonspecific DSM-IV-TR diagnosis of PDNOS when they believe that a patient meets the general criteria for a personality disorder, because they often do not have enough information to make a specific diagnosis (Widiger and Saylor 1998). Alternatively, clinicians will diagnose personality disorders hierarchically: once a patient is seen as having one (usually severe) personality disorder, the clinician will not assess whether traits of other personality disorders are present (Adler et al. 1990; Herkov and Blashfield 1995).

Reliance on interaction with the clinician for personality diagnosis runs the risk of generalizing a mode of interpersonal relating that may be limited to a particular situation or context—that is, the evaluation itself. Although the interaction of patient and clinician can be a useful and objective observation, caution should be used in interpreting its significance, and attempts must be made to integrate this information into a broader overall picture of patient functioning.

Direct Questioning

In psychiatric research, a portion of the poor reliability of personality disorder diagnosis has been assumed to be due to the variance in information resulting from unsystematic assessment of personality traits. Therefore, efforts have been made to develop various structured methods for assessing personality disorders (Kaye and Shea 2000) comparable with those that have been successful in reducing information variance in assessing Axis I disorders (Skodol and Bender 2000). These methods include both 1) self-report measures such as the Personality Disorders Questionnaire–4 (Hyler 1994), the Millon Clinical Multiaxial Inventory–III (Millon et al. 1997), and the Minnesota Multiphasic Personality Inventory–2 (Somwaru and Ben-Porath 1995); and 2) clinical interviews such as the Structured Interview for DSM-IV Personality Disorders (Pfohl et al. 1997), the International Personality Disorder Examination (Loranger 1999), the Structured Clinical Interview for DSM-IV, Axis II (First et al. 1997), the Diagnostic Interview for DSM-IV Personality Disorders (Zanarini et al. 1996), and the Personality Disorder Interview–IV (Widiger et al. 1995).

The interviews are based on the general premise that the patient can be asked specific questions that will indicate the presence or absence of each of the criteria of each of the 10 DSM-IV-TR personality disorder types. The self-report instruments are generally considered to require a follow-up interview because of a very high rate of apparently false-positive responses, but data from studies comparing self-report measures with clinical interviews suggest that the former aid in identification of personality disturbances (Hyler et al. 1990, 1992). Thus, the clinician can keep in mind that patients do not necessarily deny negative personality attributes: in fact, the evidence suggests that they may even overreport traits that clinicians might not think are very important, and that patients can, if asked, consistently describe a wide range of personality traits to multiple interviewers. A self-report inventory might be an efficient way to help focus a clinical interview on a narrower range of personality disorder psychopathology. A semistructured

interview is useful clinically when the results of an assessment might be subject to close scrutiny, such as in child custody, disability, or forensic evaluations (Widiger and Coker 2002). Instruments to assist the clinician in the assessment of personality psychopathology are presented in detail in Chapter 5, "Assessment Instruments and Standardized Evaluation."

Interviewing Informants

Frequently, a patient with a personality disorder consults a mental health professional for evaluation or treatment because another person has found his or her behavior problematic. This person may be a boss, spouse, boyfriend or girlfriend, teacher, parent, or representative of a social agency. Indeed, some people with personality disorders do not even recognize the problematic aspects of their manner of relating or perceiving except as it has a negative effect on someone with whom they interact.

Because of these "blind spots" that people with personality disorders may have, the use of a third-party informant in the evaluation can be useful (Zimmerman et al. 1986). In some treatment settings, such as a private individual psychotherapy practice, it may be considered counterproductive or contraindicated to include a third party, but in many inpatient and outpatient settings, certainly during the evaluation process, it may be appropriate and desirable to see some person close to the patient to corroborate both the patient's report and one's own clinical impressions.

Of course, there is no reason to assume that the informant is bias-free or not coloring a report about the patient with his or her own personality style. In fact, the correspondence between patient self-assessments of personality disorder psychopathology and informant assessments has been generally found to be modest at best (Klonsky et al. 2002). Agreement on pathological personality traits, temperament, and interpersonal problems appears to be somewhat better than on DSM personality disorders. Informants usually report more personality psychopathology than patients. Self/informant agreement on personality disorders is highest for Cluster B disorders (excluding narcissistic personality disorder), lower for Clusters A and C, and lowest for traits related to narcissism and entitlement, as might be expected. So the clinician must make a judgment about the objectivity of the informant and use this as a part, but not a sufficient part, of the overall data on which to base a personality disorder diagnosis (Zimmerman et al. 1988). Which source, the patient or the informant, provides information that is more useful for clinical purposes, such as choosing a treatment or predicting outcome (e.g., Klein 2003), is yet to be definitively determined.

PROBLEMS IN CLINICAL ASSESSMENT

Assessing Pervasiveness

The pervasiveness of personality disturbance can be difficult to determine. When a clinician inquires if a person "often" has a particular experience, a patient will frequently reply "sometimes," which then has to be judged for clinical significance. What constitutes a necessary frequency for a particular trait or behavior (Widiger 2002) and in how many different contexts or with how many different people the trait or behavior needs to be expressed has not been well worked out. Clinicians are forced to rely on their own judgment, keeping in mind also that maladaptivity and inflexibility are hallmarks of pathological traits.

For the clinician interviewing a patient with a possible personality disorder, data about the many areas of functioning, the interpersonal relationships with people interacting in different social roles with the patient, and the nature of the patient–clinician relationship should be integrated into a comprehensive assessment of pervasiveness. Too often, clinicians place disproportionate importance on a patient's functioning at a particular job or with a particular boss or significant other person.

State Versus Trait

An issue that cuts across all personality disorder diagnoses and presents practical problems in differential diagnosis is the distinction between clinical state and personality trait. Personality is presumed to be an enduring aspect of a person, yet assessment of personality ordinarily takes place cross-sectionally—that is, over a brief interval in time. Thus, the clinician is challenged to separate out long-term dispositions of the patient from other more immediate or situationally determined characteristics. This task is more complicated by the fact that the patient often comes for evaluation when there is some particularly acute problem, which may be a social or job-related crisis or the onset of an Axis I disorder (Shea 1997). In either case, the situation in which the patient is being evaluated is frequently a state that is not completely characteristic of the patient's life over the longer run.

Assessing an Enduring Pattern

DSM-IV-TR indicates that personality disorders are of long duration and are not "better accounted for as a manifestation or consequence of another mental disorder" (American Psychiatric Association 2000, p. 689). Making these determinations in practice is not easy. First of all, an accurate assessment requires recognition of current state. An assessment of current state, in turn, includes knowledge of the circumstances that have prompted the person to seek treatment, the consequences in terms of the decision to seek treatment, the current level of stress, and any actual Axis I psychopathology, if present.

The DSM-IV-TR multiaxial system is of considerable aid in the assessment of these problems because of its separation of Axis I disorders from Axis II disorders and its individual axes for physical disorders and psychosocial stressors. A multiaxial system forces clinicians to think about the effects of aspects of patients' current state on long-term patterns of behavior, but it does not make the distinctions for them.

It is not clear from the diagnostic criteria of DSM-IV-TR how long a pattern of personality disturbance needs to be present, or when it should become evident, for a personality disorder to be diagnosed. Earlier iterations of the DSM stated that patients were usually 18 years of age or older because it can be argued that, up to that age, a personality pattern could neither have been manifest long enough nor have become significantly entrenched to be considered a stable constellation of behavior. DSM-IV-TR states, however, that some manifestations of personality disorder are usually recognizable by adolescence or earlier and that personality disorders can be diagnosed in individuals younger than 18 years if manifestations are present for at least 1 year. Longitudinal research has shown that personality disorder symptoms evident in childhood or early adolescence may not persist into adult life (Johnson et al. 2000). Longitudinal research has also shown that there is continuity between certain disorders of childhood and adolescence and personality disorders in early adulthood (Kasen et al. 1999, 2001). Thus, a young boy with oppositional defiant or attention-deficit/hyperactivity disorder in childhood may go on to develop conduct disorder as an adolescent, which can progress to full-blown ASPD in adulthood (Bernstein et al. 1996; Lewinsohn et al. 1997; Rey et al. 1995; Zoccolillo et al. 1992). ASPD is the only diagnosis not given before age 18; an adolescent exhibiting significant antisocial behavior before age 18 is diagnosed with conduct disorder.

Regarding the course of a personality disorder, DSM-IV-TR states that personality disorders are relatively stable over time, although certain of them (e.g., ASPD and BPD) may become somewhat attenuated with age, whereas others may not or may, in fact, become more pronounced (e.g., obsessive-compulsive and schizotypal personality disorders). As mentioned earlier and discussed in greater detail in Chapter 6, "Course and Outcome of Personality Disorders," this degree of stability may not necessarily pertain to all of the features of all DSM-IV-TR personality disorders equally.

To assess stability retrospectively, the clinician must ask questions about periods of a person's life that are of various degrees of remoteness from the current situation. Retrospective reporting is subject to distortion, however, and the only sure way of demonstrating stability over time is, therefore, to do prospective follow-up evaluations. Thus from a practical, clinical point of view, personality disorder diagnoses made cross-sectionally and on the basis of retrospectively collected data would be tentative or provisional pending confirmation by longitudinal evaluation. On an inpatient service, a period of intense observation by many professionals from diverse perspectives may suffice to establish a pattern over time (Skodol et al. 1988, 1991). In a typical outpatient setting in which there are much less frequent encounters with a patient, more time may be required. Ideally, features of a personality disorder should be evident over years, but it is not practical to delay inordinate amounts of time before coming to a diagnostic conclusion. A good retrospective history confirmed by a period of prospective evaluation should make the personality pattern evident.

Assessing the Effect of Axis I Disorder

An Axis I disorder can complicate the diagnosis of a personality disorder in several ways (Widiger and Sanderson 1995; Zimmerman 1994). An Axis I disorder may cause changes in a person's behavior or attitudes that can appear to be signs of a personality disorder. Depression, for example, may cause a person to seem excessively dependent, avoidant, or self-defeating. Cyclothymia or bipolar disorder (not otherwise specified; bipolar II) may lead to periods of grandiosity, impulsivity, poor judgment, and depression that might be confused with manifestations of narcissistic or borderline personality disorders.

The clinician must be aware of the Axis I psychopathology and attempt to assess Axis II independently. This assessment can be attempted in one of two ways. First, the clinician can ask about aspects of personality functioning at times when the patient is not experiencing Axis I symptoms. This approach is feasible when the Axis I disorder is of recent onset and short duration or, if more chronic, if the course of the disorder has been characterized by relatively clear-cut episodes with complete remission and symptom-free periods of long duration. When the Axis I disorder is chronic and unremitting, then the Axis I psychopathology and personality functioning blend together to an extent that makes differentiating between them clearly artificial.

A second approach to distinguishing signs of Axis I pathology from signs of Axis II personality is longitudinal and would defer an Axis II diagnosis pending the outcome of a trial of treatment for the Axis I disorder. This strategy may be the preferred approach in the case of a long-standing and chronic Axis I disorder, like cyclothymia, that has never been previously recognized or treated. Although one always runs the risk of a partial response to treatment and some residual symptoms, this tactic may bring the clinician as close, practically speaking, as he or she will get to observing the patient's baseline functioning.

Case Example

The following case is adapted from Skodol (1989).

A 24-year-old, unemployed man sought psychiatric hospitalization because of a serious problem with depression. The man reported that he had felt mildly, but continuously, depressed since the age of 16. When he reached his twenties, he had begun to have more severe bouts that made him suicidal and unable to function.

During the most recent episode, beginning about 6 months previously, he had quit his job as a taxi driver and isolated himself from his friends. He spent his time "lying around and eating a lot" and, in fact, had gained 60 pounds. He had difficulty falling asleep, felt fatigued all day long, could not concentrate, felt worthless ("There's no purpose to my life") and guilty ("I missed my chances; I've put my family through hell"), and had taken an overdose of sleeping pills.

The man received a semistructured interview assessment of Axis II psychopathology. In describing his personality, he said that he once thought of himself as lively and good-natured, but that over the past 4 or 5 years, he felt he had changed. He said that he was very sensitive to criticism, afraid to get involved with people, fearful of new places and experiences, convinced he was making a fool of himself, and afraid of losing control. He felt very dependent on others for decision making and for initiative. He said that he was so "needy" of others that they "could do anything" to him and he would "take it."

He felt helpless when alone, was sure he would end up "alone and in the streets," and was constantly looking to others, especially family members, for comfort and reassurance.

The man also thought that people took advantage of him now and that he "let them" because he never stood up for his own self-interest. He felt like a total failure with no redeeming virtues. He said he either deliberately passed up opportunities to improve his situation because he felt "I don't deserve any better" or else undermined himself "without thinking" by failing to follow through, for example, on a job interview. He believed that no one could really be trusted, that old friends probably talked about him behind his back ("They think I'm a slob"), that he could not open up with new people because they too would eventually turn on him and reject him, and that he now carried a chip on his shoulder because he had been "burned" by others so often. He admitted that he was not blame-free in relationships because he had also used people, especially members of his family.

The patient felt that he was not improving in his outpatient treatment of the last 3 years. His reason for seeking hospitalization, in addition to the fact that he continually thought of suicide and was frightened he might actually succeed in killing himself, was that he felt "totally lost" in his life, without direction, goals, or knowing what mattered to him. He said he felt "hollow." "If they cut me open after I was dead," he said, "they'd probably find out I was all shriveled up inside."

This man's description of his "personality," the ways in which he characteristically thought about himself, saw others and his relationships to them, and behaved, actually met DSM-IV-TR criteria for avoidant, dependent, paranoid, and borderline personality disorders. He was hospitalized for long-term treatment, which was available at the time. In addition to receiving individual, psychoanalytically oriented psychotherapy sessions and participating in a variety of therapeutic groups, he was given fluoxetine, up to 80 mg/day, for treatment of Axis I MDD and dysthymia.

Six months after admission, the patient reported that he felt significantly less depressed. Measured in terms of the Hamilton Rating Scale for Depression, the initial severity of his depression was 30, and his posttreatment score was 10. A repeat semistructured assessment of his personality functioning revealed that he no longer met DSM-IV-TR criteria for any personality disorder, although he continued to exhibit some dependent traits.

Another example of the way in which Axis I and II disorders interact to obscure differential diagnosis is the case of apparent Axis II psychopathology that, in fact, is the prodrome of an Axis I disorder. Distinguishing Cluster A personality disorders, such as paranoid, schizoid, and schizotypal, from the early signs of Axis I disorders in the schizophrenia and other psychotic disorders class can be particularly difficult. If a clinician is evaluating a patient early in the course of the initial onset of a psychotic disorder, he or she may be confronted with changes in the person toward increasing suspiciousness, social withdrawal, eccentricity, or reduced functioning. Because the diagnosis of psychotic disorders, including schizophrenia, requires that the patient have an episode of active psychosis with delusions and hallucinations, it is not possible to diagnose this prodrome as a psychotic disorder. In fact, until the full-blown disorder is present, the clinician cannot be certain if it is, indeed, a prodrome.

If a change in behavior is of recent onset, then it does not meet the stability criteria for a personality disorder. In such cases, the clinician is forced to diagnose an unspecified mental disorder (nonpsychotic; DSM-IV-TR code 300.9). If, however, the pattern of suspiciousness or social withdrawal with or without eccentricities has been well established, it may legitimately be a personality disorder and be diagnosed as such.

If the clinician follows such a patient over time and the patient develops a full-fledged psychotic disorder, the personality disturbance is no longer adequate for a complete diagnosis because none of the Axis II disorders includes frankly psychotic symptoms. This fairly obvious point is frequently overlooked in practice. All of the personality disorders that have counterpart psychotic disorders on Axis I have milder symptoms in which reality testing is, at least in part, intact. For instance, a patient with paranoid personality disorder may have referential ideas but not frank delusions of reference, and a patient with schizotypal personality disorder may have illusions but not hallucinations. A possible exception is BPD, in which brief psychotic experiences (lasting minutes to an hour or two at most) are included in the diagnostic criteria. In all cases, however, when the patient becomes psychotic for even a day or two, an additional Axis I diagnosis is necessary.

For the patient with a diagnosis of schizotypal personality disorder, the occurrence of a psychotic episode of 1 month's duration almost certainly means the disturbance will meet the criteria for schizophrenia, the symptoms of schizotypal personality disorder "counting" as prodromal symptoms toward the 6-month duration requirement. Under these circumstances, the diagnosis of schizophrenia, with its pervasive effects on cognition, perception, functional ability, and so on, is sufficient, and a diagnosis of schizotypal personality disorder is redundant. When the patient becomes nonpsychotic again, he or she would be considered to have residual schizophrenia instead of schizotypal personality disorder.

Personality Traits Versus Personality Disorders

Another difficult distinction is between personality traits or styles and personality disorders. All patients—all people for that matter—can be described in terms of distinctive patterns of personality, but all do not necessarily warrant a diagnosis of personality disorder. This error is particularly common among inexperienced evaluators. The important features that distinguish pathological personality traits from normal traits are their inflexibility and maladaptiveness, as discussed earlier.

DSM-IV-TR recognizes that it is important to describe personality style as well as to diagnose personality disorder on Axis II. Therefore, instructions are included to list personality features on Axis II even when a personality disorder is absent, or to include them as modifiers of one or more diagnosed personality disorders (e.g., BPD with histrionic features). In practice, however, this option has been seldom utilized (Skodol et al. 1984), even though research has shown that, in addition to the approximately 50% of clinic patients who meet criteria for a personality disorder, another 35% warrant information descriptive of their personality styles on Axis II (Kass et al. 1985). The overlap among the features of personality disorders also becomes very evident when emphasis is placed on the assessment of traits of all personality disorders, even when one is predominant.

The following case example describes a patient with an Axis I disorder whose ongoing treatment was very much affected by Axis II personality traits, none of which met criteria for a personality disorder.

Case Example

The following case is adapted from Skodol (1989).

A 25-year-old, single female receptionist was referred for outpatient therapy following hospitalization for her first manic episode. The patient had attended college for 1 year but dropped out in order to "go into advertising." Over the next 5 years, she had held a series of receptionist, secretarial, and sales jobs, each of which she quit because she wasn't "getting ahead in the world." She lived in an apartment on the north side of Chicago, by herself, that her parents had furnished for her. She ate all of her meals, however, at her mother's house and claimed not even to have a box of crackers in her cupboard. Between her jobs, her parents paid her rent.

Her "career" problems stemmed from the fact that, although she felt quite ordinary and without talent for the most part, she had fantasies of a career as a movie star or high fashion model. She took acting classes and singing lessons but had never had even a small role in a play or show. What she desired was not so much the careers themselves but the glamour associated with them. Although she wanted to move in the circles of the "beautiful people," she was certain that she had nothing to offer them. She sometimes referred to herself as nothing but a shell and scorned herself because of it. She was unable to picture herself working her way up along any realistic career line, feeling both that it would take too long and that she would probably fail.

She had had three close relationships with men that were characterized by an intense interdependency that initially was agreeable to both parties. She craved affection and attention and fell deeply in love with these men. Eventually, however, she became overtly self-centered, demanding, and manipulative, and the man would break off the relationship. After breaking up, she would almost immediately start claiming that the particular man was "going nowhere," was not for her, and would not be missed. In between these relationships, she often had periods in which she engaged in a succession of one-night stands, having sex with a half-dozen partners in a month. Alternatively, she would frequent rock clubs and bars, "in-spots," as she called them, merely on the chance of meeting someone who would introduce her to the glamorous world she dreamed of.

The patient had no female friends other than her sister. She could see little use for such friendships. She preferred spending her time shopping for stylish clothes or watching television alone at home. She liked to dress fashionably and seductively but often felt that she was too fat or that her hair was the wrong color. She had trouble controlling her weight and would periodically go on eating binges for a few days that might result in a 10-pound weight gain. She read popular novels but had very few other interests. She admitted she was bored much of the time but would not admit that cultural or athletic pursuits were other than a waste of time.

This patient was referred for outpatient follow-up without an Axis II personality disorder diagnosis. In fact, her long-term functioning failed to meet DSM-IV-TR criteria for any specific type of personality disorder. On the other hand, she almost met the criteria for several, especially BPD: the patient showed signs of impulsivity (overeating, sexual promiscuity), intense interpersonal relationships (manipulative, overidealization/devaluation), identity disturbance, and chronic feelings of emptiness. She did not, however, display intense anger, intolerance of being alone, physically self-damaging behavior, stress-related paranoia or dissociation, or affective instability independent of her mood disorder. Similarly, she had symptoms of histrionic personality disorder: she was inappropriately sexually seductive and used her physical appearance to draw attention to herself, but she was not emotionally overdramatic. She had shallow expression of emotions and was uncomfortable when she was not the center of attention, but was not overly suggestible. She also had some features of narcissistic, avoidant, and dependent personality disorders. The attention paid to personality traits in her outpatient clinic evaluation conveyed a vivid picture of the patient's complicated personality pathology, which became the focus of her subsequent therapy.

Effects of Gender, Culture, and Age

Gender

Although definitive estimates about the sex ratio of personality disorders cannot be made because ideal epidemiological studies do not exist, some personality disorders are believed to be more common in clinical settings among men and others among women. Those listed in DSM-IV-TR as occurring more often among men are paranoid, schizoid, schizotypal, antisocial, narcissistic, and obsessive-compulsive personality disorders. Those occurring more often in women are borderline, histrionic, and dependent personality disorders. Avoidant is said to be equally common in men and women. Apparently elevated sex ratios that do not reflect true prevalence rates can be the result of sampling or diagnostic biases in clinical settings (Widiger 1998). Factors affecting the sex ratios of personality disorders are addressed in detail in Chapter 34, "Gender."

Culture

Apparent manifestations of personality disorders must be considered in the context of a patient's cultural reference group and the degree to which behaviors such as diffidence, passivity, emotionality, emphasis on work and productivity, and unusual beliefs and rituals are culturally sanctioned. Only when such behaviors are clearly in excess or discordant with the standards of a person's cultural milieu would the diagnosis of a personality disorder be considered. Certain sociocultural contexts may lend themselves to eliciting and reinforcing behaviors that might be mistaken for personality disorder psychopathology. Members of minority groups, immigrants, or refugees, for example, might appear overly guarded or mistrustful, avoidant, or hostile in response to experiences of discrimination, language barriers, or problems in acculturation. Cultural issues relevant to the diagnosis and treatment of personality disorders are the subjects of Chapter 35, "Cross-Cultural Issues."

Age

As mentioned earlier, although personality disorders are usually not diagnosed prior to the age of 18 years, certain thoughts, feelings, and behaviors suggestive of personality psychopathology may be apparent during childhood. Dependency, social anxiety and hypersensitivity, disruptive behavior, or identity problems, for example, may be developmentally expected. Follow-up studies of children have shown decreases in such behaviors over time (Johnson et al. 2000), although children with elevated rates of personality disorder–type signs and symptoms do appear to be at higher risk for both Axis I and Axis II disorders in young adulthood (Johnson et al. 1999; Kasen et al. 1999). Thus, some childhood problems may not turn out to be transitory, and personality disorder may be viewed developmentally as a failure to mature out of certain age-appropriate or phase-specific feelings or behaviors. A developmental perspective on personality disorders is presented more fully in Chapter 11, "Developmental Issues."

Other Aspects of Personality Functioning

A problem with the DSM conceptualizations of personality disorders is that the individual categories do not correspond well with existing treatment approaches. Thus, whether a clinician is a psychodynamically oriented therapist, a cognitive-behavioral therapist, or a psychopharmacologist, information in addition to that necessary for a DSM personality disorder diagnosis is needed to formulate a treatment plan. Usually, this additional information is based on the theory of why a patient has a personality disorder and/or the mechanisms responsible for perpetuating the dysfunctional patterns.

Conflicts, Ego Functions, Object Relations, and Defense Mechanisms

Psychodynamically oriented clinicians have expressed dissatisfaction with the DSM system of axes, including Axis II, since its inception. The DSM multiaxial system fails, in their opinion, to discriminate between patients according to clinical variables important for planning treatment with psychodynamic psychotherapy (Karasu and Skodol 1980). Thus, they may be more interested in exploring conflicts between wishes, fears, and moral standards; ego functions such as impulse control or affect regulation; or self and other (object) representations based on early attachment experiences than on the signs and symptoms of personality disorders. Elaborations of psychodynamic theories of personality disorders can be found in Chapter 2, "Theories of Personality and Personality Disorders"; Chapter 16, "Psychoanalysis"; and Chapter 17, "Psychodynamic Psychotherapies"; along with discussions of relevant clinical variables.

Several groups of researchers (Bond and Vaillant 1986; Perry and Cooper 1989; Vaillant et al. 1986) have been able to document empirically the clinical utility of categorizing a patient's defensive functioning. *Defense mechanisms* are automatic psychological processes that protect people against anxiety and against awareness of internal or external stressors or dangers. Although this work was considered too early in its development to justify including a separate official axis based on it, Appendix B in DSM-IV ("Criteria Sets and Axes Provided for Further Study") includes a Defensive Functioning Scale and a "Glossary of Specific Defense Mechanisms and Coping Styles." The 27 defense mechanisms defined in this glossary are acting-out, affiliation, altruism, anticipation, autistic fantasy, denial, devaluation, displacement, dissociation, help-rejecting complaining, humor, idealization, intellectualization, isolation of affect, omnipotence, passive aggression, projection, projective identification, rationalization, reaction formation, repression, self-assertion, self-observation, splitting, sublimation, suppression, and undoing. Some defense mechanisms, such as projection, splitting, or acting-out, are always maladaptive, whereas others, such as sublimation or humor, are adaptive. Patients with personality disorders have characteristic predominant defensive patterns. Thus patients with paranoid personality disorder use denial and projection, those with BPD typically rely on acting-out and splitting (among others), and those with OCPD use isolation of affect and undoing. Clinicians may note current defenses or coping styles as well as a patient's predominant current defense level using the Defensive Functioning Scale. Defensive functioning in patients with personality disorders is the topic of Chapter 33, "Defensive Functioning."

Coping Styles

Although defense mechanisms in DSM-IV-TR are said to include coping styles, the literature on coping discusses styles not included in the DSM list. *Coping* refers to specific thoughts and behaviors that a person uses to manage the internal and external demands of situations appraised as stressful (Folkman and Moskowitz 2004; Lazarus and Folkman 1984; Pearlin and Schooler 1978). Coping involves cognitive, behavioral, and emotional responses and may or may not be consistent across stressful situations or functional roles. Two major broad styles of coping are problem-focused coping and emotion-focused coping. *Problem-focused coping* refers to efforts to resolve a threatening problem or diminish its impact by taking direct action. *Emotion-focused coping*

refers to efforts to reduce the negative emotions aroused in response to a threat by changing the way the threat is attended to or interpreted. Meaning-focused and social coping are other observed coping strategies. Coping has traditionally been assessed by retrospective self-report measures (e.g., the Coping Responses Inventory [Moos 1993], the Ways of Coping Questionnaire [Folkman and Lazarus 1988], and the COPE Inventory [Carver et al. 1989])—and more recently by ecological momentary assessment (real-time) techniques (Stone et al. 1998); but the major types of coping, such as problem solving, seeking support, distancing and distracting, accepting responsibility, positive reappraisal, or self-blame, can also be assessed by clinical interview.

Cognitive Schemas

Cognitive therapists want to characterize patients with personality disorders according to patients' dysfunctional cognitive schemas (core beliefs by which they process information) or their automatic thoughts, interpersonal strategies, and cognitive distortions. Again, particular personality disorders tend to have particular core beliefs. For example, patients with BPD frequently have beliefs such as "I am needy and weak" or "I am helpless if left on my own," whereas patients with OCPD believe "It is important to do a perfect job on everything" or "People should do things my way" (Beck et al. 2004). In contrast to beliefs, which map onto personality disorders specifically, *schemas* are broader themes regarding the self and relationships with others and can cut across personality disorder categories. For example, a schema of "impaired limits" can encompass the entitlement of narcissistic personality disorder as well as the lack of self-control of ASPD or BPD. A system for assessing and characterizing cognitive schemas and dysfunctional beliefs is included in Chapter 18, "Schema Therapy."

Objective Behaviors Versus Inferential Traits

Another difficulty in diagnosing personality disorders stems from the degree of inference and judgment necessary to make many of the diagnoses. Numerous critics have noted that it is easy to disagree about symptoms such as affective instability, self-dramatization, shallow emotional expression, exaggerated fears, or feelings of inadequacy—all symptoms of DSM-IV-TR personality disorders. Only the antisocial criteria, among the personality disorders, have historically yielded acceptable levels of reliability, and those criteria have emphasized overtly criminal and delinquent acts.

These observations led several investigators to attempt to determine sets of behaviors that might serve to identify types of personality disorder. Although any one behavior might not be sufficient to indicate a particular personality trait, multiple behavioral indicators considered together would increase confidence in recognizing the trait.

Behaviors that typify a particular personality style have been referred to as *prototypical*. Livesley (1986) developed a set of prototypical behaviors for the DSM-III (American Psychiatric Association 1980) personality disorders and compared them with prototypical traits. He found that highly prototypical behaviors could be derived from corresponding traits. For example, with regard to the concepts of social awkwardness and withdrawal of the schizoid personality disorder, Livesley found that behaviors such as "does not speak unless spoken to," "does not initiate social contacts," and "rarely reveals self to others" were uniformly rated as highly prototypic. Corresponding to the overly dramatic and emotional traits of the histrionic personality disorder were behaviors such as "expressed feelings in an exaggerated way," "considered a minor problem catastrophic," and "flirted with several members of the opposite sex." Behaviors such as "has routine schedules and is upset by deviations," "overreacted to criticism," and "spent considerable time on the minutest details" corresponded to the controlled, perfectionist traits of OCPD.

DSM-IV-TR makes strides in translating the characteristic traits of the personality disorders into explicit behaviors. The criteria for each personality disorder begin with the definition of the overall style or set of traits, followed by a listing of ways this might be expressed. In some instances, for example, for dependent personality disorder, the criteria are quite behavioral. For dependent personality disorder, a pervasive and excessive need to be taken care of that leads to submissive and clinging behavior and fears of separation is indicated by such items as "has difficulty making everyday decisions without an excessive amount of advice and reassurance from others" and "needs others to assume responsibility for most major areas of his or her life" (American Psychiatric Association 2000, p. 725). For other disorders, such as OCPD, an example of the behavior is given along with the trait. For OCPD, perfectionism is indicated by the following criterion: "Shows perfectionism that interferes with task completion, e.g., is unable to complete a project because his or her own overly strict standards are not met" (American Psychiatric Association 2000, p. 729).

Not all of the DSM-IV-TR personality disorders are equally well defined or illustrated by prototypical behaviors. Yet because it seems likely that such behaviors are much more reliably recognized than more abstract and inferential traits, the clinician should make special efforts to elicit examples of behaviors, from patients or other informants, that would constitute objective evidence of the presence of particular personality traits. Such an approach to assessment is likely to result in more accurate diagnosis.

COMORBIDITY

Since the introduction of a multiaxial system for recording diagnoses in DSM-III, which provided for the diagnosis of personality disorders on an axis (II) separate from the majority of other mental disorders, it has become apparent that most patients with personality disorders also meet criteria for other disorders. Rates have ranged from about two-thirds to almost 100% (Dolan-Sewell et al. 2001). The co-occurrence of Axis I and Axis II disorders has often been referred to as *comorbidity*, although our current understanding of the fundamental nature of most mental disorders is insufficient to justify the use of the term according to its formal definition, which requires that a comorbid disorder be "distinct" from the index disease or condition (Feinstein 1970). The DSM system, with its tendency to "split" as opposed to "lump" psychopathology via its many and expanding lists of disorders, encourages the diagnosis of multiple putative disorders to describe a patient's psychopathology and virtually ensures that patients will receive more than one diagnosis. In addition to the co-occurrence of personality disorders with Axis I disorders, it is also common for patients to receive more than one personality disorder diagnosis to fully describe their personality problems (Lilienfeld et al. 1994; Oldham et al. 1992). In the sections that follow, major patterns of personality disorder "comorbidity" will be described.

Co-Occurrence of Personality Disorders and Axis I Disorders

There are a number of explanations for the high rates of co-occurrence of personality disorders and Axis I disorders (Lyons et al. 1997). Co-occurring disorders may share a common etiology and be different phenotypic expressions of a common causal factor or factors. They may also be linked by etiology or pathological mechanism, but one disorder may be a milder version of the other on a spectrum of severity of pathology or impairment. One disorder may precede and increase the risk for the occurrence of another disorder, making a person more "vulnerable" to developing the second disorder. A second disorder may arise after a first as a complication or residual phenomenon or "scar." People with certain personality disorders and related Axis I disorders may share common psychobiological substrates that regulate cognitive or affective processes or impulse control. The Axis I disorders may be the direct symptomatic expression of dysfunctions in these systems, whereas personality disorders may reflect coping mechanisms and more general personality predispositions arising from the same systems (Siever and Davis 1991). This more comprehensive model of disorder co-occurrence integrates aspects of the common cause, spectrum, and vulnerability hypotheses.

Axis I/Axis II co-occurrence may be viewed from the perspectives of the course of a person's lifetime or the current presenting illness. Lifetime rates will obviously be higher. Patients with personality disorders who are seeking treatment also tend to have elevated rates of Axis I disorder co-occurrence, because the development or exacerbation of an Axis I disorder is often the reason a personality disorder patient comes for clinical attention (Shea 1997). For disorder co-occurrence to be significant from a scientific perspective, rates must be elevated above those expected by chance, based on the rates of occurrence of the individual disorders in a given clinical setting or population. From a treatment perspective, any co-occurrence may be significant.

The personality disorders of Cluster A—paranoid, schizoid, and schizotypal—are linked by theory and phenomenology to Axis I psychotic disorders such as delusional disorder, schizophreniform disorder, or schizophrenia. Few studies have actually documented these associations, however, possibly because of problems in being able to differentiate between clinical presentations of attenuated and full-blown psychotic symptoms that warrant two diagnoses instead of just one. (This problem in differential diagnosis is discussed later.) Oldham et al. (1995) found elevated odds of a current psychotic disorder in patients with Cluster A personality disorders but also found elevated odds for Clusters B and C personality disorders as well, suggesting less disorder specificity than might be expected.

In contrast, Cluster B personality disorders, especially BPD, which is linked by theory and phenomenology to Axis I mood and impulse control disorders, have repeatedly been shown to have high rates of co-occurring MDD and other mood disorders, substance use disorders, and bulimia nervosa (Oldham et al. 1995; Skodol et al. 1993, 1999; Zanarini et al. 1989, 1998). Taking into account co-occurrence expected by chance alone, however, neither Oldham et al. (1995) nor McGlashan et al.

(2000) substantiated the relationship between BPD and MDD. In addition, several studies have shown significantly elevated rates of anxiety disorders, including panic disorder and posttraumatic stress disorder, in patients with BPD (McGlashan et al. 2000; Skodol et al. 1995). ASPD is most strongly associated with substance use disorders in clinical and general population samples (Grant et al. 2004; Kessler et al. 1997; Morgenstern et al. 1997; see also Chapter 30, "Substance Abuse"). This association supports an underlying dimension of impulsivity or externalization (acting-out and being at odds with mainstream goals and values) shared by these disorders (Krueger et al. 1998, 2002).

Cluster C personality disorders, especially avoidant and dependent personality disorders, are linked by theory and phenomenology to anxiety disorders (Tyrer et al. 1997). A number of studies have demonstrated high rates of co-occurrence of avoidant personality disorder with MDD, agoraphobia, social phobia, and obsessive-compulsive disorder (Herbert et al. 1992; Oldham et al. 1995; Skodol et al. 1995). The co-occurrence rates between avoidant personality disorder and social phobia (particularly the generalized type) have been so high in some studies that investigators have argued that they are the same disorder. Ways of deciding whether two diagnoses are warranted are discussed below under "Problems in Differential Diagnosis." Several studies have indicated that dependent personality disorder co-occurs with a wide variety of Axis I disorders, consistent with the notion of excessive dependency as a nonspecific maladaptive behavior pattern that may result from coping with other chronic mental disorders (Skodol et al. 1996). OCPD may be specifically linked to obsessive-compulsive disorder; however, an association between them has only inconsistently been found.

Paying attention to the co-occurrence of Axis I and Axis II disorders is more than an intellectual exercise. The presence of an Axis I disorder in a patient with a personality disorder may suggest a more specific treatment approach, either with pharmacological agents, psychotherapy, or self-help groups (as in the case of substance use disorders), that will favorably affect outcome in these patients. Conversely, the presence of personality disorder in a patient with an Axis I disorder often indicates greater and more widespread levels of impairment (Jackson and Burgess 2002; Skodol et al. 2002), more chronicity (Grilo et al. 2005; Hart et al. 2001), and an overall poorer response to treatment requiring more intensive and prolonged care (Reich and Vasile 1993; Shea et al. 1992).

Co-Occurrence of Personality Disorders With Other Personality Disorders

When thorough assessments of the full range of Axis II disorders are conducted, as in research studies employing semistructured interviews, approximately half of patients receive more than one personality disorder diagnosis. Patterns of co-occurrence of personality disorders generally follow the DSM cluster structure (i.e, schizotypal personality disorder occurs more frequently with paranoid and schizoid personality disorders than with personality disorders outside Cluster A). These patterns are consistent with factor-analytic studies that support the clustering of personality disorders in DSM (Kass et al. 1985; Sanislow et al. 2002). Some personality disorders, however, particularly those in Cluster C, show associations with personality disorders from other clusters. Dependent personality disorder commonly occurs in patients with BPD, which makes clinical sense because patients with BPD can display regressive, clinging, and dependent behavior in interpersonal relationships. Some personality disorders rarely co-occur. OCPD and ASPD would be an exceedingly rare combination, because the careful planning and work orientation of OCPD are the antithesis of the impulsivity and irresponsibility of ASPD.

Multiple Overlapping Personality Syndromes

Elevated rates of personality disorder co-occurrence raise questions about the appropriate application of DSM-IV-TR categories to phenomenology that rarely appears to have discrete boundaries. Although DSM-IV-TR clearly stipulates that for many patients, personality disturbance would frequently meet criteria for more than one disorder, clinicians have found the practice of diagnosing multiple disorders conceptually difficult and therefore seldom attempt such diagnoses.

Prior to DSM-III-R (American Psychiatric Association 1987), part of the problem had been that most of the personality disorders were defined as classical categories (Cantor et al. 1980)—that is, ones in which all members clearly share certain identifying features. Classical categories imply a clear demarcation between members and nonmembers, but natural phenomena rarely fit neatly into such categories.

CATEGORIES VERSUS DIMENSIONS OF PERSONALITY

Traditionally, in much of the psychological literature, personality has been described and measured along certain dimensions (Frances 1982). Dimensions of personality frequently are continuous with opposite traits at either end of a spectrum, such as dominant-submissive or hostile-friendly. People can then vary in the extent to which each of the traits describes them. Dimensional models of personality diagnosis appear to be more flexible and specific than categorical models when the phenomenology lacks clear-cut boundaries between normal and abnormal and between different constellations of maladaptive traits, as seems true of personality disturbance (Widiger et al. 1987). Scaled rating systems have been devised to transform Axis II disorders into dimensions (Kass et al. 1985; Oldham and Skodol 2000), but they are not representative of dimensional approaches currently in wide use. Dimensional models of personality disorders are being seriously considered for DSM-V. They are discussed in detail in Chapter 3, "Categorical and Dimensional Models of Personality Disorders."

CLASSICAL VERSUS PROTOTYPAL CATEGORIES

Prototypal models have been shown to be more accurate than classical models in categorizing various natural phenomena. In the prototypal model, no defining feature is considered to be absolutely necessary, nor is any combination of features sufficient. Membership is heterogeneous, and boundaries overlap. There are few, if any, pathognomonic signs. The diagnostic criteria for a prototypal model are polythetic rather than monothetic. *Monothetic classifications* are those in which categories differ by at least one feature that is shared by each of its members. In contrast, in *polythetic classifications*, members share a large proportion of features but do not necessarily share any particular feature (Widiger and Frances 1985). In the prototypal model, polythetic criteria would vary in their diagnostic value, and members would differ in terms of their prototypicality.

A prototypal approach to personality disorder classification is conceptually satisfying because of its flexibility, the inherent heterogeneity of the categories, and the acceptance of overlapping boundaries and many borderline cases. From a conceptual point of view, some of the diagnostic problems alluded to earlier would be lessened with a prototypal approach; for example, multiple diagnoses and variability within diagnostic groups would be expected.

Monothetic categories are inherently more difficult to recognize or diagnose because disagreement on any one of the required defining features results in disagreement on the diagnosis. With polythetic criteria, because no single symptom is required for a diagnosis, clinicians can disagree about an individual symptom and still agree on the diagnosis, provided the particular symptom was not the one that met the minimum threshold for the number of symptoms required for the diagnosis.

DSM-IV-TR has a prototypal model for all personality disorders, defined by polythetic criteria sets. The number of features listed varies from seven to nine, with cut-points for the diagnosis at four or five required symptoms. ASPD is an exception in that it is still a "mixed" category. A current age of 18, a childhood history of conduct disturbance, and irresponsible and antisocial behavior as an adult are necessary for an ASPD diagnosis.

All DSM-IV-TR criteria carry equal weight; in a true prototypal model, certain criteria would have more diagnostic significance. Research studies have demonstrated that for BPD, certain individual symptoms, such as chronic feelings of emptiness and boredom (Widiger et al. 1984) and suicidality or self-injury (Grilo et al. 2001, 2004a), have a higher value in predicting a diagnosis than other symptoms, such as impulsivity. Similar highly predictive individual symptoms have been suggested for schizotypal personality disorder (e.g., odd behavior, odd thinking or speech, constricted affect) and OCPD (e.g., miserliness, preoccupation with details and rules) (Grilo et al. 2001). Predictive symptoms need to be determined for all of the personality disorders and need an appropriate weighting system devised for them.

The currently required numbers of symptoms for each of the personality disorders are arbitrary. Arguments have been made that fixed cut-points for diagnosis are inappropriate and inefficient. Appropriate cut-points are actually dependent on the base rate of the syndrome—that is, how common it is in the population. For a particular symptom to be more likely to indicate the presence of a syndrome rather than its absence, the ratio of the base rate to one minus the base rate must exceed the ratio of the false-positive rate to the true-positive rate (Finn 1982). If a symptom correctly identifies 80% of patients with the disorder and misidentifies only 25% without the disorder, then at least 24% of the patients must have the disorder or the symptom will misclassify more patients than it correctly classifies. Therefore, if the disorder occurred less often, given the presence of any one symptom with the above diagnostic value, it would be more efficient never to diagnose the disorder because the clinician would then be wrong less often!

As the base rate of a syndrome changes, the efficiency of any cut-point also changes. If the base rate is high, it is more efficient to move the cut-point down because, with a high base rate, there is less chance of missing the diagnosis and more chance of correctly identifying the cases. If the base rate is low, the cut-point should be increased, because it is increasingly likely to incorrectly identify a noncase as a case. A higher threshold for the symptoms would guard against this error. Finally, the relative costs and gains of correctly or incorrectly diagnosing cases could be factored into establishing cut-points. This depends on how the diagnosis is used or the implications of a missed diagnosis and is referred to as the "utility." Studies need to be done to determine cut-points for the various personality disorders that would be optimal in a variety of clinical settings and that might take into account the utilities of the diagnostic decisions.

Some personality disorder researchers advocate a prototype matching approach to the diagnosis of personality disorders rather than the current DSM procedure, which continues to involve making present/absent judgments about individual criteria (Shedler and Westen 2004). They would replace the diagnostic criteria sets with descriptions of various personality disorder prototypes in paragraph form and ask clinicians to rate the degree of similarity between the prototypes and the patient undergoing evaluation. They argue that a prototype matching approach allows the clinician to consider individual criteria in the context of the whole personality disorder description, such that no single criterion can "make or break" the diagnosis. They also argue that a prototype matching approach is closer to the way clinicians make personality disorder diagnoses in actual practice.

PROBLEMS IN DIFFERENTIAL DIAGNOSIS

In this section, the individual personality disorders are grouped according to the three descriptive clusters in DSM-IV-TR: 1) the odd or eccentric, 2) the dramatic, emotional, or erratic, and 3) the anxious or fearful. Although these clusters were originally introduced solely to emphasize the descriptive similarities among the disorders grouped together, some empirical evidence has shown the validity of the clusters (Kass et al. 1985; Sanislow et al. 2002; Widiger et al. 1987).

Odd or Eccentric Cluster

Paranoid, schizoid, and schizotypal personality disorders constitute the odd or eccentric cluster. Disorders in this cluster share beliefs that are associated with traits of social awkwardness, being ill at ease in social situations, and social withdrawal.

Paranoid Personality Disorder

People with paranoid personality disorder are characterized by pervasive distrust and suspiciousness of others. Because of their expectation that others will exploit, harm, or deceive them in some way, they are reluctant to confide in others and therefore may seem distant and removed. This type of social discomfort or withdrawal is distinguishable from that of the schizoid patient because the schizoid patient appears not to care, whereas the paranoid patient cares a great deal. People with paranoid personality disorder are therefore the opposite of those with schizoid personality disorder in their responses to the praise or criticism of others. Whereas schizoid people are indifferent, paranoid people are extremely sensitive, very easily slighted, quick to take offense, ready to counterattack, and prone to bear grudges. Patients with paranoid personality disorder can be distinguished from those with schizotypal personality disorder by the absence of symptoms such as magical thinking, unusual perceptions, and odd speech.

Patients with BPD also may react angrily to seemingly minor provocations, but they are not generally suspicious and distrustful. Patients with narcissistic personality disorder may appear distant from others, particularly when they perceive threats to their self-esteem, but not because of general distrust. Patients with avoidant personality disorder also are reluctant to confide in others, but this reticence is based on their insecurity and not because they fear exploitation or harm.

Another point relevant to the differential diagnosis of paranoid personality disorder is the relationship of nonpsychotic suspiciousness and ideas of reference to the delusions characteristic of a delusional disorder or paranoid schizophrenia. The distinction rests on the degree to which reality testing is impaired. In brief, in paranoid personality disorder, the person can at least entertain the possibility that his or her suspicions are unfounded or that he or she is overreacting. Also, the perceived threats of the person with a paranoid personality disorder are more likely to come from known other people in the environment—a neighbor or a co-worker, for instance—or from common institutions such as the government or the utility company rather than from bizarre sources. In cases in which beliefs of expected harm or persecution are firmly held and result in extensive effects on behavior, paranoid personality disorder is not a sufficient diagnosis: the diagnosis of a psychotic disorder is warranted.

Schizoid Personality Disorder

There is some question of the validity of schizoid personality disorder as a distinct personality disorder. People who would have received the diagnosis of schizoid personality traditionally might be diagnosed as either schizoid, schizotypal, or avoidant by DSM-IV-TR criteria. In the few studies looking at the full range of personality disorders (e.g., Oldham et al. 1995; Pfohl et al. 1986), schizoid personality disorder was uncommon. It must be remembered, however, that subjects in clinical studies are selected by virtue of their seeking treatment; schizoid people, by their very nature, are less likely to seek treatment because subjective distress about their attitudes and behavior is apt to be low, and impairment would be evident only in the eyes of others, whom they typically avoid. The crucial distinguishing features of schizoid personality are that the person is detached from social relationships and has a restricted range of emotions in interpersonal settings. Although all Cluster A personality disorders are characterized by social isolation, schizoid personality disorder can be distinguished from paranoid personality disorder by a lack of general suspiciousness and from schizotypal personality disorder by a lack of cognitive and perceptual distortions. The more passive detachment and limited desire for social intimacy serves to distinguish schizoid persons from avoidant persons—who are also socially isolated because they are petrified by their fear of rejection, despite a great desire for relationships (Trull et al. 1987). Patients with OCPD are often interpersonally constricted—but this is because they use excessive devotion to their work to "protect" themselves from their discomfort with the emotions that arise in intimate relationships. Schizoid personality disorder is distinguished from psychotic disorders by the absence of delusions and hallucinations.

Schizotypal Personality Disorder

Schizotypal personality disorder was first introduced in DSM-III. The criteria for schizotypal personality disorder were developed in a study conducted by Spitzer et al. (1979). The criteria were developed from the case records of the "borderline schizophrenic" relatives of people genetically related to probands with schizophrenia in the Danish Adoption Studies of Schizophrenia (Kety 1983). They were intended to help clarify the murky diagnostic area of "borderline" patients.

The key defining features of schizotypal personality disorder are the soft, nonpsychotic symptoms that resemble those seen in more florid form in schizophrenia and make schizotypal patients appear eccentric. These include magical thinking, ideas of reference, recurrent illusions, odd speech, and paranoid ideation. Among the problems in differential diagnosis are how to distinguish these features from their psychotic counterparts and how to distinguish schizotypal patients from others in the odd, eccentric cluster.

The distinction between the soft, suggestive signs and the full-blown psychotic symptoms rests on the conviction regarding the beliefs, the vividness of the illusions, and the degree of disorganization of speech. Illusions are misperceptions of real external stimuli and are thus distinct from hallucinations, in which a sensory perception occurs without external stimulation of the sense organs. An example of a visual illusion might be mistaking a shadow for a real person or seeing one's face change in a mirror. An auditory illusion might be hearing derogatory remarks made in muffled conversation heard from a distance. In the case of an illusion, the person can usually consider the possibility that his or her perception was mistaken.

Odd speech may be tangential, circumstantial, stilted, vague, or overly metaphorical. It differs from loosening of associations in that it is generally more understandable, although coherence is obviously along a continuum. If a person with schizotypal personality disorder develops full-blown delusions or hallucinations, then the diagnosis becomes schizophrenia because the premorbid symptoms of schizotypal personality disorder almost invariably would meet the 6-month duration requirement for schizophrenia as prodromal symptoms.

The likelihood of schizotypal personality disorder's evolving into schizophrenia is not fully established. What is known about the historical forerunners of the diagnosis of schizotypal personality disorder—simple and latent schizophrenia—suggests that only a limited proportion actually develops schizophrenia on follow-up. The only long-term follow-up study of DSM-III–defined schizotypal personality disorder was conducted by McGlashan (1986). He found that pure schizotypal personality disorder had a better prognosis than schizophrenia but worse than BPD. The frequency with which schizotypal personality disorder became schizophrenia was 17% in the 15 years of follow-up (Fenton and McGlashan 1989). If a patient with a past history of schizophrenia currently displays symptoms of schizotypal personality disorder, the symptoms are usually referred to instead as residual schizophrenia.

The schizoid/schizotypal distinction is made on the basis of the presence of the psychotic-like symptoms in the latter. Schizotypal patients are more odd and eccentric than patients with paranoid personality disorder and have perceptual as well as cognitive distortions. Patients with BPD may have transient paranoid and dissociative symptoms accompanied by strong affects, such as anger or anxiety, in response to the stress of perceived abandonment. Although the psychotic-like symptoms of patients with schizotypal personality disorder may also worsen with stress, this response is less likely to occur in the context of a disruption in an interpersonal relationship and to be accompanied by strong affect. Patients with BPD periodically withdraw from social relationships in the face of disappointment, whereas patients with schizotypal personality disorder more generally avoid social involvement and are not typically impulsive.

The following vignette illustrates the case of a socially isolated person that raises differential diagnostic questions.

Case Example

A videotaped interview of a 30-year-old bachelor was shown to 133 American and 194 British psychiatrists in the late 1960s as part of the United States–United Kingdom comparative study of psychiatric diagnosis (see Skodol 1989).

Problems began for the patient when he was 13 or 14 years old. He described himself as insecure and very dependent on his mother for emotional support. Although he claimed he sometimes did well in high school—played football, boxed, acted, and played the trumpet—at other times, he said, he was afraid to go to school and would stay home with his mother. He said he was afraid other kids would pick on him and he would get into a fight. He attended several colleges but did not study and accumulated only 1½ years of credit.

He then joined the army but lasted only 5 months. He was hospitalized briefly, at age 19, at Walter Reed Hospital but claims he was told that there was nothing wrong. He states that he felt like a little boy and wanted to go home to his mother. He said he broke down and screamed and cried like a baby.

His most recent hospitalization was his fifth. The longest had been for 5 months; the others, for several days to several weeks. In all cases and on other occasions he requested hospitalization. He was often refused and told that he did not need hospitalization but should go to work. He had been treated with a variety of medicines, including phenothiazines, and had received 20 electroconvulsive treatments as an outpatient.

Other problems he describes were periodic abuse of drugs, including alcohol, barbiturates, opioids, and amphetamines. He reports periods of not being able to get out of bed, shave, or shower; he denies depressed mood or symptoms of a depressive syndrome. He also denies grandiosity or other symptoms of a manic syndrome. He has worked very sporadically and states that he purposely fails at tasks. He says he makes friends but quickly loses them. He has not seen any friend for the past 6 months.

On the videotaped interview, the patient has just described an incident in which he developed a "paralyzed arm," which his psychiatrist called a hysterical symptom.

> Interviewer: What other sorts of things have happened to your body?
> Patient: Well, one thing is that no matter how I look to you now, my facial appearance changes sometimes, unbelievably. Now, a lot of doctors thought I was exaggerating, but my own mother says it's true. Sometimes my face just blows up, my nose gets wider, my eyes close up, and (giving his cheek a twist), I can't feel nothin'—like this.
> Interviewer: What does this to you?
> Patient: Simply, if it didn't, I'd have no reason to tell myself that I'm afraid to go out into the world.
> Interviewer: You mean that your face actually does swell up, or that you imagine it?
> Patient: It actually does! I swear on my heart that I never imagined anything, or seen anything that wasn't there.
> Interviewer: How long has this been happening to you?
> Patient: Ten years.
> Interviewer: What happens if you look in the mirror?
> Patient: I don't.
> Interviewer: Why not?
> Patient: To avoid it. I try to forget about it. I know that my basic problem isn't my face—I used to think it was. Now I know it'll change when the basic problem goes away.
> Interviewer: Does it frighten you that this happens?
> Patient: It used to. I used to think that I was the owner of a fantastic symptom that was totally unbelievable, plus I couldn't get any medical man to believe me. Finally, I went to one or two psychiatrists who told me they'd seen it before, maybe not the face, but a physical change can take place.
> Interviewer: If you go out in public, do you feel self-conscious about this?
> Patient: That's what's amazing. When I'm sick like this I don't feel self-conscious. I could be as ugly as the day is long. But when I'm well, and look my best, or get attention from people, I can't stand it.
> Interviewer: What do you do then?

> Patient: I withdraw—into myself. This way nobody is going to come up to me. I won't be forced to react—"Hello; goodbye." Converse. Talk. Walk. Work.
> Interviewer: I see you wear dark glasses.
> Patient: Yeah, well in the safety of my own house I feel OK, but if I walk out onto the street, it hits me: "Where? How? Who do I go to? There's 30 billion people. Who do I speak to? Where do I go?" Next thing I know, I'm paranoid.
> Interviewer: What do you mean, paranoid?
> Patient: People look at me. They could be saying anything. "He's good-looking" or "He's ugly." But all I feel is "Oh, my God! I can't stand this! People looking at me!" You know, when I get looked at because I look terrible, that doesn't frighten me. But should I feel good and get some attention, you know, I get sick.

The patient depicted in this vignette was fascinating because there was more disagreement between American and British psychiatrists on the appropriate diagnosis than on any other case in the study (Kendell et al. 1971). Sixty-nine percent of American psychiatrists in the late 1960s diagnosed this man as having schizophrenia; only 2% of British psychiatrists did so. The most common British diagnosis was personality disorder, usually hysterical. The next most common diagnosis by British psychiatrists was neurosis. Most mental health clinicians in the United States to whom I have presented the videotape corresponding to this vignette agree that on Axis I, diagnoses of mixed substance abuse and conversion disorder are warranted. A factitious disorder is the second most frequently chosen diagnosis. On Axis II, using DSM-III criteria, most clinicians chose schizotypal personality disorder with histrionic features. With the expansion of the concept of avoidant personality disorder in DSM-IV to include more prominent fearfulness, I suspect that clinicians using DSM-IV would also note avoidant features.

Dramatic, Emotional, or Erratic Cluster

The dramatic, emotional, or erratic cluster includes antisocial, borderline, histrionic, and narcissistic personality disorders. These highly overlapping disorders share the characteristics of reactive emotionality and poor impulse control.

Antisocial Personality Disorder

ASPD is unique among personality disorders in that it can be reliably diagnosed, even in clinical settings. It is less difficult to recognize because its characteristic pattern of behaviors, which disregard or violate the rights of others, beginning in adolescence, are identified by very explicit lists of antisocial activities. DSM-defined ASPD has also been widely criticized, however, for an overemphasis on overt criminal acts at the expense of the personality traits of psychopathy, such that it is overdiagnosed in criminal or forensic settings and underdiagnosed in noncriminal settings (Widiger and Corbitt 1996).

Patients with narcissistic personality disorder share some of the arrogant, exploitative, nonempathic characteristics of patients with ASPD but usually are not impulsive or physically aggressive, nor do they have a history of childhood conduct disorder. Patients with narcissistic personality disorder who engage in criminal behavior are most likely to commit white-collar crimes. Patients with histrionic and borderline personality disorders may be impulsive and manipulative but are seeking attention and nurturance, respectively, rather than profit, power, or material gain. Patients with BPD may be overrepresented in criminal populations, especially among women (see Chapter 36, "Correctional Populations: Criminal Careers and Recidivism"). If patients with paranoid personality disorder engage in antisocial behavior, it is based on a desire for revenge over a perceived slight, rather than for personal gain or exploitation of others.

Conduct disorder is a diagnosis for a repetitive and persistent pattern of behavior among children or adolescents under 18 years of age in which the rights of others or societal norms are violated. The restriction of ASPD to persons over 18 means that the pattern has to have persisted into adult life, because many childhood conduct problems may remit or may lead to other mental disorders.

Other mental disorders such as psychotic disorders and mood disorders can lead to breaking of laws and antisocial acts. Schizophrenic or manic episodes preempt the diagnosis of ASPD. Patients with substance-related disorders (see Chapter 30, "Substance Abuse") may engage in antisocial behaviors such as illegal drug selling or theft to obtain money for drugs. Both diagnoses may be given, even if some of the criteria met for ASPD are related to drug use. When antisocial behavior occurs that is not a part of the full pattern of ASPD or is not due to another mental disorder such as schizophrenia, then the V code category of adult antisocial behavior is appropriate.

Borderline Personality Disorder

BPD has generated by far the most extensive and intensive research of all of the DSM-IV-TR personality disorders. This research interest simply reflects the intense clinical interest in borderline patients, who seem to have swelled the ranks of inpatient hospitals and outpatient practices of the past 35 years. The two major questions that have been asked are 1) What are the "borders" of borderline? and 2) What are the key clinical features of this disorder?

The criteria for BPD were originally defined by Spitzer et al. (1979) in an effort to delineate which patients clinicians referred to as "borderline." These investigators found two overlapping sets of descriptive items, a set reflecting instability of affect, identity, and impulse control and another reflecting eccentricity of thought, speech, and behavior. The former became the criteria for BPD, and the latter for schizotypal personality disorder, in DSM-III.

Although traditionally, and in psychoanalytic terms, borderline patients were thought to occupy a "border" between psychosis or schizophrenia and "neurotic" disorders, evidence accumulated, based on the validation techniques of family history, treatment response, and outcome on follow-up, that indicated that BPD bore much more of a relationship to affective disorders than to schizophrenia (e.g., Akiskal et al. 1985; Snyder et al. 1982). This led many clinicians (and researchers) into the diagnostic dilemma of attempting to distinguish whether a particular patient has BPD or an affective disorder.

This dilemma is a product of asking the wrong question. The appropriate question is which patients with BPD also have a mood disorder. The relevancy of this question for clinical practice is supported by the most recent reviews of this area of differential diagnosis. Gunderson and colleagues (Gunderson and Elliot 1985; Gunderson and Phillips 1991) examined four hypotheses about the interface between BPD and affective disorder: 1) that affective disorder is primary and that borderline character traits such as drug use and sexual promiscuity arise in an attempt to alleviate depression; 2) that BPD leads to affective disorder (depression) as a result of problems that result from primary deficits in impulse control, maintaining stable interpersonal relationships, and sense of self-esteem; 3) that the two disorders are independent, but because both occur frequently in the population, they are often seen together; and 4) that they are related, but in a nonspecific fashion. The data, the authors argued, supported none of the hypotheses as stated. They were most consistent with the independence hypothesis, but the two disorders co-occurred more frequently than would be expected by chance.

Recently, Gunderson et al. (2004) have reexamined the relationship of BPD and MDD from a longitudinal perspective. They found that although the courses of BPD and MDD could be independent, improvements in MDD were more likely to occur following improvements in BPD than the reverse. These results support the view that BPD is a fundamental form of psychopathology that accounts for co-occurring depressions and that these depressions should be understood as epiphenomena of the abnormal sensitivity and interpersonal disappointments of patients with BPD. This view is further supported by the qualitative differences in the depressive experiences (e.g., the marked reactivity of mood to identifiable events [Gunderson 1996]) of patients with BPD compared with those with MDD (Rogers et al. 1995; Westen et al. 1992); by follow-up studies that fail to show that BPD evolves into more typical mood disorders over time (Grilo et al. 1998); and by the relatively modest response of patients with BPD to antidepressant medications (Koenigsberg et al. 1999; Soloff et al. 1998).

From a clinical perspective, the important distinctions to be made, therefore, are among BPD alone, BPD in association with a mood disorder in the depressive or bipolar spectra, and affective disorder alone. These distinctions are facilitated by the DSM-IV-TR multiaxial system because Axes I and II are considered separately, and multiple diagnoses can be listed on each axis.

Case Example

The following case example is adapted from Skodol (1989).

> A 37-year-old single woman, a bookkeeper for a building restoration and waterproofing company, was evaluated for hospital treatment. She described herself as chronically and severely depressed since the age of 18 and bulimic since her early 20s. She said, "I've cried every day for the past 10 years." She had an extremely low opinion of herself: "You have never met anyone as bad as I am, I guarantee it."
>
> She had had 14 years of therapy with a halfdozen therapists. She typically became very attached to them, then reacted extremely negatively, "sooner or later," when they let her down. Once, when a therapist would not allow her to extend a session beyond her time, she picked up an ashtray and threw it at him. Another time, she waited for one of her therapists after his day was over, lay down in front of his car, and would not let him go home before he talked more to her. On still another occasion when she was angry at a therapist, she took a razor blade from her purse and cut her wrist in the therapist's office.
>
> Many medications had been tried for both the depression and the bulimia. She had been on Librium and Valium many years before, then Elavil, Tofranil, Mellaril, and lithium, followed by Xanax, Par-

nate, and Nardil; most recently she had been given Prozac, Zoloft, and Effexor. Occasionally, the depression abated slightly "for maybe 1 week." As far as her concern with her weight and her binge eating, she claimed nothing helped. Her weight had ranged from a low of 110 to a high of 130. She claimed that she had taken up to 70 laxatives in a week and had vomited every day for almost 10 years. She also had panic attacks and had abused alcohol, cannabis, and stimulants in the past.

> The patient continued to work, although she did not get along well with her coworkers. "I know people don't like me. I'm just a lazy, nasty person. Some of them probably think I'm grotesque. I'm sure they're also laughing at me. Who wouldn't? I'm an absurdity." The patient had not had a date in 8 years and had only a few female "acquaintances."
>
> A research interview indicated that the patient met DSM-IV-TR criteria for five (!) personality disorders: avoidant, obsessive-compulsive, schizotypal, histrionic, and borderline. The BPD was rated severe.

Standard treatments for major depression (or bulimia) are no match for this woman's personality psychopathology. It is not difficult to conceptualize her overall maladjustment as being so severe that minor improvements in mood would be insignificant to her— or even unacceptable, given her self-defeating tendencies. A skeptical clinician might argue that given the patient's tendencies to exaggerate, manipulate, and provoke, it would not be possible to accurately assess the state of her mood in response to treatment. This problem raises the question of which components of a mood disorder are most likely to be affected by Axis II psychopathology. Clearly, in work with patients with severe personality disorders, the subjective state of the patient is very resistant to change. Improvement may be evident only by objective criteria, from the perspective of either the clinician or of a significant other in the person's life.

Other Axis I disorders, such as anxiety disorders, substance-related disorders, eating disorders, somatoform disorders, dissociative disorders, and psychotic disorders, may also complicate the course of BPD (Zanarini et al. 1998; Zimmerman and Mattia 1999a). Co-occurrence of BPD with substance-related and eating disorders suggests that BPD lies on a spectrum of disorders of impulse control (Siever and Davis 1991). A new criterion in DSM-IV for "transient, stress-related paranoid ideation or severe dissociative symptoms" may raise new issues in differentiating dissociative and psychotic disorders from BPD (the reactive, stress-related nature of the symptoms characterize BPD [Sternbach et al. 1992]). Again, however, in these instances the clinician should not necessarily pose the differential diagnosis in terms of either/or but instead as both/and.

BPD overlaps extensively with histrionic, narcissistic, antisocial, and dependent personality disorders. Patients with histrionic personality disorder can be manipulative and experience rapidly shifting emotions but are not self-destructive, angry, or "empty" as are patients with BPD. Patients with narcissistic personality disorder often react angrily to provocation but have more stable identities and lack the problems of impulse control, self-destructiveness, and fears of abandonment seen in BPD. Patients with ASPD are manipulative for personal gain, whereas those with BPD are manipulative in order to get their needs met. Both borderline and dependent personality disorders are characterized by fears of losing the support of caretakers, but patients with BPD react to threats of loss of such a person with angry demands, whereas the patient with dependent personality disorder becomes more acquiescent and submissive.

Histrionic Personality Disorder

Histrionic personality disorder is defined in DSM-IV-TR by excessive emotionality and attention-seeking behavior. In clinical and research settings, the features of histrionic personality disorder overlap considerably with those of other disorders in this cluster, especially the narcissistic and borderline, and with dependent personality disorder. Although histrionic patients may make up a large proportion of psychotherapy patients, they have not been well studied in terms of DSM-IV-TR criteria.

The diagnostic overlap of histrionic with narcissistic personality disorder is possible because of the traits and behaviors that the two have in common. Histrionic personality disorder includes incessant drawing of attention to oneself and egocentrism; narcissistic personality disorder includes a grandiose sense of self-importance, entitlement, interpersonal exploitiveness, and lack of empathy. Patients with narcissistic personality disorder usually want recognition because of their superiority, whereas patients with histrionic personality disorder will allow themselves to be viewed as weak and dependent if doing so attracts attention. When criteria for both disorders are met, both diagnoses should be given.

Patients with BPD are frequently histrionic. Histrionic patients are demanding and manipulative. BPD patients display inappropriate, intense anger, perform physically self-damaging acts, and are demanding and manipulate others. Histrionic patients lack the more malignant characteristics of BPD. These patients, referred to in the classic literature as hysterical, may be very vain and self-indulgent, always drawing atten-tion to themselves or craving action and excitement, without having angry outbursts, making suicidal threats or gestures, or feeling empty.

Another problem in making a diagnosis of histrionic personality disorder is that the symptoms are difficult for the patient to recognize. A patient who overreacts to minor events in most cases does not consider the reaction excessive or the event minor. Few patients are aware that others consider them shallow or manipulative or that their speech is overly impressionistic. Therefore, histrionic personality disorder is a diagnosis that often requires the input of third-party informants. Fortunately, histrionic traits are usually displayed to the therapist, and observation is therefore of great diagnostic value.

Patients with histrionic personality disorder may be especially prone to Axis I disorders in the somatoform disorders class. The clinician should therefore be alert to the possible additional diagnoses of somatization disorder, conversion disorder, pain disorder, hypochondriasis, or body dysmorphic disorder.

Narcissistic Personality Disorder

The hallmark features of narcissistic personality disorder in DSM-IV-TR are a grandiose sense of self-importance or uniqueness, preoccupation with fantasies of success, an excessive need for admiration, and interpersonal relationship problems, such as feeling entitled, exploiting others for personal gain, and failing to empathize with the feelings of others.

Overlap with other disorders in Cluster B has been described previously. Both patients with narcissistic and with obsessive-compulsive personality disorders may appear perfectionistic, but patients with OCPD are self-critical, whereas those with narcissistic are not. Grandiosity is a symptom of a manic or hypomanic episode, but the absence of an abrupt onset of elevated mood and impairment in functioning help to distinguish narcissistic personality disorder from bipolar disorders. Chronic use of certain substances, such as cocaine, can also lead to grandiose, self-preoccupied behavior patterns.

The diagnosis of narcissistic personality disorder presents the difficult problem of translating concepts of psychological functioning derived largely from the psychoanalytic literature into descriptions of traits and behaviors that can be recognized by clinicians with diverse theoretical orientations. As Frances (1980) has indicated, the psychoanalytic definition of narcissistic personality disorder would include 1) deficits in object constancy, 2) incomplete internalization and maturation of psychic structures and mechanisms regulating self-esteem, and 3) immature grandiosity. These problems are not easily recognized, especially by nonanalytic clinicians, in one or two diagnostic interviews.

Deficits in object constancy are reflected in the characteristic interpersonal disturbances of narcissistic personality disorder. Narcissistic people have an inflated sense of their own self-importance and often devalue the importance of others. Despite their outward air of superiority, self-esteem problems are evident when they react with disdain, rage, humiliation, or emptiness in response to criticism or defeat. Immature grandiosity is reflected by narcissistic personality disorder criteria describing a grandiose sense of self-importance, preoccupations with fantasies of unlimited potential, beliefs in special and unique attributes, and entitlement.

Anxious or Fearful Cluster

Avoidant, dependent, and obsessive-compulsive personality disorders make up the anxious and fearful cluster. At least one factor analytic study (Kass et al. 1985) has shown that OCPD may not fit as well into this group as the others.

Avoidant Personality Disorder

Avoidant personality disorder is characterized by social inhibition due to feelings of inadequacy and a fear of being negatively evaluated by others. Both avoidant and dependent personality disorders are characterized by feelings of inadequacy, hypersensitivity to criticism, and need for reassurance. In patients with avoidant personality disorder, the concern is with avoiding embarrassment or humiliation; in patients with dependent personality disorder, it is with being taken care of. The two disorders often co-occur, however.

Items referring to exaggerating the difficulties or risks of new but ordinary activities and situations, and to embarrassment and social anxiety, make avoidant personality disorder in DSM-IV-TR close in concept to the "phobic character" style common in the psychoanalytic literature. Differentiating avoidant personality disorder from social phobia, especially generalized social phobia, can be difficult. Research has shown that although there is significant co-occurrence of social phobia and avoidant personality disorder, they are not synonymous, and patients can meet criteria for one disorder without meeting criteria for the other (Skodol et al. 1995). The concept of avoidant personality disorder is broader than that of generalized social phobia in that it includes feelings of inadequacy, infe-

riority, and ineptness and a general reluctance to take risks and engage in new activities.

Dependent Personality Disorder

Dependent personality disorder is characterized by clinging and submissive behavior and an excessive need to be taken care of. Dependent personality shares with histrionic personality disorder a covariation with gender, occurring more frequently in women (Kaplan 1983; Kass et al. 1983). It has been argued that this covariation results from a sex bias in the diagnostic criteria (Kaplan 1983), such that normal women conforming to their sex role stereotype will be labeled abnormal because of a masculine bias about what constitutes healthy behavior.

One of the real problems in the diagnosis of dependent personality disorder is its threshold for clinical significance. The earlier discussion in this chapter about personality traits versus personality disorder is germane. For dependent personality traits to indicate a personality disorder, evidence of significant distress or social or occupational impairment is necessary. If a woman subordinates her needs to those of her husband to avoid losing him, then there would have to be clear evidence that this behavior is damaging to her; for example, if she does not choose other equally viable options for herself socially—and with respect to her family and living arrangements—because of her inability to make her own decisions or act according to her own needs. Another consideration is that a particular woman's needs may be very different from her husband's; she may desire greater affiliation and need less self-determination in traditional areas of living such as economic productivity. Keeping in mind the need for strong evidence of the pathological nature of the dependency may help guard against too many false-positive diagnoses of women.

Many of the diagnostic criteria for dependent personality disorder resulted from a need to specify more explicitly the kinds of dependent behaviors indicative of the disorder and to emphasize their pathological nature, for example, "has difficulty making everyday decisions without an excessive amount of advice and reassurance from others" and "has difficulty initiating projects or doing things on his or her own" (American Psychiatric Association 2000, p. 725). The person with dependent personality disorder stays in poor relationships, goes along with others even when thinking they are wrong, does demeaning things, and feels helpless when alone all because of an inability to see himself or herself as sufficiently competent. It is not the lack of confidence per se that is significant for the person with dependent personality disorder but the pathological use of relationships to attempt to deal with the perceived deficiency. Patients with dependent personality disorder are prone to having associated depressive or adjustment disorders because they are so vulnerable to disappointments and disruptions in relationships.

Dependent personality disorder has been found to co-occur with other personality disorders (Trull et al. 1987). The dependent-avoidant combination is particularly common.

Obsessive-Compulsive Personality Disorder

The essential features of OCPD are perfectionism, inflexibility, and control. OCPD does not overlap extensively with other personality disorders in this cluster. OCPD shares with dependent and histrionic personality disorders the problem of being applied as a sex stereotype—only this time referring to stereotypic male behavior such as excessive devotion to work or insistence on getting one's way (Reich 1987). The same caution applies, therefore, for the clinician to document the pathological nature of the behaviors and the impairment that results. This documentation is somewhat easier in the case of OCPD than dependent personality disorder because the disorder items in the former, such as perfectionism, preoccupation with details, and excessive devotion to work, all explicitly refer to how these traits interfere with functioning. Perfectionism, for example, interferes with task completion, so that the patient "is unable to complete a project because his or her own overly strict standards are not being met" (American Psychiatric Association 2000, p. 729).

A significant distinction should be made between OCPD and obsessive-compulsive (anxiety) disorder. Patients with OCPD may not have true obsessions or compulsions—that is, recurrent, senseless thoughts or repetitive, stereotypic behavior rituals. Occasionally, the OCPD person's preoccupation with details, lists, schedules, and the like may approach the threshold of definition of obsessions or compulsions, but usually these behaviors will "feel" ego-syntonic and purposeful to such a person.

Other Personality Disorder Types

Passive-Aggressive (Negativistic) Personality Disorder

Passive-aggressive personality disorder is identified by passive resistance to demands for adequate social and occupational performance and by negative attitudes. Passive-aggressive personality disorder is in DSM-IV Appendix B, "Criteria Sets and Axes Provided for Further Study." Long an "official" personality disorder in DSM, passive-aggressive personality was placed in this appendix because it was not clear whether the criteria identified a pervasive pattern of thinking, feeling, and behaving characteristic of a personality disorder, or simply a single trait (i.e., resistance to external demands). Some attempt has been made to emphasize cognitive and affective aspects of the disorder. Thus, criteria refer to the person's believing that he or she "is misunderstood and unappreciated by others," being critical or scornful of people in authority, and becoming "sullen and argumentative" (American Psychiatric Association 2000, p. 791).

The other major difficulty in the diagnosis of passive-aggressive personality disorder is that the behavior must be evident even in situations in which more self-assertive behavior is possible. The military is usually given as the best example in which self-assertive behavior is frequently not permitted and compliance with the demands of others is required. Passive resistance to demands in this situation would not necessarily indicate a personality disorder. Sometimes it is more difficult for the clinician to assess the rigidity of the demands imposed by the external circumstances. An example would be a job situation in which an employer indicated that there was much latitude for individual, independent initiative while subtly exerting almost total control of the employee's behavior.

Depressive Personality Disorder

Depressive personality disorder was a new disorder introduced into DSM-IV Appendix B. This addition reflects an ongoing debate as to the appropriate characterization of chronic, mild depression as a personality disorder or a mood disorder (Hirschfeld and Holzer 1994). Depressive personality disorder is manifested by a pervasive pattern of depressive cognitions and behaviors, such as a gloomy and unhappy mood, beliefs of inadequacy or worthlessness, critical and blaming attitudes toward self and others, brooding, pessimism, and guilt. The major problem in differential diagnosis is in distinguishing depressive personality disorder from dysthymic disorder. Studies have shown rates of co-occurrence of these two disorders that vary widely, from 18% to 95%, depending on the sample and the criteria used to make the diagnoses (e.g., Klein 1999; Klein and Shih 1998; McDermut et al. 2003). Using DSM-IV-TR criteria, depressive personality disorder can be distinguished from dysthymic disorder by an emphasis on cognitive, interpersonal, and intrapsychic personality traits in the former and more physical, "vegetative" symptoms, such as sleep and appetite disturbance or fatigue, in the latter. When criteria for both disorders are present, both diagnoses can be made. Depressive personality disorder may also predispose to the development of episodes of major depressive disorder.

Self-Defeating Personality Disorder

The diagnosis of masochistic personality disorder was by far the most frequently made diagnosis under the rubric of "other personality disorder" in DSM-III. Masochistic personality disorder is thought by many clinicians to be a useful concept. In the process of revising DSM-III, it quickly became a very controversial category, however, because feminist groups in particular objected to what they viewed as its sexually discriminatory content. In part in response to these objections, the diagnosis was renamed "self-defeating personality disorder" and was included in an appendix of DSM-III-R as a proposed diagnostic category needing further study. The category was dropped completely from DSM-IV (American Psychiatric Association 1994) because its criteria described a behavior pattern common to many other personality disorders and not sufficiently distinctive to represent a separate category (Skodol et al. 1994), and data on its clinical utility and external validity were sparse (Feister 1996).

Sadistic Personality Disorder

Some critics have also objected to the preoccupation of mental health professionals with classifying the "victim" and ignoring the "victimizer" in situations in which one person takes advantage of or abuses another. This mental set may be the result of victims being more likely than victimizers to seek help with emotional problems, but this likelihood does not justify trying to understand the nature of only the victims' troubles.

Therefore, also included in the appendix of DSM-III-R were criteria for a new diagnosis that describes a pattern of behavior characterized by cruel, demeaning, and aggressive behavior for reasons other than sexual arousal. This disorder was called *sadistic personality disorder*. The important points in the differential diagnosis are to distinguish the behavior from those of the paraphilias and from those of other disorders in the differential diagnosis of violent behavior, such as ASPD (see Chapter 31, "Violence"). Sadistic personality disorder was also dropped from DSM-IV because of a paucity of empirical research to support its inclusion.

Personality Disorder Not Otherwise Specified

DSM-IV has a residual category for mixed or other personality disorders. The mixed category is to be used when a person with a personality disorder had features of several of the specific personality disorder types but does not meet the criteria for any one. "Other personality disorder" is used when the clinician wants to diagnose a specific personality disorder type that is not included in DSM-IV-TR (e.g., passive-aggressive, depressive, or self-defeating).

A common error in the use of the personality disorders section of DSM-IV-TR is assigning a diagnosis of mixed personality disorder to a patient who meets criteria for one disorder and has features of one or more other personality disorders, or to a patient who meets full criteria for more than one personality disorder. In the first instance, the clinician should diagnose, for example, BPD with narcissistic and histrionic traits; in the second instance, diagnoses of multiple individual personality disorders should be made.

SUMMARY

This chapter considers the manifestations, problems in differential diagnosis, and patterns of comorbidity of the DSM-IV personality disorders. Although considerable dissatisfaction has been expressed over the DSM approach to these disorders and a major overhaul has been recommended by many researchers and clinicians in the field (Clark et al. 1997; Shedler and Westen 2004; Widiger 1991, 1993), the DSM approach remains the official standard for diagnosing personality disorder psychopathology. Work on DSM-V has recently begun, but its publication is not anticipated until at least 2010. Therefore, even if a dimensional approach to personality disorders were to replace the categorical approach in DSM-V, these changes would not be implemented for several years.

Included in this chapter are descriptions of the clinical characteristics of the 10 DSM-IV personality disorders; discussions of problems in interviewing the patient with a suspected personality disorder in state versus trait discrimination, trait versus disorder distinctions, categorical versus alternative classificatory approaches to personality disorder diagnosis, and diagnosis based on inferential judgments; and an overview of personality disorder comorbidity. Problems in the diagnosis of each individual disorder are covered, grouped according to the three DSM-IV clusters. Despite limitations in the DSM approach, personality disorders diagnosed by this system have been shown in the past 25 years to have considerable clinical utility in predicting functional impairment over and above that associated with comorbid Axis I disorders, extensive and intensive utilization of treatment resources, and in many cases, adverse outcomes.

REFERENCES

Adler DA, Drake RE, Teague GB: Clinicians' practices in personality assessment: does gender influence the use of DSM-III Axis II? Compr Psychiatry 31:125–133, 1990

Akiskal HS, Chen SE, Davis GC, et al: Borderline: an adjective in search of a noun. J Clin Psychiatry 46:41–48, 1985

American Psychiatric Association: Diagnostic and Statistical Manual of Mental Disorders, 3rd Edition. Washington, DC, American Psychiatric Association, 1980

American Psychiatric Association: Diagnostic and Statistical Manual of Mental Disorders, 3rd Edition, Revised. Washington, DC, American Psychiatric Association, 1987

American Psychiatric Association: Diagnostic and Statistical Manual of Mental Disorders, 4th Edition. Washington, DC, American Psychiatric Association, 1994

American Psychiatric Association: Diagnostic and Statistical Manual of Mental Disorders, 4th Edition, Text Revision. Washington, DC, American Psychiatric Association, 2000

Andreoli A, Gressot G, Aapro N, et al: Personality disorders as a predictor of outcome. J Personal Disord 3:307–321, 1989

Beck AT, Freeman A, Davis DD, et al: Cognitive Therapy of Personality Disorders, 2nd Edition. New York, Guilford, 2004

Benjamin LS: Interpersonal Diagnosis and Treatment of Personality Disorders, 2nd Edition. New York, Guilford, 1996

Bernstein DP, Cohen P, Skodol AE, et al: Childhood antecedents of adolescent personality disorders. Am J Psychiatry 153:907–913, 1996

Blashfield RK, Herkov MJ: Investigating clinician adherence to diagnosis by criteria: a replication of Morey and Ochoa (1989). J Personal Disord 10:219–228,1996

Bond MP, Vaillant JS: An empirical study of the relationship between diagnosis and defense style. Arch Gen Psychiatry 43:285–288, 1986

Cantor N, Smith EE, French RS, et al: Psychiatric diagnosis as prototype categorization. J Abnorm Psychol 89:181–193, 1980

Carver CS, Scheier MF, Weintraub JK: Assessing coping strategies: a theoretically based approach. J Pers Soc Psychol 56:267–283, 1989

Casey PR, Tyrer P: Personality disorder and psychiatric illness in general practice. Br J Psychiatry 156:261–265, 1990

Clark LA, Livesley WJ, Morey L: Special feature: personality disorder assessment: the challenge of construct validity. J Personal Disord 11:205–231, 1997

Dolan-Sewell RT, Krueger RF, Shea MT: Co-occurrence with syndrome disorders, in Handbook of Personality Disorders: Theory, Research, and Treatment. Edited by Livesley WJ. New York, Guilford, 2001, pp 84–104

Drake RE, Vaillant GE: A validity study of Axis II of DSM-III. Am J Psychiatry 142:553–558, 1985

Feinstein AR: The pre-therapeutic classification of comorbidity in chronic disease. J Chronic Dis 23:455–468, 1970

Feister SJ: Self-defeating personality disorder, in DSM-IV Sourcebook, Vol 2. Edited by Widiger TA, Frances AJ, Pincus HA, et al. Washington, DC, American Psychiatric Association, 1996, pp 833–847

Fenton WS, McGlashan TH: Risk of schizophrenia in character disordered patients. Am J Psychiatry 146:1280–1284, 1989

Finn SE: Base rates, utilities, and DSM-III: shortcomings of fixed rule systems of psychodiagnosis. J Abnorm Psychol 91:294–302, 1982

First M, Gibbon M, Spitzer RL, et al: User's Guide for the Structured Clinical Interview for DSM-IV Axis II Personality Disorders. Washington, DC, American Psychiatric Press, 1997

Folkman S, Lazarus RS: The Ways of Coping Questionnaire. Palo Alto, CA, Consulting Psychologists Press, 1988

Folkman S, Moskowitz JT: Coping: pitfalls and promise. Ann Rev Psychol 55:745–774, 2004

Frances A: The DSM-III personality disorders section: a commentary. Am J Psychiatry 137:1050–1054, 1980

Frances A: Categorical and dimensional systems of personality diagnosis: a comparison. Compr Psychiatry 23:516–527, 1982

Grant BF, Stinson FS, Dawson DA, et al: Co-occurrence of 12-month alcohol and drug use disorders and personality disorders in the United States: results from the National Epidemiologic Survey on Alcohol and Related Conditions. Arch Gen Psychiatry 61:361–368, 2004

Grilo CM, McGlashan TH, Oldham JM: Course and stability of personality disorders. Journal of Practical Psychiatry and Behavioral Health 1:61–75, 1998

Grilo CM, McGlashan TH, Morey LC, et al: Internal consistency, intercriterion overlap, and diagnostic efficiency of criteria sets for DSM-IV personality disorders. Acta Psychiatr Scand 104:264–272, 2001

Grilo CM, Becker DF, Anez LM, et al: Diagnostic efficiency of DSM-IV criteria for borderline personality disorder: an evaluation in Hispanic men and women with substance use disorders. J Consult Clin Psychol 72:126–131, 2004a

Grilo CM, Shea MT, Sanislow CA, et al: Two-year stability and change in schizotypal, borderline, avoidant, and obsessive-compulsive personality disorders. J Consult Clin Psychol 72:767–775, 2004b

Grilo CM, Sanislow CA, Shea MT: Two-year prospective naturalistic study for remission from major depressive disorder as a function of personality disorder comorbidity. J Consult Clin Psychol 73:78–85, 2005

Gunderson J: Introduction to section IV: personality disorders, in DSM-IV Sourcebook, Vol 2. Edited by Widiger TA, Frances AJ, Pincus HA, et al. Washington, DC, American Psychiatric Association, 1996, pp 647–664

Gunderson JG, Elliot GR: The interface between borderline personality disorder and affective disorder. Am J Psychiatry 142:277–288, 1985

Gunderson JG, Phillips KA: A current view of the interface between borderline personality disorder and depression. Am J Psychiatry 148:967–975, 1991

Gunderson JG, Morey LC, Stout RL, et al: Major depressive disorder and borderline personality disorder revisited: longitudinal interactions. J Clin Psychiatry 65:1049–1056, 2004

Hart AB, Craighead WE, Craighead LW: Predicting recurrence of major depressive disorder in young adults: a prospective study. J Abnorm Psychol 110:633–643, 2001

Herbert JD, Hope DA, Bellack AS: Validity of the distinction between generalized social phobia and avoidant personality disorder. J Abnorm Psychol 101:332–339, 1992

Herkov MJ, Blashfield RK: Clinicians' diagnoses of personality disorder: evidence of a hierarchical structure. J Pers Assess 65:313–321, 1995

Hirschfeld RMA, Holzer CE III: Depressive personality disorder: clinical implications. J Clin Psychiatry 55 (suppl):10–17, 1994

Hyler SE: Personality Diagnostic Questionnaire–4 (PDQ-4). New York, New York State Psychiatric Institute, 1994

Hyler SE, Skodol AE, Kellman D, et al: Validity of the Personality Diagnostic Questionnaire: comparison with two structured interviews. Am J Psychiatry 147:1043–1048, 1990

Hyler SE, Skodol AE, Oldham JM, et al: Validity of the Personality Diagnostic Questionnaire–Revised (PDQ-R): a replication in an outpatient sample. Compr Psychiatry 33:73–77, 1992

Jackson HJ, Burgess PM: Personality disorders in the community: results from the Australian National Survey of Mental Health and Well-Being, part II. Relationships between personality disorder, Axis I mental disorders, and physical conditions with disability and health consultations. Soc Psychiatry Psychiatr Epidemiol 37:251–260, 2002

Johnson JG, Cohen P, Skodol AE, et al: Personality disorders in adolescence and risk of major mental disorders and suicidality during adulthood. Arch Gen Psychiatry 56:805–811, 1999

Johnson JG, Cohen P, Kasen S, et al: Age-related change in personality disorder trait levels between early adolescence and adulthood: a community-based longitudinal investigation. Acta Psychiatr Scand 102:265–275, 2000

Kaplan MA: A woman's view of DSM-III. Am Psychol 38:786–792, 1983

Karasu TB, Skodol AE: Fourth axis for DSM-III: psychodynamic evaluation. Am J Psychiatry 137:607–610, 1980

Kasen S, Cohen P, Skodol AE, et al: The influence of child and adolescent psychiatric disorders on young adult personality disorder. Am J Psychiatry 156:1529–1535, 1999

Kasen S, Cohen P, Skodol AE, et al: Childhood depression and adult personality disorder: alternative pathways of continuity. Arch Gen Psychiatry 58:231–236, 2001

Kass F, Spitzer RL, Williams JBW: An empirical study of the issue of sex bias in the diagnostic criteria of DSM-III axis II personality disorders. Am Psychol 38:799–801, 1983

Kass F, Skodol AE, Charles E, et al: Scaled ratings of DSM-III personality disorders. Am J Psychiatry 142:627–630, 1985

Kaye AL, Shea MT: Personality disorders, personality traits, and defense mechanisms measures, in Handbook of Psychiatric Measures. Edited by Task Force for the Handbook of Psychiatric Measures. Washington, DC, American Psychiatric Association, 2000, pp 713–749

Kendell RE, Cooper JE, Gourlay AJ, et al: Diagnostic criteria of American and British psychiatrists. Arch Gen Psychiatry 25:123–130, 1971

Kessler RC, Crum RM, Warner LA, et al: Lifetime co-occurrence of DSM-III-R alcohol abuse and dependence with other psychiatric disorders in the National Comorbidity Survey. Arch Gen Psychiatry 54:313–321, 1997

Kety SS: Mental illness in the biological and adoptive relatives of schizophrenic adoptees: findings relevant to genetic and environmental factors in etiology. Am J Psychiatry 140:720–727, 1983

Kiesler DJ: Contemporary Interpersonal Theory and Research: Personality, Psychopathology, and Psychotherapy. New York, Wiley, 1996

Klein DN: Depressive personality: reliability, validity, and relation to dysthymia. J Abnorm Psychol 99:412–421, 1999

Klein DN: Patients' versus informants' reports of personality disorders in predicting 7½-year outcome in outpatients with depressive disorders. Psychol Assess 15:216–222, 2003

Klein DN, Shih JH: Depressive personality disorder: associations with DSM-III-R mood and personality disorders and negative and positive affectivity, 30-month stability, and prediction of course of Axis I depressive disorders. J Abnorm Psychol 107:319–327, 1998

Klonsky ED, Oltmanns TF, Turkheimer E: Informant-reports of personality disorder: relation to self-reports and future directions. Clin Psychol Sci Pract 9:300–311, 2002

Koenigsberg HW, Anwunah I, New AS, et al: Relationship between depression and borderline personality disorder. Depress Anxiety 10:158–167, 1999

Krueger RF, Caspi A, Moffitt TE, et al: The structure and stability of common mental disorders (DSM-III-R): a longitudinal-epidemiological study. J Abnorm Psychol 106:216–227, 1998

Krueger RF, Hicks BM, Patrick CJ, et al: Etiologic connections among substance dependence, antisocial behavior, and personality: modeling the externalizing spectrum. J Abnorm Psychol 111:411–424, 2002

Lazarus RS, Folkman S: Stress, Appraisal, and Coping. New York, Springer, 1984

Lenzenweger MF: Stability and change in personality disorder features: the Longitudinal Study of Personality Disorders. Arch Gen Psychiatry 56:1009–1015, 1999

Lewinsohn PM, Rohde P, Seeley JR, et al: Axis II psychopathology as a function of Axis I disorder in childhood and adolescents. J Am Acad Child Adolesc Psychiatry 36:1752–1759, 1997

Lilienfeld SO, Waldman ID, Israel AC: A critical examination of the use of the term "comorbidity" in psychopathology research. Clin Psychol Sci Pract 1:71–83, 1994

Livesley WJ: Trait and behavioral prototypes of personality disorder. Am J Psychiatry 143:728–732, 1986

Loranger AW: International Personality Disorder Examination (IPDE). Odessa, FL, Psychological Assessment Resources, 1999

Lyons MJ, Tyrer P, Gunderson J, et al: Special feature: heuristic models of comorbidity of Axis I and Axis II disorders. J Personal Disord 11:260–269, 1997

McDermut W, Zimmerman M, Chelminski I: The construct validity of depressive personality disorder. J Abnorm Psychol 112:49–60, 2003

McGlashan TH: Schizotypal personality disorder: Chestnut Lodge follow-up study, VI. Long-term follow-up perspectives. Arch Gen Psychiatry 43:328–334, 1986

McGlashan TH, Grilo CM, Skodol AE, et al: The Collaborative Longitudinal Personality Disorders Study: baseline patterns of DSM-IV Axis I/II and II/II diagnostic co-occurrence. Acta Psychiatr Scand 102:256–264, 2000

McGlashan TH, Grilo CM, Sanislow CA, et al: Two-year prevalence and stability of individual DSM-IV criteria for schizotypal, borderline, avoidant and obsessive-compulsive personality disorders. Am J Psychiatry (in press)

Millon T, Millon C, Davis R: MCMI-III Manual, 2nd Edition. Minneapolis, MN, National Computer Systems, 1997

Modestin J, Villiger C: Follow-up study on borderline versus nonborderline personality disorders. Compr Psychiatry 30:236–244, 1989

Moos RH: Coping Responses Inventory. Odessa, FL, Psychological Assessment Resources, 1993

Morey LC, Ochoa ES: An investigation of adherence to diagnostic criteria. J Personal Disord 3:180–192, 1989

Morgenstern J, Langenbucher J, Labouvie E, et al: The comorbidity of alcoholism and personality disorders in a clinical population: prevalence rates and relation to alcohol typology variables. J Abnorm Psychol 106:74–84, 1997

Noyes R Jr, Reich J, Christiansen J, et al: Outcome of panic disorder: relationship to diagnostic subtypes and comorbidity. Arch Gen Psychiatry 47:809–818, 1990

Oldham JM, Skodol AE: Charting the future of Axis II. J Personal Disord 14:17–29, 2000

Oldham JM, Skodol AE, Kellman HD, et al: Diagnosis of DSM-III-R personality disorders by two structured interviews: patterns of comorbidity. Am J Psychiatry 149:213–220, 1992

Oldham JM, Skodol AE, Kellman HD, et al: Comorbidity of Axis I and Axis II disorders. Am J Psychiatry 152:571–578, 1995

Paris J, Brown R, Nowlis D: Long-term follow-up of borderline patients in a general hospital. Compr Psychiatry 28:530–535, 1987

Pearlin LI, Schooler C: The structure of coping. J Health Soc Behav 19:2–21, 1978

Perry JC, Cooper SH: An empirical study of defense mechanisms, I: clinical interview and life vignette ratings. Arch Gen Psychiatry 46:444–452, 1989

Pfohl B, Stangl D, Zimmerman M: The implications of DSM-III personality disorders with major depression. J Affect Disord 7:309–318, 1984

Pfohl B, Coryell W, Zimmerman M, et al: DSM-III personality disorders: diagnostic overlap and internal consistency of individual DSM-III criteria. Compr Psychiatry 27:21–34, 1986

Pfohl B, Blum N, Zimmerman M: Structured Interview for DSM-IV Personality. Washington, DC, American Psychiatric Press, 1997

Pope HG Jr, Jonas JM, Hudson JI, et al: The validity of DSM-III borderline personality disorder: a phenomenologic, family history, treatment response, and long-term follow-up study. Arch Gen Psychiatry 40:23–30, 1983

Reich J: Sex distribution of DSM-III personality disorders in psychiatric outpatients. Am J Psychiatry 144:485–488, 1987

Reich J, Vasile RG: Effect of personality disorders on the treatment outcome of Axis I conditions: an update. J Nerv Ment Dis 181:475–484, 1993

Reich J, Yates W, Nduaguba M: Prevalence of DSM-III personality disorders in the community. Soc Psychiatry Psychiatr Epidemiol 24:12–16, 1989

Rey JM, Morris-Yates A, Singh M, et al: Continuities between psychiatric disorders in adolescents and personality disorders in young adults. Am J Psychiatry 152:895–900, 1995

Roberts BW, Caspi A, Moffitt TE: Work experiences and personality development in young adulthood. J Pers Soc Psychol 84:582–593, 2003

Rogers JH, Widiger TA, Krupp A: Aspects of depression associated with borderline personality disorder. Am J Psychiatry 152:268–270, 1995

Sanislow CA, Morey LC, Grilo CM, et al: Confirmatory factor analysis of DSM-IV borderline, schizotypal, avoidant, and obsessive-compulsive personality disorders: findings from the Collaborative Longitudinal Personality Study. Acta Psychiatr Scand 105:28–36, 2002

Seivewright H, Tyrer P, Johnson T: Persistent social dysfunction in anxious and depressed patients with personality disorder. Acta Psychiatr Scand 109:104–109, 2004

Shea MT: Assessment of change in personality disorders, in Measuring Changes in Mood, Anxiety, and Personality Disorders: Toward a Core Battery. Edited by Strupp HH, Horowitz LM, Lambert MJ. Washington, DC, American Psychological Association, 1997, pp 389–400

Shea MT, Widiger TA, Klein MH: Comorbidity of personality disorders and depression: implications for treatment. J Consult Clin Psychol 60:857–868, 1992

Shea MT, Pilkonis PA, Beckham E, et al: Personality disorder and treatment outcome in the NIMH Treatment of Depression Collaborative Research Program. Am J Psychiatry 147:711–718, 1990

Shea MT, Stout RL, Gunderson J, et al: Short-term diagnostic stability of schizotypal, borderline, avoidant, and obsessive-compulsive personality disorders. Am J Psychiatry 159:2036–2041, 2001

Shedler J, Westen D: Refining personality disorder diagnosis: integrating science and practice. Am J Psychiatry 161:1350–1365, 2004

Siever LJ, Davis KL: A psychobiological perspective on the personality disorders. Am J Psychiatry 148:1647–1658, 1991

Skodol AE: Problems in Differential Diagnosis: From DSM-III to DSM-III-R in Clinical Practice. Washington, DC, American Psychiatric Press, 1989

Skodol AE, Bender DS: Diagnostic interviews for adults, in Handbook of Psychiatric Measures. Edited by Task Force for the Handbook of Psychiatric Measures. Washington, DC, American Psychiatric Association, 2000, pp 45–70

Skodol AE, Williams JBW, Spitzer RL, et al: Identifying common errors in the use of DSM-III through diagnostic supervision. Hosp Community Psychiatry 35:251–255, 1984

Skodol AE, Rosnick L, Kellman D, et al: Validating structured DSM-III-R personality disorder assessments with longitudinal data. Am J Psychiatry 145:1297–1299, 1988

Skodol AE, Oldham JM, Rosnick L, et al: Diagnosis of DSM-III-R personality disorders: a comparison of two structured interviews. Int J Methods Psychiatr Res 1:13–26, 1991

Skodol AE, Oldham JM, Hyler SE, et al: Comorbidity of DSM-III-R eating disorders and personality disorders. Int J Eating Disorders 14:403–416, 1993

Skodol AE, Oldham JM, Gallaher PE, et al: Validity of self-defeating personality disorder. Am J Psychiatry 151:560–567, 1994

Skodol AE, Oldham JM, Hyler SE, et al: Patterns of anxiety and personality disorder comorbidity. J Psychiatr Res 29:361–374, 1995

Skodol AE, Gallaher PE, Oldham JM: Excessive dependency and depression: is the relationship specific? J Nerv Ment Dis 184:165–171, 1996

Skodol AE, Oldham JM, Gallaher PE: Axis II comorbidity of substance use disorders in patients referred for treatment of personality disorders. Am J Psychiatry 156:733–738, 1999

Skodol AE, Gunderson JG, McGlashan TH, et al: Functional impairment in patients with schizotypal, borderline, avoidant, or obsessive-compulsive personality disorder. Am J Psychiatry 159:276–283, 2002

Skodol AE, Pagano MP, Bender DS, et al: Stability of functional impairment in patients with schizotypal, borderline, avoidant, or obsessive-compulsive personality disorder over two years. Psychol Med (in press)

Snyder S, Sajadi C, Pitts WM Jr, et al: Identifying the depressive border of the borderline personality disorder. Am J Psychiatry 139:814–817, 1982

Soloff PH: Algorithm for pharmacological treatment of personality dimensions: symptom-specific treatments for cognitive-perceptual, affective and impulsive-behavioral dysregulation. Bull Menninger Clin 62:195–214, 1998

Soloff PH, Ulrich RF: Diagnostic interview for borderline patients: a replication study. Arch Gen Psychiatry 38:686–692, 1981

Somwaru DP, Ben-Porath YS: Development and reliability of MMPI-2 based personality disorder scales. Paper presented at the 30th annual Workshop and Symposium on Recent Developments in the Use of the MMPI-2 and MMPI-A. St. Petersburg, FL, April, 1995

Spitzer RL, Endicott J, Gibbon M: Crossing the border into borderline personality and borderline schizophrenia: the development of criteria. Arch Gen Psychiatry 36:17–24, 1979

Sternbach S, Judd A, Sabo A, et al: Cognitive and perceptual distortions in borderline personality disorder and schizotypal personality disorder in a vignette sample. Compr Psychiatry 33:186–189, 1992

Stone AA, Schwartz JE, Neale JM, et al: A comparison of coping assessed by ecological momentary assessment and retrospective recall. J Pers Soc Psychol 74:1670–1680, 1998

Swartz M, Blazer D, George L, et al: Estimating the prevalence of borderline personality disorder in the community. J Personal Disord 4:257–272, 1990

Torgersen S: Genetic and nosological aspects of schizotypal and borderline personality disorders: a twin study. Arch Gen Psychiatry 41:546–554, 1984

Trull TJ, Widiger TA, Frances A: Covariation of criteria sets for avoidant, schizoid, and dependent personality disorders. Am J Psychiatry 144:767–771, 1987

Turner SM, Beidel DC, Borden JW, et al: Social phobia: Axis I and II correlates. J Abnorm Psychol 100:102–106, 1991

Tyrer P, Gunderson J, Lyons MJ, et al: Special feature: extent of comorbidity between mental state and personality disorders. J Personal Disord 11:242–259, 1997

Vaillant GE, Bond M, Vaillant CO: An empirically validated hierarchy of defense mechanisms. Arch Gen Psychiatry 43:786–794, 1986

Westen D: Divergences between clinical and research methods for assessing personality disorders: implications for research and the evolution of Axis II. Am J Psychiatry 154:895–903, 1997

Westen D, Moses MJ, Silk KR, et al: Quality of depressive experience in borderline personality disorder and major depression: when depression is not just depression. J Personal Disord 6:382–393, 1992

Widiger TA: Personality disorder dimensional models proposed for DSM-V. J Personal Disord 5:386–398, 1991

Widiger TA: The DSM-III-R categorical personality disorder diagnoses: a critique and an alternative. Psychological Inquiry 4:75–90, 1993

Widiger TA: Sex biases in the diagnosis of personality disorders. J Personal Disord 12:95–118, 1998

Widiger TA: Personality disorders, in Handbook of Assessment and Treatment Planning for Psychological Disorders. Edited by Antony MM, Barlow DH. New York, Guilford, 2002, pp 453–480

Widiger TA, Coker LA: Assessing personality disorders, in Clinical Personality Assessment: Practical Approaches, 2nd Edition. Edited by Butcher JN. New York, Oxford University Press, 2002, pp 407–434

Widiger TA, Corbitt EM: Antisocial personality disorder, in DSM-IV Sourcebook, Vol 2. Edited by Widiger TA, Frances AJ, Pincus HA, et al. Washington, DC, American Psychiatric Association, 1996, pp 703–716

Widiger TA, Frances A: The DSM-III personality disorders: perspectives from psychology. Arch Gen Psychiatry 42:615–623, 1985

Widiger TA, Sanderson CJ: Assessing personality disorders, in Clinical Personality Assessment: Practical Approaches. Edited by Butcher JN. New York, Oxford University Press, 1995, pp 380–394

Widiger TA, Saylor KI: Personality assessment, in Comprehensive Clinical Psychology. Edited by Bellack AS, Hersen M. New York, Pergamon, 1998, pp 145–167

Widiger TA, Hurt SW, Frances A, et al: Diagnostic efficiency and DSM-III. Arch Gen Psychiatry 41:1005–1012, 1984

Widiger TA, Trull TJ, Hurt SW, et al: A multidimensional scaling of the DSM-III personality disorders. Arch Gen Psychiatry 44:557–563, 1987

Widiger TA, Mangine S, Corbitt EM, et al: Personality Disorder Interview–IV: A Semistructured Interview for the Assessment of Personality Disorders. Odessa, FL, Psychological Assessment Resources, 1995

Wiggins JS: Paradigms of Personality Assessment. New York, Guilford, 2003

Zanarini MC, Gunderson JG, Frankenburg FR: Axis I phenomenology of borderline personality disorder. Compr Psychiatry 30:149–156, 1989

Zanarini MC, Frankenburg FR, Sickel AE, et al: Diagnostic Interview for DSM-IV Personality Disorders. Belmont, MA, McLean Hospital, 1996

Zanarini MC, Frankenburg FR, Dubo ED, et al: Axis I comorbidity of borderline personality disorder. Am J Psychiatry 155:1733–1739, 1998

Zimmerman M: Diagnosing personality disorders: a review of issues and research methods. Arch Gen Psychiatry 51:225–245, 1994

Zimmerman M, Coryell W: DSM-III personality disorder diagnosis in a nonpatient sample: demographic correlates and comorbidity. Arch Gen Psychiatry 46:682–689, 1989

Zimmerman M, Mattia JI: Axis I diagnostic comorbidity and borderline personality disorder. Compr Psychiatry 40:245–252, 1999a

Zimmerman M, Mattia JI: Differences between clinical and research practices in diagnosing borderline personality disorder. Am J Psychiatry 156:1570–1574, 1999b

Zimmerman M, Pfohl B, Stangl D, et al: Assessment of DSM-III personality disorders: the importance of interviewing an informant. J Clin Psychiatry 47:261–263, 1986

Zimmerman M, Pfohl B, Coryell W, et al: Diagnosing personality disorder in depressed patients: a comparison of patient and informant interviews. Arch Gen Psychiatry 45:733–737, 1988

Zoccolillo M, Pickles A, Quinton D, et al: The outcome of conduct disorder: implications for defining adult personality disorder and conduct disorder. Psychol Med 22:971–986, 1992

5

Assessment Instruments and Standardized Evaluation

Wilson McDermut, Ph.D.
Mark Zimmerman, M.D.

Accurate psychodiagnostic assessment of personality disorders is essential to our understanding of Axis II pathology. Personality pathology consists of a network of latent constructs for which a taxonomy and accepted nomenclature already exist. The validity of the taxonomy, and in turn its theoretical and pragmatic value, are inferred or deduced from the manner in which we measure personality pathology. Ultimately, our faith in these constructs rests, we would like to think, on the scientifically established validity of the assessments we use. Furthermore, the validity of our measurement instruments is not possible unless the test is known to be reliable as well.

For the researcher or clinician interested in assessing personality pathology, an array of interviews and paper-and-pencil tests are available. Most of these instruments measure personality pathology according to DSM-IV-TR (American Psychiatric Association 2000) taxonomy, which identifies 10 official personality disorders and 2 appendix (provisional) diagnoses. Although not without its share of controversy and detractors, the DSM-IV-TR personality disorder taxonomy is,

if nothing else, the most widely adopted system for diagnosing personality disorders. However, other conceptualizations of personality pathology have their own instruments as well. This chapter discusses the interviews and self-administered questionnaires most widely used in psychiatric research and in the clinical assessment of personality disorders and pathology.

BACKGROUND

In the bulk of this chapter, we describe the most commonly used interviews and self-administered questionnaires for the assessment of personality pathology. Currently, no data conclusively demonstrate superior reliability or validity for any one structured interview (Clark and Harrison 2001; Widiger 2002; Widiger and Coker 2002; Zimmerman 1994). Generally speaking, the assessment instruments described in the following sections have at least adequate (if not better) reliability and validity. Some assessment instruments presented may have limited psychometric data, but the data that do exist are promising. In a few cases, instruments with limited psychometric data were included because they represent novel methodologies or are derived from non–DSM-based theories of personality that are worthy of further systematic study.

Interested readers should also be aware of several other thorough and informative reviews of well-known instruments for the assessment of personality written by Clark and Harrison (2001), Kaye and Shea (2000), Rogers (2003), Widiger (2002), Widiger and Coker (2002), and Zimmerman (1994). Rogers (2003) described the most commonly used interview-based assessments of personality, the importance of incorporating them into routine clinical practice, and reasons for choosing one instrument over another depending on the circumstances and the person being interviewed. The review by Zimmerman (1994) focused only on semistructured interviews, whereas the reviews by Clark and Harrison (2001), Kaye and Shea (2000), Widiger (2002), and Widiger and Coker (2002) covered interviews and self-administered questionnaires. These review papers each summarize much of the extant reliability and validity data. They also address pragmatic concerns such as the who, what, and when of personality assessment and issues critical to interpretability, such as the effect of co-occurring Axis I disorders on self-reported personality functioning.

IMPORTANCE OF STANDARDIZED ASSESSMENTS

Standardized assessments have been developed to avoid some of the pitfalls of routine, unstructured clinical interviews (or "traditional" interviews). Clinical interviews usually begin with questions that focus on the presenting problem and then usually touch on several broad areas (e.g., psychiatric history, family background, psychosocial functioning). Most clinicians adjust their focus throughout the interview and explore some issues in considerably more detail than others (Westen 1997). Some clinical settings may have an intake form, which serves as a rough guideline for the overall interview. A relatively unstructured interview has the advantage of a high degree of responsiveness to the patient's apparent needs and can enhance rapport. Standardized assessments are quite different. In the case of fully structured interviews, all questions are provided to the interviewer, who then reads them verbatim. There is little or no room for departure from the specific set of questions. Semistructured interviews also provide a core set of questions that are asked in a particular order. Typically, questions tap less threatening areas of functioning first, then move to material that is less likely to be spontaneously disclosed. In contrast to fully structured interviews, in semistructured interviews the interviewer has the option of asking follow-up questions to clarify whether or not a symptom or trait is present. Self-report questionnaires are equivalent to "fully structured interviews that are self-administered" (Widiger 2002, p. 463). Almost without exception, standardized interviews also have highly articulated, systematized scoring criteria. Standardized assessment procedures were developed in part because of the poor reliability of clinical interviews. Poor reliability, typically indexed by lack of agreement between interviewer-raters, is a problem for researchers and theorists because it limits validity. In clinical terms, poor reliability means missed diagnoses and misdiagnoses (e.g., Rogers 2003; Zimmerman and Mattia 1999a, 1999b).

Standardized assessment procedures for assessing personality disorders have been de rigueur in research since the mid-1980s. For reasons discussed further later in this chapter, it is not recommended that clinicians rely solely on self-report questionnaires to diagnose personality disorders. Regarding the use of standardized interviews, their adoption into routine clinical practice has been hindered by several obstacles: perceived detriment to developing rapport due to the potentially perfunctory nature of conducting interviews, logistical problems, and inadequate training opportunities. To be sure, a standardized interview can degenerate into a rapid-fire symptom checklist. However, when used competently, a standardized interview can provide a reliable and valid assessment. Research suggests that most diagnostic disagreements in psychological assessment are not due to the questions but rather to discrepancies in the application of diagnostic criteria (Widiger and Spitzer 1991). Unstructured interviews and standardized interviews can coexist. In fact, clinicians could begin an initial interview in an unstructured manner to facilitate rapport and then employ a standardized interview (Rogers 2003).

The main logistical problem in clinical practice is time. Most clinicians would find it impractical to conduct a standardized interview that can take as long as 2 hours to administer. Having a client complete a self-report questionnaire first can help narrow the focus of the interview to those traits and disorders most likely to be present and shorten the length of the interview. Although a personality disorder might not be the presenting problem, research has established that patients with personality disorders are less likely to benefit from treatment for their Axis I symptoms (McDermut and Zimmerman 1997). The last impediment to the integration of standardized assessment (particularly the interviews) into routine clinical practice is lack of emphasis in clinical training programs. Doctoral students in clinical psychology often spend a semester learning projective assessment techniques but get no exposure to standardized interviews.

Historically, the development of fully structured and semistructured interviews occurred in research settings. Westen (1997) pointed out that the process of diagnosing personality disorders with semistructured interviews in research settings is very different from the way clinicians diagnose personality disorders in routine clinical practice. The main difference is that clinicians do not rely on the direct questions that form the core of diagnostic instruments. Instead, clinicians listen to the narratives of patients over time, with special attention to how the patients describe their interpersonal interactions (Westen 1997). However, although it is true that clinicians arrive at Axis II diagnoses differently than researchers, it cannot be assumed that clinical diagnoses are more valid than research diagnoses (Zimmerman and Mattia 1999a), especially given the research showing the unreliability of unstructured clinical diagnoses (Zimmerman 1994) and the evidence of validity of research diagnoses (e.g., McDermut and Zimmerman 1997).

INTERVIEWS AND CLINICIAN-RATED INSTRUMENTS

Most of the interviews described in this section are semistructured. In semistructured interviews, to assess a particular feature the interviewer typically asks a predetermined question or set of questions. The interviewer can then ask any number of additional questions to clarify what score should be assigned to rate that feature. The total number of questions in a semistructured interview can be thought of as an approximation of the number of questions one can expect to ask. However, the actual number of questions can vary depending on whether the instructions call for the interviewer to skip certain items or whether the interviewer goes beyond the core questions to ask follow-up questions.

Composite International Diagnostic Interview, Antisocial Section

The Composite International Diagnostic Interview (CIDI) was developed as part of a collaboration between the World Health Organization and the U.S. Alcohol, Drug Abuse, and Mental Health Administration (Robins et al. 1988). The purpose of this joint venture, which began in the late 1970s, was to conduct a cross-national evaluation of the scientific status of alcohol, drug abuse, and mental disorder diagnosis and classification. In 1982, a task force on instrumentation began developing diagnostic interviews that would render diagnoses congruent with widely accepted diagnostic systems such as ICD-10 (World Health Organization 1992) and DSM-III (American Psychiatric Association 1980). One of the final products of the task force was the CIDI, which was designed primarily for use with the general population. When the measure was created, it incorporated questions from the Diagnostic Interview Schedule (DIS; described below), a semistructured interview already in use. The incorporation of the DIS made the CIDI compatible with DSM-III. The CIDI covered major clinical syndromes for the most part, but it also gathered sufficient information to yield a diagnosis of antisocial personality disorder, which was one of 12 personality disorders in DSM-III. The CIDI is a fully structured interview in that questions are read essentially verbatim by examiners, and response options are easily answered by providing a number or by selecting from among predetermined choices. It is suitable for use by trained nonclinicians and clinicians alike.

Revised Diagnostic Interview for Borderlines

The Revised Diagnostic Interview for Borderlines (DIB-R; Zanarini et al. 1989) was designed to assess Gunderson's conceptualization of borderline personality pathology (Gunderson et al. 1981). Gunderson's concept of borderline personality is similar to, but not identical with, the DSM-IV-TR formulation of borderline personality. The DIB-R is a semistructured interview composed of 105 items that yield ratings on summary statements characterizing borderline pathology. These summary statements are drawn upon to assess the following four areas of functioning: impulse action patterns, affects, cognition, and interpersonal relations. The interview focuses on assessing features during the past 2 years. The four section scores are summed to yield a total score ranging from 0 to 10. A cutoff score of 8 or higher indicates the presence of borderline personality.

Diagnostic Interview for DSM-IV Personality Disorders

The Diagnostic Interview for DSM-IV Personality Disorders (DIPD-IV; Zanarini et al. 1996) is a 398-item structured interview that assesses the 10 DSM-IV-TR personality disorders as well as passive-aggressive (negativistic) and depressive personality disorders, both of which appear in Appendix B of DSM-IV-TR ("Criteria Sets and Axes Provided for Further Study"). Items are grouped by diagnosis. The DIPD-IV determines the presence of traits by focusing on the 2 years prior to the interview. The DIPD-IV was selected for use in the Collaborative Longitudinal Personality Disorders Study (Gunderson et al. 2000), the first multisite collaborative study of personality disorders, which is being conducted in four Northeastern cities.

Diagnostic Interview for Narcissism

The Diagnostic Interview for Narcissism (Gunderson et al. 1990) assesses narcissism as it is conceptualized by Gunderson and colleagues. Narcissism in this view is more heterogeneous than in DSM-IV-TR's conceptualization. The Diagnostic Interview for Narcissism generates ratings of grandiosity, interpersonal relations, reactiveness, affects and mood states, and social and moral judgments. The ratings in these areas are derived from an interview composed of 33 statements. For clinicians and researchers interested in the assessment of narcissism and narcissistic personality disorder, Hilsenroth et al. (1996) provide an excellent review of extant instruments.

Hare Psychopathy Checklist–Revised

The Hare Psychopathy Checklist–Revised (PCL-R; Hare 1991) can be used to assess psychopathy both categorically and dimensionally. It was designed for use primarily in forensic settings. The construct of psychopathy is somewhat broader than in DSM-IV-TR, in which the definition of psychopathy consists predominantly of a history of antisocial behaviors. Psychopathy also encompasses glibness and charm, grandiosity, lack of empathy, and shallow affect. The PCL-R is a 20-item checklist; thus, it is not strictly an interview. However, information for rating of items can be gleaned from a semistructured interview and/ or ancillary sources (e.g., institutional records). Clinical judgment and inference are required for scoring most of the items. Items are scored from 0 to 2, in which a 2 indicates that the item is true of the examinee. The total score ranges from 0 to 40. The scale has

two subscales (or "factors"); Factor 1 represents psychopathic personality characteristics, and Factor 2 represents socially deviant behaviors. Scoring the PCL-R involves generating scores for each of the factors and a combined total score. A cutoff score of 30 or greater can be used to signify the presence of psychopathy.

International Personality Disorders Examination

The International Personality Disorders Examination (IPDE; Loranger 1999) is a 537-question semistructured interview that evaluates personality disorders according to both DSM-IV-TR and ICD-10 criteria. Personality disorders included in the ICD-10 are as follows: paranoid, schizoid, dissocial, emotionally unstable–impulsive, emotionally unstable–borderline, histrionic, anankastic, anxious, and dependent. The interviewer inquires about age of onset of pathologic traits, and at least one trait must have been present before age 25 years. The IPDE is designed for use by professionals with substantial psychodiagnostic experience. The IPDE questions are organized by topic: work, self, interpersonal relationships, affects, reality testing, and impulse control. The IPDE has been translated into several different languages for use in a multisite international study of personality disorders (Loranger et al. 1994). The IPDE also has a 77 true/ false question screener that is completed by the subject prior to the interview.

National Institute of Mental Health Diagnostic Interview Schedule, Antisocial Section

The Diagnostic Interview Schedule (DIS; Robins et al. 1981) was developed at the request of the National Institute of Mental Health for use in the Epidemiologic Catchment Area projects (Regier et al. 1984). Its structure and features followed the general design of the Renard Diagnostic Interview (Helzer et al. 1981), which was used to make diagnoses consistent with the Washington University criteria (Feighner et al. 1972). Features of the Renard Diagnostic Interview that were incorporated into the DIS were that all questions and probes were fully specified and that diagnoses were made according to a computer algorithm to minimize clinical judgment. These features, it was hoped, would allow lay interviewers with 1–2 weeks of training to make diagnoses as accurately as psychiatrists. The use of lay interviewers was considered important to avoiding the high cost and impracticality of employing psychiatrists as interviewers in large epidemiologic studies. The DIS gathered information primarily on mood anxiety, substance, and psychotic disorders and generated diagnoses according to multiple diagnostic systems, including the DSM-III. The only personality disorder measured was antisocial personality disorder.

Personality Assessment Form

The Personality Assessment Form (Pilkonis et al. 1991) is not an interview per se, but could best be characterized as a "clinician-report" instrument (Widiger 2002). It does not provide of list of questions to ask a subject, nor does it yield categorical assignments of personality disorder diagnoses. Rather, it provides a brief description of the important features of each personality disorder and a six-point scale against which to make a diagnosis. Thus, the form requires substantial clinical judgment. Based on previous research, a cutoff score of four or higher has been established as the threshold for identifying cases of personality disorder (Shea et al. 1990).

Personality Assessment Schedule

The Personality Assessment Schedule, developed by Tyrer (1988) in Britain, is a comprehensive interview that assesses 24 traits (e.g., conscientiousness, aggression, and impulsivity) and generates dimensional ratings of five personality styles: normal, passive-dependent, sociopathic, anankastic (analogous to obsessive-compulsive), and schizoid. Regrettably, this instrument has received little attention in the United States, despite being a comprehensive interview that yields dimensional ratings of personality style.

Personality Disorder Interview–IV

The Personality Disorder Interview–IV (PDI-IV; Widiger et al. 1995) is the most current version of what was previously known as The Personality Interview Questions (versions I, II, and III). The PDI-IV has questions assessing the 94 DSM-IV-TR criteria for the 10 official DSM-IV-TR personality disorders and two appendix diagnoses. A trait is rated as present if it has been characteristic for much of the subject's adult life and present since age 18. The PDI-IV has two versions, one with items grouped by diagnosis and the other with items grouped by topic. A translated version of the PDI-IV was recently used in China (Yang et al. 2000).

Structured Clinical Interview for DSM-IV Axis II Personality Disorders

The Structured Clinical Interview for DSM-IV Axis II Personality Disorders (SCID-II; First et al. 1997) is a 119-item semistructured interview with items keyed to the DSM-IV-TR personality disorder criteria. The SCID-II evaluates traits for the past 5 years. The presence of traits and disorders is operationalized based on DSM-IV-TR's guideline that subjects describe how they have generally felt, exclusive of Axis I symptoms. The essential features of each disorder should have been present cross-contextually since early adulthood. Authors of the SCID-II recommend administration only by experienced clinicians. Items are grouped by diagnosis. The SCID-II interview is preceded by administration of the SCID-II Personality Questionnaire. Interviewers then follow up on items endorsed as present by the subject on the screener. The screener has 119 items.

Structured Interview for DSM-IV Personality Disorders

The Structured Interview for DSM-IV Personality Disorders (SIDP-IV; Pfohl et al. 1997) is a 101-item semistructured interview that assesses the 10 DSM-IV-TR official personality disorders plus the proposed depressive, self-defeating, and negativistic personality disorders. Each item is rated from 0 to 3 (0=not present, 1=subthreshold, 2=present, 3=strongly present). The items are keyed to the DSM-IV-TR personality disorder criteria. The SIDP comes in two versions: one in which items are grouped topically and another in which items are grouped by diagnosis. The interviewee is asked to focus on his or her "usual self"; and if there has been a dramatic recent change in the individual's personality, then the functioning that predominated for the greatest amount of time in the past 5 years is considered typical. For a diagnosis to be considered present, the traits endorsed must have been present for the majority of time in the past 5 years. The SIDP is designed for use by individuals with a minimum of a bachelor's degree in the social sciences, 6 months' experience interviewing psychiatric patients, and about 1 month of specific training in using the SIDP.

Structured Interview for the Five-Factor Model of Personality

The 120-item Structured Interview for the Five-Factor Model of Personality (Trull and Widiger 1997) is unique in that it is the only semistructured interview that assesses general personality. It is modeled after the NEO Personality Inventory–Revised (NEO-PI-R; Costa and McCrae 1992) in that it assesses the five domains of the five-factor model (FFM) of personality, which include neuroticism, extraversion, openness to experience, agreeableness, and conscientiousness. It also assesses the six facets of each of the five major domains. The Structured Interview for the Five-Factor Model of Personality has a slightly stronger emphasis on maladaptive components of general personality than does the NEO-PI-R.

SELF-ADMINISTERED QUESTIONNAIRES

Coolidge Axis II Inventory

The Coolidge Axis II Inventory (CATI; Coolidge and Merwin 1992) has 200 items, rated on a four-point true/false scale ranging from 1 (strongly false) to 4 (strongly true). The personality disorder items were selected or developed specifically to assess the DSM Axis II symptoms. In addition to assessing 13 DSM-III-R personality disorders (11 official personality disorders plus sadistic and self-defeating personality disorders as described in the DSM-III-R appendix) (American Psychiatric Association 1987), the CATI also has scales to assess depression, anxiety, and brain dysfunction.

Dimensional Assessment of Personality Pathology–Basic Questionnaire

The Dimensional Assessment of Personality Pathology–Basic Questionnaire (DAPP-BQ; Livesley and Jackson, in press) is a 290-item assessment instrument that assesses 18 dimensions of personality pathology. Respondents rate each item on a five-point Lykert-type scale in which a score of 1 equals "very unlike me" and a score of 5 equals "very like me." Items included were those that highlighted traits and behavioral acts characteristic of DSM-III personality disorders, but items were not explicit paraphrasings of DSM-III personality disorder criteria. Examples of some of the dimensions assessed include some that correspond to DSM personality disorder criteria (e.g., self-harming behaviors, social avoidance); some that correspond to prototypical features of particular personality disorders (e.g., narcissism); some that cover interpersonal difficulties (e.g., intimacy problems); and some that span both the traits traditionally studied in academic psychology and disordered personality, which has been the traditional emphasis of psychiatric research on personality (e.g.,

anxiousness, compulsivity). Although the DAPP-BQ covers the components of DSM personality disorders, it does not render scale scores that correspond with them.

Inventory of Interpersonal Problems

The Inventory of Interpersonal Problems is a 64-item self-administered questionnaire (Horowitz et al. 2000). The items assess a wide range of interpersonal problems. Respondents rate items in terms of how distressing the problem has been, ranging from 0 (not at all) to 4 (extremely). The interpersonal theory on which the scale is based is an adaptation of the interpersonal circumplex (IPC) model of interpersonal dispositions. According to this model, interpersonal behavior can be located in two-dimensional circular space, with dominance versus submission on one axis and hostility versus friendliness on the other axis. The scale yields information about a person's interpersonal behavior with respect to the following areas: being domineering, vindictive, cold, avoidant, unassertive, exploitable, hypernurturing, and intrusive. A 32-item short form is also available.

Millon Clinical Multiaxial Inventory–III

The Millon Clinical Multiaxial Inventory–III (MCMI-III; Millon et al. 1997) is a 175-item true/false questionnaire that assesses Axis I and II pathology. Now in its third generation, this inventory has been one of the most widely used paper-and-pencil tests in research and the most widely used paper-and-pencil test employed clinically to generate actual diagnoses. Its purpose is to operationalize the assessment of Millon's theory of psychopathology. Millon's proposed psychopathologic constructs are congruent to a great degree, but not entirely, with the disorders in DSM-IV-TR. The MCMI-III assesses many Axis I disorders and the following personality disorders in addition to those assessed by the DSM-IV-TR: aggressive (sadistic), self-defeating (masochistic), depressive, and negativistic (passive-aggressive).

Minnesota Multiphasic Personality Inventory–Personality Disorder Scales

The Minnesota Multiphasic Personality Inventory (MMPI) Personality Disorder Scales (Morey et al. 1985) were developed using a two-step, rational-empirical process. In the first step, clinical psychologist judges searched the 566 MMPI items and selected those expected to be representative of one or more of the 11 DSM-III personality disorders. In the second step, the selected items were analyzed iteratively to determine that they discriminated between high and low scorers on the scales to which they belonged. The result was 154 true/false items. Some items were common to two or more scales, so the authors developed two sets of scales, one in which items overlapped and a second set with no overlapping items. These personality disorder scales have been updated (MMPI-II, Colligan et al. 1994), but have not yet been coordinated with DSM-IV-TR.

Minnesota Multiphasic Personality Inventory—Personality and Psychopathology Five Scales

Using MMPI items, Harkness et al. (1995) developed five scales (the PSY-5) to facilitate the description of general personality and to complement the diagnosis of personality disorders. The five constructs these scales measure are aggressiveness, psychoticism, constraint, negative emotionality/neuroticism, and positive emotionality/extraversion.

Narcissistic Personality Inventory

The Narcissistic Personality Inventory (Raskin and Terry 1988) is a 40-item self-administered questionnaire that measures trait narcissism. Although many items were originally constructed to correspond to features of DSM-III narcissistic personality disorder, the instrument is not intended to yield categorical diagnoses. Each item on the inventory consists of a pair of statements (one that reflects narcissism, the other nonnarcissistic). The respondent is instructed to choose the item that is most true.

NEO Personality Inventory–Revised

The NEO-PI-R (Costa and McCrae 1992) is designed to assess general personality traits according to the FFM. The development of this instrument grew out of academic psychology's traditional interest in normal personality traits and dimensions. The five factors are thought to be fundamental and nearly ubiquitous dimensions of personality, representing higher-order traits composed of multiple lower-order traits. In addition to the putative universality of the five factors, the theory holds that individual differences in the expression of personality can be explained in terms of any given individual's location along each of the five basic dimensions. The NEO-PI-R is a 240-item self-administered questionnaire intended to assess the five

factors (see earlier discussion, "Structured Interview for the Five-Factor Model of Personality"). Within each higher-order factor, the NEO-PI-R also assesses six lower-order traits or "facets." For example, the six facets of the higher-order trait of neuroticism that are measured by the NEO-PI-R are depression, anxiety, angry hostility, self-consciousness, vulnerability, and impulsiveness. There is also a 60-item alternative to the NEO-PI-R, the NEO–Five Factor Inventory (Costa and McCrae 1992), which is designed to assess just the five factors of the FFM, not their constituent facets.

Personality Diagnostic Questionnaire–4

The Personality Diagnostic Questionnaire–4 (Hyler 1994) produces diagnoses consistent with DSM-IV-TR criteria for the 10 official and 2 appendix Axis II diagnoses. It consists of 85 items. Previous versions have shown adequate test-retest reliability. Items were selected or developed specifically to assess DSM Axis II symptoms. The questionnaire's predecessors had high sensitivity but lower specificity. It generated many false positive diagnoses, but very few false negatives. Yang et al. (2000) used a Chinese version of the Personality Diagnostic Questionnaire–4 in a large sample of psychiatric patients in the People's Republic of China.

Personality Assessment Inventory

The Personality Assessment Inventory is a self-report questionnaire consisting of 344 items (Morey 1991). It produces 22 scales that provide continuous ratings of major clinical syndromes, personality features, and factors that may compromise treatment. Among the 22 scales are also 4 validity scales. Each item is rated by respondents on a 4-point Lykert-type scale. The Personality Assessment Inventory has four personality dimensions including borderline features, antisocial features, and the interpersonal dimensions of dominance and warmth.

Psychopathic Personality Inventory

The Psychopathic Personality Inventory (Lilienfield and Andrews 1996) is a self-administered questionnaire that was developed to assess traits of psychopathy (i.e., the assessment of antisocial acts is deemphasized). The measure contains eight subscales developed using factor analysis: Machiavellian egocentricity, social potency, coldheartedness, carefree nonplanfulness, fearlessness, blame externalization, impulsive nonconformity, and stress immunity. The Psychopathic Personality Inventory also contains validity scales to detect malingering and careless responding.

Schedule for Nonadaptive and Adaptive Personality

The Schedule for Nonadaptive and Adaptive Personality (SNAP) contains 375 true/false questions (Clark 1993). Many items were selected or developed specifically to assess DSM Axis II symptoms. In addition to 12 diagnostic scales that are congruent with DSM Axis II constructs, the SNAP has validity scales and 15 trait and temperament scales. The items reflect a broad array of personality disorder descriptors, corresponding in some cases to the DSM. Other items were based on non-DSM formulations of personality disorder, and others congruent with symptoms of particular Axis I disorders with traitlike manifestations (e.g., chronic disturbances associated with dysthymia or generalized anxiety disorder). Scoring rules for making DSM-IV-TR personality disorder diagnoses have also been established.

Shedler-Westen Assessment Procedure

The Shedler-Westen Assessment Procedure (SWAP-200; Westen and Shedler 1998) is composed of 200 items representing the 94 DSM-IV-TR personality disorder diagnostic criteria, personality disorder symptomatology, defense mechanisms, and adaptive personality traits. The respondent is a clinician who rates the patient using a Q-sort procedure, in which he or she rates items according to a Lykert-style format in which ratings conform to a predetermined distribution. For example, Westen and Shedler (1998) used an eight-point scale (from 0 [not at all descriptive, irrelevant, or inapplicable] to 7 [highly descriptive]), and clinician raters were required to assign a rating of 7 on eight of the 200 items. Ten items were required to receive a score of 6, and 100 of the 200 items were required to receive a rating of 0.

Schizotypal Personality Questionnaire

The Schizotypal Personality Questionnaire (Raine 1991) is a 74-item self-administered questionnaire with items assessing each of the DSM-III-R schizotypal personality disorder criteria. The questionnaire was developed to assess schizotypal personality patterns and to screen for schizotypal personality disorder in the community. Raine and Benishay (1995) developed a brief 22-item version to be used as a screening instrument.

Structural Analysis of Social Behavior Intrex Questionnaire

The Structural Analysis of Social Behavior Intrex Questionnaire is a series of questionnaires that operationalize concepts outlined in Benjamin's Structural Analysis of Social Behavior (SASB) model (Benjamin 1996). The SASB model delineates three important aspects of inter- and intrapersonal behavior: focus, affiliation, and interdependence. It has roots in Leary's (1957) IPC model and in the work of Sullivan (1953). Similar to the IPC, the SASB model depicts a horizontal friendliness-versus-hostility *(affiliation)* axis. Unlike the IPC, in the SASB model the affiliation axis is crossed with a vertical enmeshment-versus-differentiation axis, called *interdependence. Enmeshment* refers to control and submission. Control and submission are not depicted as diametrically opposed, but rather they are conceived of as complementary, differing only in terms of their focus of action, where control is directed toward another and submission is in response to another. *Differentiation* refers to processes called *emancipation, separation,* and *assertiveness.* In the SASB model, there are three IPCs (with affiliation and interdependence axes), one for each of three foci of action: transitive, intransitive, and introjective. *Transitive, intransitive,* and *introjective* refer to whether or not social action is toward others (transitive), in reaction to others (intransitive), or toward oneself (introjective).

The SASB consists of a series of self-administered questionnaires, selected by the patient and clinician in collaboration. There is a standard series comprising versions directed toward self, significant other, mother, father, mother in relationship with father, and father in relationship with mother. Patients are asked to rate themselves or others at their best and at their worst. Items are rated from 0 to 100 in 10-point increments, ranging from 0 ("never, or not at all" applicable) to 100 ("always, perfectly" applicable). Up to 36 scores are plotted for each of the three IPCs, representing different foci of action. Numerous other scores, which are often generated by complex mathematical algorithms, are available.

Temperament and Character Inventory

The Temperament and Character Inventory (TCI; Cloninger et al. 1994) is a 240-item self-administered questionnaire designed to measure personality from the perspective of Cloninger's seven-factor model (Cloninger et al. 1993). The TCI measures four dimensions of temperament and three dimensions of character. Cloninger et al. (1993) postulated that temperament is highly heritable, remains stable throughout life, and has specific neurobiological and neuroanatomical substrates. The character dimensions, on the other hand, are more malleable. Character is postulated to be modifiable through learning and sociocultural influences and is capable of evolving throughout the lifespan. Cloninger's model contains four dimensions of temperament (novelty seeking, harm avoidance, reward dependence, and persistence) and three dimensions of character (self-directedness, cooperativeness, and self-transcendence) (see Chapter 9, "Genetics").

Wisconsin Personality Inventory

The Wisconsin Personality Inventory (Klein et al. 1993) is a 214-item self-administered questionnaire that yields dimensional as well as categorical scores for DSM-III-R personality disorders. It contains items coordinated with each personality disorder diagnostic criterion. Each item is rated on a 10-point scale from 1 (never, not at all) to 10 (always, extremely). Respondents are asked to focus on what is true of them during the past 5 years or more. Many of the items were written from the interpersonal, object relational standpoint of Benjamin's (1996) SASB model.

ADVANTAGES AND DISADVANTAGES OF PERSONALITY ASSESSMENT INSTRUMENTS

Semistructured Interviews

None of the assessment instruments described earlier has been shown to have unequivocally superior reliability and validity, and no instrument is without distinct disadvantages. Advantages of various assessment instruments are discussed later. Among the available semistructured interviews, one obvious consideration is whether the interview assesses all DSM-IV-TR personality disorders. There are five semistructured interviews developed specifically to correspond to DSM-IV-TR personality disorders: DIPD-IV, IPDE, PDI-IV, SCID-II, SIDP-IV. For clinical purposes, the IPDE and PDI-IV in particular have detailed administration and scoring manuals that can be valuable assets for clinicians. The IPDE, SCID-II, and SIDP-IV have been used in the most empirical studies. The IPDE and SIDP-IV also provide information about which questions are required to make diagnoses according to ICD-10. The IPDE is the longest to administer, with 537 questions requiring up to 2 hours. The IPDE and SCID-II have screening questionnaires that can help narrow the focus to traits and disorders most

likely to be present. However, a clinician might want to use one of the self-report questionnaires described earlier as a screening device, because there are many questionnaires whose psychometric properties are supported by much larger bodies of research. If a clinician wants to focus the interview on traits and/or disorders identified by a screening questionnaire, a standardized interview with questions arranged by disorder will be easier to use because finding the relevant questions will be easier. All standardized interviews except the IPDE have versions organized in a disorder-by-disorder format. The IPDE, PDI-IV, and SIDP-IV also have versions organized by thematic content (e.g., interpersonal relations, work, interests, and hobbies). The thematic organization of items is thought to mitigate against potential halo effects.

In addition to comprehensive semistructured interviews for the assessment of all DSM-IV-TR personality disorders, other interviews specifically target the assessment of borderline pathology, narcissism, and psychopathy. The DIB-R and Diagnostic Interview for Narcissism assess borderline pathology and narcissism, respectively, from Gunderson's conceptualization (Gunderson et al. 1981, 1990). These interviews have the advantage of furnishing rich descriptions of an individual's functioning in these areas, but they can be almost as time consuming as the comprehensive semistructured interviews covering all the DSM personality disorders. The PCL-R is a measure of Hare's concept of psychopathy, which in addition to gathering data about an individual's history of antisocial behavior includes coverage of features such as glibness, superficiality, and charm associated with psychopathy. The Structured Interview for the Five-Factor Model of Personality can be used to flesh out the description of a client's general personality functioning (e.g., extraversion vs. introversion; antagonism vs. agreeableness) from the standpoint of the FFM.

Self-Report Questionnaires

There are many advantages to using self-report questionnaires as well, although all are problematic for varying reasons. If one wants a comprehensive measure of personality disorders from the DSM perspective, there are several options: MMPI personality disorder scales, MCMI-III, Personality Diagnostic Questionnaire–4, and CATI. The MMPI personality disorder scales and the CATI have the disadvantage of not being coordinated with DSM-IV. The MMPI scales are also embedded within the 567 items of the MMPI-I, which can be time-consuming to complete. The MCMI-III has been the most heavily researched (see Craig's 1999 review of MCMI research), although research suggests that the MCMI-III is prone to gender bias, and the technical manual does not explain in sufficient detail the mathematics underlying the determination of base rates. Research indicates that self-report questionnaires assessing personality disorders tend to detect many false positives compared with interviews. However, they are highly sensitive, making self-report measures useful as screening devices. Self-report measures have also been shown to demonstrate high convergent validity, probably as a result of being so structured (Widiger 2002).

There are also self-report measures of personality functioning that grew out of non–DSM-based theoretical and or research traditions. Although the MCMI-III provides scores on DSM-IV-TR personality disorders, Millon's theory of psychopathology—rooted in evolutionary theory—provides ratings of personality pathology (depressive, negativistic, masochistic, sadistic) that are not officially part of DSM-IV-TR. The Wisconsin Personality Inventory–IV, Inventory of Interpersonal Problems, and SASB are heavily influenced by interpersonal theory. The Wisconsin Personality Inventory–IV and SASB also have strong ties to object relations theory. The SNAP and DAPP-BQ provide ratings of personality functioning that complement but are by no means identical to the DSM formulation of personality disorders. The Wisconsin Personality Inventory–IV, Inventory of Interpersonal Problems, SASB, SNAP, and DAPP-BQ have not been as heavily researched as the scales from the MMPI, MCMI-III, and Personality Diagnostic Questionnaire–4. The TCI measures personality from the perspective of a comprehensive psychobiological approach to personality functioning. For comprehensive evaluations of personality functioning from the standpoint of general personality, there are the NEO-PI-R and the NEO Five-Factor Model. The NEO-PI-R has been found to provide valuable information above and beyond pathology-laden assessment techniques based on DSM models (Garb 2003). The PSY-5 is a recently developed set of five subscales of the MMPI-II that provide scores on measures of both general personality functioning and personality pathology. There are also innovative approaches to rating personality functioning such as the SWAP-200, which uses a clinician-rated Q-sort methodology. The SWAP-200 also generates ratings of defense mechanisms, although ratings must adhere to a specified distribution and thus may result in incomplete coverage of an individual's personality functioning. For assessments that target one or two dimensions of personality pathology, there

are the Personality Assessment Inventory (borderline, antisocial), Psychopathic Personality Inventory (psychopathy), Narcissistic Personality Inventory (narcissism), and Schizotypal Personality Questionnaire (schizotypy). The Psychopathic Personality Inventory, Narcissistic Personality Inventory, and Schizotypal Personality Questionnaire are relatively short and thus are useful for targeted investigations of specific dimensions of functioning. The borderline and antisocial scales in the Personality Assessment Inventory are embedded in a larger 344-item questionnaire, which may be impractical for certain uses. It also has yet to be coordinated with DSM-IV-TR. However, the Personality Assessment Inventory has multiple subscales capturing Axis I pathology, validity scales, and measures of personality dimensions related to dominance and warmth.

IMPORTANT ISSUES IN THE ASSESSMENT OF PERSONALITY PATHOLOGY

Effect of Axis I Symptoms on Reported Personality

It is now well established that Axis I symptoms, such as acute depressive, anxious, or psychotic states, can bias the self-reported personality characteristics of patients (Hirshfeld et al. 1983; Piersma 1989; Zimmerman 1994). Depressed patients, for example, will depict themselves in a more negative light (introverted, dependent, inadequate) than they would have in a nondepressed state (Widiger 1993). However, individuals with eating disorders (Ames-Frankel et al. 1992) and obsessive-compulsive disorder (Ricciardi et al. 1992) have also been shown to report lower levels of personality pathology following treatment, relative to reported levels of personality pathology at treatment initiation. It may be tempting to think that semistructured interviews can circumvent the state-biasing effect of acute Axis I symptoms on reported personality pathology. The comprehensive semistructured interviews make a point of trying to distinguish the patient's usual personality from personality functioning at the initiation of treatment for Axis I disorders. On balance, however, the available evidence suggests that both personality disorder interviews and self-report questionnaires are prone to overreporting bias due to psychiatric state (Widiger and Coker 2002; Zimmerman 1994).

Use of Informants

Most information about personality pathology comes directly from patients and thus is vulnerable to distortions or omissions that could undermine the validity of the material provided. As previously discussed, reported traits may be affected by comorbid Axis I pathology. Alternatively, patients may deny the presence of socially undesirable behavior, lack insight, or simply be unaware of the effect their behavior has on others. Thus, there has been increased research on the degree to which informants (e.g., spouses, relatives, friends) can elucidate the presence of personality pathology in patients. From the standpoint of the researcher, obtaining consistent data from patients and informants serves as a form of convergent validity (Widiger 1993). Overviews of the state of the research on patient–informant agreement have generally noted "poor to adequate" agreement (Widiger and Coker 2002).

Despite the low to modest agreement between patients and informants, most researchers have stressed the value of including informants in Axis II assessments whenever feasible (Clark and Harrison 2001; Widiger 2002). Even when patient and informant reports do not agree at all on the presence of a personality disorder, informants may be identifying patients with personality disorders who did not self-identify in their own interviews. For example, Riso et al. (1994) pointed out that of all the personality disorder diagnoses made based on informant interview, only 18% of those disorders were also made based on patient interviews. From the standpoint of the clinician, the use of information from a collateral source (such as a significant other) may illuminate personality traits that the patient denies or is unaware of and may help clinicians mitigate the biasing effect of Axis I symptomatology on the patient's self-report.

INTERVIEW VERSUS QUESTIONNAIRE

There are fewer logistical problems associated with conducting studies that compare interviews and self-report measures, and consequently these types of comparisons are conducted far more frequently (Zimmerman 1994). In both patient and nonpatient samples, researchers have found low levels of agreement between interviews and questionnaires (i.e., mean kappas between 0.25 and 0.36) (Zimmerman 1994). The reason for the low agreement is primarily the fact that questionnaires tend to overdiagnose. In some cases, questionnaires overdiagnose the presence of a personality disorder at a rate almost 10 times higher than that of interviews (Hunt and Andrews 1992). The high sensitivity of questionnaires suggests that they may be useful as screening measures in clinical settings but are inappropriate for use in making diagnoses.

Questionnaires also have value for researchers. Assuming structured interviews demonstrate reliability, there still remains the possibility of intersite differences in terms of the unstructured follow-up questions that might be used or the interpretation of diagnostic criteria. Therefore, Zimmerman et al. (1993) proposed that self-report questionnaires be used as a paper standard. In other words, if two research centers obtain different prevalence rates for personality disorders, the validity of their respective findings could be judged against the degree of concordance between interview results and questionnaire results at the two centers. Assuming no real population differences, the questionnaire thus becomes the definitive standard.

REFERENCES

American Psychiatric Association: Diagnostic and Statistical Manual of Mental Disorders, 3rd Edition. Washington, DC, American Psychiatric Association, 1980

American Psychiatric Association: Diagnostic and Statistical Manual of Mental Disorders, 3rd Edition, Revised. Washington, DC, American Psychiatric Association, 1987

American Psychiatric Association: Diagnostic and Statistical Manual of Mental Disorders, 4th Edition. Washington, DC, American Psychiatric Association, 1994

American Psychiatric Association: Diagnostic and Statistical Manual of Mental Disorders, 4th Edition, Text Revision. Washington, DC, American Psychiatric Association, 2000

Ames-Frankel J, Devlin MJ, Walsh BT, et al: Personality disorder diagnoses in patients with bulimia nervosa: clinical correlates and changes with treatment. J Clin Psychiatry 53:90–96, 1992

Benjamin LS: Interpersonal Diagnosis and Treatment of Personality Disorders, 2nd Edition. New York, Guilford, 1996

Clark LA: Manual for the Schedule for Nonadaptive and Adaptive Personality. Minneapolis, MN, University of Minnesota Press, 1993

Clark LA, Harrison JA: Assessment instruments, in Handbook of Personality Disorders. Edited by Livesley WJ. New York, Guilford, 2001, pp 277–306

Cloninger CR, Svrakic DM, Przybeck TR: A psychosocial model of temperament and character. Arch Gen Psychiatry 50:975–990, 1993

Cloninger CR, Przybeck TR, Svrakic DM, et al: The Temperament and Character Index: A Guide to Its Development and Use. St Louis, MO, Washington University, Center for Psychobiology of Personality, 1994

Colligan RC, Morey LC, Offord KP: MMPI/MMPI-2 personality disorder scales: contemporary norms for adults and adolescents. J Clin Psychol 50:168–200, 1994

Coolidge FL, Merwin MM: Reliability and validity of the Coolidge Axis II Inventory: a new inventory for the assessment of personality disorders. J Pers Assess 59:223–238, 1992

Costa PT, McCrae RR: Revised NEO Personality Inventory (NEO PI-R) and NEO Five Factor Inventory Professional Manual. Odessa, FL, Psychological Assessment Resources, 1992

Craig RJ: Overview and current status of the Millon Clinical Multi-axial Inventory. J Pers Assess 72:390–406, 1999

Feighner JP, Robins E, Guze SB, et al: Diagnostic criteria for use in psychiatric research. Arch Gen Psychiatry 26:57–63, 1972

First MB, Gibbon RL, Spitzer RL, et al: Structured Clinical Interview for DSM-IV Axis II Personality Disorders, (SCID-II). Washington, DC, American Psychiatric Press, 1997

Garb H: Incremental validity and the assessment of psychopathology in adults. Psychol Assess 15:508–520, 2003

Gunderson JG, Kolb JE, Austin V: The Diagnostic Interview for Borderline Patients (DIB). Am J Psychiatry 138:896–903, 1981

Gunderson JG, Ronningstam E, Bodkin A: The Diagnostic Interview for Narcissistic Patients. Arch Gen Psychiatry 47:676–680, 1990

Gunderson JG, Shea MT, Skodol AE, et al: The collaborative longitudinal personality disorders study: development, aims, design, and sample characteristics. J Personal Disord 14:300–315, 2000

Hare RD: The Hare Psychopathy Checklist–Revised Manual. North Tonawanda, NY, Multi-Health Systems, 1991

Harkness AR, McNulty JL, Ben-Porath YS: The Personality Psychopathology Five (PSY-5): constructs and MMPI-2 scales. Psychol Assess 7:104–114, 1995

Helzer JE, Robins LN, Croughan JL, et al: Renard Diagnostic Interview: its reliability and procedural validity with physicians and lay interviewers. Arch Gen Psychiatry 38:393–398, 1981

Hilsenroth MJ, Handler L, Blais MA: Assessment of Narcissistic Personality Disorder: a multi-method review. Clin Psychol Rev 16:655–683, 1996

Hirshfeld RMA, Klerman GL, Clayton PJ, et al: Assessing personality: effects of the depressive state on trait measurement. Am J Psychiatry 140:695–699, 1983

Horowitz LM, Alden LE, Wiggins JS, et al: Inventory of Interpersonal Problems: IIP-64. San Antonio, TX, Harcourt Assessment, 2000

Hunt C, Andrews G: Measuring personality disorder: the use of self-report questionnaires. J Personal Disord 6:125–133, 1992

Hyler SE: Personality Diagnostic Questionnaire-4 (PDQ-4). New York, New York State Psychiatric Institute, 1994

Kaye A, Shea MT: Personality disorders, personality traits, and defense mechanisms, in Handbook of Psychiatric Measures. Edited by Pincus HA, Rush AJ, First MB, et al. Washington, DC, American Psychiatric Association, 2000, pp 713–749

Klein MH, Benjamin LS, Rosenfeld R, et al: The Wisconsin Personality Disorders Inventory: development, reliability, and validity. J Personal Disord 7:285–303, 1993

Leary T: Interpersonal Diagnosis of Personality: A Functional Theory and Methodology for Personality Evaluation. New York, Ronald Press, 1957

Lilienfield SO, Andrews BP: Development and preliminary validation of a self-report measure of psychopathic personality traits in noncriminal populations. J Pers Assess 60:488–524, 1996

Livesley WJ, Jackson DN: Dimensional Assessment of Personality Problems—Basic Questionnaire. Port Huron, MI, Sigma Assessment Systems (in press)

Loranger AW: International Personality Disorders Examination Manual. Odessa, FL, Psychological Assessment Resources, 1999

Loranger AW, Sartorius N, Andreoli A, et al: The International Personality Disorder Examination: The World Health Organization/Alcohol, Drug Abuse, and Mental Health Administration International Pilot Study of Personality Disorders. Arch Gen Psychiatry 51:215–224, 1994

McDermut W, Zimmerman M: The effect of personality disorders on outcome in the treatment of depression, in Mood and Anxiety Disorders. Edited by Rush AJ. Philadelphia, PA, Current Science, 1997, pp 321–338

Millon T, Davis R, Millon C: Manual for the MCMI-III. Minneapolis, MN, National Computer Systems, 1997

Morey LC: Personality Assessment Inventory Professional Manual. Odessa, FL, Psychological Assessment Resources, 1991

Morey LC, Waugh MH, Blashfield RK: MMPI scales for DSM-III personality disorders: their derivation and correlates. J Pers Assess 49:245–251, 1985

Pfohl B, Blum N, Zimmerman M: Structured Interview for DSM-IV Personality. Washington, DC, American Psychiatric Press, 1997

Piersma HL: The MCMI-II as a treatment outcome measure for psychiatric inpatients. J Clin Psychol 45:87–93, 1989

Pilkonis PA, Heape CL, Ruddy J, et al: Validity in the diagnosis of personality disorders: the use of the LEAD standard. Psychol Assess 3:46–54, 1991

Raine A: The SPQ: a scale for the assessment of schizotypal personality based on DSM-III-R criteria. Schizophr Bull 17:555–564, 1991

Raine A, Benishay D: The SPQ-B: a brief screening instrument for schizotypal personality disorder. J Personal Disord 9:346–355, 1995

Raskin RN, Terry H: A principal-components analysis of the narcissistic personality inventory and further evidence of its construct validity. J Pers Soc Psychol 54:890–902, 1988

Regier DA, Myers JK, Kramer M, et al: The NIMH Epidemiologic Catchment Area (ECA) program: historical context, major objectives, and study population characteristics. Arch Gen Psychiatry 41:934–941, 1984

Ricciardi JN, Baer L, Janice MA, et al: Changes in DSM-III-R Axis II diagnoses following treatment of obsessive-compulsive disorder. Am J Psychiatry 149:829–831, 1992

Riso LN, Klein DN, Anderson RL, et al: Concordance between patients and informants on the Personality Disorder Examination. Am J Psychiatry 151:568–573, 1994

Robins LN, Helzer JE, Croughan J, et al: The National Institute of Mental Health Diagnostic Interview Schedule: its history, characteristics, and validity. Arch Gen Psychiatry 42:381–389, 1981

Robins LN, Wing J, Wittchen HU: The Composite International Diagnostic Interview: an epidemiologic Instrument suitable for use in conjunction with different diagnostic systems and in different cultures. Arch Gen Psychiatry 12:1069–1077, 1988

Rogers R: Standardizing DSM-IV diagnoses: the clinical applications of structured interviews. J Pers Assess 81:220–225, 2003

Shea MT, Pilkonis PA, Beckham PA, et al: Personality disorders and treatment outcome in the NIMH Treatment of Depression: Collaborative Research Program. Am J Psychiatry 147:711–718, 1990

Sullivan HS: The Interpersonal Theory of Psychiatry. New York, WW Norton, 1953

Trull TJ, Widiger TA: Structured Interview for the Five-Factor Model of Personality. Odessa, FL, Psychological Assessment Resources, 1997

Tyrer P: Personality Disorders: Diagnosis, Management and Course. London, Wright, 1988

Westen D: Divergences between clinical research methods for assessing personality disorders: implications for research and the evolution of Axis II. Am J Psychiatry 154:895–903, 1997

Westen D, Shedler J: Refining the measurement of Axis II: a Q-sort procedure for assessing personality pathology. Assessment 5:333–353, 1998

Widiger TA: The DSM-III-R categorical personality disorder diagnoses: a critique and an alternative. Psychol Inq 4:75–90, 1993

Widiger TA: Personality disorders, in Handbook of Assessment and Treatment Planning for Psychological Disorders. Edited by Antony MM, Barlow DH. New York, Guilford, 2002, pp 453–480

Widiger TA, Coker LA: Assessing personality disorders, in Clinical Personality Assessment: Practical Approaches, 2nd Edition. Edited by Butcher JN. New York, Oxford University Press, 2002, pp 380–394

Widiger TA, Spitzer RL: Sex bias in the diagnosis of personality disorders: conceptual and methodological issues. Clin Psychol Rev 11:1–22, 1991

Widiger TA, Mangine S, Corbitt EM, et al: Personality Disorder Interview–IV: A Semi-Structured Interview for the Assessment of Personality Disorders, Professional Manual. Odessa, FL, Psychological Assessment Resources, 1995

World Health Organization: The ICD-10 Classification of Mental and Behavioural Disorders: Clinical Descriptions and Diagnostic Guidelines. Geneva, Switzerland, World Health Organization, 1992

Yang J, McCrae RR, Costa PT, et al: The cross-cultural generalizability of Axis-II constructs: an evaluation of two personality disorder assessment instruments in the People's Republic of China. J Personal Disord 14:249–263, 2000

Zanarini MC, Gunderson JG, Frankenburg FR, et al: The Revised Diagnostic Interview for Borderlines: discriminating borderline personality disorder from other Axis II disorders. J Personal Disord 3:10–18, 1989

Zanarini MC, Frankenburg FR, Sickel AE, et al: Diagnostic Interview for DSM-IV Personality Disorders. Boston, MA, Laboratory for the Study of Adult Development, McLean Hospital, and the Department of Psychiatry, Harvard University, 1996

Zimmerman M: Diagnosing personality disorders: a review of issues and research methods. Arch Gen Psychiatry 51:225–245, 1994

Zimmerman M, Mattia JI: Differences between clinical and research practices in diagnosing borderline personality disorder. Am J Psychiatry 156:1570–1574, 1999a

Zimmerman M, Mattia JI: Psychiatric diagnosis in clinical practice: is comorbidity being missed? Compr Psychiatry 40:182–191, 1999b

Zimmerman M, Coryell W, Black DW: A method to detect intercenter differences in the application of contemporary diagnostic criteria. J Nerv Ment Dis 181:130–134, 1993

6

Course and Outcome of Personality Disorders

Carlos M. Grilo, Ph.D.
Thomas H. McGlashan, M.D.

A *personality disorder* is defined in DSM-IV-TR (American Psychiatric Association 2000) as "an enduring pattern of inner experience and behavior that deviates markedly from the expectations of the individual's culture, is pervasive and inflexible, has an onset in adolescence or early adulthood, is stable over time, and leads to distress or impairment" (p. 685). The diagnostic construct of personality disorder has evolved considerably over the past few decades (see Skodol 1997 for a detailed ontogeny of the DSM system; and see Chapter 1, "Personality Disorders: Recent History and Future Directions," for a historical overview). Substantial changes have occurred in both the number and types of specific personality disorder diagnoses over time, as well as in the "admixture of criteria" (Sanislow and McGlashan 1998) representing possible manifestations of personality disorders (i.e., DSM-IV-TR specifies that the "enduring pattern" can be manifested by problems in at least two of the following areas: cognition, affectivity, interpersonal functioning, or impulse control). One central tenet—that a personality disorder reflects a persistent, pervasive, enduring, and stable pattern—has not

changed. The concept of stability is salient in both major classification systems, DSM-IV-TR and ICD-10 (World Health Organization 1992), although the two systems differ somewhat in their classification and definitions for personality disorders and thus demonstrate only moderate convergence for some diagnoses (Ottosson et al. 2002). The extent of stability of personality disorders remains uncertain (Shea and Yen 2003; Tyrer and Simonsen 2003). This chapter provides an overview of the course and outcome of personality disorders and synthesizes the empirical literature on the stability of personality disorders.

STABILITY AS THE CENTRAL TENET OF PERSONALITY DISORDERS

The concept of stability has remained a central tenet of personality disorders throughout the various editions of DSM, dating back to the first edition, published in 1952. In what some experts have referred to as a "bold step" (Tyrer and Simonsen 2003), personality disorders were placed on a separate Axis (Axis II) of the multiaxial DSM-III (American Psychiatric Association 1980), published in 1980. DSM-III stated that the separation to Axis II was intended, in part, to encourage clinicians to assess "the possible presence of disorders that are frequently overlooked when attention is directed to the usually more florid Axis I disorder." Conceptually, this separation reflected the putative stability of personality disorders relative to the episodically unstable course of Axis I psychiatric disorders (Grilo et al. 1998; Skodol 1997).

FIRST- AND SECOND-GENERATION RESEARCH STUDIES ON STABILITY

First, we provide a brief review of the empirical literature through the end of the twentieth century. This period can be thought of as including the first generation (mostly clinical-descriptive accounts) and the second generation (the emerging findings based on attempts at greater standardization of diagnoses and assessment methods) of research efforts on personality disorders. Second, we provide a brief overview of methodological problems and conceptual gaps that characterize this literature and that must be considered when interpreting ongoing research and designing future studies. Third, we summarize emerging findings from ongoing longitudinal studies that have shed light on a number of key issues about the course of personality disorders.

OVERVIEW OF THE LITERATURE THROUGH 1999

A number of previous reviews have been published addressing aspects of the course and outcome of personality disorders (Grilo and McGlashan 1999; Grilo et al. 1998; McDavid and Pilkonis 1996; Perry 1993; Ruegg and Frances 1995; Stone 1993; Zimmerman 1994). These reviews, although varied, have agreed on the pervasiveness of methodological problems that characterize much of the literature and thereby preclude any firm conclusions regarding the nature of the stability of personality disorders. The reviews, however, have also generally agreed that available research raises questions regarding many aspects of the construct validity of personality disorders (Zimmerman 1994), including their hypothesized high degree of stability (Grilo and McGlashan 1999).

The few early (pre-DSM-III era) studies of the course of personality disorders reported findings that borderline (Carpenter and Gunderson 1977; Grinker et al. 1968) and antisocial (Maddocks 1970; Robins et al. 1977) personality disorders were highly stable. Carpenter and Gunderson (1977), for example, reported that the impairment in functioning observed for borderline personality disorder (BPD) was comparable with that observed for patients with schizophrenia over a 5-year period. As previously noted (Grilo et al. 1998), the dominant clinical approach to assessing personality disorder diagnoses based partly on treatment refractoriness naturally raises the question of whether these findings simply reflect a tautology.

The separation of personality disorders to Axis II in DSM-III contributed to increased research attention to these clinical problems (Blashfield and McElroy 1987). The development and utilization of a number of structured and standardized approaches to clinical interviewing and diagnosis during the 1980s represented notable advances (Zimmerman 1994). The greater attention paid to defining the criteria required for diagnosis in the classification systems and by researchers during the development of standardized interviews greatly facilitated research efforts in this field.

In our previous reviews of the DSM-III and DSM-III-R (American Psychiatric Association 1987) studies, we concluded that the available research suggested that "personality disorders demonstrate only moderate stability and that, although personality disorders are generally associated with negative outcomes, they can improve over time and can benefit from specific treatments" (Grilo and McGlashan 1999, p. 157). In our 1998 review (Grilo et al. 1998), we noted that the 20 selected studies of DSM-III-R criteria generally found low to moderate stability of any personality disorder over relatively short follow-up periods (6 to 24 months). For example, the major studies that employed diagnostic interviews reported kappa coefficients for the presence of any personality disorder of 0.32 (Johnson et al. 1997), 0.40 (Ferro et al. 1998), 0.50 (Loranger et al. 1994), and 0.55 (Loranger et al. 1991). Especially noteworthy is that the stability coefficients for specific personality disorder diagnoses (in the few cases in which they could be calculated given the sample sizes) were generally lower. In addition, follow-up studies of adolescents diagnosed with personality disorders also reported modest stability; for example, Mattanah et al. (1995) reported a 50% rate of stability for any personality disorder at 2-year follow-up. More recently, Grilo and colleagues (2001) also found modest stability in dimensional personality disorder scores in this adolescent follow-up study. Squires-Wheeler et al. (1992), as part of the New York State High-Risk Offspring Study, reported low stability for schizotypal personality disorder and features, although the stability was higher for the offspring of patients with schizophrenia than for those with mood disorders or control subjects.

Subsequently, we (Grilo and McGlashan 1999) reviewed nine reports of longitudinal findings for personality disorder diagnoses published in 1997 and 1998. In terms of specific diagnoses, the studies generally reported moderate stability (kappa approximately 0.5) for BPD and antisocial personality disorder (ASPD). These reports, like most of the previous literature, had small sample sizes and infrequently followed more than one personality disorder.

CONCEPTUAL AND METHODOLOGICAL QUESTIONS ABOUT COURSE

Previous reviews of personality disorders have raised many methodological problems. Common limitations highlighted include small sample sizes; concerns about nonstandardized assessments, interrater reliability, blindness to baseline characteristics, and narrow assessments; failure to consider alternative (e.g., dimensional) models of personality disorder; reliance on only two assessments typically over short follow-up periods; insufficient attention to the nature and effects of co-occurring Axis I and Axis II diagnoses; and inattention to treatment effects. Diagnoses other than ASPD and BPD have received little attention. Particularly striking is the absence of "relevant" comparison or control groups in the longitudinal literature. We comment briefly on a few of these issues.

Reliability

Reliability of assessments represents a central issue for any study of course and outcome. The creation of standardized instruments for collecting data was a major development of the 1980s (Loranger et al. 1991; Zimmerman 1994). Such instruments, however, were less-than-perfect assessment methods and have been criticized for a variety of reasons (Westen 1997; Westen and Shedler 1999). It is critical to keep in mind that interrater reliability and test–retest reliability represent the limits (or ceiling) for estimating the stability of a construct.

Previous reviews (Grilo and McGlashan 1999; Zanarini et al. 2000; Zimmerman 1994) of reliabilities for Axis II diagnostic interviews have generally reported median interrater reliabilities of roughly 0.70 and short-interval test–retest reliabilities of 0.50 for diagnoses. These reliabilities compare favorably with those generally reported for diagnostic instruments for Axis I psychiatric disorders. Both interrater and test–retest reliability coefficients tend to be higher for dimensional scores than for categorical diagnoses of personality disorders. Another finding of note is that even when experts administer diagnostic interviews, the degree of convergence or agreement produced by two different interviews administered only 1 week apart is limited (Oldham et al. 1992).

Reliability and "Change"

Test–retest reliability is also relevant for addressing, in part, the well-known problem of "regression to the mean" in repeated measures studies (Nesselroade et al. 1980). It has been argued that the multiwave or repeated measures approach lessens the effects of regression to the mean (Lenzenweger 1999). This argument may be true in terms of the obvious decreases in severity with time (i.e., very symptomatic participants meeting eligibility at study entry are likely to show some improvement because, by definition, they are already reporting high levels of symptoms). However, other effects need to be considered whenever assessments are repeated within a study. As cogently noted by Shea and Yen (2003), repeated measures studies of both Axis II (Loranger et al. 1991) and Axis I (Robins 1985) disorders have found hints that participants systematically report or endorse fewer problems during repeated interviews to reduce interview time. For example, Loranger et al. (1991), in his test–retest study of the Personality Disorder Examination interview (Loranger 1988) conducted between 1 and 26 weeks after baseline, documented significant decreases in personality disorder criteria for all but two of the DSM-III-R diagnoses. Recall that the Personality Disorder Examination, which requires skilled and trained research clinicians, has a required minimum duration stipulation of 5 years for determining persistence and pervasiveness of the criteria being assessed. Thus, the magnitude of changes observed during such a short period of time, which was shown to be unrelated to "state-trait effects," reflects some combination of the following: regression to the mean, error in either or both the baseline and repeated assessments, and overreporting by patients at hospital admission and underreporting during retest at discharge (Loranger et al. 1991; Shea and Yen 2003). These phenomena were discussed further by Gunderson and colleagues (2000).

Categorical Versus Dimensional Approaches

Long-standing debate regarding the conceptual and empirical advantages to dimensional models of personality disorders (Frances 1982; Livesley et al. 1992; Loranger et al. 1994; Widiger 1992) has accompanied the DSM categorical classification system. In Chapter 3, "Categorical and Dimensional Models of Personality Disorders," Widiger and Mullins-Sweatt address this issue. We comment only briefly on the literature that applies specifically to the issue of course of personality disorders. Overall, longitudinal studies of personality disorder have reported moderate levels of stability for dimensional scores for most personality disorders, with the stability coefficients tending to be higher than for categorical or diagnostic stability (Ferro et al. 1998; Johnson et al. 1997; Klein and Shih 1998; Loranger et al. 1991, 1994).

Comorbidity

Most studies have ascertained participants who meet criteria for multiple Axis I and Axis II diagnoses. This problem of diagnostic overlap, or comorbidity, represents a well-known, long-standing major challenge (Berkson 1946) in working with clinical samples. One expert and critic of DSM (Tyrer 2001), in speaking of the "spectre of comorbidity," noted that "the main reason for abandoning the present classification is summed up in one word, comorbidity. Comorbidity is the nosologist's nightmare; it shouts, 'you have failed'" (p. 82). We suggest, however, that such clinical realities (multiple presenting problems that are especially characteristic of treatment-seeking patients) represent not only potential confounds but also potential opportunities to understand personality and dysfunctions of personality better. Comorbidity begs the question: what are the fundamental personality dimensions and disorders of personality, and how do their courses influence (and conversely, how are their courses affected by) the presence and course of Axis I psychiatric disorders?

Continuity

A related issue pertaining to course concerns "longitudinal comorbidities" (Kendell and Clarkin 1992) or "continuities." An obvious example is that conduct disorder during adolescence is required for the diagnosis of ASPD to be given to adults. This definitional isomorphism is one likely reason for the consistently strong associations between conduct disorder and later ASPD in the literature. This association is, how-ever, more than an artifactual relationship, because longitudinal research has clearly documented that children and adolescents with behavior disorders have substantially elevated risk for antisocial behavior during adulthood (Robins 1966). More generally, studies with diverse recruitment and ascertainment methods reported that disruptive behavior disorders during the adolescent years prospectively predicted personality disorders during young adulthood (Bernstein et al. 1996; Lewinsohn et al. 1997; Myers et al. 1998; Rey et al. 1995). The Yale Psychiatric Institute follow-up study found that personality disorder diagnoses in adolescent inpatients prospectively predicted greater drug use problems but not global functioning (Levy et al. 1999).

The importance of considering comorbidity is underscored in the findings of the longitudinal study by Lewinsohn et al. (1997). They found that the apparent longitudinal continuity noted for disruptive behavioral disorders during adolescence and subsequent ASPD in adulthood was accounted for, in part, by Axis I psychiatric comorbidity. A longitudinal study of young adult men found that personality disorders predicted the subsequent onset of psychiatric disorders during a 2-year follow-up, even after controlling for previous psychiatric history (Johnson et al. 1997).

Comorbidity and Continuity Models

A variation of the comorbidity concept is that certain disorders may be associated with one another in a number of possible ways over time. A variety of models have been proposed for the possible relationships between Axis II and Axis I disorders (Dolan-Sewell et al. 2001; Lyons et al. 1997; Tyrer et al. 1997). These include, for example, the predisposition or vulnerability model, the complication or scar model, the pathoplasty or exacerbation model, and various spectrum models. We emphasize that these models do not necessarily assume categorical entities. Indeed, an especially influential spectrum model proposed by Siever and Davis (1991) posits four psychobiological dimensions to account for Axis II and Axis I psychopathology. The Cloninger et al. (1993) psychobiological model of temperament and character represents another valuable approach that considers dimensions across personality and psychopathology. More broadly, Krueger (Krueger 1999; Krueger and Tackett 2003) noted that although most research has focused on pairs of constructs (i.e., Axis II and Axis I associations), it seems important to examine the "multivariate structure of the personality-psychopathology domain" (p. 109).

Age (Early Onset)

A related point, stressed by Widiger (2003), is that personality disorders need to be more clearly conceptualized and carefully characterized as having an early onset. However, the validity of personality disorders in adolescents remains controversial (Krueger and Carlson 2001). It can be argued, for example, that determining early onset of personality disorders is impossible because adolescence is a period of profound changes and flux in personality and identity. A recent critical review of the longitudinal literature on personality traits throughout the lifespan revealed that personality traits are less stable during childhood and adolescence than they are throughout adulthood (Roberts and DelVecchio 2000). Roberts and DelVecchio's (2000) meta-analysis of data from 152 longitudinal studies of personality traits revealed that rank-order consistency for personality traits increased steadily throughout the lifespan; test–retest correlations (over 6.7-year time intervals) increased from 0.31 (during childhood) to 0.54 (during college), to 0.64 (age 30), to a high of 0.74 (ages 50–70).

Nonetheless, if childhood precursors of personality disorders could be identified (as in the case of conduct disorder for ASPD), they could become part of the diagnostic criteria and thus create some degree of longitudinal continuity in the diagnostic system. Myers et al. (1998), for example, found that early onset (before 10 years of age) of conduct disorder problems predicted subsequent ASPD. More generally, temperamental vulnerabilities or precursors to personality disorders have been posited as central in a variety of models of personality disorders (Cloninger et al. 1993; Siever and Davis 1991). Specific temperamental features evident in childhood have been noted to be precursors for diverse personality disorders (Paris 2003; Rettew et al. 2003; Wolff et al. 1991) as well as for differences in interpersonal functioning (Newman et al. 1997) in adulthood. For example, studies have noted early odd and withdrawn patterns for schizotypal personality disorder in adults (Wolff et al. 1991) and shyness for avoidant personality disorder (Rettew et al. 2003). Speaking more generally, although the degree of stability for personality traits is higher throughout adulthood than throughout childhood and adolescence (Roberts and DelVecchio 2000), longitudinal analyses of personality data have revealed that the transition from adolescence to adulthood is characterized by greater personality continuity than change (Roberts et al. 2001).

Age and the Aging Process

Another age issue concerns the aging process itself. Considerable research suggests that personality remains relatively stable thorough adulthood (Heatherton and Weinberger 1994; Roberts and DelVecchio 2000) and is highly stable after age 50 (Roberts and DelVecchio 2000). Little is known, however, about personality disorders in older persons (Abrams et al. 1998). The recent 12-year follow-up of personality disorders as part of the Nottingham Study of Neurotic Disorders (Seivewright et al. 2002) documented substantial changes in personality disorder trait scores based on blind administration of a semistructured interview. Seivewright and colleagues (2002) reported that Cluster B personality disorder diagnoses (ASPD, histrionic) showed significant improvements, whereas Cluster A and Cluster C diagnoses appeared to worsen with age. Although the Seivewright et al. (2002) findings are limited somewhat by the two-point cross-sectional assessment (little is known about the intervening period), Tyrer and colleagues (1983) previously reported good reliability (weighted kappa of 0.64) for this diagnostic interview over a 3-year test–retest period. These findings echo somewhat the results of the seminal Chestnut Lodge follow-up studies (McGlashan 1986a, 1986b) that suggested distinctions between BPD and schizotypal personality disorders, decreases in impulsivity and interpersonal instability with age, and increased avoidance with age. There are other reports of diminished impulsivity with increasing age in BPD (Paris and Zweig-Frank 2001; Stevensen et al. 2003), although this type of reduction was not observed in a recent prospective analysis of individual BPD criteria (McGlashan et al. in press).

The reader is referred to Judd and McGlashan (2003) for detailed accounts of four specific cases that elucidate the course and outcome of BPD. These detailed case studies, based on rich clinical material available through the Chestnut Lodge Study, demonstrate the considerable heterogeneity in the course of BPD.

Summary and Implications

To resolve these complex issues, complementary research efforts are required, with large samples of both clinical and community populations. It is clear that prospective longitudinal studies with repeated assessments over time are needed to understand the course of personality disorders. Such studies must consider (and cut across) different developmental eras, broad domains of functioning, and multimodal approaches to personality and disorders of personality. These approaches have, in fact, been performed with personality traits (Roberts et al. 2001) and with other forms of psychiatric problems and have yielded invaluable insights. Notable are the contributions of the National Institutes of Health (NIH)–funded multisite efforts on depression (Collaborative Depression Study; Katz et al. 1979) and anxiety (Harvard/Brown Anxiety Research Program; Keller 1991).

REVIEW OF RECENT EMPIRICAL ADVANCES AND UNDERSTANDING OF STABILITY

Of particular relevance for this review are three prospective studies on the longitudinal course of adult personality disorders funded by the NIH during the 1990s. These studies included the Longitudinal Study of Personality Disorders (Lenzenweger 1999), the McLean Study of Adult Development (Zanarini et al. 2003), and the multisite Collaborative Longitudinal Personality Disorders Study (CLPS; Gunderson et al. 2000). NIH also funded a community-based prospective longitudinal study of personality, psychopathology, and functioning of children/adolescents and their mothers (Children in the Community Study; Brook et al. 2002) that began in 1983. These four studies are especially noteworthy in that they, to varying degrees, partly correct for a number of the conceptual and methodological issues noted earlier. These studies utilized multiple and standardized assessment methods, carefully considered training and reliability, and—perhaps most notably—multiwave repeated assessments that are essential for determining longitudinal change. They have employed, to varying degrees, multiple assessment methods and have considered personality and its disorders (personality disorders) as well as Axis I psychiatric disorders. Collectively, these studies have provided valuable insights into the complexities of personality (traits and disorders) and its vicissitudes over time.

Longitudinal Study of Personality Disorders

The Longitudinal Study of Personality Disorders (Lenzenweger 1999; Lenzenweger et al. 1997) assessed 250 participants drawn from Cornell University at three points over a 4-year period. It utilized a semistructured diagnostic interview (International Personality Disorders Examination; Loranger et al. 1994) and a self-report measure (Millon Clinical Multiaxial Inventory–II) to obtain complementary information on personality. Of the 250 participants, 129 met criteria for at least one personality disorder and 121 did not meet any personality disorder diagnosis. Dimensional scores for the personality disorders were characterized by significant levels of stability on both the interview and self-report measures. Stability coefficients for the total number of personality disorder features ranged from 0.61 to 0.70. Cluster B personality disorders had the highest stability coefficients and Cluster A personality disorders had the lowest. Personality disorder dimensions showed significant declines over time, and the decline was more rapid for the personality disorder group than for the nondisordered group. Axis I psychiatric disorders (diagnosed in 63% of personality disorder subjects and 26% of non–personality disorder subjects) did not significantly influence changes in personality disorder dimensions over time.

The Longitudinal Study of Personality Disorders (Lenzenweger 1999) BPD findings are generally consistent (although the three-point assessment is an important incremental contribution) with those previously reported by Trull and colleagues (1997, 1998) in a prospective study of BPD features using two different assessment instruments administered to a college student sample assessed twice over a 2-year period.

The Longitudinal Study of Personality Disorders (Lenzenweger 1999), however, is limited by its relatively homogeneous study group of college students, its narrow developmental time frame, and most importantly the insufficient frequency of any personality disorder diagnosis at a categorical (diagnostic) level to allow analysis of a clinical entity. Lenzenweger (1999) noted the need for repeated-measure longitudinal data from clinically based personality disorder samples to address the question of the course and stability of dysfunctions of personality.

McLean Study of Adult Development

The McLean Study of Adult Development (Zanarini et al. 2003) is an ongoing prospective, longitudinal study comparing the course and outcome of hospitalized patients with BPD with those of patients with other personality disorders. It utilizes repeated assessments performed every 2 years (Zanarini et al. 2003). Zanarini et al. (2003) assessed personality disorders in 362 inpatients (290 with BPD and 72 with other personality disorders) using two semistructured diagnostic interviews and administered assessments to characterize Axis I psychiatric disorders, psychosocial functioning domains, and treatment utilization. Of the patients diagnosed with BPD, remission was observed for 35% by year 2, 49% by year 4, and 74% by year 6. Recurrences were rare and were reported for only 6% of those patients who achieved a remission. The authors concluded that "symptomatic improvement is both common and stable, even among the most disturbed borderline patients, and that the symptomatic prognosis for most, but not all, severely ill borderline patients is better than previously recognized" (p. 274).

Collaborative Longitudinal Personality Disorders Study

The Collaborative Longitudinal Personality Disorders Study (CLPS; Gunderson et al. 2000; McGlashan et al. 2000) is an ongoing prospective, longitudinal, repeated measures study designed to examine the course and outcome of patients meeting DSM-IV (American Psychiatric Association 1994) criteria for one of four personality disorders: schizotypal, borderline, avoidant, and obsessive-compulsive. CLPS includes a comparison group of patients with major depressive disorder (MDD) without any personality disorder. This comparison group was selected because of its episodic and fluctuating course (thought to distinguish Axis I from Axis II) and because MDD has been carefully studied in similar longitudinal designs (e.g., Collaborative Depression Study; Katz et al. 1979; Solomon et al. 1997). CLPS has employed multimodal assessments (Gunderson et al. 2000; Zanarini et al. 2000) to prospectively follow and capture different aspects of the fluctuating nature of personality disorders and dimensions (both interviewer-based and self-report representing different conceptual models), Axis I psychiatric disorders and symptoms, various domains of psychosocial functioning, and treatment utilization.

To date, the CLPS has reported on different concepts of categorical and dimensional stability of four personality disorders over 12 months (Shea et al. 2002) and 24 months (Grilo et al. 2004) using prospective data obtained for 668 patients recruited from diverse settings at four universities. Based on the traditional test–retest approach, blind repeated administration of a semistructured interview conducted 24 months after baseline revealed "remission" rates (based solely on falling below DSM-IV diagnostic thresholds) ranging from 50% (avoidant personality disorder) to 61% (schizotypal personality disorder). Grilo et al. (2004) applied lifetable survival analyses to prospective data

obtained using an assessment methodology modeled after the Collaborative Depression Study (Keller et al. 1982) and the Longitudinal Interval Follow-Up Evaluation (Keller et al. 1987) methodology. These findings are summarized in Figures 6–1 and 6–2.

Figure 6–1 shows the times to remission for the four personality disorder groups and for the MDD comparison group, which were calculated based on parallel definitions of two consecutive months with minimal symptoms (Grilo et al. 2004). As can be seen, the MDD group had a significantly higher remission rate than the personality disorder groups. This study represents the first empirical demonstration of the central tenet that personality disorders are characterized by greater degree of stability than the hypothesized episodic course of Axis I psychiatric disorders (Grilo et al. 1998; Shea and Yen 2003.

The reader is referred to Shea and Yen (2003) for a broader discussion of this issue. These researchers, who have played roles in the CLPS as well as the longitudinal studies of depression (Collaborative Depression Study) and anxiety (Harvard/Brown Anxiety Research Program), provide an overview of the central findings that pertain to the issue of stability as a distinction between Axis II and Axis I diagnoses (Shea and Yen 2003). Briefly, comparison across the studies (which can be done given the parallel assessment instrumentation) reveals that personality disorders demonstrate greater stability than Axis I mood and anxiety disorders (as hypothesized) but show less diagnostic (categorical) stability than conceptualized. Perhaps noteworthy is that the longitudinal studies for both mood and anxiety disorders documented much greater chronicity (much lower remission rates) than previously known.

Returning to the CLPS findings (Grilo et al. 2004), Figure 6–1 reveals that although personality disorders were more stable than MDD, a substantial number of "remissions" occurred during the 24 months of follow-up. Using the arbitrarily selected 2-month definition (2 months with two or fewer criteria) adopted from the MDD field (Keller et al. 1982; Solomon et al. 1997), remission rates range from 33% (schizotypal personality disorder) to 55% (obsessive-compulsive personality disorder). Figure 6–2 shows the comparable remission rates if a very stringent definition of 12 consecutive months with two or fewer criteria is adopted. As can be seen, the remission rates using the 12-month definition range from 23% (schizotypal personality disorder) to 38% (obsessive-compulsive personality disorder). Grilo et al. (2004) concluded that these four personality disorders show substantial im-

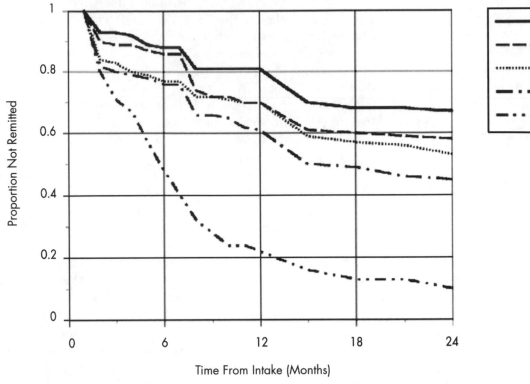
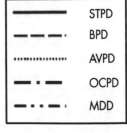

Figure 6–1.   Time to remission using a 2-month criterion.

AVPD=avoidant personality disorder; BPD=borderline personality disorder; MDD=major depressive disorder; OCPD=obsessive-compulsive personality disorder; STPD=schizotypal personality disorder.

Source.   Grilo et al. 2004. Copyright © 2004 by the American Psychological Association. Reprinted with permission.

provements in symptomatology over a 2-year period even when a stringent definition is used.

The CLPS also provided complementary analyses using dimensional approaches for 12-month (Shea et al. 2002) and 24-month (Grilo et al. 2004) follow-ups. Grilo et al. (2004) documented a significant decrease in the mean proportion of criteria met in each of the personality disorder groups over time, which is suggestive of decreased severity. However, when the relative stability of individual differences was examined across the multiwave assessments (baseline and 6-, 12-, and 24-month time points), a high level of consistency was observed as evidenced by correlation coefficients ranging from 0.53 to 0.67 for proportion of criteria met between baseline and 24 months. Grilo and colleagues (2004) concluded that patients with personality disorder are consistent in terms of their rank order of personality disorder criteria (i.e., that individual differences in personality disorder features are stable), although they may fluctuate in the severity or number of personality disorder features over time. It is worth noting that the range of the stability coefficients was

quite similar to that documented by the Longitudinal Study of Personality Disorders (Lenzenweger 1999) for a nonclinical sample.

In contrast to their symptomatic improvement, however, patients with personality disorders show less significant and more gradual improvement in their functioning, particularly in social relationships (Skodol et al. in press). In addition, depressed patients with personality disorders show longer time to remission from major depressive disorder (Grilo et al. in press). Because personality psychopathology usually begins in adolescence or early adulthood, the potential for delays in occupational and interpersonal development is great—and even after symptomatic improvement, it might take time to overcome deficits and make up the necessary ground to achieve "normal" functioning. Developmental issues for patients with personality disorders are discussed in more detail in Chapter 11, "Developmental Issues."

Several recent reports from the CLPS are also relevant here given the issue of longitudinal comorbidities and continuities. Shea and colleagues (2004) examined

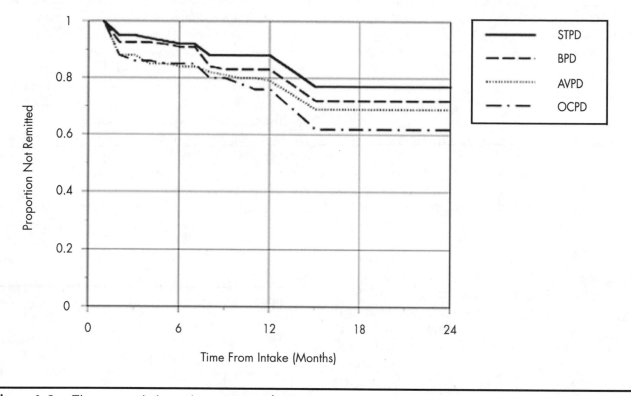

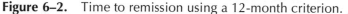

Figure 6–2. Time to remission using a 12-month criterion.

AVPD=avoidant personality disorder; BPD=borderline personality disorder; OCPD=obsessive-compulsive personality disorder; STPD=schizotypal personality disorder.

Source. Grilo et al. 2004. Copyright © 2004 by the American Psychological Association. Reprinted with permission.

the time-varying (longitudinal) associations between personality disorders and psychiatric disorders, in part guided by the Siever and Davis (1991) cross-cutting psychobiological dimension model. BPD demonstrated significant associations with certain psychiatric disorders (MDD and posttraumatic stress disorder), whereas avoidant personality disorder was significantly associated with two anxiety disorders (social phobia and obsessive-compulsive disorder). While these findings were consistent with predictions based on the Siever and Davis (1991) model, other personality disorders (schizotypal and obsessive-compulsive) did not demonstrate significant longitudinal associations. Gunderson et al. (2004) followed up on the Shea et al. (2004) findings regarding changes in BPD and MDD by performing a more fine-grained analysis of specific changes in the two disorders using 3 years of longitudinal data. Changes (improvements) in BPD severity preceded improvements in MDD but not vice versa (Gunderson et al. 2004).

Another recent report (Warner et al. 2004) examined whether personality traits are stable in patients with personality disorders and tested the hypothesis

that the stability of these personality disorders is due in part to the stability in these traits (Lyman and Widiger 2001). A series of latent longitudinal models tests whether changes in specific traits prospectively predicted changes in relevant personality disorders. Warner et al. (2004) documented significant cross-lagged relationships between changes in specific traits and subsequent (later) changes for schizotypal, borderline, and avoidant personality disorders but not for obsessive-compulsive personality disorder.

McGlashan and colleagues (in press) examined the individual criteria for schizotypal, borderline, avoidant, and obsessive-compulsive personality disorders and how they changed over a 2-year period. The individual criteria for these four personality disorders showed varied patterns of stability and change over time. Overall, within personality disorders, the relatively fixed (least changeable) criteria were generally more traitlike (and attitudinal), whereas the more fluctuating criteria were generally behavioral (or reactive). McGlashan and colleagues (in press) posited that perhaps personality disorders are hybrids of traits and symptomatic behaviors and that it is the interaction of these over time that helps to define the observable diagnostic stability. Collectively, along with the recent CLPS efforts, these findings suggest that personality disorder traits are stable over time and across developmental eras and may generate intra- and interpersonal conflicts that result in behaviors symptomatic of personality disorders (which are less stable over time).

Children in the Community Study

The Children in the Community Study (D.W. Brook et al. 2002; J.S. Brook et al. 1995) is an especially impressive longitudinal effort that has already provided a wealth of information about the course of personality and behavioral traits, psychiatric problems, substance abuse, and adversities. It is an ongoing prospective study of nearly 1,000 families with children aged 1 to 10 years originally recruited in1975 in New York State using a random sampling procedure. The study has employed repeated multimodal assessments and has followed over 700 participants since childhood and through the development eras of childhood, adolescence, and early adulthood. This landmark study has provided data that speaks to the critical issues of longitudinal comorbidities and continuities. In a series of papers, the collaborating researchers have documented important findings relevant to the issues raised in this review but especially to the critical issues of continuity of risk and functioning across developmental eras. These include documentation of the validity of certain forms of dramatic-erratic personality disorders in adolescents (Crawford et al. 2001a, 2001b); findings of age-related changes in personality disorder traits, including their moderate levels of stability throughout adolescence and early adulthood (Johnson et al. 2000b); and indications that early forms of behavioral disturbances predict personality disorders in adolescents and that personality disorders during adolescence, in addition to demonstrating significant levels of continuity into adulthood, also predict psychiatric disorders, suicidality, and violent and criminal behavior during young adulthood (Johnson et al. 2000a, 2000b). Collectively, these findings support the continuity and persistence of personality disturbances, although their development pathways are not yet understood.

SUMMARY

We have reviewed the literature regarding the course and stability of personality disorders. We once again conclude that personality disorders demonstrate only moderate stability and that they can improve over time. This conclusion is offered with less caution than during our previous reviews (Grilo and McGlashan 1999), given some notable advances in research. We also conclude that when personality disorders are considered dimensionally, the degree of stability is substantial. Emerging work has suggested that personality disorder traits, although deviant, are stable over time and across developmental eras and may generate intra- and interpersonal conflicts that result in personality disorder–symptomatic behaviors (which are less stable over time). Future research in personality disorders is necessary to dissect and understand this trait/state interaction and track its vicissitudes across time and circumstances.

REFERENCES

Abrams RC, Spielman LA, Alexopoulos GS, et al: Personality disorder symptoms and functioning in elderly depressed patients. Am J Geriatr Psychiatry 6:24–30, 1998

American Psychiatric Association: Diagnostic and Statistical Manual of Mental Disorders, 3rd Edition. Washington, DC, American Psychiatric Association, 1980

American Psychiatric Association: Diagnostic and Statistical Manual of Mental Disorders, 3rd Edition, Revised. Washington, DC, American Psychiatric Association, 1987

American Psychiatric Association: Diagnostic and Statistical Manual of Mental Disorders, 4th Edition. Washington, DC, American Psychiatric Association, 1994

American Psychiatric Association: Diagnostic and Statistical Manual of Mental Disorders, 4th Edition, Text Revision. Washington, DC, American Psychiatric Association, 2000

Berkson J: Limitations of the application of fourfold table analysis to hospital data. Biometrics Bulletin 2:47–53, 1946

Bernstein DP, Cohen P, Skodol AE, et al: Childhood antecedents of adolescent personality disorders. Am J Psychiatry 153:907–913, 1996

Blashfield RK, McElroy RA: The 1985 journal literature on the personality disorders. Compr Psychiatry 28:536–546, 1987

Brook DW, Brook JS, Zhang C, et al: Drug use and the risk of major depressive disorder, alcohol dependence, and substance use disorders. Arch Gen Psychiatry 59:1039–1044, 2002

Brook JS, Whiteman M, Cohen P, et al: Longitudinally predicting late adolescent and young adult drug use: childhood and adolescent precursors. J Am Acad Child Adolesc Psychiatry 34:1230–1238, 1995

Carpenter WT, Gunderson JG: Five year follow-up comparison of borderline and schizophrenic patients. Compr Psychiatry 18:567–571, 1977

Cloninger CR, Svrakic DM, Przybeck TR: A psychobiological model of temperament and character. Arch Gen Psychiatry 50:975–990, 1993

Crawford TN, Cohen P, Brook JS: Dramatic-erratic personality disorder symptoms, I: continuity from early adolescence into adulthood. J Personal Disord 15:319–335, 2001a

Crawford TN, Cohen P, Brook JS: Dramatic-erratic personality disorder symptoms, II: developmental pathways from early adolescence to adulthood. J Personal Disord 15:336–350, 2001b

Dolan-Sewell RT, Krueger RF, Shea MT: Co-occurrence with syndrome disorders, in Handbook of Personality Disorders. Edited by Livesley WJ. New York, Guilford, 2001, pp 84–104

Ferro T, Klein DN, Schwartz JE, et al: 30-month stability of personality disorder diagnoses in depressed outpatients. Am J Psychiatry 155:653–659, 1998

Frances A: Categorical and dimensional systems of personality diagnosis: a comparison. Compr Psychiatry 23:516–527, 1982

Grilo CM, McGlashan TH: Stability and course of personality disorders. Curr Opin Psychiatry 12:157–162, 1999

Grilo CM, McGlashan TH, Oldham JM: Course and stability of personality disorders. J Pract Psychiatry Behav Health 4:61–75, 1998

Grilo CM, Becker DF, Edell WS, et al: Stability and change of personality disorder dimensions in adolescents followed up two years after psychiatric hospitalization. Compr Psychiatry 42:364–368, 2001

Grilo CM, Shea MT, Sanislow CA, et al: Two-year stability and change in schizotypal, borderline, avoidant, and obsessive-compulsive personality disorders. J Consult Clin Psychol 72:767–775, 2004

Grilo CM, Sanislow CA, Shea MT, et al: Two-year prospective naturalistic study of remission from MDD as a function of personality disorder comorbidity. J Consult Clin Psychol (in press)

Grinker RR, Werble B, Drye RC: The Borderline Syndrome. New York, Basic Books, 1968

Gunderson JG, Shea MT, Skodol AE, et al: The Collaborative Longitudinal Personality Disorders Study, I: development, aims, designs and sample characteristics. J Personal Disord 14:300–315, 2000

Gunderson JG, Morey LC, Stout RL, et al: Major depressive disorder and borderline personality disorder revisited: longitudinal associations. J Clin Psychiatry 65:1049–1056, 2004

Heatherton TF, Weinberger JL (eds): Can Personality Change? Washington, DC, American Psychological Press, 1994

Johnson JG, Williams JBW, Goetz RR, et al: Stability and change in personality disorder symptomatology: findings from a longitudinal study of HIV+ and HIV– men. J Abnorm Psychol 106:154–158, 1997

Johnson JG, Cohen P, Smailes E, et al: Adolescent personality disorders associated with violence and criminal behavior during adolescence and early adulthood. Am J Psychiatry 157:1406–1412, 2000a

Johnson JG, Cohen P, Kasen S, et al: Age-related change in personality disorder trait levels between early adolescence and adulthood: a community-based longitudinal investigation. Acta Psychiatr Scand 102:265–275, 2000b

Judd PH, McGlashan TH: A Developmental Model of Borderline Personality Disorder: Understanding Variations in Course and Outcome. Washington, DC, American Psychiatric Publishing, 2003

Katz MM, Secunda SK, Hirschfeld R, et al: NIMH Clinical Research Branch Collaborative Program on Psychobiology of Depression. Arch Gen Psychiatry 36:765–771, 1979

Keller MB, Shapiro RW, Lavori PW, et al: Recovery in major depressive disorder: analysis with the lifetable and regression models. Arch Gen Psychiatry 39:905–910, 1982

Keller MB, Lavori PW, Friedman B, et al: The Longitudinal Interval Follow-Up Evaluation. Arch Gen Psychiatry 44:540–548, 1987

Kendell PC, Clarkin JF: Introduction to special section: comorbidity and treatment implications. J Consult Clin Psychol 60:833–834, 1992

Klein DN, Shih JH: Depressive personality: associations with DSM-III-R mood and personality disorders and negative and positive affectivity, 30-month stability, and prediction of course of axis I depressive disorders. J Abnorm Psychol 107:319–327, 1998

Krueger RF: The structure of common mental disorders. Arch Gen Psychiatry 56:921–926, 1999

Krueger RF, Carlson SR: Personality disorders in children and adolescents. Curr Psychiatry Rep 3:46–51, 2001

Krueger RF, Tackett JL: Personality and psychopathology: working toward the bigger picture. J Personal Disord 17:109–128, 2003

Lenzenweger MF: Stability and change in personality disorder features: the longitudinal study of personality disorders. Arch Gen Psychiatry 56:1009–1015, 1999

Lenzenweger MF, Loranger AW, Korfine L, et al: Detecting personality disorders in a nonclinical population: application of a 2-stage procedure for case identification. Arch Gen Psychiatry 54:110–133, 1997

Levy KN, Becker DF, Grilo CM, et al: Concurrent and predictive validity of the personality disorder diagnosis in adolescent inpatients. Am J Psychiatry 156:1522–1528, 1999

Lewinsohn PM, Rohde P, Seeley JR, et al: Axis II psychopathology as a function of Axis I disorder in childhood and adolescents. J Am Acad Child Adolesc Psychiatry 36:1752–1759, 1997

Livesley WJ, Jackson DN, Schroeder ML: Factorial structure of traits delineating personality disorders in clinical and general population samples. J Abnorm Psychol 101:432–440, 1992

Loranger AW. Personality Disorder Examination (PDE) Manual. Yonkers, NY, DV Communications, 1988

Loranger AW, Lenzenweger MF, Gartner AF, et al: Trait-state artifacts and the diagnosis of personality disorders. Arch Gen Psychiatry 48:720–728, 1991

Loranger AW, Sartorius N, Andreoli A, et al: The International Personality Disorder Examination (IPDE). Arch Gen Psychiatry 51:215–224, 1994

Lynam DR, Widiger TA: Using the five-factor model to represent the DSM-IV personality disorders: an expert consensus approach. J Abnorm Psychol 110:401–412, 2001

Lyons MJ, Tyrer P, Gunderson J, et al: Special feature: heuristic models of comorbidity of Axis I and Axis II disorders. J Personal Disord 11:260–269, 1997

Maddocks PD: A five year follow-up of untreated psychopaths. Br J Psychiatry 116:511–515, 1970

Mattanah JJ, Becker DF, Levy KN, et al: Diagnostic stability in adolescents followed up 2 years after hospitalization. Am J Psychiatry 152:889–894, 1995

McDavid JD, Pilkonis PA: The stability of personality disorder diagnoses. J Personal Disord 10:1–15, 1996

McGlashan TH: The Chestnut Lodge Follow-up Study, part III: long-term outcome of borderline personalities. Arch Gen Psychiatry 42:20–30, 1986a

McGlashan TH: The Chestnut Lodge Follow-up Study, part VI: schizotypal personality disorder. Arch Gen Psychiatry 43:329–334, 1986b

McGlashan TH, Grilo CM, Skodol AE, et al: The Collaborative Longitudinal Personality Disorders Study: baseline Axis I/II and II/II diagnostic co-occurrence. Acta Psychiatr Scand 102:256–264, 2000

McGlashan TH, Grilo CM, Sanislow CA, et al: Two-year prevalence and stability of individual DSM-IV criteria for schizotypal, borderline, avoidant, and obsessive-compulsive disorders. Am J Psychiatry (in press)

Myers MG, Stewart DG, Brown SA: Progression from conduct disorder to antisocial personality disorder following treatment for adolescent substance abuse. Am J Psychiatry 155:479–485, 1998

Nesselroade JR, Stigler SM, Baltes PB: Regression toward the mean and the study of change. Psychol Bull 88:622–637, 1980

Newman DL, Caspi A, Moffitt TE, et al: Antecedents of adult interpersonal functioning: effects of individual differences in age three temperament. Dev Psychol 33:206–217, 1997

Oldham JM, Skodol AE, Kellman HD, et al: Diagnoses of DSM-III-R personality disorders by two structured interviews: patterns of comorbidity. Am J Psychiatry 149:213–230, 1992

Ottosson H, Ekselius L, Grann M, et al: Cross-system concordance of personality disorder diagnoses of DSM-IV and diagnostic criteria for research of ICD-10. J Personal Disord 16:283–292, 2002

Paris J: Personality disorders over time: precursors, course and outcome. J Personal Disord 17:479–488, 2003

Paris J, Zweig-Frank H: A twenty-seven year follow-up of borderline patients. Compr Psychiatry 42:482–487, 2001

Perry JC: Longitudinal studies of personality disorders. J Personal Disord 7 (suppl):63–85, 1993

Rettew DC, Zanarini MC, Yen S, et al: Childhood antecedents of avoidant personality disorder: a retrospective study. J Am Acad Child Adolesc Psychiatry 42:1122–1130, 2003

Rey JM, Morris-Yates A, Singh M, et al: Continuities between psychiatric disorders in adolescents and personality disorders in young adults. Am J Psychiatry 152:895–900, 1995

Robbins E, Gentry KA, Munoz RA, et al: A contrast of the three more common illnesses with the ten less common in a study and 18-month follow-up of 314 psychiatric emergency room patients, III: findings at follow-up. Arch Gen Psychiatry 34:285–291, 1977

Roberts BW, DelVecchio WF: The rank-order consistency of personality traits from childhood to old age: a quantitative review of longitudinal studies. Psychol Bull 126:3–25, 2000

Roberts BW, Caspi A, Moffitt TE: The kids are alright: growth and stability in personality development from adolescence to adulthood. J Pers Soc Psychol 81:670–683, 2001

Robins LN: Deviant Children Grown Up: A Sociological and Psychiatric Study of Sociopathic Personality. Baltimore, MD, Williams and Wilkins, 1966

Robins LN: Epidemiology: reflections on testing the validity of psychiatric interviews. Arch Gen Psychiatry 42:918–924,1985

Ruegg R, Frances A: New research in personality disorders. J Personal Disord 9:1–48, 1995

Sanislow CA, McGlashan TH: Treatment outcome of personality disorders. Can J Psychiatry 43:237–250, 1998

Seivewright H, Tyrer P, Johnson T: Change in personality status in neurotic disorders. Lancet 359:2253–2254, 2002

Shea MT, Yen S: Stability as a distinction between axis I and axis II disorders. J Personal Disord 17:373–386, 2003

Shea MT, Stout RL, Gunderson JG, et al: Short-term diagnostic stability of schizotypal, borderline, avoidant, and obsessive-compulsive personality disorders. Am J Psychiatry 159:2036–2041, 2002

Shea MT, Stout RL, Yen S, et al: Associations in the course of personality disorders and Axis I disorders over time. J Abnorm Psychol 113:449–508, 2004

Siever LJ, Davis KL: A psychobiological perspective on the personality disorders. Am J Psychiatry 148:1647–1658, 1991

Skodol AE: Classification, assessment, and differential diagnosis of personality disorders. J Pract Psychiatry Behav Health 3:261–274, 1997

Skodol AE, Pagano ME, Bender DS, et al: Stability of functional impairment in patients with schizotypal, borderline, avoidant, or obsessive-compulsive personality disorder over two years. Psychol Med (in press)

Solomon DA, Keller MB, Leon AC, et al: Recovery from major depression: a 10-year prospective follow-up across multiple episodes. Arch Gen Psychiatry 54:1001–1006, 1997

Squires-Wheeler E, Skodol AE, Erlenmeyer-Kimling L: The assessment of schizotypal features over two points in time. Schizophrenia Res 6:75–85, 1992

Stevenson J, Meares R, Comerford A: Diminished impulsivity in older patients with borderline personality disorder. Am J Psychiatry 160:165–166, 2003

Stone MH: Long-term outcome in personality disorders. Br J Psychiatry 162:299–313, 1993

Trull TJ, Useda JD, Conforti K, et al: Borderline personality disorder features in nonclinical young adults, 2: two-year outcome. J Abnorm Psychol 106:307–314, 1997

Trull TJ, Useda JD, Doan BT, et al: Two-year stability of borderline personality measures. J Personal Disord 12:187–197, 1998

Tyrer P: Personality disorder. Br J Psychiatry 179:81–84, 2001

Tyrer P, Simonsen E: Personality disorder in psychiatric practice. World Psychiatry 2:41–44, 2003

Tyrer P, Strauss J, Cicchetti D: Temporal reliability of personality in psychiatric patients. Psychol Med 13:393–398, 1983

Tyrer P, Gunderson J, Lyons M, et al: Special feature: extent of comorbidity between mental state and personality disorders. J Personal Disord 11:242–259, 1997

Warner MB, Morey LC, Finch JF, et al: The longitudinal relationship of personality traits and disorders. J Abnorm Psychol 113:217–227, 2004

Westen D: Divergences between clinical and research methods for assessing personality disorders: implications for research and the evolution of axis II. Am J Psychiatry 154:895–903, 1997

Westen D, Shedler J: Revising and assessing axis II, Part II: toward an empirically based and clinically useful classification of personality disorders. Am J Psychiatry 156:273–285, 1999

Widiger TA: Categorical versus dimensional classification: implications from and for research. J Pers Disord 6:287–300, 1992

Widiger TA: Personality disorder and Axis I psychopathology: the problematic boundary of Axis I and Axis II. J Personal Disord 17:90–108, 2003

Wolff S, Townshend R, McGuire RJ, et al: Schizoid personality in childhood and adult life, II: adult adjustment and the continuity with schizotypal personality disorder. Br J Psychiatry 159:620–629, 1991

World Health Organization. ICD-10: Classification of Mental and Behavioral Disorders. Geneva, World Health Organization, 1992

Zanarini MC, Skodol AE, Bender D, et al: The Collaborative Longitudinal Personality Disorders Study: reliability of Axis I and II diagnoses. J Personal Disord 14:291–299, 2000

Zanarini MC, Frankenburg FR, Hennen J, et al: The longitudinal course of borderline psychopathology: 6-year prospective follow-up of the phenomenology of borderline personality disorder. Am J Psychiatry 160:274–283, 2003

Zimmerman M: Diagnosing personality disorders: a review of issues and research methods. Arch Gen Psychiatry 51:225–245, 1994

Part III

Etiology

7

A Current Integrative Perspective on Personality Disorders

Joel Paris, M.D.

MENTAL DISORDERS AND THE STRESS-DIATHESIS MODEL

By themselves, neither chemical imbalances, psychological adversities, nor troubled social environments account for the development of psychopathology. A multitude of interactions between biological, psychological, and social factors are involved in the etiology of any mental disorder. This statement may be a truism, but in practice, we find it difficult to deal with complexity. Although the real world is nonlinear and multivariate, the human mind is structured for linear thinking. Even researchers are not immune to oversimplifications.

One way to embrace complexity is to frame psychological phenomena in a systems perspective. General systems theory (Sameroff 1995) takes into account the biological roots of behavior without reducing psychology to neurochemistry. Mental processes have emergent properties that cannot be explained at other levels of analysis.

The stress-diathesis model (Monroe and Simons 1991) is a general theory of psychopathology that is both nonreductionistic and interactional. Every category of mental disorder is associated with some kind of genetic vulnerability (Paris 1999). Yet genes are not the direct causes of mental disorders; rather, they shape individual variability in temperament and traits. Some of these temperamental variants constitute a vulnerability to psychopathology. By and large, however, traits only become maladaptive under specific environmental conditions. In other words, diatheses become apparent when uncovered by stressors. For example, even in a condition such as schizophrenia, with its well-established genetic risk, only half of identical twins are concordant for the disorder (Meehl 1990).

The interactions between diatheses and stressors are bidirectional. Genetic variability influences the way individuals respond to their environment, while environmental factors determine whether genes are expressed. These relationships help explain why adverse life events by themselves do not consistently lead to pathological sequelae. Most children are resilient to all but the most severe and consistent adversities (Rutter and Maughan 1997). However, trauma, neglect, and dysfunctional families probably have greater effects on temperamentally vulnerable children (Paris 2000b).

TEMPERAMENT, TRAITS, AND PERSONALITY DISORDERS

We can now apply these principles to the development of personality disorders. To conceptualize how diatheses and stressors interact to shape personality pathology, we need to consider the hierarchical and nested relationship among personality disorders, personality traits, and temperament (Rutter 1987). Temperament reflects the genetic factors that account for a large proportion of the variance in personality traits (Plomin et al. 2001a). Personality traits—that is, individual differences in behavior that remain stable over time and context—are an amalgam of temperament and experience. Personality disorders are dysfunctional outcomes that occur when these traits are amplified and used in rigid and maladaptive ways. By themselves, trait differences are fully compatible with normality, but trait profiles determine what type of personality disorder can develop (Paris 2003).

Strong evidence supports the principle that there is no definite boundary between personality traits and personality disorders (Cloninger et al. 1993; Costa and Widiger 2001; Livesley et al. 1993; Siever and Davis 1991). For this reason disorders are best understood as pathological amplifications of traits (Millon and Davis 1995; Paris 2003). Whereas some personality disorders (particularly those in the borderline category) show symptoms that are rare in community populations, they are still rooted in trait dimensions (Siever and Davis 1991). Moreover, genetic, neuropsychological, and biological markers are not consistently associated with any of the categories of disorders described in DSM-IV-TR (American Psychiatric Association 2000) but are related to traits (Livesley 2003). Thus, traits are closer to biological bedrock than disorders, which are more colored by psychosocial influences. Similar principles can be broadly applied to all forms of psychopathology, including Axis I disorders, which are also rooted in traits and temperament (Kendell and Jablensky 2003).

Epidemiological studies (Samuels et al. 2002; Torgersen et al. 2001; Weissman 1993) have estimated that as much as 10% or more of the general population has a personality disorder. However, if there is no absolute cutoff point between personality traits and disorders, one can question these findings. Although it is probably true that one out of ten people has problematic traits, everything depends on how much dysfunction is required to diagnose a disorder.

The overall criteria for diagnosis of a personality disorder in DSM-IV-TR require an enduring pattern of inner experience and behavior that deviates markedly from the expectations of the individual's culture, affecting cognition, affect, interpersonal functioning, and impulse control. The pattern must be inflexible and pervasive across a broad range of personal and social situations, leading to clinically significant distress or impairment in social, occupational, or other important areas of functioning. Finally, the pattern must be stable and of long duration and must have an onset that can be traced back to adolescence or early adulthood.

Each of these criteria requires an informed clinical judgment. For this reason, personality disorder diagnoses may not be reliable unless pathology is severe. Moreover, only three categories of personality disorder have a large empirical literature (schizotypal, antisocial, and borderline). Given the less well-defined characteristics of the other categories, it is not surprising that many patients meet overall criteria in DSM-IV-TR for a personality disorder but do not fall into any specific category and can only be classified as personality disorder not otherwise specified. About a third of all cases in practice fall into this group (Loranger et al. 1994).

Ever since the publication of DSM-III (American Psychiatric Association 1980), psychiatry has classified mental disorders on the basis of phenomenology. This decision was the right one for its time. In the absence of solid data on etiology, it is better to categorize what clinicians can observe. However, an etiologically based classification must be our ultimate goal. In this respect, all the categories of disorder on Axis II of DSM-IV-TR can only be considered provisional. Future classifications of personality disorders may be based on the underlying neurobiological mechanisms that shape traits (Paris 2000a). This approach, which involves classifying disease on the basis of pathogenesis or etiology, is becoming standard in all areas of medicine. It would combine data at many levels of analysis: molecular genetics, behavior genetics, neurochemistry, neurophysiology, cognitive science, and developmental psychopathology. Classifying personality disorders in this way need not exclude the crucial influence of environmental factors, which ultimately affect brain circuitry and brain chemistry.

Factor and cluster analytic studies of personality traits and disorders suggest an underlying structure that is obscured by current diagnoses (Livesley 2003). Several suggestions have been made about the nature of this structure. Costa and Widiger (2001) have proposed that disorders can be accounted for by the five-factor model (FFM) of personality. Livesley and Jang (2000) have developed a somewhat similar model, with superfactors that parallel four of the five factors in the FFM. Cloninger et al. (1993) have developed a seven-factor model that also describes similar trait dimensions.

Applying any of these systems would lead to a very different classification of personality disorders. A dimensional system would help to deal with widespread comorbidity of Axis II disorders. Many (albeit not all) of these overlaps occur within the Axis II clusters (Pfohl et al. 1986), supporting the concept that trait dimensions underlie categories. The problem is that current categories of personality disorders are not well-defined phenotypes (Jang et al. 2001); this is probably why diagnoses tend to overlap.

Krueger (1999) found that almost all DSM-defined disorders can be accounted for by factors that reflect *internalizing* and *externalizing* symptoms; these are the same superfactors that emerge from studies of psychopathology in children (Achenbach and McConaughy 1997). These broad factors also correspond to the personality trait dimensions measured by the FFM in adult community populations (Costa and Widiger 2001): internalizing dimensions are associated with high levels of introversion and neuroticism, whereas externalizing dimensions are associated with high extraversion and low conscientiousness. However, this distinction fails to take into account another crucial trait for psychopathology: the cognitive dimension associated with vulnerability to psychotic disorders. Building dimensional models from psychopathology rather than from normality allows us to include phenomena rarely seen in community populations. For example, in a model linking traits and overt disorders, Siever and Davis (1991) conceptualized all categories (on both Axis I and Axis II) within four trait dimensions: cognitive, depressive, impulsive, and anxious.

The Axis II clusters described in DSM-IV-TR are rough-and-ready clinically derived concepts and need to be redefined to improve their boundaries. At this point, the Axis II clusters are only approximations of spectra that include a number of overlapping disorders. Nonetheless, the clusters show some interesting parallels with dimensional approaches to personality disorders.

The categories in Cluster A (schizoid, paranoid, and schizotypal) are related to the schizophrenia spectrum (Paris 2003; Siever and Davis 1991). Similarly, categories in Cluster B are associated with trait impulsiv-

ity and/or affective dysregulation (Siever and Davis 1991; Zanarini 1993). This is most clearly apparent for antisocial personality disorder (ASPD) and borderline personality disorder (BPD), but histrionic and narcissistic personality also show these features, albeit in attenuated form (Looper and Paris 2000). The situation for Cluster C is more complex: although avoidant and dependent personality disorders are clearly associated with trait anxiety (Kagan 1994; Paris 1997), the compulsive category may reflect a separate compulsivity trait dimension (Livesley and Jang 2000).

GENES, ENVIRONMENT, AND PERSONALITY TRAITS

It is difficult to separate the influence of genes from that of environment on personality. It has been consistently shown that personality traits are heritable, with genetic factors accounting for nearly half of the variance (Plomin et al. 2001a). However, single genes are not associated with single temperamental characteristics. Rather, the heritable component of personality emerges from complex and interactive polygenetic mechanisms associated with variations in multiple alleles—that is, quantitative trait loci (Rutter and Plomin 1997). Thus, attempts to find genetic associations between genes and traits have been disappointing, and research needs to take environmental effects on gene expression into account (Rutter et al. 2001).

The existence of a genetic component in personality suggests that traits may be linked to biological markers. These relationships have remained rather obscure. The most robust finding in the literature is a relationship between low levels of central serotonin activity and impulsivity (Mann 1998). Again, the problem lies in the lack of precisely defined phenotypes. Livesley (2003) suggested that genes and biological markers are more likely to correlate with narrowly defined traits (which may be affected by fewer alleles) than with broader traits.

In behavioral genetic research, half of the variance in personality traits derives from the environment, but this portion is almost entirely "unshared" (Plomin et al. 2001a, 2001b). These findings show that environmental influences on traits do not necessarily derive from being raised in the same family. This finding has been the subject of great controversy, because it contradicts many classical ideas in developmental and clinical psychology that focus on parenting as a primary factor shaping personality development (Harris 1998; Paris 2000b).

There are several possible reasons why unshared (but not shared) environmental factors are important in personality (Plomin et al. 2001b). The first is that a child's temperament affects the response of other people in the child's environment. In a large-scale study of adolescents (Reiss et al. 2000) that used a combination of twin and family methods, multivariate analyses showed that the temperament of the child was the underlying factor driving differential parenting and differential behavioral outcomes.

A second explanation is that even when the family provides a similar environment for siblings, each child may perceive experiences differently and respond to them with different behavioral patterns. Again, temperamental differences can make environmental influences unshared.

A third explanation is that some environmental factors affecting personality are extrafamilial. Every child has shaping experiences with peers, with teachers, or with community leaders (Rutter and Maughan 1997). Harris (1998) proposed that peer groups might be even more crucial than parents for personality development.

A final possibility is that personality might be affected by intrauterine factors, a biological environment that is not shared. However, there is little research supporting this hypothesis.

Whatever the ultimate explanation, almost all the empirical literature claiming to establish links between childhood experiences and personality has to be questioned on the grounds that genetic factors may be latent variables accounting for some of these relationships (Harris 1998). This difficulty also affects the validity of research measures. Plomin and Bergeman (1991) reported that behavioral genetic studies of standard measures of life experience, past and present, have a heritable component that correlates with personality trait differences.

Genetic Factors

If personality disorders are pathologically amplified traits, it would be logical for them to show heritability levels similar to personality dimensions. This expectation has been confirmed empirically. Torgersen et al. (2000) located a large sample of twins in Norway in which one proband met criteria for at least one categorical Axis II diagnosis (except for the antisocial category). All personality disorders had heritabilities resembling those observed for traits (i.e., close to half the variance). Although the findings cannot be considered quantitatively precise (in view of small sample size

and local variations in base rates), they were consistent across disorders. Moreover, even in personality disorders that have not traditionally been considered heritable (such as the borderline and narcissistic categories), genetic factors accounted for more than half of the variance. Although there were no patients with ASPD in the Norwegian cohort, other lines of research (Cloninger et al. 1982) have pointed to heritable influences on that disorder.

Genetic factors influencing both traits and disorders have been supported by family history studies examining spectra of disorders across Axis I and Axis II. Thus, first-degree relatives of patients with disorders in Cluster A show pathology in the schizophrenic spectrum (Siever and Davis 1991); those of patients in Cluster B tend to have other impulsive disorders (Zanarini 1993) in some cases and other affective disorders in other cases (Siever and Davis 1991); relatives of patients in Cluster C often have anxiety disorders (Paris 1997). These findings support the relationship of trait dimensions to disorders. Moreover, if these same traits underlie all forms of psychopathology, it should not be surprising that patients with Axis II disorders can have wide-ranging Axis I comorbidity (McGlashan et al. 2000; Zanarini et al. 2001).

The influence of genetic factors on personality disorders supports a continued search for biological markers associated with Axis II disorders and their underlying traits. In Cluster A disorders, biological markers, such as abnormal eye tracking, are found that are also common in schizophrenia (Siever and Davis 1991). In Cluster B disorders, we see the same relationship between central serotonin activity and impulsive aggression that has been studied on the trait level (Coccaro et al. 1989). The most consistent results in neurophysiological and neuropsychological research on Cluster B disorders are also related to impulsive traits. Thus, functional abnormalities in prefrontal cortex are associated with impulsive aggression, as shown by decreases in the mass of frontal gray matter in subjects with ASPD (Raine et al. 2000). Patients with ASPD and BPD have deficits in executive function as measured by the Wisconsin Card Sorting Test (O'Leary 2000). Although we know much less about Cluster C disorders, the physiological correlates of trait anxiety have been measured in longitudinal designs (Kagan 1994).

Psychological Factors

A large body of evidence supports the concept that childhood adversities are risk factors for personality disorders (Paris 2003). The problem is that there is insufficient evidence to establish a direct causal relationship. For example, research on patients with BPD has documented that histories of sexual abuse, physical abuse, and gross neglect are common (Paris 1994; Zanarini 2000). One current theory of BPD is that children who develop this disorder have abnormal patterns of attachment that emerge from exposure to adversity (Fonagy et al. 1995). However, longitudinal studies are needed to determine the origins of these patterns as well as their impact on development.

It has been consistently shown that the impact of childhood adversities is different in clinical and community samples. Community surveys of the effects of childhood sexual abuse (Browne and Finkelhor 1986; Rind and Tromofovitch 1997), as well as of physical abuse (Malinovsky-Rummell and Hansen 1993), have found that only a minority of children exposed to abuse and trauma suffer measurable sequelae. One explanation could be that adverse life experiences lead to psychopathology only in the presence of specific trait profiles associated with temperamental vulnerability.

Finally, single traumatic events are rarely, by themselves, associated with pathological sequelae; instead, continuously adverse circumstances have cumulative effects associated with the development of symptomatology (Rutter 1989). For this reason, one cannot understand the impact of childhood adversities without placing events within a longitudinal and developmental context.

Another problem with the existing research literature is that most studies have examined childhood risk factors using retrospective methodologies. Reports of life experiences occurring many years in the past tend to be colored by recall bias—that is, the tendency for individuals with symptoms in the present to remember more adversities in the past (Robins et al. 1985; Schacter 1996). To address this problem we need longitudinal data.

A good example of the kind of study we require is the follow-back study by Robins (1966) of children with conduct disorder. Here it was observed that the strongest predictor of adult ASPD among children with conduct disorder was parental psychopathy (usually in the father), an association later supported by Farrington (1998). Several studies have demonstrated that first-degree relatives of patients with BPD have increased levels of impulsive spectrum disorders (Links et al. 1988; Zanarini 1993).

Yet even here, causality is unclear. Because the mechanism behind these relationships could involve inheritance, modeling, or pathological parenting, one needs to separate the effects of personality traits common between parents and children from the effects of family dysfunction. For this reason, research methods are needed in which temperament is controlled for using behavior-genetic designs. An ongoing study (Dionne et al. 2003) has been prospectively following large cohorts of monozygotic and dizygotic twins from infancy, but these cohorts have only reached middle childhood.

Community studies avoid the problems in studying clinical populations because clinical samples are already biased toward psychopathology. One large-scale prospective longitudinal project, the Albany-Saratoga study, has been following a cohort of children from middle childhood to early adulthood and examining the predictors of pathological sequelae. Johnson et al. (1999) reported that early adversities, including neglect, physical abuse, and sexual abuse, were associated with a higher number of personality disorder symptoms. This study is important and unique, but the researchers had to use a continuous variable to measure outcome because there were not enough subjects with a diagnosable personality disorder. Also, the research design lacked data on temperamental factors in early childhood that might have preceded environmental adversities and affected their impact.

With all these caveats, it is impossible to escape the conclusion that adversity in childhood, as well as in later life, is a crucial factor affecting the development of personality disorders. The impact of negative life events tends to amplify temperamental vulnerability (Paris 1996) but can often be modulated by resilience factors (Rutter 1989).

Social Factors

The role of social factors on personality disorders has not been widely researched. Yet, like other forms of psychopathology, personality disorders develop in a sociocultural context. There are two ways to test this relationship. First, one could look for cross-cultural differences in personality disorders (Paris 1996). Second, one could determine whether personality disorders vary in prevalence over time (Paris 2004).

Mental disorders can present with different symptoms in different cultures, and some categories of illness are seen only in specific social settings (Murphy 1982). Personality disorders are "socially sensitive" (Paris 2004) because their symptoms reflect behaviors and feelings that could be shaped and molded by culture. Moreover, if traits themselves show sociocultural variation, personality disorders might present with different symptoms in different social contexts, and some categories might even be culture bound.

The broader dimensions of personality have been shown to be similar in different societies (McCrae and Costa 1999), but this may not be the case for personality disorders. Whereas Loranger et al. (1994) showed that the categories in DSM-IV-TR and ICD-10 (World Health Organization 1992) can be identified in clinical settings around the world, there are no epidemiological data concerning possible differences in prevalence between cultures and societies. This lacuna may be partially filled by the upcoming International Comorbidity Study, which will be a replication of the National Comorbidity Survey (Kessler et al. 1994) in several countries. The largest community surveys, such as the Epidemiological Catchment Area Study (Robins and Regier 1991) as well as the National Comorbidity Survey, have examined only ASPD (which has behavioral symptoms that are readily measured). The International Comorbidity Study will make use of a reliable instrument, the International Personality Disorder Examination (Loranger et al. 1994), that will also determine the prevalence of BPD.

At this point, cross-cultural studies support the role of social factors in ASPD. This category is relatively rare in traditional societies such as Taiwan (Hwu et al. 1989) and Japan (Sato and Takeichi 1993), but prevalence reaches North American and European levels in Korea (Lee et al. 1987). The East Asian cultures that have a low prevalence of ASPD have cultural and family structures that are protective against antisocial behavior. Thus, families are a mirror image of the risk factors for the disorder described by Robins (1966): fathers are strong and authoritative, expectations of children are high, and family loyalty is prized. In addition, communities outside the family have high social cohesion, further containing those with impulsive temperament. One might also hypothesize that less well-structured family and social structures are among the factors that make ASPD more common in Western societies.

The strongest evidence thus far for sociocultural factors in personality disorders comes from cohort effects (changes in prevalence over short periods of time). ASPD (as well as other impulsive spectrum disorders such as substance abuse) has become more common in adolescents and young adults, both in North America and Europe, since World War II (Rutter and Smith 1995).

There may also be cohort effects on the prevalence of BPD (Millon 2000; Chapter 14, "Sociocultural Factors"). Expanding on this thesis, Paris (1996) pointed to several lines of supportive evidence: recent increases in the prevalence of parasuicide and completed suicide (Bland et al. 1998) and the observation that a third of youths who commit suicide can be diagnosed with BPD (Lesage et al. 1994).

One likely mechanism for an increase of prevalence in BPD may derive from the breakdown of traditional structures guiding the development of adolescents and young adults (Millon 2000). Traditional societies have long been defined in the sociological literature (e.g., Lerner 1958) as having high social cohesion, fixed social roles, and high intergenerational continuity; these characteristics stand in contrast to modern societies, which have lower social cohesion, fluid social roles, and lower continuity between generations. Although traditional societies could carry a different set of risks for psychopathology, the problem of identity is often associated with personality disorders and may be exacerbated by the conditions of modernity in which individuals must develop their own social roles (Paris 1996).

Impulsive disorders (substance abuse, eating disorders, ASPD, BPD) may be particularly responsive to social context because they are contained by structure and limits and amplified by the absence of these. However, these conditions would only be expected to develop in individuals who also have the biological and psychological risk factors for impulsive disorders. Linehan (1993) suggested that patients with BPD act impulsively as way of dealing with emotional dysregulation and that decreases in social support in modern society amplify these traits by interfering with a buffering mechanism.

The relationship of social factors is less clear for other personality disorders. In narcissistic personality disorder, one might hypothesize that underlying traits may no longer be channeled into fruitful ambition due to breakdowns in family and social structures (Kohut 1977; Paris 2003). Similarly, avoidant personality disorder might be understood as reflecting the outcome of social anxiety in modern society. Kagan (1994) has studied "behavioral inhibition" in infants, a temperamental syndrome that increases the risk for anxiety disorders later in life. In a traditional society, anxious traits would be buffered by family and community structures, whereas in modern society, the same traits are more likely to become disabling and lead to disorders (Paris 1997).

IMPLICATIONS OF A STRESS-DIATHESIS MODEL OF PERSONALITY DISORDERS

The biological, psychological, and social risk factors for personality disorders can be integrated within a stress-diathesis model. Both genetic-temperamental and psychosocial factors would be necessary conditions for the development of personality disorders, but neither would be sufficient. A combination of risks—that is, a "two-hit" or "multiple-hit" mechanism—is required. The effects of psychosocial adversity will be greatest in individuals who are temperamentally predisposed to psychopathology. The cumulative effects of multiple risk factors, rather than single adversities, will determine whether psychopathology develops. Finally, the specific disorder that emerges depends on temperamental profiles specific to the individual.

Gene–environment interactions would further mediate the pathogenesis of personality disorders. Abnormal temperament is associated with a greater sensitivity to environmental risk factors, and children with problematic temperaments are more likely to experience adversities (Rutter and Maughan 1997). Vulnerable children also elicit responses from others that tend to amplify their most problematic characteristics, creating a positive feedback loop. These adverse experiences further amplify traits, increasing the risk for further adversities.

An integrative model also helps to account for the course of personality disorders over time (Paris 2003). Early onset of pathology probably tends to reflect abnormal temperament. ASPD is a good example: even as early as age 3, behavioral disturbances predict its development in adulthood (Caspi et al. 1996; Kim-Cohen et al. 2003; Zoccolillo et al. 1992). However, the development of conduct symptoms in childhood is clearly related to family pathology (Patterson and Yoerger 1997; Robins 1966). Similarly, children with unusual shyness and reactivity may be at higher risk for anxious cluster personality disorders (Paris 1998), but these traits may be amplified by family experience (Head et al. 1991).

By adolescence, when personality trait patterns become stable (Costa and McCrae 2001), one can diagnose typical cases of personality disorder (Kernberg et al. 2000), although specific categories tend to shift over time (Bernstein et al. 1993). In adult life, most personality disorders have a chronic course (Seivewright et al. 2002), possibly due to continuing interactions between temperament and experience. However, Cluster B disorders are the exception because they tend to "burn out" by middle age (Paris 2003), possibly reflecting the evolution of traits, with impulsivity leveling out over time.

A stress-diathesis model of personality disorders also has important implications for treatment. It suggests that neither a purely biological or a purely psychosocial perspective is a useful guide to effective treatment of personality disorders. A strictly biological perspective tends to support a strongly pharmacological approach to these patients. Yet clinical trials do not show specific efficacy for existing drugs, even if some produce a certain degree of symptomatic relief (Paris 2003; Soloff 2000). The limitations of pharmacotherapy are shown by evidence that patients with BPD may be given as many as four or five drugs (Zanarini et al. 2001) despite the fact that polypharmacy rarely yields dramatic results.

A psychosocial perspective on personality disorders has generally supported psychotherapy as a primary form of treatment. However, maladaptive traits, established in childhood and reinforced during adult life, are often difficult to change. The efficacy of long-term therapies has not been established in clinical trials. Patients with personality disorders are generally less responsive to standard forms of psychotherapy than are patients with Axis I disorders without any Axis II comorbidity (Shea et al. 1990). Psychodynamic therapy has been tested in selected patient populations, most particularly those with BPD (Bateman and Fonagy 1999; Stevenson and Meares 1992), but it is not known whether these results are specific to the techniques used and whether they are generalizable to ordinary practice. Cognitive approaches to personality disorders (Beck and Freeman 1990) have generated investigation, and dialectical behavior therapy for BPD (Linehan 1993) has been consistently shown to reduce impulsive behavior in BPD but has not been examined for long-term efficacy.

Personality disorders will probably remain difficult to treat until we understand their etiology and pathogenesis. As we obtain more knowledge concerning the diatheses and stressors driving both traits and disorders, we will be in a better position to develop more specific and more useful forms of treatment for these patients—more targeted biological interventions and more targeted forms of psychotherapy.

REFERENCES

Achenbach TM, McConaughy SH: Empirically Based Assessment of Child and Adolescent Psychopathology: Practical Applications, 2nd Edition. Thousand Oaks, CA, Sage, 1997

American Psychiatric Association: Diagnostic and Statistical Manual of Mental Disorders, 3rd Edition. Washington, DC, American Psychiatric Association, 1980

American Psychiatric Association: Diagnostic and Statistical Manual of Mental Disorders, 4th Edition, Text Revision. Washington, DC, American Psychiatric Association, 2000

Bateman A, Fonagy P: Effectiveness of partial hospitalization in the treatment of borderline personality disorder: a randomized controlled trial. Am J Psychiatry 156:1563–1569, 1999

Beck AT, Freeman A: Cognitive Therapy of Personality Disorders. New York, Guilford, 1990

Bernstein DP, Cohen P, Skodol A, et al: Prevalence and stability of the DSM-III personality disorders in a community-based survey of adolescents. Am J Psychiatry 150:1237–1243, 1993

Bland RC, Dyck RJ, Newman SC, et al: Attempted suicide in Edmonton, in Suicide in Canada. Edited by Leenaars AA, Wenckstern S, Sakinofsky I, et al. Toronto, Canada, University of Toronto Press, 1998, pp 136–150

Browne A, Finkelhor D: Impact of child sexual abuse: a review of the literature. Psychol Bull 99:66–77, 1986

Caspi A, Moffitt TE, Newman DL, et al: Behavioral observations at age three predict adult psychiatric disorders: longitudinal evidence from a birth cohort. Arch Gen Psychiatry 53:1033–1039, 1996

Cloninger CR, Sigvardsson S, Bohman M, et al: Predisposition to petty criminality in Swedish adoptees, II: cross-fostering analysis of gene–environment interactions. Arch Gen Psychiatry 39:1242–1247, 1982

Cloninger CR, Svrakic DM, Pryzbeck TR: A psychobiological model of temperament and character. Arch Gen Psychiatry 50:975–990, 1993

Coccaro EF, Siever LJ, Klar HM, et al: Serotonergic studies in patients with affective and personality disorders. Arch Gen Psychiatry 46:587–599, 1989

Costa PT, Widiger TA (eds): Personality Disorders and the Five-Factor Model of Personality, 2nd Edition. Washington, DC, American Psychological Association, 2001

Dionne G, Tremblay R, Boivin M, et al: Physical aggression and expressive vocabulary in 19-month-old twins. Dev Psychol 39:261–273, 2003

Farrington DP: Youth crime and antisocial behavior, in The Social Child. Edited by Campbell A, Muncer S. Hove, England, Psychology Press, 1998, pp 353–392

Fonagy P, Steele M, Steele H, et al: Attachment, the reflective self, and borderline states, in Attachment Theory: Social, Developmental and Clinical Perspectives. Edited by Goldberg S, Muir R, Kerr J. Hillsdale, NJ, Analytic Press, 1995, pp 233–278

Harris JR: The Nurture Assumption. New York, Free Press, 1998

Head SB, Baker JD, Williamson DA: Family environment characteristics and dependent personality disorder. J Personal Disord 5:256–263, 1991

Hwu HG, Yeh EK, Change LY: Prevalence of psychiatric disorders in Taiwan defined by the Chinese Diagnostic Interview Schedule. Acta Psychiatr Scand 79:136–147, 1989

Jang K, Vernon PA, Livesley WJ: Behavioural Genetic Perspectives on Personality Function. Can J Psychiatry 46:234–244, 2001

Johnson JJ, Cohen P, Brown J, et al: Childhood maltreatment increases risk for personality disorders during early adulthood. Arch Gen Psychiatry 56:600–606, 1999

Kagan J: Galen's Prophecy. New York, Basic Books, 1994

Kendell R, Jablensky A: Distinguishing between the validity and utility of psychiatric diagnoses. Am J Psychiatry 160:4–12, 2003

Kernberg PF, Weiner AS, Bardenstein KK: Personality Disorders in Children and Adolescents. New York, Basic Books, 2000

Kessler RC, McGonagle KA, Nelson CB, et al: Lifetime and 12-month prevalence of DSM-III-R psychiatric disorders in the United States. Arch Gen Psychiatry 51:8–14, 1994

Kim-Cohen J, Caspi A, Moffitt TE, et al: Prior juvenile diagnoses in adults with mental disorder: developmental follow-back of a prospective-longitudinal cohort. Arch Gen Psychiatry 60:709–717, 2003

Kohut H: The Restoration of the Self. New York, International Universities Press, 1977

Krueger RF: The structure of common mental disorders. Arch Gen Psychiatry 56:921–926, 1999

Lee KC, Kovac YS, Rhee H: The national epidemiological study of mental disorders in Korea. J Korean Med Sci 2:19–34, 1987

Lerner D: The Passing of Traditional Society. New York, Free Press, 1958

Lesage AD, Boyer R, Grunberg F, et al: Suicide and mental disorders: a case control study of young men. Am J Psychiatry 151:1063–1068, 1994

Linehan MM: Cognitive Behavioral Therapy of Borderline Personality Disorder. New York, Guilford, 1993

Links PS, Steiner B, Huxley G: The occurrence of borderline personality disorder in the families of borderline patients. J Personal Disord 2:14–20, 1988

Livesley WJ: Personality Disorders: A Practical Approach. New York, Guilford, 2003

Livesley WJ, Jang KL: Toward an empirically based classification of personality disorder. J Personal Disord 14:137–151, 2000

Livesley WJ, Jang KL, Jackson DN, et al: Genetic and environmental contributions to dimensions of personality disorders. Am J Psychiatry 150:1826–1831, 1993

Looper K, Paris J: What are the dimensions underlying Cluster B personality disorders? Compr Psychiatry 41:432–437, 2000

Loranger AW, Sartori N, Andreoli A, et al: The International Personality Disorder Examination. Arch Gen Psychiatry 51:215–224, 1994

Malinovsky-Rummell R, Hansen DJ: Long-term consequences of physical abuse. Psychol Bull 114:68–79, 1993

Mann JJ: The neurobiology of suicide. Nat Med 4:425–430, 1998

McCrae RR, Costa PT: A five-factor theory of personality, in Handbook of Personality: Theory and Research, 2nd Edition. Edited by Pervin LA, John OP. New York, Guilford, 1999, pp 139–153

McGlashan TH, Grilo CM, Skodol AE, et al: The Collaborative Longitudinal Personality Disorders Study: baseline Axis I/II and II/II diagnostic co-occurrence. Acta Psychiatr Scand 102:256–264, 2000

Meehl PE: Toward an integrated theory of schizotaxa, schizotypy, and schizophrenia. J Personal Disord 4:1–99, 1990

Millon T: Sociocultural conceptions of the borderline personality. Psychiatr Clin North Am 23:123–136, 2000

Millon T, Davis R: Personality Disorders: DSM-IV and Beyond. New York, Wiley, 1995

Monroe SM, Simons AD: Diathesis-stress theories in the context of life stress research. Psychol Bull 110:406–425, 1991

Murphy HBM: Comparative Psychiatry. New York, Springer, 1982

O'Leary KM: Neuropsychological testing results. Psychiatr Clin North Am 423:1–60, 2000

Paris J: Borderline Personality Disorder: A Multidimensional Approach. Washington, DC, American Psychiatric Press, 1994

Paris J: Social Factors in the Personality Disorders. Cambridge, England, Cambridge University Press, 1996

Paris J: Childhood trauma as an etiological factor in the personality disorders. J Personal Disord 11:34–49, 1997

Paris J: Anxious traits, anxious attachment, and anxious cluster personality disorders. Harv Rev Psychiatry 6:142–148, 1998

Paris J: Nature and Nurture in Psychiatry. Washington, DC, American Psychiatric Press, 1999

Paris J: The classification of personality disorders should be rooted in biology. J Personal Disord 14:127–136, 2000a

Paris J: Myths of Childhood. Philadelphia, PA, Brunner/Mazel, 2000b

Paris J: Personality Disorders Over Time. Washington, DC, American Psychiatric Publishing, 2003

Paris J: Sociocultural factors in the management of personality disorders, in Treatment of Personality Disorders. Edited by Magnavita T. New York, Wiley, 2004, pp 135–147

Patterson GR, Yoerger K: A developmental model for late-onset delinquency. Nebr Symp Motiv 44:119–177, 1997

Pfohl B, Coryell W, Zimmerman M, et al: DSM-III personality disorders: diagnostic overlap and internal consistency of individual DSM-III criteria. Compr Psychiatry 27:21–34, 1986

Plomin R, Bergeman CS: The nature of nurture: genetic influence on "environmental" measures. Behav Brain Sci 14:373–427, 1991

Plomin R, DeFries JC, McClearn GE, et al: Behavioral Genetics, 4th Edition. New York, Freeman, 2001a

Plomin R, Asbury K, Dunn J: Why are children in the same family so different? Nonshared environment a decade later. Can J Psychiatry 46:225–233, 2001b

Raine A, Lencz T, Bilhul S: Reduced prefrontal gray matter and reduced autonomic activity in antisocial personality disorder. Arch Gen Psychiatry 37:119–127, 2000

Reiss D, Hetherington EM, Plomin R: The Relationship Code. Cambridge, MA, Harvard University Press, 2000

Rind B, Tromofovitch P: A meta-analytic review of findings from national samples on psychological correlates of child sexual abuse. J Sex Res 34:237–255, 1997

Robins LN: Deviant Children Grown Up. Baltimore, MD, Williams and Wilkins, 1966

Robins LN, Regier DA (eds): Psychiatric Disorders in America. New York, Free Press, 1991

Robins LN, Schoenberg SP, Holmes SJ: Early home environment and retrospective recall: a test for concordance between siblings with and without psychiatric disorders. Am J Orthopsychiatry 55:27–41, 1985

Rutter M: Temperament, personality, and personality development. Br J Psychiatry 150:443–448, 1987

Rutter M: Pathways from childhood to adult life. J Child Psychol Psychiatry 30:23–51, 1989

Rutter M, Maughan B: Psychosocial adversities in psychopathology. J Personal Disord 11:19–33, 1997

Rutter M, Plomin R: Opportunities for psychiatry from genetic findings. Br J Psychiatry 171:209–219, 1997

Rutter M, Smith DJ: Psychosocial Problems in Young People. Cambridge UK, Cambridge University Press, 1995

Rutter M, Pickles A, Murray R, et al: Testing hypotheses on specific environmental causal effects on behavior. Psychol Bull 127:291–324, 2001

Sameroff AJ: General systems theories and developmental psychopathology, in Developmental Psychopathology: Theory and Methods. Edited by Ciccheti D, Cohen DJ. New York, Wiley, 1995, pp 659–699

Samuels J, Eaton WW, Bienvenu J, et al: Prevalence and correlates of personality disorders in a community sample. Br J Psychiatry 180:536–542, 2002

Sato T, Takeichi M: Lifetime prevalence of specific psychiatric disorders in a general medicine clinic. Gen Hosp Psychiatry 15:224–233, 1993

Schacter DL: Searching for Memory: The Brain, the Mind, and the Past. New York, Basic Books, 1996

Seivewright H, Tyrer P, Johnson T: Change in personality status in neurotic disorders. Lancet 359:2253–2254, 2002

Shea MT, Pilkonis PA, Beckham E: Personality disorders and treatment outcome in the NIMH Treatment of Depression Collaborative Research Program. Am J Psychiatry 147:711–718, 1990

Siever LJ, Davis KL: A psychobiological perspective on the personality disorders. Am J Psychiatry 148:1647–1658, 1991

Soloff P: Psychopharmacological treatment of borderline personality disorder. Psychiatr Clin North Am 23:169–192, 2000

Stevenson J, Meares R: An outcome study of psychotherapy for patients with borderline personality disorder. Am J Psychiatry 149:358–362, 1992

Torgersen S, Lygren S, Oien PA, et al: A twin study of personality disorders. Compr Psychiatry 41:416–425, 2000

Torgersen S, Kringlen E, Cramer V: The prevalence of personality disorders in a community sample. Arch Gen Psychiatry 58:590–596, 2001

Weissman MM: The epidemiology of personality disorders: a 1990 update. J Personal Disord 3 (suppl 7):44–62, 1993

World Health Organization: International Classification of Diseases, 10th Edition. Geneva, Switzerland, World Health Organization, 1992

Zanarini MC: Borderline personality as an impulse spectrum disorder, in Borderline Personality Disorder: Etiology and Treatment. Edited by Paris J. Washington, DC, American Psychiatric Press, 1993, pp 67–86

Zanarini MC: Childhood experiences associated with the development of borderline personality disorder. Psychiatr Clin North Am 23:89–101, 2000

Zanarini MC, Frankenburg FR, Khera GS, et al: Treatment histories of borderline inpatients. Compr Psychiatry 42:144–150, 2001

Zoccolillo M, Pickles A, Quinton D, et al: The outcome of childhood conduct disorder: implications for defining adult personality disorder and conduct disorder. Psychol Med 22:971–986, 1992

8

Epidemiology

Svenn Torgersen, Ph.D.

From clinical work we get an impression of which personality disorders are more common and which are rarer. However, people with some types of personality disorders may be more likely to seek treatment and obtain treatment compared with people with other types of personality disorders. Consequently, if we are interested in how prevalent different personality disorders are in the general population, we have to study representative samples of the general population. Epidemiological research does just that.

Clinical work also gives us ideas about relationships between socioeconomic and sociodemographic factors and personality disorders. However, in a clinical setting we only meet those from an unfavorable environment who have developed a personality disorder. We do not meet those from an unfavorable environment who have *not* developed a disorder. Furthermore, the combination of a specific personality disorder and specific sociodemographic features may increase the likelihood of a particular person to seek treatment. These complexities mean that only population (epidemiological) studies can demonstrate the "true" relationship between personality disorders and socioeconomic and sociodemographic variables, or any other variables such as traumata, disastrous events, upbringing, or partner relationships.

PREVALENCE

We know much about the prevalence of Axis I disorders in the general population (Kringlen et al. 2001). As to personality disorders, however, less is known. Some studies have been performed, but few of them adequately represent the general population (Torgersen et al. 2001). In this chapter I review published studies that are closest to what one might call an epidemiological population study. These individual studies are discussed below in view of different elements of epidemiology, beginning with a discussion of sample selection for each study.

Sample Selection

The sample studied by Zimmerman and Coryell (1989, 1990) included first-degree relatives of normal subjects (23%) and of psychiatric patients (mood disorders and schizophrenia) as well as a smaller group of first-degree relatives of nonpsychotic psychiatric patients. Thus, even if this is a "nonpatient sample" it is not an average population sample. However, the prevalence of mania was not higher than 2%, and the prevalence of schizophrenia was not higher than 1%. Twenty-seven percent of the interviews were conducted in person and the remainder by telephone. The Structured Interview for DSM-III Personality Disorders was applied (Stangl et al. 1985). The study took place in Iowa City.

The sample reported on by Black et al. (1993) consisted of 120 relatives of 32 outpatients with obsessive-compulsive disorder and 127 relatives of a comparison group screened for Axis I disorders. Strangely, no difference was found between the prevalence of personality disorders in the two relative groups. More than half of the sample were siblings, a quarter were parents, and the rest were children. A little more than half were women. The mean age was 42 years. More than half were interviewed in person and the rest by telephone.

Maier et al. (1992) conducted one of the few reported studies in which the sample is relatively representative of the general population. Control probands were selected by a marketing company to match patients older than age 20 on sex, age, residential area, and educational level. The participants had to have at least one living first-degree relative who also had agreed to be interviewed. Otherwise, this sample represented the general population of a mixed urban/rural German residential area near Mainz. No screening for medical or psychiatric history was performed. The control probands, their spouses, and first-degree relatives constituted the sample.

The sample studied by Moldin et al. (1994) consisted of parents and their offspring in two control groups used in the New York High Risk Project. One of the groups was recruited from two schools in the New York metropolitan area. The other group came from the pool of a population sampling firm. The subjects were white, English-speaking families screened for psychiatric disorder.

In the study by Klein et al. (1995), the sample comprised relatives of a control group screened for Axis I disorders in Stony Brook, New York. The interviews were partly conducted in person and partly by telephone.

Lenzenweger et al. (1997) examined a sample consisting initially of 1,684 undergraduate students from Cornell University in New York. They were screened by means of a questionnaire; a sample of those expected and those not expected to have a personality disorder was interviewed. The total number of subjects interviewed was 258. In this overview (Table 8–1), I apply the actual numbers. The estimated prevalence for any personality disorder is a little different.

The study by Torgersen et al. (2001) was conducted in Oslo, the capital of Norway. A random sample of names of 3,590 citizens between 18 and 65 years of age was selected from the National Register of Oslo. Some had moved out of town, some were impossible to trace,

and some were dead. Others refused to participate or postponed the interview beyond the period of the study (18%). Of the original sample, 2,053 (57%) delivered interviews of sufficient quality for the study. All interviews were performed in person. The sampling procedure made it possible to identify all causes of reduction in the sample from the initial to the final sample. There were almost equal numbers of men and women.

The sampling procedure used by Samuels et al. (2002) was very complicated. Initially, a sample of 3,481 adult household residents in Baltimore was studied in the 1980s. About 10 years later, a subsample was selected that included individuals previously evaluated by psychiatrists or those who appeared to have an Axis I diagnosis based on the Diagnostic Interview Schedule. In addition, a random sample was selected. A number of subjects could not be traced, refused, were too ill to participate, or were deceased. The remaining sample consisted of 742 individuals. Their ages varied between 34 and 94 years, and two-thirds were women.

Results

Table 8–1 presents the prevalences in the published studies discussed above, including all personality disorders. So-called mixed personality disorders, defined by the absence of one criterion for two or more personality disorders and not having the required number of criteria for any disorder, are excluded. Unweighted prevalences (rather than weighted prevalences based on questionable weighting procedures) are presented, because the prevalences among those not reached cannot be known. The qualified, although questionable, guesswork gives one an impression of increased accuracy. A nonweighted rate is transparent and does not claim more than it can stand for.

The prevalence of any personality disorder varies between 3.9% and 22.7%. If the small samples of 303 and under are disregarded, the variation is much less, from 10.0% to 14.3%. The median prevalence of all the studies for any personality disorder is 11.55%, and the pooled prevalence is 12.26%.

As to the specific disorders, the prevalence of obsessive-compulsive and passive-aggressive personality disorders is around 2%, regardless of whether the median or pooled prevalence is used. For avoidant personality disorder, the result for median and pooled prevalence is somewhat different (1.23% vs. 2.92%) because of the high prevalence in the large Norwegian study (Torgersen et al. 2001), perhaps consistent with the low genetic loading of avoidant personality disorder in Norway (Torgersen et al. 2000) (see Chapter 9,

Table 8–1. Prevalences of personality disorders in eight epidemiological studies

	Zimmerman and Coryell 1989	Black et al. 1992	Maier et al. 1992	Moldin et al. 1994	Klein et al. 1995	Lenzenweger et al. 1997	Torgersen et al. 2001	Samuels et al. 2002	Range	Median	Pooled
Place	Iowa	Iowa	Mainz	NYC	New York	New York	Oslo	Baltimore			
Method	SIDP	SIDP	SCID-II	PDE	PDE	PDE	SIDP-R	IPDE			
System	DSM-III	DSM-III	DSM-III-R	DSM-III-R	DSM-III-R	DSM-III-R	DSM-III-R	DSM-IV			
Personality disorder											
Paranoid	0.9	1.6	1.8	0.0	1.8	0.4	2.2	0.7	0.0–2.2	1.25	1.48
Schizoid	0.9	0.0	0.4	0.0	0.9	0.4	1.6	0.7	0.0–1.6	0.65	0.96
Schizotypal	2.9	3.2	0.7	0.7	0.0	0.0	0.6	1.8	0.0–3.2	0.70	1.20
Antisocial	3.3	0.8	0.2	2.6	2.6	0.8	0.6	4.5	0.2–4.5	1.70	1.77
Borderline	1.7	3.2	1.1	2.0	1.8	0.0	0.7	1.2	0.0–3.2	1.45	1.16
Histrionic	3.0	3.2	1.3	0.3	1.8	1.9	1.9	0.4	0.4–3.2	1.85	1.77
Narcissistic	0.0	0.0	0.0	0.0	4.4	1.2	0.8	0.1	0.0–4.4	0.05	0.61
Avoidant	1.3	2.0	1.1	0.7	5.7	0.4	5.0	1.4	0.4–5.0	1.35	2.91
Dependent	1.8	1.6	1.6	1.0	0.4	0.4	1.5	0.3	0.4–1.8	1.30	1.24
Obsessive-compulsive	2.0	9.3	2.2	0.7	3.1	0.0	1.9	1.2	0.0–9.3	1.95	2.09
Passive-aggressive	3.3	10.5	1.8	1.7	1.8	0.0	1.6	—	0.0–10.5	1.80	1.99
Self-defeating	—	—	—	—	—	0.0	0.8	—	0.0–0.83	0.40	0.74
Sadistic	—	—	—	—	—	0.0	0.2	—	0.0–0.19	0.10	0.17
Any personality disorder	14.3	22.7	10.0	7.3	14.8	3.9	13.1	10.0	3.9–22.7	11.55	12.26
Number	797	247	452	303	229	258	2,053	742		5,081	5,081

Note. IPDE=International Personality Disorders Examination; NYC=New York City; PDE=Personality Disorder Examination; SCID-II=Structured Clinical Interview for DSM-IV Axis II Personality Disorders; SIDP=The Structured Interview for DSM-III Personality Disorders; SIDP-R=The Structured Interview for DSM-III-R Personality Disorders.

"Genetics"). If there is cultural pressure in the direction of avoidant behavior, then the prevalence will increase and the genetic estimate will decrease as the environmental estimate increases. However, three of eight studies have found a prevalence above 2%, so the "true" prevalence is probably not much lower. The prevalence of histrionic and antisocial personality disorder is between 1.5% and 2%.

The prevalence of paranoid, dependent, and borderline personality disorder seems to be between 1% and 1.5%. As to schizotypal personality disorder, the difference between median and pooled prevalence is mostly due to large variation among the studies. However, an estimate of 1% may be quite good. Finally, the prevalence of schizoid and self-defeating personality disorder is between 0.5% and 1%, and the prevalence of narcissistic and sadistic personality disorder appears to be even smaller.

Table 8–2 shows a comparison between the prevalences in a large outpatient clinic in Oslo (Alnæs and Torgersen 1988) and in the general population of that city (Torgersen et al. 2001). The ratio between the prevalence in the clinic and that in the population is calculated separately for women and men and in the total sample. There are relatively small differences in the range of the ratios between women and men, even if the ratios are a little larger for the specific personality disorder among men (not for all personality disorders). Those with dependent, borderline, avoidant, and obsessive-compulsive personality disorder are strongly overrepresented among the patients based on prevalence rates in the general population, whereas those with antisocial, schizoid, and paranoid personality disorder are less common in the clinical compared with the general population. To have a borderline, avoidant, or schizotypal personality disorder implies pain and dysfunction, as I discuss later in the chapter. One may speculate that those who are dependent seek help, whereas obsessive-compulsive patients want to do something with their problems, even if they do not suffer as much. In the other direction, those who are antisocial do not want psychological help and are also refused help. Schizoid individuals keep their distance, whereas paranoid subjects do not believe in any cure.

SOCIODEMOGRAPHIC CORRELATES

Gender

Gender differences are common among mental disorders. Women more often have mood and anxiety disorders, and men more often have substance-related disorders (Kringlen et al. 2001). For personality disorders, women and men also differ (Chapter 34, "Gender").

With regard to personality disorders, Zimmerman and Coryell (1989) observed a higher prevalence of personality disorders among males, as did Jackson and Burgess (2000) for ICD-10 screening when regression analysis was applied. However, differences between genders were very small, and Torgersen et al. (2001) did not observe any differences.

As to the personality disorder clusters, Samuels et al. (2002) and Torgersen et al. (2001) reported that Cluster A (odd/eccentric) and Cluster B (dramatic/emotional) personality disorders or traits were more common among men. Among the specific Cluster A disorders, both Torgersen et al. (2001) and Zimmerman and Coryell (1990) found that schizoid personality disorder or traits were more common among men. Zimmerman and Coryell (1990) found this also for paranoid traits, and neither Zimmerman and Coryell (1989, 1990) nor Torgersen et al. (2001) observed any difference for schizotypal personality disorder. Among the Cluster B personality disorders, antisocial disorder is much more common among men (Torgersen et al. 2001; Zimmerman and Coryell 1989, 1990). Those with histrionic personality disorder or traits appear more often to be women (Torgersen et al. 2001; Zimmerman and Coryell 1990). Narcissistic traits are found more often among men, and there are no statistically significant gender differences for borderline personality disorder or traits (Torgersen et al. 2001; Zimmerman and Coryell 1990). Among the Cluster C (anxious/fearful) personality disorders, dependent personality disorder is much more common among women, and obsessive-compulsive personality disorder or traits are found more often among men (Torgersen et al. 2001; Zimmerman and Coryell 1989, 1990); only Zimmerman and Coryell (1989, 1990) reported more avoidant personality disorder and traits among women.

Regarding personality disorders "provided for further study" (American Psychiatric Association 2000), Torgersen et al. (2001)—(but not Zimmerman and Coryell 1989, 1990)—found that men more often had passive-aggressive personality disorder. Torgersen and colleagues also found that women more often presented with self-defeating traits, and men more often presented with sadistic traits.

The most clear-cut results from the studies are that men tend to be antisocial and women tend to be dependent. These results are perhaps not surprising. However, more surprising is a lack of gender difference for borderline traits; in patient samples border-

Table 8–2. Prevalences of personality disorders in the common population and among outpatients in Oslo, Norway

Personality disorder	Females			Males			Total		
	Torgersen et al. 2001	Alnæs and Torgersen 1988	Ratio (range)	Torgersen et al. 2001	Alnæs and Torgersen 1988	Ratio (range)	Torgersen et al. 2001	Alnæs and Torgersen 1988	Ratio (range)
Paranoid	2.2	3.9	1.8 (9)	2.3	7.6	3.3 (9)	2.2	5.0	2.3 (9)
Schizoid	1.1	0.0	0.0 (10)	2.2	5.4	2.5 (10)	1.6	1.7	1.1 (10)
Schizotypal	0.6	3.9	6.5 (6)	0.5	12.0	24.0 (3)	0.6	6.4	10.7 (4)
Antisocial	0.0	0.0	0.0 (10)	1.3	0.0	0.0 (11)	0.6	0.0	0.0 (11)
Borderline	0.9	17.0	18.9 (2)	0.4	9.8	24.5 (2)	0.7	14.8	21.1 (2)
Histrionic	2.5	15.0	6.0 (7)	1.2	10.9	9.1 (7)	1.9	13.8	7.3 (6)
Narcissistic	0.8	1.9	2.4 (8)	0.9	10.9	12.1 (6)	0.8	4.7	5.9 (8)
Avoidant	5.0	53.4	10.7 (3)	4.9	59.8	12.2 (5)	5.0	55.4	11.1 (3)
Dependent	2.0	47.6	23.8 (1)	0.9	45.7	50.8 (1)	1.5	47.0	31.3 (1)
Obsessive-compulsive	1.3	13.6	10.5 (4)	2.6	33.7	13.0 (4)	1.9	19.8	10.4 (5)
Passive-aggressive	0.9	6.3	7.0 (5)	2.2	18.5	8.4 (8)	1.6	10.1	6.3 (7)
Any personality disorder	12.6	76.7	6.1	13.7	90.2	6.6	13.1	80.9	6.2
Number	1,142	206	—	911	92	—	2,053	298	—

line personality disorder is not more prevalent among women than among men (Alnæs and Torgersen 1988; Fossati et al. 2003; Golomb et al. 1995). In one study borderline personality disorder was, in fact, more common among men than among women (Carter et al. 1999). In our unsystematic impression of people, we are more likely to "see" borderline features in women than in men. That schizotypal personality disorder does not show any gender bias will more easily be recognized. A trend in the direction of men being schizoid, narcissistic, and obsessive-compulsive and women being more histrionic is in accordance with common opinion.

Age

To diagnose a personality disorder in an individual under the age of 18 years, the features must have been present at least 1 year (American Psychiatric Association 2000). At the same time, it is assumed that personality disorders start early in life and are relatively stable. For some personality disorders, especially the dramatic types, it is also assumed that they are typical for young people. On the other hand, the older people are, the longer they have had to develop personality disorders, even though personality disorders may also disappear. Suicide and fatal accidents also may happen more often among those with personality disorders than among other individuals. This fact will influence the rate of specific personality disorders in older age.

What does empirical research show? Zimmerman and Coryell (1989) observed that those with personality disorders were younger than those without. Jackson and Burgess (2000) found the same using a short ICD-10 screening instrument (International Personality Disorders Examination screener). Torgersen et al. (2001), however, observed the opposite. This opposite finding can be explained by the high prevalence of introverted and low prevalence of impulsive personality traits in Norway as compared with the United States.

As to the clusters of personality disorders, Torgersen et al. (2001) found that individuals with odd/eccentric personality disorders were older, whereas Samuels et al. (2002) did not find any age variation. For the dramatic/emotional cluster, Samuels et al. (2002) found a higher prevalence among the younger subjects, whereas Torgersen et al. (2001) found that the dramatic/emotional trait dimensions decreased with age. As to the anxious/fearful cluster, neither group observed any age trend.

Among the odd/eccentric personality disorders, schizoid personality disorder or traits seem to be asso-

ciated with being older (Torgersen et al. 2001; Zimmerman and Coryell 1989, 1990). Paranoid personality disorder is unrelated to age (Torgersen et al. 2001; Zimmerman and Coryell 1989, 1990), whereas Zimmerman and Coryell (1989, 1990) observed that those with schizotypal personality disorder were younger, and Torgersen et al. (2001) found that they were older.

Among the dramatic/emotional personality disorders, those with antisocial and borderline personality disorder or traits are younger (Torgersen et al. 2001; Zimmerman and Coryell 1989, 1990), and Zimmerman and Coryell (1990) observed that those with histrionic and narcissistic traits are younger as well. These results are not confirmed by Torgersen et al. (2001).

Zimmerman and Coryell (1989, 1990) did not find any age trend for any of the fearful disorders, whereas Torgersen et al. (2001) observed that individuals with obsessive-compulsive disorder and avoidant traits are older. No difference was found for dependent personality disorders.

Among the proposed personality disorders, Zimmerman and Coryell (1989) found that those with passive-aggressive personality disorder are younger, and Torgersen et al. (2001) observed also that such traits were negatively correlated with age. The latter study also examined self-defeating and sadistic traits and found that sadistic traits were associated with being younger.

To summarize, persons with schizoid personality disorder appear to be older, and persons with antisocial and borderline personality disorder seem to be younger. Perhaps individuals with obsessive-compulsive and avoidant disorders also are older, and those with histrionic and narcissistic disorders are younger. The reason for this age difference in disorders is that people become more introverted and obsessive and less impulsive and overtly aggressive as they age. Thus, the basic relative frequency of odd/eccentric and anxious/fearful versus dramatic/emotional personality disorders in a population will determine whether having any personality disorder is more frequent in younger or older age.

Marital Status

Most of the results concerning marital status are from Zimmerman and Coryell (1989). Some of the data from Torgersen et al. (2001) have been calculated for this chapter to fit the tables in Zimmerman and Coryell (1989) (see Table 8–3).

As illustrated in Table 8–3, subjects with personality disorder have more often been separated or di-

Table 8–3. Marital status and personality disorders, calculated from Torgersen et al. (2001)

Personality disorder	Number	Single (never married)	Married	Separated	Divorced	Widowed	Ever separated[e]	Ever divorced[d]
Paranoid	46	34.8	34.8	6.5	21.7[a]	2.2	15.8	36.7
Schizoid	32	56.3	31.3	0.0	6.3	6.3	20.0	28.6
Schizotypal	12	50.0	33.3	0.0	8.3	8.3	20.0	16.7
Antisocial	12	75.0[a]	8.3[a]	0.0	16.7	0.0	0.0	66.7
Borderline	14	57.1	35.7	7.1	0.0	0.0	20.0	16.7
Histrionic	39	46.2	35.9	0.0	17.9	0.0	0.0	47.6[a]
Narcissistic	17	35.6	52.9	0.0	5.9	5.9	10.0	9.1
Avoidant	102	45.1	36.3	1.0	14.7	2.9	7.5	28.6
Dependent	31	58.1[a]	25.8[a]	3.2	12.9	0.0	11.1	30.8
Obsessive-compulsive	39	41.6	43.6	0.0	10.3	5.1	5.6	21.7
Passive-aggressive	32	35.3	31.3	6.3	9.4	3.1	18.2	31.3
Self-defeating	17	35.3	17.6[a]	0.0	41.2[c]	5.9	25.0	63.6
Sadistic	4	50.0	56.0	0.0	0.0	0.0	0.0	0.0
Eccentric	80	45.6	33.8[a]	3.8	15.0	2.5	13.8	34.1
Dramatic	62	49.3	35.2	1.4	12.7	1.4	8.3	33.3
Fearful	189	45.5	36.5[a]	1.3	14.1	2.6	8.2	28.2
Any personality disorder	269	43.9	36.8[b]	2.2	15.6[a]	1.5	7.9	33.1[b]
No personality disorder	1,784	38.8	46.5	2.4	10.4	1.8	5.1	23.2
Number	2,053	693	830	43	185	33	43	253

[a]X^2–test, $P<0.05$
[b]X^2–test, $P<0.01$
[c]X^2–test, $P<0.001$
[d]Excluding those who are never married
[e]Excluding those who are never married, and those who are divorced

vorced compared with those without a personality disorder, and they are more often divorced at the time of the interview (Zimmerman and Coryell 1989). They are less frequently married (Jackson and Burgess 2000; Zimmerman and Coryell 1989), and they are more often never married (Zimmerman and Coryell 1989). If we include living nonmarried persons with a partner, subjects with personality disorder live more often alone without a partner compared with those without a personality disorder in the general population (Torgersen et al. 2001).

However, as the risk of having a personality disorder is related to gender and age, the real effect of other sociodemographic variables such as marital status is difficult to determine. Younger people are less often married, and education is related to gender and age. The best way to determine the independent effect of other sociodemographic variables is to apply multivariate methods. However, to apply such methods one needs large samples. Thus multivariate methods have been used in very few studies. In the study of Torgersen et al. (2001), such multivariate analyses have been carried out for living alone versus living with a partner.

Those with eccentric personality disorders have more often been divorced or separated, they are more often divorced when interviewed, and are seldom married (Samuels et al. 2002) (Table 8–3). Those with dramatic personality disorders are also often unmarried and live more often alone (Torgersen et al. 2001). Those with fearful personality disorders are also less often married (Samuels et al. 2002) and live more often alone (Torgersen et al. 2001).

When we examine the specific personality disorders, we find little correspondence between the studies by Zimmerman and Coryell (1989) and Torgersen et al. (2001). Marital status does not seem to be as important in the Norwegian study, perhaps because many Norwegians live in stable relationships without being married. When we include "living together with a partner" from the study of Torgersen et al. (2001) and consider this life situation as analogous to marriage, we find more similarity between the two studies. It is important to note that the relationships in the Torgersen et al. study are based on logistic and linear regression analysis, taking into account a number of other sociodemographic variables.

Among the odd/eccentric personality disorders, those with paranoid personality disorder are more often divorced (Table 8–3) and living alone (Torgersen et al. 2001). Those with schizoid personality disorder are more *seldom* separated (Zimmerman and Coryell

1989), less often married (Torgersen et al. 2001), and more often living alone (Torgersen et al. 2001). Those with schizotypal personality disorder have more often been separated (Zimmerman and Coryell 1989) and live more often alone (Torgersen et al. 2001).

The only personality disorder for which the American and Norwegian studies have reached the same conclusion is for one of the dramatic/emotional personality disorders, namely histrionic personality disorder. Persons with histrionic personality disorder have more often been separated or divorced (Zimmerman and Coryell 1989). They are also more often not married when interviewed (Zimmerman and Coryell 1989) and live more often alone (Torgersen et al. 2001). Those with antisocial personality disorder have also more often been divorced or separated (Zimmerman and Coryell 1989), are less often married when interviewed, and live more often alone (Torgersen et al. 2001). Persons with borderline personality disorder also have more often been separated if married, are more often divorced, and are not married when interviewed (Zimmerman and Coryell 1989). They are more often never married, and live more often alone (Torgersen et al. 2001). Finally, those with narcissistic personality disorder also more often live alone (Torgersen et al. 2001).

Among persons with anxious/fearful personality disorders, those with avoidant personality disorder and dependent personality disorder have more often been separated (Zimmerman and Coryell 1989). They are more often separated (Zimmerman and Coryell 1989) and not married when interviewed and live more often alone (Torgersen et al. 2001). Those with obsessive-compulsive traits are less often married (Torgersen et al. 2001).

Among the proposed personality disorders, persons with passive-aggressive personality disorder have more often been divorced and are less often married when interviewed (Zimmerman and Coryell 1989) and live more often alone (Torgersen et al. 2001). Those with self-defeating personality disorder have more often been divorced, are more often divorced and not married when interviewed, and live more often alone (Torgersen et al. 2001).

Education and Income

Very few studies have investigated the relationship between personality disorders and education and income. Torgersen et al. (2001) observed that those with any personality disorder had less education. The same was observed for those with odd/eccentric personality disorders, and those with dramatic/emotional as well as anxious/fearful personality disorder traits. Samuels et al. (2002) confirmed that those with dramatic/emotional personality disorders had less education but not those with odd/eccentric or anxious/fearful personality disorders.

As to the specific personality disorders, results are published only from the study of Torgersen et al. (2001). They observed, applying logistic regression analysis and taking into account a number of other sociodemographic variables, that only those with paranoid and avoidant personality disorders had less education than those without the disorders. Interestingly, those with obsessive-compulsive disorder in fact had *higher* education than those without the disorder.

If the personality disorders are treated as continuous variables by adding traits, we find that all personality disorder traits, except histrionic, narcissistic, and passive-aggressive, are related to education by applying linear regression analysis. All are negatively related except obsessive-compulsive, which is positively related.

Samuels et al. (2002) also investigated the relationship between income and personality disorders but did not find any association. Jackson and Burgess (2000) did not find any relationship to unemployment. It is important to note that all of these studies applied multivariate methods while taking into account other sociodemographic variables.

Urban Location

The study of Torgersen et al. (2001) showed that those living in the populated center of the city more often had a personality disorder. The same was true for all clusters of personality disorders and all specific disorders except antisocial, sadistic, avoidant, and dependent personality.

One may speculate about why there are more personality disorders in the center than in the outskirts of the city. Quality of life is generally lower in the center of the city (Cramer et al. 2004), and there is a higher rate of symptom disorders in the city or in the center of the city (Kringlen et al. 2001; Lewis and Booth 1992, 1994; Marcelis et al. 1998; Sundquist et al. 2004; van Os et al. 2001). One reason may be that the concentrated urban life creates stress leading to personality disorders. Another reason may be that individuals with personality problems drift to the center, where they can lead an anonymous life. A third explanation may be that less social control simply makes it easier to express the less socially acceptable aspects of one's personality. We used to think that excessive social control creates mental problems. Perhaps social control hinders the development of problems—not only aggressive, antisocial personality styles but also accentuated eccentric, narcissistic, impulsive, and extraverted personality styles.

QUALITY OF LIFE AND DYSFUNCTION

Central to the definition of personality disorder are the interpersonal problems, reduced well-being, and dysfunction that personality disorders imply. Only one study has investigated reduced quality of life among those with personality disorders (Cramer et al. 2003). In the sample studied by Torgersen et al. (2001), quality of life was assessed by interview and included the following aspects: subjective well-being, self-realization, relation to friends, social support, negative life events, relation to family of origin, and neighborhood quality. All aspects were integrated in a global quality-of-life index.

The results showed that among the odd/eccentric personality disorders, schizotypal personality disorder implied the most reduced quality of life, followed by schizoid and paranoid personality disorders. Among the dramatic/emotional personality disorders, those with borderline personality disorder had the most reduced quality of life, followed by narcissistic and antisocial personality disorders. Those with histrionic personality disorder had only a slightly reduced quality of life. Among the anxious/fearful personality disorders, those with avoidant personality disorder had the lowest quality of life, followed by dependent personality disorder. Those with obsessive-compulsive personality disorder had only slightly reduced quality of life. Among the personality disorders "provided for further study," those with self-defeating personality disorder (American Psychiatric Association 1987) had somewhat reduced quality of life, whereas those with passive-aggressive personality disorder (American Psychiatric Association 2000) had only slightly reduced quality of life.

A dysfunction index was created by combining quality of life (reversed); the answer to the Structured Interview for DSM-III Personality Disorders–Revised question "do you feel that the way you usually deal with people and handle situations causes you problems?"; the number of lifetime Axis I diagnoses; and any incidence of seeking treatment with varying degrees of seriousness, from private psychologist and psychiatrist—via outpatient and inpatient clinics—to psychiatric hospitals. The dysfunction index was re-

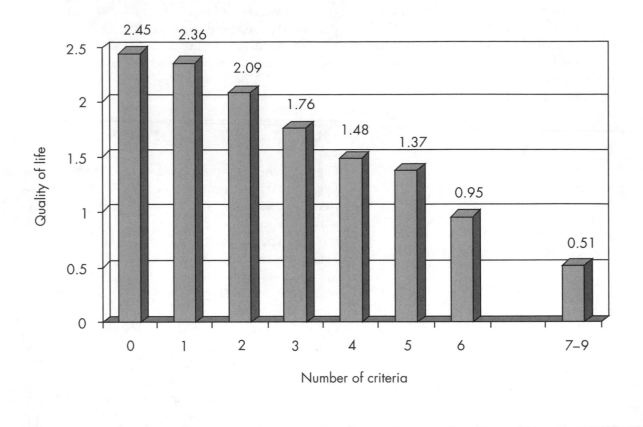

Figure 8–1.   The relationship between maximum number of criteria fulfilled on any personality disorder and quality of life.

As explained in text, the ordinate (quality of life) is a composite of subjective well-being, self-realization, social support, lack of negative life-events, and relation to family, friends and neighbors. The mean is set to 2 and the standard deviation is 1.

lated to personality disorder much as the global quality-of-life index was. The only differences found in comparing results derived from the dysfunction index with those from the global quality-of-life index for dramatic/emotional personality disorders were that those persons with borderline and histrionic personality disorder appeared more dysfunctional, and those persons with antisocial personality disorder appeared less dysfunctional. Among the anxious/fearful personality disorders, those persons with dependent personality disorder became more similar to those with avoidant personality disorder, and among the proposed personality disorders the difference between self-defeating and passive-aggressive personality disorders increased strongly. The reason for the differences is mainly that those with borderline, histrionic, dependent, and self-defeating personality disorders are more likely to seek treatment and those with antisocial and passive-aggressive personality disorders are less likely to seek treatment.

However, the most important result in this study was that for both quality of life and dysfunction, there was a perfect linear dose–response relationship to numbers of criteria fulfilled for all personality disorders together and to the number of criteria fulfilled for any specific personality disorder. Thus, if a person has one criterion fulfilled for any personality disorder, the quality of life is lower and dysfunction is higher than among those with no criteria fulfilled. Those with two criteria fulfilled on any disorder or a specific disorder have more problems than those with one, those with three criteria have more problems than those with two, and so on. When those with zero criteria on all disorders are grouped together—that is, those with a maximum of one criterion on any disorder, those with a maximum of two, and so on—the relationship to global quality of life and dysfunction was perfectly linear (Figures 8–1 and 8–2). This result means that there are no arguments for any specific number of criteria to define a personality disorder if one uses quality of life or dysfunction as validation variables. There is no natural cutoff point.

A high level of dysfunction and disability was also observed among those with schizotypal, borderline,

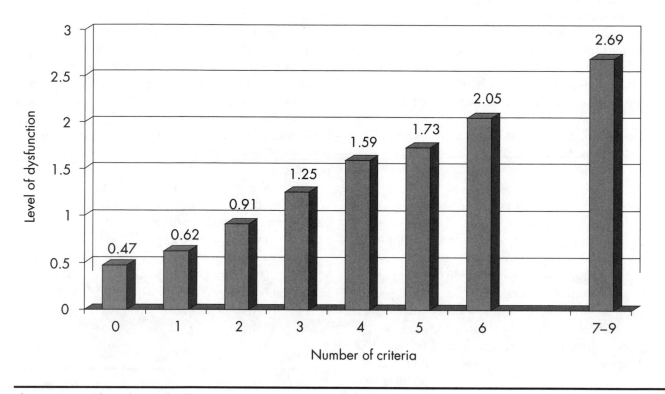

Figure 8–2. The relationship between maximum number of criteria fulfilled on any personality disorder and dysfunction.

As explained in text, the ordinate (dysfunction) is a composite of life quality (reversed), treatment seeking, comorbid Axis I disorders, and the notion that one's behavior causes problems. The mean and standard deviation is 1.

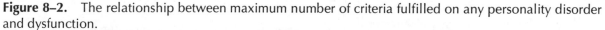

and avoidant personality disorders in a large-scale multicenter study of patients with personality disorders (Skodol et al. 2002). It was also observed that those with obsessive-compulsive personality disorder showed much less disability.

Zimmerman and Coryell (1989) also found a high frequency of psychosexual dysfunction among persons with avoidant personality disorder. Surprisingly, this dysfunction was infrequent for persons with borderline personality disorder, and, not surprisingly, it was also infrequent for those with antisocial personality disorder.

In the future, there is reason to believe that we will see more studies of quality of life, dysfunction, and disability among subjects with personality disorders, either in the general population or in patient samples.

CONCLUSIONS

Personality disorders are prevalent: more than 1 in 10 adult individuals has a personality disorder.

The average prevalence of the specific personality disorders is a little above 1%, somewhat higher for ob-

sessive-compulsive, passive-aggressive, avoidant, histrionic, and antisocial personality disorders, and somewhat lower for sadistic, narcissistic, and self-defeating personality disorders. Two of these low-prevalence disorders, sadistic and self-defeating, are only "provided for further study" in DSM-III-R (American Psychiatric Association 1987), and none of the three exists in ICD-10.

Those with dependent, borderline, obsessive-compulsive, avoidant, and schizotypal personality disorders are overrepresented in patient populations, both overall and when gender is controlled for, whereas those with antisocial, schizoid, and paranoid personality disorders are underrepresented.

The highest prevalences of personality disorders in the general population are observed among subjects with lower education living in populated areas, for example in the city center. They often have a history of divorce and separation and are more often living without a partner.

Men have typically a schizoid, antisocial, or obsessive-compulsive personality disorder, whereas women are more inclined toward a dependent or histrionic personality disorder. Antisocial, borderline, and passive-aggressive personality disorders are more often observed among younger persons, whereas older individuals more often have a schizoid personality disorder. Typical for those with histrionic personality disorder is to have a history of divorces and separations. These individuals—together with those with other dramatic/emotional personality disorders, such as borderline and antisocial personality disorders—are often unmarried, divorced, or generally live alone without a partner. The same is also true for those with passive-aggressive personality disorder.

Lower education is most typical for those with paranoid and avoidant personality disorders, whereas those with obsessive-compulsive personality disorder in fact have higher education than those without the disorder. Those with paranoid, schizotypal, histrionic, and passive-aggressive personality disorders are most inclined to live in the city center.

Personality disorders imply dysfunction and reduction in quality of life, including reduced subjective well-being and self-realization, relational problems, lack of social support, and frequent negative life events.

Among the personality disorders, individuals with schizotypal, borderline, and avoidant personality disorders tend to have the most reduced quality of life, dysfunction, and disability. Individuals with obsessive-compulsive, histrionic, and passive-aggressive personality disorders tend to have the least reduction in quality of life, dysfunction, and disability.

There is an even reduction in quality of life and an even increase in dysfunction for each criterion manifested. Thus, there is a continuous relationship between those with no or small personality problems, those with moderate problems, and those with severe problems. No natural cutoff point exists. Any definition of how many criteria are required for a personality disorder is arbitrary. Even so, to have a definition is important for communication. However, a change in criteria will immediately change the prevalence estimates in the society. Consequently, correlations between personality disorders and other variables are more important than prevalence rates. These correlations appear to be independent of how strictly personality disorders are defined.

Epidemiological research has perhaps changed some stereotypic notions about personality disorders. Personality disorders are more frequent in the general population than we generally believed, especially the introverted personality disorders. Borderline personality disorder is not a "female disorder." Living without a partner is a risk factor for personality disorders, but being unmarried is less a risk factor than many would

have believed. Those living in a partnership without being married function well.

Care must be taken to avoid believing that these correlations display one-directional causal relationships. Personality disorders may hinder obtaining higher levels of education and may be created by socioeconomic difficulties. Problematic personality traits may prevent a person from going into a relationship or may lead to the breaking-up of relationships, rather than having relationship issues and problems causing problematic personality traits.

Personality disorders are not something that a person has for life. Impulsive, aggressive, and extraverted features may decrease with age, whereas obsessive-introverted traits increase as people get older.

Perhaps one of the most important aspects of personality disorders is the reduction of quality of life that is implied. However, a low quality of life does not necessarily create a personality disorder; the opposite is just as likely.

REFERENCES

Alnæs R, Torgersen S: DSM-III symptom disorders (Axis I) and personality disorders (Axis II) in an outpatient population. Acta Psychiatr Scand 78:348–355, 1988

American Psychiatric Association: Diagnostic and Statistical Manual of Mental Disorders, 3rd Edition. Washington, DC, American Psychiatric Association, 1980

American Psychiatric Association: Diagnostic and Statistical Manual of Mental Disorders, 3rd Edition, Revised. Washington, DC, American Psychiatric Association, 1987

American Psychiatric Association: Diagnostic and Statistical Manual of Mental Disorders, 4th Edition. Washington, DC, American Psychiatric Association, 1994

American Psychiatric Association: Diagnostic and Statistical Manual of Mental Disorders, 4th Edition, Text Revision. Washington, DC, American Psychiatric Association, 2000

Black DW, Noyes R Jr, Pfohl B, et al: Personality disorder in obsessive-compulsive volunteers, well comparison subjects, and their first-degree relatives. Am J Psychiatry 150:1226–1232, 1993

Carter JD, Joyce PR, Mulder RT, et al: Gender differences in the frequency of personality disorders in depressed outpatients. J Personal Disord 13:67–74, 1999

Cramer V, Torgersen S, Kringlen E: Personality disorders, prevalence, sociodemographic correlations, quality of life, dysfunction, and the question of continuity. Persønlichkeitsstørungen. Theorie und Therapie 7:189–198, 2003

Cramer V, Torgersen S, Kringlen E: Quality of life in a city: the effect of population density. Social Indicator Research 69:103–116, 2004

Fossati A, Feeney JA, Donati D, et al: Personality disorders and adult attachment dimensions in a mixed psychiatric sample: a multivariate study. J Nerv Ment Dis 191:30–37, 2003

Golomb M, Fava M, Abraham M, et al: Gender differences in personality disorders. Am J Psychiatry 152:579–582, 1995

Jackson HP, Burgess PM: Personality disorders in the community: a report from the Australian National Survey of Mental Health and Well Being. Soc Psychiatry Psychiatr Epidemiol 35:531–538, 2000

Klein DN, Riso LP, Donaldson SK, et al: Family study of early onset dysthymia: mood and personality disorders in relatives of outpatients with dysthymia and episodic major depressive and normal controls. Arch Gen Psychiatry 52:487–496, 1995

Kringlen E, Torgersen S, Cramer V: A Norwegian psychiatric epidemiological study. Am J Psychiatry 158:1091–1098, 2001

Lenzenweger MF, Loranger AW, Korfine L, et al: Detecting personality disorders in a nonclinical population: application of a 2-stage procedure for case identification. Arch Gen Psychiatry 54:345–351, 1997

Lewis G, Booth M: Regional differences in mental health in Great Britain. J Epidemiol Community Health 46:608–611, 1992

Lewis G, Booth M: Are cities bad for your mental health? Psychol Med 24:913–915, 1994

Maier W, Lichtermann D, Klingler T, et al: Prevalences of personality disorders (DSM-III-R) in the community. J Personal Disord 6:187–196, 1992

Marcelis M, Navarro-Mateu F, Murray R: Urbanization and psychosis: a study of 1942–1978 birth cohorts in the Netherlands. Psychol Med 28:1197–1203, 1998

Moldin SO, Rice JP, Erlenmeyer-Kimling L, et al: Latent structure of DSM-III-R Axis II psychopathology in a normal sample. J Abnorm Psychol 103:259–266, 1994

Samuels J, Eaton WW, Bienvenu OJ III, et al: Prevalences and correlates of personality disorders in a community sample. Br J Psychiatry 180:536–542, 2002

Skodol AE, Gunderson JG, McGlashan TH, et al: Functional impairment in patients with schizotypal, borderline, avoidant, or obsessive-compulsive personality disorder. Am J Psychiatry 159:276–283, 2002

Stangl D, Pfohl B, Zimmerman M, et al: A structured interview for the DSM-III personality disorders. Arch Gen Psychiatry 42:591–596, 1985

Sundquist K, Frank G, Sundquist J: Urbanisation and incidence of psychosis and depression. Br J Psychiatry 184:293–298, 2004

Torgersen S, Kringlen E, Cramer V: The prevalence of personality disorders in a community sample. Arch Gen Psychiatry 58:590–596, 2001

Torgersen S, Lygren S, Øien PA, et al: A twin study of personality disorders. Compr Psychiatry 41:416–425, 2000

van Os J, Hanssen M, Bijl RV, et al: Prevalence of psychotic disorder and community level of psychotic symptoms: an urban-rural comparison. Arch Gen Psychiatry 58:663–668, 2001

Zimmerman M, Coryell W: DSM-III personality disorder diagnoses in a nonpatient sample: demographic correlates and comorbidity. Arch Gen Psychiatry 46:682–689, 1989

Zimmerman M, Coryell WH: Diagnosing personality disorders in the community: a comparison of self-report and interview measures. Arch Gen Psychiatry 47:527–531, 1990

9

Genetics

C. Robert Cloninger, M.D.

MEASUREMENT OF PERSONALITY AND ITS DISORDERS

Measurement is the crux of scientific analysis, so nothing can be stated rigorously about the genetics of personality without initial consideration of fundamental measurement issues that are often ignored in clinical research and practice. Traditionally, personality disorders have been described as a set of discrete categories, as in DSM-IV-TR (American Psychiatric Association 2000) and ICD-10 (World Health Organization 1992), but taxonomic analyses have long shown that such categorical descriptions are inadequate (Eysenck 1986). Efforts to demonstrate the discreteness of different psychiatric disorders have led to inconsistent results both for psychoses and for milder anxiety and depressive disorders (Cloninger et al. 1985; Kendell 1982). Even when it is found that intermediate or combined syndromes are relatively rare, the separation of groups (e.g., patients with schizophrenia versus patients with bipolar disorder) has been incomplete (Cloninger et al. 1985; Sigvardsson et al. 1986). For personality disorders, there is no evidence whatsoever of discrete boundaries between categories or even clusters, and most patients with any personality disorder satisfy criteria for two or more putative categories (Cloninger 1987, 2002b, 2004; Cloninger and Svrakic 2000; Cloninger et al. 1993).

Fortunately, individual differences in personality can be measured well in terms of multiple quantitative dimensions of personality. Essentially the same dimensions of personality are observed whether one begins with normal personality variation in the general community or with symptoms of personality disorder in treatment samples, as described in detail in the next section. Different investigators have described personality traits with differing content depending on their methods and understanding of personality development, but the alternative systems overlap extensively (Cloninger et al. 1994; Livesley et al. 1998; Svrakic et al. 1993; Zuckerman and Cloninger 1996). Fine-grained descriptions are based on 20–30 subscales and higher-order descriptions are based on 5–7 scales resulting from the grouping of the subscales. One comprehensive model is the seven-factor model of temperament and character as assessed by the Temperament and Character Inventory (TCI; Cloninger et al. 1993). The TCI includes dimensions neglected in alternative five-factor models (Svrakic et al. 1993; Zuckerman and Cloninger 1996), particularly Self-Transcendence, which is important in the development of well-being (Cloninger 2004). The TCI distinguishes between *temperament*, defined as individual differences biasing the associative conditioning of responses to simple emotional stimuli, and *character*, defined as individual differences in the supervisory cognitive processes that modulate emotional conflicts. The four TCI temperament dimensions are Harm Avoidance (i.e., anxious vs. risk taking), Novelty Seeking (i.e., impulsive vs. rigid), Reward Dependence (i.e., sociable vs. aloof), and Persistence (i.e., overachieving vs. underachieving). The three TCI character dimensions are Self-Directedness (i.e., purposeful vs. aimless), Cooperativeness (i.e., helpful vs. hostile), and Self-Transcendence (i.e., insightful vs. repressive). Each of these seven dimensions has unique genetic determinants that modulate specific brain circuitry carrying on distinct information-processing tasks (Cloninger 2002a; Gillespie et al. 2003; Gusnard et al. 2003; Turner et al. 2003). Initially temperament traits were expected to be more heritable than character traits, but nothing about the model required this to be so. Empirical studies have now shown that temperament and character differ in terms of their psychological functions and brain circuitry but not in their degree of heritability (Cloninger 2004).

Extensive clinical research has shown that putative categories of personality disorder have a characteristic multidimensional profile that allows diagnoses to be made without the redundancy that results from lists of categorical items (Cloninger 2000b). For example, Cluster A personality disorders are distinguished by low Reward Dependence (e.g., aloofness), Cluster B by high Novelty Seeking (e.g., anger), and Cluster C by high Harm Avoidance (e.g., anxiety). Empirically, when a fourth cluster is identified, it is distinguished by high Persistence as seen in anankastic or obsessional personality disorders. Individuals often satisfy criteria for disorders in multiple clusters because the four temperaments are nearly uncorrelated with one another phenotypically and have little or no genetic overlap. The clinical and genetic independence of the temperament dimensions means that all possible combinations of high or low scores occur. For example, individuals with borderline or explosive temperament configurations are defined as those individuals high in both Harm Avoidance and Novelty Seeking and low in Reward Dependence. Such explosive individuals have strong approach-avoidance conflicts and emotional instability, which is characteristic of both Clusters B and C in DSM-IV-TR (Cloninger 1987; Cloninger and Svrakic 2000). Such multidimensional patterns of temperament and character influence susceptibility to specific patterns of comorbid psychopathology (Cloninger 2002b; Cloninger et al. 1998). Personality configurations are predictive of susceptibility to illness and patterns of comorbidity throughout the full range of psychopathology (Battaglia et al. 1996; Cloninger et al. 1994), including anxiety disorders (Jiang et al. 2003), eating disorders (Anderson et al. 2002), substance dependence (Howard et al. 1997), somatoform disorders (Cloninger 1986), mood disorders (Cloninger et al. 1998), and schizophrenia (Szoke et al. 2002).

John Livesley and his colleagues (1993) developed the Dimensional Assessment of Personality Pathology (DAPP) to measure the self-report of a hierarchy of dimensions of personality problems. The questionnaire is composed of 560 items measuring 18 dimensions derived by factor analysis, each with at least three specific facet scales. Factor analysis of the 18 basic scales yields four higher-order factors labeled Emotional Lability or Dysregulation, Antagonism or Dissocial Behavior, Interpersonal Unresponsiveness or Inhibition, and Compulsivity (Jang et al. 1996; Livesley et al. 1998). These higher-order dimensions of abnormal personality resemble the dimensions of normal personality, such as the dimensions of the five-factor model (FFM), which includes Neuroticism, Extraversion, Openness to Experience, Agreeableness, and Conscientiousness as assessed in the NEO personality inventory (Costa and McCrae 1990). For example, DAPP Emotional Lability or Dysregulation is similar to high Neuroticism in the FFM and low Self-Directedness in the TCI. Antagonism or Dissocial Behavior is similar to low Agreeableness in the FFM and low Cooperativeness in the TCI. Hence these dimensions define healthy personality at one extreme (namely, high TCI Self-Directedness and Cooperativeness, or low DAPP Emotional Dysregulation and Dissocial Behavior, or low NEO Neuroticism and Agreeability) and personality disorder at the other extreme (e.g., low TCI Self-Directedness and Cooperativeness) (Livesley et al. 1998; Svrakic et al. 1993).

CORRESPONDENCE BETWEEN NORMAL AND ABNORMAL PERSONALITY STRUCTURE

One of the most robust findings about personality, but one that is surprising to many psychiatrists, is that the same dimensions of personality observed in the general population account well for the personality variation observed in psychiatric patients. Patients with personality disorders and other forms of psychopathology have extreme values on one or more personality dimensions, but the dimensional structure is the same in samples from the general community and from psychiatric treatment facilities (Cloninger et al. 1994; Krueger 1996, 1999a, 1999b; Livesley et al. 1998; Sigvardsson et al. 1987; Svrakic et al. 1993). This shared structure is surprising to those who assume that personality only colors the expression of mental disorders, which are assumed to be independent and discrete entities. Rather, many studies have demonstrated either strong correlations among measures of normal and abnormal personality (Cloninger and Svrakic 1994; Costa and McCrae 1990; Duggan et al. 2003) or joint loadings of measures of normal and abnormal personality on the same factors (DiLalla et al. 1993). The genetic structure of normal and abnormal personality traits in studies of twins is indistinguishable, suggesting that influences on normal and abnormal personality act through systems common to both, whether the twins are reared together (Livesley et al. 1998) or apart (Markon et al. 2002). Furthermore, the genetic and environmental structure of personality is indistinguishable from that of common mental disorders (Krueger 1996, 1999b). In other words, the risk of common mental disorders can be well explained as clinical manifestations of personality traits. Childhood personality is also moderately predictive of adult personality and psychopathology, suggesting that personality measures susceptibility to psychopathology to the degree that personality and psychopathology are heritable (Krueger 1996, 1999a; Sigvardsson et al. 1987). Together, these replicable findings show that normal personality, abnormal personality, and common mental disorders share a common causal foundation. In other words, the same biopsychosocial systems influence individual differences in normal personality and its disorders.

THE INHERITANCE OF PERSONALITY DISORDER SYMPTOMS AND CATEGORIES

Prior to 1993, most work on the inheritance of personality disorders was carried out with categorical diagnoses, as reviewed elsewhere (Thapar and McGuffin 1993). Family, twin, and adoption studies provided clear evidence for the moderate heritability of schizotypal personality disorder and antisocial personality disorder (ASPD), which were the most studied personality disorders up to that time. The most thoroughly studied personality disorder is ASPD, which is commonly ascertained through studies of convicted criminals. Adoption studies of ASPD (Crowe 1972, 1974), psychopathy (Schulsinger 1972), and criminality (Cloninger et al. 1975c; Mednick et al. 1984) were carried out in the United States and Scandinavia, all showing substantial heritable influences. Interactions between genetic predisposition and childhood rearing in an unstable environment were also demonstrated for petty criminality and ASPD (Cadoret et al. 1985; Cloninger et al. 1975c). Monozygotic (MZ) twins were also more often concordant for criminality than were

dizygotic (DZ) twins, as reviewed in detail elsewhere (Cloninger and Gottesman 1987). The concordances for criminality and ASPD were predicted by differences in severity of liability by a function proportional to the inverse of the prevalence in the general population, indicating that susceptibility was inherited to an underlying quantitative variable like personality (Cloninger et al. 1975a, 1975b). For example, ASPD is less frequent in women than in men, so antisocial women have a stronger genetic loading (measured by more antisocial relatives) than do antisocial men.

Schizotypal personality disorder has also been extensively studied as a categorical diagnosis in family, twin, and adoption studies of schizophrenia. There is a consistently greater incidence of schizotypal individuals among the relatives of schizophrenic probands than among normal control subjects but less consistent evidence of an excess of schizophrenic individuals among the relatives of schizotypal probands, as reviewed elsewhere (Thapar and McGuffin 1993). This asymmetry in results may be explained by the lower severity of liability represented by schizotypal probands or heterogeneity within schizotypal personality disorder. More recent work using quantitative multidimensional measures of schizotypy indicates that schizotypy is multidimensional and genetically heterogeneous. For example, the positive and negative components of schizotypy are both moderately heritable and genetically independent, although each may contribute to cognitive disorganization (Linney et al. 2003). Only the eccentric, affect-constricted aspect of schizotypal personality disorder may be within the heritable spectrum of schizophrenia (Lyons et al. 1994; Squires-Wheeler et al. 1989; Torgersen et al. 2000).

Since 1993, the inheritance of personality disorders has been studied primarily through use of quantitative scales that measure individual differences in the number of symptoms of personality disorder, because quantitative scales contain more information than is present when a categorical diagnosis is made. Quantitative measurement has also led to information about the full range of symptoms observed in personality disorders as defined in international classifications. An excellent set of studies has been carried out by John Livesley and his colleagues using the DAPP. This questionnaire, briefly described earlier in the chapter, was developed on the basis of linear factor analyses that identified a stable structure underlying personality disorders in clinical and nonclinical subjects (Jang et al. 1996, 1998; Livesley et al. 1993, 1998). The median heritability estimates from these twin studies was 45%. Most dimensions of personality disorder symp-

Table 9–1.   A study of categorical personality disorders assessed by SCID-II interviews in 92 MZ twin pairs and 129 DZ twin pairs in Norway

Diagnoses	MZ correlation	DZ correlation	Heritability
Any personality disorder	0.58 ± 0.10	0.36 ± 0.10	0.44 ± 0.20
Any Cluster A	0.37 ± 0.14	0.09 ± 0.11	0.37 ± 0.25
Any Cluster B	0.60 ± 0.11	0.31 ± 0.12	0.59 ± 0.23
Any Cluster C	0.61 ± 0.09	0.23 ± 0.11	0.59 ± 0.20

Note.   DZ=dizygotic; MZ=monozygotic; SCID-II=Structured Clinical Interview for DSM-IV Axis II Personality Disorders.
Source.   Adapted from Torgersen et al. 2000

toms show moderate heritability (40%–60%), as shown in Table 9–1 (Jang et al. 1996). Moderate heritability was also observed for most traits even after regression on the four higher-order factors previously described, suggesting that each basic scale measures genetic variability not explained by the higher-order dimensions (Livesley et al. 1998). Overall, the genetic and environmental structure of personality disorder symptoms was indistinguishable from that of normal personality, suggesting a continuity between normal and disordered personality (Livesley et al. 1993, 1998). Other studies using other instruments and age groups have obtained similar results indicating both the moderate heritability of personality disorder symptoms and continuity between normal and disordered personality (Coolidge et al. 2001; Markon et al. 2002; Samuels et al. 2000).

One twin study based on a wide range of categorical diagnoses has been carried out in Norway by Svenn Torgersen and his colleagues (Torgersen et al. 2000). They identified 92 MZ twin pairs and 129 DZ twin pairs in which at least one proband had a diagnosis of personality disorder, and they divided the cases according to DSM clusters and categories. The probandwise concordances for any definite personality disorder were 40% for MZ pairs and 29% for DZ pairs, indicating substantial genetic influences ($P<0.01$), as summarized in Table 9–2. Concordance for membership in personality disorder clusters also could not be explained without taking genetic variability into account. Estimates of heritability for the clusters and specific categories were moderate (i.e., between 40% and 60%), much as observed for quantitative measures of normal and abnormal personality traits (Eaves et al. 1989; Jang et al. 1996). The correlations between DZ twins were usually less than half of those of MZ pairs, suggesting that gene–gene and gene–environment interactions are as important for categorical diagnoses as they are for personality dimensions in twins reared apart (Bergeman et al. 1993; Pedersen et al. 1991; Plomin et al. 1998;

Tellegen et al. 1988). The small number of individuals with particular categorical diagnoses made any conclusions about the heritability of individual categories of personality in Torgersen's twin study imprecise, as shown by the large standard errors even for broad clusters of diagnoses shown in Table 9–2. For example, most of the individuals with a Cluster B personality disorder in Torgersen's study had borderline personality disorder. As a result, the authors found significant evidence that genetic factors influence vulnerability to borderline personality disorder, but the estimate of the magnitude of its heritability is imprecise due to the small number of cases. Nevertheless, the consistency of the overall results with those of studies of personality models derived by linear factor analysis indicates that personality and its disorders are moderately heritable and approximately equally influenced by genetic factors and other factors unique to each individual. The influence of environmental influences shared by siblings reared together accounts for less than 10% of the variance in personality and its disorders (Eaves et al. 1989; Jang et al. 1996; Livesley et al. 1993, 1998; Pedersen et al. 1988).

THE INHERITANCE OF GENERAL PERSONALITY DIMENSIONS

The personality dimensions relevant to the regulation of gene expression in the brain are expected to be interactive with one another because of the nonlinear nature of complex adaptive systems and extensive evidence that the extremes of personality dimensions are reproductively disadvantageous (Cloninger 2000a). The nonlinear nature of personality was foreseen in the development of the seven-factor model of personality assessed by the TCI (Cloninger et al. 1993). The TCI was developed as a set of scales measuring specific psychological constructs. No effort was made to

Table 9–2. Heritability and concordances in 236 MZ twin pairs and 247 DZ twin pairs for the 18 basic scales of the Differential Assessment of Personality Pathology in Canada

Scale label	MZ correlation	DZ correlation	Heritability
Affective lability	0.49	0.12	0.45
Anxiousness	0.42	0.25	0.44
Callousness	0.56	0.32	0.56
Cognitive distortion	0.48	0.31	0.49
Compulsivity	0.40	0.19	0.37
Conduct problems	0.53	0.36	0.56
Identity problems	0.51	0.28	0.53
Insecure attachment	0.45	0.27	0.48
Intimacy problems	0.47	0.24	0.48
Narcissism	0.51	0.22	0.53
Oppositionality	0.41	0.29	0.46
Rejection	0.33	0.19	0.35
Restricted expression	0.48	0.26	0.41
Self-harm	0.39	0.26	0.41
Social avoidance	0.52	0.27	0.53
Stimulus-seeking	0.38	0.21	0.40
Submissiveness	0.41	0.29	0.45
Suspiciousness	0.42	0.29	0.45

Note. DZ=dizygotic; MZ=monozygotic.
Source. Adapted from Jang et al. 1996.

select or combine items in such a way as to give the appearance that the relations between the dimensions were linear or functionally independent, as is done in tests derived by factor analytic methods. Each of the seven dimensions can be described as unique because most of the correlation coefficients among dimensions are negligible (<0.25) and none is strong (>0.70). Nevertheless, each dimension has a correlation with at least one other dimension, and these vary in magnitude from weak (0.25–0.39) to moderate (0.40–0.59).

Initial twin studies were carried out using only measures of temperament (Heath et al. 1994; Stallings et al. 1996). More recent studies have used the TCI and show that each of the seven TCI dimensions has a unique genetic variance that is not explained by the other dimensions (Gillespie et al. 2003). The TCI includes heritable dimensions of personality that are neglected in five-factor models, including TCI Self-Transcendence and TCI Reward Dependence (Svrakic et al. 1993; Zuckerman and Cloninger 1996). A sample of 2,517 Australian twins aged 50 years or older between 1993 and 1995 completed the TCI. The correlation between each of the seven TCI dimensions of personality was higher in MZ twin pairs than in DZ twin pairs, suggesting significant genetic effects for each dimension. Heritability was derived using a standard multivariate model that is similar to estimating total genetic

effects from twice the difference between the correlations of MZ minus DZ twin pairs. For example, for Harm Avoidance the correlations in female MZ twins was 0.47 and that in female DZ twins was 0.21, so twice the difference of 0.26 gives an estimate of 52% heritability. The estimates of heritability for each TCI dimension based on both male and female twins are summarized in Table 9–3. Total genetic effects or heritability varied from 27%–45%, without correcting for the reliability of the short forms of the TCI used in this study, and correction for reliability showed that each dimension was moderately heritable. Each dimension still had significant unique genetic variance when any overlap with other dimensions was taken into account. Both additive genetic and environmental influences unique to each individual were significant. Environmental influences shared by twin pairs reared together did not improve the fit of the model to the data. Hence, higher cognitive processing, as measured by TCI character traits, was found to be as heritable as emotional processing, as measured by TCI temperament traits. Nongenetic influences unique to each individual influence each dimension of personality as much as do genetic factors.

These studies of twins did suggest substantial genetic effects on human personality, warranting subsequent molecular genetic studies of linkage and associ-

Table 9–3.   Total genetic effects (heritability) of each of the seven TCI personality dimensions estimated in 2,517 twins in Australia

Personality dimension	Genetic effects	
	Total percentage	Unique percentage
Harm Avoidance	42	29
Novelty Seeking	39	32
Reward Dependence	35	20
Persistence	30	23
Self-Directedness	34	25
Cooperativeness	27	16
Self-Transcendence	45	26

Note. Unique effects exclude genetic contributions shared with other personality dimensions.
TCI = Temperament and Character Inventory.
Source. Adapted from Gillespie et al. 2003.

ation (Benjamin et al. 2002; Cloninger 1998). Many twin studies suggest heritabilities of about 50% for most complex personality and cognitive traits, including the dimensions of the three-, five-, and seven-factor models of personality (Eaves et al. 1989; Gillespie et al. 2003; Heath et al. 1994; Pedersen et al. 1988; Stallings et al. 1996). However, these estimates of additive genetic effects are inflated by gene–gene and gene–environmental interactions that have a greater influence on MZ than on DZ twins (Cloninger et al. 1979). These interactions indicate that particular combinations of genetic and environmental factors interact in ways that cannot be explained by their average effects—that is, the whole is more than the sum of its parts. Adoption studies indicate that the heritability of personality is about 20%–30% (Cloninger 1998; Loehlin 1992; Plomin et al. 1998) rather than 50%. The discrepancy between twin and adoption studies suggests that the estimates of heritability in twin studies are inflated by gene–gene and gene–environment interactions or that the estimates in adoption studies are reduced by the effects that distinguish the members of two generations, such as age and cohort effects. Either explanation involves nonadditive interactions among multiple genetic and environmental factors; thus, the whole personality is more than the sum of its individual parts. Unfortunately, twin studies have little or no power to test their Mendelian assumptions, such as the assumption that the total genetic effects are additive (Gillespie et al. 2003; Plomin et al. 1998; Torgersen et al. 2000). A practical consequence of these limitations is that the probable nonadditive interactions between genes must be examined directly by measuring

specific genetic polymorphisms in molecular genetic studies of linkage and association (Benjamin et al. 2002) and then carrying out studies of gene–environment interaction (Caspi et al. 2003; Keltikangas-Jarvinen et al. 2004). There is now substantial direct evidence that personality development depends on the nonadditive effects of gene–gene (Benjamin et al. 2000; Strobel et al. 2003; Van Gestel et al. 2002) and gene–environment (Caspi et al. 2003; Keltikangas-Jarvinen et al. 2004) interactions.

The interactions among a few genes that have been extensively studied in relation to personality illustrate the complex interactions among variables influencing the development of personality and its relationship to psychopathology. Serotonin and dopamine are phylogenetically ancient neurotransmitters that play basic roles in brain function and behavior (Cravchik and Goldman 2000). Extensive diversity in the regulation of serotonin and dopamine function has been studied sufficiently in relation to personality to identify some general epigenetic principles. Some of the genetic polymorphisms that have been studied most extensively are genes that promote, transport, and catabolize these key neurotransmitters. The marked differences in such neurotransmitter functions between individuals is of special interest because they modulate individual differences in personality (Borg et al. 2003; Cloninger 1987; Ding et al. 2002; Hamer et al. 1999; Strobel et al. 2003).

In the human prefrontal cortex, the enzyme catechol-*O*-methyltransferase (COMT) is critical in the metabolic degradation of dopamine, and by regulating dopamine availability, it can influence personality and cognitive function. The *COMT* gene has a common variant (i.e., polymorphism) involving the substitution of valine (Val) by methionine (Met) at position 158. Individuals who are homozygous *Met/Met* have fourfold less activity than *Val/Val* or *Val/Met* individuals. Individuals with the low-activity form of COMT (i.e., *Met/Met* homozygotes) have been found to have higher scores in TCI Harm Avoidance and to have low-voltage alpha activity on electroencephalography more frequently than others (Enoch et al. 2003).

The expression of the serotonin transporter is regulated by a promoter polymorphism that is unique in humans and simian primates (Reif and Lesch 2003). Its low-activity form (i.e., short allele) interacts nonlinearly with stressful life events to increase susceptibility to depression, illustrating the importance of gene–environment interaction (Caspi et al. 2003). The short allele has been associated with anxiety-related traits such as neuroticism, which confound high Harm Avoidance with the low Self-Directedness and low Cooperativeness seen in personality disorders. The less active short allele of the serotonin transporter promoter may be more strongly associated with low TCI Self-Directedness and low TCI Cooperativeness than with the temperament trait of Harm Avoidance (Hamer et al. 1999; Thierry et al. 2004).

Furthermore, the high-activity forms of COMT (*Val/Val* or *Val/Met*) have increased dopamine catabolism in the prefrontal cortex, which impairs prefrontal brain physiology and increases perseverative errors in the Wisconsin Card Sorting Test, and which has been found to slightly increase the risk of schizophrenia (Egan et al. 2001). The genotype explained 4% of the variance in perseverative errors—that is, having difficulty switching strategies when an error is made. The relationship was further supported by studies of prefrontal physiology on functional magnetic resonance imaging during a working memory task and by a family study showing the increased transmission of the *Val* allele to schizophrenic offspring (Egan et al. 2001).

Such findings about a single gene have often proven to be inconsistently replicable when they are studied by many independent groups, as has been the case with the association of the dopamine receptor gene *DRD4* and Novelty Seeking (Kluger et al. 2002; Schinka et al. 2002). Such inconsistent results need to be evaluated within the general context of the role of personality dimensions as moderator variables in nonlinear adaptive systems. As a result of their nonlinear function as moderators, the inheritance of personality is expected to involve gene–gene and gene–environment interactions (Keltikangas-Jarvinen et al. 2004; Kluger et al. 2002). For most quantitative traits, individuals with intermediate values are usually adapted better than individuals with extremely high or low values. In contrast, individuals at the each extreme of a quantitative trait are more prone to disorders and are less well adapted than intermediate individuals. For example, type 1 and type 2 alcoholism may be at opposite extremes of the epigenetic regulation of alcohol consumption, with type 1 alcoholics being mature but excessively Harm Avoidant and type 2 alcoholics being immature and excessively Novelty Seeking (Cloninger 2004). Other intermediate personality profiles provide sufficient checks and balances to maintain normative drinking, but both extremes increase susceptibility to problems. Unless the relevant interacting biopsychosocial variables are simultaneously measured, results with individual variables in different samples are expected to be inconsistent despite their validity in some contexts.

Molecular genetic studies on Novelty Seeking confirm the importance of nonlinear gene–gene and gene–environment interactions in Novelty Seeking. A polymorphism of the dopamine transporter is associated with individual differences in initiating and continuing to smoke cigarettes, effects which are mediated by the joint association of cigarette smoking and the dopamine transporter with Novelty Seeking (Sabol et al. 1999). In addition, the *DRD4* exon 2 seven-repeat allele has been associated with high Novelty Seeking and increased risk of opiate dependence (Kotler et al. 1997). Other work has shown that Novelty Seeking is associated with the ten-repeat allele of the dopamine transporter DAT1 when the *DRD4* seven-repeat allele is absent (Van Gestel et al. 2002).

Novelty Seeking also depends on the three-way interaction of *DRD4* with *COMT* and the serotonin transporter locus promoter's regulatory region (*5-HTTLPR*). In the absence of the short *5-HTTLPR* allele (*5-HTTLPR L/L* genotype) and in the presence of the high-activity COMT *Val/Val* genotype, Novelty Seeking scores are higher in the presence of the *DRD4* seven-repeat allele than its absence (Benjamin et al. 2000). Furthermore, within families, siblings who shared identical genotype groups for all three polymorphisms (*COMT, DRD4,* and *5-HTTLPR*) had significantly correlated Novelty Seeking scores (intraclass correlation=0.39 in 49 subjects, $P<0.008$). In contrast, siblings with dissimilar genotypes in at least one polymorphism showed no significant correlation for Novelty Seeking (intraclass coefficient=0.18 in 110 subjects, $P=0.09$). Similar interactions were also observed between these three polymorphisms and Novelty Seeking in an independent sample of unrelated subjects (Benjamin et al. 2000) and have been replicated by independent investigators (Strobel et al. 2003). A similar three-way interaction has been described for the temperament dimension Persistence with *D4DR* and *D3DR* and the serotonin receptor gene type 2c (*5-HT2c*) (Ebstein et al. 1997).

Gene–environment interaction has also been demonstrated for TCI Novelty Seeking in prospective population-based studies (Ekelund et al. 1999; Keltikangas-Jarvinen et al. 2003, 2004). The TCI was administered to two large birth cohorts of Finnish men and women, and the individuals who scored in the top 10% and bottom 10% of TCI Novelty Seeking were genotyped for the exon 3 repeat polymorphism of *DRD4*. The four-repeat and seven-repeat alleles were most common in the Finnish sample (Ekelund et al. 1999; Keltikangas-Jarvinen et al. 2003), as is usual throughout the world (Ding et al. 2002). The two-repeat and five-repeat alleles, which are rare in the Americas and Africa, were more than three times as frequent (16% vs. 5%) in Finns who were very high in Novelty Seeking than in those who were very low in Novelty Seeking (Ekelund et al. 1999; Keltikangas-Jarvinen et al. 2003), and this difference was replicated in an independent sample (Keltikangas-Jarvinen et al. 2003). The association with the two-repeat and five-repeat alleles was strongest for the two most adaptive aspects of Novelty Seeking, exploratory excitability and impulsive decision making (Keltikangas-Jarvinen et al. 2003). Finnish men and women with the two-repeat and five-repeat alleles of the exon 3 *DRD4* polymorphism were higher in Novelty Seeking as adults if they experienced a hostile childhood environment, as measured by maternal reports of emotional distance and a strict authoritarian disciplinary style with physical punishment (Keltikangas-Jarvinen et al. 2004). The mother's reports of childhood environment were obtained when the children were aged 18–21 years, and genotyping and personality assessment of Novelty Seeking was done independently 15 years later. If children had the two-repeat or five-repeat alleles of the *DRD4* polymorphism, their TCI Novelty Seeking scores were high if they were reared in a hostile childhood environment and their Novelty Seeking was low if they were reared in a kind and cooperative environment. Children with certain genotypes are likely to evoke a characteristic pattern of responses from their parents and others, and to select for themselves certain aspects from the available environments (Scarr and McCartney 1983). However, therapeutic environments, such as kind and cooperative parenting, can evoke positive adaptation by modifying gene expression, which depends on the orchestrated interaction of many genes and environmental influences (Keltikangas-Jarvinen et al. 2004). Such complex gene–gene and gene–environment interactions are well documented for other common diseases, such as coronary artery disease and hypertension (Sing et al. 1996; Zerba et al. 2000). For example, a hostile childhood environment is correlated with many variables that are associated with coronary artery disease, such as marital dissatisfaction, type A personality, emotional distance, and a high level of job involvement among fathers (Keltikangas-Jarvinen et al. 2004).

What are the consequences of such complex epigenetic effects for brain activity? Fortunately, the relationship between individual differences in Persistence and the activity of related brain networks has been worked out in detail recently (Gusnard et al. 2003). Persistence was found to be strongly correlated ($r=0.79$) with activation of a well-known circuit for regulation of reward-seeking behavior in a recent functional magnetic resonance imaging study (Gusnard et al. 2003). The circuit includes the ventral striatum, anterior cingulate (Brodmann area 24), and orbitofrontal cortex (Brodmann area 47) bilaterally. Subjects were asked to rate pictures as pleasant, unpleasant, or neutral. As the percentage of neutral pictures in the picture set increased, subjects who were more persistent rated more pictures as pleasant at the expense of neutral pictures ($r=0.34$, $P<0.05$). This selection bias was independent of the percentage of neutral pictures in the sets. There was also a nonlinear interaction between the percentage in brain activity change and the percentage of neutral pictures. The same distributed neural circuit was upregulated (i.e., became more metabolically active) when persistent individuals viewed a high percentage of neutral pictures, but it was downregulated in nonpersistent individuals when they viewed a high percentage of neutral pictures.

These findings show that the regulation of gene expression by personality is mediated by complex adaptive systems made up of multiple genetic and environmental factors. Personality is made up of multiple heritable dimensions composed of unique but partially overlapping sets of epistatic genes (i.e., genes that interact nonadditively with other genes). These developmental systems modulate brain states by modifying the transitory connections between changing distributed networks of neurons. The prominence of gene–gene and gene–environment interactions is characteristic of most common diseases and quantitative phenotypes such as personality traits (Cloninger 2004).

IMPLICATIONS FOR DIAGNOSIS AND CLINICAL PRACTICE

A substantial body of research now shows that personality and its disorders are complex biopsychosocial phenomena influenced by multiple genetic and environmental variables. The psychobiological systems that regulate personality are under "stabilizing" selection in which intermediate phenotypes are favored under most circumstances. Consequently, individuals in the extremes of these complex adaptive networks are vulnerable to psychopathology. To be more specific, the TCI measures seven major dimensions of personality that account for individual differences in both normal and disordered personality traits. Each of these dimensions of personality is influenced by different genes and by variables unique to each individual. Extreme configurations of these dimensions are vulnerable to personality disorders and related psychopathology. Consequently, clinicians can efficiently assess personality and susceptibility to other psychopathology by measurement of variables that can be assessed in every patient as part of an adequate mental status examination and psychiatric history (Cloninger 2000b).

Temperament is moderately stable regardless of treatment but is modulated by character traits that determine the level of a person's maturity and integration. Antidepressants and cognitive behavioral therapy have been shown to increase a person's Self-Directedness (Anderson et al. 2002; Cloninger 2000b; Tome et al. 1997). Such increases in self-awareness initiate a self-organizing spiral of development leading to increasing maturity and well-being (Cloninger 2004). A unified biopsychosocial approach to personality and its disorders is possible by understanding the normal path of personality development along with the genetic and environmental influences that may lead to deviations from that path. The study of the psychobiology of human personality provides the foundation for any coherent understanding of mental disease and mental health.

REFERENCES

American Psychiatric Association: Diagnostic and Statistical Manual of Mental Disorders, 4th Edition, Text Revision. Washington, DC, American Psychiatric Association, 2000

Anderson CB, Joyce PR, Carter FA, et al: The effect of cognitive-behavioral therapy for bulimia nervosa on temperament and character as measured by the temperament and character inventory. Compr Psychiatry 43:182–188, 2002

Battaglia M, Przybeck TR, Bellodi L, et al: Temperament dimensions explain the comorbidity of psychiatric disorders. Compr Psychiatry 37:292–298, 1996

Benjamin J, Osher Y, Kotler M, et al: Association of tridimensional personality questionnaire (TPQ) traits and three functional polymorphisms: dopamine receptor D4 (DRD4), serotonin transporter promoter region (5-HTTLPR) and catechol O-methyltransferase (COMT). Mol Psychiatry 5:96–100, 2000

Benjamin J, Ebstein RP, Belmaker RH (eds): Molecular Genetics and the Human Personality. Washington, DC, American Psychiatric Publishing, 2002

Bergeman CS, Chipur HM, Plomin R, et al: Genetic and environmental effects on openness to experience, agreeableness, and conscientiousness: an adoption/twin study. J Pers 61:159–179, 1993

Borg J, Andree B, Soderstrom H, et al: The serotonin system and spiritual experiences. Am J Psychiatry 160:1965–1969, 2003

Cadoret RJ, O'Gorman TW, Troughton E, et al: Alcoholism and antisocial personality: interrelationships, genetics and environmental factors. Arch Gen Psychiatry 42:162–167, 1985

Caspi A, Sugden K, Moffitt TE, et al: Influence of life stress on depression: moderation by a polymorphism in the 5-HTT gene. Science 301:386–389, 2003

Cloninger CR: A unified biosocial theory of personality and its role in the development of anxiety states. Psychiatr Dev 3:167–226, 1986

Cloninger CR: A systematic method for clinical description and classification of personality variants: a proposal. Arch Gen Psychiatry 44:573–587, 1987

Cloninger CR: The genetics and psychobiology of the seven factor model of personality, in The Biology of Personality Disorders. Edited by Silk KR. Washington, DC, American Psychiatric Press, 1998, pp 63–84

Cloninger CR: Biology of personality dimensions. Curr Opin Psychiatry 13:611–616, 2000a

Cloninger CR: A practical way to diagnose personality disorder: a proposal. J Personal Disord 14:99–108, 2000b

Cloninger CR: Functional neuroanatomy and brain imaging of personality and its disorders, in Biological Psychiatry, Vol 2. Edited by D'Haenen H, den Boer JA, Willner P. Chichester, England, Wiley, 2002a, pp 1377–1385

Cloninger CR: Implications of comorbidity for the classification of mental disorders: the need for a psychobiology of coherence, in Psychiatric Diagnosis and Classification. Edited by Maj M, Gaebel W, Lopez-Ibor JJ, et al. Chichester, England, Wiley, 2002b, pp 79–106

Cloninger CR: Feeling Good: The Science of Well Being. New York, Oxford University Press, 2004

Cloninger CR, Gottesman II: Genetic and environmental factors in antisocial behavior disorders, in Causes of Crime: New Biological Approaches. Edited by Mednick SA, Moffitt TE, Stack SA. Cambridge, England, Cambridge University Press, 1987, pp 92–109

Cloninger CR, Svrakic DM: Differentiating normal and abnormal personality by the seven-factor personality model, in Differentiating Normal and Abnormal Personality. Edited by Strack S, Lorr M. New York, Springer, 1994

Cloninger CR, Svrakic DM: Personality disorders, in Comprehensive Textbook of Psychiatry. Edited by Sadock BJ, Sadock VA. New York, Lippincott Williams and Wilkins, 2000, pp 1723–1764

Cloninger CR, Reich T, Guze SB: The multifactorial model of disease transmission, II: sex differences in the familial transmission of sociopathy (antisocial personality). Br J Psychiatry 127:11–22, 1975a

Cloninger CR, Reich T, Guze SB: The multifactorial model of disease transmission, III: familial relationship between sociopathy and hysteria (Briquet's syndrome). Br J Psychiatry 127:23–32, 1975b

Cloninger CR, Sigvardsson S, Bohman M, et al: Predisposition to petty criminality in Swedish adoptees, II: cross-fostering analysis of gene-environment interaction. Arch Gen Psychiatry 39:1242–1247, 1975c

Cloninger CR, Rice J, Reich T: Multifactorial inheritance with cultural transmission and assortative mating, II: a general model of combined polygenic and cultural inheritance. Am J Hum Genet 31:176–198, 1979

Cloninger CR, Martin RL, Guze SB, et al: Diagnosis and prognosis in schizophrenia. Arch Gen Psychiatry 42:12–25, 1985

Cloninger CR, Svrakic DM, Przybeck TR: A psychobiological model of temperament and character. Arch Gen Psychiatry 50:975–990, 1993

Cloninger CR, Przybeck TR, Svrakic DM, et al: The Temperament and Character Inventory: A Guide to Its Development and Use. St. Louis, MO, Washington University Center for Psychobiology of Personality, 1994

Cloninger CR, Bayon C, Svrakic DM: Measurement of temperament and character in mood disorders: a model of fundamental states as personality types. J Affect Disord 51:21–32, 1998

Coolidge FL, Thede LL, Jang KL: Heritability of personality disorders in childhood: a preliminary investigation. J Personal Disord 15:33–40, 2001

Costa PT, McCrae RR: Personality disorders and the five-factor model of personality. J Personal Disord 4:362–371, 1990

Cravchik A, Goldman D: Neurochemical individuality: genetic diversity among human dopamine and serotonin receptors and transporters. Arch Gen Psychiatry 57:1105–1114, 2000

Crowe RR: The adopted offspring of women criminal offenders: a study of their arrest records. Arch Gen Psychiatry 27:600–603, 1972

Crowe RR: An adoption study of antisocial personality. Arch Gen Psychiatry 31:785–791, 1974

DiLalla DL, Gottesman II, Carey G: Assessment of normal personality in an abnormal sample, in Progress in Experimental Personality and Psychopathology Research, Vol 16. Edited by Chapman LJ, Chapman JP, Fowles D. New York, Springer, 1993, pp 137–162

Ding YC, Chi HC, Grady DL, et al: Evidence for positive selection acting at the human dopamine receptor D4 gene locus. Proc Natl Acad Sci U S A 99:309–314, 2002

Duggan C, Milton J, Egan V, et al: Theories of general personality and mental disorder. Br J Psychiatry 182 (suppl 44):S19–S23, 2003

Eaves LJ, Eysenck HJ, Martin NG: Genes, Culture and Personality: An Empirical Approach. London, England, Academic Press, 1989

Ebstein RP, Segman R, Benjamin J, et al: 5-HT$_{2C}$ serotonin receptor gene polymorphism associated with the human personality trait of reward dependence: interaction with dopamine D4 receptor (D4DR) and dopamine D3 receptor (D3DR) polymorphisms. Am J Med Genet 74:65–72, 1997

Egan MF, Goldberg TE, Kolachana BS, et al: Effect of COMT Val108/158Met genotype on frontal lobe function and risk for schizophrenia. Proc Natl Acad Sci U S A 98:6917–6922, 2001

Ekelund J, Lichtermann D, Jaervelin M-R, et al: Association between novelty seeking and the type 4 dopamine receptor gene in a large Finnish cohort sample. Am J Psychiatry 156:1453–1455, 1999

Enoch MA, Xu K, Ferro E, et al: Genetic origins of anxiety in women: a role for a functional catechol-*O*-methyltransferase polymorphism. Psychiatr Genet 13:33–41, 2003

Eysenck HJ: A critique of contemporary classification and diagnosis, in Contemporary Directions in Psychopathology. Edited by Millon T, Klerman G. New York, Guilford, 1986, pp 73–98

Gillespie NA, Cloninger CR, Heath AC, et al: The genetic and environmental relationship between Cloninger's dimensions of temperament and character. Pers Individ Dif 35:1931–1946, 2003

Gusnard DA, Ollinger JM, Shulman GL, et al: Persistence and brain circuitry. Proc Natl Acad Sci U S A 100:3479–3484, 2003

Hamer DH, Greenberg BD, Sabol SZ, et al: Role of the serotonin transporter gene in temperament and character. J Personal Disord 13:312–327, 1999

Heath AC, Cloninger CR, Martin NG: Testing a model for the genetic structure of personality: a comparison of the personality systems of Cloninger and Eysenck. J Pers Soc Psychol 66:762–775, 1994

Howard MO, Kivlahan D, Walker RD: Cloninger's tridimensional theory of personality and psychopathology: applications to substance use disorders. J Stud Alcohol 58:48–66, 1997

Jang KL, Livesley WJ, Vernon PA, et al: Heritability of personality disorder traits: a twin study. Acta Psychiatr Scand 94:438–444, 1996

Jang KL, Livesley WJ, Vernon PA: A twin study of genetic and environmental contributions to gender differences in traits delineating personality disorder. Eur J Pers 12:331–344, 1998

Jiang N, Sato T, Hara T, et al: Correlations between trait anxiety, personality and fatigue: study based on the Temperament and Character Inventory. J Psychosom Res 55:493–500, 2003

Keltikangas-Jarvinen L, Elovainio M, Kivimaeki M, et al: Association between the type 4 dopamine receptor gene polymorphism and novelty seeking. Psychosom Med 65:471–476, 2003

Keltikangas-Jarvinen L, Raeikkoenen K, Ekelund J, et al: Nature and nurture in novelty seeking. Mol Psychiatry 9:308–311, 2004

Kendell RE: The choice of diagnostic criteria for biological research. Arch Gen Psychiatry 39:1334–1339, 1982

Kluger AN, Siegfried Z, Ebstein RP: A meta-analysis of the association between DRD4 polymorphism and novelty seeking. Mol Psychiatry 7:712–717, 2002

Kotler M, Cohen H, Segman R: Excess dopamine D4 receptor (D4DR) exon III seven repeat allele in opioid-dependent subjects. Mol Psychiatry 2:251–254, 1997

Krueger RF: Personality traits are differentially linked to mental disorders: a multitrait-multidiagnosis study of an adolescent birth cohort. J Abnorm Psychol 105:299–312, 1996

Krueger RF: Personality traits in late adolescence predict mental disorders in early adulthood: a prospective epidemiological study. J Pers 67:39–65, 1999a

Krueger RF: The structure of common mental disorders. Arch Gen Psychiatry 56:921–926, 1999b

Linney YM, Murray RM, Peters ER, et al: A quantitative genetic analysis of schizotypal personality traits. Psychol Med 33:803–816, 2003

Livesley WJ, Jang KL, Jackson DN, et al: Genetic and environmental contributions to dimensions of personality disorder. Am J Psychiatry 150:1826–1831, 1993

Livesley WJ, Jang KL, Vernon PA: Phenotypic and genetic structure of traits delineating personality disorder. Arch Gen Psychiatry 55:941–948, 1998

Loehlin JC: Genes and Environment in Personality Development. Newbury Park, CA, Sage, 1992

Lyons MJ, Toomey R, Faraone SV, et al: Comparison of schizotypal relatives of schizophrenia versus affective probands. Am J Med Genet 54:279–285, 1994

Markon KE, Krueger RF, Bouchard TJJ, et al: Normal and abnormal personality traits: evidence for genetic and environmental relationships in the Minnesota Study of Twins Reared Apart. J Pers 70:661–693, 2002

Mednick SA, Gabrielli WFJ, Hutchings B: Genetic influences in criminal convictions: evidence from an adoption cohort. Science 22:891–894, 1984

Pedersen NL, Plomin R, McClearn GE, et al: Neuroticism, extraversion, and related traits in adult twins reared apart and reared together. J Pers Soc Psychol 55:950–957, 1988

Pedersen NL, McClearn GE, Plomin R, et al: The Swedish Adoption Twin Study of Aging: an update. Acta Genet Med Gemellol (Roma) 40:7–20, 1991

Plomin R, Corley R, Caspi A, et al: Adoption results for self-reported personality: evidence for nonadditive genetic effects? J Pers Soc Psychol 75:211–218, 1998

Reif A, Lesch KP: Toward a molecular architecture of personality. Behav Brain Res 139:1–20, 2003

Sabol SZ, Nelson ML, Fisher C, et al: A genetic association for cigarette smoking behavior. Health Psychol 18:7–13, 1999

Samuels J, Nestadt G, Bienvenu OJ, et al: Personality disorders and normal personality dimensions in obsessive-compulsive disorder. Br J Psychiatry 177:457–462, 2000

Scarr S, McCartney K: How people make their own environments: a theory of genotype greater than environment effects. Child Dev 54:424–435, 1983

Schinka JA, Letsch EA, Crawford FC: DRD4 and novelty seeking: results of meta-analyses. Am J Med Genet 114:643–648, 2002

Schulsinger F: Psychopathy, heredity and environment. Int J Ment Health 1:190–206, 1972

Sigvardsson S, Bohman M, von Knorring AL, et al: Symptom patterns and causes of somatization in men. Genet Epidemiol 3:153–169, 1986

Sigvardsson S, Bohman M, Cloninger CR: Structure and stability of childhood personality: prediction of later social adjustment. J Child Psychol Psychiatry 28:929–946, 1987

Sing CF, Haviland MB, Reilly SL: Genetic architecture of common multifactorial diseases. Ciba Foundation Symposium 197:211–229, 1996

Squires-Wheeler E, Skodal A, Bassett A, et al: DSM-III-R schizotypal personality traits in offspring of schizophrenic disorder, affective disorder, and normal control parents. J Psychiatr Res 23:229–239, 1989

Stallings MC, Hewitt JK, Cloninger CR, et al: Genetic and environmental structure of the Tridimensional Personality Questionnaire: three or four temperament dimensions? J Pers Soc Psychol 70:127–140, 1996

Strobel A, Lesch KP, Jatzke S, et al: Further evidence for a modulation of Novelty Seeking by DRD4 exon III, 5-HTTLPR, and COMT val/met variants. Mol Psychiatry 8:371–372, 2003

Svrakic DM, Whitehead C, Przybeck TR, et al: Differential diagnosis of personality disorders by the seven factor model of temperament and character. Arch Gen Psychiatry 50:991–999, 1993

Szoke A, Schurhoff F, Ferhadian N, et al: Temperament in schizophrenia: a study of the tridimensional personality questionnaire. Eur Psychiatry 17:379–383, 2002

Tellegen A, Lykken TD, Bouchard TJJ, et al: Personality similarity in twins reared apart and together. J Pers Soc Psychol 54:1031–1039, 1988

Thapar A, McGuffin P: Is personality disorder inherited? An overview of the evidence. J Psychopathol Behav Assess 15:325–345, 1993

Thierry N, Willeit M, Praschak-Rieder N, et al: Serotonin transporter promoter gene polymorphic region (5-HTTLPR) and personality in female patients with seasonal affective disorder and in healthy controls. Eur Neuropsychopharmacol 14:53–58, 2004

Tome MB, Cloninger CR, Watson JP, et al: Serotonergic autoreceptor blockade in the reduction of antidepressant latency: personality and response to paroxetine and pindolol. J Affect Disord 44:101–109, 1997

Torgersen S, Lygren S, Oien PA, et al: A twin study of personality disorders. Compr Psychiatry 41:416–425, 2000

Turner RM, Hudson IL, Butler PH, et al: Brain function and personality in normal males: a SPECT study using statistical parametric mapping. Neuroimage 19:1145–1162, 2003

Van Gestel S, Forsgren T, Claes S, et al: Epistatic effects of genes from the dopamine and serotonin systems on the temperament traits of novelty seeking and harm avoidance. Mol Psychiatry 7:448–450, 2002

World Health Organization: International Statistical Classification of Diseases and Related Health Problems, 1989 Revision, Geneva, Switzerland, World Health Organization, 1992

Zerba KE, Ferrell RE, Sing CF: Complex adaptive systems and human health: the influence of common genotypes of the apolipoprotein E (ApoE) gene polymorphism and age on the relational order within a field of lipid metabolism traits. Hum Genet 107:466–476, 2000

Zuckerman M, Cloninger CR: Relationships between Cloninger's, Zuckerman's, and Eysenck's dimensions of personality. Pers Individ Dif 21:283–285, 1996

10

Neurobiology

Emil F. Coccaro, M.D.
Larry J. Siever, M.D.

The study of personality disorder involves the study of both disordered character and disordered temperament. *Character* relates to how we see and operate in our world and is based on how we develop and what we are taught about how to go through life. *Temperament*, in contrast, relates to our innate tendency to behave and to react to any of a variety of challenges presented by other people and our environment. Although both aspects of personality may be studied empirically, the study of temperament is uniquely suited to biological study because temperament has known genetic and neurobiological correlates, both of which are linked to critical processes involving cognition, emotion, and behavior.

The neurobiology of temperament, as it appears in personality disorders, can be studied in a variety of ways, including those that involve behavioral genetics, neuropsychopharmacology and molecular genetics, and psychophysiology and neuroimaging. Behavioral genetic study informs us about the degree to which personality (or temperamental) traits are under genetic influence. This work largely involves studies of families and twins and is designed to document familial, if not genetic, components to behavior. Previous work defining the genetic underpinnings of temperament has been critical to our current understanding that temperament is in-

herently biological in nature. Neuropsychopharmacological study informs us about the nature of brain chemistry and how the regulation of any of a variety of brain neurotransmitters influences temperament. Work in this area has led to the understanding that brain serotonin, for example, is critical in modulating impulsive aggressive behavior in individuals with personality disorder. Consequently, work in neuropsychopharmacology leads to work in molecular genetics whereby the presence of a specific copy of a specific gene (e.g., for a component of the brain serotonin system) influences a temperamental trait. For example, individuals carrying a specific gene for the serotonin transporter may be more anxious than other individuals who do not carry this gene. Finally, work in psychophysiology and neuroimaging brings investigative work up to a level that integrates genes, neuropsychopharmacology, and networks of neural transmission. In this methodology, both brain structure and brain function are examined regarding their contribution to the expression of various temperamental traits. In some groups of patients with personality disorder, neuroimaging has revealed differences in the size and function of specific structures.

Ultimately, the study of the neurobiology of personality disorders is conducted to lead to a more comprehensive understanding of the biological substrates of personality disorder so that better treatments may be discovered and/or so that existing treatments may be improved. Uncovering the biological substrate for a specific temperamental trait naturally leads to treatment strategies aimed at this specific substrate. The best example of this approach is the use of serotonin uptake inhibitors in the treatment of impulsive aggression in personality-disordered individuals. Curiously, work in this area revealed the likely presence of two treatment response groups: one responsive to serotonin uptake inhibitors, the other responsive to mood stabilizers.

In this chapter, we discuss the various aspects of the neurobiology of personality disorder on a cluster-by-cluster basis. We have chosen this organization because the prototypical personality disorders of interest tend to break out into one of the three personality disorder clusters. Despite this type of organization, we should note that research has clearly shown the relevance of a dimensional approach to the study of personality. Each section begins with a brief summary of the phenomenology characteristic of each personality disorder cluster and follows with a summary of data relevant to behavioral genetics, neuropsychopharmacology (and molecular genetics where relevant), and neuropsychology and neuroimaging. Each of the first two sections ends with a brief vignette illustrating some of the points made about the psychobiology of prototypical patients with selected personality disorders.

CLUSTER A PERSONALITY DISORDERS

The Cluster A personality disorders include schizotypal, paranoid, and schizoid personality disorder. The criteria of these disorders capture shared characteristics of social isolation, detachment, suspiciousness, and in the case of schizotypal personality disorder, psychotic-like cognitive/perceptional distortion. Schizotypal personality was formulated in part on the clinical profile observed in relatives of schizophrenic probands, whereas the other two were defined more in a clinical tradition. A high degree of overlap exists between schizotypal and paranoid personality disorder, whereas schizoid personality disorder is not frequently diagnosed in the clinical setting and may represent a milder version of the Cluster A personality disorders. These disorders can be perceived as consisting of a dimension of social deficits (no friends, detached affect) and cognitive impairment, and in the case of schizotypal personality disorder, a psychotic-like dimension. Because of its relationship to schizophrenia and its more common prevalence in clinical populations, most of the neurobiological research on this cluster has focused on schizotypal personality disorder and is summarized here in relation to these dimensions.

Behavioral Genetics

Schizotypal personality disorder is found more frequently in the relatives of schizophrenic probands than in the relatives of control subjects, and this association is grounded in genetics rather than shared familial environment as suggested by adoptive and twin studies (Siever 1991). The genetics of paranoid personality disorder are less well understood, but it has a high overlap with schizotypal personality disorder, and its presence may be greater in families of patients with schizophrenia or delusional disorder (Webb and Levinson 1993). Schizoid personality disorder has received little or no genetic study but is more common in the relatives of patients with schizophrenia (Kalus et al. 1993).

Neuropsychopharmacology

Dopamine System

The dopamine system has been extensively studied in patients with schizophrenia and particularly associated with the psychotic symptoms of this disorder, consistent with the antipsychotic effects of the neuroleptics, which act as dopamine antagonists. Accordingly, given the phenomenological and genetic relationships between schizophrenia and schizotypal personality disorder, the dopaminergic system has been the primary neurotransmitter system studied in schizotypal personality disorder.

Neurochemistry. Plasma homovanillic acid (HVA), a major metabolite of dopamine, has been found to be elevated in clinically selected patients with schizotypal personality disorder, and this elevation is significantly correlated with psychotic-like criteria for this disorder, such that statistical correction for the presence of psychotic-like symptoms abolishes the difference between groups (Siever et al. 1991). An identical configuration of results is found with respect to cerebrospinal fluid (CSF) HVA (Siever et al. 1993). On the other hand, among relatives of patients with schizophrenia, who are generally characterized more by the social and cognitive deficit-like symptoms of schizotypal personality disorder, plasma HVA is lower in subjects with schizotypal personality disorder than control subjects (Amin et al. 1999). In these studies, plasma HVA was negatively correlated with the negative or deficit-like symptoms of schizotypal personality disorder. Interestingly, however, when the negative symptoms were entered as a covariant, the positive relationship with psychotic-like symptoms in plasma HVA emerged (Amin et al. 1997). Reduced plasma HVA concentrations have been associated with impairment in tests of frontally mediated executive function such as the Wisconsin Card Sort Test (Siever et al. 1991). Thus, these results suggest that dopaminergic activity may be relatively increased or decreased depending on the predominance of psychotic-like versus deficit-like symptoms, respectively. This distinction is consistent with formulations that increased dopaminergic activity, particularly in striatum, is associated with psychotic-like symptoms and that decreased dopaminergic activity, particularly in prefrontal regions, is especially associated with deficit-like symptoms (Siever and Davis 2004).

Acute Pharmacological Interventions. Amphetamine, which stimulates the release of the monoamines, particularly dopamine and norepinephrine, has been shown to improve the cognitive performance of schizotypal personality disorder subjects on tests of executive function, working memory, and to a lesser extent, sustained attention and verbal learning (Kirrane et al. 2000; Siegel et al. 1996). These improvements are more consistent than those observed in schizophrenic subjects given amphetamine and are not accompanied by the behavioral worsening—that is, increased psychotic symptoms—found after amphetamine administration in schizophrenic patients. Indeed, the deficit-like symptoms of schizotypal personality disorder tend to improve following amphetamine administration (Laruelle et al. 2002; Siegel et al. 1996). These results suggest that agents that enhance catecholamines, including dopamine, may have beneficial effects on cognition, presumably through stimulation of D_1 receptors in prefrontal cortex.

Similarly, the administration of a glucopyruvic stressor, 2-deoxyglucose, which activates stress-sensitive subcortical systems such as the dopamine system and the hypothalamic-pituitary-adrenal (HPA) axis, results in greater stress-related (i.e., plasma cortisol and HVA) responses in patients with schizophrenia than in normal subjects. In contrast, patients with schizotypal personality disorder show normal (plasma HVA) or even reduced (cortisol) activation compared with control subjects, suggesting that patients with schizotypal personality disorder have better-buffered subcortical stress-responsive systems than patients with schizophrenia. Consequently, it is possible that this buffer provides a protective factor against psychosis in patients with schizotypal personality disorder (Siever and Davis 2004).

Longer-term pharmacological interventions have been evaluated in individuals with schizotypal personality disorder to determine their effects on cognitive function. Preliminary data from studies of guanfacine, an α_2-adrenergic agonist, and pergolide, a D_1/D_2 agonist, suggest improvement in cognitive function, particularly working memory, with these catecholaminergic interventions, consistent with the facilitatory effects of the catecholamines on cognitive function and prefrontal cortex. Cognitive function may also improve with risperidone (Koenigsberg et al. 2003), possibly due to the effects that 5-HT$_2$ blockade has on facilitating dopaminergic activity in frontal lobe. Antipsychotic effects have been documented in a number of clinical trials of atypical and typical neuroleptics in individuals with schizotypal personality disorder (Hymowitz et al. 1986; Schulz et al. 2003).

DNA Polymorphisms. Catechol-O-methyltransferase (COMT) plays a critical role in inactivation of dopamine in the frontal lobe, where the dopamine transporter is not the primary mode of inactivation of dopamine. Recently, a single nucleotide polymorphism in the *COMT* gene has been discovered. With this polymorphism, the allele for the *COMT* gene codes for the amino acid valine (Val), as opposed to methionine (Met), in the COMT enzyme. The substitution of Val for Met leads to a COMT enzyme that has far more activity than a COMT enzyme coded by the *MET* allele. Thus, individuals with *VAL* alleles should have increased activity of COMT compared with those with the *MET* allele. Because increased COMT activity is associated with increased destruction of catecholamines, individuals with *VAL* alleles should have less central dopamine activity than those with *MET* alleles. Consistent with this idea, cognitive impairment, particularly evident in dopamine-dependent working memory, has been associated with the presence of the *VAL* allele in patients with schizophrenia (Weinberger et al. 2001) as well as their healthy siblings and control subjects (Goldberg et al. 2003). Preliminary studies in patients with schizotypal personality disorder also suggest an association between cognitive impairment and the *VAL* allele, consistent with the role of reduced dopaminergic activity hypothesized to contribute to the cognitive dysfunction in the schizophrenia spectrum disorders such as schizotypal personality disorder.

Cognitive Function and Psychophysiology

Although cognitive dysfunction may exist in subtle forms in a variety of personality disorders, the most consistent and robust changes are found in people with Cluster A personality disorders, more specifically schizotypal personality disorder. Patients with schizotypal personality disorder show attenuated patterns of cognitive impairment similar to those of patients with schizophrenia but somewhat more specific. For example, overall intelligence may not be impaired (Mitropoulou et al. 2002; Trestman et al. 1995), whereas specific disturbances in sustained attention, in verbal learning, and particularly in working memory have been reported in patients with schizotypal personality disorder compared with patients with other non-schizophrenia-related personality disorders, the latter of whom are generally not impaired in these indices, and with normal control subjects (Mitropoulou et al. 2002). Although patients with schizophrenia showed deviations from normal control subjects on the order of two standard deviations, patients with schizotypal personality disorder have more on the order of one standard deviation below the mean or less (Mitropoulou et al. 2002). The deficits in working memory and attention may contribute to the impaired rapport and misreading of verbal and facial cues in patients with schizotypal personality disorder, who often clinically complain that they have a hard time focusing on others, which detracts from their ability to engage. Indeed, performances on working memory tasks have been reported to be correlated with interpersonal impairment (Mitropoulou et al. 2002; Siever et al. 2002).

A variety of psychophysiological endophenotypes that may reflect genetic substrates to the schizophrenia spectrum disorders have been found to be abnormal in patients with schizotypal personality disorder as well as in patients with chronic schizophrenia. Many of these psychophysiological abnormalities have also been found in relatives of patients with schizophrenia, who may have mild schizophrenia-spectrum symptoms or may even appear to be clinically healthy, raising the possibility that these abnormalities reflect an underlying genetic susceptibility to the schizophrenia spectrum that is variably expressed. Although a detailed review of psychophysiological abnormalities is beyond the scope of this chapter, abnormalities in eye movement, visual processing, and inhibition of startle response are among the most consistently replicated. Thus, individuals with schizotypal personality disorder showed impaired smooth-pursuit eye movement, antisaccade generation, and velocity discrimination. Furthermore, they show less capacity for inhibition on a prepulse inhibition paradigm and P_{50}-evoked potential paradigm. The latter finding is of particular interest because it has been linked to a specific allele of the nico-

tinic receptor in families of patients with schizophrenia.

Backward masking, reflecting early visual processing, has also been reported to be abnormal in patients with schizotypal personality disorder and schizophrenia (Siever and Davis 2004; see Braff and Friedman [2002] for an overview of these psychophysiologic abnormalities).

Neuroimaging

(See also Chapter 38, "Brain Imaging.")

Structural Imaging

Patients with schizotypal personality disorders show ventricular enlargement and reduced volumes of several brain regions, as do patients with schizophrenia. In studies of patients with schizotypal personality disorder, ventricular volume is increased, although studies of relatives of patients with schizotypal personality disorder are mixed (Shihabuddin et al. 1996; Siever 1995). Temporal volume reductions in patients with schizotypal personality disorder appear to be comparable with those observed in schizophrenic patients and occur in both superior temporal gyrus and other temporal regions. However, some data suggest that frontal volumes are relatively preserved, suggesting that greater frontal capacity may serve as a buffer against the severe cognitive and social deterioration we see in schizophrenia. Whereas striatal volumes of patients with schizophrenia are enlarged secondary (in large part) to neuroleptic medications, the striatal volumes (including putamen [Shihabuddin et al. 2001] and caudate [Levitt et al. 2002]) of patients with schizotypal personality disorder are reduced in comparison with normal control subjects and unmedicated patients with schizophrenia. Reduced striatal volumes are consistent with the possibility of reduced dopaminergic activity, which may be protective against the emergence of psychosis.

Functional Imaging

Both positron emission tomography (PET) and single photon emission computed tomography (SPECT) functional imaging studies suggest that patients with schizotypal personality disorder do not activate regions such as dorsolateral prefrontal cortex in response to an executive function or learning task to the same degree as control subjects, but do so to a greater degree than do patients with schizophrenia. However, patients with schizotypal personality disorder are able to activate other compensatory regions, including the anterior pole of frontal cortex (Brodmann area 10), which is believed to be a high-level executive region (Buchsbaum et al. 2002). A recent functional magnetic resonance imaging (fMRI) study (Koenigsberg et al. 2001) using a visuospatial working-memory task also showed increased activation in patients with schizotypal personality disorder in Brodmann area 10, but lesser activation in dorsolateral prefrontal cortex than in normal control subjects. Thus, patients with schizotypal personality disorder may have compensatory mechanisms available to them that patients with schizophrenia do not have in the face of diminished capacity to use dorsolateral prefrontal cortex. The compensatory mechanisms may involve using higher executive regions than are required for normal individuals.

An IBZM SPECT study measuring dopamine released by displacement of [^{11}C] iodine-methoxybenzamide (IBZM) demonstrated that subjects with schizotypal personality disorder released significantly more dopamine in response to amphetamine administration than did normal control subjects but less than did acute schizophrenic patients (Siever et al. 2002). These results are consistent with functional imaging studies suggesting increased activation of ventral striatum, which is normally inhibited by dopamine, in unmedicated schizotypal patients compared with control subjects and unmedicated schizophrenic patients as well as the reduced plasma HVA responses to 2-deoxyglucose and striatal volumes noted earlier in these studies, suggesting dopaminergic activity that is better buffered than that of schizophrenic patients.

Case Example

Mr. C is a 56-year-old common-law married male, employed in his extended family's business, whose current complaint is that "people at work are accusing me of saying things that I am not saying." Mr. C has been seen by the psychiatry service for more than 20 years, after he was admitted to medicine for complaints of back pain. He was transferred to psychiatry because he "couldn't stand up." He was first psychiatrically hospitalized when he was in the Navy for an episode of "going crazy" after a dispute with his captain. He had symptoms of depersonalization, irritability, and difficulty getting along with his peers. Six years after his tour in the Navy, he saw a therapist but would have vivid dreams that were disturbing to both the therapist and himself, at which point Mr. C states his therapy ended. He has had paranoid ideation, thinking that people at work are against him, although this suspiciousness and ideation are responsive to reality testing, as are his ideas of reference. He has prolonged periods of anhedonia and demoralization but, other than insomnia at times, does not have extensive vegetative symptoms of depression. He has experienced epi-

sodes of depersonalization described as looking down at himself. He complains of low self-esteem but denies worthlessness, hopelessness, or helplessness. Mr. C notes that he was always a loner and had no close friends since the fifth grade. He went to college just before he went to Vietnam. He smokes one pack of cigarettes per day, does not use recreational drugs, and drinks up to three drinks per night, although he goes for periods without drinking significantly.

Mr. C underwent a research evaluation in the Mood and Personality Disorders Program. Research diagnostic evaluation revealed the presence of a schizotypal personality disorder with traits of paranoid and narcissistic personality disorder; he was also found to meet DSM-IV-TR (American Psychiatric Association 2000) criteria for alcohol abuse (past). Neurobiological evaluation uncovered a number of abnormalities. First, he displayed modestly impaired eye-movement accuracy (3.38 on a 1=best to 5=worst scale) and mild cognitive impairment. His dopaminergic indices were high, with a plasma HVA level of 14.5 ng/mL (mean for normal subjects is 7.4 ± 1.8 ng/mL) and a CSF HVA level of 38.0 ng/mL (mean for normal control subjects = 24.1 ± 6 ng/mL). In addition, Mr. C showed hypofrontality on a PET scan during a verbal memory task. Finally, he showed modest improvement following administration of amphetamine. Since evaluation, Mr. C has been treated with low-dose neuroleptic medication that helps him control multiple symptoms, including an olfactory hallucination-like experience of the smell of "cordite," a feeling that others are staring at him, a feeling of being detached or "separated by a bubble" from other people, a lack of any close friends other than a common-law wife, feelings in the past that his wife might be "following around," and a feeling in the past that he has seen future events.

Summary

These studies suggest that patients with schizotypal personality disorder have at least a profile of cognitive impairment and structural brain abnormalities, particularly in temporal cortex, similar to that found in patients with schizophrenia, but a combination of better prefrontal reserves and more subdued dopaminergic activity subcortically protect them from the emergence of psychosis. Their more subtle cognitive impairments are reflected in their eccentricity and interpersonal disengagement but do not reach the threshold of overt psychosis. For these reasons, they present more in the context of their disturbed interpersonal style and coping mechanisms rather than in the context of overt psychosis as in schizophrenia. However, this disorder provides an example of a spectrum that in its more extreme forms manifests as an Axis I disorder (schizophrenia) but in milder forms as an Axis II disorder. There are few biological data regarding paranoid personality disorder when it is not comorbid with schizotypal personality disorder.

CLUSTER B PERSONALITY DISORDERS

The Cluster B personality disorders include antisocial, borderline, histrionic, and narcissistic personality disorder. Individuals with these disorders present with varied degrees of impulsivity, aggression, and emotional dysregulation. As in other clusters, there is a high degree of overlap among the disorders in Cluster B, particularly between antisocial personality disorder (ASPD) and borderline personality disorder (BPD). ASPD and BPD are the best studied of the cluster, due to clear and reliable criteria for the former and the high prevalence of the latter in clinical populations.

Behavioral Genetics

Twin studies suggest that the genetic influence underlying personality disorders is at least as high as that underlying personality traits that underlie the various personality disorders. In a relatively small twin study (Torgersen et al. 2000) that may tend to overestimate the underlying genetic influence of any of a variety of personality disorders, the heritability for Cluster B personality disorders was 0.60. The heritabilities of the specific Cluster B disorders in this study were 0.79 for narcissistic personality disorder, 0.69 for BPD, and 0.67 for histrionic personality disorder. The best-fitting models did not include shared familial environment effects, although such effects may influence the development of BPD. Adoption studies of ASPD confirm a strong genetic, although a less strong environmental, influence for this disorder (Cadoret et al. 1985). Although adoption studies of other Cluster B personality disorders have not been conducted, the results of family history studies suggest a complex pattern of familial aggregation in which traits related to impulsive aggressiveness and mood dysregulation, rather than BPD itself, are transmitted in families (Silverman et al. 1991).

Neuropsychopharmacology

The serotonin (5-HT) system has been extensively studied in individuals with personality disorder in general and in particular as an inverse correlate of im-

pulsive aggressive behavior. Other neurotransmitters and/or modulators have also been studied in this regard, but to a much lesser degree.

Serotonin

There is a clear and consistent role for 5-HT in the regulation of aggression and/or impulsivity, particularly in individuals with personality disorder. Most data suggest an inverse relationship between any of a variety of measures of 5-HT levels and levels of aggression or impulsivity. Although some studies suggest a primary relationship with impulsivity, most studies report a 5-HT relationship more consistent with the construct of "impulsive aggression."

Neurochemical Studies. Inverse relationships between human aggression and measures of central 5-HT function have been reported since 1979, when Brown and colleagues reported an inverse relationship between CSF levels of the main central 5-HT metabolite, 5-hydroxyindoleacetic acid (5-HIAA), and life history of actual aggressive behavior in males with a variety of DSM-II (American Psychiatric Association 1968) personality disorder diagnoses (Brown et al. 1979). This finding was extended (Brown et al. 1982) to include a trivariate relationship between history of aggression, suicide attempts, and reduced CSF 5-HIAA, whereby history of aggression and suicide attempts were correlated directly with each other and inversely with CSF 5-HIAA. Later work with violent offenders (Linnoila et al. 1983) found reduced CSF 5-HIAA in impulsive, but not nonimpulsive, violent offenders with a variety of DSM-II personality disorder diagnoses, suggesting that impulsive aggression was the form most associated with reduced CSF 5-HIAA concentration. Although these findings have been replicated, an inverse relationship between CSF 5-HIAA and aggression has not been reported in samples of individuals with personality disorder without a prominent history of criminal activity (Coccaro et al. 1997a, 1997b; Gardner et al. 1990; Simeon et al. 1992). It is likely that CSF 5-HIAA, being a relatively insensitive index of 5-HT activity, is most reduced in the most severely aggressive individuals and that it is difficult to detect this relationship in less severely aggressive individuals.

Acute Pharmacological Interventions. There are a variety of 5-HT acute pharmacological challenge studies that have been performed in individuals with personality disorder in the context of the study of aggression. Typically, hormonal (e.g., prolactin) responses to the 5-HT selective agents are reported to correlate inversely with various measures of aggression and impulsivity (Coccaro et al. 1989, 1997a, 1997b; Dolan et al. 2001; Moss et al. 1990; O'Keane et al. 1992; Paris et al. 2004; Siever and Trestman 1993). Pharmacological challenge studies using putatively receptor-selective 5-HT agents also seem to support the hypothesis of an inverse relationship between 5-HT and measures of aggression and suggest a role for at least the 5-HT_{1A} receptor in particular (Cleare and Bond 2000; Coccaro et al. 1990, 1995; Hansenne et al. 2002). A more complex picture in regard to central 5-HT_{1A} receptors has been suggested recently by the observation of reduced 5-HT_{1A} receptor–mediated responses in females with BPD with a history of sustained child abuse (Rinne et al. 2000). Because childhood abuse has been linked to impulsive aggression in later adolescence and adulthood (Crick and Dodge 1996), it remains to be determined whether the relationships between 5-HT and aggression are linked to this environmental/developmental variable. Although behavioral responses to 5-HT stimulation in individuals with personality disorder have not received much attention, at least one study reported a significant reduction in anger in 12 patients with BPD after administration of the mixed 5-HT agonist *meta*-chlorophenylpiperazine (m-CPP) but not placebo (Hollander et al. 1994); a reduction in fear was also observed in the males with BPD.

Platelet Receptor Markers.   Despite considerable platelet receptor work in other psychiatric populations, relatively little research in this area has been published on subjects with personality disorder. Inverse correlations between the number of platelet ^{3}H-imipramine (5-HT transporter) binding sites and self-mutilation and impulsivity have been reported in individuals with personality disorder but not in patients without a history of self-mutilation (Simeon et al. 1992). Similarly, an inverse correlation between the number of platelet ^{3}H-paroxetine (5-HT transporter) binding sites (Coccaro et al. 1996), and the quantity of platelet serotonin (Goveas et al. 2004), and life history of aggression has been reported in individuals with personality disorder.

DNA Polymorphism Studies.   Work in this area began with an examination of DNA polymorphisms in the gene for tryptophan hydroxylase (TPH). TPH is the rate-limiting step for the synthesis of serotonin, and it was thought that polymorphisms in TPH would lead to TPH enzymes of different activities. Although this *TPH* polymorphism was not found to have a clear functional consequence regarding serotonin synthesis, the presence of the L allele (L referred to the "lower band" on the genotyping gel) was found to have some

association with clinically relevant variables. For example, impulsive violent offenders (nearly all with a personality disorder) with at least one copy of the L *TPH* allele have been reported to have significantly lower CSF 5-HIAA compared with impulsive violent offenders with the UU genotype (U referred to the "upper band" on the genotyping gel) in at least one study (Neilson et al. 1994). This finding did not generalize to nonimpulsive violent offenders (many of whom also had a personality disorder) or to normal control subjects and was not replicated in a later study by the same authors (Neilson et al. 1998). The presence of the L allele was associated with an increased risk of suicidal behavior in all violent offenders in this and in a later study by these authors (Neilson et al. 1994, 1998). New et al. (1998) have also reported that the self-reported tendency toward aggression varies as a function of *TPH* genotype whereby subjects with the LL genotype had higher aggression scores than those with the UU genotype. Curiously, however, the reverse finding was reported by Manuck et al. (1999) in a sample of healthy volunteers from the community: higher aggression scores were associated with the presence of the U allele. These disparate findings may be due to critical differences in the subject samples. As such, the relationship between the *TPH* allele and 5-HT function may be dependent on the *TPH* allele's relationship with some other gene depending on the subject sample. Lappalainen et al. (1998) reported an association between "antisocial alcoholism" (i.e., alcoholism with ASPD or intermittent explosive disorder) and the C allele for the 5-HT_{1D} beta-receptor polymorphism. Because the 5-HT_{1D} beta receptor is a critical receptor involved in the regulation of 5-HT release on neuronal impulse, this finding could be highly relevant to the understanding of ASPD comorbid with alcoholism.

Catecholamines

Compared with serotonin, far fewer data have been published regarding the role of other neurotransmitters and behavioral dimensions of relevance to the Cluster B personality disorders.

Neurochemical Studies.   A positive correlation between CSF methoxyhydroxyphenylglycol (MHPG, the major metabolite of norepinephrine) concentrations and life history of aggression has been reported in males with personality disorder, although further analysis revealed that CSF 5-HIAA concentration accounted for most (80%) of the variance in aggression scores. Similarly, one study reported a small positive correlation between plasma norepinephrine and self-reported impulsivity in males with personality disorder (Siever and Trestman 1993). In contrast, at least one study (Virkkunen et al. 1987) reported a significant reduction in CSF MHPG concentration in males who have committed violent offenses. Finally, a recent study reports an inverse relationship between plasma free MHPG and life history of aggression in males with personality disorder (Coccaro et al. 2003). Compared with patients with nonborderline personality disorders, patients with BPD had lower plasma free MHPG compared with the nonborderline control subjects; a finding that disappeared after differences in aggression scores were accounted for. Evidence for the role of dopamine in aggression in individuals with personality disorder is limited and contradictory. Although some studies demonstrate no relationship between CSF HVA concentration and aggression (Brown et al. 1979; Virkkunen et al. 1987), other studies demonstrate an inverse relationship between these variables (Linnoila et al. 1983; Virkkunen et al. 1989). Given the consistent observation of a strong correlation between CSF 5-HIAA and CSF HVA concentrations, it is possible that findings with CSF HVA may be related to similar findings with CSF 5-HIAA concentration. If so, a specific assessment of CSF HVA may not be made unless the effect of CSF 5-HIAA concentration is accounted for, a statistical adjustment that has not been made in published studies to date.

Acute Pharmacological Interventions.   Early studies of the acute administration of amphetamine in patients with BPD demonstrated a greater behavioral sensitivity to amphetamine challenge among the patients with personality disorder than among control subjects (Schulz et al. 1985). Replication studies found that global worsening in psychopathology after amphetamine was typical of patients with both borderline and schizotypal personality disorder whereas global improvement was typical of borderline subjects without comorbid schizotypal personality disorder (Schulz et al. 1988). This finding suggests important biological differences among patients with BPD as a function of comorbid schizotypy (perhaps because of preexisting dopaminergic hyperactivity in mesolimbic dopamine circuits). In other studies of amphetamine challenge relevant to Cluster B personality disorder, a direct relationship with affective lability has been noted in healthy volunteers, suggesting that increases in norepinephrine and/or dopamine may play a role in the moment-to-moment dysregulation of affect seen in patients with BPD (Kavoussi et al. 1993). Only limited data are available regarding the study of norepinephrine receptor–mediated responses related to the features of Cluster B personality disorder. One study reported a positive correlation between the growth hormone response to the α_2 norepinephrine agonist clonidine and self-reported "irritability" (a correlate of aggression) in a small sample of males with personality disorder and healthy volunteers (Coccaro et al. 1991). A more recent study of females with BPD, however, reported no difference in growth hormone responses to clonidine (Paris et al. 2004).

DNA Polymorphism Studies.   The presence of the low-functioning *MAO-A* allele in young men combined with a history of childhood maltreatment has recently been shown to be associated with an increased risk of aggressive and criminal offending (e.g., antisocial) behavior (Caspi et al. 2002). This specific *MAO-A* allele is associated with reduced catabolism of catecholamines (and serotonin) and accordingly with higher levels of these neurotransmitters that may be associated with aggressive behavior. These data suggest that although the presence of this allele may be important in increasing the risk of antisocial behavior, the co-occurrence of childhood maltreatment in vulnerable individuals is also needed to meaningfully increase the risk of antisocial behavior.

Acetylcholine and Other Neurotransmitters/ Neuromodulators

Studies of acetylcholine function in personality disorder have been limited to two studies. In the first (Steinberg et al. 1997), patients with BPD reported greater self-rated depression scores in response to the cholinomimetic agent physostigmine than did patients with nonborderline personality disorders or healthy volunteer control subjects. Peak physostigmine-induced depression scores correlated positively with the number of "affective instability," but not with the number of "impulsive aggression," borderline personality traits. This finding suggests that the trait of affective lability in patients with BPD may be mediated in part by a heightened sensitivity to acetylcholine. In the second study (Paris et al. 2004), however, no differences in hormonal responses to a different cholinomimetic agent, pyridostigmine, were seen between females with BPD and control subjects. These divergent findings suggest the possibility that the cholinergic receptors mediating behavioral and hormonal responses to cholinergic agents in these subjects may be very different by virtue of brain location.

Other neurotransmitters or neuromodulators that may play a role in Cluster B–related features include vasopressin, which may have a direct relationship with aggression (Coccaro et al. 1998); substances related to limbic-hypothalamic-pituitary adrenal axis functioning (corticotropin releasing factor, adrenocorticotropic hormone, cortisol), which may have varied relationships regarding aggressive behavior dependent on social context and stress (Rinne et al. 2002); testosterone, which is variably correlated with aggression, particularly in violent offenders with ASPD (Virkkunen et al. 1994); and cholesterol and fatty acids, which may play a role in both aggression (both: Atmaca et al. 2002; New et al. 1999) and mood regulation (fatty acids: Zanarini and Frankenberg 2003).

Neuroimaging

(See also Chapter 38, "Brain Imaging.")

Structural Imaging

Reduced prefrontal gray matter (e.g., by 11%) has been associated with autonomic deficits in individuals with ASPD characterized by aggressive behaviors (Raine et al. 2000). Conversely, increases in corpus callosum white matter volume and length have recently been described in similar subjects (Raine et al. 2003), where larger callosal volumes were also associated with affective/interpersonal deficit, low autonomic stress reactivity, and spatial ability. Given the complex role these structures play in mediating cognitive and affective processes, these findings may represent anatomical correlates of the complex behaviors seen in ASPD. A confounding role for alcoholism in these matters must always be addressed, however, because it also has been shown that volume changes may be correlated with duration of alcoholism (Laakso et al. 2002).

Similar structural imaging studies of females with BPD report reductions in the volume of subcortical structures such as the amygdala (Rusch et al. 2003; Schmahl et al. 2003; Tebartz van Elst et al. 2003) and hippocampus (Schmahl et al. 2003; Tebartz van Elst et al. 2003). One study also reports reductions in the volumes of both cortical (right orbitofrontal) and other limbic structures including right anterior cingulated and amygdala/hippocampal volumes (Tebartz van Elst et al. 2003). Given the role these structures are thought to play in emotional information processing, it is tempting to speculate that these structures represent anatomical correlates of the emotional dysregulation (including impulsive aggression) seen in patients with BPD.

Functional Imaging (PET and SPECT)

Whereas structural imaging yields only a static picture of the brain, SPECT or PET scanning can yield functional information related to cerebral blood flow or cerebral glucose metabolism, respectively. For example, SPECT studies have demonstrated reduced perfusion in prefrontal cortex as well as focal abnormalities in left temporal lobe and increased activity in anteromedial frontal cortex in limbic system in aggressive individuals with ASPD and alcoholism (Amen et al. 1996). A more recent study using SPECT reported significant correlations between reduced cerebral blood flow in frontal and temporal brain regions and the "disturbed interpersonal attitude" factor from the Psychopathy Checklist (Soderstorm et al. 2002). In homicide offenders (many of whom presumably had ASPD), a bilateral diminution of glucose metabolism has been reported in both medial frontal cortex and at a trend level in orbital frontal cortex (Raine et al. 1994). In a study of patients with a variety of personality disorders, an inverse relationship was found between life history of aggressive impulsive behavior and regional glucose metabolism in orbital frontal cortex and right temporal lobe (Goyer et al. 1994). Patients meeting criteria for BPD had decreased metabolism in frontal regions corresponding to Brodmann areas 46 and 6 and increased metabolism in superior and inferior frontal gyrus (Brodmann areas 9 and 45; Goyer et al. 1994). More-recent PET studies in females with BPD reported hypometabolism in both frontal and prefrontal regions as well as in the hippocampus and cuneus (Juengling et al. 2003), supporting previous structural studies that demonstrated reductions in the volumes of these brain areas. Although most of these PET studies were performed in the resting condition, a recent PET study in females with BPD showed that the replay of abandonment scripts prior to PET scan are associated with greater increases in activity in dorsolateral prefrontal cortex (bilaterally) and in cuneus, but with reductions in activity in the right anterior cingulate (Schmahl et al. 2003). Given that several of these structures have been shown to be smaller in these subjects compared with control subjects, the increased activity in these regions after the abandonment task is quite notable.

PET studies may also be performed after the administration of neurotransmitter-specific agents so that the activity of brain regions in response to activation of specific receptors by these agents can be assessed. To date, at least four studies of patients with personality disorder have been performed in this way. Two utilized the indirect 5-HT agonist fenfluramine, one utilized the more direct postsynaptic 5-HT agonist m-CPP, and one examined the trapping of a ^{11}C analogue of tryptophan. In the first fenfluramine study, patients with prominent histories of impulsive aggression and BPD demonstrated blunted responses of glucose metabolism in orbital frontal, ventral medial frontal, and cingulate cortex compared with normal subjects (Siever et al. 1999). A similar result was reported in the second fenfluramine study, in which patients with BPD displayed reduced glucose metabolism (relative to placebo) compared with control subjects in right medial and orbital frontal cortex, left middle and superior temporal gyri, left parietal lobe, and left caudate (Soloff et al. 2000). In the PET study involving *m*-CPP, patients with prominent histories of impulsive aggression and personality disorder were found to have reduced activation of the anterior cingulate and increased activation of the posterior cingulate compared with control subjects (New et al. 2002). Given the role of the anterior cingulate in emotional information processing, it is noteworthy that this area is underactivated by 5-HT stimulation. In the PET study examining the unilateral trapping of a ^{11}C analogue of tryptophan, evidence for a reduction in 5-HT synthesis was present in the corticostriatal (e.g., medial frontal, anterior cingulate, superior temporal gyri, and corpus striatum) brain areas of subjects with BPD (Leyton et al. 2001). Reduction in 5-HT synthesis in these regions was reported to correlate with a laboratory measure of behavioral disinhibition.

Functional Imaging (fMRI)

Unlike PET or SPECT, fMRI does not require the injection of a radiolabeled agent. Instead, fMRI assesses changes in cerebral blood flow using changes in the blood oxygenation level–dependent signal in the magnetic resonance imaging scanner. This offers a much greater spatial and temporal resolution compared with either PET or SPECT and allows a finer assessment of the activation and deactivation of discrete regions of the brain in response to specific stimuli. To date, at least three studies using fMRI in patients with personality disorder have been published. In one study using fMRI, males with (psychopathic) ASPD activated preselected frontal and temporal regions of interest less than did control subjects during trials of negatively charged emotional words (Kiehl et al. 2001), suggesting an important deficit in emotional information processing. In a similar fMRI study in females with BPD, the study group demonstrated greater activation of the amygdala bilaterally (as well as activation of selected frontal regions) while viewing emotionally aversive images (e.g., crying children) than did control subjects (Herpertz et al. 2001). The most recent fMRI study in females with BPD reported a generally similar finding (left amygdala as opposed to bilateral activation) using emotional faces (Donegan et al. 2003). Given the clear differences in known emotional information processing between psychopathic antisocial subjects on the one hand and borderline subjects on the other, these data suggest the brain sites of these differences.

Case Example

Mr. D is a 29-year-old married male computer technician referred for treatment of his impulsive aggressive outbursts in the context of a threatened separation from his wife of 4 years. Mr. D reports impulsive aggressive outbursts since his mid-teens. These outbursts typically involve screaming, shouting, and throwing things around; he has only occasionally physically hit anyone. However, these aggressive outbursts occur several times a month and usually several times a week, particularly when Mr. D is "held up" in traffic. Most recently, he has been having serious marital difficulty, and his wife is now threatening to leave him if he does not get help for his anger problem. He reports that his relationship with his wife is often "stormy," with frequent fighting that sometimes goes on for hours. Sometimes in the aftermath of these fights Mr. D runs off and gets exceedingly drunk and drives recklessly around town while high. At other times, he reports, he beats his head so hard against a wall that his forehead bleeds (once he needed stitches). Still, at other times he frantically pleads with his wife not to leave him; once he took an overdose of aspirin, in front of his wife, to get her to stay with him. Mr. D reports a history of alcohol abuse in his late teens and early twenties and a history of gambling to excess up until 1 year prior to evaluation.

Mr. D underwent a research evaluation in the Mood and Personality Disorders Program. Diagnostic evaluation revealed the presence of BPD with traits of histrionic, narcissistic, and obsessive-compulsive personality disorder. He was also found to meet DSM-IV-TR criteria for two episodes of major depression in the past and for alcohol abuse (past) and pathological gambling (past). He underwent a variety of research-related studies including *d*-fenfluramine (*d*-FEN) challenge and was found to have a blunted, but not absent, prolactin response to *d*-FEN (2.3 ng/mL compared with 6.3 ± 3.4 ng/mL for healthy male control subjects); his CSF 5-HIAA level was not abnormal (23.9 ng/mL compared with 20.0 ± 4.9 ng/mL for healthy male control subjects). The modest magnitude of his prolactin response to *d*-FEN suggests a limited degree of central serotonin system dysfunction. Mr. D entered a treatment trial of fluoxetine and experienced a reduction in overt aggressive behavior over a period of several weeks. Over this time his relationship with his wife somewhat improved, and he is now in dialectical behavioral therapy to work on other aspects of his interpersonal difficulties with others in his life.

Summary

The studies discussed in this section suggest that patients with Cluster B personality disorder have dysfunction in a variety of neurobiological areas that may underlie their clinical presentation. Dysfunction can occur in multiple monoaminergic systems (e.g., serotonin, norepinephrine, vasopressin for impulsivity and aggression, possibly acetylcholine for mood reactivity) and in brain structures related to behavioral inhibition and emotional information processing (e.g., orbitofrontal cortex, amygdala). Although patients with borderline personality are often the most extreme in these features and in related biological dysfunction, specific biological dysfunction related to specific traits (e.g., serotonin dysfunction with impulsive aggression) can be seen in patients with other, nonborderline personality disorders. As such, it is doubtful that any assessment of specific neurobiological function will be specific to patients with BPD.

CLUSTER C: ANXIOUS CLUSTER PERSONALITY DISORDERS

The Cluster C personality disorders include avoidant, dependent, and compulsive personality disorders. Individuals with these disorders present with varied degrees of anxiety sometimes expressed as "rigidity," particularly in the case of compulsive personality disorder. Of the three disorders, avoidant personality disorder is most like generalized social phobia in Axis I, and a great degree of comorbidity occurs between the two diagnoses (Dahl 1996). As in other personality disorder clusters, there is overlap among the disorders in this cluster and with those in other personality disorder clusters, particularly Cluster B. To date, there has been much less empirical neurobiological research with patients in Cluster C.

Behavioral Genetics

As with the Cluster B personality disorders, twin studies suggest substantial genetic influence for each of the Cluster C personality disorders (Torgersen et al. 2000). Heritability for Cluster C personality disorders as a group was estimated at 0.62; heritabilities for each disorder in the study were 0.78 for obsessive-compulsive, 0.57 for dependent, and 0.28 for avoidant personality disorder. The best-fitting models did not include shared familial environment effects, although a model consisting only of shared familial and unique environmental effects could not be definitively ruled out for dependent personality disorders. Family studies suggest a familial association between social anxiety disorder and avoidant personality disorder (Schneier et al. 2002). Avoidant, dependent, and anxious cluster personality disorders show significant familiarity (Reich 1989), and both avoidant and independent personality traits are found in relatives of patients with panic disorder (Reich 1991).

Neuropsychopharmacology

There has been little biological study of the Cluster C personality disorders. However, low dopamine metabolites in CSF have been identified in patients with social anxiety disorder (Johnson et al. 1994), which overlaps to a great extent with avoidant personality disorder, whereas nonselective monoamine oxidase inhibitors (which increase dopamine transmission) or dopaminergic antidepressants improve social anxiety (Schneier et al. 2002). Imaging studies are also consistent with this finding, with low dopamine transporter binding demonstrated in generalized social anxiety disorder (Tiihonen et al. 1997) and lower D_2 receptor binding in a SPECT study of generalized social anxiety disorder (Schneier et al. 2000). In addition, three PET studies support a relationship of reduced D_2 binding associated with detachment, which correlates with social avoidance consistent with that observed both in patients with Cluster C personality disorders and in patients with schizoid personality disorder (Schneier et al. 2000). Genetic studies of these types of behaviors have been found in association with the dopamine transporter gene *DAT1* (Blum et al. 1997). These studies cumulatively suggest low dopaminergic activity in social anxiety disorder and likely in avoidant personality disorder as well.

In the serotonergic system, on the other hand, patients with social anxiety have increased cortisol responses to serotonergic agents (Tancer et al. 1999), and social anxiety disorders respond to selective serotonin reuptake inhibitors that re-regulate serotonergic activity (Schneier et al. 2003). Shyness (related to avoidant traits) has been associated with the serotonin transporter reporter region L allele but not to *COMT*, *MAO-A*, or *DRD4* alleles. Growth hormone regulation has also been associated with social anxiety (Schneier et al. 2002).

Neuropsychologic and Psychophysiologic Correlates

Increased amygdala activation in fMRI has been shown in social phobia in one study (Schneier et al.

1999) as well as in recognition bias for recall of disapproving faces in another (Foa et al. 2000). However, skin conductance and heart rate change and startle response during viewing of slides with emotionally charged themes did not distinguish patients with avoidant personality disorder from control subjects (Herpertz et al. 2000). Psychophysiologic studies have not been extensively undertaken in the other Cluster C personality disorders.

Summary

Genetic and neurobiologic research has been limited in patients with Cluster C personality disorders but reductions in dopaminergic activity and increases in serotonergic activity are hinted at in the data available.

FUTURE DIRECTIONS

Research in the psychobiology of personality disorder has advanced much since the 1980s. Although there is clear evidence of a number of biogenetic correlates of personality disorder traits, future efforts need to be directed along a variety of lines to increase our understanding of how alterations in brain function lead to the development and manifestation of these traits. Such lines of investigation may be aimed at 1) how genetic and environmental influences interact with neurotransmitter function to lead to specific traits; 2) how neurotransmitter function interacts with the regulation of cognitive and emotional function across distributed neural networks to lead to specific traits; and 3) how understanding brain function at these levels can enable us to devise more effective ways to treat personality disorder traits both pharmacologically and psychotherapeutically.

REFERENCES

Amen DG, Stubblefield M, Carmicheal B: Brain SPECT findings and aggressiveness. Ann Clin Psychiatry 3:129–137, 1996

American Psychiatric Association: Diagnostic and Statistical Manual of Mental Disorders, 2nd Edition. Washington, DC, American Psychiatric Association, 1968

American Psychiatric Association: Diagnostic and Statistical Manual of Mental Disorders, 4th Edition, Text Revision. Washington, DC, American Psychiatric Association, 2000

Amin F, Coccaro EF, Mitropoulou V, et al: Plasma HVA in schizotypal personality disorder, in Plasma Homovanillic Acid Studies in Schizophrenia: Implications for Presynaptic Dopamine Dysfunction. Edited by Friedhoff AJ, Amin F. Washington, DC, American Psychiatric Press, 1997, pp 133–149

Amin F, Silverman JM, Siever LJ, et al: Genetic antecedents of dopamine dysfunction in schizophrenia. Biol Psychiatry 45:1143–1150, 1999

Atmaca M, Kuloglu M, Tezcan E, et al: Serum cholesterol and leptin levels in patients with borderline personality disorder. Neuropsychobiology 45:167–171, 2002

Blum K, Braverman ER, Wu S: Association of polymorphisms of dopamine D2 receptor (DRD2), and dopamine transporter (DAT1) genes with schizoid/avoidant behaviors (SAB). Mol Psychiatry 2:239–246, 1997

Braff DL, Freedman R: Endophenotypes in studies of the genetics of schizophrenia, in Neuropsychopharmacology: The Fifth Generation of Progress. Edited by Davis KL, Charney D, Coyle JT, et al. Philadelphia, PA, Lippincott Williams and Wilkins, 2002, pp 703–716

Brown GL, Goodwin FK, Ballenger JC, et al: Aggression in humans correlates with cerebrospinal fluid amine metabolites. Psychiatry Res 1:131–139, 1979

Brown GL, Ebert MH, Goyer PF, et al: Aggression, suicide, and serotonin: relationships to CSF amine metabolites. Am J Psychiatry 139:741–746, 1982

Buchsbaum MS, Nenadic I, Hazlett EA, et al: Differential metabolic rates in prefrontal and temporal Brodmann areas in schizophrenia and schizotypal personality disorder. Schizophr Res 54:141–150, 2002

Cadoret RJ, O'Gorman TW, Troughton E, et al: Alcoholism and antisocial personality: interrelationships, genetic and environmental factors. Arch Gen Psychiatry 42:161–167, 1985

Caspi A, McClay J, Moffitt TE, et al: Role of genotype in the cycle of violence in maltreated children. Science 297:851–854, 2002

Cleare AJ, Bond AJ: Ipsapirone challenge in aggressive men shows an inverse correlation between 5-HT1A receptor function and aggression. Psychopharmacology 148:344–349, 2000

Coccaro EF, Siever LJ, Klar HM, et al: Serotonergic studies in affective and personality disorder: correlates with suicidal and impulsive aggressive behavior. Arch Gen Psychiatry 46:587–599, 1989

Coccaro EF, Gabriel S, Siever LJ: Buspirone challenge: preliminary evidence for a role for 5-HT-1A receptors in impulsive aggressive behavior in humans. Psychopharmacol Bull 26:393–405, 1990

Coccaro EF, Lawrence T, Trestman R, et al: Growth hormone responses to intravenous clonidine challenge correlates with behavioral irritability in psychiatric patients and in healthy volunteers. Psychiatry Res 39:129–139, 1991

Coccaro EF, Kavoussi RJ, Hauger RL: Physiologic responses to d-fenfluramine and ipsapirone challenge correlate with indices of aggression in males with personality disorder. Int Clin Psychopharmacol 10:177–180, 1995

Coccaro EF, Kavoussi RJ, Sheline YI, et al: Impulsive aggression in personality disorder: correlates with 3H-Paroxetine binding in the platelet. Arch Gen Psychiatry 53:531–536, 1996

Coccaro EF, Kavoussi RJ, Cooper TB, Hauger RA. Central serotonin and aggression: inverse relationship with prolactin response to d-fenfluramine, but not with CSF 5-HIAA concentration in human subjects. Am J Psychiatry 154:1430–1435, 1997a

Coccaro EF, Kavoussi RJ, Trestman RL, et al: Serotonin function in personality and mood disorder: intercorrelations among central indices and aggressiveness. Psychiatry Res 73:1–14, 1997b

Coccaro EF, Kavoussi RK, Hauger RL, et al: Cerebrospinal fluid vasopressin: correlates with aggression and serotonin function in personality disordered subjects. Arch Gen Psychiatry 55:708–714, 1998

Coccaro EF, Lee R, McCloskey M: Norepinephrine function in personality disorder: plasma free MHPG correlates inversely with life history of aggression. CNS Spectr 8:731–736, 2003

Crick NR, Dodge KA: Social information-processing mechanisms in reactive and proactive aggression. Child Dev 67:993–1002, 1996

Dahl AA: The relationship between social phobia and avoidant personality disorder: workshop report 3. Int Clin Psychopharmacol 11(suppl 3):109–112, 1996

Dolan M, Anderson IM, Deakin JF: Relationship between 5-HT function and impulsivity and aggression in male offenders with personality disorders. Br J Psychiatry 178:352–359, 2001

Donegan NH, Sanislow CA, Blumberg HP, et al: Amygdala hyperreactivity in borderline personality disorder: implications for emotional dysregulation. Biol Psychiatry 54:1284–1293, 2003

Foa EB, Gilboa-Schechtman E, Amir N: Memory bias in generalized social phobia: remembering negative emotional expressions. J Anxiety Disord 14:501–519, 2000

Gardner DL, Lucas PB, Cowdry RW: CSF metabolites in borderline personality disorder compared with normal controls. Biol Psychiatry 28:247-54, 1990

Goldberg TE, Egan MF, Gscheidle T, et al: Executive subprocesses in working memory: relationship to catechol-O-methyltransferase Val158Met genotype and schizophrenia. Arch Gen Psychiatry 60:889–896, 2003

Goveas JS, Csernansky JG, Coccaro EF: Platelet serotonin content correlates inversely with life history of aggression in personality-disordered subjects. Psychiatry Res 126:23–32, 2004

Goyer PF, Andreason PJ, Semple WE, et al: Positron-emission tomography and personality disorders. Neuropsychopharmacology 10:21–28, 1994

Hansenne M, Pitchot W, Pinto E, et al: 5-HT1A dysfunction in borderline personality disorder. Psychol Med 32:935–941, 2002

Herpertz SC, Schwenger UB, Kunert HJ, et al: Emotional responses in patients with borderline as compared with avoidant personality disorder. J Personal Disord 14:339–351, 2000

Herpertz SC, Dietrich TM, Wenning B, et al: Evidence of abnormal amygdala functioning in borderline personality disorder: a functional MRI study. Biol Psychiatry 50:292–298, 2001

Hollander E, Stein D, DeCaria CM, et al: Serotonergic sensitivity in borderline personality disorder: preliminary findings. Am J Psychiatry 151:277–280, 1994

Hymowitz P, Frances A, Jacobsberg LB, et al: Neuroleptic treatment of schizotypal personality disorders. Compr Psychiatry 27:267–271, 1986

Johnson MR, Lydiard RB, Zealberg JJ: Plasma and CFS levels in panic patients with comorbid social phobia. Biol Psychiatry 36:426–427, 1994

Juengling FD, Schmahl C, Hesslinger B, et al: Positron emission tomography in female patients with borderline personality disorder. J Psychiatr Res 37:109–115, 2003

Kalus O, Bernstein DP, Siever LJ: Schizoid personality disorder: a review of its current status. J Personal Disord 7:43–52, 1993

Kavoussi RJ, Coccaro EF: The amphetamine challenge test correlates with affective lability in healthy volunteers. Psychiatry Res 48:219–228, 1993

Kiehl K, Smith AM, Hare RD, et al: Limbic abnormalities in affective processing by criminal psychopaths as revealed by functional magnetic resonance imaging. Biol Psychiatry 50:677–684, 2001

Kirrane RM, Mitropoulou V, Nunn M, et al: Effects of amphetamine on visuospatial working memory performance in schizophrenia spectrum personality disorder. Neuropsychopharmacology 22:14–18, 2000

Koenigsberg HW, Buchsbaum MS, Harvey P, et al: Regional brain activation in schizotypal personality disorder patients during visuospatial working memory task as measured by fMRI. Abstract of the Fifty-sixth Annual Meeting of the Society of Biological Psychiatry, Vol 49, abstract 327, 2001

Koenigsberg HW, Reynolds D, Goodman M, et al: Risperidone in the treatment of schizotypal personality disorder. J Clin Psychiatry 64:628–634, 2003

Laakso MP, Gunning-Dixon F, Vaurio O, et al: Prefrontal volumes in habitually violent subjects with antisocial personality disorder and type 2 alcoholism. Psychiatry Res 114:95–102, 2002

Lappalainen J, Long JC, Eggert M, et al: Linkage of antisocial alcoholism to the serotonin 5-HT1B receptor gene in two populations. Arch Gen Psychiatry 55:989–994, 1998

Laruelle M, Kegeles L, Zea-Pance Y, et al: Amphetamine-induced dopamine release in patients with schizotypal personality disorders studies by SPECT and [123] IBZM. Neuroimage 16:S61, 2002

Levitt JJ, McCarley RW, Dickey CC, et al: MRI study of caudate nucleus volume and its cognitive correlates in neuroleptic-naïve patients with schizotypal personality disorder. Am J Psychiatry 159:1190–1197, 2002

Leyton M, Okazawa H, Diksic M, et al: Brain regional alpha-[11C]methyl-L-tryptophan trapping in impulsive subjects with borderline personality disorder. Am J Psychiatry 158:775–782, 2001

Linnoila M, Virkkunen M, Scheinin M, et al: Low cerebrospinal fluid 5-hydroxyindolacetic acid concentration differentiates impulsive from nonimpulsive violent behavior. Life Sci 33:2609–2614, 1983

Manuck SB, Flory JD, Ferrell RE, et al: Aggression and anger-related traits associated with a polymorphism of the tryptophan hydroxylase gene. Biol Psychiatry 45:603–614, 1999

Mitropoulou V, Harvey PD, Maldari LA, et al: Neuropsychological performance in schizotypal personality disorder: evidence regarding diagnostic specificity. Biol Psychiatry 52:1175–1182, 2002

Moss HB, Yao JK, Panzak GL: Serotonergic responsivity and behavioral dimensions in antisocial personality disorder with substance abuse. Biol Psychiatry 28:325–338, 1990

New AS, Gelernter J, Yovell Y, et al: Tryptophan hydroxylase genotype is associated with impulsive aggression measures. Am J Med Genet 81:13–17, 1998

New AS, Sevin EM, Mitropoulou V, et al: Serum cholesterol and impulsivity in personality disorders. Psychiatry Res 85:145–150, 1999

New AS, Hazlett EA, Buchsbaum MS, et al: Blunted prefrontal cortical [18]fluorodeoxyglucose positron emission tomography response to *meta*-chlorophenylpiperazine in impulsive aggression. Arch Gen Psychiatry 59:621–629, 2002

Nielsen DA, Goldman D, Virkkunen M, et al: Suicidality and 5-hydroxyindoleacetic acid concentration associated with a tryptophan hydroxylase polymorphism. Arch Gen Psychiatry 51:34–38, 1994

Nielsen DA, Virkkunen M, Lappalainen J, et al: A tryptophan hydroxylase gene marker for suicidality and alcoholism. Arch Gen Psychiatry 55:593–602, 1998

O'Keane V, Moloney E, O'Neill H, et al: Blunted prolactin responses to d-fenfluramine in sociopathy: Evidence for subsensitivity of central serotonergic function. Br J Psychiatry 160:643–646, 1992

Paris J, Zweig-Frank H, Kin NM, et al: Neurobiological correlates of diagnosis and underlying traits in patients with borderline personality disorder compared with normal controls. Psychiatry Res 121:239–252, 2004

Raine A, Buchsbaum M, Stanley J, et al: Selective reductions in prefrontal glucose metabolism in murderers. Biol Psychiatry 36:365–373, 1994

Raine A, Lencz T, Bihrle S, et al: Reduced prefrontal gray matter volume and reduced autonomic activity in antisocial personality disorder. Arch Gen Psychiatry 57:119–127, 2000

Raine A, Lencz T, Taylor K, et al: Corpus callosum abnormalities in psychopathic antisocial individuals. Arch Gen Psychiatry 60:1134–1142, 2003

Reich JH: Familiality of DSM-III dramatic and anxious personality clusters. J Nerv Ment Dis 177:96–100, 1989

Reich JH: Avoidant and dependent personality traits in relatives of patients with panic disorder, patients with dependent personality disorder, and normal controls. Psychiatry Res 39:89–98, 1991

Rinne T, Westenberg HG, den Boer JA, et al: Serotonergic blunting to *meta*-chlorophenylpiperazine (m-CPP) highly correlates with sustained childhood abuse in impulsive and autoaggressive female borderline patients. Biol Psychiatry 47:548–556, 2000

Rinne T, de Kloet ER, Wouters L, et al: Hyperresponsiveness of hypothalamic-pituitary-adrenal axis to combined dexamethasone/corticotropin-releasing hormone challenge in female borderline personality disorder subjects with a history of sustained childhood abuse. Biol Psychiatry 52:1102–1112, 2002

Rusch N, van Elst LT, Ludaescher P, et al: A voxel-based morphometric MRI study in female patients with borderline personality disorder. Neuroimage 20:385–392, 2003

Schmahl CG, Vermetten E, Elzinga BM, et al: Magnetic resonance imaging of hippocampal and amygdala volume in women with childhood abuse and borderline personality disorder. Psychiatry Res 122:193–198, 2003

Schneier F, Weiss U, Kessler C: Subcortical correlates of differential classical conditioning of aversive emotional reactions in social phobia. Biol Psychiatry 45:863–871, 1999

Schneier FR, Liebowitz MR, Abi-Dargham A: Low dopamine D2 receptor binding potential in social phobia. Am J Psychiatry 157:457–459, 2000

Schneier FR, Blanco C, Smita XA, et al: The social anxiety spectrum. Psychiatr Clin North Am 25:757–774, 2002

Schneier FR, Blanco C, Campeas R, et al: Citalopram treatment of social anxiety disorder with comorbid major depression. Depress Anxiety 17:191–196, 2003

Schulz SC, Schulz PM, Dommisse C, et al: Amphetamine response in borderline patients. Psychiatry Res 15:97–108, 1985

Schulz SC, Cornelius J, Schulz PM, et al: The amphetamine challenge test in patients with borderline personality disorder. Am J Psychiatry 145:809–814, 1988

Schulz SC, Thomson R, Brecher M: The efficacy of quetiapine vs. haloperidol and placebo: a meta-analytic study of efficacy. Schizophr Res 62:1–12, 2003

Shihabuddin L, Silverman JM, Buchsbaum MS, et al: Ventricular enlargement associated with linkage marker for schizophrenia-related disorders in one pedigree. Mol Psychiatry 1:215–222, 1996

Shihabuddin L, Buchsbaum MS, Hazlett EA, et al: Striatal size and relative glucose metabolic rate in schizotypal personality disorder and schizophrenia. Arch Gen Psychiatry 58:877–884, 2001

Siegel BV, Trestman RL, O'Flaithbheartaigh SO, et al: D-amphetamine challenge effects on Wisconsin Card Sort Test performance in schizotypal personality disorder. Schizophr Res 20:29–32, 1996

Siever LJ: The biology of the boundaries of schizophrenia, in Advances in Neuropsychiatry and Psychopharmacology, Vol 1: Schizophrenia Research. Edited by Tamminga CA, Schulz SC. New York, Raven, 1991, pp 181–191

Siever LJ: Brain structure/function and the dopamine system in schizotypal personality disorder, in Schizotypal Personality. Edited by Raine A, Lencz T, Mednick F. New York, Cambridge University Press, 1995, pp 272–286

Siever LJ, Davis KL: The pathophysiology of the schizophrenic disorders: perspective from the spectrum. Am J Psychiatry 161:398–413, 2004

Siever LJ, Trestman RL: The serotonin system and aggressive personality disorder. Int Clin Psychopharmacol 8 (suppl 2):33–39, 1993

Siever LJ, Amin F, Coccaro EF, et al: Plasma homovanillic acid in schizotypal personality disorder patients and controls. Am J Psychiatry 148:1246–1248, 1991

Siever LJ, Amin F, Coccaro EF, et al: CSF homovanillic acid in schizotypal personality disorder. Am J Psychiatry 150:149–151, 1993

Siever LJ, Buchsbaum M, New A, et al: D,L-fenfluramine response in impulsive personality disorder assessed with [18]-fluorodeoxyglucose positron emission tomography. Neuropsychopharmacology 20:413–423, 1999

Siever LJ, Koenigsberg HW, Harvey P, et al: Cognitive and brain function in schizotypal personality disorder. Schizophr Res 54:157–167, 2002

Silverman JM, Pinkham L, Horvath TB, et al: Affective and impulsive personality disorder traits in the relatives of patients with borderline personality disorder. Am J Psychiatry 148:1378–1385, 1991

Simeon D, Stanley B, Frances A, et al: Self-mutilation in personality disorders: psychological and biological correlates. Am J Psychiatry 149:221–226, 1992

Soderstrom H, Hultin L, Tullberg M, et al: Reduced frontotemporal perfusion in psychopathic personality. Psychiatry Res 114:81–94, 2002

Soloff PH, Meltzer CC, Greer PJ, et al: A fenfluramine-activated FDG-PET study of borderline personality disorder. Biol Psychiatry 47:540–547, 2000

Steinberg BJ, Trestman R, Mitropoulou V, et al: Depressive response to physostigmine challenge in borderline personality disorder patients. Neuropsychopharmacology 17:264–273, 1997

Tancer ME, Mailman RB, Stein MB, et al: Subcortical correlates of differential classical conditioning of aversive emotional reactions in social phobia. Biol Psychiatry 45:863–871, 1999

Tebartz van Elst L, Hesslinger B, Thiel T, et al: Frontolimbic brain abnormalities in patients with borderline personality disorder: a volumetric magnetic resonance imaging study. Biol Psychiatry 54:163–171, 2003

Tiihonen J, Kuikka J, Bergstrom K: DA reuptake site densities in patients with social phobia. Am J Psychiatry 154:239–242, 1997

Torgersen S, Lygren S, Oien PA, et al: A twin study of personality disorders. Compr Psychiatry 41:416–425, 2000

Trestman RL, Keefe RSE, Harvey PD, et al: Cognitive function and biological correlates of cognitive performance in schizotypal personality disorder. Psychiatry Res 59:127–136, 1995

Virkkunen M, Nuutila A, Goodwin FK, et al: Cerebrospinal fluid monoamine metabolite levels in male arsonists. Arch Gen Psychiatry 44:241–247, 1987

Virkkunen M, DeJong J, Bartko J, et al: Relationship of psychobiological variables to recidivism in violent offenders and impulsive fire setters. Arch Gen Psychiatry 46:600–603, 1989

Virkkunen M, Rawlings R, Tokola R: CSF biochemistries, glucose metabolism, and diurnal activity rhythms in alcoholic, violent offenders, fire setters, and healthy volunteers. Arch Gen Psychiatry 51:20–27, 1994

Webb CT, Levinson DF: Schizotypal and paranoid personality disorder in the relatives of patients with schizophrenia and affective disorders: a review. Schizophr Res 11:81–92, 1993

Weinberger DR, Egan MF, Bertolino A, et al: Prefrontal neurons and the genetics of schizophrenia. Biol Psychiatry 50:825–844, 2001

Zanarini MC, Frankenburg FR: Omega-3 Fatty acid treatment of women with borderline personality disorder: a double-blind, placebo-controlled pilot study. Am J Psychiatry 160:167–169, 2003

11

Developmental Issues

Patricia Cohen, Ph.D.
Thomas Crawford, Ph.D.

Aside from well-documented developmental links between early conduct disorder and antisocial personality disorder (ASPD), there are large gaps in our knowledge about childhood antecedents of other DSM-IV-TR personality disorders (American Psychiatric Association 2000; Widiger and Sankis 2000). In this chapter we discuss how developmental processes and selected risk factors lead to the emergence and persistence of personality disorders in young people. We highlight changes in how children and adolescents construct mental representations of themselves and other people and then consider how distortions in this developmental process manifest in personality disorder. We outline what we have learned about early trajectories of personality disorders and discuss how clinicians and researchers can evaluate the normative and clinical significance of symptoms in children and adolescents. Finally, we address problems in assessing these disorders in young people based on the limited number of measurement instruments currently available.

ETIOLOGICAL AND DEVELOPMENTAL FACTORS

In an early paper on the "borderline-child-to-be," Pine (1986) identified three key factors in his developmental model of borderline personality disorder (BPD) in young people. First, he hypothesized how early abuse or trauma overwhelms the child, especially when the trauma is ongoing or experienced from a variety of sources. Second, childhood trauma may interfere with the development of how trust, libidinous attachments, anxiety, aggression, and self-esteem are experienced and expressed. Third, young people may fasten onto immature defenses almost as though these defenses were survival techniques for desperate situations. More recent empirical research points to other factors that contribute to the emergence and persistence of personality disorders over time, including genetic effects and co-occurring Axis I disorders (Crawford et al. 2001b; Livesley et al. 1998).

When individual risk factors occur in isolation, they often may be offset by normative maturational factors in social or cognitive domains. Conduct disorder in childhood, for instance, does not usually lead to ASPD in adulthood. When risk factors occur in combination, however, they may overwhelm the young person's ability to cope, thus leading immature defenses to become inflexible and maladaptive over time. On the other hand, even a child who has experienced a significant trauma may be protected from lasting damage to personality functioning if he or she is securely attached to parents who can buffer the impact of the trauma. If traumatized children are anxiously attached to parents instead, thus reducing the protective effects, they may be at greater risk for lasting personality dysfunction (Alexander 1992). Because genetic, interpersonal, and early trauma risk factors are all addressed elsewhere in this textbook (see Chapter 9, "Genetics"; Chapter 12, "Attachment Theory and Mentalization-Oriented Model of Borderline Personality Disorder"; and Chapter 13, "Role of Childhood Experiences in the Development of Maladaptive and Adaptive Personality Traits"), we focus here on disturbances in how children perceive themselves and the people around them and how developmental changes in cognitive ability may play a role in the formation of personality disorders. In this context we draw on the theoretical literature on attachment in infancy and childhood (e.g., Cassidy and Shaver 1999; Fonagy et al. 2003) and identity development in adolescence (Erikson 1968) and seek to bridge the two using Harter's (1998) work on development of self-representation.

Early Working Models of Self and Other

Attachment theory (Bowlby 1969, 1973) focuses on developmental experiences reflecting secure and insecure relationships between infants and caregivers and emphasizes how young people come to perceive themselves and others. A secure attachment typically occurs when the caregiver has been available and sensitive to the needs of the infant or toddler, especially in times of distress. Young children can better manage negative emotions, such as anger or fear, within a secure relationship because these feelings have been associated with soothing and effective responses by the caregiver (Sroufe 1996). By providing this external form of affect regulation, caregivers prevent infants from being overwhelmed and help them gradually develop the ability to regulate their own affect. When caregivers are inconsistent or rejecting, infants and

toddlers instead may underregulate their own affect or restrict it excessively.

As hypothesized in attachment theory, very basic mental representations of self and others are thought to emerge during infancy through affective experiences characterizing the child–caregiver relationship. These preverbal experiences are labeled "internal working models" and broadly reflect whether infants expect caregivers to be available or helpful when needed. Young children may also internalize a basic sense of whether they are worthy of love and whether other people can be trusted to provide love and emotional support. Individuals who have predominately negative self-representations usually have anxious attachment styles, and those who have predominantly negative representations of others tend to have avoidant attachment styles. Avoidant attachment is thought to stem from cool, rejecting, and distant treatment by attachment figures, and anxious attachment is traced to inconsistent and unpredictable treatment by early attachment figures (Ainsworth et al. 1978; Rothbard and Shaver 1994).

As a guide to behavior, internal working models influence whether young children seek to regulate affective distress by approaching or by avoiding attachment figures, or even by alternating between these opposing strategies for managing negative emotions. With growth in cognitive capacity, these basic mental representations of self and other ("schemas") are subject to elaboration, refinement, and increasing differentiation from affective experiences that occur in close relationships. Nevertheless, these schemas appear to have a remarkably enduring impact on interpersonal strategies used to regulate emotional distress (e.g., Waters et al. 2000). Developmental changes often reflect heterotypic continuity in how attachment styles are expressed in different relationships across developmental stages. That is, a negative self-schema may generate anxious preoccupation with changing attachment figures—a primary caregiver in early childhood, a peer group in adolescence, a romantic partner in adulthood—but nevertheless reflect the same basic difficulty regulating affect across the different relationships.

Although distorted working models accompanying insecure attachment are not pathological by themselves, they nevertheless may contribute to the formation of Axis II psychopathology, especially when combined with other risks or biological vulnerability. Markedly negative representations of others, for instance, may explain higher levels of distrust and suspiciousness in avoidant preadolescents when compared with more securely attached age peers. From this developmental starting point, a variety of pathways leading to pathological and nonpathological outcomes may depend on heritable and environmental risk factors that also influence how personality unfolds. A negative working model of others, reinforced by a hostile and secretive family environment and combined with a biological vulnerability to Cluster A disturbances, may foster a developmental trajectory leading toward paranoid or schizotypal disturbances in adolescence and adulthood. In the absence of biological vulnerability, negative schemas regarding others and corresponding behaviors may gradually be modified as young people learn that their family is not typical of the broader social environment. Normal maturation processes thus may reduce the likelihood that early Cluster A disturbances persist over time.

Early maltreatment by caregivers may produce a serious disturbance called *disorganized attachment* (Solomon and George 1999). Abused infants and children often experience sharp conflicts when approaching caregivers for comfort and support when they also expect maltreatment from them—thus provoking unstable fluctuations between conflicting attachment strategies and behavior. Furthermore, children may fear the loss of the caregivers they depend on, thus limiting their ability to experience or express any age-appropriate anger or aggression toward that person. This phenomenon probably pertains most to the development of the marked instability in interpersonal relationships associated with borderline psychopathology (Fonagy et al. 2000).

Developmental Changes in How the Self and Others Are Perceived

Harter (1998) described how cognitive development in infancy, childhood, and adolescence leads to changes in how young people experience their sense of self. Harter characterized the *self* as a cognitive structure around which behavior is organized, thus anchoring it squarely within the larger framework of personality. As a product of the interaction of biological and social forces, the self undergoes progressive change throughout development. Despite these changes, the self provides a sense of continuity and a source for scripts to organize behavior, thereby creating a foundation for later identity.

Harter emphasized how self-representation often reflects self-evaluation, a process of comparing oneself with other people or with an ideal self, which evolves over time as new cognitive abilities emerge during development. Self-evaluation may be filled with inflated self-worth at one end of the spectrum or laden with self-contempt at the other, and both ends of the spectrum may play an early role in the formation of personality disorders. Even at these extremes, however, cognitive development may nevertheless allow gradual movement toward a more accurate self-representation with a balanced integration of positive and negative attributes. Although not addressed in self-perception literature, per se, changes in cognitive development probably influence how others are perceived in an analogous manner.

One aspect of the cognitive development of the self can be seen in how children describe themselves at different ages. At early ages children typically describe themselves by their physical characteristics, typical behaviors, or material possessions. Self-perception thus lacks much coherence or integration and self-representation is organized instead around all-or-none thinking (all good or all bad). Because negative and positive characteristics are polar opposites, the child cannot recognize that a single person can have both. Given their inability to distinguish real and ideal selves, young children typically have unrealistically positive self-perceptions that often shade into childhood grandiosity. Older children can admit to negative characteristics in one domain while retaining a positive self-representation in another. Vacillation between positive and negative self-image in early adolescence is gradually replaced by a more integrated sense of self and a greater awareness of the importance of the context to behavior. Early grandiosity thus subsides as young people gain the ability to integrate conflicting self-perceptions into a coherent whole in adolescence and early adulthood.

Inaccurate but age-appropriate self-perceptions in young children thus may resemble later symptoms of narcissistic personality disorder. If unrealistically positive self-representations become inflexible and persist over time, they may limit the young person's ability to abandon immature self-representations as their cognitive resources and perceptual skills increase during the course of normal development. When serving defensive functions against childhood adversity, early grandiosity may persist and harden into personality disorder symptoms. Furthermore, grandiosity may be pathological when asserted aggressively as a way to prevent "all good" self-representations from shifting and suddenly becoming "all bad." This defensive style may lead young people with narcissistic disturbances to have dismissing or derogatory perceptions of others. In BPD, young people may lack sufficient internal defenses to prevent self-representations from alternating frequently between the extremes of all good and all bad. Their perception of others similarly alternates between extremes of idealization and devaluation, thus constituting the clinical phenomenon called "splitting."

Among severely abused children, negative self-perceptions may predominate over positive self-images and lead those children to feel profoundly unworthy and unlovable (Fischer and Ayoub 1994). In abusive family environments, caregivers typically reinforce negative evaluations of the child that are then incorporated into the child's self-representations. As a result, there may be little foundation for any cognitive structure of self that would allow the child to develop and integrate both positive and negative self-evaluations. Furthermore, negative self-evaluations may become automatic (Siegler 1991) in ways that make them even more resistant to change.

Formal operational thinking, including logical and abstract reasoning abilities, normally emerges in adolescence (Keating 1990). Dramatic increases in differentiation between self and other also occur during adolescence (Bowlby 1973) and thus increase young people's ability to view themselves as distinct from caregivers. Because differentiation facilitates greater autonomy, dependence on parental attachment figures normally declines during adolescence as young people instead identify more with peer groups. At present we know little about how peer relationships influence personality maturation during adolescence, but this important social factor may reinforce self-perceptions that are more internally based and less centered around the parent–child relationship. Although elevated dependency might not necessarily be pathological earlier in adolescence, it may become a symptom of dependent personality disorder if it persists past late adolescence and on into early adulthood.

The advent of formal operational thinking provides adolescents with a greater capacity to evaluate and compare their relationships with different attachment figures, not just with one another but also against hypothetical ideals. The adolescent's ability to consider attachment relationships in the abstract may bring with it recognition that parents are deficient in some ways (Kobak and Cole 1994), perhaps provoking a dismissive rejection of the parents or angry preoccupation with their shortcomings. Gains in adolescent insight into parent–child relationships will ideally lead to greater openness, objectivity, and flexibility as young people reevaluate attachment relationships and attain a more realistic and integrated perception of parents. This developmental process may reduce dismissing behaviors or dramatic outbursts of anger that might appear earlier in adolescence to be symptoms of narcissism or histrionic personality disorder. If parents respond to these adolescent behaviors in maladaptive ways based on their own interpersonal disturbances, they may not facilitate the resolution of parent–child conflicts and may instead reinforce narcissistic and histrionic tendencies past developmental stages when they normally decline. Linehan (1993) emphasized how invalidating responses from parents can contribute substantially to the formation of BPD, and Bezirganian et al. (1993) have documented that kind of relationship empirically.

Self-Understanding, Self-Direction, and Identity

Erikson (1968) argued that once young people gain greater awareness of themselves and more accurate perceptions of others, they often experience a normative crisis of identity during adolescence and early adulthood. This identity crisis is one of eight age-specific normative crises that occur in human development from infancy through old age. According to Erikson, a crisis is a turning point when development must move in one direction or another. In adolescence, young people either move toward consolidating a secure and stable sense of self or they experience diffuse identities that provide limited direction or sense of continuity over time. When the developmental crisis of identity is successfully resolved, it normally leads to increased integration of personality. When an identity crisis goes unresolved, it may result in potentially pathological delays in maturation instead.

Identity consolidation during adolescence primarily entails establishing a clear sense of self and finding a place in the community. *Identity* is broadly defined in Erikson's theory to encompass self-esteem, satisfaction with personal and occupational goals, and confidence in coping skills. Group membership and sexual identity represent other important domains in a young person's identity. Identity diffusion, on the other hand, is typically expressed in the inability to select clear occupational goals or the adoption of roles deviating from conventional social norms. Erikson notes that identity diffusion may at times include delinquent behavior or psychotic-like symptoms but cautions that these disturbances are often transient during adolescence. Any significant disturbances in social and emotional development may act to distort or interfere with normative identity consolidation, perhaps thereby contributing to the persistence of early personality disorder symptoms that otherwise might resolve through normal maturational processes.

As defined by Erikson, identity diffusion shares many characteristics with Axis II symptoms (Cloninger et al. 1993; Kernberg 1975; Taylor and Goritsas 1994). Indeed, identity disturbances are explicitly included in diagnostic criteria for BPD. Identity disturbances are strongly implied in the suggestibility to other people's influence in histrionic personality disorder, idealized but unrealistic self-perceptions in narcissistic personality disorder, marked worry about other people's criticism in avoidant personality disorder, and difficulties in making everyday decisions in dependent personality disorder. Moreover, identity diffusion and personality disorder symptoms share similar developmental trajectories: both decline with age during adolescence and early adulthood (Johnson et al. 2000a; Meeus et al. 1999).

Distinctions between normal identity diffusion and more enduring personality disorder symptoms in adolescence may be difficult to make in clinical evaluations. Erikson noted that it is normal for young people to "try on" different identities during adolescence and later abandon them when they fail to fit comfortably with their sense of identity. For instance, early attempts to express sexuality may manifest in provocative dress during adolescence without necessarily being a symptom of histrionic personality disorder. After trying out that overt expression of sexuality, young people may subsequently opt for less provocative attire that corresponds more with their internal sense of self. On the other hand, if provocative dressing co-occurs with poorly regulated affect and maladaptive preoccupation with interpersonal relationships, it may signal a more lasting disturbance of personality.

Despite the broad overlap between personality disorder symptoms and Erikson's construct of identity diffusion, relatively little research has investigated the association between the two. It thus remains unclear whether identity disturbances contribute to the emergence of personality disorders in adolescence and later persistence into adulthood or if personality disorder symptoms delay the consolidation of identity. Consistent with Erikson's epigenetic theory of development, Cluster B symptoms do appear to interfere with the formation of lasting and committed romantic relationships that represent the key developmental task of early adulthood (Crawford et al. 2004). Identity consolidation may occur at a critical stage in the development of personality disorders because it coincides with a period when parental influence declines and youths increasingly assert their independence. As young people gradually separate from the family, the identity they choose plays that much greater a role in defining their personality. If adolescents are unable to clearly differentiate themselves from their parents or to resolve any ongoing disturbances in their relationship, they are likely to carry internalized versions of those difficulties with them in how they perceive themselves and others, perhaps even recapitulating those disturbances in new relationships in adulthood. In other words, if identity remains poorly differentiated as young people separate from their family, any corresponding interpersonal disturbances may become self-perpetuating during adulthood.

PERSONALITY MATURATION AND AXIS II PSYCHOPATHOLOGY

Personality traits reflect a complex adaptive system to internal and environmental conditions, including changes in affective and cognitive structures during development (Caspi 1998). Specific affects, behaviors, and cognitions that are age appropriate or normative at one stage of personality development may reflect immaturity or psychopathology at subsequent ages. As young people gain emotional and cognitive skills, they usually abandon immature ways of experiencing and interacting with the world around them. On the other hand, when young people continue to experience affects, behaviors, or cognitions that their peers have outgrown, they may encounter interpersonal difficulties that in some cases accumulate over time. Interpersonal difficulties may be traced to various deficits in the development of affect regulation during infancy, the formation of conscience during early childhood, the establishment of age-appropriate impulse control in childhood and adolescence, or the consolidation of identity in late adolescence and early adulthood. Although deficits or delays in emotional development do not necessarily signify Axis II pathology, they may indicate that an individual is on a deviant pathway with increased risk for further maladaptive behavior. Persistence on a deviant pathway is related to increasing difficulty in returning to a more normal developmental trajectory. Maturational change remains possible, but given the organizational function of personality, developmental change will be constrained by the individual's previous history. (For a further discussion of developmental considerations, see Geiger and Crick 2001 and Kernberg et al. 2000.)

Emotional and Behavioral Problems and Personality Disorder Symptoms

Children and adolescents appear to outgrow many problem behaviors that are reflected in current symptom criteria for personality disorder diagnoses. For instance, parent reports on the Child Behavior Checklist (CBCL; Achenbach 1991) show a significant linear decline in withdrawn behavior from age 4 to age 18 (Bongers et al. 2003). Withdrawn behavior pertains not just to Cluster A personality disorders (paranoid, schizoid, and schizotypal personality disorders) but also to avoidant personality disorder. Parent reports on individual CBCL items associated with Cluster B personality disorders (borderline, histrionic, and narcissistic personality disorders and conduct disorder that precedes ASPD) similarly indicate declines in bragging, showing off, demanding attention, getting into fights, lying, cheating, having a hot temper, crying a lot, feeling excessive dependence, having problems with peers, and experiencing jealousy (Achenbach 1991). Despite broad normative reductions in emotional and behavioral problems, parents report average increases in some childhood and adolescent symptoms such as being suspicious, secretive, and obsessively preoccupied with certain thoughts. Furthermore, age changes in symptoms in normative samples do not necessarily follow the same trajectories as children and adolescents brought in for clinical evaluation or treatment (Achenbach 1991). Parents may take normative age changes into account when assessing the well-being of their children and thus become concerned only when the expected normative decline does not appear, at least for some problems.

It may be useful to put these changes in symptom levels in the context of changes in the prevalence of Axis I symptoms and disorders over childhood and adolescence. Disruptive behavior shows a standard inverted U-shaped prevalence distribution in a wide range of studies (see Moffitt 1993 for a review), with large increases from childhood to adolescence and a sharp drop in young adulthood. Based on parent reports, there are different curvilinear trajectories for mean levels of anxious and depressive symptoms for boys and girls over the full age range from 4–18 years, with higher rates of problems for boys in childhood followed by an adolescent decline (Bongers et al. 2003). For girls these problems increase until the transitional stage of puberty and then level off. Using teachers as informants in a large national epidemiological study, McDermott (1996) found means on every symptom cluster changing with age between ages 5 and 17 years, often quite differently for males and females.

Normal and Abnormal Personality Traits

Many researchers view personality disorder symptoms as extreme variants of personality traits that are continuously distributed in the population (Costa and Widiger 2002; Livesley et al. 1998). We currently have only partial information on developmental changes in trait levels and no information in childhood because of problems in conceptualizing and measuring personality before adolescence (Shiner and Caspi 2003).

Perhaps the most complete information available on age changes is based on the five-factor model (FFM) and its component facets that attempt to measure variation in the full normative range of personality. These broad dimensions and more narrowly defined facets have also been proposed as a way of understanding and potentially measuring personality disorder (Costa and Widiger 2002; see also Chapter 3, "Categorical and Dimensional Models of Personality Disorders"). The dimension labeled neuroticism is especially pertinent because it is hypothesized to reflect many of the criteria for personality disorder. Age changes in self-reported scores on the Revised NEO Personality Inventory (NEO-PI-R; Costa and McCrae 1992) were recently evaluated in a longitudinal sample of gifted children at ages 12 and 16 years and in a much larger cross-sectional sample of Flemish adolescents between 14 and 18 years (McCrae et al. 2002). Most age changes were very small and did not follow previously established adult trajectories that show a gradual decline in neuroticism from the college years to age 30 (e.g., McCrae et al. 1999). When evaluated in younger adolescent samples, neuroticism showed an elevation in girls up to about age 14 and stability thereafter, and there were no significant age changes in boys. Within each broader factor of the FFM, individual facet–age correlations were sometimes different in direction in this study, with some neuroticism facets increasing with age, some stable over the age span, and some declining.

Although knowledge of normative age changes in personality disorder symptoms is limited, the available data clearly show that nearly every Axis II disorder has a gradual linear decrease in the mean number of symptoms between ages 10 and 25 (Johnson et al. 2000a). Based on combined maternal and child reports, Figure 11–1 depicts normative declines in mean symptom levels for approximately 800 youths in the Children in the Community random sample (Cohen and Cohen 1996), which has been studied longitudinally since 1975. Mean scores shown indicate the presence of symptoms without saying anything about how scores are dispersed. Individual scores in the clinical range, for instance, fall well above mean values displayed in Figure 11–1. When mean levels are higher overall, more youths are likely to meet fixed diagnostic criteria that do not take changing age norms into account, thereby possibly increasing the rate of false-positive diagnoses during adolescence. These data suggest that age-specific norms may be desirable for an assessment instrument in this age range. However, they also make clear that the problem of changing normative symptom levels is not limited to childhood and adolescence. Despite changes in symptom level norms, adolescent psychiatric disorders warrant clinical attention even in developmental periods when they are most prevalent. In keeping with this realization, it is important to determine the association of childhood and adolescent personality disorder with impairment and negative prognosis, as is discussed later.

On the whole, normative data do not show any clear congruence between average age changes in normal personality dimensions measured on the NEO-PI-R and normative changes observed using personality disorder measures based on combined youth and parent reports or parent-reported measures of clinically relevant emotional and behavior symptoms. Some of the discrepancy may reflect how the NEO-PI-R assesses personality traits in the normal range and may be limited by ceiling effects at the extreme range of functioning assessed by personality disorder measures or the CBCL. Once again, the direction of age-related changes in symptoms in normative community samples may not always correspond to age-related change in symptoms in children from clinical populations.

CHANGE AND STABILITY IN CHILDHOOD

Given our knowledge that the prevalence of particular behaviors changes with age, what can be said about the correlational or rank-order stability of personality or its temperamental precursors over childhood and adolescence? In particular, to what extent may we expect that the same individuals who manifest the most extreme personality problems at one age will be among those who do so at another age?

Temperament

Often regarded as an early precursor to personality, temperament reflects basic biological differences in childhood characteristics such as activity level, fearful withdrawal, ability to be soothed, responsiveness to stimuli, and affective intensity. Temperament is typically measured by observational ratings or maternal report. Cloninger and his colleagues have developed a measure assessing temperament dimensions in preschool children that are posited to be related to later

personality disorder (Constantino et al. 2002).

In general, temperament shows significant but low stability in early childhood (Rothbart and Bates 1998) for reasons that may be intrinsic to the developmental process. For example, there may be effects specific to maturational levels due to genetic or other constitutional influences. The impact of contextual factors may vary at different maturational levels. Constitutional–environmental interactions also may be a more important source of variation in early childhood, when strong behavioral habits have not yet become firmly established. There may be more error in observation-based measures of temperament in infants and preschool children than in older children due to their greater reactivity to fatigue, hunger, and other temporary influences. Increased measurement error thus contributes to lower stability estimates in younger children.

An additional problem has been an absence of consensus on how to define the major temperament dimensions, an issue that has only recently begun to be resolved. Some dimensions of temperament and the measures devised to assess them have been theoretically derived (Rothbart et al. 2001; Tellegen 1985), including predicted relationships with specific personality disorders (Cloninger 1987; Cloninger et al. 1993). However, theoretically derived dimension names sometimes do not clearly correspond to the content of items. Despite an array of unique construct-derived names, certain dimensions of temperament can be viewed in the frame of the FFM (Shiner and Caspi 2003). This frame has the advantage of uniting the personality and temperament literatures but does only partial justice to the original conceptions of the important individual differences in early childhood such as executive control and emotional reactivity. Research linking temperament measured in early childhood to later personality disorder is only beginning to appear (Constantino et al. 2002).

Personality Dimensions

There is clear evidence that, on average, a personality dimension assessed by a self-report instrument will show lower correlation over equivalent time for younger persons than for older persons (Roberts and DelVecchio 2000). Because instability in personality dimensions continues throughout life, stability coefficients reach a maximum at about age 50 and remain far below the reliabilities of the measures even then. Stabilities for symptom measures of personality disorder are very likely to show a similar pattern. Although we have no preadolescent data, correlations measur-

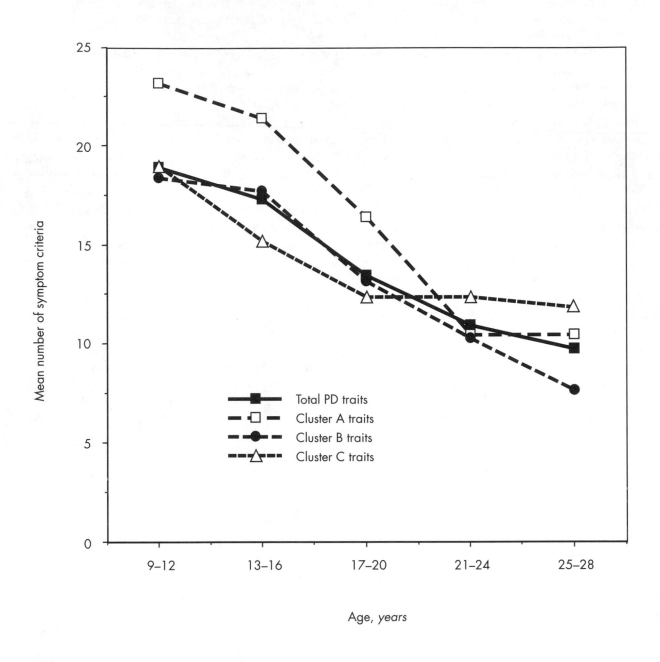

Figure 11–1. Declining personality disorder (PD) symptoms by age.
Source. Adapted from Johnson et al. 2000a.

ing stability are moderate in adolescence (Crawford et al. 2001a), and it is not clear that they increase from adolescence into young adulthood (Johnson et al. 2000a). General stability may not be the issue if disorders are outcomes of gene–environment interactions, so that it is expected that there may be lower stability on extreme scores than over the full range of relevant dimensions (DiLalla et al. 2000).

Axis II diagnoses, on the other hand, tend to be much less stable in clinical and community samples of adolescents (Bernstein et al. 1993; Mattanah et al. 1995). Axis II diagnoses in adults similarly tend to be unstable even in clinical samples (Shea et al. 2002; Zanarini et al. 2003). This instability is likely to be a consequence not only of the generally poorer measurement quality of dichotomized continuous measures (MacCallum et al. 2002) but also of somewhat arbitrary decisions about diagnostic cut-points. Despite the relative instability of categorically defined diagnoses, there is increasing evidence of long-term impairment and poor prognosis associated with adolescent personality disorder or high personality disorder symptoms independent of Axis I disorders or symptoms (Crawford et al. 2001b; Johnson et al. 1999, 2000b; Kasen et al. 1999; Lofgren et al. 1991; Rey et al. 1997). We are thus accumulating evidence that the criteria for adult disorders may be useful indicators of Axis II pathology even in young samples and not necessarily less predictive at times when they are more normative. However, there are no current studies large enough to investigate these issues for individual diagnostic criteria, and thus at present this question remains unanswered at the criterion level.

Case Examples

Given what we know about developmental trajectories of personality disorder symptoms in adolescents, it appears unwise to make categorical diagnoses during initial clinical assessment except perhaps in extreme cases. Nevertheless, it is meaningful to consider youths at risk for subsequent personality disorder based on how they present for treatment and based on collateral risk factors in close family members, as illustrated by the following vignette.

> A 15-year-old boy from an intact family was brought for individual psychotherapy to address uncontrolled anger, a pervasive hatred toward age peers, and oppositional and self-defeating behavior (e.g., threatening to drop out of high school). His self-image reflected grandiosity or self-contempt depending on different social contexts, and he tended to be avoidant and dismissive of others. During treatment it became evident that one parent tried to cope with excessive anxiety by becoming overinvolved in the patient's long-term plans in ways that provoked stubborn and oppositional behavior. The other parent had recurrent depressive episodes, an explosive and unpredictable temper, identity diffusion, and a dismissive interpersonal style.
>
> On initial evaluation, this 15-year-old youth appeared at increased risk for lasting BPD based on persistent symptoms of uncontrolled anger, marked antipathy for others, and poorly integrated representations of self and others. The long-term risk may be compounded by the presence of parental anxiety and mood disturbances, especially as they are woven into parent–child relationships. Personality disturbances thus appeared to be reinforced by defensive reactions to one parent's overinvolvement and also by identification with the other parent's angry and dismissive interpersonal style. Despite poor social adjustment with peers, this youth nevertheless reported having a positive relationship with his parents. Given this protective factor and an absence of key risk factors such as childhood trauma, his personality disorder symptoms may well subside over

time as he gains maturity. Treatment in this case focused on assisting the youth to regulate angry affect more adaptively and to articulate how peers upset him so much. Treatment also helped the parents to become more aware of how their own anxiety and mood disturbances contributed to maladaptive parent–child interactions in ways that inhibited the youth's gradual movement toward independent adult functioning.

Just as maturational factors appear to confound the assessment of personality disorders in adolescents, they may also obscure the presence of personality disorder in adults who have outgrown some earlier manifestations of the disorder. Knowledge of normative trajectories of personality disorder thus can inform the assessment and treatment of personality disturbances in adult patients whose symptoms fall short of current diagnostic criteria:

> A 42-year-old woman presented for treatment with complaints of loneliness and an enduring inability to establish a stable romantic relationship. She recalled adolescence and early adulthood as periods characterized by labile mood, frequent abandonment fears, volatile and unpredictable romantic relationships, reactive anger toward parents and peers, and a series of suicidal gestures. During childhood she witnessed violent conflicts between mother and father before they divorced and experienced significant emotional neglect afterward. When presenting for treatment, this patient denied any mood lability or suicidal ideation and functioned well at work. However, abandonment fears, reactive anger, and mood lability recurred whenever she became involved in new romantic relationships, thereby prompting a general avoidance of close relationships and reinforcing unwanted feelings of loneliness.

Even allowing for inaccuracies that distort retrospective clinical reports, this patient undoubtedly met full criteria for BPD during adolescence and early adulthood. Although her symptoms have since fallen below diagnostic threshold, either due to maturational factors or the effects of prior individual psychotherapies, she nevertheless continues to experience significant borderline psychopathology in ways that become painfully apparent whenever new romantic attachments evoke long-standing abandonment fears she otherwise seeks to avoid. Treatment in this case focused on clarifying and then reducing abandonment fears and addressing how her reactive anger undermined the stability of her romantic relationships. Treatment also addressed the disorganizing effects of childhood trauma and neglect.

WHAT IS THE BEST MEASUREMENT STRATEGY FOR ASSESSING EARLY PERSONALITY DISORDERS?

Three overall issues pose problems for the assessment of personality disorders in children and adolescents. As indicated earlier, DSM-IV-TR does not take into account normative developmental changes in the prevalence of certain problems and the consequent possibility that certain diagnostic criteria should not be seen as abnormal behavior at some ages. Second, there is a shortage of appropriate and validated diagnostic instruments for children and adolescents and unresolved questions about the best measurement strategy. Third, aspects of personality are less stable in childhood and adolescence, thus raising concern that early diagnosis of personality disorders might lead to premature labeling.

Choice of Informant

In clinical assessment of adults the patient is usually the primary informant, although the corroboration and independent perspectives of knowledgeable sources such as family members are welcome and often useful. Research measures designed for use with adults in clinical or other samples generally are confined to self-report. In the child mental health field, there is still little consensus about which informants should be considered primary and which should be seen as auxiliary at different points in childhood development. It is often assumed that the primary caretaker should be the principal informant for preschool children. As such, instruments measuring temperament, personality, and psychopathology in children younger than age 9 or 10 years are most often based on information supplied by parents—for example, the Children's Behavior Questionnaire (Rothbart et al. 2001), the Personality Inventory for Children (PIC-2; Lachar 1999a), and the CBCL. For young children in preschool or day care, teachers or childcare leaders may provide the best data based on greater familiarity with normative patterns of behavior for the age.

Similarly, parents and teachers are both thought to provide relevant data for older children in elementary school, although in general, agreement on the child's problems is poor across these informants (Achenbach et al. 1987). Sometime in childhood, at least by age 9 or 10, most children are able to provide data on their own characteristics and problems. For instance, the youth-reported version of the Diagnostic Interview Schedule for Children—IV (Shaffer et al. 2000) assesses psychopathology in children as young as 9 years old. Similarly, the Personality Inventory for Youth (PIY; Lachar and Gruber 1995) uses self-reports to assess personality in children starting at the same age. Most self-report measures of normal personality, however, are used only with adolescents and adults (Shiner and Caspi 2003).

Agreement between parent and offspring on youth behaviors and problems is not very good (e.g., Achenbach et al. 1987), and age changes in prevalence based on youth self-report look different from those based on parent report or teacher report. Agreement between self and informant reports on personality disorder measures for adults is similarly poor (Klonsky et al. 2002). Despite these difficulties, the research field has reached general consensus that all informants add usefully to the assessment of Axis I disorders in children and adolescents. As a consequence, the preferred strategy is to obtain data from at least two informants and consider any symptomatic report to be valid providing there is evidence of associated impairment. If only a single informant can be used, evidence indicates that adolescents are better informants about emotions and often acknowledge disruptive or antisocial behaviors that may be unknown to the parent. Parents or teachers are thought to be better informants on issues where normative comparisons are relevant.

Where does this leave us when deciding which informants to assess for personality disturbances in children and adolescents? At present we do not know whether diagnostic criteria for Axis II are intrinsically more difficult to assess in youth than most criteria for Axis I. All things considered, it appears prudent to gather data from multiple sources whenever possible when assessing children and adolescents.

RESEARCH AND CLINICAL MEASURES OF CHILD OR ADOLESCENT PERSONALITY DISORDER

As interest in early Axis II disturbances in young people has grown, a variety of instruments designed to measure normal and abnormal personality in adults have been evaluated for use in adolescent samples. Certain personality disorder instruments for adults have been specifically adapted to be age appropriate for child or adolescent respondents. Among self- and parent-reported instruments, Axis II scales are typically combined with various measures of Axis I disturbances and thus facilitate the assessment of co-occurrence between these psychiatric constructs. On the whole, individual scales for these instruments have internal consistency reliability comparable with or favorable to adult instruments recently evaluated by Clark and Harrison (2001).

The largest full assessment of Axis II disorders in a general community sample of children was undertaken in the Children in the Community Study (Cohen and Cohen 1996) long before any Axis II scales were developed for children or adolescents. Prior to assessing this large sample of youths (ranging in age between 9 and 19 years) and their mothers in 1983, Drs. Cohen and Kasen selected relevant items from scales included in the research protocol that corresponded to DSM-III (American Psychiatric Association 1980) diagnostic criteria and then added items or adapted items from then-current adult instruments to assess diagnostic criteria not already covered elsewhere (Bernstein et al. 1993). After data collection was complete, a team of clinical researchers reviewed these youth- and parent-reported items and wrote algorithms for Axis II symptom scales and categorical diagnoses. Drs. Schwab-Stone and Cohen updated this assessment by adding items relevant to DSM-III-R (American Psychiatric Association 1987) for a follow-up assessment 2.5 years later at mean age 16 (Bernstein et al. 1993). A new set of DSM-IV (American Psychiatric Association 1994) algorithms was developed to be consistent across these two waves of data collection and an additional assessment of the sample 6 years later at a mean age of 22 (Johnson et al. 1999, 2000a). Validity information on these Axis II scales and diagnoses comes from a series of analyses of the longitudinal data showing prediction of both long-term impairment and dysfunction independently of Axis I disorders (Bernstein et al. 1993, 1996; Johnson et al. 1999, 2000b; Kasen et al. 2001). Despite the utility of this research instrument, it has only recently been adapted for use by other researchers and is not designed to be a clinical instrument.

Structured Clinical Interviews

Of the structured interviews designed to assess DSM-defined personality disorders in adults, the Personality Disorder Evaluation (Loranger 1988) has been most thoroughly evaluated and appears to be a valid measure of Axis II disturbance in adolescents. Nevertheless, more work is needed to identify age-related differences in adolescent and adult manifestations of personality disorders. In a longitudinal comparison of

adolescent and adult inpatient samples, personality disorders assessed with the Personality Disorder Evaluation were less stable over a 2-year interval in adolescents than in adults (Mattanah et al. 1995). However, threshold effects often add unreliability to stability estimates of categorically defined personality disorders, thus making comparisons across age groups more difficult to interpret. When assessed as dimensional constructs, stability estimates for personality disorders usually appear higher than when assessed as categorical constructs.

Self-Report Instruments

Although self-report instruments are easier and more cost-efficient to administer than structured interviews, questions are raised about whether respondents have sufficient self-awareness or willingness to acknowledge Axis II symptoms that might stigmatize them. Given problems in setting reliable thresholds, the available instruments for children and adolescents tend to assess Axis II symptoms using continuous scales instead of making formal diagnoses.

The Millon Adolescent Clinical Inventory (MACI) is a well-known instrument modeled on the Millon Clinical Multiaxial Inventory designed for adults (see Davis et al. 1999). Intended for adolescents as young as age 13, the MACI uses 160 self-report items to measure personality disorder constructs congruent with DSM-defined personality disorders but also reflecting Millon's (1990) theory of personality. The MACI thus measures 12 personality styles labeled Introversive, Inhibited, Doleful, Submissive, Dramatizing, Egotistic, Unruly, Forceful, Conforming, Oppositional, Self-Demeaning, and Borderline Tendency. Computer-generated scores on the MACI make adjustments for age and gender differences in Axis II disturbances based on norms from separate samples of normal and disturbed adolescents. Standardized scores are further adjusted to take estimated base rates of psychopathology into account even though the prevalence of Axis II disturbances in adolescents has yet to be established. These built-in adjustments are not readily transparent and effectively preclude their use for investigating the population prevalence of adolescent Axis II disturbances or for assessing developmental change.

Parallel Parent- and Youth-Reported Instruments

The PIC-2 and PIY were both originally modeled on the Minnesota Multiphasic Personality Inventory and thus do not correspond directly to DSM-IV Axis II disorders. The parent-reported PIC-2 uses 275 forced-choice items to measure constructs labeled Cognitive Impairment, Impulsivity and Distractibility, Delinquency, Family Dysfunction, Reality Distortion, Somatic Concern, Psychological Discomfort, Social Withdrawal, and Social Skills Deficits. The youth-reported PIY uses 270 forced-choice items to measure the same constructs. As suggested by the labels, the PIY and PIC-2 measure constructs that probably tap a mixture of Axis I and Axis II disturbances. Despite substantial similarity on the PIY and PIC-2, youth and parent informants show moderate agreement (median correlation=0.43, range 0.28–0.53) (Lachar 1999b). These concordance rates appear better than the 0.25 correlation between youth and parent reports for comparable age groups on the CBCL (Achenbach et al. 1987).

Additional Instruments for DSM-IV/ DSM-IV-TR Personality Disorders

The Adolescent Psychopathology Scale (Reynolds 1998) is a self-report measure designed for adolescents between 12 and 19 years old. It measures five of the ten DSM-IV personality disorders (borderline, avoidant, obsessive-compulsive, paranoid, and schizotypal personality disorders) along with conduct disorder as the childhood precursor of ASPD. The Coolidge Personality and Neuropsychological Inventory for Children (CPNI; Coolidge 1998) assesses DSM-IV Axis II disorders in children and adolescents from 5–17 years old by parent report. The CPNI assesses symptoms of all DSM-IV personality disorders as well as conduct disorder symptoms. The Shedler-Westen Assessment Procedure–200 for Adolescents (SWAP-200-A; Westen et al. 2003) is a newly developed Q-sort instrument designed for use by skilled clinical observers to assess Axis II pathology in adolescent patients they see in treatment. Q-sort is a method by which items are arrayed by the clinician from most descriptive of the adolescent to least descriptive of the adolescent. This measure was adapted from the Shedler-Westen Assessment Procedure–200, a Q-sort designed for adults that has shown evidence of validity, reliability, and utility in taxonomic research with adult samples (e.g., Shedler and Westen 1998). At present none of the available instruments has demonstrated clear superiority in clinical and research applications, and there are limited validity data available for newly developed scales measuring DSM-IV and DSM-IV-TR personality disorders.

CONCLUSIONS

During the past 15 years there has been accumulating evidence that clinically meaningful personality disorders occur in adolescents. Adolescent personality disorders are associated with emotional distress and psychosocial impairment in community samples (Golombek et al. 1987; Lewinsohn et al. 1997; Marton et al. 1987; Stein et al. 1987) and clinical samples in inpatient and outpatient settings (Brent et al. 1994; Grilo et al. 1996; Pinto et al. 1996; Westen et al. 2003). When adolescent and adult personality disorders are compared, many similarities have been observed. Just as adult personality disorders are associated with co-occurring Axis I disturbances (Bienvenu and Stein 2003; Farmer and Nelson-Gray 1990), adolescent personality disorders also have been shown to co-occur with Axis I disturbances (Becker et al. 2000; Crawford et al. 2001a). However, more work is needed on age-related differences in adolescent and adult manifestations of personality disorders.

Although elevated personality disorder scores in adolescence represent a risk for subsequent psychiatric and psychosocial disturbances, early personality disorder symptoms are also likely to decline over time. Caution is thus warranted in evaluating their clinical significance during adolescence. On the other hand, there is almost universal agreement that prevention of mental disorders is best accomplished at a very young age and in collaboration with parents, particularly when other risk factors are also present. Therefore, children with elevated symptoms or their precursors are prime targets for secondary prevention—that is, for prevention of further developmental delays or elevation to frank disorder. Regardless of how childhood and adolescent personality disorders are defined—either as an early version of adult disorder or an early indicator of elevated risk of adult disorder—it appears appropriate to consider interventions to alleviate Axis II disturbances when they manifest in young people.

REFERENCES

Achenbach TM: Manual for the Child Behavior Checklist, Ages 4–18 and 1991 Profile. Burlington, VT, University of Vermont, Department of Psychiatry, 1991
Achenbach TM, McConaughy SH, Howell CT: Child/adolescent behavioral and emotional problems: implications of cross-informant correlations for situational specificity. Psychol Bull 101:213–232, 1987

Ainsworth MDS, Blehar MC, Waters E, et al: Patterns of attachment: a psychological study of the Strange Situation. Hillsdale, NJ, Erlbaum, 1978

Alexander PC: Application of attachment theory to the study of sexual abuse. J Consult Clin Psychol 60:185–195, 1992

American Psychiatric Association: Diagnostic and Statistical Manual of Mental Disorders, 3rd Edition. Washington, DC, American Psychiatric Association, 1980

American Psychiatric Association: Diagnostic and Statistical Manual of Mental Disorders, 3rd Edition, Revised. Washington, DC, American Psychiatric Association, 1987

American Psychiatric Association: Diagnostic and Statistical Manual of Mental Disorders, 4th Edition. Washington, DC, American Psychiatric Association, 1994

American Psychiatric Association: Diagnostic and Statistical Manual of Mental Disorders, 4th Edition, Text Revision. Washington, DC, American Psychiatric Association, 2000

Becker DF, Grilo CM, Edell WS, et al: Comorbidity of borderline personality disorder with other personality disorders in hospitalized adolescents and adults. Am J Psychiatry 157:2011–2016, 2000

Bernstein DP, Cohen P, Velez CN, et al: Prevalence and stability of the DSM-III-R personality disorders in a community-based survey of adolescents. Am J Psychiatry 150:1237–1243, 1993

Bernstein DP, Cohen P, Skodol A, et al: Childhood antecedents of adolescent personality disorders. Am J Psychiatry 153:907–913, 1996

Bezirganian S, Cohen P, Brook JS: The impact of mother–child interaction on the development of borderline personality disorder. Am J Psychiatry 150:1836–1842, 1993

Bienvenu OJ, Stein MB: Personality and anxiety disorders: a review. J Personal Disord 17:139–151, 2003

Bongers IL, Koot HM, van der Ende J, et al: The normative development of child and adolescent problem behavior. J Abnorm Psychol 112:179–192, 2003

Bowlby J: Attachment and Loss, Vol 1: Attachment. New York, Basic Books, 1969

Bowlby J: Attachment and Loss, Vol 2: Separation. New York, Basic Books, 1973

Brent DA, Johnson B, Perper J, et al: Personality disorder, personality traits, impulsive violence and completed suicide in adolescents. J Am Acad Child Adolesc Psychiatry 33:1080–1086, 1994

Caspi A: Personality development across the life course, in Handbook of Child Psychology, Vol 3: Social, Emotional, and Personality Development, 5th Edition. Edited by Damon W, Eisenberg N. New York, Wiley, 1998, pp 311–388

Cassidy J, Shaver PR: Handbook of Attachment: Theory, Research, and Clinical Applications. New York, Guilford, 1999

Clark LA, Harrison JA: Assessment instruments, in Handbook of Personality Disorders. Edited by Livesley WJ. New York, Guilford, 2001, pp 277–306

Cloninger CR: A systematic method for clinical description and classification of personality variants: a proposal. Arch Gen Psychiatry 44:573–588, 1987

Cloninger CR, Svrakic DM, Przybeck TR: A psychobiological model of temperament and character. Arch Gen Psychiatry 50:975–990, 1993

Cohen P, Cohen J: Life Values and Adolescent Mental Health. Mahwah, NJ, Lawrence Erlbaum, 1996

Constantino JN, Cloninger CR, Clarke AR, et al: Application of the seven-factor model of personality to early childhood. Psychiatr Res 109:229–244, 2002

Coolidge FL: Coolidge Personality and Neuropsychological Inventory for Children Manual: CPNI. Colorado Springs, CO, FL Coolidge, 1998

Costa PT Jr, McCrae RR: Revised NEO Personality Inventory (NEO-PI-R) and NEO Five-Factor Inventory (NEO-FFI) Professional Manual. Odessa, FL, Psychological Assessment Resources, 1992

Costa PT Jr, Widiger TA (eds): Personality Disorders and the Five-Factor Model of Personality, 2nd Edition. Washington, DC, American Psychological Association, 2002

Crawford TN, Cohen P, Brook JS: Dramatic erratic personality disorder symptoms, I: continuity from early adolescence into adulthood. J Personal Disord 15:319–335, 2001a

Crawford TN, Cohen P, Brook JS: Dramatic erratic personality disorder symptoms, II: developmental pathways from early adolescence to adulthood. J Personal Disord 15:336–350, 2001b

Crawford TN, Cohen P, Johnson JG, et al: The course and psychosocial correlates of personality disorder symptoms in adolescence: Erikson's developmental theory revisited. J Youth Adolesc 33:373–387, 2004

Davis RD, Woodward M, Goncalves A, et al: Treatment planning and outcome in adults: the Millon Clinical Multiaxial Inventory-III, in The Use of Psychological Testing for Treatment Planning and Outcomes Assessment, 2nd Edition. Edited by Maruish ME. Mahwah, NJ, Erlbaum, 1999, pp 1051–1081

DiLalla DL, Gottesman II, Carey G: Madness beyond the threshold? Associations between personality and psychopathology, in Temperament and Personality Development Across the Life Span. Edited by Molfese VJ, Molfese DL. Mahwah, NJ, Erlbaum, 2000, pp 177–210

Erikson EH: Identity: Youth and Crisis. New York, WW Norton, 1968

Farmer R, Nelson-Gray RO: Personality disorders and depression: hypothetical relations, empirical findings, and methodological considerations. Clin Psychol Rev 10:453–476, 1990

Fischer KW, Ayoub C: Affective splitting and dissociation in normal and maltreated children: developmental pathways for self in relationships, in Disorders and Dysfunctions of the Self: Rochester Symposium on Developmental Psychopathology, Vol 5. Edited by Cicchetti D, Toth SL. New York, Plenum Press, 1994, pp 149–222

Fonagy P, Target M, Gergely G: Attachment and borderline personality disorder: a theory and some evidence. Psychiatr Clin North Am 23:103–122, 2000

Fonagy P, Target M, Gergely G, et al: The developmental roots of borderline personality disorder in early attachment relationships: a theory and some evidence. Psychoanalytic Inquiry 23:412–459, 2003

Geiger TC, Crick NR: A developmental psychopathology perspective on vulnerability to personality disorders, in Vulnerability to Psychopathology. Edited by Ingram RE, Price JM. New York, Guilford, 2001, pp 57–102

Golombek H, Marton P, Stein B, et al: Personality functioning status during early and middle adolescence. Adolesc Psychiatry 14:365–377, 1987

Grilo CM, Becker DF, Fehon DC, et al: Gender differences in personality disorders in psychiatrically hospitalized adolescents. Am J Psychiatry 153:1089–1091, 1996

Harter S: The development of self-representations, in Handbook of Child Psychology, Vol 3: Social, Emotional, and Personality Development, 5th Edition. Edited by Damon W, Eisenberg N. New York, Wiley, 1998, pp 553–617

Johnson JG, Cohen P, Skodol AE, et al: Personality disorders in adolescence and risk of major mental disorders and suicidality during adulthood. Arch Gen Psychiatry 56:805–811, 1999

Johnson JG, Cohen P, Kasen S, et al: Age-related change in personality disorder trait levels between early adolescence and adulthood: a community-based longitudinal investigation. Acta Psychiatr Scand 102:265–275, 2000a

Johnson JG, Cohen P, Smailes E, et al: Adolescent personality disorders associated with violence and criminal behavior during adolescence and early adulthood. Am J Psychiatry 157:1406–1412, 2000b

Kasen S, Cohen P, Skodol AE, et al: Influence of child and adolescent psychiatric disorders on young adult personality disorder. Am J Psychiatry 156:1529–1535, 1999

Kasen S, Cohen P, Skodol AE, et al: Childhood depression and adult personality disorder: alternative pathways of continuity. Arch Gen Psychiatry 58:231–236, 2001

Keating D: Adolescent thinking, in At the Threshold: The Developing Adolescent. Edited by Feldman SS, Elliott G. Cambridge, MA, Harvard University Press, 1990, pp 54–90

Kernberg OF: Borderline Conditions and Pathological Narcissism. Northvale, NJ, Jason Aronson, 1975

Kernberg OF, Weiner AS, Bardenstein KK: Personality Disorders in Children and Adolescents. New York, Basic Books, 2000

Klonsky ED, Oltmanns TF, Turkheimer E: Informant reports of personality disorders: relation to self-reports and future research directions. Clinical Psychology: Science and Practice 9:300–311, 2002

Kobak R, Cole C: Attachment and metamonitoring: implications for adolescent autonomy and psychopathology, in Rochester Symposium on Development and Psychopathology, Vol 5: Disorders of the Self. Edited by Cicchetti D. Rochester, NY, University of Rochester Press, 1994, pp 267–297

Lachar D: Personality Inventory for Children-2 (PIC-2) Manual. Los Angeles, CA, Western Psychological Services, 1999a

Lachar D: Personality Inventory for Children, 2nd Edition (PIC-2), Personality Inventory for Youth (PIY), and Student Behavior Survey (SBS), in The Use of Psychological Testing for Treatment Planning and Outcomes Assessment, 2nd Edition. Edited by Maruish ME. Mahwah, NJ, Lawrence Erlbaum Associates, 1999b, pp 399–427

Lachar D, Gruber CP: Personality Inventory for Youth (PIY) Manual. Los Angeles, CA, Western Psychological Services, 1995

Lewinsohn PM, Rohde P, Seeley JR, et al: Axis II psychopathology as a function of Axis I disorders in childhood and adolescence. J Am Acad Child Adolesc Psychiatry 36:1752–1759, 1997

Linehan MM: Cognitive Behavioral Treatment of Borderline Personality Disorder. New York, Guilford, 1993

Livesley WJ, Jang KL, Vernon PA: The phenotypic and genetic architecture of traits delineating personality disorder. Arch Gen Psychiatry 55:941–948, 1998

Lofgren DP, Bemporad J, King J, et al: A follow-up study of so-called borderline children. Am J Psychiatry 148:1541–1547, 1991

Loranger AW: Personality Disorder Examination (personality disorder E) Manual. Yonkers, NY, DV Communications, 1988

MacCallum RC, Zhang S, Preacher KJ, et al: On the practice of dichotomization of quantitative variables. Psychol Methods 7:41–63, 2002

Marton P, Golombek H, Stein B, et al: Behavior disturbance and changes in personality dysfunction from early to middle adolescence. Adolesc Psychiatry 14:394–406, 1987

Mattanah JJF, Becker DF, Levy KN, et al: Diagnostic stability in adolescents followed 2 years after hospitalization. Am J Psychiatry 152:889–894, 1995

McCrae RR, Costa PT, de Lima MP, et al: Age differences in personality across the adult life span: parallels in five cultures. Dev Psychol 35:466–477, 1999

McCrae RR, Costa PT, Terracciano A, et al: Personality trait development from age 12 to age 18: longitudinal, cross-sectional, and cross-cultural analyses. J Pers Soc Psychol 83:1456–1468, 2002

McDermott PA: A nationwide study of developmental and gender prevalence for psychopathology in childhood and adolescence. J Abnorm Child Psychol 24:53–66, 1996

Meeus W, Iedema J, Helsen M, et al: Patterns of adolescent identity development: review of literature and longitudinal analysis. Dev Rev 19:419–461, 1999

Millon T: Toward a New Personology: An Evolutionary Model. New York, Wiley, 1990

Moffitt T: Adolescence-limited and life-course-persistent antisocial behavior: a developmental taxonomy. Psychol Rev 100:674–701, 1993

Pine F: On the development of the "borderline-child-to-be." Am J Orthopsychiatry 56:450–457, 1986

Pinto A, Grapentine WL, Francis G, et al: Borderline personality disorder in adolescents: affective and cognitive features. J Am Acad Child Adolesc Psychiatry 35:1338–1343, 1996

Rey JM, Singh M, Morris-Yates A, et al: Referred adolescents as young adults: the relationship between psychosocial functioning and personality disorder. Aust N Z J Psychiatry 31:219–226, 1997

Reynolds WM: Adolescent Psychopathology Scale. Odessa, FL, Psychological Assessment Resources, 1998

Roberts BW, DelVecchio WF: The rank-order consistency of personality traits from childhood to old age: a quantitative review of longitudinal studies. Psychol Bull 126:3–25, 2000

Rothbard JC, Shaver PR: Continuity of attachment across the life span, in Attachment in Adults: Clinical and Developmental Perspectives. Edited by Sperling MB, Berman WH. New York, Guilford, 1994, pp 31–71

Rothbart MK, Bates JE: Temperament, in Handbook of Child Psychology, 5th Edition, Vol 3: Social, Emotional, and Personality Development. Edited by Damon M, Eisenberg N. New York, Wiley, 1998, pp 105–176

Rothbart MK, Ahadi SA, Hershey KL, et al: Investigations of temperament at three to seven years: the Children's Behavior Questionnaire. Child Dev 72:1394–1408, 2001

Shaffer D, Fisher P, Lucas CP, et al: NIMH Diagnostic Interview Schedule for Children Version IV (NIMH DISC-IV): description, differences from previous versions, and reliability of some common diagnoses. J Am Acad Child Adolesc Psychiatry 39:28–38, 2000

Shea MT, Stout R, Gunderson J, et al: Short-term diagnostic stability of schizotypal, borderline, avoidant, and obsessive-compulsive personality disorders. Am J Psychiatry 159:2036–2041, 2002

Shedler J, Westen D: Refining the measurement of Axis II: a Q-sort procedure for assessing personality pathology. Assessment 5:335–355, 1998

Shiner R, Caspi A: Personality differences in childhood and adolescence: measurement, development, and consequences. J Child Psychol Psychiatry 44:2–32, 2003

Siegler RS: Children's Thinking, 2nd Edition. Englewood Cliffs, NJ, Prentice Hall, 1991

Solomon J, George C: Attachment Disorganization. New York, Guilford, 1999

Sroufe LA: Emotional Development: The Organization of Emotional Life in the Early Years. New York, Cambridge University Press, 1996

Stein B, Golombek H, Marton P, et al: Personality functioning and change in clinical presentation from early to middle adolescence. Adolesc Psychiatry 14:378–393, 1987

Taylor S, Goritsas E: Dimensions of identity diffusion. J Personal Disord 8:229–239, 1994

Tellegen A: Structure of mood and personality and their relevance to assessing anxiety, with an emphasis on self-report, in Anxiety and the Anxiety Disorders. Edited by Tuma AH, Maser JD. Hillsdale, NJ, Erlbaum, 1985, pp 681–706

Waters E, Merrick S, Treboux D, et al: Attachment security in infancy and early adulthood: a longitudinal study. Child Dev 71:684–689, 2000

Westen D, Shedler J, Glass S, et al: Personality diagnoses in adolescence: DSM-IV Axis II diagnoses and an empirically derived alternative. Am J Psychiatry 160:952–966, 2003

Widiger TA, Sankis L: Adult psychopathology: issues and controversies. Ann Rev Psychol 51:377–404, 2000

Zanarini MC, Frankenburg FR, Hennen J, et al: The longitudinal course of borderline psychopathology: 6-year prospective follow-up of the phenomenology of borderline personality disorder. Am J Psychiatry 160:274–283, 2003

12

Attachment Theory and Mentalization-Oriented Model of Borderline Personality Disorder

Peter Fonagy, Ph.D., F.B.A.
Anthony W. Bateman, M.A., F.R.C.Psych.

Borderline personality disorder (BPD) is a dysfunction of self-regulation particularly in the context of social relationships. Both the regulation of emotion and the catastrophic reaction to the loss of intensely emotionally invested social ties place BPD in the domain of attachment. A number of theorists have drawn on Bowlby's ideas in explanation of borderline pathology. Most specifically, Gunderson (1996) suggested that intolerance of aloneness was at the core of borderline pathology, and the inability of those with BPD to invoke a "soothing introject" was a consequence of early attachment failures. He carefully described typical patterns of borderline dysfunction in terms of exaggerated reactions of the insecurely attached infant; for example, clinging, fearfulness about dependency needs, terror of abandonment, and constant monitoring of the proximity of the caregiver. Lyons-Ruth and Jacobovitz (1999) focused on the disorganization of the attachment system in infancy as predisposing to later borderline pathology. Notably, they identified an insecure, as opposed to a secure, disorganized pattern as predisposing to conduct problems. Crittenden (1997) was particularly concerned with incorporating borderline individuals' deep ambivalence and fear of close relationships in her representation of adult attachment disorganization. Fonagy and colleagues (Fonagy 2000; Fonagy et al. 2000) also used the framework of attachment theory but emphasized the role of attachment in the development of symbolic function and the way in which insecure disorganized attachment may generate vulnerability in the face of further turmoil and challenges. All of these, and other, theoretical approaches predict that representations of attachment will be seriously insecure and arguably disorganized in patients with BPD.

In this chapter we briefly outline the theory of attachment and some empirical work linking BPD with dysfunctions of the attachment system. We consider BPD from an attachment theory perspective, introducing some modifications of classical attachment theory that have helped us understand the disordered attachment of individuals with BPD. In particular, we link the development of the capacity of mentalization (the ability to represent the behavior of self and others in terms of underlying mental states) with the quality of attachment relationships—and link the failure of mentalization with symptoms of BPD. Finally, the treatment implications of our attachment theory–based model of BPD are discussed.

Brief Outline of Attachment Theory

Bowlby's attachment theory has a biological focus (Bowlby 1969). Attachment readily reduces to a "molecular" level of infant behaviors, such as smiling and vocalizing, that alert the caregiver to the child's interest in socializing and bring the caregiver close to the child. Smiling and vocalizing are attachment behaviors, as is crying, which is experienced by most caregivers as aversive, and they engage the caregiver in caretaking behaviors. Bowlby emphasized the survival value of attachment in enhancing safety through proximity to the caregiver in addition to feeding, learning about the environment, and social interaction, as well as protection from predators. Bowlby (1969) considered the latter to be the biological function of attachment behavior. Attachment behaviors were seen as part of a "behavioral system" (a term Bowlby borrowed from ethology).

In the second volume of his *Attachment and Loss* trilogy, Bowlby established the set goal of the attachment system as maintaining the caregiver's accessibility and responsiveness, which he covered with a single term: *availability* (Bowlby 1973). *Availability* means confident expectation—gained from "tolerably accurately" (p. 202) represented experience over a significant time period—that the attachment figure will be available. The attachment behavioral system thus came to be underpinned by a set of cognitive mechanisms, discussed by Bowlby as representational models or by Craik (1943) as internal working models (Bretherton and Munholland 1999; Crittenden 1994; Main 1991; Sroufe 1996). Four representational sys-

tems are implied by the internal working models: 1) expectations of interactive attributes of early caregivers created in the first year of life and subsequently elaborated; 2) event representations by which general and specific memories of attachment-related experiences are encoded and retrieved; 3) autobiographical memories by which specific events are conceptually connected because of their relation to a continuing personal narrative and developing self-understanding; and 4) understanding of the psychological characteristics of other people and differentiating them from the characteristics of the self. It is in this last layer of the internal working models that we consider the dysfunctions of individuals with BPD to be most profound.

The second great pioneer of attachment theory, Mary Ainsworth (1969, 1985; Ainsworth et al. 1978), developed the well-known laboratory-based procedure of the Strange Situation for observing infants' internal working models in action. When infants are briefly separated from their caregivers in an unfamiliar situation, they show one of four patterns of behavior. Infants who display *secure* attachment explore readily in the presence of the caregiver, are anxious in the presence of the stranger and avoid her, are distressed by the caregiver's brief absence, rapidly seek contact with the caregiver afterward, and are reassured by this contact and return to their exploration. Some infants, designated as *anxious/avoidant*, appear to be made less anxious by separation, may not seek contact with the caregiver following separation, and may not prefer her over the stranger. *Anxious/resistant* infants show limited exploration and play, tend to be highly distressed by separation from the caregiver, and have great difficulty in settling afterward, showing struggling, stiffness, continued crying, or fuss in a passive way. The caregiver's presence or attempts at comforting fail to reassure, and the infant's anxiety and anger appear to prevent him from deriving comfort from proximity.

A fourth group of infants who show seemingly undirected behavior are referred to as *disorganized/disoriented* (Main and Solomon 1990). They show freezing, hand clapping, head banging, and a wish to escape the situation even in the presence of the caregiver (Lyons-Ruth and Jacobovitz 1999; Van IJzendoorn et al. 1999). It is generally held that for such infants the caregiver has served as a source of both fear and reassurance, and thus arousal of the attachment behavioral system produces strong conflicting motivations.

Prospective longitudinal research has demonstrated that children with a history of secure attachment are independently rated as more resilient, self-reliant, socially oriented (Sroufe 1983; Waters et al.

1979), and empathic to distress (Kestenbaum et al. 1989), with deeper relationships and higher self-esteem (Sroufe 1983; Sroufe et al. 1990). Bowlby proposed that internal working models of the self and others provide prototypes for all later relationships. Such models are relatively stable across the lifespan (Collins and Read 1994).

Because internal working models function outside of awareness, they are change resistant (Crittenden 1990). The stability of attachment is demonstrated by longitudinal studies of infants assessed with the strange situation and followed up in adolescence or young adulthood with the Adult Attachment Interview (AAI; George C, Kaplan N, Main M: "The Adult Attachment Interview." Unpublished manuscript, Department of Psychology, University of California at Berkeley, 1985). This structured clinical instrument elicits narrative histories of childhood attachment relationships—the characteristics of early relationships, experiences of separation, illness, punishment, loss, maltreatment, or abuse. The AAI scoring system (Main M, Goldwyn R: "Adult Attachment Rating and Classification System, Manual in Draft, Version 6.0." Unpublished manuscript, University of California at Berkeley, 1994) classifies individuals into secure/autonomous, insecure/dismissing, insecure/preoccupied, or unresolved with respect to loss or trauma, which are categories based on the structural qualities of narratives of early experiences. Whereas *autonomous* individuals value attachment relationships, coherently integrate memories into a meaningful narrative, and regard these as formative, *insecure* individuals are poor at integrating memories of experience with the meaning of that experience. Those individuals who are *dismissing* of attachment show avoidance by denying memories and by idealizing or devaluing (or both idealizing and devaluing) early relationships. *Preoccupied* individuals tend to be confused, angry, or passive in relation to attachment figures, often still complaining of childhood slights, echoing the protests of the resistant infant. *Unresolved* individuals give indications of significant disorganization in their attachment relationship representation; this disorganization manifests in semantic or syntactic confusions in their narratives concerning childhood trauma or a recent loss.

Many studies have demonstrated that the AAI, administered to the mother or father, will predict not only the child's security of attachment to that parent but even more remarkably the precise attachment category that the child manifests in the strange situation (Van IJzendoorn 1995). Thus, a dismissing AAI interview predicts avoidant strange-situation behavior, whereas a preoccupied interview predicts anxious/resistant infant attachment. Lack of resolution of mourning (unresolved interviews) predicts disorganization in infant attachment (discussed later). Temperament (child-to-parent effects) seems an inadequate account of the phenomena, because the AAI of each parent, collected and coded before the birth of the child, predicts the attachment classification of the infant at 12 and 18 months (Fonagy et al. 1991b; Steele et al. 1996).

Evidence by Slade et al. (1999) provided an important clue about the puzzle of intergenerational transmission of attachment security. They demonstrated that autonomous (secure) mothers on the AAI represented their relationship with their toddlers in a more coherent way than dismissing and preoccupied mothers. Mothers interviewed with the AAI who demonstrated a strong capacity to reflect on their own and their own caregiver's mental states in the context of recollecting their own attachment experiences were far more likely to have children securely attached to them—a finding that we have linked to the parent's capacity to foster the child's self-development (Fonagy et al. 1993). We have also found that mothers in a relatively high-stress (deprived) group characterized by single-parent families, parental criminality, unemployment, overcrowding, and psychiatric illness would be far more likely to have securely attached infants if their capacity to be reflective (psychologically minded) in relation to their attachment histories was high (Fonagy et al. 1994).

The disorganized/disoriented infant category appears to have the strongest predictive significance for later psychological disturbance (Carlson 1998; Lyons-Ruth 1996; Lyons-Ruth et al. 1993; Ogawa et al. 1997). A number of studies (Lyons-Ruth 1995; Lyons-Ruth et al. 1989; Shaw and Vondra 1995; Shaw et al. 1997) have suggested that disorganized attachment is a vulnerability factor for later psychological disturbance in combination with other risk factors. A study with a large sample ($N = 223$) confirmed that those whose attachment classification was disorganized in infancy or atypical at age 24 months were most likely to be rated high on externalizing behavior at 3.5 years (Vondra et al. 2001). A meta-analysis of studies of disorganized attachment based on 2,000 mother–infant pairs (Van IJzendoorn et al. 1999) estimated its prevalence at 14% in middle-income samples and 24% in low-income groups. Similarly, adolescent mothers tended to have an overrepresentation of disorganized infants (23%) as well as fewer secure infants (40% versus 62%) and more avoidant infants (33% versus 15%). The stability of the classification of disorganized attachment is fair ($r = 0.36$) (Van IJzendoorn et al. 1999), with some indication that lack of stability may be accounted for by increases in the number of disorganized infants between 12 and 18 months (Barnett et al. 1999; Vondra et al. 1999).

Quite a lot is known about the causes of disorganized attachment. The prevalence of attachment disorganization is strongly associated with family risk factors such as maltreatment (Carlson et al. 1989) and major depressive disorder (Lyons-Ruth et al. 1990; Teti et al. 1995). In addition, there is an extensively proven association between disorganization of attachment in the baby and unresolved mourning or abuse in the mother's own personal experience, revealed in the AAI (Van IJzendoorn 1995). Three studies have helped to clarify this superficially mysterious association between slips in the mother's narrative about past trauma and bizarre behavior by the infant in the strange situation with her. Jacobovitz et al. (1997) reported a strong association between such slips in the AAI before the child was born and observations of frightened or frightening behavior toward the baby at 8 months. These behaviors included extreme intrusiveness, baring teeth, and entering apparently trance-like states. If the mother's unresolved trauma happened before she was 17 years old, her frightened or frightening behavior was more evident. Interestingly, these unresolved mothers did not differ from the rest of the sample in terms of other measures of parenting such as sensitivity and warmth. Maternal frightened or frightening behavior predicted infant attachment disorganization, but the strongest predictor was maternal dissociated behavior (Schuengel et al. 1999). In an independent investigation, Lyons-Ruth et al. (1999b) also found that frightened and frightening behavior predicted infant disorganization, particularly when the mother strongly misinterpreted the baby's attachment cues and when the mother gave conflicting messages that both elicited and rejected attachment.

Both cross-sectional and longitudinal investigations indicate that disorganized infant attachment shifts into controlling attachment behavior in middle childhood (Van IJzendoorn et al. 1999). Observational studies suggest that disorganized children are less competent in playing with other children, in conflict resolution (Wartner et al. 1994), and in consistency of interaction with different peers (Jacobovitz and Hazen 1999).

In terms of the long-term consequences of attachment classification from childhood, studies only partially confirm initial hopes of theorists and researchers. There can be little doubt that something is carried forward. Prediction from insecure-disorganized attachment is particularly powerful for various adverse outcomes, including psychiatric disorder. The path-

ways of association are by no means straightforward (Sroufe et al. 1999). For individuals with extremely harsh or chaotic early caregiving, the process of attentional, emotional, and symbolic regulation might be derailed, and the integration of self-states across behavioral states may never be fully achieved. Because early attachment disturbance makes itself felt as a dysfunction of self-organization (stress regulation, attention regulation, and mentalization)—and because these capacities are needed to deal with social stress—relationship disturbance in the early years, together with additional social pressures, does predict psychological disturbance.

EMPIRICAL STUDIES OF BORDERLINE PERSONALITY DISORDER USING MEASURES OF ATTACHMENT

Adult Attachment Interview

To our knowledge, five studies have used the AAI with BPD (Fonagy et al. 1996; Frodi et al. 2001; Patrick et al. 1994; Rosenstein and Horowitz 1996; Stalker and Davies 1995). All of these studies report that individuals with BPD diagnoses according to structured interview or diagnostic criteria are more likely to be classified as preoccupied on the AAI. Interview transcripts that are classified as preoccupied tend to be long, confusing, incoherent, angry, passive, or fearful accounts of childhood attachment experiences. In addition, in one study (Patrick et al. 1994), almost all BPD subjects were classified as the somewhat unusual E3 (fearful of losing attachment) subcategory. The AAI permits the assignment of an "unresolved" (U) for experiences of trauma or loss on the basis of subtle signs of cognitive disorganization that are described as experiences of maltreatment or loss of attachment figures. In these studies, individuals with BPD diagnosis were more likely than Axis I or Axis II control subjects to receive U classifications. In the Frodi et al. (2001) study, psychopathic criminal offenders were contrasted with AAI norms. This study showed that the offenders were more likely to be categorized as dismissing or unresolved but not preoccupied. This finding is consistent with the results of a study from our laboratory (Levinson and Fonagy in press).

Self-Report Measures of Attachment

Several measures of attachment have been used, and to make matters worse, many of these measures are versions of each other that offer slightly different classifications or dimensional scoring indicators. Two studies have used the Attachment Rating Scale (Nickell et al. 2002; Sack et al. 1996). This scale (Hazan and Shaver 1987) employs a three-category scheme of secure, preoccupied, and dismissing. The BPD groups emerge from these studies as more likely to be anxious/ambivalent or avoidant than a normal sample or those with other psychiatric disorders. "Ambivalent" on the Attachment Rating Scale is the self-description of an individual who is lonely in romantic relationships, craves intimacy, and fears dependency. The Nickell et al. (2002) study is particularly important because it controlled for adverse childhood events as well as Axis I and non-BPD Axis II pathology. Thus the ambivalent attachment style predicted BPD scores after physical or sexual abuse, Axis I and Axis II symptoms, and perceived abnormal parenting attitudes were controlled for.

Two studies (Brennan and Shaver 1998; Dutton et al. 1994) have used the Relationship Questionnaire (Bartholomew and Horowitz 1991) or Relationship Scales Questionnaire (Griffin and Bartholomew 1994). These questionnaires use a four-category attachment typology that includes secure, preoccupied, fearful, and dismissing attachment. In this scheme, "fearful" describes an individual longing for intimacy but mistrustful and afraid of rejection. In both of these studies, the BPD group emerged as fearful relative to normal subjects and as preoccupied relative to other personality disorder groups, but Axis I comorbidity was not controlled for. The Attachment Styles Questionnaire (Fossati et al. 2001) and the Reciprocal Attachment Questionnaire (Sack et al. 1996) were used in one study each. The Attachment Styles Questionnaire (Feeney and Noller 1990) is a derivative of the Attachment Rating Scale and the Reciprocal Attachment Questionnaire and has five factors: confidence, discomfort with closeness, need for approval, preoccupation with relationships, and relationships as secondary. BPD patients relative to normal subjects, those with other personality disorders, and those with no personality disorder were more insecure but were not distinguished by a specific pattern. These conclusions must be qualified by the fact that concurrent Axis I diagnoses were not fully controlled for. The investigation reported by Fossati et al. (2001) is unusually well controlled. Although the investigation showed differences in attachment style in the directions indicated, controlling for attachment styles did not reduce the difference between BPD and other groups in terms of impulsiveness-related traits. Given that in at least one longitudinal study impulsiveness-related traits turned out to be significant and substantial pre-

dictors of BPD diagnosis at a 7-year follow-up, Fossati et al. suggest that the independence of attachment classification from this important dimension of impulsivity questions the centrality of the attachment construct (Links et al. 1999).

Another well-controlled study with a far more appropriate measure of attachment (Meyer et al. 2001) found that changes in psychosocial functioning over a 6-month period were uniquely predicted by attachment classifications at intake using Pilkonis's (1988) attachment prototype interview assessment, particularly in clinician-rated scales of depression and anxiety rather than self-report scales. This finding highlighted the particular problems associated with using self-report measures of attachment in BPD. Furthermore, the Meyer et al. (2001) study confirmed the close association between BPD features and prototypes for preoccupied and insecure attachment and the stability of attachment styles over a 1-year period. The associations between attachment prototypes and treatment success were also reported in other studies using the Pilkonis prototype method, work that has been replicated by a large-scale German investigation (Mosheim et al. 2000).

Summary of Empirical Data

Studies using varying and mostly quite limited methodologies are nevertheless consistent in showing borderline patients as seeking close, intimate relationships at the same time as being alert to signs of rejection and undervaluation. The ambivalent, preoccupied, dysfunctional attachment pattern perhaps reflects difficulties in managing anxiety and distress that arise from interpersonal challenges and may be manifested in emotional instability, extreme rage, and suicidal behavior aimed at achieving one's interpersonal needs (Bartholomew et al. 2001). It should be noted, however, that not all studies find an association between BPD and ambivalent preoccupied attachment patterns. For example, Salzman and colleagues (1997) found that all participants meeting diagnostic criteria for BPD demonstrated ambivalent attachment in their first study, but in their replication study BPD participants were classified as demonstrating avoidant attachment.

The fearful subtype of preoccupied attachment in the AAI appears to coincide with the diagnosis of BPD in some studies (Patrick et al. 1994) and not others (Fonagy et al. 1996). It should be noted that subcategories of the AAI are not normally part of reliability tests for coders. Nevertheless, there is a clear indication that

BPD diagnosis is linked with insecure, preoccupied, ambivalent, and perhaps fearful attachment patterns. Implicitly or explicitly, Bowlby's (1973) suggestion that early experience with the caregiver serves to organize later attachment relationships has been used in many attempted explanations of psychopathology in BPD. For example, it has been suggested that the borderline person's experiences of interpersonal attack, neglect, and threats of abandonment may account for the perception of current relationships as attacking and neglectful (Benjamin 1993). Others have suggested that individuals with BPD are specifically characterized by a fearful and preoccupied attachment style reflecting "an emotional template of intimacy anxiety/anger" (Dutton et al. 1994). In studies of AAI narratives of patients with personality disorder, preoccupied is the most frequently assigned classification, (Fonagy et al. 1996) and within this, the confused, fearful, and overwhelmed subclassification (E3) appears to be most common (Patrick et al. 1994).

Past attempts at linking work on attachment with theories of borderline pathology have stressed the common characteristic shared by the ambivalently attached/preoccupied and borderline groups to check for proximity, signaling to establish contact by pleading or other calls for attention or help, and clinging behaviors (Gunderson 1996). Borderline patients also tend to be unresolved with regard to their experience of trauma or abuse (Fonagy et al. 1996; Patrick et al. 1994).

Problems With a Simple Attachment Model

There is no doubt that borderline individuals are insecure in their attachment, but descriptions of insecure attachment from infancy or adulthood provide an inadequate clinical account for several reasons: 1) Anxious attachment is very common; in working-class nonclinical population samples, the majority of children are classified as anxiously attached, with a high proportion classified as disorganized (Broussard 1995). 2) Anxious patterns of attachment in infancy correspond to relatively stable adult strategies (Main et al. 1985), yet the hallmark of the disordered attachments of borderline individuals is the absence of stability (Higgitt and Fonagy 1992). 3) In both delinquent and borderline individuals there are variations across situations or types of relationships; the delinquent adolescent is, for example, aware of the mental states of others in his gang, and the borderline individual is at times hypersensitive to the emotional states of mental health professionals and family members. 4) The clinical presentation of borderline patients frequently includes a violent attack on the patient's own body or that of another human being. It is likely that the propensity for such violence must include an additional component that predisposes such individuals to act upon bodies rather than upon minds.

To the extent that we assume that abnormal patterns of attachment arise as a consequence of abnormalities in child rearing, it is somewhat of an embarrassment that prospective studies of maltreatment often fail to yield powerful personality effects beyond the contextual (e.g., life events; Widom 1999). A more important problem is that all adult attachment measures are hopelessly confounded with symptoms and traits. Thus, for example, in Meyer et al.'s (2001) study of Pilkonis's borderline attachment prototype, the correlation between the attachment prototype and symptomatology was so high that only one of these variables could be used in the regression because of colinearity problems. Similarly, the AAI coding for fearful preoccupied categories calls for statements about fear of loss that are also symptomatic of a diagnosis of BPD.

The model of attachment in use by attachment theorists places greatest importance on early experience, yet the social experiences of individuals with BPD are likely to be distorted by later rather than earlier social encounters. It is unclear in most theories proposing attachment as an explanatory variable how early attachment and later maltreatment might interact. As we have seen, controlling for attachment styles does not account for temperamental and characterological differences between BPD and non-BPD patients. Impulsivity and negative affectivity/emotional dysregulation characterize BPD best (Gurvits et al. 2000; Paris 2000; Silk 2000; Trull 2001a). Many attachment measures such as the AAI rely on autobiographical memory. In fact, in the AAI specific memories are coded as indicators of insecurity. Studies of autobiographical memory of borderline patients suggest that they have a tendency to produce overly general memories (Startup et al. 2001), which again underscores the difficulty of establishing independent measures of BPD status and attachment.

AN ATTACHMENT THEORY OF BORDERLINE PERSONALITY DISORDER

Disorganization of Attachment

As we have seen, the caregiver's sensitivity to the child's mental state is strongly associated with secure attachment and the development in the child of the capacity to mentalize—that is, to represent the behavior of self and others in terms of underlying mental states (Fonagy and Target 1997; Fonagy et al. 1991a; Meins and Fernyhough 1999; Meins and Russell 1997; Meins et al. 1998, 2001). *Mentalizing* is a relatively new term for a concept as ancient as philosophy of mind. Mentalizing is akin to what Olson (1994) construes as subjectivity—that is, "the *recognition* that what is in the mind is in the mind…the recognition of one's own and others' mental states as mental states" (p. 234). The term *mentalizing* was introduced into the psychoanalytic literature some decades ago (Brown 1977; Compton 1983; De M'Uzan 1973; Lecours and Bouchard 1997) and came to be applied to the understanding of autism as a neurobiologically based failure of psychosocial development (Frith et al. 1991; Morton 1989). Fonagy and colleagues opened the door to wider clinical applications of this developmental research in showing how mentalizing plays a significant role in diverse forms of developmental psychopathology (Fonagy 1991a, 1995; Fonagy and Target 1997; Fonagy et al. 2002; Target and Fonagy 1996), and we continue expanding these clinical applications here.

True to its origins in psychoanalysis, mentalizing intertwines with the related concepts of psychological mindedness (Appelbaum 1973; Namnum 1968), observing ego, and potential space (Bram and Gabbard 2001; Ogden 1985; Winnicott 1971). Mentalizing also overlaps with the venerable concepts of empathy and insight. We do not propose replacing these traditional concepts with mentalizing but rather argue that theory and research on mentalizing anchor this network of clinical concepts in evolutionary biology, neurobiology, contemporary developmental research, and attachment theory.

High levels of parental reflective function (capacity for mentalization) are associated with good outcomes in terms of secure attachment in the child. The converse, then, is that low levels of reflective function generate insecure and perhaps disorganized attachment. The latter category of attachment in infancy is most likely to be associated with self-harming or aggressive and potentially violent behavior later in development. A study by Grienenberger et al. (2001) showed that mothers with low levels of mentalization (or reflective function) on the Parent Development Interview (an interview assessing the parent's mental representation of the child) are more likely to show intrusiveness, fearfulness, withdrawing, and other behaviors shown to generate disorganized attachment in the infant (Lyons-Ruth et al. 1999b). The suggestion here is that poor mentalization of the infant in the

mother permits behaviors that undermine the healthy development of the infant's representational capacities (particularly the organization of affect and the organization of focused attention or effortful control) (Fonagy and Target 2002), which in turn can undermine attachment processes, leading to the development of a disorganized self, parts of which are experienced as "alien" or not really belonging to the self. In the absence of the capacity for mentalization, the coherence of this self can only be ensured by primitive psychological strategies such as projective identification. It is the impact of attachment disorganization on the self that might be most important for us in understanding BPD.

Establishment of the "Alien Self"

An important complication arises if the processes that normally generate an agentive self fail. In early childhood the failure to find another being behaving contingently with one's internal states can create a desperation for meaning as the self seeks to find itself in the other. This desperation leads the individual to take in noncontingent reflections from the object. Unfortunately, as these reflections do not map onto anything within the child's own experience, they cannot function as totally effective experiences of the self. As Winnicott (1967) noted, inaccurate mirroring leads the child to internalize representations of the parent's state rather than a usable version of his own experience. This creates what we have termed an *alien experience* within the self: ideas or feelings are experienced as part of the self that do not seem to belong to the self (Fonagy et al. 1995, 2000). These representations of the other internalized as part of the self probably originate in early infancy, when the mother's reflective function at least partially but regularly failed the infant.

This alien other, the residue of maternal nonresponsiveness, probably exists in seed form in all our self-representations, because we have all experienced neglect to a greater or lesser extent (Tronick and Gianino 1986). Normally, however, parts of the self-representation that are not rooted in the internalized mirroring of self-states are nevertheless integrated into a singular, coherent self-structure by the capacity for mentalization. The representational agentive self creates an illusion of coherence within our representations of ourselves by attributing agency, accurately or inaccurately assuming that mental states invariably exist to explain experience. Dramatic examples of this capacity for mentalization were noted long ago in studies of individuals with neural lesions, such as individuals with surgical bisections of the corpus callosum, so-called split-brain patients (Gazzaniga 1985). When presented with emotionally arousing pictures in the hemifield without access to language, they would find improbable mentalized accounts for their heightened emotional state.

Controlling Internal Working Model

The normal process of attributing agency through putative mental states preconsciously works in the background of our minds to lend coherence and psychological meaning to our lives, our actions, and our sense of self. Individuals whose capacity for mentalization is not well developed may need to use controlling and manipulative strategies to restore coherence to their sense of self. The alien aspects of the self may be externalized into an attachment figure. Using processes often described in the clinical literature as "projective identification," the attachment figure is manipulated into feeling the internalized emotions as part of the self but not entirely "of the self." These are not self-protective maneuvers in the sense of needing to shed feelings that the individual cannot acknowledge; rather, they protect the self from the experience of incongruence or incoherence that has the potential to generate far deeper anxieties (see Kernberg 1982, 1983; Kohut 1977). Apparently coercive, manipulative behavior reflects the individual's inability to contain the incoherence of his self-structure. Unfortunately, in performing this function—in becoming, for example, angry and punitive in response to unconscious provocation—the attachment figure is in the worst possible state to help restore the afflicted individual's mentalizing function because he or she has lost touch with the individual's mental world. Thus the controlling internal working model further undermines the child's capacity to establish an agentive self-structure.

To state it simply, disorganized attachment is rooted in a disorganized self. Attachment research has demonstrated the sequelae of disorganized attachment in infancy to be extreme controlling and dominating behavior in middle childhood (see Solomon and George 1999). The individual, when alone, feels unsafe and vulnerable because of the proximity of a torturing and destructive representation from which he or she cannot escape because it is experienced from within rather than from without the self. Unless the individual's relationship permits externalization, he or she feels almost literally at risk of disappearance, psychological merging, and the dissolution of all relationship boundaries. The need to externalize the alien part

of the self may serve inadvertently to re-create relationships in which the persecutor is "generated" outside, in the shape of relationships of emotional turmoil and significant negativity.

Failure of Mentalization

Disturbed interpersonal relatedness is a key aspect of BPD related to temperamental attributes of negative affectivity and impulsivity (Gurvits et al. 2000; Paris 2000; Silk 2000; Trull et al. 2000) and psychosocial experiences of maltreatment (e.g., Trull 2001b; Zanarini et al. 1997; Zlotnick et al. 2001). Studies that have attempted to find the underlying dimensions of borderline phenomenology tended to identify either two (Rosenberg and Miller 1989) or three factors (Clarkin et al. 1993; Sanislow et al. 2000). These factors normally include a dimension of disturbed relatedness, emotional dysregulation and impulsivity, or behavioral dyscontrol. At least the first of these may be related to a deficit in the capacity for accurate perception of the respective mental states of self and other and self–other differentiation (Fonagy et al. 2000; Gunderson 2001). Deficits of this aspect of interpersonal perception have been demonstrated in analogue studies using film clips (e.g., Arntz and Veen 2001), affect recognition and alexithymic symptoms (e.g., Sayar et al. 2001), and narratives of childhood experiences (Fonagy et al. 1996; Vermote et al. 2004).

A deficit of interpersonal awareness implies an underlying failure of effective and stable self–other differentiation at the level of distinguishing respective mental states. Some of the brain abnormalities identified in BPD patients correspond to a failure of representation of self-states being a key dysfunction. Some evidence suggests that the anterior cingulate cortex plays a key role in mentalizing the self, at least in the domain of emotional states (Damasio 1999; Frith and Frith 1999; Lane et al. 1997, 1998). Lane (2000) proposed more specifically that implicit self-representations (i.e., phenomenal self-awareness) can be localized to the dorsal anterior cingulate, whereas explicit self-representations (i.e., reflection) can be localized to the rostral anterior cingulate. Moreover, intriguing findings regarding mirror neurons suggest that representations of self and others bearing on interpretation of intentional action promote mentalization by virtue of shared anatomical circuitry (Brothers 1997; Gallese 2000, 2001; Jeannerod 1997). Activation of the medial prefrontal cortex (including the ventromedial prefrontal cortex overlapping the orbitofrontal cortex) has been demonstrated in a series of neuroimaging studies in conjunction with a wide range of theory of mind inferences in both visual and verbal domains (Fletcher et al. 1995; Gallagher et al. 2000; Goel et al. 1995; Happe et al. 1996; Klin et al. 2000). It appears likely that extensive prefrontal cortex (i.e., orbitofrontal extending into more dorsal medial cortex) is involved in mentalizing interactively in a way that requires implicitly representing the mental states of others.

Impact of Trauma

Key to understanding severe personality disorder is the inhibition of mentalization, perhaps prototypically in response to trauma. Patients with BPD defensively avoid thinking about the mental states of self and others, because these experiences have led them to experiences of unbearable pain in the course of maltreatment (Fonagy 1991). Especially in individuals in whom the capacity for mentalization is already weak, trauma may bring about a complete collapse.

Both clinical and experimental evidence supports the view that trauma commonly brings about a partial and temporary collapse of mentalization. The disorganizing effects of trauma on attention and stress regulation are well known (Allen 2001). The capacity for mentalization is undermined in a significant proportion of individuals who have experienced trauma. Maltreated toddlers have difficulty in learning to use internal state words (Beeghly and Cicchetti 1994; Cicchetti and Beeghly 1987). Neglected children have greater difficulty in discriminating facial emotional expression, and physically abused children show a response bias toward angry expression and greater variance in their interpretation of facial affect (Pollak et al. 2000). A study of sexually abused Canadian girls demonstrated that children with sexual abuse histories had lower reflective functioning (RF) scores on the childhood attachment interviews in relation to self than demographically matched control subjects (Normandin et al. 2002). In the same study, dissociation was shown to be closely related to the low RF of abused children. Whereas 75% of those with low RF on the child attachment interview scored high in dissociation, only 20% of those with high RF could be said to be dissociating. Young adults who have been maltreated experience greater difficulty with the Reading the Mind in the Eyes Test (a relatively simple measure of implicit mentalization that involves identifying photographs with one of four mental states) (Fonagy et al. 2001).

Considerable evidence supports the claim that individuals with a history of abuse who are also limited in their capacity to think about mental states in them-

selves and others in the AAI are highly likely to have a diagnosis of BPD (Fonagy et al. 1996). Other researchers have replicated this finding with other samples showing trauma. For example, in the Kortenberg-Leuven Process-Outcome Study of inpatient treatment of personality disorder (Vermote et al. 2004), a significant negative correlation was reported between RF measured on the Object Relations Inventory (Blatt et al. 1996) and Structured Clinical Interview for DSM-IV Axis II Personality Disorders diagnosis of BPD, and an even stronger correlation was found with clinical observation of self-harm.

Although psychological trauma is a functional route to impaired mentalizing, neurobiological approaches underscore how trauma may compromise the development of cerebral structures that support mentalizing. As noted earlier, Schore (2001) reviewed extensive evidence that secure attachment relationships are essential to the normal development of the prefrontal cortex and thus to affect regulation. Hence, early maltreatment, which is associated with extremely compromised (disorganized) attachment (Barnett et al. 1999; Lyons-Ruth and Jacobovitz 1999; Lyons-Ruth et al. 1999a, 1999b), is most likely to undermine the development of cortical structures key to mentalization.

Arnsten (1998; Arnsten et al. 1999) and Mayes (2000, 2002) have linked extreme stress to altered dynamics in arousal regulation in a way that is highly pertinent to trauma. They described how increasing levels of norepinephrine and dopamine interact with each other and differentially activate receptor subtypes so as to shift the balance between prefrontal executive control and posterior-subcortical automatic control over attention and behavior. Mild to moderate levels of arousal are associated with optimal prefrontal functioning and thus with employment of flexible mental representations and response strategies conducive to complex problem solving. On the other hand, extreme levels of arousal trigger a neurochemical switch that shifts the individual into posterior cortical-subcortical dominance such that vigilance, the fight-or-flight response, and amygdala-mediated memory encoding predominate. In effect, high levels of excitatory stimulation (at α-1 adrenergic and D_1 dopaminergic receptors) take the prefrontal cortex offline. This switch in attentional and behavioral control is adaptive in the context of danger that requires rapid automatic responding. Yet Mayes (2000) pointed out that early stressful and traumatic experiences may permanently impair the dynamic balance of arousal regulation, altering the threshold for this switch process. Thus, sensitized individuals may be prone to impaired prefrontal functioning in the face of stress, with automatic posterior-subcortical responding taking control of attention and behavior and undermining flexible mental representations and coping. In line with this suggestion is the observation that *N*-acetyl-aspartate, a marker of neural integrity, is lowered in the anterior cingulated region of the medial prefrontal cortex of maltreated children and adolescents (De Bellis et al. 2000).

These proposals regarding impaired arousal regulation and shifting the balance of prefrontal-posterior cortical functioning are consistent with neuroimaging studies employing symptom provocation in persons with posttraumatic stress disorder (PTSD). Such induced posttraumatic states are associated with diminished medial prefrontal and anterior cingulate activity (Bremner et al. 1999a, 1999b; Lanius et al. 2001; Rauch et al. 1996; Shin et al. 2001). A similar observation was reported in a positron emission tomography study comparing sexually abused women who had PTSD with women with a similar history who did not. The women with PTSD were found to have lower levels of anterior cingulate blood flow during traumatic imagery (Shin et al. 1999). This finding suggests that some BPD symptoms may be connected to an impairment of medial prefrontal cortical functioning (Zubieta et al. 1999). Van der Kolk and colleagues (1996) viewed findings showing deactivation in Broca's area in posttraumatic states as indicative of "speechless terror" and concluded that in such states, "the brain is 'having' its experience. The person may feel, see, or hear the sensory elements of the traumatic experience, but he or she may be physiologically prevented from translating this experience into communicable language" (p. 131). Thus, dysfunctional arousal may play a part in the reemergence of the subjective state we have described as psychic equivalence. *Psychic equivalence* is a developmentally primitive mode of experiencing the subjective world before mentalization has fully developed. The 2-year-old child is convinced that all that is in his mind is equivalent to that which exists outside and all that is outside must by definition exist in his mind, because his mind is functionally equivalent to the material world (Fonagy and Target 1996; Target and Fonagy 1996). The complement to this state is the pretend mode of experiencing subjectivity, in which the child feels that nothing that he experiences as subjective has any possible connection with reality.

We propose a synergy among psychological defenses, neurobiological development, and shifts in brain activity during posttraumatic states such that mentalizing activity is compromised. The shift in the balance of cortical control locks the traumatized person either into 1) the psychic equivalence mode, associated with an inability to employ alternate representations of the situation (i.e., functioning at the level of primary rather than secondary representations), much less the ability to explicate the state of mind (metarepresentation); or 2) the pretend mode, associated with states of dissociative detachment.

Exposure of the "Alien Self"

When mirroring fails in infancy, the child internalizes a noncontingent mental state as part of a representation within the psychological self. These internalizations sit within the self without being connected to it by a set of meanings. It is this incoherence within the self-structure that we referred to as an "alien self" (Fonagy and Target 2000). As we have said, such incoherencies in self-structure may not only characterize profoundly neglected children. The coherence of self that we all experience is somewhat illusory. This illusion is normally maintained by the continuous narrative commentary on behavior that mentalization provides, which fills in the gaps and makes us feel that our experiences are meaningful. In the absence of a robust mentalizing capacity, with disorganized patterns of attachment, the disorganization of the self-structure is clearly revealed.

When trauma inhibits mentalization, the self is suddenly experienced as incoherent. Parts within the trauma survivor feel like the self yet also feel substantively different, sometimes even persecutory. The persecutory nature of the alien part of the self arises as a sequel to maltreatment in childhood, adolescence, or even adulthood. Anna Freud (1936) described the process by which the child aims to gain control over powerful, hostile external forces through identification with the aggressor. If the cohesion of the self-structure has been weakened by limited interpersonal interpretive function and the discontinuity within the self represented by the alien part of the self is well established, identification with the maltreater is most likely to occur with the help of this alien part of the self-structure. In slight disagreement with Anna Freud, we do not look at this process as an identification, because that would imply (following Sandler's [1987] clarification of the concept) a change in the shape of the self in the direction of achieving more significant similarities with the abusive figure. It is more like a kind of "colonization" of the alien part of the self by the child's or adolescent's image of the mental state of the abuser.

The aim of the strategy is to gain a sense of control over the uncontrollable. This attempt at control is ultimately a highly maladaptive solution, because the persecution from the maltreating person is now experienced from within. A part of the self-structure is thought to wish to destroy the rest of the self. This experience of persecution from within may be one aspect of the massive impact that maltreatment can have on the self-esteem of those subject to abuse (e.g., Mullen et al. 1996). They feel that they are evil because they have internalized evil into the part of the self that is most readily decoupled from the self but nevertheless is felt as part of the self. A way of coping with the intolerable pain that this self-persecutory self-within-the-self represents is through externalization into the physically proximal other. The part of the self that is so painful is forced outside and another physical being is manipulated and cajoled until they behave in a way that enables the individual to feel that they no longer own the persecutory alien part of the self. At the simplest level, the world then becomes terrifying because the persecutory parts are experienced as outside. At a more complex level, it is felt essential that the alien experiences are owned by another mind, so that another mind is in control of these parts of the self. This defensive externalization might help to explain why, strikingly, persons with BPD frequently find themselves in interpersonal situations in which they are maltreated or abused by their partners.

Given that the relationship between childhood maltreatment and BPD is complex, the statistics on the sequelae of childhood sexual abuse seem quite relevant to this point. Victims of childhood abuse who are revictimized are most likely to have severe mental health problems, including (as we have seen frequently) BPD. According to one study, 49% of abused women compared with 18% of women without the experience of sexual abuse had been battered by their partners (Briere and Runtz 1987). In a large study with a sample representative of San Francisco (Russell 1986), between 38% and 48% of abused women (depending on the severity of abuse) had physically abusive husbands compared with 10%–17% of nonabused women. This finding should in no sense be taken to mean that the men involved in the battering are any less culpable. Individuals with experiences of maltreatment appear to be drawn to individuals who are likely to maltreat them, we would argue, in order to increase the opportunity of externalizing intolerable mental states concerning themselves. As thus might be expected, many sexual assaults experienced by college-age survivors of sexual abuse occur at the hands of a known individual (Gidycz et al. 1995). Indeed, one survey demonstrated that 81% of the adult sexual assaults experienced by revictimized women were perpetrated by male acquaintances of the survivors (Cloitre et al. 1997).

Another person is essential to create the illusion of coherence. BPD patients require rather than enjoy relationships. Relationships are necessary to stabilize the self-structure but are also the source of greatest vulnerability because in the absence of the other, when the relationships break down or if the other shows independence, the alien self returns to wreak havoc (persecute from within) and to destabilize the self-structure. Vulnerability is greatest in the context of attachment relationships. Past trauma leaves an impoverished internal working model from the point of view of clear and coherent representations of mental states in self and other. This representational system is activated by the attachment relationship with the consequence that the mental states of the other are no longer clearly seen. The physical other is desperately needed to free the self from its inwardly directed violence, but only as long as it acts as the vehicle for the patient's self-state. When this process occurs, dependence on the other is total. Substitution is inconceivable, no matter how destructive or hopeless the relationship might seem from the outside.

Self-Harm

We can now begin to understand the violence committed by certain individuals with BPD against others or themselves. For such individuals, self-harm may entail a fantasy of eradicating the alien part of the self unconsciously imagined to be part of their body. Self-mutilators report a range of conscious motivations, including self-punishment, tension reduction, improvement in mood, and distraction from intolerable affects (Favazza 1992; Herpertz 1995). Following the act of self-harm, the individual mostly reports feeling better and relieved (Favazza 1992; Herpertz 1995; Kemperman et al. 1997). We suggest that in the absence of a person who may act as a vehicle for the alien part of the self, a person with BPD achieves self-coherence through the externalization of this part of the self into a part of their body. Attempts at self-harm are acts carried out in a mode of psychic equivalence when a part of the body is considered isomorphic with the alien part of the self at the same time as creating a respite from intolerable affects. Attempts at self-mutilation are more common when the patient is in isolation or after the loss of an other who, up to that point, could fulfill the task of being a vehicle for the persecuting alien part of the self.

Suicide

Clinical and epidemiological studies have demonstrated that between 55% and 85% of those who self-mutilate also attempt suicide (Dulit et al. 1994; Stanley et al. 1992), and BPD carries a suicide risk of around 5%–10% (Fyer et al. 1988; Stone et al. 1987). Most consider attempted suicide to be on a continuum of lethality with other types of deliberate self-harm (e.g., Linehan 1986). We understand suicide attempts as at the extreme of attempts at self-mutilation often consequent on experience of loss of the other. In such states, feelings of despair, hopelessness, and depression predominate. The loss of the other as a vehicle for the alien parts of the self—the disruption of the process of externalization—signals the destruction of the constitutional, or real, part of the self. Hence, the sense of despair is not from the loss of the object who normally would not have been a genuine attachment figure in the first place but the anticipated loss of self-cohesion. The act of suicide is at least in part an act in the psychic equivalence mode aimed at destroying the alien part of the self (hence the continuum with self-harm). When BPD patients attempt suicide, their subjective experience is decoupled from reality (in the pretend mode of subjectivity), and in a sense they believe they (or their true selves) will survive the attempt but their alien selves will be destroyed forever. Consistent with our view is evidence that suicide attempters with BPD features perceive their suicidal attempts as less lethal, with a greater likelihood of rescue and with less certainty of death (Stanley et al. 2001). In fact, in some patients suicide is felt as "a secure base," a reunion with a state that can reduce existential fear.

Impulsive Acts of Violence

The same models of pathology that account for self-harming behavior are generally held to be applicable to certain categories of acts of interpersonal violence (Dutton 1995; Fonagy 1999; Fonagy et al. 1997; Gilligan 1997; Meloy 1992). In BPD we see interpersonal violence of an explosive or affective type (Vitiello and Stoff 1997) that is often associated with antisocial personality disorder. Identification with the aggressor leads to the colonization of the alien part of the self by the maltreating figure, and vulnerability to a malevolent mind brings with it the defensive inhibition of mentalizing capacity. Acts of violence themselves are usually the consequence of a failure of the externalization of the alien self. When the other refuses to be a vehicle for intolerable self-states—he or she refuses to be

cowed or humiliated—the vulnerable mind of such an individual turns to interpersonal destruction. An important trigger for violence is the experience of "ego-destructive shame." The lack of a coherent sense of agentive self creates a massive vulnerability to humiliation in such individuals. This humiliation is felt when the other refuses to accept a role of complete passivity and through manifesting agency presents unbearable humiliation to the violent mind. The challenge is unbearable in the mode of psychic equivalence, in which shame is experienced not just as an idea or feeling but as having the actual power to destroy the self. The destruction of the other through violence is an expression of the hoped-for destruction of the alien self; it is an act of hope or liberation and is often associated with elation and only later with regret. The absence of mentalization at these moments is of course of further assistance.

TREATMENT IMPLICATIONS OF THE ATTACHMENT MODEL

It should be apparent from this discussion about attachment and BPD that the focus in treatment needs to be on stabilizing the sense of self and helping the patient maintain an optimal level of arousal. To this end, we have defined some core underpinning techniques to be used in the context of group and individual therapy and labeled them Mentalization-Based Treatment (MBT; Bateman and Fonagy 2004). The initial task in MBT is to stabilize emotional expression because without improved control of affect there can be no serious consideration of internal representations. Although the converse is true to the extent that without stable internal representations there can be no robust control of affects, identification and expression of affect are targeted first simply because they represent an immediate threat to continuity of therapy as well as potentially to the patient's life. Uncontrolled affect leads to impulsivity, and only once this affect is under control is it possible to focus on internal representations and to strengthen the patient's sense of self.

To implement MBT effectively, greater activity on the part of the therapist is required, with more collaboration and openness than is implied in the classical analytic stance. In psychodynamic treatment of BPD patients, the therapist has to become what the patient needs him or her to be—the vehicle for the alien self, the carrier of alternative but not destabilizing perspectives. Yet to become the alien self is to be lost to the patient as a provider of different perspectives and therefore to be of no help to the patient. The therapist must aim to achieve a state of equipoise between the two—allowing him- or herself to do as required yet trying to retain as clearly and coherently as possible an image of his or her own state of mind alongside that of the patient. This mental attitude is what we have called the mentalizing stance of the therapist.

Enhancing Mentalization, Retaining Mental Closeness, and Working With Current Mental States

A therapist needs to maintain a mentalizing stance in order to help a patient develop a capacity to mentalize. Self-directed mentalistic questions are a useful way of ensuring that a focus on mentalizing is maintained. Why is the patient saying this now? Why is the patient behaving like this? What might I have done that explains the patient's state? Why am I feeling as I do now? What has happened recently in the therapy or in our relationship that may justify the current state? The therapist will be asking him- or herself these typical questions within the mentalizing therapeutic stance and is perfectly at liberty to ask these out loud in a spirit of inquiry. This approach pervades the entire treatment setting. Thus in group therapy, techniques focus on encouraging patients to consider the mental states and motives of other members as well as their own: "Why do you think that she is feeling as she does?" The therapist is not looking for complex "unconscious" reasons but rather the answers that common sense or folk psychology would suggest to most reasonable people.

Focusing the therapist's understanding of his or her interactions with the patient on the patient's current mental state will allow the therapist to link external events, however small, to powerful internal states that are otherwise experienced by the patient as inexplicable, uncontrollable, and meaningless. A focus on psychological process and the "here and now" rather than on mental content in the present and past is implicit in this approach. Little therapeutic gain results from continually focusing on the past. Recovering memories is now recognized as a somewhat risky aim with BPD patients (Brenneis 1997; Sandler and Fonagy 1997). We would wish to add that another risk involves the possibility of encouraging BPD patients to enter a pretend-psychic equivalent mode of relating, in which they (unbeknownst to the therapist) no longer use the same circumspect subjective criteria of historical accuracy that most of us use but rather assume that because they experience something in relation to a childhood (usually adult) figure, it is bound to be true. To avoid these risks, the focus of MBT needs to be on the present state and how it remains influenced by events of the past rather than on the past itself. If the patient persistently returns to the past, the therapist needs to link back to the present, move the therapy into the here and now, and consider the present experience.

An important indicator of underlying process and the here and now is the manifest affect that is specifically targeted, identified, and explored within an interpersonal context in MBT. The challenge for the professional working with the patient is to maintain a mentalizing therapeutic stance in the context of countertransference responses that may provoke the therapist to react rather than to think. Understanding within an interpersonal context why the situation arose in the first place, why such an externalization became necessary, is the likely immediate solution to this challenge. Retaining mental closeness is done simply by representing accurately the current or immediately past feeling state of the patient and its accompanying internal representations and by strictly and systematically avoiding the temptation to enter into conversation about matters not directly linked to the patient's beliefs, wishes, and feelings.

It could be argued that the focus on mentalization in MBT is akin to the emphasis on cognitions in cognitive-behavioral treatments and that the exploration of affects is similar to the stress on affect control in dialectical behavior therapy (Linehan et al. 1991, 1999, 2002). There is some truth in this observation, but we would argue that the techniques used in those therapies are often effective because they enhance mentalizing; the success that they have is through the stimulation of exploration of the mind and the joint attention given to mental processes. Our interventions are more firmly rooted within the interpersonal context and understood within that framework, and they are perhaps more inherently integrative in taking not only the specific mental processes and behavior of the patient into account but also the relational context. Furthermore, we explicitly use transference to explore the meaning of the patient's experience, and we now turn to discuss this approach.

Transference, Interpretation, and Bearing in Mind the Deficits

Bearing in mind the limited processing capacities of BPD patients in relation to attachment issues, patients cannot be assumed to have a capacity to work with conflict, to express feelings through verbalization, to use metaphor, to resist actions, and to reflect on content, all of which form part of standard psychoanalytic process. These attributes depend on a stable self-structure and ability to form secondary (symbolic) and perhaps tertiary representations (e.g., your feelings about my thoughts about your wishes) that buffer feelings, explain ideas, and give context and meaning to interpersonal and intrapsychic processes. Borderline patients' enfeebled mentalizing capacity and emergence of psychic equivalence means that feelings, fantasies, thoughts, and desires are experienced with considerable force because they cannot be symbolized, held in a state of uncertainty, or given secondary representation with meaning. Under these circumstances the use of metaphor and the interpretation of conflict are more likely to induce bewilderment and incomprehension than to heighten the underlying meaning of the discourse, so the use of these techniques is minimized in MBT. This technical stance has important implications for the use of transference.

Our overall approach owes much to that of Otto Kernberg, John Clarkin, Frank Yeomans, and their groups (Clarkin et al. 1996, 1998, 1999; Kernberg 1992; Kernberg et al. 2002). In many respects, the model of the mind that underpins our approach is the one brilliantly advanced by Kernberg over the past few decades (Kernberg 1975, 1976, 1980, 1984). However, there are also important differences, and nowhere are these differences more apparent than in our approach to the transference. In the Transference Focused Psychotherapy (TFP) model, patients are seen as reestablishing dyadic relations with their therapists that reflect rudimentary representations of self–other relationships of the past (so-called part–object relationships). Thus, TFP considers the externalization of these self-object-affect triads to be at the heart of therapeutic interventions. We do not differ from the TFP therapist in emphasizing the externalization process, but we are far less concerned with the apparent relationship that is thus established between patient and therapist. In our model, the role relationships established by the patient through the transference relationship are considered preliminary to the externalization of the parts of the self the patient wishes to disown. In order to achieve a state of affairs where the alien part of the self is experienced as outside rather than within, the patient needs to create a "relationship" with the therapist through which this externalization may be achieved. The patient subtly and unconsciously manipulates the therapist to experience

particular intense feelings, sometimes quite specific thoughts. These originally belong to the patient, but after a period of coercive interactions they are reassuringly seen by him to be outside, in the therapist's mind. Once the externalization is achieved, the patient has no interest in the relationship with the therapist and may in fact wish to repudiate it totally. At these moments the therapist may feel abandoned. Some instances of boundary violations may be related to the therapist's difficulty in coping with the implicit rejection entailed by the patient's wish to distance himself from the disowned part of his mind. Focusing the patients' attention on the dyad that is established through the externalization can be seen as undermining their attempts to separate from the disowned part of themselves. This focus can be counterproductive, leading the patient to prematurely terminate the treatment.

Effectiveness of Mentalization-Based Treatment

Our initial study (Bateman and Fonagy 1999) of MBT compared its effectiveness in the context of a partial hospital program with routine general psychiatric care for patients with BPD. Treatment took place within a routine clinical service and was implemented by mental health professionals without full psychotherapy training who were offered expert supervision. Results showed that patients in the partial hospital program showed a statistically significant decrease on all measures in contrast with the control group, which showed limited change or deterioration over the same period. Improvement in depressive symptoms, decrease in suicidal and self-mutilatory acts, reduced inpatient days, and better social and interpersonal function began after 6 months and continued to the end of treatment at 18 months.

The 44 patients who participated in the original study were assessed at 3-month intervals after completion of the trial using the same battery of outcome measures (Bateman and Fonagy 2001). Results demonstrated that patients who had received partial hospital treatment not only maintained their substantial gains but also showed a statistically significant continued improvement on most measures in contrast with the control group of patients who showed only limited change during the same period. Because of continued improvement in social and interpersonal function, these findings suggest that longer-term rehabilitative changes were stimulated.

Finally, an attempt was made to assess health care

costs associated with partial hospital treatment compared with treatment within general psychiatric services (Bateman and Fonagy 2003). Health care utilization of all patients who participated in the trial was assessed using information from case notes and service providers. Costs were compared 6 months prior to treatment, during 18 months of treatment, and at 18-month follow-up. No cost differences were found between the groups during pretreatment or treatment. During the treatment period, the costs of partial hospital treatment were offset by less psychiatric inpatient care and reduced emergency department treatment. The trend for costs to decrease in the experimental group during follow-up was not duplicated in the control group, suggesting that specialist partial hospital treatment for BPD is no more expensive than general psychiatric care and leads to considerable cost savings after the completion of 18 months' treatment.

A number of important questions have arisen from this research. First, although we operationalized treatment for research purposes, a more detailed manual was required if we were to demonstrate that treatment was generalizable across settings and practitioners and could be applied with fidelity by generically trained mental health staff. Second, in common with other treatments of BPD, it remains unclear what exactly are the effective ingredients of treatment. The partial hospital program is a complex, multifaceted intervention including analytic and expressive therapies, and there is inevitably a "milieu" effect. We were unable to show that the target of our interventions, mentalization, had been enhanced in patients treated within the partial hospital program compared with control patients because of the complexity of measuring reflective function. For research purposes Fonagy and colleagues (1998) have now operationalized the ability to apply a mentalizing interpretational strategy as reflective function. Individuals are not expected to articulate this theoretically but to demonstrate it in the way they interpret events within attachment relationships. Individuals differ in the extent to which they are able to go beyond observable phenomena to give an account of their own or others' actions in terms of beliefs, desires, plans, and so on, and in BPD patients this capacity is reduced.

We have operationalized MBT as an outpatient adaptation to answer some of these questions. Outpatient treatment removes the milieu aspect of therapy and focuses solely on mentalization within individual and group analytic therapy. Treatment consists of an individual and group psychoanalytic session once a week, a total of 2.5 hours of psychotherapy, and is part

of a randomized controlled trial that is under way at present. Again, treatment is implemented by generic mental health practitioners trained in MBT who are offered expert supervision. Even if this program turns out to be reasonably effective, the research into MBT and other treatments for BPD is only just beginning.

CONCLUSIONS

MBT may not be radically different from other forms of intervention widely practiced by psychotherapists and other mental health professionals in the various contexts in which individuals with BPD are being treated. We claim no originality for the intervention. How could we? MBT represents the relatively unadulterated implementation of a combination of developmental processes readily identified in all our histories: a) the establishment of an intense (attachment) relationship based on contingent mirroring of the mental states of patients, and b) the coherent re-presentation of their feelings and thoughts so that patients are able to identify themselves as thinking and feeling in the context of powerful bonds and high levels of emotional arousal. In turn, the recovery of mentalization helps patients regulate their thoughts and feelings, which then makes relationship and self-regulation a realistic possibility. Although we would claim to have identified a particular method that makes the delivery of this therapeutic process possible, we make no claims of uniqueness. Many situations can likely bring about symptomatic and personality change by this mechanism. The goal of further research is to identify increasingly effective and cost-effective methods for generating change in this excessively difficult group. In pursuing this goal there may indeed be nothing quite so practical as a good theory, such as the theory of human bonding.

REFERENCES

Ainsworth MDS: Object relations, dependency and attachment: a theoretical review of the infant–mother relationship. Child Dev 40:969–1025, 1969

Ainsworth MDS: Attachments across the lifespan. Bull N Y Acad Med 61:792–812, 1985

Ainsworth MDS, Blehar MC, Waters E, et al: Patterns of Attachment: A Psychological Study of the Strange Situation. Hillsdale, NJ, Erlbaum, 1978

Allen JG: Interpersonal Trauma and Serious Mental Disorder. Chichester, England, Wiley, 2001

Appelbaum SA: Psychological-mindedness: word, concept and essence. Int J Psychoanal 54:35–46, 1973

Arnsten AFT: The biology of being frazzled. Science 280:1711–1712, 1998

Arnsten AFT, Mathew R, Ubriani R, et al: Alpha-1 noradrenergic receptor stimulation impairs prefrontal cortical cognitive function. Biol Psychiatry 45:26–31, 1999

Arntz A, Veen G: Evaluations of others by borderline patients. J Nerv Ment Dis 189:513–521, 2001

Barnett D, Ganiban J, Cicchetti D: Maltreatment, emotional reactivity and the development of type D attachments from 12 to 24 months of age. Monogr Soc Res Child Dev 64:172–192, 1999

Bartholomew K, Horowitz LM: Attachment styles among young adults: a test of a four-category model. J Pers Soc Psychol 61:226–244, 1991

Bartholomew K, Kwong MJ, Hart SD: Attachment, in Handbook of Personality Disorders: Theory, Research, and Treatment. Edited by Livesley WJ. New York, Guilford, 2001, pp 196–230

Bateman A, Fonagy P: The effectiveness of partial hospitalization in the treatment of borderline personality disorder: a randomized controlled trial. Am J Psychiatry 156:1563–1569, 1999

Bateman A, Fonagy P: Treatment of borderline personality disorder with psychoanalytically oriented partial hospitalization: an 18-month follow-up. Am J Psychiatry 158:36–42, 2001

Bateman A, Fonagy P: Health service utilization costs for borderline personality disorder patients treated with psychoanalytically oriented partial hospitalization versus general psychiatric care. Am J Psychiatry 160:169–171, 2003

Bateman A, Fonagy P: Psychotherapy for Borderline Personality Disorder: Mentalization Based Treatment. Oxford, England, Oxford University Press, 2004

Beeghly M, Cicchetti D: Child maltreatment, attachment, and the self system: emergence of an internal state lexicon in toddlers at high social risk. Dev Psychopathol 6:5–30, 1994

Benjamin LS: Interpersonal Diagnosis and Treatment of Personality Disorder. New York, Guilford, 1993

Blatt SJ, Stayner D, Auerbach JS, et al: Change in object and self representations in long-term, intensive, inpatient treatment of seriously disturbed adolescents and young adults. Psychiatry: Interpersonal and Biological Processes 59:82–107, 1996

Bowlby J: Attachment and Loss, Vol 1: Attachment. London, Hogarth Press and the Institute of Psycho-Analysis, 1969

Bowlby J: Attachment and Loss, Vol 2: Separation: Anxiety and Anger. London, Hogarth Press and the Institute of Psycho-Analysis, 1973

Bram AD, Gabbard GO: Potential space and reflective functioning: towards conceptual clarification and preliminary clinical implications. Int J Psychoanal 82:685–699, 2001

Bremner JD, Staib LH, Kaloupek D, et al: Neural correlates of exposure to traumatic pictures and sound in Vietnam combat veterans with and without posttraumatic stress disorder: a positron emission tomography study. Biol Psychiatry 45:806–816, 1999a

Bremner JD, Narayan M, Staib LH, et al: Neural correlates of memories of childhood sexual abuse in women with and without posttraumatic stress disorder. Am J Psychiatry 156:1787–1795, 1999b

Brennan KA, Shaver PR: Attachment styles and personality disorders: their connections to each other and to parental divorce, parental death, and perceptions of parental caregiving. J Pers 66:835–878, 1998

Brenneis CB: Recovered Memories of Trauma: Transferring the Present to the Past. Madison, CT, International Universities Press, 1997

Bretherton K, Munholland KA: Internal working models in attachment relationships: a construct revisited, in Handbook of Attachment: Theory, Research and Clinical Applications. Edited by Cassidy J, Shaver PR. New York, Guilford, 1999, pp 89–114

Briere J, Runtz M: Post-sexual abuse trauma: data and implications for clinical practice. J Interpers Violence 2:367–397, 1987

Brown DG: Drowsiness in the countertransference. Int Rev Psychoanal 4:481–492, 1977

Brothers L: Friday's Footprint: How Society Shapes the Human Mind. New York, Oxford University Press, 1997

Broussard ER: Infant attachment in a sample of adolescent mothers. Child Psychiatry Hum Dev 25:211–219, 1995

Carlson EA: A prospective longitudinal study of attachment disorganization/disorientation. Child Dev 69:1107–1128, 1998

Carlson V, Cicchetti D, Barnett D, et al: Disorganised/disoriented attachment relationships in maltreated infants. Dev Psychol 25:525–531, 1989

Cicchetti D, Beeghly M: Symbolic development in maltreated youngsters: an organizational perspective, in Atypical Symbolic Development: New Directions for Child Development, Vol 36. Edited by Cicchetti D, Beeghly M. San Francisco, CA, Jossey-Bass, 1987, pp 5–29

Clarkin JF, Hull JW, Hurt SW: Factor structure of borderline personality disorder criteria. J Personal Disord 7:137–143, 1993

Clarkin J, Foelsch PA, Kernberg OF: Manual for the Inventory of Personality Organization. Ithaca, NY, Cornell University Medical College, 1996

Clarkin JF, Yeomans F, Kernberg OF: Psychodynamic Psychotherapy of Borderline Personality Organization: A Treatment Manual. New York, Wiley, 1998

Clarkin JF, Kernberg OF, Yeomans F: Transference-Focused Psychotherapy for Borderline Personality Disorder Patients. New York, Guilford, 1999

Cloitre M, Scarvalone P, Difede J: Posttraumatic stress disorder self and interpersonal dysfunction among sexually retraumatized women. J Trauma Stress 10:437–452, 1997

Collins NR, Read SJ: Representations of attachment: the structure and function of working models, in Advances in Personal Relationships, Vol 5: Attachment Process in Adulthood. Edited by Bartholomew K, Perlman D. London, Jessica Kingsley, 1994, pp 53–90

Compton A: The current status of the psychoanalytic theory of instinctual drives, I: drive concept, classification, and development. Psychoanal Q 52:364–401, 1983

Craik K: The Nature of Explanation. Cambridge, England, Cambridge University Press, 1943

Crittenden PM: Internal representational models of attachment relationships. Infant Ment Health J 11:259–277, 1990

Crittenden PM: Peering into the black box: an exploratory treatise on the development of self in young children, in Rochester Symposium on Developmental Psychopathology, Vol 5: Disorders and Dysfunctions of the Self. Edited by Cicchetti D, Toth SL. Rochester, NY, University of Rochester Press, 1994, pp 79–148

Crittenden PM: Toward an integrative theory of trauma: a dynamic-maturation approach, in Rochester Symposium on Developmental Psychopathology, Vol 8: Developmental Perspectives on Trauma. Edited by Cicchetti D, Toth SL. Rochester, NY, University of Rochester Press, 1997, pp 33–84

Damasio A: The Feeling of What Happens: Body and Emotion in the Making of Consciousness. New York, Harcourt Brace, 1999

De Bellis MD, Keshavan MS, Spencer S, et al: N-acetyl-aspartate concentration in the anterior cingulate of maltreated children and adolescents with PTSD. Am J Psychiatry 157:1175–1177, 2000

De M'Uzan M: A case of masochistic perversion and an outline of a theory. Int J Psychoanal 54:455–467, 1973

Dulit RA, Fyer MR, Leon AC, et al: Clinical correlates of self-mutilation in borderline personality disorder. Am J Psychiatry 151:1305–1311, 1994

Dutton DG: Male abusiveness in intimate relationships. Clin Psychol Rev 15:567–581, 1995

Dutton DG, Saunders K, Starzomski A, et al: Intimacy-anger and insecure attachment as precursors of abuse in intimate relationships. J Appl Soc Psychol 24:1367–1386, 1994

Favazza AR: Repetitive self-mutilation. Psychiatr Ann 22:60–63, 1992

Feeney JA, Noller P: Attachment style as a predictor of adult romantic relationships. J Pers Soc Psychol 58:281–291, 1990

Fletcher PC, Happe F, Frith U, et al: Other minds in the brain: a functional imaging study of "theory of mind" in story comprehension. Cognition 57:109–128, 1995

Fonagy P: Thinking about thinking: some clinical and theoretical considerations in the treatment of a borderline patient. Int J Psychoanal 72:1–18, 1991

Fonagy P: Playing with reality: the development of psychic reality and its malfunction in borderline patients. Int J Psychoanal 76:39–44, 1995

Fonagy P: Male perpetrators of violence against women: an attachment theory perspective. Journal of Applied Psychoanalytic Studies 1:7–27, 1999

Fonagy P: Attachment and borderline personality disorder. J Am Psychoanal Assoc 48:1129–1146, 2000

Fonagy P, Target M: Playing with reality, I: theory of mind and the normal development of psychic reality. Int J Psychoanal 77:217–233, 1996

Fonagy P, Target M: Attachment and reflective function: their role in self-organization. Dev Psychopathol 9:679–700, 1997

Fonagy P, Target M: Playing with reality, III: the persistence of dual psychic reality in borderline patients. Int J Psychoanal 81:853–874, 2000

Fonagy P, Target M: Early intervention and the development of self-regulation. Psychoanal Inq 22:307–335, 2002

Fonagy P, Steele H, Moran G, et al: The capacity for understanding mental states: the reflective self in parent and child and its significance for security of attachment. Infant Ment Health J 13:200–217, 1991a

Fonagy P, Steele H, Steele M: Maternal representations of attachment during pregnancy predict the organization of infant-mother attachment at one year of age. Child Dev 62:891–905, 1991b

Fonagy P, Steele M, Moran GS, et al: Measuring the ghost in the nursery: an empirical study of the relation between parents' mental representations of childhood experiences and their infants' security of attachment. J Am Psychoanal Assoc 41:957–989, 1993

Fonagy P, Steele M, Steele H, et al: Theory and practice of resilience. J Child Psychol Psychiatry 35:231–257, 1994

Fonagy P, Leigh T, Kennedy R, et al: Attachment, borderline states and the representation of emotions and cognitions in self and other, in Rochester Symposium on Developmental Psychopathology, Vol 6: Cognition and Emotion. Edited by Cicchetti D, Toth SL. Rochester, NY, University of Rochester Press, 1995, pp 371–414

Fonagy P, Leigh T, Steele M, et al: The relation of attachment status, psychiatric classification, and response to psychotherapy. J Consult Clin Psychol 64:22–31, 1996

Fonagy P, Target M, Steele M, et al: The development of violence and crime as it relates to security of attachment, in Children in a Violent Society. Edited by Osofsky JD. New York, Guilford, 1997, pp 150–177

Fonagy P, Target M, Steele H, et al: Reflective-Functioning Manual, Version 5.0, for Application to Adult Attachment Interviews. London, University College London, 1998

Fonagy P, Target M, Gergely G: Attachment and borderline personality disorder: a theory and some evidence. Psychiatr Clin North Am 23:103–122, 2000

Fonagy P, Stein H, White R: Dopamine receptor polymorphism and susceptibility to sexual, physical and psychological abuse: preliminary results of a longitudinal study of maltreatment. Paper presented at the 10th Biannual Meeting of the Society for Research in Child Development, Minneapolis, MN, April 2001

Fonagy P, Gergely G, Jurist E, et al: Affect Regulation, Mentalization and the Development of the Self. New York, Other Press, 2002

Fossati A, Donati D, Donini M, et al: Temperament, character, and attachment patterns in borderline personality disorder. J Personal Disord 15:390–402, 2001

Freud A: The Ego and the Mechanisms of Defence. New York, International Universities Press, 1936

Frith CD, Frith U: Interacting minds: a biological basis. Science 286:1692–1695, 1999

Frith U, Morton J, Leslie AM: The cognitive basis of a biological disorder: autism. Trends Neurosci 14:433–438, 1991

Frodi A, Dernevik M, Sepa A, et al: Current attachment representations of incarcerated offenders varying in degree of psychopathy. Attach Hum Dev 3:269–283, 2001

Fyer MR, Frances AJ, Sullivan T, et al: Suicide attempts in patients with borderline personality disorder. Am J Psychiatry 145:737–739, 1988

Gallagher HL, Happe F, Brunswick N, et al: Reading the mind in cartoons and stories: an fMRI study of "theory of mind" in verbal and nonverbal tasks. Neuropsychologia 38:11–21, 2000

Gallese V: The acting subject: toward the neural basis of social cognition, in Neural Correlates of Consciousness. Edited by Metzinger T. Cambridge, MA, MIT Press, 2000, pp 325–333

Gallese V: The "shared manifold" hypothesis: from mirror neurons to empathy. Journal of Consciousness Studies 8:33–50, 2001

Gazzaniga MS: The Social Brain: Discovering the Networks of the Mind. New York, Basic Books, 1985

Gidycz CA, Hanson K, Layman MJ: A prospective analysis of the relationships among sexual assault experiences: an extension of previous findings. Psychol Women Q 19:5–29, 1995

Gilligan J: Violence: Our Deadliest Epidemic and Its Causes. New York, Grosset/Putnam, 1997

Goel V, Grafman N, Sadato M, et al: Modeling other minds. Neuroreport 6:1741–1746, 1995

Grienenberger J, Kelly K, Slade A: Maternal reflective functioning and the caregiving relationship: the link between mental states and mother–infant affective communication. Paper presented at the Biennial Meetings of the Society for Research in Child Development, Minneapolis, MN, April 2001

Griffin DW, Bartholomew K: The metaphysics of measurement: the case of adult attachment, in Advances in Personal Relationships, Vol 5: Attachment Processes in Adulthood. Edited by Bartholomew K, Perlman D. London, Jessica Kingsley, 1994, pp 17–52

Gunderson JG: The borderline patient's intolerance of aloneness: insecure attachments and therapist availability. Am J Psychiatry 153:752–758, 1996

Gunderson JG: Borderline Personality Disorder: A Clinical Guide. Washington, DC, American Psychiatric Publishing, 2001

Gurvits IG, Koenigsberg HW, Siever LJ: Neurotransmitter dysfunction in patients with borderline personality disorder. Psychiatr Clin North Am 23:27–40, 2000

Happe F, Ehlers S, Fletcher P, et al: "Theory of mind" in the brain: evidence from a PET scan study of Asperger syndrome. Neuroreport 8:197–201, 1996

Hazan C, Shaver P: Romantic love conceptualized as an attachment process. J Pers Soc Psychol 52:511–524, 1987

Herpertz SC: Self-injurious behavior: psychopathological and nosological characteristics in subtypes of self-injurers. Acta Psychiatr Scand 91:57–68, 1995

Higgitt A, Fonagy P: The psychotherapeutic treatment of borderline and narcissistic personality disorder. Br J Psychiatry 161:23–43, 1992

Jacobovitz D, Hazen N: Developmental pathways from infant disorganization to childhood peer relationships, in Attachment Disorganization. Edited by Solomon J, George C. New York, Guilford, 1999, pp 127–159

Jacobovitz D, Hazen N, Riggs S: Disorganized mental processes in mothers, frightening/frightened caregiving and disoriented/disorganized behavior in infancy. Paper presented at the Biennial Meeting of the Society for Research in Child Development, Washington, DC, April 1997

Jeannerod M: The Cognitive Neuroscience of Action. Oxford, England, Blackwell, 1997

Kemperman I, Russ MJ, Shearin E: Self-injurious behavior and mood regulation in borderline patients. J Personal Disord 11:146–157, 1997

Kernberg OF: Borderline Conditions and Pathological Narcissism. New York, Jason Aronson, 1975

Kernberg OF: Object Relations Theory and Clinical Psychoanalysis. New York, Jason Aronson, 1976

Kernberg OF: Internal World and External Reality: Object Relations Theory Applied. New York, Jason Aronson, 1980

Kernberg OF: Self, ego, affects and drives. J Am Psychoanal Assoc 30:893–917, 1982

Kernberg OF: Object relations theory and character analysis. J Am Psychoanal Assoc 31:247–271, 1983

Kernberg OF: Severe Personality Disorders: Psychotherapeutic Strategies. New Haven, CT, Yale University Press, 1984

Kernberg OF: Aggression in Personality Disorders and Perversions. New Haven, CT, Yale University Press, 1992

Kernberg OF, Clarkin JF, Yeomans FE: A Primer of Transference Focused Psychotherapy for the Borderline Patient. New York, Jason Aronson, 2002

Kestenbaum R, Farber E, Sroufe LA: Individual differences in empathy among preschoolers' concurrent and predictive validity, in Empathy and Related Emotional Responses: New Directions for Child Development. Edited by Eisenberg N. San Francisco, CA, Jossey-Bass, 1989, pp 51–56

Klin A, Schultz R, Cohen DJ: Theory of mind in action: developmental perspectives on social neuroscience, in Understanding Other Minds: Perspectives From Developmental Cognitive Neuroscience, 2nd Edition. Edited by Baron-Cohen S, Tager-Flusberg H, Cohen DJ. New York, Oxford University Press, 2000, pp 357–388

Kohut H: The Restoration of the Self. New York, International Universities Press, 1977

Lane RD: Neural correlates of conscious emotional experience, in Cognitive Neuroscience of Emotion. Edited by Lane RD, Nadel L. New York, Oxford University Press, 2000, pp 345–370

Lane RD, Ahern GL, Schwartz GE, et al: Is alexithymia the emotional equivalent of blindsight? Biol Psychiatry 42:834–844, 1997

Lane RD, Reiman EM, Axelrod B, et al: Neural correlates of levels of emotional awareness: evidence of an interaction between emotion and attention in the anterior cingulate cortex. J Cogn Neurosci 10:525–535, 1998

Lanius RA, Williamson PC, Densmore M, et al: Neural correlates of traumatic memories in posttraumatic stress disorder: a functional MRI investigation. Am J Psychiatry 158:1920–1922, 2001

Lecours S, Bouchard M-A: Dimensions of mentalisation: outlining levels of psychic transformation. Int J Psychoanal 78:855–875, 1997

Levinson A, Fonagy P: Offending and attachment: the relationship between interpersonal awareness and offending in a prison population with psychiatric disorders. Can J Psychiatry (in press)

Linehan M: Suicidal people: one population or two? Ann N Y Acad Sci 487:16–33, 1986

Linehan MM, Armstrong HE, Suarez A, et al: Cognitive-behavioural treatment of chronically parasuicidal borderline patients. Arch Gen Psychiatry 48:1060–1064, 1991

Linehan MM, Schmidt H, Dimeff LA, et al: Dialectical behavior therapy for patients with borderline personality disorder and drug dependence. Am J Addict 8:279–292, 1999

Linehan MM, Dimeff LA, Reynolds SK, et al: Dialectical behavior therapy versus comprehensive validation therapy plus 12-step for the treatment of opioid dependent women meeting criteria for borderline personality disorder. Drug Alcohol Depend 67:13–26, 2002

Links PS, Heslegrave R, van Reekum R: Impulsivity: core aspect of borderline personality disorder. J Personal Disord 13:1–9, 1999

Lyons-Ruth K: Broadening our conceptual frameworks: can we reintroduce relational strategies and implicit representational systems to the study of psychopathology? Dev Psychol 31:432–436, 1995

Lyons-Ruth K: Attachment relationships among children with aggressive behavior problems: the role of disorganized early attachment patterns. J Consult Clin Psychol 64:32–40, 1996

Lyons-Ruth K, Jacobovitz D: Attachment disorganization: unresolved loss, relational violence and lapses in behavioral and attentional strategies, in Handbook of Attachment Theory and Research. Edited by Cassidy J, Shaver PR. New York, Guilford, 1999, pp 520–554

Lyons-Ruth K, Zoll D, Connell DB, et al: Family deviance and family disruption in childhood: associations with maternal behavior and infant maltreatment during the first two years of life. Dev Psychopathol 1:219–236, 1989

Lyons-Ruth K, Connell DB, Grunebaum HU: Infants at social risk: maternal depression and family support services as mediators of infant development and security of attachment. Child Dev 61:85–98, 1990

Lyons-Ruth K, Alpern L, Repacholi B: Disorganized infant attachment classification and maternal psychosocial problems as predictors of hostile-aggressive behavior in the preschool classroom. Child Dev 64:572–585, 1993

Lyons-Ruth K, Bronfman E, Atwood G: A relational diathesis model of hostile-helpless states of mind: expressions in mother–infant interaction, in Attachment Disorganization. Edited by Solomon J, George C. New York, Guilford, 1999a, pp 33–70

Lyons-Ruth K, Bronfman E, Parsons E: Atypical attachment in infancy and early childhood among children at developmental risk, IV: maternal frightened, frightening, or atypical behavior and disorganized infant attachment patterns. Monogr Soc Res Child Dev 64:67–96, 1999b

Main M: Metacognitive knowledge, metacognitive monitoring, and singular (coherent) vs. multiple (incoherent) model of attachment: findings and directions for future research, in Attachment Across the Life Cycle. Edited by Parkes CM, Stevenson-Hinde J, Marris P. London, Tavistock/Routledge, 1991, pp 127–159

Main M, Solomon J: Procedures for identifying infants as disorganized/disoriented during the Ainsworth strange situation, in Attachment During the Preschool Years: Theory, Research and Intervention. Edited by Greenberg M, Cicchetti D, Cummings EM. Chicago, IL, University of Chicago Press, 1990, pp 121–160

Main M, Kaplan N, Cassidy J: Security in infancy, childhood and adulthood: a move to the level of representation. Monogr Soc Res Child Dev 50:66–104, 1985

Mayes LC: A developmental perspective on the regulation of arousal states. Semin Perinatol 24:267–279, 2000

Mayes LC: A behavioral teratogenic model of the impact of prenatal cocaine exposure on arousal regulatory systems. Neurotoxicol Teratol 24:385–395, 2002

Meins E, Fernyhough C: Linguistic acquisitional style and mentalising development: the role of maternal mind-mindedness. Cogn Develop 14:363–380, 1999

Meins E, Russell J: Security and symbolic play: the relation between security of attachment and executive capacity. Br J Dev Psychol 15:63–76, 1997

Meins E, Fernyhough C, Russell J, et al: Security of attachment as a predictor of symbolic and mentalising abilities: a longitudinal study. Soc Dev 7:1–24, 1998

Meins E, Ferryhough C, Fradley E, et al: Rethinking maternal sensitivity: mothers' comments on infants mental processes predict security of attachment at 12 months. J Child Psychol Psychiatry 42:637–648, 2001

Meloy RJ: Violent Attachments. Northvale, NJ, Jason Aronson, 1992

Meyer B, Pilkonis PA, Proietti JM, et al: Attachment styles and personality disorders as predictors of symptom course. J Personal Disord 15:371–389, 2001

Morton J: The origins of autism. New Scientist 1694:44–47, 1989

Mosheim R, Zachhuber U, Scharf L, et al: Quality of attachment and interpersonal problems as possible predictors of inpatient therapy outcome. Psychotherapeut 45:223–229, 2000

Mullen PE, Martin JL, Anderson JC, et al: The long-term impact of the physical, emotional, and sexual abuse of children: a community study. Child Abuse Negl 20:7–21, 1996

Namnum A: The problem of analyzability and the autonomous ego. Int J Psychoanal 49:271–275, 1968

Nickell AD, Waudby CJ, Trull TJ: Attachment, parental bonding and borderline personality disorder features in young adults. J Personal Disord 16:148–159, 2002

Normandin L, Ensink K, Kernberg P: The role of trauma in the development of borderline personality disturbance in children. Paper presented at the Transference Focused Psychotherapy for Borderline Personality Disorder Symposium, New York, November 2002

Ogawa JR, Sroufe LA, Weinfield NS, et al: Development and the fragmented self: longitudinal study of dissociative symptomatology in a nonclinical sample. Dev Psychopathol 9:855–879, 1997

Ogden T: On potential space. Int J Psychoanal 66:129–141, 1985

Olson DR: The World on Paper. Cambridge, UK, Cambridge University Press, 1994

Paris J: Childhood precursors of borderline personality disorder. Psychiatr Clin North Am 23:77–88, 2000

Patrick M, Hobson RP, Castle D, et al: Personality disorder and the mental representation of early social experience. Dev Psychopathol 6:375–388, 1994

Pilkonis P: Personality prototypes among depressives. J Personal Disord 2:144–152, 1988

Pollak SD, Cicchetti D, Hornung K, et al: Recognizing emotion in faces: developmental effects of child abuse and neglect. Dev Psychol 36:679–688, 2000

Rauch SL, van der Kolk BA, Fisler RE, et al: A symptom provocation study of posttraumatic stress disorder using positron emission tomography and script-driven imagery. Arch Gen Psychiatry 53:380–387, 1996

Rosenberg PH, Miller GA: Comparing borderline definitions: DSM-III borderline and schizotypal personality disorders. J Abnorm Psychol 98:161–169, 1989

Rosenstein DS, Horowitz HA: Adolescent attachment and psychopathology. J Consult Clin Psychol 64:244–253, 1996

Russell DEH: The Secret Trauma: Incest in the Lives of Girls and Women. New York, Basic Books, 1986

Sack A, Sperling MB, Fagen G, et al: Attachment style, history, and behavioral contrasts for a borderline and normal sample. J Personal Disord 10:88–102, 1996

Salzman J, Salzman C, Wolfson AN: Relationship of childhood abuse and maternal attachment to the development of borderline personality disorder, in Role of Sexual Abuse in the Etiology of Borderline Personality Disorder. Edited by Zanarini MC. Washington, DC, American Psychiatric Press, 1997

Sandler J: From Safety to the Superego: Selected Papers of Joseph Sandler. New York, Guilford, 1987

Sandler J, Fonagy P (eds): Recovered Memories of Abuse: True or False? London, Karnac Books, 1997

Sanislow CA, Grilow CM, McGlashan TH: Factor analysis of DSM-III-R borderline personality criteria in psychiatric inpatients. Am J Psychiatry 157:1629–1633, 2000

Sayar K, Ebrinc S, Ak I: Alexithymia in patients with antisocial personality disorder in a military hospital setting. Isr J Psychiatry Relat Sci 38:81–87, 2001

Schore AN: Effects of a secure attachment relationship on right brain development, affect regulation, and infant mental health. Infant Ment Health J 22:7–66, 2001

Schuengel C, Bakermans-Kranenburg M, Van IJzendoorn M: Frightening maternal behaviour linking unresolved loss and disorganised infant attachment. J Consult Clin Psychol 67:54–63, 1999

Shaw DS, Vondra JI: Infant attachment security and maternal predictors of early behavior problems: a longitudinal study of low-income families. J Abnorm Child Psychol 23:335–357, 1995

Shaw DS, Owens EB, Vondra JI, et al: Early risk factors and pathways in the development of early disruptive behavior problems. Dev Psychopathol 8:679–700, 1997

Shin LM, McNally RJ, Kosslyn SM, et al: Regional cerebral blood flow during script-driven imagery in childhood sexual abuse-related PTSD: a PET investigation. Am J Psychiatry 156:575–584, 1999

Shin LM, Whalen PJ, Pitman RK, et al: An fMRI study of anterior cingulate function in posttraumatic stress disorder. Biol Psychiatry 50:932–942, 2001

Silk KR: Borderline personality disorder: overview of biologic factors. Psychiatr Clin North Am 23:61–75, 2000

Slade A, Belsky J, Aber JL, et al: Mother's representation of their relationships with their toddlers links to adult attachment and observed mothering. Dev Psychol 35:611–619, 1999

Solomon J, George C: Attachment Disorganization. New York, Guilford, 1999

Sroufe LA: Infant–Caregiver Attachment and Patterns of Adaptation in Preschool: The Roots of Maladaption and Competence, Vol 16. Hillsdale, NJ, Erlbaum, 1983

Sroufe LA: Emotional Development: The Organization of Emotional Life in the Early Years. New York, Cambridge University Press, 1996

Sroufe LA, Egeland B, Kreutzer T: The fate of early experience following developmental change: longitudinal approaches to individual adaptation in childhood. Child Dev 61:1363–1373, 1990

Sroufe LA, Carlson E, Levy AK, et al: Implications of attachment theory for developmental psychopathology. Dev Psychopathol 11:1–13, 1999

Stalker CA, Davies F: Attachment organization and adaptation in sexually abused women. Can J Psychiatry 40: 234–240, 1995

Stanley B, Winchel R, Molcho A, et al: Suicide and the self-harm continuum: phenomenological and biochemical evidence. Int Rev Psychiatry 4:149–155, 1992

Stanley B, Gameroff MJ, Michalsen V, et al: Are suicide attempters who self-mutilate a unique population? Am J Psychiatry 158:427–432, 2001

Startup M, Heard H, Swales M, et al: Autobiographical memory and parasuicide in borderline personality disorder. Br J Clin Psychol 40:113–120, 2001

Steele H, Steele M, Fonagy P: Associations among attachment classifications of mothers, fathers, and their infants. Child Dev 67:541–555, 1996

Stone MH, Hurt SW, Stone DK: The PI 500: long-term follow-up of borderline inpatients meeting DSM-III criteria, I: global outcome. J Personal Disord 1:291–298, 1987

Target M, Fonagy P: Playing with reality, II: the development of psychic reality from a theoretical perspective. Int J Psychoanal 77:459–479, 1996

Teti D, Gelfand D, Isabella R: Maternal depression and the quality of early attachment: an examination of infants, preschoolers and their mothers. Dev Psychol 31:364–376, 1995

Tronick EZ, Gianino AF: The transmission of maternal disturbance to the infant, in Maternal Depression and Infant Disturbance. Edited by Tronick EZ, Field T. San Francisco, CA, Jossey Bass, 1986, pp 5–11

Trull TJ: Relationships of borderline features to parental mental illness, childhood abuse, Axis I disorder, and current functioning. J Personal Disord 15:19–32, 2001a

Trull TJ: Structural relations between borderline personality disorder features and putative etiological correlates. J Abnorm Psychol 110:471–481, 2001b

Trull TJ, Sher KJ, Minks-Brown C, et al: Borderline personality disorder and substance use disorders: a review and integration. Clin Psychol Rev 20:235–253, 2000

van der Kolk PA, McFarlane AC, Weisaeth L (eds): Traumatic Stress: The Effects of Overwhelming Experience on Mind, Body, and Society. New York, Guilford, 1996

Van IJzendoorn MH: Adult attachment representations, parental responsiveness, and infant attachment: a meta-analysis on the predictive validity of the Adult Attachment Interview. Psychol Bull 117:387–403, 1995

Van IJzendoorn MH, Scheungel C, Bakermans-Kranenburg MJ: Disorganized attachment in early childhood: meta-analysis of precursors, concomitants and sequelae. Dev Psychopathol 22:225–249, 1999

Vermote R, Vertommen H, Corveleyn J, et al: The Kortenberg-Louvain Process-Outcome Study. Paper presented at the IPA Congress, New Orleans, LA, March 2004

Vitiello B, Stoff DM: Subtypes of aggression and their relevance to child psychiatry. J Am Acad Child Adolesc Psychiatry 36:307–315, 1997

Vondra JI, Hommerding KD, Shaw DS: Atypical attachment in infancy and early childhood among children at developmental risk, VI: stability and change in infant attachment in a low-income sample. Monogr Soc Res Child Dev 64:119–144, 1999

Vondra JI, Shaw DS, Swearingen L, et al: Attachment stability and emotional and behavioral regulation from infancy to preschool age. Dev Psychopathol 13:13–33, 2001

Wartner UG, Grossman K, Fremmer-Bombrik E, et al: Attachment patterns at age six in South Germany: predictability from infancy and implications for pre-school behaviour. Child Dev 65:1014–1027, 1994

Waters E, Wippman J, Sroufe LA: Attachment, positive affect, and competence in the peer group: two studies in construct validation. Child Dev 50:821–829, 1979

Widom CS: Posttraumatic stress disorder in abused and neglected children grown up. Am J Psychiatry 156:1223–1229, 1999

Winnicott DW: Mirror-role of the mother and family in child development, in The Predicament of the Family: A Psycho-Analytical Symposium. Edited by Lomas P. London, Hogarth Press, 1967, pp 26–33

Winnicott DW: Playing and Reality. London, Tavistock, 1971

Zanarini MC, Williams AA, Lewis RE, et al: Reported pathological childhood experiences associated with the development of borderline personality disorder. Am J Psychiatry 154:1101–1106, 1997

Zlotnick C, Mattia J, Zimmerman M: Clinical features of survivors of sexual abuse with major depression. Child Abuse Negl 25:357–367, 2001

Zubieta JK, Chinitz JA, Lombardi U, et al: Medial frontal cortex involvement in PTSD symptoms: a SPECT study. J Psychiatr Res 33:259–264, 1999

13

Role of Childhood Experiences in the Development of Maladaptive and Adaptive Personality Traits

Jeffrey G. Johnson, Ph.D.
Elizabeth Bromley, M.D.
Pamela G. McGeoch, M.A.

During the past century, clinical experience and research have provided considerable support for the hypothesis that interpersonal experiences during childhood and adolescence play an important role in personality development (e.g., Erikson 1963). Childhood adversities such as maladaptive parenting and childhood abuse and neglect may be likely to have an adverse impact on personality development because they interfere with or alter the trajectory of normative socialization processes during childhood and adolescence (Cohen 1999; Johnson et al. 2001a). Positive experiences during childhood and adolescence, such as parental warmth and support, may be likely to promote the development of adaptive traits such as trust, altruism, and optimism, due to social learning processes and

development of a secure attachment style during childhood (e.g., Erikson 1963; Sroufe et al. 1999). This chapter presents a summary of research findings that are currently available regarding the role that childhood experiences may play in the development of maladaptive and adaptive personality traits. We begin by summarizing the evidence that is currently available from retrospective and prospective studies regarding the hypothesized association between childhood adversities and personality disorders. The association of childhood abuse and neglect with risk for the development of personality disorders is examined in particular depth because this association is of considerable interest to clinicians and because comparatively little information is available regarding other adversities that may contribute to the development of maladaptive traits. The chapter concludes with an examination of the available evidence regarding the association of positive childhood experiences with the development of adaptive traits.

CHILDHOOD ADVERSITIES ASSOCIATED WITH DEVELOPMENT OF PERSONALITY DISORDERS

A large body of research has provided findings that are indirectly consistent with the hypothesis that some types of childhood adversities may contribute to the development of maladaptive personality traits and personality disorders. Retrospective studies, the majority of which have been conducted with clinical samples, have demonstrated that individuals with personality disorders tend to be more likely than individuals without personality disorders to report a history of childhood maltreatment and other traumatic childhood experiences. These findings have also been of interest because they have provided evidence of specificity, indicating that patients with personality disorders are particularly likely to report having experienced specific types of childhood abuse or neglect. However, retrospective studies cannot rule out the alternative hypotheses that the association of childhood adversities with maladaptive personality traits is attributable to recall bias or to preexisting childhood traits that may contribute to the onset of some types of childhood adversities (Maughan and Rutter 1997; Paris 1997).

Both of these alternative hypotheses have presented significant challenges to researchers in this field. Although there have been findings supporting the validity of retrospective reports of childhood adversities (e.g., Bifulco et al. 1997; Robins et al. 1985), and although retrospective studies have promoted the formulation of developmental hypotheses, it is nevertheless problematic to make strong causal inferences based on retrospective data. In addition, a number of studies have supported the hypothesis that genetic and prenatal factors may play an important role in the development of behavioral and emotional problems that may become evident during childhood (Livesley et al. 1993; Neugebauer et al. 1999; Thomas and Chess 1984). Furthermore, research has indicated that maladaptive childhood traits may have an adverse influence on parenting behavior, potentially increasing risk for childhood maltreatment (Kendler 1996). Such findings have contributed to skepticism about the hypothesis that childhood adversities play an important role

in the development of maladaptive personality traits and personality disorders.

However, in recent years, investigations utilizing a number of different research paradigms have provided new and compelling evidence in support of the hypothesis that childhood experiences have an important influence on personality development. Research has indicated that maladaptive personality traits are likely to be caused by the interaction of genetic and environmental risk factors (Caspi et al. 2002), including maternal behavior, health, and environmental characteristics affecting prenatal development (Neugebauer et al. 1999). Epidemiological studies and co-twin analyses that have controlled for genetic factors have indicated that childhood abuse is likely to be causally related to an increased risk for a broad spectrum of psychiatric symptoms (Kendler et al. 2000). Neurobiological studies have provided considerable evidence suggesting that childhood maltreatment may cause persistent deficits in brain activity associated with a wide range of psychiatric symptoms (Teicher et al. 2003). Prospective longitudinal studies and investigations that obtained evidence of childhood maltreatment from official records have supported the hypothesis that childhood abuse and neglect may contribute to increased risk for the development of personality disorders. (Drake et al. 1988; Guzder et al. 1996; Johnson et al. 1999a, 2000, 2001a, 2001b; Luntz and Widom 1994). The findings of these studies and those that have provided relevant retrospective data are described in greater detail below.

Childhood Physical Abuse

Research conducted with clinical, forensic, and epidemiological samples has indicated that indices of childhood physical abuse may be associated with antisocial, borderline, and other personality disorder traits. Patients with antisocial personality disorder (ASPD) have been found to be more likely than patients with other psychiatric disorders to report a history of physical abuse during childhood (e.g., Norden et al. 1995; see also Bernstein et al. 1998). Confirmatory findings have indicated that individuals identified as having experienced childhood physical abuse are likely to have problems with aggressive, criminal, or antisocial behavior (Pollock et. al. 1990; Widom 1989). Patients with borderline personality disorder (BPD) have also been found to be likely to report a history of physical abuse during childhood (e.g., Brown and Anderson 1991; Goldman et al. 1992). Other studies have yielded findings indicating that paranoid, schizoid, and schizotypal traits were associated with reports of childhood physical abuse in clinical samples (Bernstein et al. 1998; Yen et al. 2002).

Data from the Children in the Community Study (CICS; for detailed information about the study methodology, please see http://nyspi.org/childcom), a community-based longitudinal study, indicated that documented physical abuse was associated with elevated antisocial, borderline, dependent, depressive, passive-aggressive, and schizoid personality disorder traits after parental education and parental psychopathology were controlled statistically (Johnson et al. 1999a). Antisocial and depressive personality disorder traits remained significantly associated with documented physical abuse after other personality disorder traits were controlled statistically. Evidence of physical abuse, obtained from either official records or retrospective self-reports, was associated with elevated antisocial, borderline, passive-aggressive, and schizotypal personality disorder traits after controlling for parental education, parental psychopathology, sexual abuse, and neglect (Johnson et al. 1999a).

In summary, prospective epidemiological studies and retrospective clinical studies have provided considerable evidence in support of the hypothesis that childhood physical abuse may contribute to the onset of ASPD, independent of the effects of other types of childhood maltreatment (Table 13–1). Epidemiological studies that relied on prospective and retrospective data and retrospective clinical findings have suggested that childhood physical abuse may be associated with elevated risk for the development of borderline and schizotypal personality disorders after other kinds of childhood maltreatment are accounted for. In addition, prospective or retrospective studies have provided evidence suggesting that childhood physical abuse may be associated with the development of depressive, paranoid, passive-aggressive, and schizoid personality disorder traits.

Childhood Sexual Abuse

Many studies have provided evidence indicating that patients with personality disorders are significantly more likely than patients without personality disorders to report a history of sexual abuse. Patients with BPD are more likely than other patients to report a history of childhood sexual abuse (Brown and Anderson 1991; Laporte and Guttman 1996; Westen et al. 1990). Evidence also has suggested that patients with BPD may tend to have experienced chronic (as opposed to episodic) sexual abuse during childhood (Weaver and Clum 1993). Systematic studies have suggested that other personality disorders may also be associated

with a history of reported sexual abuse. Norden et al. (1995) found that reports of childhood sexual abuse were associated with borderline, histrionic, narcissistic, and schizotypal personality disorders. Shea et al. (1999) obtained convergent findings from both inpatient and outpatient samples indicating that reported childhood sexual abuse in both samples was associated with elevated avoidant, paranoid, and schizotypal personality disorder symptom levels. Ruggiero et al. (1999) found that military veterans who reported severe childhood sexual abuse had higher antisocial, avoidant, passive-aggressive, schizoid, and schizotypal personality disorder symptom levels than did men who reported minimal childhood maltreatment. Reports of childhood sexual abuse have also been found to be associated with depressive symptoms and interpersonal difficulties (Browne and Finkelhor 1986).

Community-based research findings have indicated that documented sexual abuse was associated with elevated BPD traits after parental education and parental psychopathology were controlled statistically (Johnson et al. 1999a). Evidence of sexual abuse, obtained from either official records or retrospective self-reports, was associated with elevated borderline, depressive, and histrionic personality disorder traits after controlling for parental education, parental psychopathology, physical abuse, and neglect (Johnson et al. 1999a).

In summary, prospective epidemiological studies and retrospective clinical studies have provided considerable support for the hypothesis that childhood sexual abuse may contribute to the onset of BPD, independent of the effects of other types of childhood maltreatment (Table 13–1). Epidemiological studies that relied on prospective and retrospective data and retrospective clinical findings have suggested that childhood sexual abuse may be associated with elevated risk for the development of histrionic and depressive personality disorder traits after other kinds of childhood maltreatment are accounted for. In addition, prospective or retrospective studies have provided evidence suggesting that childhood sexual abuse may be associated with the development of antisocial, avoidant, narcissistic, paranoid, passive-aggressive, schizoid, and schizotypal personality disorder traits.

Childhood Emotional Abuse

Research has suggested that emotional abuse (including verbal abuse, humiliation, and other psychological maltreatment) may contribute, independently, to the development of personality disorder traits during childhood and adolescence. Childhood emotional

Table 13–1. Prospective and retrospective associations between specific types of childhood maltreatment and personality disorder traits

Personality disorder	Physical abuse	Sexual abuse	Emotional abuse	Emotional neglect	Physical neglect	Supervision neglect	Any neglect
Antisocial	P, C*, R	R		R	R		P, C*, R
Avoidant		R	R	P*, R			P*, C*, R
Borderline	C*, R	P, C*, R	P*, R	R	R	P*, R	P*, C*, R
Dependent				R			- P*, C*
Depressive	P	C*	R				P
Histrionic		C*, R					
Narcissistic		R	P*				P, C*
Obsessive-compulsive			P*				
Paranoid	R	R	P*	P*, R		P*	P*
Passive-aggressive	C*	R				P*	P*, C*, R
Schizoid	R	R	P*	R			R
Schizotypal	C*, R	R	P*		P*		P*, C*, R

Note. Each of the associations in this table has been investigated by one or more prospective studies. Associations of retrospectively reported childhood physical and sexual abuse with specific types of personality disorder symptoms have been studied among patients with antisocial and borderline personality disorders. However, the associations of retrospective reports of childhood emotional abuse and childhood neglect with specific types of personality disorder traits have not yet been investigated systematically.

C=Combined prospective and retrospective reports of childhood physical abuse, sexual abuse, or any childhood neglect yielded significant findings after controlling for co-occurring personality disorder symptoms, parental education, and parental psychiatric symptoms. P=Prospective epidemiological findings, based on documented evidence of childhood maltreatment, were significant after controlling for co-occurring personality disorder symptoms, parental education, and parental psychiatric symptoms. R=Retrospective clinical studies have obtained a significant association after covariates were controlled statistically.

*Association remained significant after controlling for other types of childhood abuse and neglect.

abuse may increase risk for the development of personality disorders in part by increasing the likelihood that youths will experience maladaptive thoughts and feelings, such as excessive guilt, resentment, social anxiety, shame, and mistrust of others during their most critical years of psychosocial development. Severe childhood verbal abuse may leave deeper scars than other types of abuse, because children tend to internalize verbally abusive statements and to self-inflict these abusive thoughts against themselves throughout their lives (Ney 1987).

Clinical studies have indicated that many patients with BPD and other personality disorders report a history of childhood verbal abuse (Laporte and Guttman 1996; Oldham et al. 1996; Zanarini et al. 1997). Childhood emotional abuse and intolerant, shaming parental behavior have been found to be associated with avoidant personality traits among psychiatric patients (Grilo and Masheb 2002; Stravynski et al. 1989). Bernstein et al. (1998) reported that Cluster B and C personality disorders were significantly associated with retrospective reports of childhood emotional abuse. When sexual and physical abuse have been statistically controlled, emotional abuse has also been found to be independently associated with depressive personality traits, including poor self-esteem and suicidality (Briere and Runtz 1990; Mullen et al. 1996).

Longitudinal research has indicated that verbal abuse during childhood, assessed in a series of maternal interviews, was associated with increased risk for borderline, narcissistic, obsessive-compulsive, and paranoid personality disorders and with elevated borderline, narcissistic, paranoid, schizoid, and schizotypal personality disorder symptom levels during adolescence and early adulthood (Johnson et al. 2001b). These findings were obtained after behavioral and emotional problems during childhood, physical abuse, sexual abuse, neglect, physical punishment, parental education, parental psychopathology, and co-occurring psychiatric disorders were controlled statistically. Such findings have suggested that childhood verbal abuse may contribute to the development of some types of personality disorders, independent of the effects of other types of childhood maltreatment.

When the available data from prospective epidemiological studies and retrospective clinical studies are considered together, considerable evidence supports the hypothesis that childhood emotional abuse may contribute to the onset of BPD, independent of the effects of other types of childhood maltreatment (Table 13–1). In addition, prospective or retrospective studies have provided evidence suggesting that childhood emotional abuse may be associated with the development of avoidant, depressive, narcissistic, obsessive-compulsive, paranoid, schizoid, and schizotypal personality disorder traits.

CHILDHOOD NEGLECT

The association of childhood neglect with the development of personality disorders has been investigated less extensively than the corresponding associations regarding childhood sexual and physical abuse. Nevertheless, the available evidence suggests that childhood neglect may contribute as or more strongly than physical and sexual abuse to the development of personality disorder symptoms and other maladaptive personality traits (Gauthier et al. 1996; Johnson et al. 1999a). Many patients with personality disorders report a history of childhood neglect (Oldham et al. 1996), and reports of a lack of parental affection during childhood have been found in clinical samples to be associated with antisocial, avoidant, borderline, dependent, paranoid, and schizoid personality disorder symptoms (Arbel and Stravynski 1991; Carter et al. 1999; Norden et al. 1995). Reports of severe childhood neglect have been found to be associated with elevated avoidant, schizoid, and schizotypal personality disorder symptom levels among military veterans (Ruggiero et al. 1999). Childhood neglect has also been found to be associated with a wide range of other maladaptive personality traits, including antisocial or avoidant behavior, attachment difficulties, hostility, paranoia, and self-destructive behavior (Dubo et al. 1997; Gauthier et al. 1996; Robins 1966; Sroufe et al. 1999).

Longitudinal research has suggested that childhood neglect may increase risk for the development of personality disorders. Evidence of childhood neglect (i.e., lack of parental affection and supervision during early adolescence) has been found to be associated with risk for dependent and passive-aggressive personality disorders during adulthood (Drake et al. 1988). CICS findings indicated that documented childhood neglect was associated with elevated antisocial, avoidant, borderline, dependent, narcissistic, paranoid, passive-aggressive, and schizotypal personality disorder traits after parental education and parental psychopathology were controlled statistically (Johnson et al. 1999a). Antisocial, avoidant, borderline, narcissistic, and passive-aggressive personality disorder traits remained significantly associated with documented neglect after other personality disorder traits were controlled statistically. Evidence of childhood neglect, obtained from either official records or retrospective self-reports, was associated with elevated antisocial, avoidant, borderline, dependent, narcissistic, passive-aggressive, and schizotypal personality disorder traits after controlling for parental education, parental psychopathology, sexual abuse, and neglect (Johnson et al. 1999a).

In recent years, research has suggested that specific types of childhood neglect may be differentially associated with specific types of personality disorder traits. Patients with BPD have been found to be more likely than patients with other personality disorders to report a history of childhood emotional, physical, and supervision neglect (Zanarini et al. 1997). Patients with antisocial, avoidant, dependent, and paranoid personality disorders have been found to be more likely than other patients to report a history of childhood emotional neglect (Carter et al. 1999). Patients with elevated schizoid personality disorder symptom levels have been found to be particularly likely to report a history of childhood emotional neglect (Bernstein et al. 1998). Dubo et al. (1997) found that symptoms of self-mutilation and suicidality were associated with retrospective reports of childhood emotional neglect among patients with BPD. Johnson et al. (2000) reported that childhood emotional neglect was independently associated with increased risk for avoidant personality disorder and elevated paranoid personality disorder symptom levels, physical neglect was independently associated with elevated schizotypal symptom levels, and supervision neglect was independently associated with elevated borderline, paranoid, and passive-aggressive personality disorder symptom levels. In addition, emotional, physical, and supervision neglect were independently associated with elevated overall personality disorder symptom levels and overall risk for personality disorders during adolescence or early adulthood after other types of childhood maltreatment were accounted for (Johnson et al. 2000). These findings suggest that specific types of childhood neglect may contribute in unique ways, in combination with other childhood adversities, to the development of different types of personality disorder symptoms.

In summary, prospective epidemiological studies and retrospective clinical studies have provided considerable evidence in support of the hypothesis that childhood neglect may contribute to the onset of avoidant, borderline, passive-aggressive, and schizotypal personality disorders, independent of the effects of other types of childhood maltreatment (Table 13–1). In addition, epidemiological studies that relied on prospective and retrospective data and retrospective clinical findings have

suggested that childhood neglect may be associated with risk for ASPD after other kinds of childhood maltreatment are accounted for. Furthermore, prospective or retrospective studies have provided evidence suggesting that childhood neglect may be associated with the development of dependent, narcissistic, paranoid, and schizoid personality disorder traits.

Prospective epidemiological studies have suggested that specific types of childhood neglect may be differentially associated with elevated risk for specific types of personality disorder symptoms.

Case Example

Ms. E was a 19-year-old psychiatric outpatient diagnosed with depressive, obsessive-compulsive, and borderline personality disorder symptoms and severe narcissistic personality disorder symptoms. During psychotherapy sessions, she reported that she had been molested and sexually abused by an older half-brother from age 4 years until early adolescence, when she became aware of the meaning of sexual activity. The sexual abuse began with episodic molestation but became more severe from age 7 onward, occurring during lengthy periods of time when she and her half-brother were left alone and unsupervised by her parents. Ms. E tried to tell her mother about the sexual abuse—she wrote a suicide note that her mother found—but her mother did not put an end to her half-brother's behavior.

Ms. E also reported that her father frequently relied on harsh physical punishment to discipline her, for example, using a belt to whip her when she received poor grades in school. At times, this punishment was so severe that it resulted in bruises or lacerations, including an open gash in her leg, indicative of physical abuse. Ms. E also reported that her father abused her emotionally, calling her names like "stupid," "lazy," and a "whore." In addition, she reported that her mother was emotionally and physically abusive, although this abuse was not as severe as that perpetrated by her father.

Ms. E frequently witnessed physical violence between her parents, who were often verbally or physically combative. Her father often drank heavily and had a number of extramarital affairs. Ms. E informed her mother about one of her father's indiscretions, and her mother became so enraged that she shot Ms. E's father. There was abundant evidence indicating that Ms. E's history of maltreatment and problematic parenting contributed to the development and persistence of her depressive, obsessive-compulsive, borderline, and narcissistic personality disorder traits, which were associated with considerable impairment and distress.

Case Example

Ms. F was a 22-year-old psychiatric inpatient with severe BPD, dependent personality disorder traits, and posttraumatic stress disorder, with a history of dissociative symptoms, severe insomnia, depressed mood, and psychotic episodes. Ms. F reported that she had been emotionally abused and "scapegoated" by her mother throughout her childhood. For example, she reported that her mother frequently forced her to wait until the other family members had finished their meals before allowing her to eat. She also reported that her mother made her spend substantially more of her time than her siblings doing housework and other chores. Ms. F reported that her mother often humiliated her by doing things such as making her wear boys' clothing to school, and that her mother punished her severely for any appearance of sexual behavior. In addition, Ms. F reported that her mother neglected her emotionally and that her mother rarely, if ever, was affectionate, nurturing, or supportive toward her.

Ms. F reported that she was forced to leave the family home at age 17 and soon afterward became homeless. She became involved in an abusive relationship with a man who beat and raped her repeatedly. She ran away from him and asked her mother to take her in, but her mother told her, "You chose your bed. Now you can lie in it." Ms. F went to a homeless shelter, where she was beaten by some other young women on the day she arrived. During her stay at the shelter, Ms. F began receiving psychiatric treatment for the first time. However, her sense of well-being was frequently threatened while she lived there, and she reported that she constantly felt endangered during that time. She reported that on one occasion she was raped by a stranger while at the shelter. Prior to her initial hospitalization, Ms. F reported having cut her wrists on several occasions when she found the adversities of life in the homeless shelter to be overwhelming. She received several years of treatment that enabled her to recover sufficiently to be able to live semi-independently. However, many of her symptoms were so severe and unremitting that she was eventually classified as chronically disabled.

HYPOTHESIZED ASSOCIATIONS OF SPECIFIC TYPES OF CHILDHOOD MALTREATMENT AND PERSONALITY DISORDERS

Research on the association between childhood maltreatment and personality disorders has advanced significantly in recent years. Interestingly, the findings that are currently available suggest that specific types or combinations of childhood emotional abuse, physical abuse, sexual abuse, emotional neglect, physical neglect, and supervision neglect may be associated with the development of specific types of personality disorder traits. Although much research remains to be done, evidence from prospective studies that have

controlled for co-occurring childhood maltreatment and personality disorder symptoms, and from retrospective studies, supports the following hypotheses:

1. Youths who experience physical abuse and one or more types of childhood neglect may be at particularly elevated risk for ASPD.
2. Youths who experience emotional neglect may be at elevated risk for avoidant personality disorder.
3. Youths who experience sexual abuse and emotional abuse, physical abuse, or one or more types of childhood neglect may be at particularly elevated risk for BPD.
4. Youths who experience one or more types of childhood neglect may be at elevated risk for dependent personality disorder.
5. Youths who experience physical and/or sexual abuse may be at elevated risk for poor self-esteem and other traits associated with depressive personality disorder.
6. Youths who experience sexual abuse may be at elevated risk for histrionic personality disorder.
7. Youths who experience emotional abuse and/or one or more types of childhood neglect may be at particularly elevated risk for narcissistic personality disorder.
8. Childhood emotional abuse may contribute to the development of obsessive-compulsive personality disorder.
9. Childhood emotional abuse, in combination with emotional or supervision neglect, may contribute to the development of paranoid personality disorder.
10. Youths who experience physical abuse and/or supervision neglect may be at elevated risk for passive-aggressive personality disorder.
11. Youths who experience any emotional abuse and one or more other types of childhood maltreatment may be at particularly elevated risk for schizoid personality disorder.
12. Youths who experience emotional abuse, physical abuse, and/or physical neglect may be at elevated risk for schizotypal personality disorder.

CLINICAL IMPLICATIONS OF RESEARCH ON CHILDHOOD MALTREATMENT AND RISK FOR PERSONALITY DISORDER

It may be possible to prevent the onset of chronic personality disorders among some youths by providing high-risk parents with services that assist them in developing more adaptive parenting behaviors. Research has indicated that it is possible to reduce the likelihood that children will develop psychiatric disorders by helping parents to learn more effective child-rearing techniques (Redmond et al. 1999). In addition, because treatment of parental disorders may help to reduce the likelihood of childhood maltreatment and problematic parenting, it may be possible to decrease offspring risk for personality disorders by improving the recognition and treatment of psychiatric disorders among parents in the community (Chilcoat et al. 1996).

OTHER CHILDHOOD ADVERSITIES ASSOCIATED WITH THE DEVELOPMENT OF PERSONALITY DISORDERS

Although childhood abuse and neglect are likely to play a particularly important role in the development of personality disorder symptoms, a number of studies have indicated that problematic parenting (e.g., parenting behavior that, although problematic, is not sufficiently severe to be classified as "abuse" or "neglect") is likely to be associated with the development of maladaptive personality traits and personality disorders (see Chapter 11, "Developmental Issues"). Research has indicated that a lack of parental affection during childhood, low family communication and expressiveness, a lack of parental time with the child, and harsh, controlling parenting behavior are associated with elevated personality disorder traits among adolescent nonpatients and adult psychiatric patients (Baker et al. 1996; Head et al. 1991; Johnson et al. 1997; Parker et al. 1999; Stravynski et al. 1989). Retrospective reports of a lack of parental affection during childhood by patients with personality disorders have been found, in a patient sample, to be associated with ASPD and schizoid personality disorder symptoms while paternal overprotection was associated with schizoid personality disorder symptoms (Norden et al. 1995). Community-based longitudinal research has also indicated that a wide range of problematic parenting behaviors may be associated with risk for personality disorders (Drake et al. 1988; Johnson et al. 2001a). In addition, research has indicated that a number of other childhood adversities including parental death, parental separation or divorce, socioeconomic adversities, traumatic life events, and victimization (e.g., assault, bullying) may be associated with elevated risk for personality disorders (Coid 1999; Johnson et al. 1999b; Zanarini and Frankenburg 1997).

PROTECTIVE FACTORS ASSOCIATED WITH THE DEVELOPMENT OF ADAPTIVE TRAITS

Research has identified a wide variety of experiences, relationships, and community resources that may promote the development of adaptive personality traits, such as hardiness or resiliency during childhood and adolescence. Familial warmth, extrafamilial support, and other facilitative environmental characteristics have been found to be associated with the development of adaptive traits. These traits, in turn, are likely to play an important mediating role in determining whether individuals are able to adapt effectively to adversities during adulthood (Garmezy 1985; Shiner 2000; Werner and Smith 1982).

Familial Protective Factors

A wide range of parenting behaviors (e.g., affection, communication, time spent with children) and characteristics of the family and home environment play an important role in healthy child development (Johnson et al. 2001a; see also Chapter 11, "Developmental Issues"). Parental empathy, support, and warmth have been found to help children and adolescents cope effectively with many types of adversities (Cowen et al. 1997; Luthar and Zigler 1991; Wyman et al. 1991). Research has also indicated that children who develop a close, strong, and mutually respectful relationship with their parents tend to be particularly resilient and to have adaptive coping skills (Kobak and Sceery 1988). Furthermore, strong and supportive relationships with parents and family members tend to be associated with healthy interpersonal functioning during adulthood and successful adaptation to adult responsibilities (Werner and Smith 1982; see also Chapter 11, "Developmental Issues"). Young adults who perceive their family as warm and supportive tend to be relatively confident and adaptable and to have high self-esteem, whereas those who perceive their parents as authoritarian tend to be more uncertain about themselves and the future (Strage 1998).

It is important to note that a variety of parenting styles may lead to positive outcomes (Baldwin et al. 1990) and that the child-rearing behavior of the parent is determined, in part, by the disposition or temperament of the child (Cohen 1999; Kendler 1996). For example, youths with externalizing behavior problems may need extra parental supervision, and youths with internalizing problems may be in particular need of parental warmth and support. However, research has indicated that most youths benefit from having responsible, nurturing, supportive parents who gradually encourage them to function in an increasingly autonomous manner as they mature (Cowen et al. 1997; Luthar and Zigler 1991; Strage 1998; Wyman et al. 1991).

Extrafamilial Protective Factors

Many different types of community and neighborhood resources may help to promote healthy personality development during childhood and adolescence. Supportive community organizations that help young people to develop ethics and values; mentors such as teachers, godparents, and adult role models; and confidants in the form of highly functioning and supportive peers may facilitate the development of adaptive personality traits (Werner 1989). The presence of a mentor during adolescence has been found to be associated with improved academic achievement, attitudes about school, insight, relationships with parents and peers, and self-esteem, and with reductions in aggressive behavior and psychoactive substance use (Wolkow and Ferguson 2001; Zimmerman et al. 2002).

Participation in community activities and organizations may also have a variety of beneficial consequences. Community involvement may help to provide a sense of purpose, to increase the availability of social support, and to foster resiliency (Vaillant 1977). Youths who have a strong sense of membership in and identification with the community may adapt more effectively to stressful life events (Heath et al. 1999). Extracurricular activities, such as participation in athletic activities, arts and crafts, hobbies, musical ensembles, and organized recreational activities may also promote healthy adaptation to adversity (Bell and Suggs 1998). Thus, communities and schools that provide young people with a wide range of opportunities to engage in such activities may help to promote healthy personality development during childhood and adolescence.

Resiliency and Other Adaptive Personality Traits

The research findings cited earlier are consistent with Erik Erikson's (1963) hypothesis that personality development during childhood and adolescence is determined, in large measure, by the child's upbringing, chronic adversities, and other important interpersonal experiences. Although each child begins life with behavioral tendencies that are influenced by genetic and prenatal factors (Livesley et al. 1993; Neugebauer et al. 1999; Thomas and Chess 1984), life experiences appear to play a critical role in determining how these temperamental characteristics are expressed (Caspi et al. 2002; Cohen 1999). Research has also supported Erikson's hypothesis that children who grow up in a supportive environment are more likely to develop character strengths such as trust in others, autonomy, industriousness, and self-esteem (see Chapter 11, "Developmental Issues"). These and other personality traits have been found to promote the development of strong, supportive relationships with others and to facilitate adaptation to adversities later in life (Garmezy 1985; Rutter 1987; Shiner 2000; Werner and Smith 1982).

Resiliency

Research has identified personality traits, such as optimism and productivity, that tend to be associated with an adaptive, resilient response to stress (Pengilly and Dowd 2000; Rutter 1987). The development of resiliency may stem in part from experiences that teach individuals how to cope effectively with difficulties, thereby "inoculating" them so that they are able to deal with future adversities more effectively (Rutter 1987). Adaptive traits referred to as "ego resiliency" (confident optimism, insight and warmth, productive activity, and skilled expressiveness) have been found to be associated with positive outcomes, such as the ability to arouse liking and acceptance by others (Block and Gjerde 1990; Klohnen 1996; Klohnen et al. 1996).

Hardiness

Kobasa (1979) identified a similar set of adaptive traits as being indicative of hardiness. Individuals with a high level of hardiness tend to view stressful events as being potentially meaningful and interesting, to view themselves as capable of changing the events and circumstances in their lives, and to believe that planning and preparation can mitigate or prevent future problems (Kobasa 1979). In addition, hardy individuals have been found to view changing circumstances as opportunities for growth (Pengilly and Dowd 2000; Werner 1989, 1992).

Self-Efficacy

Children and adults who believe that they are in control of their lives tend to remain well in the face of adversity. Longitudinal research has indicated that children with high self-efficacy scores who experienced a high level of family stress were more likely than other children to have positive outcomes, such as being competent and caring (Werner 1989, 1992). Similarly, self-mastery and an internal locus of control have also been found to be associated with positive outcomes (Wyman et al. 1991). Longitudinal research has indicated that successful peer and school adaptation are particularly evident among children who work enthusiastically, creatively, and persistently and who strive to achieve high standards (Shiner 2000).

PRO-SOCIAL TRAITS

Pro-social traits, including communication skills, confidence, empathy, perceptiveness, and warmth, appear to play an important role in the development of adaptive functioning during childhood and adolescence (Shiner 2000). Resilient youths tend to interact with and reach out to others, rather than withdrawing, in both adverse and normal circumstances. Longitudinal research has shown that adolescents with pro-social tendencies tend to have better long-term psychosocial outcomes (Shiner 2000). This may be attributable in part to the familial and extrafamilial support that may be made particularly abundant to individuals with pro-social personality traits (Garmezy 1985).

OTHER ADAPTIVE TRAITS

Conscientiousness, impulse control, integrity, and persistence have been found to be associated with the development of resiliency during adolescence (Funder and Block 1989; Klohnen et al. 1996; Luthar and Zigler 1991; Rutter 1990; Shiner 2000). The ability to respond to humor and to share it with others has been found to promote positive outcomes (Klohnen et al. 1996; Luthar and Zigler 1991; Vaillant 1977). Humor is viewed as an adaptive defense or coping style by psychoanalytic theorists, as are altruism, suppression (i.e., the conscious postponement of attention to disturbing circumstances), anticipation (i.e., consciously planning how to cope with stressful circumstances), and sublimation (Vaillant 1977).

Case Example

Ms. G was a 31-year-old woman with metastatic adenocarcinoma. At the time of her diagnosis, she was living with her boyfriend and working as a painter with some commercial success. She had graduated from a prestigious university and attended graduate art school. The oncologist described Ms. G as a "real fighter, all the way through the chemotherapy and surgery." She learned what she could about the illness and treatment. Ms. G brought small, bright paintings for the nurses and patients every week. She came to the hospital each week with a variety of close friends and loved ones. Her parents were helpful with the treatment arrangements.

When seen by the psychiatrist, Ms. G's boyfriend, mother, and father were sitting around her bed. Flowers and small paintings were on the bedside table. Ms. G, bald and thin, smiled weakly. She said that at the time of her diagnosis, "my career was really taking off, and my boyfriend and I were engaged. It was such a shock, but I had no choice but to learn what I could from the horror." She described how she coped. She grew closer to her father and learned more about his illness experience. She took a long-wished-for trip to Italy to visit her high school art teacher. She committed herself to finishing her work on a large painting exhibit with a friend, saying "I just knew my work and my community would keep me upbeat and give my days hope." Referring to how she coped with a friend's death as a teen, she said she learned at the time that "I had the strength to find some meaning in hardship." Ms. G was also able to explore her anger, sense of loss, and sorrow for those she would leave behind.

Ms. G's story illustrates how community, activity, self-efficacy, parents, and loved ones are called on in times of profound stress. She not only coped with the difficulties of cancer treatment but also found generative ways to help others. The love and encouragement that she received from her parents and mentors, her insight into her own feelings, her perseverance, and her ability to rally others around her were important aspects of her successful coping.

CLINICAL IMPLICATIONS OF RESEARCH ON PROTECTIVE FACTORS AND ADAPTIVE PERSONALITY TRAITS

The present literature review supports the recommendation to assess protective factors and personality strengths as well as symptoms and maladaptive traits. Assessing protective factors and adaptive personality traits may increase the effectiveness of a clinical intervention, in part, by making it clear to the patient that the clinician is interested in developing a well-rounded understanding of the patient's strengths and weaknesses, thereby fostering the development of a strong therapeutic alliance. In addition, there are many ways that clinicians and other professionals who work with young people can help to promote the development of adaptive personality traits during childhood and adolescence. Some examples include promoting extracurricular activities, encouraging youths to take on age-appropriate challenges and responsibilities, facilitating the development of appropriate relationships with suitable adult mentors, and assisting the youth and family in taking advantage of community resources and in participating actively in the life of the community. Furthermore, it may be important to assist parents in improving their child-rearing skills, developing a closer and more supportive relationship with their children, and encouraging parents to minimize reliance on disciplinary methods that have been found to be problematic if utilized too frequently (e.g., harshly controlling, punishing, or shaming offspring; see Redmond et al. 1999).

REFERENCES

Arbel N, Stravynski A: A retrospective study of separation in the development of adult avoidant personality disorder. Acta Psychiatr Scand 83:174–178, 1991

Baker JD, Capron EW, Azorlosa J: Family environment characteristics of persons with histrionic and dependent personality disorders. J Personal Disord 10:82–87, 1996

Baldwin AL, Baldwin C, Cole RE: Stress-resistant families and stress-resistant children, in Risk and Protective Factors in the Development of Psychopathology. Edited by Rolf J, Masten AS, Cicchetti D, et al. Cambridge, England, Cambridge University Press, 1990, pp 257–280

Bell CC, Suggs H: Using sports to strengthen resiliency in children: training heart. Child Adolesc Psychiatr Clin N Am 7:859–865, 1998

Bernstein DP, Stein JA, Handelsman L: Predicting personality pathology among adult patients with substance use disorders: effects of childhood maltreatment. Addict Behav 23:855–868, 1998

Bifulco A, Brown GW, Lillie A, et al: Memories of childhood neglect and abuse: corroboration in a series of sisters. J Child Psychol Psychiatry 38:365–374, 1997

Block J, Gjerde PF: Depressive symptoms in late adolescence: a longitudinal perspective on personality antecedents, in Risk and Protective Factors in the Development of Psychopathology. Edited by Rolf J, Masten AS, Cicchetti D, et al. Cambridge, England, Cambridge University Press, 1990, pp 334–360

Briere J, Runtz M: Differential adult symptomatology associated with three types of child abuse histories. Child Abuse Neglect 14:357–364, 1990

Brown GR, Anderson B: Psychiatric morbidity in adult inpatients with childhood histories of sexual and physical abuse. Am J Psychiatry 148:55–61, 1991

Browne A, Finkelhor D: Impact of child sexual abuse: a review of the research. Psychol Bull 99:66–77, 1986

Carter JD, Joyce PR, Mulder RT, et al: Early deficient parenting in depressed outpatients is associated with personality dysfunction and not with depression subtypes. J Affect Disord 54:29–37, 1999

Caspi A, McClay J, Moffitt TE, et al: Role of genotype in the cycle of violence in maltreated children. Science 297:851–854, 2002

Chilcoat HD, Breslau N, Anthony JC: Potential barriers to parent monitoring: social disadvantage, marital status, and maternal psychiatric disorder. J Am Acad Child Adolesc Psychiatry 35:1673–1682, 1996

Cohen P: Personality development in childhood: old and new findings, in Personality and Psychopathology. Edited by Cloninger CR. Washington, DC, American Psychiatric Press, 1999, pp 101–127

Coid JW: Aetiological risk factors for personality disorders. Br J Psychiatry 174:530–538, 1999

Cowen EL, Wyman PA, Work WC, et al: Follow-up study of young stress-affected and stress-resilient urban children. Dev Psychopathol 9:565–577, 1997

Drake RE, Adler DA, Vaillant GE: Antecedents of personality disorders in a community sample of men. J Personal Disord 2:60–68, 1988

Dubo ED, Zanarini MC, Lewis RE, et al: Childhood antecedents of self-destructiveness in borderline personality disorder. Can J Psychiatry 42:63–69, 1997

Erikson EH: Childhood and Society, 2nd Edition. New York, WW Norton, 1963

Funder DC, Block J: The role of ego-control, ego-resiliency, and IQ in delay of gratification in adolescence. J Pers Soc Psychol 57:1041–1050, 1989

Garmezy N: Stress-resistant children: the search for protective factors, in Recent Research in Developmental Psychopathology. Edited by Stevenson JE. Oxford, England, Pergamon Press, 1985, pp 213–233

Gauthier L, Stollak G, Messé L, et al: Recall of childhood neglect and physical abuse as differential predictors of current psychological functioning. Child Abuse Neglect 20:549–559, 1996

Goldman SJ, D'Angelo EJ, DeMaso DR, et al: Physical and sexual abuse histories among children with borderline personality disorder. Am J Psychiatry 149:1723–1726, 1992

Grilo C, Masheb RM: Childhood maltreatment and personality disorders in adult patients with binge eating disorder. Acta Psychiatr Scand 106:183–188, 2002

Guzder J, Paris J, Zelkowitz P, et al: Risk factors for borderline pathology in children. J Am Acad Child Adolesc Psychiatry 35:26–33, 1996

Head SB, Baker JD, Williamson DA: Family environment characteristics and dependent personality disorder. J Personal Disord 5:256–263, 1991

Heath AC, Madden PA, Grant JD, et al: Resiliency factors protecting against teenage alcohol use and smoking: influences of religion, religious involvement and values, and ethnicity in the Missouri Adolescent Female Twin Study. Twin Res 2:145–155, 1999

Johnson JG, Quigley JF, Sherman MF: Adolescent personality disorder symptoms mediate the relationship between perceived parental behavior and Axis I symptomatology. J Personal Disord 11:381–390, 1997

Johnson JG, Cohen P, Brown J, et al: Childhood maltreatment increases risk for personality disorders during early adulthood. Arch Gen Psychiatry 56:600–606, 1999a

Johnson JG, Cohen P, Dohrenwend BP, et al: A longitudinal investigation of social causation and social selection processes involved in the association between socioeconomic status and psychiatric disorders. J Abnorm Psychol 108:490–499, 1999b

Johnson JG, Smailes EM, Cohen P, et al: Associations between four types of childhood neglect and personality disorder symptoms during adolescence and early adulthood: findings of a community-based longitudinal study. J Personal Disord 14:171–187, 2000

Johnson JG, Cohen P, Kasen S, et al: Association of maladaptive parental behavior with psychiatric disorder among parents and their offspring. Arch Gen Psychiatry 58:453–460, 2001a

Johnson JG, Cohen P, Smailes EM, et al: Childhood verbal abuse and risk for personality disorders during adolescence and early adulthood. Compr Psychiatry 42:16–23, 2001b

Kendler KS: Parenting: a genetic-epidemiologic perspective. Am J Psychiatry 153:11–20, 1996

Kendler KS, Bulik CM, Silberg J, et al: Childhood sexual abuse and adult psychiatric and substance use disorders in women: an epidemiological and co-twin control analysis. Arch Gen Psychiatry 57:953–959, 2000

Klohnen EC: Conceptual analysis and measurement of the construct of ego-resiliency. J Pers Soc Psychol 70:1067–1079, 1996

Klohnen EC, Vandewater EA, Young A: Negotiating the middle years: ego-resiliency and successful midlife adjustment in women. Psychol Aging 11:431–442, 1996

Kobak RR, Sceery A: Attachment in late adolescence: working models, affect regulation, and representations of self and others. Child Dev 59:135–146, 1988

Kobasa SC: Stressful life events, personality and health: an inquiry into hardiness. J Pers Soc Psychol 37:1–11, 1979

Laporte L, Guttman H: Traumatic childhood experiences as risk factors for borderline and other personality disorders. J Personal Disord 10:247–259, 1996

Livesley WJ, Jang KL, Jackson DN, et al: Genetic and environmental contributions to dimensions of personality disorder. Am J Psychiatry 150:1826–1831, 1993

Luntz BK, Widom CS: Antisocial personality disorder in abused and neglected children grown up. Am J Psychiatry 151:670–674, 1994

Luthar SS, Zigler E: Vulnerability and competence: a review of research on resilience in childhood. Am J Orthopsychiatry 61:6–22, 1991

Maughan B, Rutter M: Retrospective reporting of childhood adversity: Issues in assessing long-term recall. J Personal Disord 11:19–33, 1997

Mullen PE, Martin JL, Anderson JC, et al: The long-term impact of the physical, emotional and sexual abuse of children: a community study. Child Abuse Neglect 20:7–21, 1996

Neugebauer R, Hoek HW, Susser E: Prenatal exposure to wartime famine and development of antisocial personality disorder in early adulthood. JAMA 282:455–462, 1999

Ney PG: Does verbal abuse leave deeper scars: a study of children and their parents. Can J Psychiatry 32:371–378, 1987

Norden KA, Klein DN, Donaldson SK, et al: Reports of the early home environment in DSM-III-R personality disorders. J Personal Disord 9:213–223, 1995

Oldham JM, Skodol AE, Gallagher PE, et al: Relationship of borderline symptoms to histories of abuse and neglect: a pilot study. Psychiatr Q 67:287–295, 1996

Paris J: Childhood trauma as an etiological factor in the personality disorders. J Personal Disord 11:34–49, 1997

Parker G, Roy K, Wilhelm K, et al: An exploration of links between early parenting experiences and personality disorder type and disordered personality functioning. J Personal Disord 13:361–374, 1999

Pengilly JW, Dowd ET: Hardiness and social support as moderators of stress. J Clin Psychol 56:813–820, 2000

Pollock VE, Briere J, Schneider L, et al: Childhood antecedents of antisocial behavior: parental alcoholism and physical abusiveness. Am J Psychiatry 147:1290–1293, 1990

Redmond C, Spoth R, Shin C, et al: Modeling long-term parent outcomes of two universal family focused preventive interventions: one-year follow-up results. J Consult Clin Psychol 67:975–984, 1999

Robins LN: Deviant Children Grow Up: A Sociological and Psychiatric Study of Sociopathic Personality. Baltimore, MD, Williams and Wilkins, 1966

Robins LN, Schoenberg SP, Holmes SJ, et al: Early home environment and retrospective recall: a test for concordance between siblings with and without psychiatric disorders. Am J Orthopsychiatry 55:27–41, 1985

Ruggiero J, Bernstein DP, Handelsman L: Traumatic stress in childhood and later personality disorders: a retrospective study of male patients with substance dependence. Psychiatr Ann 29:713–721, 1999

Rutter M: Psychosocial resiliency and protective mechanisms. Am J Orthopsychiatry 57:316–329, 1987

Rutter M: Psychosocial resilience and protective mechanisms, in Risk and Protective Factors in the Development of Psychopathology. Edited by Rolf J, Masten AS, Cicchetti D, et al. Cambridge, England, Cambridge University Press, 1990, pp 181–214

Shea MT, Zlotnick C, Weisberg RB: Commonality and specificity of personality disorder profiles in subjects with trauma histories. J Personal Disord 13:199–210, 1999

Shiner RL: Linking childhood personality with adaptation: evidence for continuity and change across time into late adolescence. J Pers Soc Psychol 78:310–325, 2000

Sroufe LA, Carlson EA, Levy AK, et al: Implications of attachment theory for developmental psychopathology. Dev Psychopathol 11:1–13, 1999

Strage AA: Family context variables and the development of self-regulation in college students. Adolescence 33:17–31, 1998

Stravynski A, Elie R, Franche RL: Perception of early parenting by patients diagnosed with avoidant personality disorder: a test of the overprotection hypothesis. Acta Psychiatr Scand 80:415–420, 1989

Teicher MH, Andersen SL, Polcari A, et al: The neurobiological consequences of early stress and childhood maltreatment. Neurosci Biobehav Rev 27:33–44, 2003

Thomas A, Chess S: Genesis and evolution of behavioral disorders: from infancy to early adult life. Am J Orthopsychiatry 141:1–9, 1984

Vaillant GE: Adaptation to Life. Cambridge, MA, Harvard University Press, 1977

Weaver TL, Clum GA: Early family environments and traumatic experiences associated with borderline personality disorder. J Consult Clin Psychol 61:1068–1075, 1993

Werner EE: High-risk children in young adulthood: a longitudinal study from birth to 32 years. Am J Orthopsychiatry 59:72–81, 1989

Werner EE: The children of Kauai: resiliency and recovery in adolescence and adulthood. J Adolesc Health 13:262–268, 1992

Werner EE, Smith RS: Vulnerable But Invincible: A Study of Resilient Children. New York, McGraw-Hill, 1982

Westen D, Ludolph P, Misle B, et al: Physical and sexual abuse in adolescent girls with borderline personality disorder. Am J Orthopsychiatry 60:55–66, 1990

Widom CS: The cycle of violence. Science 244:160–166, 1989

Wolkow KE, Ferguson HB: Community factors in the development of resiliency: considerations and future directions. Community Ment Health J 37:489–498, 2001

Wyman PA, Cowen EL, Work WC, et al: Developmental and family milieu correlates of resiliency in urban children who have experienced major life stress. Am J Community Psychol 19:405–426, 1991

Yen S, Shea MT, Battle CL, et al: Traumatic exposure and posttraumatic stress disorder in borderline, schizotypal, avoidant, and obsessive-compulsive personality disorders: findings from the Collaborative Longitudinal Personality Disorders Study. J Nerv Ment Dis 190:510–518, 2002

Zanarini MC, Frankenburg FR: Pathways to the development of borderline personality disorder. J Personal Disord 11:93–104, 1997

Zanarini MC, Williams AA, Lewis RE, et al: Reported pathological childhood experiences associated with the development of borderline personality disorder. Am J Psychiatry 154:1101–1106, 1997

Zimmerman MA, Bingenheimer JB, Notaro PC: Natural mentors and adolescent resiliency: a study with urban youth. Am J Community Psychol 30:221–243, 2002

14

Sociocultural Factors

Theodore Millon, Ph.D., D.Sc.
Seth D. Grossman, Psych.D.

The interface between personality disorders and sociocultural contexts is an extremely complex and variable one. Numerous biological, psychological, and cultural factors give shape to the development of personality characteristics and general psychopathology. Symptomatological pictures presented by patients are multidetermined in an intricately interwoven pattern of causality. The ways in which social and cultural influences give rise to the traits and disorders of personality are many, complicated, and divergent.

Sociocultural processes can be themselves a source of psychic stress, giving form and quality to the nature of life experiences as well. Additionally, social influences furnish a framework for how individuals learn to cope with the nature of their distress. The manner in which the symptoms of personality disorders will be interpreted is also a product of social and cultural value systems. No less relevant is the influence of culture in guiding how patients seek assistance therapeutically, as well as the modes of treatment that characterize the orientation of society's healers.

The value systems and nosological schemas generated in Western societies, such as those seen in ICD-10 (World Health Organization 1992) and DSM-IV-TR (American Psychiatric Association 2000), reflect particular models of thought that may be at variance with numerous cultures and subcultures around the world. More specifically, the perspective of Western schemas is oriented specifically to an individual's personal experiences and is largely grounded in an infectious disease medical model, one driven by contemporary biomedical technologies and, more particularly, those of pharmacological therapies. Western cultural perspectives contrast with numerous cultural orientations that are centered more on social contexts and relational networks, as well as interpersonal methods of intervention that reflect broad-ranging social health systems. Care must be taken, therefore, not to generalize findings generated in Western concepts and research to those of other cultures (Alarcón et al. 1998).

HISTORICAL REFLECTIONS

The sociocultural orientation to the mind represents a striking departure from most other traditions. Instead

223

of the individual being the prime focus, the wider social setting and the forces that impinge on the person—and that he or she in turn influences—take center stage. Support for this "public health" approach to physical disorders has grown consistently since the mid-1800s. With success in overcoming infectious diseases such as tuberculosis and yellow fever, it was merely a matter of time before a social-preventive approach would draw the interest of sophisticated mental health professionals. Beginning in the late nineteenth century, theoretical and practical innovations emerged to reflect this changing orientation, which led to a full manifestation of new paradigms by the mid-twentieth century. The clinical model was supplanted in many mental health settings by the public health model, along with a shift toward preventive programs and a renewed concern for the underprivileged. These social and community approaches did not have their origins in psychiatric and psychological thought but reflected the demands of public spokespersons, on the one hand, and the compelling data of anthropological and sociological theorists, on the other.

It stands to reason that a sociocultural approach would emerge to answer mental health needs. Historically, it has been the function of cultural traditions to give meaning and order to social life, to define the tasks and responsibilities of existence, and to guide group members with a system of shared beliefs, values, and goals. Such cultural forces serve as a common framework of formative influences that sets limits and establishes guidelines for members of a social group. These traditions, transmitted from parents to child, provide the young with a blueprint for organizing thoughts, behaviors, and aspirations.

The mind is therefore shaped by the institutions, traditions, and values that compose the cultural context of societal living. Methods by which social rules and regulations are transmitted between people and from generation to generation are often emotionally charged and erratic, entailing persuasion, seduction, coercion, deception, and threat. Feelings of anxiety and resentment are generated as a function of environmental stress, leaving pathological residues that linger and serve to distort future relations. Bear in mind, however, that it is not cultural and social conditions that directly shape the mind or cause personality disorders; rather, these conditions serve as a context within which the more direct and immediate experiences of interpersonal and family life take place. Sociocultural conditions not only color but may degrade personal relationships, establishing maladaptive styles of coping and pathogenic models for imitation.

In this chapter, we address in part the forces that characterize "society as the patient," as Frank (1948) suggested several decades ago:

> Instead of thinking in terms of a multiplicity of so-called social problems, each demanding special attention and a different remedy, we can view all of them as different symptoms of the same disease. That would be a real gain even if we cannot entirely agree upon the exact nature of the disease. If, for example, we could regard crime, mental disorders, family disorganization, juvenile delinquency, prostitution and sex offenses, and much that now passes as the result of pathological processes (e.g., gastric ulcer) as evidence, not of individual wickedness, incompetence, perversity or pathology, but as human reactions to cultural disintegration, a forward step would be taken. (p. 42)

In much the same way as the paired strands of the DNA double helix unwind and each selects environmental nutrients to duplicate its discarded partner, so too does each culture fashion its constituent members to fit an existing template. Those societies whose customs and institutions are fixed and traditional will generally produce a psychically structured and formal citizenry, and those societies whose values and practices are highly fluid and inconsistent will likely evolve so that its citizens develop deficits in psychic solidity and stability.

Although it would be naïve to state that sociocultural factors are directly responsible for individual pathology, responsible scientists would be lax in ignoring the role of cultural dynamics in the well-being of individuals. Whether or not one is inclined to attribute our increased incidence in youthful affective disorders, for example, to the waxing and waning of population parameters, it is both intuitively and observationally self-evident that sweeping cultural changes can affect innumerable social practices. Among those social practices most evidently affected by cultural dynamics are those of an immediate and personal nature, such as patterns of child nurturing and rearing, marital affiliation, family cohesion, leisure style, entertainment content, diminution of the role of organized religion, and so on.

The notion that many of the mind's pathological patterns observed today can best be ascribed to the perverse, chaotic, or frayed conditions of our cultural life has been voiced by many commentators of the social scene. These demographic conditions have been characterized in phrases such as "the age of anxiety," "growing up absurd," and "the lonely crowd." It is not within the scope of this chapter, however, to elaborate the themes implied in these slogans.

CONCEPTUAL AND METHODOLOGICAL CONCERNS

Numerous theoretical and research difficulties should be stated at the outset. Paris (1996) noted that empirical efforts to assess social risk factors for psychiatric disorders are difficult to measure. Moreover, there are few if any practical ways to engage in controlled experimental studies that can tease out the role of pathogenic sociocultural factors in personality disorders. Prospective methods are ideal but almost impossible to execute. Retrospective methods provide a multitude of data in which the sequential effects of several influences cannot be isolated and quantified.

The concept of etiology itself is a fuzzy notion that not only requires the careful separation of constituent empirical elements but also calls for differentiating diverse conceptual meanings, ranging from strong influences that are both causally necessary and/or sufficient, through progressively weaker levels of specificity in which causal factors exert consistent, although quantitatively marginal, differences—to those factors that are merely coincidental or situationally circumstantial.

The premise that social experience plays a central role in shaping personality attributes is one shared by numerous theorists. To say this, however, is not to agree on which specific factors during early development are critical in generating particular attributes—nor to agree that known formative influences are either necessary or sufficient. There is reason to ask whether etiologic analyses are even possible in personality pathology, given the complex and variable character of developmental influences. Can this most fundamental of scientific activities be achieved? Researchers must grapple with the interactive and sequential chain of "causes" composed of inherently inexact and probabilistic data in which the slightest variation in antecedent conditions, often of a minor or random character, produces highly divergent outcomes. Because this "looseness" in the causal network of variables is unavoidable, are there any grounds for believing that such endeavors could prove more than illusory?

Consistent findings on causal factors for specific clinical entities would be extremely useful, were only such knowledge in hand. Unfortunately, our etiologic database is both scanty and unreliable and is likely to remain so, owing to the obscure, complex, and interactive nature of influences that shape psychopathological phenomena. The yearning among researchers for a neat package of pathogenic attributes simply cannot be reconciled with the complex philosophical issues, methodological quandaries, and entanglement of subtle and random influences that shape personality disorders. In the main, almost all etiologic theses today are, at best, perceptive conjectures that ultimately rest on tenuous empirical grounds, reflecting the views of divergent schools of thought positing their favorite hypotheses. These speculative notions should be conceived as questions that deserve research evaluation rather than promulgated as the gospel of confirmed fact.

Arguments pointing to thematic or logical continuities between the nature of social experience and personality features, no matter how intuitively rational such arguments appear to be, do not provide unequivocal evidence for the causal connections between experience and personality features. Different, and equally convincing, sociocultural hypotheses can be and are posited. Each contemporary explication of the origins of most personality disorders is persuasive, yet remains but one among several plausible possibilities.

Among other troublesome aspects of contemporary etiologic proposals are the diverse syndromal consequences attributed to specific experiential or sociocultural causes. Not only is it unlikely that singular origins would be as ubiquitous as clinicians often posit them, but even if these origins were common, their ultimate psychological impact would differ substantially, depending on the configuration of other concurrent or later influences to which individuals were exposed. "Identical" causal factors cannot be assumed to possess the same import, nor can their consequences be traced without reference to the larger context of each individual's life experiences.

Because it is impossible to design an experiment in which relevant variables can systematically be controlled or manipulated, it will be impossible to establish unequivocal cause-effect relationships among sociocultural variables and personality pathology. Investigators cannot arrange, no less subvert and abuse, an individual or a social group for purposes of scientific study; research in this field must, therefore, continue to be of a naturalistic and correlational nature. The problem that arises with naturalistic studies is the difficulty of inferring causality; correlations do not give us a secure base for determining which factors were the cause and which were the effect. For example, correlations between socioeconomic class and personality disorders may signify both that deteriorated social conditions produce mental disorders and that mental disorders result in deteriorated social conditions.

Personality disorders clearly are an outgrowth of

the interplay of biological forces, psychological experiences, and sociocultural influences. As such, efforts to trace the pattern of pathogenic influences must contend with the concepts and complications inherent in each of these disciplines—those of biochemistry, psychology, sociology, and cultural anthropology. Hence, the role of context moderators must be considered, because any one finding may have different meanings, depending on the larger set of coexisting elements surrounding it.

No less important are definitional ambiguities that characterize our language. Thus, is depression an existential state of being or is it a neurological abnormality? If the latter, is it a synaptically deficient chemical or a metabolic imbalance? Furthermore, how do we separate overlapping symptomatologies—for example, how do we deal with the coexistence of several personality disorders or with their comorbidity with clinical syndromes? The multidimensional attributes of most clinical pathologies are well recognized, but which specific dimensions should be chosen for quantitative assessment—those of Cloninger's (1987) neurological model, that of one of the five-factor schemas, or perhaps Millon's evolutionary polarities? Complexities and choices such as these are not matters of mere philosophical hairsplitting. They are central to evaluating the difficulties and intricacies of determining and answering questions concerning which and how sociocultural factors influence the character of personality disorders. These semiphilosophical quandaries are complicated further by the numerous empirical tools that must be employed to identify and measure relevant variables. Not only are the many instruments employed to generate and appraise data frequently unreliable, as well as inconsistently when compared with one another, but few have been normed on diverse cultural and ethnic populations.

As the editors of the recent *Research Agenda for DSM-V*, Kupfer et al. (2002) noted that not one laboratory marker has been found to be specific to identify any DSM syndrome. Moreover, epidemiological and clinical studies show not only extreme comorbidities but also a high degree of short-term diagnostic instability. Although few will question the value of having a universally accepted diagnostic system, evidence clearly indicates that DSM's rigidly formulated syndromes may never lend themselves to uncovering specific clinical etiologies and well-defined pathogenic courses.

Nevertheless, we have no choice but to continue to pursue the suggestive leads provided us both by plausible speculation and exploratory research. Difficulties

notwithstanding, we must caution against inclinations to revert to past simplifications or to abandon research out of dismay or cynicism. Our increasing knowledge of the multideterminant and circular character of pathogenesis, as well as the inextricable developmental sequences through which it proceeds, should prevent us from falling prey to simplifications that led early investigators to attribute personality pathology to single factors. Innumerable pathogenic roots are possible; the causal elements are so intermeshed that we must plan our research strategies to disentangle not isolated determinants but their convergences, their interactions, and their continuities.

DIRECT INTERPERSONAL EXPERIENCES

Numerous demographic, political, and international changes, as well as advances in science and technology of recent decades, have stimulated a growing awareness of the role of sociocultural factors in public health and illness prevention (Kleinman 1980, 1988a, 1988b; Littlewood and Lipsedge 1987; Mezzich et al. 1996). We focus our attention in this section, however, on some of the more direct and personal elements of experience that reflect the impact of social life upon the individual.

Of the many factors that contribute to the persistence of early learned behaviors, none plays a more significant role than interpersonal relationships. These can be viewed fruitfully from the perspective taken by sociologists and social psychologists. To these scientists, the varied cultural and institutional forces of a society promote continuity by maintaining a stable and organized class of experiences to which most individuals of a particular group are repeatedly exposed. Reference to these determinants of continuity are made occasionally in later paragraphs. For the present, our focus is on the more private side of interpersonal experience. As is well known, ingrained personality patterns develop as a consequence of experiences generated in intimate and subtle relationships with members of one's immediate family.

Although exceptions certainly exist in atypical families, the daily activity of the typical young child is rather restricted and repetitive; there is not much variety in the routine experience to which the child is exposed. Day in and day out, the child eats the same kind of food, plays with the same toys, remains essentially in the same physical environment and relates to the same people. This constricted environment, this repeated exposure to a narrow range of family attitudes and training methods, not only builds in deeply etched habits and expectations but prevents the child from new experiences that are so essential to change. The helplessness of infants, and the dependency of children, keeps them restricted to a crabbed and tight little world with few alternatives for learning new attitudes and responses. Early behaviors fail to change, therefore, not because they may have gelled permanently but because the same slender band of experiences that helped form them initially continue and persist as influences for many years.

The notion that a child's early behaviors may be accentuated by the parents' response has been raised in early books by the senior author (Millon 1969, 1981); we noted that a circular interplay often arises that intensifies the child's initial biological reactivity pattern. Thus, unusually passive, sensitive, or cranky infants frequently elicit parallel reactions on the part of their mothers; this maternal reaction then perpetuates the child's original tendencies. This model of circular or reciprocal influences may be applied not only to the perpetuation of biological dispositions but also to behavior tendencies that are acquired by learning. Whatever the initial roots may have been—constitutional or learned—certain forms of behaviors provoke or "pull" from others reactions that result in a repetition of these behaviors.

The dominant features of a child's early behavior form a distinct impression on others. Once this early impression is established, people expect that the child will continue to behave in this distinctive manner; in time, they develop a fixed and simplified image of what kind of person the child is. The term *stereotype*, borrowed from social psychology, represents this tendency to simplify and categorize the attributes of others. People no longer view a child passively and objectively once they have formed a stereotype of the individual; they now are sensitized to those distinctive features they have learned to expect. The stereotype begins to take on a life of its own; it operates as a screen through which the child's behaviors are selectively perceived so as to fit the characteristics attributed to him or her. Once cast in this mold, the child will experience a consistency in the way in which others react, one that fails to take cognizance of the natural varieties and complexities of the individual's actual behaviors.

By intruding stereotyped behaviors into new situations, individuals will provoke, with unfailing regularity, reactions from others that reinforce their old responses. Almost all forms of generalized behavior set up reciprocal reactions that intensify these behaviors;

docile, ingratiating, or fearful interpersonal actions, for example, draw domineering and manipulative responses; confident and self-assured attitudes elicit admiration and submissiveness. In short, not only is interpersonal generalization a form of perpetuation itself, but it also creates conditions that promote perpetuation.

GENERAL SOCIOCULTURAL INFLUENCES

We would be remiss in our presentation if we failed to recognize that personality pathology may be shaped by the institutions, traditions, and values that compose the cultural context of societal living. These cultural forces serve as a common framework of formative influences that sets limits and establishes guidelines for members of a social group. However, we must be careful not to view the concepts of "society" and "culture" as concrete entities. Instead, it is important that these be viewed as convenient abstractions that attempt to characterize the pattern of relationships and responsibilities shared among group members.

The continuity and stability of cultural groups depend largely on the success with which their young are imbued with common beliefs and customs. To retain what has been wrought through history, each group must devise ways of molding its children to "fit in"—that is, to accept and perpetuate the system of prohibitions and sanctions that earlier group members have developed to meet the persistent tasks of life. During this socialization process, infants progressively surrender innate impulsive and naïve behaviors and regulate or supplant them with the rules and practices of the larger social group. This maturation process continues through adolescence, with a changing emphasis away from the exact actions and mores of the "adult" expectations toward identification with the common social expectations of the peer group (Harris 1999).

Attention in the following paragraphs focuses on Western sociocultural groups of the recent century. Furthermore, attention is not on the more private experiences of children in their families but on those broad public experiences that are shared in common among members of these societal groups.

Few characterizations of Western life are more apt than those that portray their societies as upwardly mobile. Stated differently, Western cultures have sought in the past century to maximize the opportunity of its members to progress, to succeed, and to achieve material rewards once considered the province only of the aristocracy and well-to-do. With certain notable and distressing exceptions, the young of Western societies have been free to rise, by dint of their wits and their talents, above the socioeconomic status of their parents. Implicit in this well-publicized option to succeed, however, is the expectancy that each person will pursue opportunities and will be measured by the extent to which he or she fulfills them. Thus, these societies not only promote ambition but also expect each of its members to meet the challenge successfully. Each aspiring individual is confronted, then, with a precarious choice; along with the promising rewards of success are the devastating consequences of failure.

Striving for achievement refers to the need to surpass one's past attainments; *competition* describes the struggle among individuals to surpass each other in these achievements. What happens, however, if the standards by which people gauge their achievements keep changing or are ambiguous? What happens if people cannot find dependable and unequivocal standards to guide their aspirations?

One of the problems modern Western societies face increasingly today is the pace of social change and the increasingly contradictory standards to which members of the society are expected to subscribe. Under the cumulative impact of rapid industrialization, immigration, urbanization, mobility, technology, and mass communication, there has been a steady erosion of traditional values and standards. Instead of a simple and coherent body of customs and beliefs, people of the Western world find themselves confronted with constantly shifting and increasingly questioned standards whose durability is uncertain and precarious. No longer can they find the certainties and absolutes that guided earlier generations. The complexity and diversity of everyday experience play havoc with simple archaic beliefs and render them useless as instruments to deal with contemporary realities. There have been few times in the history of humanity when so many people have faced the tasks of life without the aid of accepted and durable traditions.

Large segments of "third-world" societies find themselves out of the mainstream of their culture's life; isolated by the unfortunate circumstance of social prejudice or economic deprivation, they struggle less with the problem of achieving in a changing society than with managing the bare necessities of survival. To them, the question is not which of the changing social values they should pursue but whether there are any social values that are worthy of pursuit. These youngsters may be exposed to poverty and destitution and provided with inadequate schools and poor housing provisions set within decaying communities.

Deteriorating and alienated communities feed on themselves; not only do they perpetuate their decay by destroying the initiative and promise of their young, but they attract the outcast and unstable who drift into their midst. Caught in this web of disintegration, the young and the downwardly mobile join those who already have retreated from the values of the larger society. Delinquency, prostitution, broken homes, crime, violence, and addiction increasingly characterize these communities, and the vicious circle of decay and disintegration not only persists but is intensified.

We must keep in mind, however, that harsh cultural and social conditions rarely cause personality pathology; rather, they serve as a context within which the more direct and immediate experiences of interpersonal life take place. They color and degrade personal relationships and establish maladaptive and pathogenic models for imitation. These exacerbating conditions may also elicit genetic pathological predispositions that may otherwise lie dormant.

SOME EPIDEMIOLOGICAL FINDINGS

A few words should be said about broad sociocultural categories that are the basis of systematic research studies into the nature of clinical syndromes, including those of personality. Clearly, the construct of race is a central issue considered in epidemiological research, not necessarily to reflect its physiognomy but rather its emotional and social significance for individuals as well as researchers and practitioners (Witzig 1996). Similarly, ethnicity and minority status have served to crystallize a cultural characteristic that provides a context for understanding shared historical beliefs and traditions as well as socioeconomic employment and economic considerations (Pinderhughes 1989). Religious beliefs clearly influence the character of illness and disease experiences, styles of coping, and possibly clinical outcomes; they comprise epidemiological variables other than those of race and ethnicity (Lukoff et al. 1995). Language differences are another variable that may provide a significant cultural element of clinical relevance in shaping a patient's perceptions and styles of coping (Westermeyer and Janca 1997). Of increasing significance are studies of gender and sexual orientation as significant variables not only in patients' perceptions and experiences but in the stereotyped attitudes that characterize the values in different cultures (Cabaj and Stein 1996). The need to develop "internationally" sensitive models, methods, and instruments that counter the traditional Western-centrism and Eurocentrism that typify most epidemiological studies is increasingly important, given the history of recent decades in which global economies have become distinctly integrated. A few research findings of a more or less traditional epidemiological character are noted in the following paragraphs (Weiss 2001; Weissman 1993).

Recent articles in major newspapers and popular national magazines have asked a series of questions about mental health, violence, and criminality. For example: What proportion of murders is related to drug trafficking? How often do suicide victims act out immediately after a marital split, loss of a job, or any other personal crisis? Are teenagers who randomly shoot others likely to be mentally ill or have they been prompted by the degradations of their social and community life? According to public and mental health authorities, no one has accurate answers to these and other critical questions about the thousands of emotionally driven or violent behaviors that occur annually throughout the world, even though this knowledge could assist health and judicial agencies to establish wiser preventive policies and programs.

Despite popular assertions to the contrary, epidemiological research has shown that there are no consistent findings to assert whether or not mental illness, in its varied forms, is substantially more prevalent in urban than rural areas (Robins and Regier 1991). Although evidence remains supporting a belief in what Srole and Fischer (1980) called this "myth of paradise lost," much of this idea is homage to the once widely held belief that the larger the city and the more centrally congested and overpopulated the region within it, the higher the incidence. Differences between urban and rural rates have often been attributed primarily to the more benign environment of country life and to the ability of rural dwellers to care for their mentally ill at home. Yet another popular explanation is that there may be significant differences in access to services or in beliefs about seeking those services (e.g., Jian Li Wang 2004). Many other incidental interpretations are possible, but none has provided definitive answers to this inquiry. It becomes important, then, to look to more specific factors characteristic of urban settings versus rural settings rather than to make larger assumptions regarding the nature of city versus country life in general. Higher rates of mental illness in central city areas may be related to community characteristics; specific areas of large, urban settings are often poverty stricken, physically decayed, and socially disorganized. These conditions are not only conducive to generating personality disorders, but they

also tend to attract and serve as a haven of anonymity for the unstable and ineffectual who drift into the city from other regions of society.

Epidemiological studies indicate also that married persons have a lower incidence of mental disorders than single people, especially single males, who in turn have lower rates than those who are divorced (Weissman 1993). These findings have been interpreted in several ways; the two most common assert that 1) marriage protects the individual from distresses associated with loneliness and disaffection and that 2) those inclined to mental illness either are ill-disposed or incapable of establishing a marital relationship or precipitate difficulties that result in the termination of an existent relationship. Both explanations seem reasonable and together are likely to account for the obtained findings.

The high rate of mental illness among divorced persons may be explained by several factors. Emotionally impaired individuals are likely to provoke conflict with their mates, thereby increasing the likelihood of divorce. Once cut off from support and cast into isolation and disaffiliation, their pathological dispositions may be precipitated into a manifest disorder. Different incidence rates associated with marital status probably reflect both initial dispositions to pathology and the effects of lost affection and affiliation.

Numerous demographic studies have sought to demonstrate relationships between socioeconomic conditions and prevalence and type of mental disorder. Despite a sprinkling of negative data, two findings appear to hold up fairly consistently. First, members of the lowest socioeconomic class more often are diagnosed as severely impaired than those of the upper classes. Second, the manifest patterns of mental illness differ among these classes (Dohrenwend and Dohrenwend 1969).

Essentially, three interpretations have been proposed to account for the greater prevalence of severe personality pathology in lower socioeconomic classes (Paris 1996). First, some investigators suggest that the childhood environment of lower-class children contains relatively little love, protection, and stability; this lack of nurturing establishes a lifelong feeling of rejection that is confirmed by the neglectful and hostile attitude of the larger society. To this overall sense of rejection is added the persistent stress during adulthood of economic hardship, occupational insecurity, and marital instability, conditions that arise from personal histories of poor educational and vocational training as well as the malignant customs and values often found among lower-class groups. Second, lower-class patients are less likely to be identified early and less likely to gain the benefits of treatment than those who are well-off financially. Differences in income, a major criterion defining socioeconomic class, relate to the probability that a disorder will be spotted and reversed before attaining serious proportions. Because less effective steps are taken in the lower socioeconomic groups, a greater number of these individuals will succumb to severe disorders. The third reason offered for the disproportionate number of severely impaired lower-class patients relates to the notion of drift—that is, the proclivity of disturbed members of higher social classes to deteriorate to lower socioeconomic states.

Let us next turn to explanations offered for relationships between class and type of personality disorder; Paris (1996) provides a useful and detailed review that should be referenced by those interested in these findings.

Generally, the tendency for the upper class to develop disorders characterized by interpersonal anxiety, guilt, and depression (e.g., depressive, borderline, and compulsive personality disorders) as well as arrogance (narcissistic personality disorder) and theatricality (histrionic personality disorder), as contrasted with the characteristic withdrawal, aggressive, or antisocial patterns found in the lower classes (schizoid, schizotypal, avoidant, and paranoid personality disorders), is generally viewed to be a function of training differences in these subcultural groups. Some theorists suggest that middle- and upper-class youngsters are oversocialized—that is, they learn to inhibit and feel guilt for wasteful, aggressive, and sexual behaviors and experience severe conflict between their impulses and desires and the achievement standards demanded by their parents. Acceptance of these imposed values results in an inner tension; failure to fulfill parental demands results in guilt and depression. In contrast, lower-class children, faced with deprivation and neglect, learn either to withdraw and become indifferent to their surroundings or to assert themselves and exploit others who possess what they want, because they are exposed to models of aggressive and irresponsible behavior in their environment and are often admired by peers for their success in using these behaviors. In the next section, we elaborate the relationship between a number of these cultural influences on personality.

IMPACT ON SPECIFIC PERSONALITY DISORDERS

As Kupfer et al. (2002) have noted, beyond the question of boundaries between normality and abnormal-

ity, there is the question of whether personality disorders should be considered autonomous mental disorders or whether some are best considered variants of those on Axis I. Also, it is on Axis II that the issue of whether the current categorical implementation of personality disorders should be retained. This worthy issue transcends the focus and boundaries of this brief chapter. On the assumption that the current psychiatric nosology will retain at least a modicum of the categorical approach, we address a few notable personality disorders, attempting to track their etiopathogenetic course from a sociocultural perspective.

The interpersonal and sociocultural perspectives on personality disorders have become major directions of thought in recent years (Alarcón et al. 1998; Benjamin 1999; Kiesler 1996; Kleinman 1988b; Paris 1996; Weissman 1993). Despite variations among theorists in the specific constructs and rationales employed, there is agreement that personality disorders can best be understood in terms of recurrent interpersonal and social relationships that shape and perpetuate styles of behavior, thought, and feeling. Those theorists of the interpersonal point of view usually suggest that a sociocultural model can serve best as a framework for organizing the fundamental dimensions of personality. All theorists share the view that there are maladaptive causal sequences between interpersonal perceptions, behavioral enactments, and psychosocial reactions. These interpersonal sequences are rigid and extreme, being activated regardless of their ultimate inappropriateness across numerous social situations.

As instrumental styles of coping, interpersonal behaviors prove self-defeating because they are adaptively inflexible and tend to perpetuate and foster difficulties rather than resolve them. The avoidant personality, for example, enacts a consistently fearful and self-effacing stance toward an environment that resists exhibiting the very experiences of acceptance and intimacy that are so desperately desired. Such avoidant behaviors usually elicit rejection or allow others to be ignoring and hence reinforce the person's avoidant tendencies.

A major example, although related in some ways to the first, focuses instead on irresolute and readily changing sociocultural systems, presumably contributing to a marked increase in affective disorders. This amorphous cultural state, so characteristic of modern Western societies, is clearly mirrored in the interpersonal vacillations and affective instabilities that typify such longitudinal affective distress as is seen in patients presenting a borderline personality. Central to today's Western culture are the increased pace of social change and the growing pervasiveness of ambiguous and discordant customs to which children are expected to subscribe.

The impact of much of what has been described previously might be substantially lessened if concurrent or subsequent personal encounters and social customs were compensatory or restitutive—that is, if they served as buffers in preventing or repairing the destabilizing and destructive effects of problematic interpersonal experiences. Unfortunately, the converse appears to be the case in Western societies today. Whereas the cultural institutions of most societies have retained practices that furnish reparative buffers and stabilizing experiences, thereby remedying disturbed parent–child relationships, the sociocultural changes of the past four to five decades have not only fostered an increase in psychic diffusion and splintering but have also resulted in the discontinuation of psychically reparative institutions and customs, contributing thereby to both the incidence and exacerbation of features that typify recent forms of borderline pathology. Without the corrective effects of undergirding and focusing social mentors and practices, the diffusing or divisive consequences of unfavorable earlier experience take firm root and unyielding form, displaying their structural weaknesses in clinical signs under the press of even modestly stressful events.

Transformations in family patterns and relationships have evolved fairly continuously in Western societies over the past century, but the speed and nature of transitions since the Second World War have been so radical as to break the smooth line of earlier trends, and the most recent 15–20 years have seen almost exponential social change. Hence, the typical child today no longer has a clear sense of either the character or the purpose of her or his parent's work activities, much less a detailed image of the concrete actions that compose that work. Beyond the little there is of the traditional father's daily routines to model oneself after, mothers of young children have shifted their activities increasingly outside the home, seeking career fulfillments or needing dual incomes to sustain family aspirations. Not only are everyday adult activities no longer available for direct observation and modeling, but traditional gender roles, once distinct and valued, have become blurred. Today, there is little in everyday life for children to see and emulate that is clearly esteemed and rewarded by the larger society.

With the growing dissolution of the traditional family structure, there has been a marked increase in parental separation, divorce, and remarriage. Children subject to persistent parental bickering and family restructuring not only are exposed to changing and destructive models for imitative learning but also develop the internal schisms that typify the borderline personality behaviors. The stability of life, so necessary for the acquisition of a consistent pattern of feeling and thinking, is shattered when erratic conditions or marked controversy prevail. There may be an ever-present apprehension that a parent will be totally lost through divorce; dissension may lead to the undermining of one parent by the other, and a nasty and cruel competition for the loyalty and affections of children may ensue. Constantly dragged into the arena of parental schisms, the child not only loses a sense of security and stability but is subjected to paradoxical behaviors and contradictory role models. Raised in such settings, a child not only feels the constant threat of family dissolution but is also often forced to serve as a mediator to moderate conflicts between the parents. Forced to switch sides and divide loyalties, the child cannot be an individual but must internalize opposing attitudes and emotions to satisfy antagonistic parental desires and expectations. The different roles the child must assume to placate the parents are markedly divergent: as long as the parents remain at odds, the child persists with behaviors, thoughts, and emotions that are intrinsically irreconcilable.

Other "advances" in contemporary Western societies have stamped deep and distinct impressions as well as ones that are equally affectively loaded, erratic, and contradictory. The rapidly moving, emotionally intense, and interpersonally capricious character of television role models, displayed in swiftly progressing half-hour vignettes that encompass a lifetime, add to the impact of disparate, highly charged, and largely inimical value standards and behavior models. What is incorporated is not only a multiplicity of selves, but an assemblage of unintegrated and discordant roles, displayed indecisively and fitfully, especially among those youngsters bereft of secure moorings and internal gyroscopes. The striking images created by our modern-day flickering parental surrogate have replaced all other sources of cultural guidance for many; hence, by age 18, the typical American child will have spent more time watching television than in going to school or relating directly to his or her parents.

Television may be nothing but simple pabulum for those with comfortably internalized models of stable human relationships, but for those who possess a world of diffuse values and standards, or one in which parental precepts and norms have been discarded, the impact of these substitute prototypes is especially powerful, even idealized and romanticized. What these television characters and story plots present to vulnerable youngsters is the stuff of which successful half-hour or hourlong "life stories" must be composed to capture the attention and hold the fascination of their audiences—violence, danger, agonizing dilemmas, and unpredictability, each expressed and resolved in an hour or less. These ingredients of entertainment are precisely those features of social behavior and emotionality that come to characterize affective and interpersonal instabilities.

Aimless floundering and disaffiliated stagnation may be traced in part to the loss in Western society of mitigating and reparative customs and institutions that once ensured a second chance to those who had been deprived or abused, through exposure to compensatory sponsors and institutions exhibiting values and purposes around which social life could be focused and oriented. The scattering of the extended family, as well as the rise of single-parent homes and shrinkage in sibling number, adds further to the isolation of families as they migrate in and out of transient communities. Each of these changes undermines the once powerful cushioning effects of kinship support and caring relationships. Thus, in the past several decades, estranged and denigrated children have no longer found nurturing older siblings, aunts, or grandparents; nor are there the once accessible and nurturing neighbors. With increased mobility, kinship separation, single parenting, and reduced sibling numbers, our society has few surrogate parents to pick up the pieces of what real parents may have fragmented and discarded, let alone restore the developmental losses engendered thereby.

Problematic children today are rebels without a cause. Earlier generations of disaffected Western youth were bound together by their resentments, their opposition to economic or political oppression, motivated by discernible and worthy common causes that provided both group camaraderie and a path to action. Today, this is true of many of the young of Middle Eastern cultures, but middle-class Western-oriented youngsters have no shared causes to bring them together. Materially well-nourished and clothed, unconstrained in an open society to follow their talents and aspirations freely, the purposelessness and emptiness they experience are essentially an internal matter, a private rather than a collective affair, with no external agents against whom they can join with others. It is these rebels without a cause—unable to forego the material comforts of home, ineffective in externalizing their inner discontents on the larger scene, yet empty and directionless—who make up a good share of today's borderline and disaffected Western youth.

As noted previously, for some underprivileged

youngsters in the third world, the question is not which of the changing social values they should pursue, but whether there are any social values that are worthy of pursuit. Youngsters in underprivileged societies that have been exposed to poverty and destitution, provided with inadequate schools, lived in poor housing set within decaying communities, raised in chaotic and broken homes, deprived of parental models of success and attainment, and immersed in a pervasive atmosphere of hopelessness, futility, and apathy cannot help but question the validity of the "good society." Reared in these settings, one quickly learns that there are few worthy standards to which one can aspire successfully. Whatever efforts are made to raise oneself from these bleak surroundings run hard against the painful restrictions of poverty, the sense of a meaningless and empty existence, and an indifferent, if not hostile, world. Moreover, and in contrast to earlier minority generations whose worlds rarely extended beyond the shared confines of ghetto poverty, the disparity between everyday contemporary realities—seen so evidently available to others in television commercials and shopping malls—is not only frustrating but painfully disillusioning and immobilizing. Why make a pretense of accepting patently false values or seeking the unattainable goals of the larger society when reality undermines every hope and social existence is so pervasively hypercritical and harsh?

Nihilistic resolutions such as these leave such youngsters bereft of a core of inner standards and customs to stabilize and guide their future actions, exposing them to the capricious power of momentary impulse and passing temptation. Beyond being merely anomic—in Durkheim's (1951) sense of lacking socially sanctioned means for achieving culturally encouraged goals—these youngsters have incorporated neither the approved customs and practices nor the institutional aspirations and values of modern advanced societies. In effect, they are both behaviorally norm-less and existentially purposeless.

Such also is the background of many antisocial personality disorders in contemporary Western societies. As pointed out by Paris (1996), antisocial behaviors are strongly correlated with several demographic variables such as age, gender, and socioeconomic status. Several studies have noted that antisocial behaviors are most common in youth, in males, and in lower socioeconomic classes. Paris noted that East Asian cultures show a low prevalence of this disorder, suggesting that the values and the traditions of these cultures strongly protect against the pathogenesis of antisocial personality patterns. Furthermore, according to Robins (1966, 1978, 1991), membership in adolescent gangs was a major risk factor for delinquent behavior in Western societies, but primarily for those who already came from dysfunctional families. The author found that special problems follow from a lack of parental models. In these cases, parents provide little or no guidance for their children, and the children are left to fend for themselves, to observe and to emulate whatever models they can find to guide them.

Many youths from outside the dominant Euro-American culture drift into antisocial patterns, rejecting outright the idea of finding a niche in American society; they question whether a country that has preached equality but has degraded their parents and deprived them of their rights and opportunities is worth conforming to at all. Broken families, especially those in which the father has abandoned his wife and children, typically characterize this state of affairs. With the model and authority of the breadwinner out of sight, and the mother harassed by overwork and financial insecurity, the youngster often is left to roam the streets, unguided and unrestrained by the affection and controls of an attending parent. The disappearance of the father and the preoccupations of a distracted mother are felt implicitly as signs of rejection. To find a model, a credo by which fate may be mobilized and given meaning, these youngsters often turn to peers, to those other barren and lost souls who also are bereft of parental attention, and wander anomically in what they see as a hostile world.

Together with their fellow outcasts, these youngsters quickly learn that they are viewed by many as misfits in society, that their misfortunes will be compounded by the deprecatory and closed-minded attitudes of much of the larger community. Many learn also that it is only by toughness and cunning that they will find a means of survival. However, this adaptive strategy sets into play a vicious circle; as the youngster ventures into society's deviant remains, such as drug dealing, that very same society voices further castigations and condemnations. Resentments mount, and the circle of hostility and counterhostility gains momentum. With no hope of a change of fate, no promise of advancement, and struggling throughout to keep a foothold in what they see as a dog-eat-dog world, these youngsters are driven further into what is judged an antisocial, if not vindictive, lifestyle.

Again, it should be kept in mind that these harsh cultural and social conditions rarely "cause" personality disorders; rather, they serve as a context within which the more direct and immediate experiences of interpersonal life take place. They not only color and

degrade immediate personal relationships but establish time and again antisocial models for imitation.

EXPLORATORY THEORETICAL MODELS

Theory is difficult to articulate in so complex a nexus of influences as those that encompass sociocultural variables. Two models are worth noting, however. The first, articulated by Paris (1993, 1996), is his integrated theory of the etiology of personality disorders. Paris hypothesizes that only the cumulative and interactive effects of numerous biopsychosocial risk factors can explain how personality disorders develop. Included in his model is the influence of protective factors, those biological, psychological, and social influences that make the development of these disorders less likely. Paris specifies the numerous interactions among these risk factors, involving several circuitous sequences, some of a random nature, as well as feedback loops that reflect reciprocal effects as well as buffers.

Another theoretical framework was formulated by Escovar (1997), in which he extends Millon's evolutionary model to include parallel sociocultural constructs. Escovar's thesis provides strong support for how clinicians' concepts of personality and psychopathology may fruitfully be set within a wider sociocultural frame of reference. He draws upon the research of numerous social psychological thinkers, such as Triandis (1994), who have studied international cultures in depth. Escovar elaborates Millon's evolutionary bipolarities, such as self/other, pain/pleasure, and passive/active, within a broad social system of interpersonal transactions. In this context, Millon's individual or personality evolutionary concepts parallel sociocultural constructs such as individualism/collectivism, malevolence/benevolence, and agrarian-ness/industriousness, respectively.

FUTURE RESEARCH DIRECTIONS

The concepts of personality styles and disorders across cultures pose a series of significant challenges to future researchers, and there is much work to be done. The utility of contemporary diagnostic systems and nomenclatures, as well as the meaning of clinical criteria, vary in different parts of the world. Localistic conceptions are not sufficient to encompass the vast range of cultural perspectives on the highly malleable personality disorders. There is need to open up every diagnostic system to subcultural variants in construct definition and symptomatic manifestation. Studies should be undertaken to delineate the nature, meaning, and relevance of different forms of psychic distress and coping behavior. Explanatory models of personality, which may vary from culture to culture, must also be studied from an anthropological perspective.

More specifically, research needs to be done to specify those variations in personality disorder that reflect the diversity of cultural influences, the permissible range in cultures of behavioral expression, as well as the idiomatic interpretation of what is and is not considered to be a disorder. Similarly, the cultural environment of different societies should be articulated so as to portray experiential areas in which they impose risks on personality development and adaptive functioning.

To achieve the preceding "map of risk," cultural biases among existing personality measures should be reshaped and revised to maximize their utility and comparability among diverse cultures. Epidemiological methods, employing suitable structured interviews and formal assessment techniques, should be employed to characterize typical dimensional trait patterns as well as their overall prevalence and demographic correlates. Finally, to provide insight into differential sources of risk, systematic studies should be undertaken to appraise family support systems, to identify the impact of cultural styles of child rearing, and to formulate specific and local explanatory models of sociocultural pathogenesis.

REFERENCES

Alarcón RD, Foulks EF, Vakkur M: Personality Disorders and Culture: Clinical and Conceptual Interactions. New York, Wiley, 1998

American Psychiatric Association: Diagnostic and Statistical Manual of Mental Disorders, 4th Edition, Text Revision. Washington, DC, American Psychiatric Association, 2000

Benjamin LS: Psychosocial factors in the development of personality disorders, in Personality and Psychopathology. Edited by Cloninger CR. Washington, DC, American Psychiatric Press, 1999, pp 309–342

Cabaj R, Stein T (eds): Textbook of Homosexuality and Mental Health. Washington, DC, American Psychiatric Press, 1996

Cloninger CR: A systematic method for clinical description and classification of personality variants. Arch Gen Psychiatry 44:573–588, 1987

Dohrenwend BP, Dohrenwend BS: Social Status and Psychological Disorder: A Causal Inquiry. New York, Wiley, 1969

Durkheim E: Suicide: A Study in Sociology. Translated by Spaulding JA, Simpson G. New York, Free Press, 1951

Frank LK: Society as the Patient: Essays on Culture and Personality. New York, Ronald Press, 1948

Escovar L: The Millon inventories: Sociocultural considerations, in The Millon Inventories. Edited by Millon T. New York, Guilford, 1997, pp 264–285

Harris JR: How to succeed in childhood, in The Nature–Nurture Debate: The Essential Readings. Edited by Ceci SJ, Williams WM. Oxford, England, Blackwell, 1999, pp 84–95

Jian Li Wang E: Rural-urban differences in the prevalence of major depression and associated impairment. Soc Psychiatry Psychiatr Epidemiol 39:19–26, 2004

Kiesler DJ: Contemporary Interpersonal Therapy and Research. New York, Wiley, 1996

Kleinman A: Patients and Healers in the Context of Culture. Berkeley, CA, University of California Press, 1980

Kleinman A: The Illness Narratives: Suffering, Healing and the Human Condition. New York, Basic Books, 1988a

Kleinman A: Rethinking Psychiatry: From Cultural Category to Personal Experience. New York, Free Press, 1988b

Kupfer D, First M, Regier D (eds): A Research Agenda for DSM-V. Washington, DC: American Psychiatric Publishing, 2002

Littlewood R, Lipsedge M: The butterfly and the serpent: culture, psychopathology and biomedicine. Cult Med Psychiatry 11:289–336, 1987

Lukoff D, Lu FG, Turner R: Cultural considerations in the assessment and treatment of religious and spiritual problems. Psychiatr Clin North Am 18:467–485, 1995

Mezzich JE, Kleinman A, Fabrega H, et al (eds): Culture and Psychiatric Diagnosis: A DSM-IV Perspective. Washington, DC, American Psychiatric Press, 1996

Millon T: Modern Psychopathology. Philadelphia, PA, WB Saunders, 1969

Millon T: Disorders of Personality. New York, Wiley, 1981

Paris J: Personality disorders: a biopsychosocial model. J Personal Disord 7:255–264, 1993

Paris J: Social Factors in the Personality Disorders. Cambridge, England, Cambridge University Press, 1996

Pinderhughes E: Understanding Race, Ethnicity and Power. New York, Free Press, 1989

Robins LN: Deviant Children Grown Up. Baltimore, MD, Williams & Wilkins, 1966

Robins LN: Sturdy childhood predictors of adult outcome. Psychol Med 8:611–622, 1978

Robins LN, Regier DA (eds): Psychiatric Disorders in America. New York, Free Press, 1991

Srole L, Fischer AK: The Midtown Manhattan Longitudinal Study vs. "The Mental Paradise Lost Doctrine." Arch Gen Psychiatry 36:17–24, 1980

Triandis HC: Major cultural syndromes and emotion, in Emotion and Culture. Edited by Kitayama S, Markus H. Washington, DC, American Psychological Association, 1994, pp 285–306

Weiss MG: Cultural epidemiology: an introduction and overview. Anthropology and Medicine 8:5–30, 2001

Weissman MM: The epidemiology of personality disorders: a 1990 update. J Personal Disord 7 (suppl):44–62, 1993

Westermeyer J, Janca A: Language, culture and psychopathology: conceptual and methodological issues. Transcult Psychiatry 34:291–311, 1997

Witzig R: The medicalization of race: scientific legitimization of a flawed social construct. Ann Intern Med 125:675–679, 1996

World Health Organization: The ICD-10 Classification of Mental and Behavioural Disorders: Clinical Descriptions and Diagnostic Guidelines. Geneva, Switzerland, World Health Organization, 1992

Part IV

Treatment

15

Levels of Care in Treatment

John G. Gunderson, M.D.
Kim L. Gratz, Ph.D.
Edmund C. Neuhaus, Ph.D.
George W. Smith, M.S.W.

In this chapter, we describe the indications, goals, structures, and empirical evidence related to the use of four different and decreasingly intensive levels of care: IV—hospital; III—partial hospital/day treatment; II—intensive outpatient; and I—outpatient. Although we are concerned primarily with the roles these levels of care play in treating personality disorders, we recognize that patients who have a personality disorder often will be placed in levels of care due to a treatment primarily directed at comorbid Axis I conditions. For example, major depression has a comorbidity of about 50% with Cluster B and C disorders (Dolan-Sewell et al. 2001), anxiety disorders have a comorbidity of about 25% with Cluster C disorders (Dyck et al. 2001), and substance abuse is associated with a comorbid Cluster B disorder more than 50% of the time (Oldham et al. 1995). The presence of a comorbid personality disorder often complicates the treatment of an Axis I disorder (Tyrer et al. 1997); for example, the patient with

avoidant personality disorder may not attend group sessions; the patient with borderline personality disorder (BPD) may refuse family contacts; the patient with histrionic personality disorder may express sensitivity to the side effects of medications, and so on. In such ways, personality disorders may diminish the prognosis for the treatment of Axis I disorders.

DEFINITIONS

Treatments can be organized according to the four different levels of care (see Table 15–1). Those personality disorders associated with the most severe crises and highest levels of dysfunction are more apt to require higher levels of care. The four levels of care are hierarchical in terms of containment, intensity, structure, and costs per day, and they are inversely related to usual length of stay.

Table 15–1. Levels of care

IV	Hospital; 24 hours/day with option of locked doors and seclusion
III	Partial hospital/day treatment; 2–8 hours/day, 3–5 days/week, 6–30 hours/week; usually heavily involving group therapies
II	Intensive outpatient; 3–6 hours/week of specifically prescribed, scheduled, and integrated therapies
I	Outpatient; 1–5 hours/week of scheduled therapies

GENERAL PRINCIPLES GOVERNING LEVELS OF CARE

The least restrictive level of care possible is usually best—this maximizes and requires use of one's personal strengths, increases the likelihood of being able to apply new capabilities and skills to community settings (i.e., generalization), and decreases the likelihood of regressive aspects of treatment (e.g., reinforcement of dysfunctional behavior).

Availability of all levels is clinically desirable (most treatment settings include only IV and I) and possibly cost beneficial (Quaytman and Scharfstein 1997). The availability of levels II and III decreases use of hospitalizations, decreases dropouts, and increases social rehabilitation interventions.

With each decrease in level of care, the treatments become more specific for different types of personality disorders.

EVIDENTIARY BASE

Several meta-analytic reports have affirmed the value of psychotherapy, which really includes all psychosocial therapies, for personality disorders (Leichsenring and Leibing 2003; Perry and Bond 2000). The extant research involving specified levels of care is shown in Table 15–2. Many of these studies have examined personality disorders in general, and these studies vary in the extent to which they control for or examine the specific impact of particular personality disorders or a personality disorder cluster on treatment efficacy. Most research examining treatment for specific personality disorders involves BPD and antisocial personality disorder (ASPD), with a growing number of studies examining the effectiveness of treatments at different levels of care on Cluster C disorders—in particular, avoidant personality disorder. Cluster A disorders have received the least systematic attention from researchers. Fur-

thermore, empirical support for the comparative efficacy of different levels of care is rare.

OVERALL THEORY FOR USE OF DIFFERENT LEVELS OF CARE

The intended goals for therapeutic change are often classified within four domains: subjective distress, maladaptive behaviors, interpersonal, and intrapsychic (i.e., psychological). These domains are identified in the sequence in which change can be expected (Gabbard et al. 2002; Gunderson and Gabbard 1999; Howard et al. 1986; Kopta et al. 1994; Lanktree and Briere 1995) as well as a sequence that generally should be prioritized in treatment planning. Table 15–3 indicates the relative capacity for the different levels of care to effect change in these four domains. Of course, this profile is tied to the expected lengths of stay.

Another way to classify goals is by the priority they should be assigned in planning treatment interventions (Gunderson 2001). Here, for example, goals include crisis management, behavioral stabilization, social rehabilitation, and psychological growth (Table 15–4). These goals naturally map onto those in Table 15–3 and vary in the extent to which they can and should be addressed within each level of care. For example, crises are often managed by hospitalizations because of the hospital's role in providing containment, asylum from stress, and the potential for rapid medication changes that offer immediate symptom relief. Behavioral stabilization and social rehabilitation are achieved through corrective social learning experiences, as well as the continued opportunities for the acquisition and generalization of coping skills that are central to partial hospital (level III) and intensive outpatient (level II) programs. Psychological growth change requires longer-term and often repetitious learning experiences available only in stable longer-term settings—that is, in level I outpatient care.

Table 15–2. Studies on level of care for personality disorders

	Hospital	Partial hospital	Intensive outpatient	Outpatient
All personality disorders	Dolan et al. 1992, 1997	Karterud et al. 1992, 2003 Mehlum et al. 1991 Vaglum et al. 1990 Wilberg et al. 1998b, 1999	NA	NA
Cluster A	NA	NA	NA	NA
Cluster B	NA	NA	NA	NA
BPD	Barley et al. 1993 Bohus et al. 2000 Silk et al. 1994	Bateman and Fonagy 1999, 2001	Linehan et al. 1991, 1993, 1994	Blum et al. 2002 Munroe-Blum and Marziali 1995 Stevenson and Meares 1992 Wilberg et al. 1998a
ASPD	Cacciola et al. 1995 Gabbard and Coyne 1987 Harris et al. 1994) Hildebrand et al. 2004 Messina et al. 1999, 2002 Ogloff et al. 1990 Reiss et al. 1999 Rice et al. 1992 Richards et al. 2003	Cacciola et al. 1995	NA	Brooner et al. 1998 Compton et al. 1998 Messina et al. 2003
Clusters B and C	NA	Krawitz 1997	NA	Hoglend 1993 Winston et al. 1994
Cluster C	Gude and Vaglum 2001	NA	NA	Hardy et al. 1995
AVPD	NA	NA	NA	Alden 1989

Note. ASPD=antisocial personality disorder; AVPD=avoidant personality disorder; BPD=borderline personality disorder; NA=not available.
Source. Search engine used: PsycINFO.

Table 15–3.   Goals and their relationship to levels of care

	Distress	**Behavioral**	**Interpersonal**	**Intrapsychic**
Hospital	++	+	−	−
Partial hospital	++	++	+	−
Intensive outpatient	+	++	++	+
Outpatient	+	+	++	++

Note.   Effectiveness: ++=strong; +=possible; −=unlikely.

CASE EXAMPLE

The following case example portrays the challenges involved in selecting or changing a level of care:

> Ms. H, a 26-year-old single white woman, was referred from another state for treatment of personality disorder not otherwise specified with borderline, schizotypal, and avoidant features. With an excellent high school grade point average, she had been accepted into a very competitive college. However, her completion of college was repeatedly delayed due to angry conflicts with peers and teachers usually followed by self-endangering behaviors of variable seriousness. For the past several years, she has been living at home doing minimal work.
>
> On arrival, Ms. H was angry at her parents for bringing her but desperate about needing help. She refused to enter the residential program, insisting that she wasn't that "sick." When advised it would provide a way to develop peer relationships, she angrily denied the need for that and claimed she could make friends whenever she wanted. Her parents' effort to correct that claim only made her resistance to entering the partial hospital more resolute. She nonetheless reiterated that she was desperate to receive an intensive outpatient program (IOP, level II) that had been unavailable at home.
>
> A clinical decision needed to be made: either accept Ms. H in an IOP (level II) as she insisted or not (under which circumstances she claimed returning home was not an option, and she would go to the streets of Boston).
>
> At her parents' urging, Ms. H was accepted into IOP and quickly found residence with someone she met there. She got attached to her individual therapist but became preoccupied with her roommate who had her own problems. After 6 months, the therapist and group therapy leaders in the IOP concluded that Ms. H was making no progress—that she had insufficient social supports or structure to use treatment for other than crisis management. The therapist felt that to insist on residential care would be experienced as rejection and might precipitate suicidal danger.

Ms. H's case illustrates several common and difficult problems. One is making a concession on level of care to accommodate a patient's insistence. Making a concession is sometimes necessary but is best done with the proviso that the patient agrees to accept your recommendations if he or she has not achieved some reasonable progress in some agreed upon time (e.g., has not achieved a job, has not attended therapies regularly, has not established a social support system, or has not diminished high-risk activities). A second problem illustrated by this case is that once treatments are under way, it can be very difficult to change them without breaking the relational alliance with the patient and/or precipitating a potentially dangerous flight. In Ms. H's case, the IOP team called for a consultation. Use of outside consultants to oversee changes helps depersonalize what often looms as a very difficult confrontation. To do this required time-consuming communications by the treaters. It is more easily done within hospitals. How to make such confrontations (advising patients of information that they do not want to hear) and how to impose limits (prohibiting behavior[s] that a patient wishes to continue) without patients becoming self-destructive or leaving treatment is not easy (see Gunderson 2001 for discussion).

LEVELS OF CARE

What follows is an elaboration of indications, goals, and structures for each of the four levels of care (see Table 15–4). Where available, relevant empirical evidence is noted.

Level IV: Hospital

Given that hospitalizations are almost always 2–14 days in duration in practice, the following discussion is geared to those lengths of stay. Still, research that has been done on hospitalizations of longer durations (e.g., 2–3 months) suggests that they can be useful in ways that are not feasible in 2–14 days. That research is described at the end of this section.

Table 15–4. Levels of care: modalities, goals, duration, and therapeutic processes

Level	Modalities	Goals and procedures	Duration	Therapeutic processes

IV. Hospital	Medication
	Milieu
	Group
	Case management
		Crisis management
		  Decrease distress
		  Decrease suicide risk
		
		Assessments
		  Neurological evaluations
		  Psychological evaluations
		
		Plan/Change treatment
		  Develop treatment plan
		  Identify primary therapist
		  Initiate medication changes
		  Expert consultation
			2–10 days
			24 hours/day
				Containment
				Support

III. Partial hospital	Milieu
	Group
	Case management
	Family
	Individual
		Skills training
		  Stabilize daily living skills
		  Structure daily activities
		  Identify maladaptive patterns
		
		Behavioral stabilization
		  Decrease impulsive behavior
		  Increase coping skills
		
		Social rehabilitation
		  Improve social functioning
		  Vocational rehabilitation
		  Community reentry
			1–2 weeks
			6–20 hours/week
			
			3–12 weeks
			6–10 hours/week
			
			16+ weeks
				Structure
				Support
				Involvement

II. Intensive outpatient	Group
	Family
	Individual
		Social (behavioral) adaptation
		  Vocational
		  Behavioral
		  Affective
		  Interpersonal
			3–18 months
			3–6 hours/week
				Support
				Involvement

I. Outpatient	Individual
	Group
		Psychological growth
		  Interpersonal
		  Intrapsychic
			12–36 months
			1–3 hours/week
				Involvement
				Validation

Potential risks associated with inpatient hospitalization include reinforcement of maladaptive behaviors (e.g., parasuicidal, attention seeking, control struggles) and/or passive problem solving. Clinicians should consider these issues for the particular patient. Nonetheless, the role of hospitalization should be appreciated, because personality disorder patients treated in community-oriented treatments (level I or II) with an aggressive emphasis on keeping patients out of the hospital have worse outcomes than patients for whom hospitals were used as needed (Tyrer and Simmonds 2003).

Indications

Hospitalization may be clinically indicated during acute crises and in response to increasingly severe behavioral dysfunction, especially with regard to suicidal behaviors and violence toward others. Perhaps also worth noting is that hospitalization may be used as an asylum to permit patients with personality disorders to leave abusive or otherwise harmful situations or relationships. Hospitalizations can also enable patients to leave treatments that were not helpful but that they would otherwise have had difficulty leaving.

Many people with personality disorders enter hospitals because of comorbid psychiatric disorders to which the personality disorder may predispose them. Indeed, more than half of psychiatrically hospitalized patients have a personality disorder, with the most common types being borderline, avoidant, and dependent personality disorders (Loranger 1990). Attention to and consideration of the personality disorder may affect treatment efficacy for the Axis I disorders and should influence treatment decisions.

Given that BPD is the predominant personality disorder found in inpatient hospital services (constituting about 15% of hospitalizations (Koenigsberg et al. 1985); Loranger 1990; Widiger and Weissman 1991), it is worth noting a common clinical situation for which hospitalizations should be used with caution. Hospitalization should rarely be used in response to self-injurious behavior without suicidal intent. Furthermore, although inpatient stays may be warranted for BPD patients who are acutely suicidal, such hospitalizations may not decrease the likelihood of future suicide attempts (Van der Sande et al. 1997).

Despite the widespread belief that hospitalization is generally contraindicated for patients with ASPD, research on the effectiveness of inpatient therapeutic community drug treatment programs and inpatient substance abuse programs suggests that ASPD patients may respond positively to certain types of inpatient programs (Cacciola et al. 1995; Messina et al.

1999, 2002). Of course, the generalizability of these results to other, less specialized inpatient hospital programs is indeterminable. With regard to contraindications to hospitalization, Gabbard and Coyne (1987) noted that negative responses to hospitalization are likely for ASPD patients with a history of felony arrests or convictions; a history of repeated lying, aliases, and conning; an unresolved legal situation at admission; forced hospitalization as an alternative to incarceration; and a history of violence toward others. Moreover, research suggests that psychiatric hospitalization is relatively contraindicated for those ASPD patients (approximately 25%–65%; see Widiger and Corbitt 1996) who are psychopathic (i.e., display a lack of remorse, lack of empathy, and shallow affect; Harris et al. 1994; Hart and Hare 1997; Hildebrand et al. 2004; Reiss et al. 1999; Richards et al. 2003; see also Salekin 2002). In contrast, there is evidence to suggest that ASPD patients without psychopathy may respond positively to forensic hospitals with therapeutic community programs (Rice et al. 1992) and that the presence of comorbid anxiety and/or depression may also be associated with a positive response to hospitalization among ASPD patients (see Gabbard and Coyne 1987).

Although level IV care is rarely indicated for Cluster C personality disorders, it is worth noting that hospitalization may offer useful exposures for patients with avoidant personality disorder. For instance, hospitalization may expose avoidant patients to typically avoided social situations (e.g., seeing others in distress) or internal experiences (e.g., of feeling helpless or anxious). Although hospitalization may result in initial improvements in symptoms for these patients, however, research suggests that patients with pure Cluster C personality disorders (especially avoidant personality disorder) may be at greater risk for relapsing after discharge than patients with Cluster B personality disorders (see Gude and Vaglum 2001).

Goals: Crisis Management, Assessments, and Planning and Implementing Treatment Changes

Following are the major goals of hospitalizations and the usual time required for meeting them:

- Crisis management (2–6 days): Hospitalization can diminish acute suicidal or violent dangers.
- Extensive neurological or psychological evaluations (2–6 days): These evaluations are more easily coordinated, and may only be feasible, in hospital settings.

- Development of a treatment plan and personnel (3–14 days): Such plans usually require arranging for continuity through appropriate step-downs and assessing the suitability of new therapy personnel. An essential part of these processes is to identify the primary clinician who will be responsible for the patient's treatment. For primary clinicians, an essential first step is to define roles and goals—that is, establish a "contractual alliance"—and to contract with the patient about participation in aftercare services.
- Changes in prior therapies (3–14 days): These changes are often indicated, but they may require expert consultation and the introduction of new therapists. If the changes are considered undesirable by the patient, working through resistance may be possible only in the hospital, where the options for flight from the proposed changes are reduced.
- Hospitalizations may allow therapists to review prior impasses or establish a clearer framework for their ongoing work. For many patients with personality disorder, hospitalization serves as an environment to initiate medication changes and evaluate medication benefits.

Structures

A businesslike, practical, supportive, and task-oriented atmosphere and orientation is useful. Harmful is a milieu that encourages long one-to-one talks or the development of personal relationships with staff or other patients. Community meetings or group therapies that emphasize cohesion or bonding among patients are relatively contraindicated. Care should be taken not to reinforce maladaptive behaviors or increasingly intense/ severe expressions of distress and suicidality. Furthermore, emphasizing the short-term nature of the treatment, retaining a focus on impending discharge, and making after-care plans for less-restrictive levels of care may be useful strategies for preventing lengthy or contraindicated hospitalizations (see Bohus et al. 2000; Silk et al. 1994). Given that it is easy for staff to feel trapped by escalating suicidal ideation as patients approach discharge, a consultant can help alleviate unrealistic liability fears.

In regard to staffing, a case manager should be assigned. The case manager should keep the patient oriented toward the problems preceding the hospitalization that the patient will need to cope with on discharge. A primary task of the case manager is to bring in relatives or other significant people to help understand precipitating events and diminish the likelihood of their recurrence after discharge, to receive psycho-

education about the personality disorder, and to coordinate aftercare plans.

The psychiatrist should oversee medications and involve the patient in any changes. As important, the psychiatrist should caution patients about the relatively modest benefits they can expect. In addition, the psychiatrist should evaluate coexisting Axis I disorders and give them appropriate priority in aftercare planning. For example, comorbid substance or alcohol abuse almost always should be assigned high priority in aftercare, and coexisting depression may not respond well to medications (Gunderson et al. 2004; Koenigsberg et al. 1999; Kool et al. 2003; Shea et al. 1987; Soloff 1998) and may require further monitoring at a less-restrictive level of care.

Longer-Term Hospitalizations: Empirical Lessons

Longer-term hospitalizations may address additional goals. Dolan et al. (1997) found that long-term (i.e., average of 7 months) therapeutic community inpatient treatment was associated with decreased borderline psychopathology. Furthermore, hospitalizations of 2–3 months may result in behavioral stabilization (a goal usually reached in level III and generally not addressed in the 2–10 day hospitalizations described above). Dialectical behavior therapy (DBT)–based inpatient programs in particular may be more effective in fulfilling this goal than other inpatient programs with equally long stays (see Barley et al. 1993). The advantages shown for such programs are presumably due to the emphasis on skills training (in particular, distress tolerance skills), behavioral analyses of problem behaviors (with the goal of identifying precipitants and consequences of problem behaviors so as to determine appropriate interventions), and the use of contingency strategies, potentially minimizing unintended reinforcement of maladaptive behaviors (Barley et al. 1993; Bohus et al. 2000). Moreover, the milieu can be used to practice, and begin to generalize, the skills being learned.

These studies of 2–3 month hospitalizations can be used to inform the development of hospital programs with shorter lengths of stay. For instance, Silk et al. (1994) developed a DBT-based inpatient treatment for BPD with an average length of stay of 10–17 days. In assessing patients' perceptions of improvement at the time of discharge, they found that patients in the DBT-based program (compared with patients assigned to a non-DBT discussion group) felt that the lessons they learned would help them to better handle difficult or painful situations. Although the same level of change found with longer-term hospital stays would not be expected with short-term hospitalizations, a similar structure can be utilized with beneficial results.

Level III: Partial Hospital/Day Treatment

The literature presents a diverse picture of partial hospital treatments for personality disorders, varying extensively with regard to treatment duration (i.e., length of stay) and treatment intensity (i.e., hours per week). These programs offer more structure, containment, and intensive treatment than outpatient care while providing the opportunity for behavioral stabilization—and for skills building and generalization—that are not usually available in typical short-term inpatient settings. Our discussion of partial hospital treatment is oriented toward the levels of duration and intensity—that is, the shorter-term partial hospital programs (2–4 weeks in duration) that are usually available in the current health care system. A discussion of the lessons that can be learned from the longer-term partial programs that have been the primary recipients of empirical attention can be found at the end of this section.

Indications

For some patients with a personality disorder, partial hospital programs offer an optimal level of care. They can diminish the likelihood of substance/alcohol abuse relapses or suicide attempts (although they do not have enough monitoring or containment to prevent these behaviors). Moreover, partial hospital programs may be indicated for patients who lack either the social supports or vocational options to make community living viable. Whether as an alternative to or step-down from hospitalization, partial hospital programs are needed for personality disorder patients with marked social or behavioral impairment. Karterud et al. (2003) operationalized the need for partial hospitalization by suggesting that it was indicated for patients with Global Assessment of Functioning scores below 50. Partial hospital programs can assess the types of, and reasons for, social disability and introduce rehabilitative efforts. This level of care can also be used to introduce or stabilize new treatments when close supervision and evaluations are needed.

As with level IV, BPD is the personality disorder most likely to use level III. Although patients with ASPD are also socially impaired, there is some evidence to suggest that they may be likely to drop out of partial hospital programs (Karterud et al. 2003; Wilberg et al. 1998b). However, given evidence of a positive response to level III therapeutic community drug treatment programs among ASPD patients (Cacciola et al. 1995), it is

possible that certain specialized partial hospital programs may be effective in the treatment of ASPD patients. Patients with schizotypal personality disorder are unlikely to be helped by partial hospital programs (see Karterud et al. 1992; Vaglum et al. 1990). Surprisingly, however, patients with paranoid personality disorder treated in an 18-week day treatment program evidenced significant improvements in global functioning, symptom severity, and interpersonal functioning—improvements comparable with those seen among patients with other personality disorders (Wilberg et al. 1998b).

Goals: Skills Training, Stabilization, and Social Rehabilitation

A pragmatic and theoretically grounded approach conceptualizes treatment in stages, each of which has its own goals and interventions. Stages are organized with respect to their duration and intensity as well as to the changes that can reasonably be expected to occur within a given time frame. Based on clinical experience, a high-intensity "front-loaded" treatment is optimal initially, followed by treatment at a titrated intensity over several months. Given that most programs can offer only short-term treatment (what we refer to here as stage 1 of treatment), this titration is particularly relevant. The following are goals for each stage:

Stage 1 (1–2 Weeks)

- Develop a therapeutic alliance and the patient attaches to treatment. This process is assisted by defining goals and establishing an initial treatment contract that gets reviewed and refined over time.
- Psychoeducation. This helps patients frame goals and understand treatment options, and enlists family support.
- Stabilize or teach daily living skills (eating, sleeping, hygiene). The need for this goal varies, as does the optimal approach to achieving it. Most patients need consistent monitoring and education about the importance of eating and sleeping in regular patterns. Sleep medications may prove useful for patients who have trouble falling asleep because of fearfulness.
- Schedule and structure time and activities. This assists with the management and planning of daily activities, promotes self-care routines (e.g., sleep, hygiene, good eating habits), and aids in overall stress management.
- Begin to identify typical patterns (e.g., interpersonal conflicts, loneliness) that lead to maladaptive behaviors. Although maladaptive patterns cannot

be expected to change in stage 1, it is often useful to introduce basic behavioral strategies at this point, including chain analyses and impulse control skills.

Stage 2 (3–8 Weeks)

- Behavioral stabilization. This goal involves attaining better impulse control, resulting in a decrease in the frequency and severity of impulsive and self-destructive behaviors (e.g., self-harm, suicide attempts, substance use). This stabilization is often a nonspecific effect of asylum, structure, and support.

- Initiate vocational rehabilitation. This goal is not easily accomplished and typically gets overlooked due to the fact that patients with a personality disorder rarely seek vocational rehabilitation. Young or inexperienced staff are unlikely to give this goal adequate value and importance. Program administrators or staff involved with families are more apt to determine whether it is addressed.

- Reevaluate the treatment contract on the basis of the extent to which patients are working collaboratively and responsibly in treatment. In stage 2 treatment, after patients have achieved more competency with regard to coping skills (e.g., better impulse control, improved anxiety management), a greater emphasis is placed on interpersonal relationships.

Structures

Partial hospital and day treatment programs rely heavily on group therapy and the positive effects of a therapeutic milieu. Such structure must be actively constructed, proactively maintained, and updated as needed. With a 1- or 2-week length of stay, patients do not have the luxury of time to "settle-in" to treatment. Clear and concise information (e.g., description of the program and treatment philosophy, expectations of patients, roles of treatment team members) provided upon entry can diminish a patient's anxiety and facilitate immediate involvement in treatment. Handouts with daily schedules and brief descriptions of groups may further orient patients and promote memory of what to expect. The structure of the partial hospital program may become a template for structuring their lives outside the program.

As with hospitals, a case manager responsible for implementing the treatment and monitoring progress should be assigned. This person should work directly with the patient, treatment team members both within and outside of the program, and family members. To be an effective case manager with personality disorder patients requires clinical savvy to set limits, confront when necessary (e.g., when patients are missing groups), and stay connected with a patient despite being vilified as not understanding or caring. An effective case manager must also be willing and able to negotiate with treatment team members outside of the program (e.g., the patient's outpatient therapist). In short-term treatment the case manager may be invaluable to the family system in providing information, support, and the framework of an overall treatment plan (e.g., anticipating the issues involved in less intensive levels of care).

Given the potential for treatment noncompliance at this level of care (because patients may have difficulty attending treatment when feeling bad), the structure of the program should include provisions for addressing noncompliance through program expectations, policies, and an explicit emphasis on therapy-interfering behaviors. Noncompliance is best addressed by the case manager and then followed up in groups. It is useful to utilize a combination of validation, confronting, limit-setting (e.g., patients cannot stay in the program unless attendance improves), and the teaching of coping skills to facilitate improved attendance despite emotional distress.

High-intensity short-term treatment at this level of care should be front-loaded with skills training and psychoeducation to promote stabilization and safety. It is essential to select and prioritize elemental skills that are feasible for patients to learn quickly. This bottom-up approach draws heavily from cognitive-behavioral therapy (CBT) principles and simplifies the treatment program for patients (Levendusky et al. 1994). Notably, even the psychoanalytic partial hospital program developed by Bateman and Fonagy (2004) is heavily cognitive-behavioral and especially so in early phases. As such, a core constellation of groups within stage 1 treatment may include treatment contracting, community meeting (a forum for addressing therapy interfering behaviors), personality disorder psychoeducation (with additional information about the influence of Axis I disorders), basic behavioral skills groups (including behavioral scheduling, impulse control, distress tolerance, and anxiety management), self-assessment groups that teach patients how to identify maladaptive behavioral patterns (including the emotional and cognitive precipitants of maladaptive behaviors), and rudimentary interpersonal groups (e.g., assertiveness training, interpersonal effectiveness, and the impact of personality styles on relationships).

Groups during stage 2 of treatment may follow the framework of stage 1, although with greater depth and further opportunities for patients to practice skills and achieve some competency in their use. At this stage of treatment, as patients begin to feel like part of the milieu, there is a natural progression to focus more explicitly on the patient's interpersonal relationships. This stage may see an intensification of treatment relationships and attachments, which offers challenges to both patients and treaters alike. Any honeymoon phase would likely be over by this stage of treatment, necessitating that the frustrations, disappointments, and realities of treatment be addressed. For effective treatment to continue, the therapeutic alliance must be strong enough to endure these obstacles.

Longer-Term Partial Hospital/Day Treatment Programs: Empirical Lessons

Research on longer-term partial hospital and day treatment programs suggests that they may provide the opportunity for behavioral stabilization (including decreased parasuicidal behavior) and symptom improvement and, unlike shorter-term programs, can also positively affect social and interpersonal functioning. For example, Bateman and Fonagy (1999) found that BPD patients treated in a psychoanalytic partial hospital program, compared with BPD patients in standard outpatient care, evidenced significantly fewer suicide attempts after 6 months, significant reductions in depression and anxiety after approximately 9 months, and significantly fewer acts of self-harm after 12 months. Moreover, partial hospital program patients not only maintained their gains but reported further improvements at follow-up (Bateman and Fonagy 2001).

Global symptom severity of patients with Cluster B and C disorders has been shown to decrease significantly after approximately 4 months of level III treatment (Karterud et al. 1992; Krawitz 1997; Vaglum et al. 1990; Wilberg et al. 1998b). These same improvements may also be found for patients with paranoid personality disorder (Wilberg et al. 1998b). Research also suggests that patients with Cluster C personality disorders may experience improvements in social functioning after 4 months (Karterud et al. 1992; Vaglum et al. 1990). For patients with BPD, on the other hand, significant improvements in social adjustment and interpersonal functioning may require up to 18 months of treatment (Bateman and Fonagy 1999).

Moreover, even in these longer-term partial hospital/day treatment programs, vocational rehabilitation is difficult to achieve. Following a 4-month day treatment program, unemployment rates of patients with Cluster B and C disorders did not change during the 2-year follow-up period despite other significant improvements in global functioning and symptom severity (Krawitz 1997). Similarly, in another study, patients with personality disorder (primarily borderline, avoidant, and paranoid) treated in a variety of day treatment programs (ranging from 18–41 weeks and from 8–16 hours/week) did not evidence any improvements in work functioning at 1-year follow-up (Karterud et al. 2003).

Finally, although it is often assumed that more treatment (i.e., greater intensity) will result in greater improvements, research suggests that when it comes to the day treatment of patients with BPD, "less is more." Karterud et al. (2003) found that lower intensity (i.e., 8–10 hours per week) partial hospital treatment was more effective (i.e., fewer dropouts and greater improvements in global functioning and symptom severity) for patients with BPD than high-intensity treatments (approximately 16 hours per week). This finding is consistent with the level of intensity found to be effective in Bateman and Fonagy's (1999, 2001) randomized controlled trial.

Level II: Intensive Outpatient Program

When described as a level of care, an IOP differs from an intensive schedule of individual psychotherapy. For purposes of this review, we define IOP as an integration of two or more modalities in which efforts are coordinated and patients receive 3–10 hours of services per week. Thus, at its higher end, IOPs overlap with low-intensity partial hospital programs. When patients need fewer than 3 hours of service per week and/or the services do not need to regularly coordinate their efforts, the treatment becomes level I. IOP or level II care is of particular value for BPD patients (Gunderson 2001; Smith et al. 2001). Although Linehan's (1993) DBT treatment has been identified as an outpatient service, it involves both individual and group therapy provided by collaborating clinicians at a level of 3.5 hours per week—thus, it could be classified as an IOP.

Indications

IOPs are indicated for personality disorder patients whose problems with living in the community are not acutely self-endangering but are sufficiently severe that only daily, or otherwise unusually intensive, care can bring about changes. IOPs can provide a gradual transition from higher levels of care (i.e., inpatient and partial hospital programs). Because patients often experience this transition as happening too quickly or before they are ready, treatment modalities at this level of care should recognize and validate patients' subjective distress while simultaneously encouraging the use of their personal strengths and skills.

Case Example

Ms. I, a 38-year-old single white woman with BPD and posttraumatic stress disorder (PTSD), was hospitalized for increased PTSD symptoms and reckless behavior following a serious accident in which her son was injured. Previous hospitalizations had lasted weeks longer than anticipated and were followed by 2–3 months in partial hospital without obvious benefit. On the inpatient unit, the patient was disappointed not to have the case manager and psychiatrist she had worked with in the past and also was eager to go home to spend Christmas with her son. Her therapist was leaving for vacation and seemed worried about the patient returning to outpatient care in her absence. The patient and therapist negotiated with the leaders of the IOP groups about how she could use the groups to manage emotional distress and to monitor any reckless behavior. The patient was discharged to an IOP, resumed her functioning as a mother, and survived her therapist's absence.

This vignette illustrates both the value of an IOP as a step-down from hospital (level IV) care and the ways it can assist during crises (in this case, the absence of a therapist) while in outpatient (level I) care.

Goals: Social (Behavioral) Adaptation

- Vocational (4–12 weeks): Enlist in needed vocational training or develop skills and initiative required to obtain work.
- Behavioral (4–12 months): Improve abilities to control impulsive behaviors and out-of-control (i.e., ineffective) expressions of feelings. Improve ability to engage in goal-directed, valued behaviors.
- Affective (6–52 weeks): Recognize feeling states in self and others and learn to associate them with behaviors (what Fonagy [1991] has termed *mentalization*). This recognition is especially important for the feelings of fear and anger in avoidant personality disorder and BPD, respectively. Increase emotional acceptance.
- Interpersonal (6 months–2 years): Recognize dependent needs as part of self and others. This goal initially involves recognition of such needs; becoming comfortable with them follows (Gunderson et al. 1993). Increase interpersonal effectiveness.

Structures

In addition to individual psychotherapy, IOPs offer complementary groups that meet three to five times per week and promote the resumption of functional capacities within the community. Groups are best offered in the morning or late afternoon to allow time in the patients' schedules to pursue nonclinical activities such as work or volunteering. Offering several different types of groups, each with a different format and function, will help patients meet the various goals of this level of care.

For instance, daily self-assessment groups can provide a structured format for each patient, in turn, to discuss the transition, identify maladaptive behaviors and/or interpersonal difficulties, and obtain support. Daily groups, by virtue of their frequency, enable patients to become familiar with the details of each others' lives, contributing to their sense of being heard and understood. The format of these groups also enables group members to hold each other accountable for managing maladaptive behaviors and interpersonal problems. DBT or CBT skills groups in an IOP provide patients with the opportunity to further develop and refine skills learned in more intensive levels of care (e.g., skills to control impulses, regulate emotions, tolerate distress, and improve their capacity to negotiate relationships). These groups are more rigorous than supportive groups (such as self-assessment ones) and require a serious commitment to homework assignments and behavioral change. Interpersonal groups are process-oriented psychotherapy groups that have a longer-term focus. These groups encourage patients to examine how they relate to others, both within the group and in their lives. Conflicts between members are expected to be frequent and may reflect ambivalence about dependency needs and competitiveness for attention.

The nature and function of these groups provides useful information as to how best to incorporate them within the structure of the IOP. Whereas self-assessment groups may be invaluable during the initial period of transition, lasting as little as a few weeks, interpersonal and DBT/CBT skills groups have a longer-term focus and may be expected to continue after the patient leaves the IOP for outpatient care (level I), thereby assisting in this new transition.

Finally, it is essential that the groups of the IOP be coordinated and integrated with the overall goals of the patient's treatment. When a patient's primary clinician works outside the IOP setting, the responsibility for coordination and implementation of the treatment plan can be handicapped. Regular communication between the patient's psychotherapist and group leaders, as well as among the group leaders themselves, is critical. For instance, Linehan's (1993) DBT includes a weekly 2-hour consultation team meeting, considered to be one of the necessary components of the treatment.

Level I: Outpatient

Level I is the level of care in which most of the treatment for personality disorders occurs. In a previous generation, psychoanalytic therapies were considered the treatment of choice for all personality disorders, even though the literature mainly consisted of negative accounts about the resistances encountered. Some of the problems traditionally encountered in outpatient care can be addressed by utilizing higher levels of care—especially IOPs. Other problems were due to applying psychoanalysis to patients who needed more structure, more of a here-and-now focus, and more support. To some extent, psychoanalytic theory has been modified to address these problems, acknowledging the importance of the "real relationships" and putting insight into perspective. Moreover, outpatient treatments for personality disorders have diversified to include a much stronger place for CBTs and medications.

Indications

There are no specific indications or contraindications for outpatient care. There are generic issues; because outpatient care requires conscious willful effort, such care is limited de facto to those who seek it and who can be sufficiently reliable to attend scheduled sessions. Beyond these considerations, some patients primarily seek support or direction, and their motivation to work on changing their personality may not be present. The absence of this motivation may be a relative contraindication for outpatient treatment.

Research on the effectiveness of outpatient treatments for personality disorders has focused primarily on relatively high-functioning clients. For instance, Winston et al. (1994) required that clients with a personality disorder have no suicidal behavior, no history of destructive impulse control problems, no use of psychotropic medications in the past year, and the presence of one close interpersonal relationship; Alden (1989) excluded participants who had ever been hospitalized for psychiatric difficulties, and most of the participants were employed or in school; in Hoglend's (1993) study, most participants were employed and none had severe acting-out behaviors. Because we do not know what fraction of the personality disorder patients in outpatient services meet these requirements, the generalizability of this research is unclear. What may be concluded is that the results will not apply to patients with severe social dysfunction.

Goals: Interpersonal and Intrapsychic Growth

Goals for level I are often the same as those identified for an IOP. Indeed, because most treatments for patients with a personality disorder are delivered in this nonintensive outpatient level of care, the goals identified for an IOP are usually initiated in level I. However, in outpatient care, achieving these goals is more apt to involve active selection and motivation by the particular patient.

An important discontinuity with the IOP is that outpatient care is rarely directed at vocational rehabilitative needs; this may be especially true for psychodynamic individual therapies. CBT- or DBT-based approaches may be more likely to accommodate this lack of vocational rehabilitation through role playing and problem-solving issues related to applying for school or work. Still, because outpatient therapies depend on what patients identify as goals, and because vocational rehabilitation is rarely a reason for which patients with a personality disorder seek therapy, this arena is often neglected.

- Enhance social involvement. Improve level of, and satisfaction from, social and recreational activities (as demonstrated by Winston et al. 1994).
- Improve impulse control. Although often begun at higher levels of care, impulse control can also occur in, or be strengthened by, outpatient care.
- Changes in interpersonal relatedness and intrapsychic structures. These are the primary targets of psychodynamic (and psychoanalytic) psychotherapies. Although the attention given to diagnoses is often limited and idiosyncratic, there is a body of evidence relevant to their effectiveness with personality disorders (see Gunderson and Gabbard 1999). The results published by Knight (1941) indicated that psychoanalytic psychotherapies are more effective for "neurosis" (63%) and character disorders (57%) than for psychosis (25%). A review of available literature suggests that such therapy is particularly likely to help patients with obsessive-compulsive, narcissistic, and dependent personality disorders (Gunderson 2003). The effectiveness of psychodynamic psychotherapy for BPD has received the most attention. Although a study conducted at McLean Hospital found that it was rare for a patient with BPD to remain in long-term treatment and get dramatically better (Waldinger and Gunderson 1989), such cases could be identified and the processes of change seemed to occur in a predictable sequence (Gunderson et al. 1993). Moreover, three studies with larger samples of BPD

patients have added credibility to the claim that long-term psychodynamic psychotherapy can be effective for patients with BPD and have significant cost offsets (Hoke LA: "Longitudinal Patterns of Behaviors in Borderline Personality Disorder," Doctoral dissertation, Boston University, 1989; Howard et al. 1986; Stevenson and Meares 1992). Of particular note, the psychoanalytic psychotherapy offered in the Stevenson and Meares (1992) study (a 1-year manualized treatment conducted by trainees) was followed by continued improvement. However, it is important to note that these studies do not show that the psychoanalytic components distinguish effective psychotherapy, nor do they indicate to what extent the favorable outcomes can be generalized to the larger universe of BPD patients.

Structures

Individual psychotherapy assumes the central role in most outpatient treatments for personality disorders. Still, split treatments (i.e., adding a suitable second modality to accompany the individual psychotherapy) have advantages (Gunderson 2001; Chapter 28, "Collaborative Treatment"). At this level of care, the split treatment may involve medications (e.g., for schizotypal, borderline, or avoidant personality disorders; Chapter 25, "Somatic Treatments"). The second modality could also include a social rehabilitative component, including a CBT (Blum et al. 2002), an interpersonal therapy group (Marziali and Munroe-Blum 1995; Munroe-Blum and Marziali 1995), a self-help group (e.g., Alcoholics Anonymous, Narcotics Anonymous; Chapter 30, "Substance Abuse"), and/or some continuation of family involvement (Chapter 23, "Family Therapy"). These therapies are often indicated for dependent, borderline, histrionic, avoidant, or schizoid personality disorders. Moreover, a meta-analysis of treatment studies on psychopathy suggests that the augmentation of individual psychotherapy with group or family therapy may enhance its effectiveness (see Salekin 2002).

Case Example

Mr. J was a 34-year-old man who sought help because he wanted to reconcile with his wife, who had kicked him out. He was "obsessed" with his wife and claimed he did not understand why she had rejected him. She had refused couples therapy, saying he, Mr. J, needed to change himself. Prior efforts to assuage his agitation and insomnia with medications had proven helpful—but he now "needs to change himself," although he could offer no ideas about what he wanted to change. In the ensuing sessions, Mr. J described a very disturbed childhood with a punitive mother.

He became quite devoted to the therapist, a woman, and began calling her frequently for what to her seemed trivial reasons. He was deeply hurt by her efforts to interpret his calls or to set limits on them, and she eventually sought consultation. The consultant suggested an interpersonal group therapy be added. In the group, his anxieties about rejection were seen as unrealistic, and the maladaptive nature of his intrusive wishes for reassurance were confronted. The patient resisted, but after starting the group, his behavior in therapy changed dramatically. He was able to clearly see his reactions to his therapist (and wife) as transference phenomena.

Impasses in individual psychotherapy with patients with a personality disorder often derive from the fact that such patients are often unaware of how they create problems for others and then can feel unjustifiably criticized by therapists who point this out. This obstacle often can be overcome by the addition of a second modality. In this case, the group therapy diminished the transference and provided a source of feedback to Mr. J that was less personalized.

Some evidence suggests that patients with a personality disorder may require longer-term treatments to reach normative levels of functioning or to maintain treatment gains. For instance, Alden (1989) found that although three different behaviorally based treatments for avoidant personality disorder resulted in greater improvements than a waiting list control group, the patients remained significantly more symptomatic than normative samples. Similarly, in a study of the long-term outcomes of 45 patients with and without personality disorders treated with outpatient dynamic psychotherapy, Hoglend (1993) found that for the patients with personality disorders, the number of sessions in treatment was significantly related to acquired insight (i.e., new emotional self-understanding) and to overall personality change at 2- and 4-year follow-up.

CONCLUSIONS

Because personality disorders are defined by enduring social maladaptations, they are intrinsically tied to social contingencies. To bring about change, good treatments across all levels of care must embody coherent and repetitious interventions with a primary initial focus on the here and now.

The interventions offered by any level of care will only be effective if patients develop an alliance with treaters. For patients with personality disorders, forming an alliance will be complicated by the obstacles created by their personalities, for example, avoidance, deceit, or attention seeking. This chapter emphasized that establishing an alliance begins with establishing agreed-upon goals, selecting the level of care appropriate to (i.e., best able to fulfill) these goals, and clarifying what is expected of patients. These activities establish a contractual alliance. This form of alliance may be sufficient for hospitals but is also a necessary prerequisite for all other levels of care. The relational alliance (i.e., an alliance based on liking or trusting the treaters) also is necessary. Such alliances usually develop from supportive attention, and in some cases respectful listening may be all that is required. When such an alliance is not formed with clinicians, progress is unlikely. Beyond this relational alliance, the value of many specific forms of intervention depends on what has been termed the *working alliance*—that is, an alliance that is needed for collaborative work toward the patient's goals (e.g., acquiring new skills and capabilities). Although such a mutual task orientation is often assumed when contractual alliances are made, for patients with personality disorders, a working alliance can be hard to achieve. Clinicians working at all levels of care need to be vigilant about whether personality disorder patients are working with the therapist for purposes of changing themselves (i.e., their identity or self).

Earlier in this review, we noted a relationship between the four levels of care and the domains of psychopathology that patients are best able to change. Table 15–3 reflects this progression as it relates to goals. Another way to understand the distinctive effectiveness of the four levels of care is via a hierarchy of therapeutic processes (Gunderson 1978, 2001). Viewed through this lens, the levels of care move from most to least containment, with an attendant increase in reliance on internal controls and self-agency. There is also a progressive decrease in the level of structure across the levels of care, such that the organization of time and activities imposed by the treatment setting is reduced at each step down. Even within the least-structured treatment setting—that is, outpatient psychotherapies—there is a hierarchy in which more directive and active interventions give way to lesser ones as patients progress. Support in the form of reassurance, advice, and expressions of concern are important elements of all levels of care. Because support often bonds people, it becomes an essential element for interpersonal attachments. Such attachments may be a negative factor in the highest

levels of care because they can form a resistance to leaving, but they become more important, like the relational alliance noted earlier, as patients move into longer-term settings.

Winnicott (1965) identified a "holding environment" as a social context that is a necessary prerequisite for the development of an internal sense of safety and security. Everyone requires a feeling of being securely contained, but the degree to which this feeling depends on external factors varies. Although Winnicott originally conceptualized the holding environment as a function served by mothers early in development, it has been transformed into a term that is used to describe a function offered by therapies. As one moves through the levels of care, the "holding" action depends progressively less on imposed constraints and structures and more on internal resources. This shift has implications for the levels of care that may be most appropriate for specific personality disorders.

Although the role of hospitalization tends to be limited for the treatment of personality disorders, many patients with personality disorders use hospitalizations to treat comorbid conditions or crises. Hospitalizations may be most useful for those patients whose sense of self is most disorganized or unstable (BPD) or whose unintegrated behaviors pose a danger to self or others (e.g., BPD and nonpsychopathic ASPD). Such patients may need more containment and structure to feel "held." Partial hospital (day treatment) care (level III) is used primarily for stabilizing mental states and initiating longer-term therapies within the 2 weeks usually allotted by the modern managed care environment. However, there is good evidence that longer-term stays can add substantial benefits. The limited durations of stay available in partial hospitals have helped create the need for a relatively new level of care, IOPs (level II). This level of care may be needed for at least 1 year and requires theoretically and structurally integrated individual and group components. These programs have been demonstrated to be useful for BPD, but in principle they should be just as applicable to any personality disorder with severe social functioning handicaps (e.g., schizoid, avoidant, dependent, and antisocial personality disorders). Ironically, this level of care, arguably the most useful for dysfunctional personality disorders, is the least available in the present health care system. Outpatient care is the primary setting for the treatment of most personality disorders. Here, long-term individual psychotherapy by itself is thought to be the treatment of choice for patients with narcissistic, histrionic, and obsessive-compulsive personality disorders. Although it is thought that significant personality change may be possible in outpatient care, availability of this treatment is largely dependent on private pay and thus is frequently inaccessible.

There is very little research relevant to systems of health care services for personality disorders. What little there is supports the value of graduated step-down levels of care. Not surprisingly, the two personality disorders for which higher levels of care are most needed and that have the most public health significance, BPD and ASPD, have generated the most research attention (see Table 15–2). This research has generally shown that BPD can be responsive to well-structured programs at all levels of institutional services. The results for ASPD are more complicated. Specialized programs at inpatient, partial hospital, and outpatient levels of care have been shown to be useful for nonpsychopathic ASPD patients. Although the higher levels of care are generally contraindicated for psychopathic ASPD patients, the aforementioned meta-analysis of treatments for psychopathy suggests that long-term, intensive individual psychotherapy may have positive results for this population (see Salekin 2002). However, the extent to which these research findings generalize to standard practices in outpatient settings is unclear, given the potential for problems related to treatment retention and compliance at this level of care.

Because research suggests that well-structured and theoretically consistent programs are more useful for patients with a personality disorder than programs that are not, these qualities should become standards for care. More attention should now be given to whether programs with different theoretical models (e.g., dynamic vs. cognitive-behavioral) have different effects. Research should also look at the relative cost-effectiveness of different treatments using follow-up data, and to the extent indicated, reimbursement policies should be changed accordingly. Another area that would benefit from research attention is how well the therapeutic alliance (and what type of alliance) predicts patients' subsequent benefits from treatment. Furthermore, increased research attention should focus on the intensive outpatient level of care (level II), a relatively new level that seems particularly promising for BPD patients. Finally, given the apparent differences in effective treatments for psychopathic and nonpsychopathic ASPD, research should continue to distinguish between these two groups when examining treatments for ASPD as well as begin to identify the extent to which the positive results found for specialized drug treatment programs (at all levels of care) are generalizable to other treatment programs for ASPD patients.

This chapter provides an overview of the structures and goals of different levels of care as well as their relative appropriateness for the treatment of different personality disorders. Attention to and consideration of personality disorder diagnosis will aid clinicians in determining the levels of care likely to be most effective and clinically indicated and should be used to inform treatment decisions. In particular, preliminary evidence suggests the value of using graduated, step-down levels of care, although more research is needed to determine the specific structure and timeline most likely to be effective within such a step-down system.

REFERENCES

Alden L: Short-term structured treatment for avoidant personality disorder. J Consult Clin Psychol 57:756–764, 1989

Barley WD, Buie SE, Peterson EW, et al: Development of an inpatient cognitive-behavioral treatment program for borderline personality disorder. J Personal Disord 7: 232–240, 1993

Bateman A, Fonagy P: Effectiveness of partial hospitalization in the treatment of borderline personality disorder: a randomized controlled trial. Am J Psychiatry 156:1563–1569, 1999

Bateman A, Fonagy P: Treatment of borderline personality disorder with psychoanalytically oriented partial hospitalization: an 18-month follow-up. Am J Psychiatry 158:36–42, 2001

Bateman A, Fonagy P: Psychotherapy for Borderline Personality Disorder. New York, Oxford University Press, 2004

Blum N, Pfohl B, St. John D, et al: STEPPS: a cognitive-behavioral systems-based group treatment for outpatients with borderline personality disorder. A preliminary report. Compr Psychiatry 43:301–310, 2002

Bohus M, Haaf B, Stiglmayr C, et al: Evaluation of inpatient dialectical behavior therapy for borderline personality disorder: a prospective study. Behav Res Ther 38:875–887, 2000

Brooner RK, Kidorf M, King VL, et al: Preliminary evidence of good treatment response in antisocial drug abusers. Drug Alcohol Depend 49:249–260, 1998

Cacciola JS, Alterman AI, Rutherford MJ, et al: Treatment response of antisocial substance abusers. J Nerv Ment Dis 183:166–171, 1995

Compton WM, Cottler LB, Spitznagel EL, et al: Cocaine users with antisocial personality improve HIV risk behaviors as much as those without antisocial personality. Drug Alcohol Depend 49:239–247, 1998

Dolan BM, Evans C, Wilson J: Therapeutic community treatment for personality disordered adults: changes in neurotic symptomatology on follow-up. Int J Soc Psychiatry 38:243–250, 1992

Dolan B, Warren F, Norton K: Change in borderline symptoms one year after therapeutic community treatment for severe personality disorder. Br J Psychiatry 171:274–279, 1997

Dolan-Sewell RT, Krueger RF, Shea MT: Co-occurrence with syndrome disorders, in Handbook of Personality Disorders: Theory, Research and Treatment. Edited by Livesley WJ. New York, Guilford, 2001, pp 84–104

Dyck IR, Phillips KA, Warshaw MG, et al: Patterns of personality pathology in patients with generalized anxiety disorders, panic disorder with and without agoraphobia, and social phobia. J Personal Disord 15:60–71, 2001

Fonagy P: Thinking about thinking: some clinical and theoretical considerations in the treatment of a borderline patient. Int J Psychoanal 72:1–18, 1991

Gabbard GO, Coyne L: Predictors of response of antisocial patients to hospital treatment. Hosp Community Psychiatry 38:1181–1185, 1987

Gabbard GO, Gunderson JG, Fonagy P: The place of psychoanalytic treatments within psychiatry. Arch Gen Psychiatry 59:505–510, 2002

Gude T, Vaglum P: One-year follow-up of patients with Cluster C personality disorders: a prospective study comparing patients with "pure" and "comorbid" conditions within Cluster C, and "pure" C with "pure" Cluster A or B conditions. J Personal Disord 15:216–228, 2001

Gunderson JG: Defining the therapeutic processes in psychiatric milieus. Psychiatry 41:327–335, 1978

Gunderson JG: Borderline Personality Disorder: A Clinical Guide. Washington, DC, American Psychiatric Press, 2001

Gunderson JG: Treatment of personality disorders: an overview. Paper presented at the annual meeting of the American Psychiatric Association, San Francisco, CA, May 2003

Gunderson JG, Gabbard GO: Making the case for psychoanalytic therapies in the current psychiatric world. J Am Psychoanal Assoc 47:679–703, 1999

Gunderson JG, Waldinger R, Sabo A: Stages of change in dynamic psychotherapy with borderline patients: clinical and research implications. J Psychother Pract Res 2:64–72, 1993

Gunderson JG, Morey LC, Stout RL, et al: Major depressive disorder and borderline personality disorder revisited: longitudinal interactions J Clin Psychiatry 65:1049–1056, 2004

Hardy GE, Barkham M, Shapiro DA, et al: Impact of Cluster C personality disorders on outcome of contrasting brief psychotherapies for depression. J Consult Clin Psychol 63:997–1004, 1995

Harris GT, Rice ME, Cormier CA: Psychopaths: is a therapeutic community therapeutic? Therapeutic Communities 15:283–299, 1994

Hart SD, Hare RD: Psychopathy: assessment and association with criminal conduct, in Handbook of Antisocial Behavior. Edited by Stoff DM, Breiling J, Maser JD. New York, Wiley, 1997, pp 22–35

Hildebrand M, de Ruiter C, Nijman H: PCL-R psychopathy predicts disruptive behavior among offenders in a Dutch forensic psychiatric hospital. J Interpers Violence 19:13–29, 2004

Hoglend P: Personality disorders and long-term outcome after brief dynamic psychotherapy. J Personal Disord 7:168–181, 1993

Howard KI, Kopta SM, Krause MS, et al: The dose-response relationship in psychotherapy. Am Psychol 41:159–164, 1986

Karterud S, Vaglum S, Friis S, et al: Day hospital therapeutic community treatment for patients with personality disorders: an empirical evaluation of the containment function. J Nerv Ment Dis 180:238–243, 1992

Karterud S, Pederson G, Bjordal E, et al: Day treatment of patients with personality disorders: experiences from a Norwegian treatment research network. J Personal Disord 17:243–262, 2003

Knight R: Evaluation of the results of psychoanalytic therapy. Am J Psychiatry 98:434–446, 1941

Koenigsberg HW, Kaplan RD, Gilmore MM, et al: The relationship between syndrome and personality disorder in DSM-III: experience with 2,464 patients. Am J Psychiatry 142:207–212, 1985

Koenigsberg HW, Anwunah I, New AS, et al: Relationship between depression and borderline personality disorder. Depress Anxiety 10:158–167, 1999

Kool S, Dekker J, Duijsens IJ, et al: Efficacy of combined therapy and pharmacotherapy for depressed patients with or without personality disorders. Harv Rev Psychiatry 11:133–141, 2003

Kopta SM, Howard KI, Lowry JL, et al: Patterns of symptomatic recovery in psychotherapy. J Clin Consult Psychol 62:1009–1016, 1994

Krawitz R: A prospective psychotherapy outcome study. Aust N Z J Psychiatry 31:465–473, 1997

Lanktree CB, Briere J: Outcome of therapy for sexual abused children: a repeated measures study. Child Abuse Negl 19:1145–1155, 1995

Leichsenring F, Leibing E: The effectiveness of psychodynamic therapy in the treatment of personality disorders: a meta-analysis. Am J Psychiatry 160:1223–1232, 2003

Levendusky PG, Willis BS, Ghinassi FA: The therapeutic contracting program: a comprehensive continuum of care model. Psychiatr Q 65:189–207, 1994

Linehan MM: Cognitive-Behavioral Treatment of Borderline Personality Disorder. New York, Guilford, 1993

Linehan MM, Armstrong HE, Suarez A, et al: Cognitive-behavioral treatment of chronically parasuicidal borderline patients. Arch Gen Psychiatry 48:1060–1064, 1991

Linehan MM, Heard HL, Armstrong HE: Naturalistic follow-up of a behavioral treatment for chronically parasuicidal borderline patients. Arch Gen Psychiatry 50:971–974, 1993

Linehan M, Tutek DA, Heard HL, et al: Interpersonal outcome of cognitive behavioral treatment for chronically suicidal borderline patients. Am J Psychiatry 151:1771–1776, 1994

Loranger AW: The impact of DSM-III on diagnostic practice in a university hospital. Arch Gen Psychiatry 47:672–675, 1990

Marziali E, Munroe-Blum H: An interpersonal approach to group psychotherapy with borderline personality disorder. J Personal Disord 9:179–189, 1995

Mehlum L, Friis S, Irion T, et al: Personality disorders 2–5 years after treatment: a prospective follow-up study. Acta Psychiatr Scand 84:72–77, 1991

Messina NP, Wish ED, Nemes S: Therapeutic community treatment for substance abusers with antisocial personality disorder. J Subst Abuse Treat 17:121–128, 1999

Messina NP, Wish ED, Hoffman JA, et al: Antisocial personality disorder and therapeutic community treatment outcomes. Am J Drug Alcohol Abuse 28:197–212, 2002

Messina N, Farabee D, Rawson R: Treatment responsivity of cocaine-dependent patients with antisocial personality disorder to cognitive-behavioral and contingency management interventions. J Consult Clin Psychol 71:320–329, 2003

Munroe-Blum H, Marziali E: A controlled trial of short-term group treatment for borderline personality disorder. J Personal Disord 9:190–198, 1995

Ogloff JR, Wong S, Greenwood A: Treating criminal psychopaths in a therapeutic community program. Behav Sci Law 8:181–190, 1990

Oldham JM, Skodol AE, Kellman HD, et al: Comorbidity of Axis I and Axis II disorders. Am J Psychiatry 152:571–578, 1995

Perry JC, Bond M: Empirical studies of psychotherapy for personality disorders, in Psychotherapy for Personality Disorders. Edited by Gunderson JG, Gabbard GO (Review of Psychiatry Series, Vol 19; Oldham JM and Riba MB, series eds). Washington, DC, American Psychiatric Press, 2000, pp 1–31

Quaytman M, Scharfstein SS: Treatment for severe borderline personality disorder in 1987 and 1997. Am J Psychiatry 154:1139–1144, 1997

Reiss D, Grubin D, Meux C: Institutional performance of male "psychopaths" in a high-security hospital. Journal of Forensic Psychiatry 10:290–299, 1999

Rice ME, Harris GT, Cormier CA: An evaluation of maximum security therapeutic community for psychopaths and other disordered offenders. Law Hum Behav 16:399–412, 1992

Richards HJ, Casey JO, Lucente SW: Psychopathy and treatment response in incarcerated female substance abusers. Crim Justice Behav 30:251–276, 2003

Salekin RT: Psychopathy and therapeutic pessimism: clinical lore or clinical reality? Clin Psychol Rev 22:79–112, 2002

Shea MT, Glass DR, Pilkonis PA, et al: Frequency and implications of personality disorders in a sample of depressed inpatients. J Personal Disord 1:27–41, 1987

Silk KR, Eisner W, Allport C, et al: Focused time-limited inpatient treatment of borderline personality disorder. J Personal Disord 8:268–278, 1994

Smith G, Ruis-Sancho A, Gunderson JG: An intensive outpatient program for patients with borderline personality disorder. Psychiatr Serv 52:532–533, 2001

Soloff PH: Algorithm for pharmacological treatment of personality dimensions: symptom-specific treatments for cognitive-perceptual, affective and impulsive-behavioral dysregulation. Bull Menninger Clin 62:195–214, 1998

Stevenson J, Meares R: An outcome study of psychotherapy for patients with borderline personality disorder. Am J Psychiatry 149:358–362, 1992

Tyrer P, Simmonds S: Treatment models for those with severe mental illness and comorbid personality disorder. Br J Psychiatry 182:44(suppl):15–18, 2003

Tyrer P, Gunderson JG, Lyons M, et al: Special feature: extent of comorbidity between mental state and personality disorders. J Personal Disord 11:242–259, 1997

Vaglum P, Friis S, Irion T, et al: Treatment response of severe and nonsevere personality disorders in a therapeutic community day unit. J Personal Disord 4:161–172, 1990

Van der Sande R, van Rooijen L, Buskens E, et al: Intensive in-patient and community intervention versus routine care after attempted suicide: a randomised controlled intervention study. Br J Psychiatry 171:35–41, 1997

Waldinger RJ, Gunderson JG: Effective Psychotherapy with Borderline Patients: Case Studies. Washington, DC, American Psychiatric Press, 1989

Widiger TA, Corbitt EM: Antisocial personality disorder, in DSM-IV Source Book, Vol 2. Edited by Widiger TA, Frances AJ, Pincus HA. Washington, DC, American Psychiatric Association, 1996, pp 703–716

Widiger TA, Weissman MM: Epidemiology of borderline personality disorder. Hosp Community Psychiatry 42:1015–1021, 1991

Wilberg T, Friis S, Karterud S, et al: Outpatient group psychotherapy: a valuable continuation treatment for patients with borderline personality disorder treated in a day hospital. A 3-year follow-up study. Nord J Psychiatry 52:213–221, 1998a

Wilberg T, Karterud S, Urnes O, et al: Outcomes of poorly functioning patients with personality disorders in a day treatment program. Psychiatr Serv 49:1562–1467, 1998b

Wilberg T, Urnes O, Friis S, et al: One-year follow-up of day treatment for poorly functioning patients with personality disorders. Psychiatr Serv 50:1326–1330, 1999

Winnicott DW: The Maturational Process and the Facilitating Environment. London, Hogarth Press, 1965

Winston A, Laikin M, Pollack J, et al: Short-term psychotherapy of personality disorders. Am J Psychiatry 151:190–194, 1994

16

Psychoanalysis

Glen O. Gabbard, M.D.

The field of psychoanalysis emerged in the last decade of the nineteenth century as a means of treatment for hysterical symptoms. However, in a relatively short time the focus of psychoanalysis shifted toward long-standing character pathology. As early as 1908, Freud was inaugurating that shift when he wrote his classic paper on "Character and Anal Eroticism" (Freud 1908/1959). Freud linked specific character traits, such as miserliness, obstinancy, and orderliness, with the anal psychosexual stage of development. Whereas he regarded neurotic symptoms as reflecting the return of repressed unconscious material, he viewed character traits as the end result of the successful use of repression as well as other defenses such as sublimation and reaction formation. As he moved in the direction of the structural model, he became aware that identification was of great importance in the formation of character. He recognized that some people can give up a lost object only by identifying with the lost person, suggesting that one seminal aspect of the development of personality is identification with parents and others in the course of development.

Freud's work was expanded by Karl Abraham (1923/1948) when he developed a system of classifying character traits according to their linkage with oral, anal, and genital eroticism. However, it was Wilhelm Reich (1931) who was the true trailblazer in the psychoanalytic understanding of character. He developed the term *character armor* to describe the unconscious and ego-syntonic defensive style of patients who come to analytic treatment. He postulated that childhood conflicts were mastered with specific defense mechanisms. These defenses subsequently emerged in the psychoanalytic setting in the way patients entered the office, reclined on the couch, related to the analyst, and resisted the psychoanalytic process. Although neurotic symptoms were regarded as compromise formations that produced distress, Reich stressed that character traits were rarely sources of anxiety or emotional pain. This distinction continues into the present, when clinicians often remark how the character traits in patients with personality disorders often cause more distress in others than in the patient. However, this generalization understates the great extent to which many people with personality disorders suffer as a result of their character pathology.

CONCEPTUAL MODEL

Contemporary psychoanalysis is primarily geared to address character. The symptomatic neuroses of

Freud's day are rare in today's clinical setting. Analysts focus on how distortions of self, compromises between wishes and defenses that oppose those wishes, and internal representations of self and others have forged the patient's personality (Gabbard 2000b).

Moreover, the psychoanalysts who treat personality disorders today must be biologically informed (Gabbard 2001). There is now abundant evidence that some personality traits are heritable (Cloninger et al. 1993; Livesley et al. 1993; Svrakic et al. 1993). The psychobiological model of Cloninger et al. (1993), for example, suggests that about 50% of personality is genetically based temperament, whereas another 50% is environmentally based character. These investigators stressed that the character variables, based on interactions with family members and peer groups, traumatic experiences, intrapsychic fantasy, and the cultural setting in which one develops, are highly influential in determining the subtype of personality disorder. Although not everyone agrees with this particular model, psychoanalysts must accept the limitations of the treatment they undertake. Genetically based temperament is unlikely to be altered by psychoanalytic efforts, but the areas of self-development, internal object relations, and the patient's effectiveness in coping with the environment may be profoundly affected by psychoanalysis. Temperament is highly stable over time, whereas the character dimensions tend to be malleable and undergo development throughout life (Svrakic et al. 1993).

From a psychoanalytic perspective, personality can be viewed as having five major components: 1) a biologically based temperament, 2) a set of internalized object relations, 3) an enduring sense of self, 4) a specific constellation of defense mechanisms, and 5) a characteristic cognitive style. Analysts would regard the achievement of a stable and positive sense of self and the establishment of mutually gratifying and enduring relationships as perhaps the two fundamental tasks of personality development (Blatt and Ford 1994). These two fundamental features of character evolve in a synergistic and dialectical relationship throughout the life cycle. Blatt (1992; Blatt and Ford 1994) has stressed that character pathology often divides into two broad subgroups: the *anaclitic* type is mainly concerned with relationships with others, and these individuals have longings to be nurtured, protected, and loved. The *introjective* subtype, on the other hand, is primarily focused on self-development, and these individuals struggle with feelings of unworthiness, failure, and inferiority. They are highly self-critical, exceedingly perfectionistic, and competitive.

Because the work of psychoanalysis is heavily influenced by transference and countertransference developments in the treatment process, psychoanalytic clinicians tend to place a great deal of emphasis on how the patient's internal object relations are externalized in interpersonal relationships with others. The psychoanalytic setting is seen as a laboratory in which analysts can directly observe how their patients recreate their internal object world in the relationships they forge in the course of their daily lives. Hence, psychoanalysts tend to conceptualize the nature of the patient's psychopathology less in terms of DSM-IV-TR (American Psychiatric Association 2000) criteria and more in terms of what unfolds in the analytic relationship (Gabbard 1997a, 2001).

The character dimension of personality is usefully conceptualized as involving an ongoing attempt to actualize certain patterns of relatedness that largely reflect unconscious wishes. Through interpersonal behavior, patients try to impose on the analyst a particular way of responding and experiencing. Character traits, therefore, must be viewed as playing a fundamental role in actualizing an internal object relationship that is central to a wish-fulfilling fantasy in the patient (Sandler 1981). The key to understanding the patient's relationships outside the analysis, then, may be the observation of what develops in the transference-countertransference dimensions of the analytic process.

Developmental themes are at the heart of all psychoanalytic theories. Part of the conceptual model of personality disorders assumes that a child internalizes a self-representation in interaction with an object representation connected by an affect state. If, for example, a father repeatedly yells at his son, the child internalizes an object relations unit involving a critical, angry object, an inadequate and beleaguered self, and an affect of shame and smoldering resentment. At other times, when the father praises his son, the little boy may internalize a loving and admiring object, a good and praiseworthy self, and an affect state of glowing self-regard. These interactions are etched in neural networks and become repetitive patterns of relatedness (Westen and Gabbard 2002). The psychoanalyst understands the psychoanalytic setting as one in which patients attempt to re-create their internal object relationships through the externalization of these relatedness patterns formed in childhood.

The wish-fulfilling nature of actualizing internal object relationships is clear in the example of an internal self wishing to be loved and admired by an internal object. The wish is less apparent in those patients who establish one conflictual and self-defeating relationship after another. However, even a "bad" or tormenting object may provide safety and affirmation to a patient for a variety of reasons (Gabbard 2001; Sandler 1981). For abused children, for example, an abusive relationship may be safe in the sense that it is preferable to having no object at all or to being abandoned. A basic paradoxical situation arises in the lives of abused children, where the person to whom they look for safety and protection is also the abuser. They may have no alternative, then, but to seek safety in the shadow of one who has abused them. They may also assume that the only way of remaining connected to a significant figure of safety is to maintain an abuser–victim paradigm in the relationship. These relationships may be sought out by patients who were abused as children because they are reliable, predictable, and provide the patient with an ongoing sense of continuity and meaning. The devil one knows is generally perceived as better than the devil one does not know.

Some of the repetitive relationship patterns seen in patients with personality disorder are approximations of actual relationships these individuals had with real figures in the past. However, in some cases they involve wished-for relationships that never actually existed. Patients with severe childhood trauma, for example, often develop elaborate fantasies about a rescuer who will save them from abuse.

The mode of actualization within the analytic relationship is often referred to as projective identification (Gabbard 1995; Ogden 1979). Within this model, patients behave in a characterologically driven way that exerts interpersonal pressure on the analyst to conform to what is being projected onto him or her. In other words, a patient may "nudge" the analyst into assuming the role of an abuser in response to the patient's "victim" role. A patient who treats the analyst with contempt, for example, may engender countertransference anger or hate and lead the analyst to make sarcastic or devaluing comments to the patient.

Case Example

A patient with narcissistic personality disorder had been in analysis for 5 weeks with a young analytic candidate. The patient began one session by complaining about the analyst's relative youth. He asserted that the analyst seemed to be a beginner who probably did not know what he was doing. "Am I your first analytic case?" he taunted. The candidate replied, "What makes you ask that?" The patient laughed and said, "I'll bet your supervisor told you not to answer my questions, right?" The candidate, feeling he was being treated with contempt, became

defensive and said, "No, I'm able to think for myself." The patient responded with further contempt, "I don't see much evidence of that." Without considering the potential consequences of his comment, the analyst blurted out, "Maybe you're too busy insulting me to notice." As soon as the words came out of his mouth, the candidate felt a deep sense of shame. He had allowed himself to be nudged into sarcasm by the patient's contempt.

In this model the patient's self-representation elicits a corresponding object representation in the analyst. This model of character is closely related to the role relationship model of Horowitz (1988, 1991, 1998). In his theory, a person's schemas reflect unconscious self-other organizational units. These units are driven by powerful internal motives that lead away from feared outcomes and toward desired ends. Another way to view these schemas is as belief structures that have both form and content. They are often characterized, however, by conflicting desires and beliefs that become expressed in the transference relationship with the analyst.

In addition to the development of self in relation to objects in the formation of character, a psychoanalyst studies the unique set of defense mechanisms found in each patient as a key to diagnostic understanding and treatment. Defenses ward off awareness of unpleasant affect states and unacceptable aggressive or sexual wishes and preserve a sense of self-esteem in the face of narcissistic vulnerability. They may also serve to ensure safety when one is feeling threatened. A contemporary analytic perspective, however, would recognize that defense mechanisms do not merely change the relationship between an emotional state and an idea. They also influence the relationship between self and object (Vaillant and Vaillant 1999). Patients may be able to manage unresolved conflicts with important figures in their lives or with old objects from the past that haunt them in the present through the use of defenses. In patients with personality disorder for whom relationship difficulties are one of the major reasons for seeking treatment, analysts conceptualize defenses as embedded in relatedness. Vaillant and Vaillant (1999) emphasized that the symptoms of patients with personality disorder often are designed to cope with unbearable relationships or unbearable people, whether in the present or in the past.

Psychoanalysts would view the specific constellation of defenses that work in concert with characteristic patterns of object relations as having enormous importance for the diagnostic understanding of the patient. For example, someone with obsessive-compulsive personality disorder (OCPD) would use defensive operations such as reaction formation, intellectualization, undoing, and isolation of affect (Gabbard 2000c). These defenses tone down powerful affect states so that the patient is not in danger of losing control. These patients may be responsible, dutiful, and unfailingly courteous toward the analyst to be sure that no trace of aggression is revealed in their analytic interactions.

The fifth component of character—cognitive style—is intimately related to the patient's characteristic defenses. Persons with OCPD, for example, will come across as lacking flexibility and spontaneity in their thought processes because they are directed toward the control of all affect states. They will also address every detail of a situation in their pursuit of a perfect solution. Histrionic personality disorder patients, on the other hand, have a cognitive style that is directly linked to their excessive emotionality. Hence they avoid detail and will give impressionistic and global responses to questions that reflect the "feel" of a situation. These cognitive styles appear to be reasonably consistent across personality types (Shapiro 1965).

MAJOR PRINCIPLES OF TECHNIQUE

Psychoanalysis is traditionally conducted in 45- to 50-minute sessions four or five times a week and may last for several years. Most patients recline on the analyst's couch, although some prefer to sit for parts of the treatment when visual contact with the analyst is seen as necessary. The patient is asked to say whatever comes to mind in an effort to facilitate the process of free association. Patients generally have difficulty saying what comes to mind because of anxieties about what the analyst will think as well as shame about certain aspects of themselves that they find unacceptable.

The difficulties encountered in lying on a couch and saying whatever comes to mind four or five times a week inevitably lead to the development of transference and resistance, two of the major foci of psychoanalytic treatment. Resistance is not simply the reluctance to say what comes to mind. It is also a manifestation of the patients' unique defense mechanisms as they enter into the treatment process. In other words, defenses are intrapsychic mechanisms, but they become interpersonalized as resistances in the relationship with the analyst (Gabbard 2000c). Resistance also reveals significant internal object relationships. A contemporary view of resistances would include the fact that they are forces that oppose the optimal state of consciousness sought

in analysis. In an ideal analytic process, patients develop a dual consciousness in which they relive certain experiences from their past in the transference to the analyst while also reflecting on those experiences and being curious about their meanings and origins (Friedman 1991).

Psychoanalysts view resistances not simply as obstacles to be avoided but as a major source of significant information about patients' characteristic defensive operations and their deeply ingrained personality traits. Analysts no longer spend most of their time in an archeological search for buried relics from the patient's past. Contemporary analysts focus more on the relationship between analyst and patient as a privileged view of how the patient's past has created certain patterns of conflict and problematic object relations in the present. In his 1914 paper, "Remembering, Repeating, and Working-Through," Freud (1914/1958) noted that what the patient cannot remember will be repeated in action in the patient's here-and-now behavior with the analyst, the original meaning of the term *acting-out*. Hence the patient's characterological pattern of internal object relations and the conflicts about those relationships unfold in front of the analyst without necessarily digging into childhood traumas to unlock hidden secrets.

While transference reflects the patient's past experiences with similar figures, it also incorporates the *real* aspects of the analyst. Hence transference is now considered to be a mixture of old relationships from the past and the new and real relationship with the analyst in the present. In other words, if an analyst chooses to be aloof, silent, and emotionally remote, the patient may well develop a transference to the analyst as a cold and unfeeling figure.

As the patient repeats long-standing patterns of relatedness during the sessions, the analyst is gradually drawn into a "dance." Through the process of projective identification described earlier, the analyst is transformed into a transference object. Not all analysts will react in the same way, and the specific features of the analyst's intrapsychic world will work in concert with what is being projected by the patient to shape the unique form of the analyst's countertransference. Some analysts may ignore the role being thrust on them or reject it. Others may defend against the role by assuming an opposite stance. Some analysts who are being pressured to take on the characteristics of a projected abusive object, for example, may become overly kind and empathic as a reaction formation to their growing feelings of sadism or anger.

In any case, a key aspect of the psychoanalytic treatment of patients with personality disorders is to maintain a free-floating responsiveness (Sandler 1981) to what is being evoked by the patient and to use this re-created "dance" as a way of understanding the patient's usual mode of object relatedness outside the treatment situation. When the role being evoked by the patient is unfamiliar and distressing to the analyst, such as the role of an abusive parent, some analysts may feel that an alien force has taken them over, and their subjective experience may be something along the lines of "I'm not behaving like myself" (Gabbard 2001). If the wished-for interaction being actualized by the patient is that of an idealized parent who is nurturing and understanding toward a needy child, the analyst may feel quite comfortable in the role and be unaware of its countertransference origins. One of the key components of technique, then, is for the analyst to clarify the nature of these unconscious relational patterns, acknowledging that they are jointly created, and then make them understandable to the patient. Transference-countertransference enactments may need to repeat themselves a number of times before they are apparent and can be interpreted to the patient.

Analysts listen to the development of themes in the associations of the patient. They carefully track patterns in the transference relationship that also emerge in narrative accounts of the patient's life in the present and in the past. As recurrent themes emerge, they begin to make these unconscious patterns more available to the patient's conscious awareness. A primary intervention is interpretation, which seeks to make connections or linkages for the patient that are largely outside the patient's awareness. The following case example will illustrate.

Case Example

Mr. K was a 24-year-old graduate student who was struggling in his academic setting because he appeared to be threatened by success. He had all of the primary symptoms of OCPD, and his highly perfectionistic expectations of himself led him to feel that he was always failing. In the course of the analysis, he talked at great length about what a harsh taskmaster his father had been and how he was never able to live up to what his father expected of him. Eventually this pattern emerged in the transference, when the patient revealed that he feared that his analyst saw him as a failure as well. He felt the analyst was heavily invested in having him succeed in graduate school, and the patient was feeling that he could not possibly measure up to what his analyst expected. The analyst drew his attention to how he had re-created with the analyst the same relationship he had with his father. The patient could readily see the connection, and he thanked the analyst for pointing it out. However, the analyst also recognized that the patient's deferential and ingratiating quality was a reaction formation to a good deal of resentment about feeling driven by others to succeed. The analyst thus interpreted that the patient had found a way to indirectly express his resentment at both his analyst and his father by thwarting their perceived hopes for his success in graduate school. By failing to pass his oral examinations, he could have the fantasy of making his dad and his analyst suffer. Eventually the analyst was also able to point out to Mr. K that his graduate student advisor, another male about the age of his father, was also part of this same pattern of relatedness. Through interpretation, the analyst made the patient aware that he had placed this paternal figure in the same role as his father and his analyst.

Depending on the nature of the psychopathology, some patients are more suited for interpretation of conflict-based pathology than others. Patients with deficit-based pathology have often had extensive childhood deprivation or trauma. They may hear interpretations as attacks and feel shamed by them. In those situations, the analyst may need to use affirmative interventions (Killingmo 1989) that confirm exactly the way the patient is feeling and empathically validate the patient's right to feel that way. Many patients with this type of background may ultimately be able to use interpretations if the way is paved for them by validating and affirming interventions (Gabbard et al. 1994).

The goals of the treatment vary according to the patient's presenting complaints and the analyst's theoretical model. Among those goals that are commonly established are resolution of conflict (Brenner 1976); a search for an authentic or *true self*, as Winnicott (1962) suggested; improved relationships as a result of a gain in understanding about one's internal object relationships (Gabbard 1996); an improved capacity to seek out appropriate selfobjects (Kohut 1984); the generation of new meanings within the therapeutic dialogue (Mitchell 1997); and an improved capacity for mentalization (Fonagy and Target 1996). (*Selfobjects* and *mentalization* are defined and discussed later in the chapter.) Regardless of the diverse goals, all analytic treatment probably works through several modes of therapeutic action, of which one is the provision of insight through interpretation.

Another mode of therapeutic action is simply making observations from an outside perspective on what one sees in the patient (Gabbard 1997b). Patients cannot know how they come across to others because they are inside themselves. The analyst has the perspective of an object and therefore can help them see things that they do not see. Moreover, the "how to" of relatedness that is internalized in the earliest childhood relationships is embedded in implicit procedural memory (Gabbard and Westen 2003). Analysts can see the automatic and unconscious patterns of relatedness in action and help the patient become aware of these patterns. An analyst may observe, for example, that the patient looks ashamed whenever talking about his mother and will thus point that out to the patient. Fonagy (1999) stresses that a crucial avenue for therapeutic change may lie in a patient's increasing capacity to "find himself" in the therapist's mind. By consistently observing and commenting on the patient's feeling states and nonverbal communications, the patient may begin to assemble a portrait of himself or herself based on the analyst's observation and thereby develop increased capacity for mentalization. Consistent observations about the characterological patterns of the patient also make ego-syntonic character traits more ego-dystonic as the patient recognizes the problematic aspects of the traits as well as the interpersonal impact that the traits have on others.

In all forms of psychoanalysis, another source of therapeutic action is internalization of the analyst and the analytic relationship. Internalizing does not necessarily require the use of a conscious, declarative representation. The analytic relationship itself is accompanied by unconscious affective connections that have been referred to by Lyons-Ruth et al. (1998) as *implicit relational knowing*. This phenomenon refers to moments of meeting between analyst and patient that are not symbolically represented or dynamically unconscious in the ordinary sense. Some change occurs in the realm of procedural knowledge involving how to act, feel, and think in a particular relational context. As patients internalize the analyst's accepting and tolerant attitude, their superego is also modified so they are less self-critical and more accepting of their humanness.

From a cognitive neuroscience perspective, the internalization of the analytic relationship gradually builds a new neural network with a different type of object representation and a corresponding self-representation. The old networks are not completely obliterated by the analytic treatment, but they are relatively weakened or deactivated while the new networks based on the analytic relationship are strengthened (Gabbard and Westen 2003).

All of these techniques and modes of therapeutic action are adapted to the individual patient and the type of personality disorder that most closely fits that patient. There is inevitably a trial-and-error component to this approach as one finds out which types of interventions are most suited to the patient's capacity to use psychoanalytic treatment.

RESEARCH

Randomized, controlled trials of psychoanalysis for personality disorders do not exist. The Research Committee of the International Psychoanalytical Association prepared a comprehensive review of the studies of psychoanalytic treatment carried out in North America and in Europe (Fonagy et al. 2002). The existing studies have significant limitations, including failure to use standardized diagnoses, failure to control for selection biases and sampling, the absence of analyses of subjects who joined the study but later dropped out (intent to treat), inadequate description of treatment procedures, little homogeneity in patient groups, the use of inexperienced therapists, the lack of random assignment, the lack of treatment manualization, and lack of statistical power (Gabbard et al. 2002). Nevertheless, 66 investigations are reviewed, and whenever effectiveness is fairly assessed, psychoanalysis produces effect sizes equal to those of other therapeutic approaches.

A growing body of research confirms that psychodynamic psychotherapy approaches derived from psychoanalysis are efficacious, both in the form of brief psychodynamic therapy (Anderson and Lambert 1995) and in the form of long-term psychoanalytic psychotherapy (Leichsenring and Leibing 2003). Some of these latter studies are randomized, controlled trials suggesting that the psychoanalytic approach is useful in the treatment of severe personality disorders when modified in psychotherapeutic versions.

The paucity of randomized, controlled trials of psychoanalysis with patients with personality disorder reflects the formidable challenges faced by psychoanalytic researchers (Gabbard et al. 2002). Psychoanalysis is a lengthy and expensive treatment that by its nature does not lend itself to random assignment. Moreover, the nature of a suitable control for a treatment that lasts several years is highly problematic. In addition, the sheer cost of a study ranging over so many years would be prohibitive in the current climate of research funding. Whereas in a 16-week trial of brief psychotherapy, a 10% dropout rate would not significantly affect statistical analysis, a 10% dropout rate every several months over a multiyear trial of psychoanalytic treatment could be disastrous for demonstrating statistical power. Finally, intermittent life events, such as death, serious illness, divorce, bankruptcy, and other major stressors come into play much more in an investigation involving several years of treatment as compared with one of several months. These challenges and others have made it difficult to collect rigorous efficacy data on psychoanalysis of patients with personality disorders.

INDICATIONS AND CONTRAINDICATIONS

In determining for whom psychoanalysis is indicated, two separate but related perspectives are necessary: 1) suitability according to the psychological characteristics of the patient, and 2) suitability according to diagnoses. Regardless of whether a patient meets diagnostic criteria for a specific personality disorder, the patient's psychological features may contraindicate the use of psychoanalysis.

Foremost among the psychological characteristics necessary to recommend psychoanalysis is psychological-mindedness. Although there are various components to this construct, the key components are the capacity to see meaningful connections between one's difficulties and one's inner world. The capacity to think in terms of analogy and metaphor is also crucial to psychological-mindedness. In addition, there must be a curiosity about the origins of one's suffering and a strong motivation to endure anxiety and discomfort in the process of learning more about oneself.

Another feature that is necessary for analytic work is the capacity to regress in the service of the ego. Patients must be able to let down their guard, relax their defenses, and get in touch with primitive and unpleasant emotional states to learn about what drives them to behave or think in the way they do. They must also have high tolerance for frustration, intact reality testing, reasonably good impulse control, and enough suffering to motivate them for the treatment.

Other signs of ego strength that make a person a reasonable candidate for psychoanalysis are the ability to sustain a job over a long period of time despite encountering difficulties and the capacity for enduring meaningful relationships with others. Finally, the presence of the capacity for mentalization based on secure attachment also is a positive sign for analyzability. *Mentalization* refers to one's ability to differentiate inner from outer states and to recognize that one's perceptions are only representations rather than accurate replicas of external reality. In other words, the patient is aware that his own and other people's ways of viewing the world are influenced by inner beliefs, feelings, and past experiences. This capacity may be present to a greater or lesser extent and exists on a continuum

that is influenced by the nature of the relationship and the patient's early experience. Some patients with impaired mentalization may nevertheless be amenable to psychoanalysis (Fonagy 2001).

Patients in a severe life crisis are rarely suited for psychoanalysis, although it may ultimately be appropriate after the crisis is over. Other contraindications are poor reality testing, poor impulse control, lack of psychological-mindedness, little capacity for self-observation, cognitive impairment based on neurological dysfunction, extreme concreteness, and poor frustration tolerance (Gabbard 2004). These guidelines are helpful in assessing analyzability, but analysts recognize that they must retain a certain degree of humility because prediction of how a particular patient will do in the psychoanalytic process is less than perfect. Kantrowitz (1987), in a study of 22 patients in analysis, concluded that even with highly sophisticated psychological testing, clinicians cannot reliably predict who will do well in psychoanalysis. The following sections describe the indications and contraindications for psychoanalysis in patients with specific personality disorders.

Determining the appropriateness of psychoanalysis is also influenced by one's diagnostic understanding of the personality disorder, but this method, too, is imperfect in predicting outcomes. In the absence of randomized controlled trials of psychoanalytic treatment for the various personality disorders, clinicians must rely on clinical wisdom and the psychological characteristics favoring analyzability described above. Moreover, the presence of various comorbid conditions on Axis I, such as affective disorder, anxiety disorder, eating disorder, or substance abuse may complicate psychoanalytic treatment even if the personality disorder itself is likely to be amenable to this approach. As a general principle, the Cluster C personality disorders appear to be amenable to psychoanalysis. Only a very small subgroup of patients with Cluster A personality disorders are likely to respond well to psychoanalytic efforts. Those patients with Cluster B personality disorders respond variably, depending on the diagnosis and the psychological characteristics.

Paranoid Personality Disorder

In a study of 100 patients who applied for psychoanalysis at the Columbia Psychoanalytic Center, Oldham and Skodol (1994) noted that 12 met research criteria for the diagnosis of paranoid personality disorder. Of those, only four were selected for analysis, and two of the four did not finish the analytic treatment. Their data suggested that most patients with paranoid personality disorder are not suited, but for a very small number with exceptional characteristics analysis may be worth a try. In general, paranoid patients do not have sufficient trust to allow for the development of an analytic process.

Schizoid and Schizotypal Personality Disorders

Schizotypal personality disorder is thought to be genetically linked with schizophrenia, and patients with schizotypal personality disorder are rarely, if ever, suitable for psychoanalysis. Schizoid patients, on the other hand, may in some cases be appropriate for analytic treatment but rarely seek it. In the study by Oldham and Skodol (1994), only one person applying for psychoanalysis was diagnosed with schizoid personality disorder. The British psychoanalytic literature suggests that there may be a small number of patients who can be reached by psychoanalytic approaches, and a number of British analysts have reported on work with these patients (Balint 1979; Fairbairn 1954; Winnicott 1963/1965).

Borderline Personality Disorder

After surveying the entire literature on the treatment of borderline personality disorder, the American Psychiatric Association practice guideline concluded that psychotherapy, rather than psychoanalysis, in concert with medication, is probably the treatment of choice for the great majority of patients with borderline personality disorder. Problems of impulsivity and difficulties in maintaining a therapeutic alliance make psychoanalytic treatment extremely challenging for patients in this category. There are reports in the literature (Abend et al. 1983; Boyer 1977; Fonagy and Target 1996; Gabbard 1991) of patients with borderline pathology who were analyzed using the couch with somewhat modified forms of psychoanalytic technique. Borderline patients who can use an analytic process represent a very small subgroup and are probably closer to the Kernberg construct of borderline personality organization (Kernberg 1975) than a DSM-IV-TR borderline personality disorder. These patients are often conceptualized as part of the "widening scope" of psychoanalysis and generally require supportive interventions to make interpretation acceptable to the patient (Horwitz et al. 1996).

Narcissistic Personality Disorder

Most experts in the treatment of narcissistic personality disorder agree that psychoanalysis is the treatment of choice if the patient has the psychological and financial resources to undertake a commitment to psychoanalysis. Although the treatments are long and arduous, sometimes nothing short of this in-depth approach will touch a patient.

Antisocial Personality Disorder

Because of lack of motivation, insufficient superego development, general dishonesty, and impulsivity, patients with antisocial personality disorder represent a contraindication to psychoanalysis.

Histrionic and Hysterical Personality Disorders

The DSM-IV-TR construct of histrionic personality disorder represents a particular type of patient with personality disorder who is very close to the borderline diagnosis. In clinical practice, one frequently encounters a higher level of histrionic personality disorder that has traditionally been referred to as hysterical personality disorder (Gabbard 2000c). These patients represent a neurotically organized individual with reasonably good impulse control, mature triangular object relations, and an intact superego. Therefore, they are considered good candidates for psychoanalysis, whereas patients on the other end of the spectrum with histrionic personality disorder may require modified versions of psychoanalytic psychotherapy because they often cannot tolerate the intense affective states that are brought about in analytic treatment. Some histrionic patients, however, appear to be able to make use of psychoanalysis.

Obsessive-Compulsive Personality Disorder

Patients with OCPD, who must be differentiated from those with obsessive-compulsive disorder, are generally good candidates for psychoanalysis. In fact, psychoanalysis may be the treatment of choice.

Avoidant Personality Disorder

Some patients with avoidant personality disorder appear to respond well to behavioral or cognitive-behavioral techniques (Alden 1989; Brown et al. 1995; Stravynski et al. 1982). However, when patients do not respond to brief behavioral or cognitive-behavioral treatments for avoidant personality disorder, they may do well in analysis, particularly if they are motivated to understand the origins of their anxieties about intimate relationships with others.

Table 16–1. Indications and contraindications for psychoanalysis according to personality disorder diagnosis

Diagnosis	Suitability for psychoanalysis
Paranoid personality disorder	Rarely indicated
Schizoid personality disorder	May be indicated in exceptional circumstances
Schizotypal personality disorder	Contraindicated
Borderline personality disorder	Generally contraindicated except for a small group of higher-level borderline patients with exceptional strengths
Narcissistic personality disorder	Strong indication for psychoanalysis
Antisocial personality disorder	Contraindicated
Histrionic/hysterical personality disorders	Strongly indicated for hysterical personality disorders, but only occasionally indicated for histrionic personality disorder
Obsessive-compulsive personality disorder	Strong indication for psychoanalysis
Avoidant personality disorder	Indicated for cases that do not respond to brief cognitive-behavioral or behavior therapy treatments
Dependent personality disorder	Likely to do well in psychoanalysis if motivation is sufficient
Masochistic or self-defeating personality disorder	Strong indication for psychoanalysis

Dependent Personality Disorder

Patients with dependent personality disorder may do well in either psychoanalysis or psychodynamic psychotherapy depending on their psychological-mindedness, the extent of their suffering, and their motivation to change and understand themselves.

Masochistic or Self-Defeating Personality Disorder

Although not in the official DSM-IV-TR nomenclature, patients with predominantly self-defeating or masochistic symptom patterns are widely seen in clinical practice. For most of these patients, psychoanalysis is the treatment of choice, provided they have the psychological characteristics necessary for the treatment.

The indications and contraindications for psychoanalysis according to personality disorder are summarized in Table 16–1.

PSYCHOANALYTIC APPROACHES TO SPECIFIC PERSONALITY DISORDERS

As noted above, the psychoanalyst's technique needs to be tailored to the specific type of personality disorder. Although most personality disorders are mixed, in that they have traits of several different personality disorders, here we consider each of the personality disorders

amenable to psychoanalysis in its pure form for the sake of clarity. In actual practice, several technical approaches may need to be combined for patients who have different personality features in mixed personality disorder. The discussion here is confined to those personality disorders that are likely to benefit from psychoanalytic approaches at least some of the time.

Schizoid Personality Disorder

Much of our understanding of the inner world of a schizoid patient derives from the work of the British object relations theorists. Balint (1979) viewed these patients as having a fundamental deficit in their ability to relate—a "basic fault" caused by significant inadequacies in the mothering they received as infants. He believed that the schizoid patient's difficulty in relating to others stems from this basic incapacity rather than from neurotic conflict. Fairbairn (1954), perhaps the foremost contributor to our understanding of schizoid patients, viewed the schizoid retreat from object relations as a defense against a conflict between a wish to relate to others and a fear that one's neediness would harm others. The child who initially perceives its mother as rejecting may withdraw from the world; however, the infant's greed and neediness grow until they are experienced as insatiable. The child then fears that its greed will devour the mother, resulting in her disappearance. Relationships are experienced as dangerous and to be avoided.

The analyst who endeavors to treat schizoid patients must recognize that their fear of relationships will manifest itself in the transference and allow the patient the opportunity to retreat without making demands for more active participation. Winnicott (1963/1965) believed that the isolation of the schizoid patient preserves an important authenticity that is absolutely sacred to the evolving self of the patient: "There is an intermediate stage in healthy development in which the patient's most important experience in relation to the good or potentially satisfying object is the refusal of it" (p. 182). Hence the analyst must recognize that the schizoid withdrawal is a way to communicate with the "true self" within the patient instead of sacrificing that authenticity to artificial interactions with others, including the analyst, that would lead to a "false self" adaptation.

Although patients with schizoid personality disorder do not commonly seek psychoanalytic help, when they do, the analyst must provide the patient with a holding environment in which their frozen internal object relations will eventually "thaw" through the provision of a new experience of relatedness. The goal of the psychoanalytic approach, then, is more to provide a new relationship for internalization than to interpret unconscious conflict. Extraordinary patience is required for the treatment to take effect, and the patient must be allowed to go at his or her own pace. Analysts must recognize that their own agenda for change may get in the way of the patient's timetable for venturing out into a world of potentially dangerous relationships.

Narcissistic Personality Disorder

The technical approaches to narcissistic personality disorder tend to diverge along a dividing line marked by whether the analyst views the pathology as based on deficit, according to the self psychology of Kohut (1971), or as related to conflict, as described by Kernberg (1974a, 1974b, 1984). The differences between the two approaches are summarized in Table 16–2.

Kohut's approach to the psychoanalysis of narcissistic personality disorders used empathy as the cornerstone of the technique (Ornstein 1974, 1998). Kohut stressed the need to empathize with the patient's experiences of having numerous empathic failures at the hands of parents. In this regard, he advised analysts to accept the patient's comments in a "straight" manner, just as the patient experiences them, rather than to interpret hidden meanings (Miller 1985). Kohut would accept this *idealizing transference* as a normal developmental need rather than interpreting what might lie beneath it. He viewed the mirror and idealizing trans-

ferences as the major developments in the analysis of narcissistic personality disorder. The *mirror transference* is an effort on the patient's part to capture the "gleam" in mother's eye by trying to impress the analyst. Sensitive to the patient's potential for self-fragmentation, Kohut would empathize with the patient's need to be affirmed and validated.

Kohut (1984) later postulated a third transference, the *twinship transference*. All three of these were regarded as the *selfobject* transferences typical of narcissistic personality disorders. The analysis of those transferences is the major part of the technical approach. Kohut also strongly endorsed calling attention to the positive aspects of the patient's experience to avoid shaming or criticizing the patient and repeating the traumas of childhood. He would not hesitate to call attention to the patient's progress. The goal of the analysis was to help the patient acquire more appropriate and mature selfobjects with the full recognition that the patient could not possibly outgrow the need for selfobject responses, such as idealization, affirmation, and validation.

Kernberg's (1974a, 1974b) approach differs in that he sees the patient's grandiose self as a highly pathological and conflict-based solution that is not to be regarded as simply an arrested development of the normal self. He regards idealization as a defense against rage, contempt, and envy, and he advocates active interpretation of idealization. In general, Kernberg's approach is more confrontational than Kohut's, and he stresses the patient's greed and demandingness rather than his or her longings for affirmation. He also focuses to a greater extent on envy and how it prevents the patient from acknowledging and receiving help. Whereas Kohut views resistances as healthy psychic activities designed to safeguard the self, Kernberg confronts and interprets resistances as defensive maneuvers. He would see the goal of psychoanalysis as much broader than Kohut's. He would hope that the patient would develop a greater sense of guilt and concern while integrating idealization and trust with rage and contempt.

In actual practice, many psychoanalysts use elements of both Kernberg and Kohut in their approach to narcissistic patients. An empathic perspective, as described by Kohut, is often extremely helpful early in the analysis to form a therapeutic alliance with the patient so that the patient is willing to explore his or her inner world. Over time, patients often are more capable of responding to interpretation and confrontation when they feel a stable relationship has been established with the analyst. Both Kohut and Kernberg

Table 16–2.   Psychoanalytic technique for narcissistic personality disorders: Kohut versus Kernberg

Kohut	Kernberg
Views mirror and idealizing transferences as two different poles of bipolar (Kohut 1977) or tripolar (Kohut 1984) self	Views mirror and idealizing as aspects of transference related to projection and reintrojection of patient's grandiose self
Accepts idealization of patient as normal developmental need	Interprets idealization as a defense
Empathizes with patient's feeling as an understandable reaction to failures of parents and others	Helps patient see his or her own contribution to problems in relationships
Accepts patient's comments at face value, viewing resistances as healthy psychic activities that safeguard the self	Confronts and interprets resistances as defensive maneuvers
Looks at the positive side of patient's experience	Examines both positive and negative aspects of patient's experience (if only positive experiences are emphasized, the patient may develop an increased fear of internal envy and rage)
Calls attention to patient's progress	Focuses on envy and how it prevents patient from acknowledging and receiving help
Has treatment goal of helping patient acquire ability to identify and seek out appropriate selfobjects	Has treatment goal of helping patient to develop guilt and concern and to integrate idealization and trust with rage and contempt

Source.   Based on Gabbard 2000c.

identify valid aspects of narcissistic pathology, but different types of narcissistic patients require different emphases.

Regardless of which technical strategy is chosen, analysts treating narcissistic patients encounter formidable countertransference difficulties. They often have a sense that they are being used as a sounding board rather than a person with a separate internal world. They may need to tolerate long periods in which they feel they are peripheral to the narcissistic patient's associations. They may also note that with the hypervigilant variety of narcissistic personality disorder (Gabbard 2000c), they feel coerced into focusing their attention completely on the patient during every moment of the session, and they may feel controlled into meeting the patient's unrealistic expectations of perfect attunement. If they fall short, they risk an explosion of narcissistic rage by a patient who sees a slight around every corner. Narcissistic patients may erupt with barrages of contempt and hatred when they feel they have not been given the attention they are due.

Hysterical/Histrionic Personality Disorders

Patients with hysterical personality disorder generally are ideal analytic patients. They have internalized conflicts about relationships that can be examined in a solid therapeutic alliance with the analyst. They are generally committed to change and to improving their chronic difficulties in forming intimate relationships. The analyst may need to focus initially on the global and impressionistic cognitive style that prevents these patients from reflecting in detail on what is happening inside. Their displays of emotionality can be highly appealing and lead the analyst to feel a sense of obligation to rescue the patient. Nevertheless, for the analyst to be useful, the patient first needs to provide more details of the situations that create distress.

Superficial and shallow feelings may defend against more disturbing and more deeply experienced affects. Patients may need assistance in identifying their true feelings and the thoughts and events linked to them. They often feel buffeted by powerful feeling states and by external events. The analyst can help them to identify patterns in their lives that lead to particular types of emotional responses. Horowitz (1977) pointed out that these patients start to develop new patterns of perceiving relationships when they attend in more detail to themselves and others in their personal context. The analyst helps them see how they play an active role in perpetuating certain patterns of relating to others. They develop a capacity to compare the actual facts in an interpersonal situation with the internal patterns they superimpose on external situations.

Hysterical patients generally work well within the transference and use it as a primary vehicle for change. They may see the solution to their problem as simple identification with the analyst, and the analyst needs to confront the wish to bypass painful self-examination in the service of identification with the analyst. They also may fall in love with the analyst and feel that a loving relationship is in itself curative. However, the transference love needs to be carefully deconstructed in terms of its multiple meanings. It functions not only as a resistance to a deepening of the analytic process but also as an indirect expression of aggression, because it may create a frustrating situation for both analyst and patient. Hysterical patients often find themselves in triangular relationships in which they constantly repeat an oedipal romance that places them in the role of the excluded party. This pattern of longing for an unavailable romantic partner deserves a good deal of scrutiny in the course of the analysis, as it often reveals conflicts about truly separating from parents and establishing a life with a partner outside the family unit. Women with hysterical personality disorder are often "Daddy's girls," whereas men with the diagnosis are often called "Mama's boys." This attachment to the opposite-sex parent may keep them in a state of extended adolescence that prevents them from coming fully into their own. The analyst must systemically analyze their loyalty conflicts of this nature.

Histrionic personality disorder is an entity that is related to the hysterical configuration, but the primitive defenses, overwhelming separation anxiety, and lax superego create difficulties when these patients enter analysis. Some may be able to tolerate the frustration of the analytic setting if they have high intelligence, some degree of impulse control, and an ability to mentalize. However, most patients with histrionic personality disorder have much in common with patients who have borderline personality disorder and lack the requisite ego strengths to tolerate the process. If they can engage in analysis, much of what applies to the technique required with hysterical patients also applies to histrionic patients. However, they will require more ego support and greater postponement of interpretation to be effectively treated.

Obsessive-Compulsive Personality Disorder

Patients with OCPD are generally well suited for psychoanalysis, but they must first overcome their anxieties about being out of control. Lying on a couch and free associating presents them with a situation in which they must be spontaneous. Most obsessive-compulsive individuals have a host of rigid defenses to avoid spontaneity so they can avoid loss of control. Hence they will use resistances that reflect defensive operations such as isolation of affect, intellectualization, and reaction formation. Analysts may need to confront the tendency to use factual information as a way of avoiding emotional expression in the analysis.

OCPD patients may also attempt to be perfect, saying exactly the right thing and thereby pleasing the analyst. This wish to please the analyst may be a reaction formation against hostility about the power differential inherent in the analytic setting, the time constraints, and the fee. The analyst carefully analyzes elements of hostility and resentment and tries to bring them into the patient's awareness when possible.

Moreover, patients with OCPD are driven by harsh superego pressures, and they frequently externalize that superego onto the analyst. They assume the analyst will react with disapproval and criticism to any expressions of sexuality or aggression, and the analyst must interpret those fears as they emerge as resistances to being open with the analyst about what is happening in their lives and in their internal affective life. As the analyst conveys a sense of acceptance and tolerance, the patient gradually enters into a process of self-acceptance so that the superego is modified in the course of the analytic work.

Another major thrust in the analytic work with these patients is helping them see that their compromise formations against aggression generally do not work. As they describe interactions with coworkers or intimate family members, the analyst needs to observe problematic patterns of relationships in which the patient tries to avoid any implications of anger. The analyst points out how their reaction formation against anger is imperfect, in that others sense the hostility and resentment below the surface, no matter how defended they are in their efforts to conceal anger. Part of the analytic work also focuses on helping the patient realize the futility of pursuing perfection. As self-acceptance increases, expectations can be lowered and the patient can understand that the perfectionistic ideals come from long-standing feelings of being unloved as a child and no longer address the original situation that fostered them. Persons with OCPD are by nature competitive. They want to be the best at whatever they do, and they are constantly finding fault with the shortcomings of others. This pattern may well emerge in the transference, no matter how conscientiously the patient tries to conceal it from the analyst. Analysts treating such patients may find themselves evoked into competitive power struggles with the patient about the amount of the bill, who is correct about a literary reference, and whose interpretation of a psychological situation is more accurate. Analysts need to be prepared to interpret this process (rather than enact it repeatedly) through the systematic interpretation of the rivalry. Obsessive-compulsive patients will then begin to recognize traces of sibling and oedipal rivalries of the past in contemporary relationships and will gain understanding of how these rivalries interfere with harmonious intimate relationships.

Avoidant Personality Disorder

Patients with avoidant personality disorder may be reluctant to seek help because the analytic relationship presents the same threats as other intimate relationships. They are prone to feeling shame, embarrassment, and humiliation associated with exposure. Shame is etymologically derived from the verb "to hide" (Nathanson 1987), and the avoidant patient often withdraws from interpersonal relationships and situations of exposure out of a wish to "hide out" from the highly unpleasant affect of shame. Hence, when they come to analysis, avoidant patients may "hide out" from the analyst and try to avoid discussions of their fears.

This form of resistance, of course, is the crux of the treatment. The analyst needs to patiently explore what it is that the patient fears from engaging the analyst in sharing his or her anxieties and fantasies. What does the patient imagine the analyst will think about the patient's fears? Initially, this exploration may meet with clichés such as "rejection." As the analyst encourages the patient to elaborate more specific fantasies, core conflicts in the patient's internal object relationships begin to emerge. One may learn of experiences of humiliation from childhood that the patient is convinced will be repeated again and again. Another common theme in avoidant patients is that they are secretly thrilled with the possibility of "showing off," but they worry that their exhibitionistic display is self-centered and destructive to others. They may fear that they will become intoxicated with themselves if they are "center stage." They may also fear deep-seated resentment and anger at parents who shamed them. The inhibition of anger is frequently connected with the shame experience (Gabbard 2000c).

When psychoanalysts treat avoidant personality disorder, they may need to combine other measures as adjuncts. For example, patients who are reluctant to expose themselves to a feared situation may need to be encouraged to do so (Gabbard and Bartlett 1998;

Sutherland and Frances 1995). In addition, a selective serotonin reuptake inhibitor may also help the patient overcome anxieties by addressing the biological temperament known as *harm avoidance.*

Dependent Personality Disorder

Insecure attachment is a hallmark of dependent personality disorder, and studies of these patients (West et al. 1994) have found a pattern of enmeshed attachment. Many of these patients grew up with parents who communicated in one way or another that independence was fraught with danger. They may have been rewarded for maintaining loyalty to their parents, who seemed to reject them in the face of any move toward independence. The central motivation of such patients is to obtain and maintain nurturing, supportive relationships.

Patients with dependent personality disorder who enter into analysis may present a formidable resistance that takes the form of transference longing. They may secretly or overtly hope that they can attach themselves forever to the analyst and solve their problem of having to face life as an independent individual. Hence the analytic setting poses a paradox: the patient must first develop dependency on the analyst to overcome problems with dependency (Gabbard 2000c).

Another variation on this dependence is that some of these patients will do whatever they can to get the analyst to tell them what to do. Their goal is often to continue a dependent attachment rather than to analyze. Analysts must systematically help them examine the underlying anxieties associated with becoming independent.

These patients may also develop idealization of the analyst (Perry 1995). The transference serves as a resistance in this way because the portrayal of the analyst as omniscient is a way of turning over all responsibility for important decisions to the analyst. Dependency may also be a way of managing anger and aggression—the so-called hostile dependency. Dependent clinging often masks aggression and can be regarded as a compromise formation in the sense that it defends against hostility while also expressing it. As many analysts know from firsthand experience, the person who is the object of the dependent patient's clinging may experience the patient's demands as hostile and tormenting (Gabbard 2000c).

The dependent patient's "dance" may evoke a number of countertransference reactions in the analyst. Some may bask in the patient's idealizing transference and fail to confront the patient's lack of real change

(Perry 1995). Others may try to take over for the patient and become authoritarian and directive as a response to frustration with the patient's failure to become independent. Some analysts may struggle with countertransference contempt or disdain. Termination may be a particularly problematic time in which transference-countertransference impasses and enactments occur. Analysts must steer a course between coercing the patient to terminate and avoiding the topic for fear of upsetting the patient.

Masochistic or Self-Defeating Personality Disorder

Even though masochistic or self-defeating personality disorder is not one of the DSM-IV-TR diagnostic entities on Axis II, it has a time-honored tradition in psychoanalysis. Masochistic character features are found in patients of both genders with striking frequency. Psychoanalytic practice is replete with examples of individuals who engage in self-defeating relationships, undermine their possibilities of vocational or financial success, and repeatedly evoke negative responses from others. The origins of this self-defeating pattern usually involve multiple determinants. Some patients are defending against dangerous competitive impulses, whereas others are presenting themselves as suffering and helpless in order to ensure care from others (Cooper 1993). Others may be actively mastering passively experienced childhood trauma by bringing on the adverse event through their own omnipotent control. They also may be reestablishing traumatic relationships as a way of maintaining familiarity and predictability instead of facing new anxieties.

Psychoanalytic work with masochistic patients attempts to lay bare the underlying psychodynamic themes and help patients see how their role as victim is one they repeatedly set up in their interactions with others. Many masochistic individuals are "grievance collectors" who wallow in self-pity but ultimately blame someone else for their predicament. They also have a secret omnipotence that shares a lot in common with narcissistic personality—namely, they feel that because they have suffered more extensively and more severely than others, they are therefore deserving of special treatment. This sense of entitlement to special martyred status may be tenaciously held on to despite the analyst's repeated interpretation of the wish.

A masochist requires a sadist to be complete, and a frequent development in the analysis of masochistic patients is that the analyst begins to enact "sadistic" attacks on the patient. These may take the form of accurately worded but aggression-fueled interpretations that make the patient worse, an example of negative therapeutic reaction (Gabbard 2004). Because the patient is deteriorating, the analyst may escalate the interpretive efforts, thus making the patient feel shamed and punished. The roles may be reversed as well—the patient may identify with the internal sadistic object and torment the analyst.

Analysts working with masochistic patients must be attuned to this development and help the patient see the gratification he or she derives from thwarting the analyst's efforts. This pleasure can often be traced back to a revenge fantasy in which the patient wishes to retaliate against parents who had excessive expectations (Gabbard 2000a). In some cases, patients may have felt that their parents wished to have them succeed so they would reflect well on the parents. Many masochistic patients seek to deprive their parents of that pleasure by repeatedly failing. In this way these patients may sacrifice their own lives because of the pleasure they take in vengeance against their parents. Analysts must help them see that they have re-created that situation in the analytic relationship and that it is ultimately self-defeating rather than "other-defeating."

Envy may also be a key component to the impasses that masochistic patients produce. To acknowledge receiving help from the analyst may make these patients riddled with envy that is tormenting to them. If they can simply collect one more grievance against the analyst as someone who is failing them, they can then avoid the envy of somebody who has the capacity to give and to be positive about life. Some masochistic patients do not want to reveal how much they have changed until after termination to ensure that the analyst derives no gratification from therapeutic success (Gabbard 2000a). Hence analysts must be wary of too much enthusiasm about changing the patient because that countertransference wish for success will activate the patient's self-defeating spiral. Often the optimal analytic posture is to help the patient understand what is happening while making it clear that how the patient chooses to apply the insight is ultimately up to the patient.

CONCLUSIONS

Psychoanalysis is a long and expensive treatment, but because of its intensity and duration, it may be capable of far-reaching changes that briefer therapies cannot approach. Defense mechanisms and representations of self and other may tenaciously resist change, and for some patients, only a systematic working through of these resistances will allow for structural, long-lasting change. The field of psychoanalysis must develop a greater research base to gain full credibility among the host of other treatments for personality disorders. A research design that will yield significant results has been outlined (Gabbard et al. 2002), but sources of funding in the current era remain scarce.

REFERENCES

Abend S, Porder M, Willick M: Borderline Patients: Psychoanalytic Perspectives. New York, International Universities Press, 1983

Abraham K: Contributions to the theory of anal character (1923), in Selected Papers of Karl Abraham. London, Hogarth Press, 1948, pp 370–392

Alden L: Short-term structured treatment for avoidant personality disorder. J Consult Clin Psychol 56:756–764, 1989

American Psychiatric Association: Diagnostic and Statistical Manual of Mental Disorders, 4th Edition, Text Revision. Washington, DC, American Psychiatric Association, 2000

Anderson EM, Lambert MJ: Short-term dynamically oriented psychotherapy: a review and meta-analysis. Clin Psychol Rev 15:504–514, 1995

Balint M: The Basic Fault: Therapeutic Aspects of Regression. New York, Brunner/Mazel, 1979

Blatt SJ: The differential effect of psychotherapy and psychoanalysis with anaclitic and introjective patients: The Menninger Psychotherapy Research Project revisited. J Am Psychoanal Assoc 40:691–724, 1992

Blatt SJ, Ford TQ: Therapeutic Change: An Object Relations Perspective. New York, Plenum, 1994

Boyer LB: Working with a borderline patient. Psychoanal Q 46:386–424, 1977

Brenner C: Psychoanalytic Technique and Psychic Conflict. New York, International Universities Press, 1976

Brown EJ, Heimberg RG, Juster HR: Social phobias subtype and avoidant personality disorder: effect on severity of social phobia, impairment, and outcome of cognitive behavioral treatment. Behav Ther 26:467–486, 1995

Cloninger CR, Svrakic DM, Pryzbeck TR: A psychobiological model of temperament and character. Arch Gen Psychiatry 50:975–990, 1993

Cooper AM: Therapeutic approaches to masochism. J Psychother Pract Res 2:51–63, 1993

Fairbairn WRD: An Object-Relations Theory of the Personality. New York, Basic Books, 1954

Fonagy P: The process of change, and the change of processes: what can change in a "good" analysis? Keynote address to the spring meeting of Division 39 of the American Psychological Association, New York, April 16, 1999

Fonagy P: Attachment Theory and Psychoanalysis. Other Press, New York, 2001

Fonagy P, Target M: Playing with reality, I: theory of mind in the normal development of psychic reality. Int J Psychoanal 77:217–233, 1996

Fonagy P, Jones E, Kächele H, et al: An open door review of outcome studies in psychoanalysis. Report prepared by the research committee of the IPA at the request of the president, 2nd Revised Edition. London, International Psychoanalytical Association, 2002

Freud S: Character and anal eroticism (1908), in The Standard Edition of the Complete Psychological Works of Sigmund Freud, Vol 9. Translated by Strachey J. London, Hogarth Press, 1959, pp 167–175

Freud S: Remembering, repeating and working-through (further recommendations on the technique of psychoanalysis II) (1914), in The Standard Edition of the Complete Psychological Works of Sigmund Freud, Vol 14. Translated by Strachey J. London, Hogarth Press, 1958, pp 145–156

Friedman L: A reading of Freud's papers on technique. Psychoanal Q 60:564–595, 1991

Gabbard GO: Technical approaches to transference hate in borderline patients. Int J Psychoanal 72:625–638, 1991

Gabbard GO: Countertransference: the emerging common ground. Int J Psychoanal 76:475–485, 1995

Gabbard GO: Love and Hate in the Analytic Setting. Northvale, NJ, Jason Aronson, 1996

Gabbard GO: Finding the "person" in personality disorders. Am J Psychiatry 154:891–893, 1997a

Gabbard GO: A reconsideration of objectivity in the analyst. Int J Psychoanal 78:15–26, 1997b

Gabbard GO: On gratitude and gratification. J Am Psychoanal Assoc 48:697–716, 2000a

Gabbard GO: Psychoanalysis, in Comprehensive Textbook of Psychiatry, 6th Edition, Vol 1. Edited by Kaplan HI, Sadock BJ. Baltimore, MD, Williams & Wilkins, 2000b, pp 431–478

Gabbard GO: Psychodynamic Psychiatry in Clinical Practice, 3rd Edition. Washington, DC, American Psychiatric Publishing, 2000c

Gabbard GO: Psychoanalysis and psychoanalytic psychotherapy, in Handbook of Personality Disorders. Edited by Livesley J. New York, Guilford, 2001, pp 359–376

Gabbard GO: Long-Term Psychodynamic Psychotherapy: A Basic Text. Washington, DC, American Psychiatric Publishing, 2004

Gabbard GO, Bartlett AB: Selective serotonin reuptake inhibitors in the context of an ongoing analysis. Psychoanalytic Inquiry 18:657–672, 1998

Gabbard GO, Westen D: Rethinking therapeutic action. Int J Psychoanal 84:823–841, 2003

Gabbard GO, Horwitz L, Allen JG, et al: Transference interpretation in the psychotherapy of borderline patients: a high-risk, high-gain phenomenon. Harv Rev Psychiatry 2:59–69, 1994

Gabbard GO, Gunderson JG, Fonagy P: The place of psychoanalytic treatments within psychiatry. Arch Gen Psychiatry 59:505–510, 2002

Horowitz MJ: Structure and the processes of change, in Hysterical Personality. Edited by Horowitz MJ. New York, Jason Aronson, 1977, pp 329–399

Horowitz MJ: Introduction to Psychodynamics: A New Synthesis. New York, Basic Books, 1988

Horowitz MJ: Person Schemas and Maladaptive Interpersonal Patterns. Chicago, IL, University of Chicago Press, 1991

Horowitz MJ: Cognitive Psychodynamics: From Conflict to Character. New York, Wiley, 1998

Horwitz L, Gabbard GO, Allen JG, et al: Borderline Personality Disorder: Tailoring the Psychotherapy to the Patient. Washington, DC, American Psychiatric Press, 1996

Kantrowitz JL: Suitability for psychoanalysis. Yearbook of Psychoanalysis and Psychotherapy 2:403–415, 1987

Kernberg OF: Contrasting viewpoints regarding the nature and psychoanalytic treatment of narcissistic personalities: a preliminary communication. J Am Psychoanal Assoc 22:255–267, 1974a

Kernberg OF: Further contributions to the treatment of narcissistic personalities. Int J Psychoanal 55:215–240, 1974b

Kernberg OF: Borderline Conditions and Pathological Narcissism. New York, Jason Aronson, 1975

Kernberg OF: Severe Personality Disorders: Psychotherapeutic Strategies. New Haven, CT, Yale University Press, 1984

Killingmo B: Conflict and deficit: implications for technique. Int J Psychoanalysis 70:65–79, 1989

Kohut H: The Analysis of the Self. New York, International Universities Press, 1971

Kohut H: How does Analysis Cure? Edited by Goldberg A. Chicago, IL, University of Chicago Press, 1984

Leichsenring, Leibing E: The effectiveness of psychodynamic therapy and cognitive behavior therapy in the treatment of personality disorders: a meta-analysis. Am J Psychiatry 160:1223–1232, 2003

Livesley WJ, Jang KL, Jackson DN, et al: Genetic and environmental contributions of dimensions of personality disorder. Am J Psychiatry 150:1826–1831, 1993

Lyons-Ruth K and Members of the Change Process Study Group: Implicit relational knowing: its role in development and psychoanalytic treatment. Infant Ment Health J 19:282–289, 1998

Miller JP: How Kohut actually worked. Progress in Self Psychology 1:13–30, 1985

Mitchell SA: Influence and Autonomy in Psychoanalysis. Hillsdale, NJ, Analytic Press, 1997

Nathanson DL: A timetable for shame, in The Many Faces of Shame. Edited by Nathanson DL. New York, Guilford, 1987, pp 1–63

Ogden TH: On projective identification. Int J Psychoanal 60:357–373, 1979

Oldham J, Skodol A: Do patients with paranoid personality disorder seek psychoanalysis? in New Psychoanalytic Perspectives. Edited by Oldham JM, Bohn S. Madison, CT, International Universities Press, 1994, pp 151–166

Ornstein PH: On narcissism: beyond the introduction, highlights of Heinz Kohut's contributions to the psychoanalytic treatment of narcissistic personality disorders. Annual of Psychoanalysis 2:127–149, 1974

Ornstein PH: Psychoanalysis of patients with primary self-disorder: a self psychological perspective, in Disorders of Narcissism: Diagnostic, Clinical, and Empirical Implications. Edited by Ronningstam EF. Washington, DC, American Psychiatric Press, 1998, pp 147–169

Perry JC: Dependent personality disorder, in Treatments of Psychiatric Disorders, Vol 2, 2nd Edition. Edited by Gabbard GO. Washington, DC, American Psychiatric Press, 1995, pp 2355–2366

Reich W: The characterological mastery of the oedipus complex. Int J Psychoanal 12:452–463, 1931

Sandler J: Character traits and object relationships. Psychoanal Q 50:694–708, 1981

Shapiro D: Neurotic Styles. New York, Basic Books, 1965

Stravynski A, Marks I, Yule W: Social skills, problems, and neurotic outpatients. Arch Gen Psychiatry 39:1378–1385, 1982

Sutherland SM, Frances A: Avoidant personality disorder, in Treatments of Psychiatric Disorders, Vol 2, 2nd Edition. Edited by Gabbard GO. Washington, DC, American Psychiatric Press, 1995, pp 2345–2353

Svrakic DM, Whitehead C, Pryzbeck TR, et al: Differential diagnosis of personality disorders by the seven-factor model of temperament and character. Arch Gen Psychiatry 50:991–999, 1993

Vaillant GE, Vaillant LM : The role of ego mechanisms of defense in the diagnosis of personality disorders, in Making Diagnosis Meaningful: Enhancing Evaluation and Treatment of Psychological Disorders. Edited by Barron J. Washington, DC, American Psychological Association, 1999, pp 139–158

West M, Rose S, Sheldon-Keller A: Assessment of patterns of insecure attachment in adults and application to dependent and schizoid personality disorders. J Personal Disord 8:249–256, 1994

Westen D, Gabbard G: Developments in cognitive neuroscience, II: implications for theories of transference. J Am Psychoanal Assoc 50:99–134, 2002

Winnicott DW: The aims of psychoanalytic treatment, in The Maturational Processes and the Facilitating Environment. London, Hogarth Press, 1962, pp 166–170

Winnicott DW: Communicating and not communicating leading to a study of certain opposites, in The Maturational Processes and the Facilitating Environment: Studies in the Theory of Emotional Development. New York, International Universities Press, 1963/1965, pp 179–192

17

Psychodynamic Psychotherapies

Frank E. Yeomans, M.D.
John F. Clarkin, Ph.D.
Kenneth N. Levy, Ph.D.

Psychodynamic theoreticians and clinicians have given increasing attention to the nature and treatment of personality disorders. In this chapter, we explore the psychodynamic models most relevant to understanding these disorders and then describe the application of these models in treatment. The psychodynamic literature has traditionally focused more on describing the underlying dynamics of personality disorders than on describing treatment techniques in detail. Following the psychoanalytic model, therapists tended to avoid setting a specific agenda, followed the patient's associations, and kept the treatment open-ended with little attention to specific treatment goals. However, psychodynamic therapists have increasingly realized that effective treatment of personality disorders requires specific treatment modifications. This awareness has come both from clinical experience and from the role of empirical research.

Early psychodynamic literature often assumed that an understanding of the characteristic unconscious conflicts in a given personality disorder al-

lowed the therapist to use the traditional psychoanalytic method of free association and interpretation to treat the disorder. More recently, there has been increased emphasis on clear explanation of techniques, including the development of treatment manuals. This trend began with the detailed description of psychodynamic treatments for patients with interpersonal difficulties (Luborsky 1984; Strupp 1984) and recently has been expanded with descriptions of psychodynamic treatments for those with severe personality disorders (Bateman and Fonagy 2003; Clarkin et al. 1999).

Psychoanalytic explorations of character pathology not only predate but also attempt to go beyond the phenomenological approach of DSM-III (American Psychiatric Association 1980) and its successors. In fact, DSM-III started the trend of taking the American Psychiatric Association's diagnostic system away from descriptions based on a psychoanalytic understanding of psychiatric illnesses toward a system based on phenomenological considerations, with the goal of increasing the reliability of diagnosis. However, a side effect of this approach has been to increase the number of Axis II diagnoses per patient. From the phenomenological vantage point of DSM-IV-TR (American Psychiatric Association 2000), there are 10 different and supposedly distinct personality disorders. We do not think it is conceptually valid to describe psychodynamic treatments for each of the 10 personality disorders as though they are separate and distinct. Many patients who appear for evaluation with personality disorder have multiple personality disorders according to DSM-IV-TR, Axis II. Thus, in most cases, it is not clinically relevant to think of assessment and treatment for one of the 10 personality disorders. It is more fruitful to consider the underlying psychological structures that subtend many of the personality disorders and to discuss the therapeutic approach to these pathological structures.

PSYCHODYNAMIC PERSPECTIVES ON THE NATURE OF THE PERSONALITY PATHOLOGY

The psychodynamic models of psychological development most relevant to the treatment of character pathology are ego psychology, object relations theory, self psychology, and attachment theory (see also Chapter 2, "Theories of Personality and Personality Disorders"). These psychodynamic models can be contrasted with and complemented by other models of pathology, such as the cognitive, interpersonal, evolutionary, and neurocognitive models (Lenzenweger and Clarkin 1996). Psychodynamic approaches do not espouse a purely "psychological" model at the expense of a biological understanding of psychopathology. Psychodynamic concepts such as affects and drives have a clear grounding in biology (Valzelli 1981). What distinguishes a psychodynamic approach is the further elaboration of mental functioning that focuses on both the conscious and unconscious meanings of experience as biological forces interact with interpersonal (social, cultural, and linguistic) influences.

The elements that link psychodynamic models are 1) an emphasis on the role of unconscious mental forces (e.g., drives, wishes, prohibitions); 2) the notion that the individual's conscious mind is only a partial slice of his mental activity and that unconscious forces influence his feelings, thoughts, and actions in ways that are not known to him (referred to as "psychic determinism"); 3) an emphasis, to varying degrees, on the past—as filtered through and registered in the mind—as determining the individual's experience of the present (this third tenet includes the concept of transference: the unconscious reexperiencing of past relationships, as registered in the individual's mind, in a present relationship); and 4) the goal of deep change in the personality that goes beyond symptomatic improvement to improve the overall quality of the patient's life experience. Beyond these commonalities, the various schools of psychodynamic thinking lend different emphases to libidinal/affiliative drives or to aggressive drives, to drives as a whole or to defenses, and to the role of conflict among intrapsychic forces versus deficits in the development of psychic structures. Most of these are not "either/or" debates but rather "degree of emphasis" debates.

Ego Psychology

Ego psychology stems directly from the Freudian "structural model" (Freud 1923/1961). This model provides many basic concepts incorporated into other psychoanalytically based therapies, but it also provides the least specific formulation of personality disorders. In this model the id, ego, and superego are the key psychic structures that interact in ways that lead either to successful or unsuccessful resolution of competing interests. Unsuccessful resolution results in psychopathology. The *id* is the seat of the drives and strives for their immediate satisfaction. The *ego* is the more-largely conscious system that mediates contact with the constraints of reality, involving perception and the use of reason, judgment, and other "ego functions." The ego also includes defense mechanisms, which are unconscious ways of attempting to resolve or deal with anxiety stemming from the conflicts between the competing psychic agencies. Certain defense mechanisms are more mature and successful, whereas others are more primitive and provide inadequate reduction in anxiety at the expense of successful adaptation to life. If the defense mechanism is "mature"—such as humor or sublimation—the conflict may be dealt with in a way that does not interfere with the individual's functioning or feeling state. However, less mature, or neurotic, defense mechanisms, such as repression or reaction formation, tend to result in psychological symptoms, such as anxiety, or in impaired functioning, as in compulsive behaviors. The most primitive defenses—such as splitting or projective identification—characterize the rigid and distortion-prone psychological structures found in severe personality disorders. The *superego* is the largely unconscious set of rules (a combination of ideals and prohibitions) that often oppose the strivings of the id for drive satisfaction. Broadly speaking, ego psychology addresses the question of what are the individual's psychological resources—ego functions and defenses—for adapting to internal and external demands. It views character pathology as the result of the habitual use of maladaptive defense mechanisms, with corresponding problems in functioning such as impulsive behavior, poor affect control, and an impaired capacity for accurate self-reflection.

Object Relations Theory

Object relations theory brought psychoanalysis from a one-person system concerned primarily with drive forces and prohibitions against them to a more complex system considering the drives in relation to their objects (Fairbairn 1954; Jacobson 1964; Kernberg 1975, 1980, 1995; Klein 1946/1975). Within this model, internalized representations of relationships are referred to as *object relation dyads*. Each dyad is composed of a particular representation of the self as it experiences an affect (related to a libidinal or aggressive drive) in relation to a particular representation of the other. An example is the contented, satisfied self in relation to a nurturing other linked by an affect of warmth and love. An opposite example is the abandoned self in relation to the neglectful other linked by an affect of fear and anger. These dyads become the building blocks of psychic structure that guide the individual's perceptions of the world and, in particular, of relationships. In normal psychological development, representations of self and others become increasingly more differentiated and integrated. These mature, integrated representations allow for the realistic blending of good and bad, positive and negative, and the tolerance of ambivalence, difference, and contradiction in oneself and others.

For Kernberg (1984), the degree of differentiation and integration of these representations of self and other, along with affective valence, constitutes personality organization. He distinguished between three levels of personality organization: neurotic, borderline, and psychotic. Borderline organization is based on simplistic representations of self and other, in contrast to more integrated and complex ones. It is characterized by the use of primitive defense mechanisms (e.g., splitting, projective identification, dissociation), identity diffusion (an inconsistent view of self and others), and unstable reality testing. The borderline level of organization includes the paranoid, schizoid, schizotypal, borderline, narcissistic, antisocial, histrionic, and dependent personality disorders of DSM-IV-TR as well as

the sadomasochistic, hypochondriacal, cyclothymic, and hypomanic personality disorders (Kernberg 1996). In this system of classification, the obsessive-compulsive, hysterical, and depressive-masochistic personality disorders are at the neurotic level. This classification system has treatment implications, because the therapeutic approach is guided by the *level* of personality organization.

We can understand how psychic structure leads to symptoms by considering the primitive defense mechanisms that devolve from the split psychic structure: splitting, idealization/devaluation, primitive denial, projective identification, and omnipotent control. These defense mechanisms are attempts to wall off intense feelings, affects, and impulses that the individual has difficulty accepting in him- or herself. This "walling off" does not eliminate awareness of these feelings but leads to experiencing/dealing with them in ways that interfere with functioning. For instance, because the split prevents the integration of aggressive feelings and libidinal/affectionate feelings into a more complex whole, the individual may alternate abruptly between extremely positive and extremely negative feelings toward other people in his or her life. This defensive split underlies the instability in interpersonal relations seen in many personality disorders. Alternatively, an individual may deal with split-off feelings by subtly inducing them in another person and then experiencing an awareness of them as though they originated in the other person (projective identification). This process of projective identification leads to chaos and confusion in relationships as well as in one's ability to deal with one's own feelings.

Self Psychology

The self psychology model, developed by Kohut (1971, 1977, 1984), is distinguished by an emphasis on the centrality of the self as the fundamental psychic structure and by the view of narcissistic and most other character pathologies as resulting exclusively from a deficit in the structure of the self without giving a role to conflict among structures within the psyche (Ornstein 1998). Adler and Buie (Adler 1985; Buie and Adler 1982) applied this model specifically to patients with borderline personality. Self psychology focuses on the cohesiveness and vitality versus weakness and fragmentation of the self and on the role that external relationships play in helping maintain the cohesion of the self. It posits that primary infantile narcissism, or love of self, is disturbed in the course of development by inadequacies in caregiving. In an effort to safeguard a primitive experience of perfection, the infant places the sense of perfection both in an image of a *grandiose self* and in an *idealized parent imago*, which are considered the archaic but healthy nuclei of the "bipolar self" that is the normal product of the evolution of these two nuclei. In the development of the bipolar self, the grandiose self evolves into self-assertive ambitions and involves self-esteem regulation, goal-directedness, and the capacity to enjoy physical and mental activities. The idealized parental imago becomes the individual's internalized values and ideals that function as self-soothing, self-calming, affect-containing structures that maintain internal psychological balance. Problems in either of these evolutions lead to psychopathology. Inadequate development of the grandiose self results in low self-esteem, lack of motivation, anhedonia, and malaise. Inadequate development of the idealized parental imago results in difficulty regulating tension and the many behaviors that can attempt to achieve this function (e.g., addictions, promiscuity) as well as a sense of emptiness, depression, and chronic despair. Pathology stems from deficits in the development of the bipolar self. The individual responds to these deficits in psychic structure by developing defensive structures that attempt to fill that gap and lead to the manifest pathology. The anger and rage that often accompany narcissistic pathology are seen as reactions either to attacks on the grandiose self or to disillusionment in the idealized imago. Because the rage is not considered a primary part of the psyche, the therapeutic focus is not on the rage itself but on the circumstances that occasioned it.

Kohut (1971, 1977) introduced the concept of *self-object*: the other seen as the "self's object." It includes the individual's intrapsychic experience of the other and emphasizes the role that the other serves in the development and structuralization of the self (the attainment and maintenance of the cohesion of the self and the unfolding of its capacities). In the course of treatment, selfobject transferences represent the revival of infantile and childhood developmental needs that were never adequately met. Behind the manifestations of psychopathology, the unextinguished hopes and needs of the patient have to be perceived in order to allow the patient a chance to belatedly build up the faulty structures and attain fulfillment.

Attachment Theory

Attachment theory, first formulated by John Bowlby (1969, 1973, 1980), emerged from the object relations tradition. However, in contrast to object relations theorists who retained much of Freud's emphasis on sexual and aggressive drives and fantasies, Bowlby stressed the centrality of the affective bond developed in close interpersonal relationships. Although his work fell within the framework of psychoanalysis, he also turned to other scientific disciplines, including ethology, cognitive psychology, and developmental psychology, to explain affectional bonding between infants and their caregivers and the long-term effects of early attachment experiences on personality development and psychopathology.

Central to attachment theory is the concept of internal working models or mental representations that are formed through repeated transactions with attachment figures (Bretherton 1987; Shaver et al. 1996). These working models subsequently act as heuristic guides in relationships, organizing personality development and the regulation of affect. They include expectations, beliefs, emotional appraisals, and rules for processing or excluding information. These working models can be partly conscious and partly unconscious and need not be completely consistent or coherent. Bowlby postulated that insecure attachment lies at the center of disordered personality traits, and he tied the overt expression of felt insecurity to specific characterological disorders. For instance, he connected anxious ambivalent attachment to "a tendency to make excessive demands on others and to be anxious and clingy when they are not met, such as is present in dependent and hysterical personalities," and avoidant attachment to "a blockage in the capacity to make deep relationships, such as is present in affectionless and psychopathic personalities" (Bowlby 1973, p. 14). Many of the symptoms of borderline personality disorder (BPD), such as the unstable, intense interpersonal relationships, feelings of emptiness, chronic fears of abandonment, and intolerance of aloneness, have been reinterpreted as sequelae of insecure internal working models of attachment (Blatt and Levy 2003; Diamond et al. 1999; Fonagy et al. 1995; Gunderson 1996; Levy and Blatt 1999).

A recent development within attachment theory has been the work of Fonagy and colleagues (Fonagy and Target 1998; Fonagy et al. 2003), who have outlined the concept of reflective function or *mentalization*, defined as the capacity to think about mental states in oneself and in others. Their evidence suggests that the capacity for reflective awareness in a child's caregiver increases the likelihood of the child's secure attachment, which in turn facilitates the development of mentalization in the child. They further proposed that a secure attachment relationship with the caregiver gives the child a chance to explore his or her own mind and the mind of the caregiver. In this way the caregiver has the child's mind in mind, and the caregiver's thinking of the child contributes to the child's understanding of himself or herself as a thinker. This model includes an understanding of the relationship between personality disorders and childhood abuse. Individuals who experience early trauma may defensively inhibit their capacity to mentalize to avoid having to think about their caregiver's wish to harm them. This inhibition of mentalizing is associated with an absence of adequate symbolic representations of self-states and creates a continuous and intense desire for understanding what is experienced as internal chaos. Some characteristics of severe BPD may be rooted in developmental pathology associated with this inhibition. Even in cases of maltreatment, the child internalizes the self-directed attitudes of the attachment figure into the self-structure. In this case, however, the internalized other remains alien and unconnected to the structure of the self. Although lodged within the self, this "alien" representation is projected outside—both because it does not match the rest of the self and because, in the worst cases, it is persecutory. This projection and attempt to control the object of the projection underlie many BPD symptoms.

INDICATIONS FOR PSYCHODYNAMIC TREATMENT

In general, patients with the less severe personality disorders, such as obsessive-compulsive, hysterical, narcissistic,[1] avoidant, and dependent, are suited for psychodynamic treatment (Gabbard 2000, 2001). These patients would be seen as neurotically organized, as compared with the more severe personality disorders with borderline organization (Kernberg 1984). The decision to recommend dynamic therapy rather than psychoanalysis for these disorders can be difficult. One major consideration entering into this decision is the patient's motivation for deep change influencing all areas of his or her life versus more specific relief from anxiety or resolution of problems in certain areas. Other considerations include psychological-minded-

ness, capacity for transference work,[2] propensity to regress, impulse control, frustration tolerance, and financial resources.

Patients with the more severe personality disorders are seen as potentially responsive to a modified, more highly structured psychodynamic treatment (Bateman and Fonagy 2003, 2004; Clarkin et al. 1999; Kernberg 1984), and there is empirical evidence to support this notion (Bateman and Fonagy 1999, 2001; Clarkin et al. 2001). Kernberg (1984) suggested that borderline patients with a high level of narcissistic, paranoid, and antisocial traits, a syndrome termed *malignant narcissism*, are the most challenging to treat and that even with a highly structured treatment have a poorer prognosis than other patients organized at the borderline level. Patients with antisocial personality disorder (those with no capacity for remorse or for nonexploitive relationships) may be beyond the reach of psychodynamic, or any, psychotherapy.

Across the spectrum of the personality disorders, psychodynamic clinicians utilize nondiagnostic patient variables as indicators of psychodynamic treatment, such as quality of object relations, degree of psychopathy, nature of attachment status, capacity for mentalization, level of secondary gain, and capacity for reflection and insight. In general, the presence and capacity for meaningful relationships and attachments to others, investment in work at the level of one's capacities and training, the capacity to reflect on one's experience, relatively good impulse control, and intact reality testing would be positive signs for psychodynamic psychotherapy (Gabbard 2001). Those patients with low intelligence, those who lack psychological-mindedness, and those who have significant secondary gain of illness (i.e., whose illness results in practical benefits such as disability payments) may be referred to a psychodynamically informed supportive treatment (Rockland 1989, 1992).

ASSESSMENT

Clinicians should be alert not only to symptoms but also to the long-standing character of the patient as manifested in the typical ways the patient conceptual-

---

[1] The reader should distinguish between the higher-level narcissistic personality disorder, per se, and the more challenging BPD with narcissistic features or with malignant narcissism.

[2] Assessing patients for psychological-mindedness and capacity for transference work may require a period of working with the patient, because apparent lack of these capacities may serve as an initial defense against insight and may change with interpretation.

izes self and others and relates to others in work, friendship, family, and intimate relationships. Experienced clinicians do not limit assessment for character pathology to reviewing the criteria in Axis II but explore the nature of relationships with others and observe the patient's behavior with the interviewer as the core of their assessment (Westen 1997). The clinical interview is a time-honored approach to the assessment of character pathology. However, a number of more structured assessments of character pathology can enrich the clinical evaluation. In addition to the International Personality Disorder Examination (Loranger et al. 1997) and the Structured Clinical Interview for DSM-III-R Personality Disorders (First et al. 1995) that assess each diagnostic criterion, there are the Diagnostic Interview for Borderlines (Zanarini et al. 1989), Kernberg's (1981) structural interview (so-called because it investigates the patient's psychological structure), and the Structured Interview of Personality Organization (Clarkin JF, Caligor E, Stern B, et al.: "Structured Interview of Personality Organization (STIPO)," unpublished manuscript, 2004).

DESCRIPTIONS OF PSYCHODYNAMIC TREATMENTS OF PERSONALITY DISORDERS

We described the principal psychodynamic models of personality pathology earlier in this chapter in order of their historical development. In this section, we describe some specific treatments that have derived from these models and the more eclectic expressive-supportive model of therapy. The most fully articulated treatments include a clinical description, a treatment manual, and empirical research. However, although there are differences in these treatments, they have many commonalities. Psychodynamic thinking about character pathology and its treatment has historically centered on narcissistic (Kernberg 1975, 1984; Kohut 1971), borderline (Fonagy et al. 1995, 2003; Gunderson 1984; Kernberg 1975, 1984), hysterical (Kernberg 1975; Zetzel 1968), obsessive-compulsive (Reich 1972), and schizoid (Fairbairn 1954) character pathology. Others (Gabbard 2000) have more specifically addressed the individual personality disorders as defined by DSM-IV-TR (American Psychiatric Association 2000), sometimes gearing treatment techniques to the Clusters A, B, and C groupings of the disorders. At present there are few controlled studies of psychotherapy for personality disorders, although there are many case reports and a number of uncontrolled trials. Overall, there is evidence for the effectiveness of psychody-

namic therapy (American Psychiatric Association 2001; Leichsenring and Leibling 2003). Most research to date has focused on a mix of personality disorders, avoidant personality disorder, or BPD. This situation makes it difficult to address treatment of the specific DSM-IV-TR Axis II diagnoses separately. Therefore, the therapist should have both an understanding of the basic psychological structure that underlies severe personality disorders (based on primitive defense mechanisms) and of the particular dynamic issues that distinguish the different disorders.

Waldinger (1987) described a set of common characteristics of dynamic therapies for patients with BPD that generalize to those with borderline organization or Axis II Cluster B disorders other than antisocial personality disorder: 1) an emphasis on the stability of the frame of the treatment; 2) an increase in the therapist's participation during sessions as compared with therapy with neurotic patients; 3) tolerance of the patient's hostility as manifested in the negative transference; 4) use of clarification and confrontation to discourage self-destructive behaviors and render them ego-dystonic and ungratifying; 5) use of interpretation to help the patient establish bridges between actions and feelings; 6) blocking acting-out behaviors by setting limits on actions that endanger the patient, others, or the treatment; 7) focusing early therapeutic work and interpretations on the here-and-now rather than on material from the past; and 8) careful monitoring of countertransference feelings.

Within these common modifications to general psychodynamic technique, we now review how different models address the treatment of personality disorders. We provide a vignette typical of each model and follow with a series of more general clinical vignettes. We take this approach for pedagogical and research reasons, knowing that many clinicians will creatively combine theory and techniques across these models.

Object Relations Models of Therapy

Among object relations models of therapy (Gabbard 2000; Strupp 1984), the most fully manualized is transference-focused psychotherapy (TFP) (Clarkin et al. 1999; Kernberg et al. 1989, Koenigsberg et al. 2000; Yeomans et al. 1992, 2002). Emerging data support this treatment (Clarkin et al. 2001; Levy KN, Clarkin JF, Foelsch PA, Kernberg OF, "Transference-Focused Psychotherapy for Borderline Personality Disorder: A Comparison With a Treatment-as-Usual Cohort," unpublished data, 2004), and it is the only object relations model currently being tested in a randomized, controlled study (Clarkin et al. 2004). TFP considers an explicit contract, a clear set of therapeutic tactics and techniques, a focus on a hierarchy of acting-out behaviors, and a highly engaged therapeutic relationship as prerequisites for transference analysis with patients with severe character disorders. Because patients with character pathology have chronic difficulties in their relationships with others, including the therapist, this model emphasizes the need for a clear understanding of the conditions of treatment to be established between therapist and patient before beginning the actual therapy. The verbal contract is the foundation both for containing acting-out and for interpreting deviations from the contract and distortions of it that will inevitably be introduced in the interaction between patient and therapist.

In TFP, building the therapeutic alliance comes first through the collaboration in discussing the treatment contract and then through the therapist's empathy with the entire range of the patient's affective responses, including the negative transference as soon as it arises. Although addressing the negative transference early on may elicit angry and hostile feelings, it is felt to create a fuller alliance with the patient by indicating that the therapist welcomes and can tolerate the full expression of the patient's most difficult internal feeling states. To avoid the negative transference would be to participate in supporting the split internal world and, perhaps, to unwittingly signal that the patient's negative feelings are not welcome in the therapeutic arena.

Mutative Techniques

TFP advocates early interpretation of transference as well as the interpretation of both the positive and negative transference. This strategy is based on the immediacy of the affect in the relationship with the therapist, whereas early interpretation of the patient's past often becomes an exercise in intellectualization. However, because poorly delivered interpretations, particularly of aggressive feelings, may result in patients feeling attacked, the ground for interpretation is set by clarification of the patient's feeling states and by exploring any contradictions in the patient's discourse or actions. These contradictions are considered reflections of the split, unintegrated internal world underlying borderline pathology.

The goal of psychotherapy for borderline personality organization is the change from a state of identity diffusion to an integrated identity. The therapist perceives the patient's principal representations of self and of others as they unfold in the transference. The

therapist brings these dyads more fully into the patient's awareness and explores the unconscious motivations for keeping distinctly different, often opposite, dyads separated. Key moments in therapy occur when the patient becomes aware of an aspect of himself that, up to now, he had only expressed in behavior, with no awareness, and/or had projected and seen in others. For example, at a time when the patient is violently accusing the therapist of being an uncaring tyrant whose only interest is in sadistically controlling her, the therapist might say: "I see the conviction with which you hold your ideas, but I'd like to suggest that you think of someone looking in on this scene. They would see you getting up out of your chair and gesturing at me in a menacing fashion. With that in mind, could you consider that you may be capable within yourself of some of the harsh, aggressive feelings that you are attributing to me?"

The working through consists of repeatedly analyzing the dyads that appear first in the transference and then as they appear in the patient's life outside the therapy and in the patient's past. In the course of this process, transference interpretations are consistently linked with material regarding the patient's relationships, behavior control, work functioning, and sense of self.

Mechanisms of Change

Change comes both from interpretations that increase the patient's awareness of aspects of him- or herself that are split off rather than integrated—and from the patient's eventual ability to experience the relationship with the therapist as different from his or her earlier "repertoire" of relations and to generalize this awareness to other relationships outside the therapeutic setting.

Attachment-Based Treatment

Attachment-based treatment has been developed for Cluster B personality disorders. The emotional instability of these disorders is seen as secondary to the instability in the self-structure. Therefore, the goal, as described by Bateman and Fonagy (2003), is to "stabilize the self-structure through the development of stable internal representations, formation of a coherent sense of self, and capacity to form secure relationships" (p. 195). To achieve this goal, the therapist must help the patient "move from a disorganized attachment in which affects are volatile and unpredictable toward a more secure attachment in which they are less capricious and more stable" (pp. 195–196). Identifying and fostering appropriate expression of affect is integral to this process. Anger and aggression are seen as responses to neglect and abuse rather than primary affects.

Mutative Techniques

The key therapy tactics are 1) agreeing clearly on the purpose and expectations of therapy; 2) using the therapist's appreciation of how the patient is stabilizing self-structure (e.g., through self-harm or substance abuse)[3] to guide the therapist's understanding, interpretations, and other interventions; 3) maintaining mental closeness, especially by the use of interventions that are "contingent" and "marked";[4] 4) accepting aspects of the "alien self" (through projection and countertransference); and 5) using brief here-and-now statements recognizing the patient's current absence of symbolic representation.

Mechanisms of Change

The mechanism of therapeutic action is based on developing the patient's ability to evolve an awareness of mental states and thus find meaning in his or her own and other people's behavior. The transference is seen as the emergence of latent meanings and beliefs that are evoked by the therapeutic relationship: "It [transference] is a new experience influenced by the past rather than a repetition of an earlier one" (Batman and Fonagy 2003, p. 200). Wary that direct transference interpretation is at too high a level of abstraction for borderline patients, the authors recommend using transference tracers, comments that predict likely future action based on the patient's previous experience in a way that heightens the patient's ability to begin to see transference patterns. In this sense, one difference between this approach and the TFP approach described earlier is that the therapist following this model would tend to "hold the projection" within him- or herself longer before directly interpreting it to the patient.

The core of the work is helping patients understand their intense emotional reactions in the context of the treatment relationship. The patient is urged to consider who engendered the feeling and how and to

ask: "What feeling may I have engendered in someone else, even if I am not conscious of it, that may have made him behave that way toward me?" An important part of this process is focusing the patient's attention on the therapist's experience, with the goal of the exploration of a mind *by* a mind within an interpersonal context. This interpersonal focusing involves *mental closeness*, which is "to represent accurately the feeling state of the patient and its accompanying internal representations, to distinguish [the] state of mind of self and other [to 'mark' the difference], and to demonstrate this distinction to the patient" (Bateman and Fonagy 2003, p. 202).

An example from this model involves a patient who came into a session looking agitated and frightened and remained silent. The therapist proposed, "You appear to see me as frightening today." The patient replied, in a challenging way: "What makes you say that?" The therapist provided the immediate evidence: "You had your head down and avoided looking at me," to which the patient responded, "Well, I thought that you were cross with me." The therapist then proposed to explore a bit more deeply within the patient, saying, "I am not aware of being cross with you, so it may help if we think about why you were concerned that I was" (Bateman and Fonagy 2003, pp. 198–199).

Self Psychology

Self psychology is described (Kohut 1971; Ornstein 1998) as a form of psychoanalysis whose principles can be applied to therapy as well. The main emphasis at the beginning of therapy is facilitating the development of the selfobject transference, which creates the precursors of a therapeutic alliance. This model sees the patient's eventual capacity for a true therapeutic alliance as evidence that he or she has resolved a borderline or narcissistic personality disorder and has advanced to a neurotic level of difficulty (Adler 1985). The model does not emphasize establishing the treatment frame through contracting as a separate process, but in the case of acting-out borderline patients, it describes the therapist's need to set limits and participate in protecting the patient.

---

[3] In accordance with the primitive defense mechanisms, self-destructive acting-out can stabilize the self-structure by satisfying intense and poorly integrated aggressive affects rather than dealing with them in more mature ways.

[4] "Marking" involves reflecting back to the patient that you understand his affect but also indicating that your affect is distinct from it.

Mutative Techniques

The self psychology model emphasizes the role of therapist empathy in facilitating selfobject transferences that can lead to developing a more adequate sense of self. These transferences are the *mirror transference* and the *idealizing transference*. The former involves experiencing the therapist as an affirming, approving, validating, and admiring presence and is believed to provide a "psychic glue" that holds the patient's fragile self together. The therapist helps the patient analyze his reactions to inevitable empathic failures on the therapist's part. These failures can lead to disruptions in this transference that result in the fragmenting of the self and the return of symptomatology. In the idealizing transference, the therapist is put on a pedestal so that the patient may borrow some of the therapist's "perfectness." This transference also provides some cohesiveness to the patient's experience of self. Again, therapeutic attention is focused on inevitable disappointments and the rage and symptomatology that may follow.

Mechanisms of Change

The selfobject's responsiveness (in the case of treatment, the therapist's) catalyzes this transformation by activating the individual's innate potential. Empathy is at the center of the therapeutic process. The patient's transference is seen as including a positive striving for a new beginning (Ornstein 1998) in addition to the repetition and distortion based on past experiences. Therapy proceeds not by challenging or focusing on the specific features of the patient's psychopathology but by focusing on the matrix, the vulnerable self, from which it emerged. The therapist's role is seen as that of facilitating the therapeutic reactivation of the patient's original need for appropriate selfobject responses. The therapist generally empathizes with the patient's need for resistances rather than interpreting them. The therapist addresses defenses by helping to see what function the defense/defensive behavior serves in maintaining some degree of cohesiveness in the fragile, fragmentation-prone self. After experiencing appropriate selfobject responses, the patient will be able to end therapy and establish appropriate selfobjects in life outside therapy.

The following example illustrates limit setting, confrontation, and interpretation as they might be carried out in a self psychology model. The therapist's intervention follows a patient's report of dangerous acting-out:

"[Y]ou must not allow yourself to take such risks again. You felt so intensely because you believed I did not care. Anytime you feel this way and are in danger of acting on it, contact me instead. It would be much better, much safer, to talk with me on the phone.... See that I exist and that this relationship is real." (Adler 1985, p. 137)

Expressive-Supportive Therapy

The most widely practiced version of psychodynamic psychotherapy for personality disorders is probably expressive-supportive therapy (Gabbard 2000; Gunderson 2001; Luborsky 1984). Wallerstein (1986), in analyzing the Menninger Foundation Psychotherapy Research Project, concluded that most therapy included a mix of the more formal elements of psychoanalysis, termed *expressive* (e.g., the therapist's neutrality and use of interpretation), and of elements described as *supportive* (e.g., the therapist at times supporting rather than interpreting the patient's current defenses). *Expressive-supportive therapy* refers to an eclectic therapeutic stance of selecting interventions from any of the more specific theoretical models according to what seems to be the best fit with a given patient at a given moment in the treatment. Therapeutic goals can vary from more analytic (e.g., gaining insight and achieving resolution of internal psychological conflict, increasing the cohesiveness of the self, improving the quality of interpersonal relationships) to more supportive (e.g., helping the patient to adapt to stresses while not directly addressing unconscious wishes and defenses). This form of therapy proposes the "expressive-supportive continuum of interventions" (Gabbard 2000, p. 96): Interpretation → Confrontation → Clarification → Encouragement to elaborate → Empathic validation → Advice and praise → Affirmation.

The expressive-supportive approach has the advantage of allowing the therapist to modulate between more analytic exploration and more supportive involvement. Yet there is a risk of countertransference enactments as the therapist shifts between an analytic focus and a supportive one. For example, the therapist could deviate from the analytic objective if he or she regularly responds to the patient's anxiety about internal conflicts by changing to a more supportive mode. Awareness of this risk and appropriate supervision are the best guarantees against countertransference enactments.

Expressive-supportive therapy emphasizes establishing the alliance as the *sine qua non* of the therapeutic process, a view that is supported by research (Luborsky et al. 1980). Therefore, the central task, especially early in therapy, is primarily supportive and relationship building, with the fostering of positive or even idealizing aspects of the transference (Buie and Adler 1982; Chessick 1974). Alliance building takes precedence over focusing on the contract and conditions of treatment out of concern that emphasis on these might elicit negative transference or too quickly challenge the patient's defenses. Luborsky's (1984) manual for expressive-supportive therapy summarizes many aspects of the treatment.

Mutative Techniques

Depending on the relative expressiveness versus supportiveness of the therapy, the therapist would either directly offer interpretations to the patient (addressing transference, defenses, impulses, and/or the patient's past) or use the therapist's own awareness to guide an understanding of the patient while avoiding interpretation. Similarly, a more expressive approach to resistance is to interpret and help the patient understand its function, whereas a supportive approach might call for bolstering resistances in the service of reinforcing weak defensive structures in the patient.

The expressive-supportive therapist gears interventions to the particular defensive structure of the patient. For instance, when treating a patient with paranoid personality disorder (Gabbard 2000), the therapist would be informed by an awareness of the patient's tendency to perceive attack from the therapist and thus to evoke the therapist's defensive responses. Resisting such responses, the therapist would leave the patient's suspicious accusations and projections "hanging," neither denying nor interpreting them. In this way, the projections of hatred and badness are contained by the therapist. As this lack of defensiveness, combined with empathy for the patient's subjective state, creates a sense of alliance, the patient will (it is hoped) become more open and revealing. In this process, the therapist helps the patient label feelings and better distinguish between emotions and reality (Meissner 1976). Therapists also guide the patient's perceptions of reality by questioning assumptions ("You assumed that when your friend didn't wave back from the other side of the theater that he was trying to avoid you. But are you sure that he saw you in that crowd?").

The fact that the therapist does not respond in the way anticipated, and provoked, by the patient is meant to lead the patient to a "creative doubt" (Meissner 1986) about the way the patient perceives the world. This questioning of his or her own way of thinking will help the patient develop a better capacity to accurately reflect on and perceive him- or herself in relation to others.

Mechanisms of Change

The traditional psychoanalytic principle of bringing subconscious aspects of the patient's mind into consciousness still holds. However, the expressive-supportive model emphasizes both the role of increasing the patient's understanding through interpretation *and* the role of the experience of a new type of relationship with the therapist as mechanisms of change.

Illustrative Vignettes

Any single vignette of a psychodynamic therapy must be understood as part of a more complex whole involving a process between patient and therapist. Maintaining a flexible approach is crucial, and it is often the case that a therapist will draw on different psychodynamic models of treatment at different times. This process extends from the evaluation phase, through the setting of the treatment frame, through the development of the therapeutic alliance, into the interpretation and working through of conflicts, and into the termination phase. The following vignettes provide a small sample of interventions with patients with personality disorder. Fuller clinical illustrations can be found in other texts (e.g., Clarkin et al. 1999; Gabbard 2000; Yeomans et al. 2002).

Addressing Omnipotent Control in a Patient With Obsessive-Compulsive Personality Disorder

An obsessive-compulsive patient, typically anxious about experiencing intense affect, filled each session with lengthy monologues full of obsessive details. A main theme was having to submit to his aggressive boss. The therapist's attempts to intervene were overridden with comments such as, "But I haven't told you…" that led to more obsessive details. After many such sessions, the therapist commented on the overall process (seeing the patient's behavior as a character defense):

> Therapist: I have a thought about what's going on here that may help explain some of the problems you've had getting close to people, keeping jobs, and so on. It's striking how you fill our sessions with talk.
> Patient: But you told me to say whatever comes to mind.
> Therapist: That's true, and yet, even with that arrangement, therapy usually has the feeling of an exchange, a dialogue. The feeling here is that you need to keep control and can't let me exist independently in the room. It is interest-

ing because what you are doing could be seen as a domination of me, similar to the domination you complain about from your boss. Yet I don't think you have any awareness of this. It may be that your fear of your own aggressive and domineering strivings leaves you unaware of them and thus unable to deal with them. This in turn could explain the stiffness, rigidity, and distance in your relations with others.

Addressing Narcissistic Defenses

A narcissistic patient, typically preoccupied with and defending against an inadequate sense of self, presented with the chief complaint of feeling depressed and anxious because he believed he should be married at his age but had not succeeded in finding a wife. In the next session, the therapist summarized the complaints:

> Therapist: So you've been depressed and anxious?
> Patient: No, not really...maybe a little, but not more than anyone feels at times.
> Therapist [attempting to find his bearings]: You said you've been frustrated because you haven't succeeded in getting married?
> Patient: That's not really going so badly. I've had a lot of dates lately.
> Therapist [somewhat confused, but thinking of his diagnostic impression of narcissism, offers a therapeutic confrontation and interpretation]: Something seems to be going on right here that may be central to the problems you have described. After telling me about some problems, you have taken them back. While one possibility is that your problems have gone away, it may also be that you feel I am judging you critically when I state your problems...seeing you as less than perfect, and you may feel you have to present me with a positive image of yourself. Yet, if we look further, we may find that the harsh judge and the demand for perfection are in you and make it impossible to ever feel good about yourself. This could be part of your difficulty in relationships, because it is very difficult to get close to someone if you feel a constant pressure to be perfect. The question is where this pressure is coming from.

Addressing Splitting in a Borderline Patient

A patient, typically torn between desperately needing others and attacking them, presented with a history of violent destructive and self-destructive behaviors. She began therapy saying, "I don't want to be here. I just need help with my stupid symptoms so I can be independent and go live by myself. People are no good and I hate everyone."

The first months of therapy were stormy, with continued self-destructive behaviors outside the sessions and much anger and devaluing of the therapist in sessions. However, the therapist noted moments when the patient would calm down, and there would be a sense of being together with a modicum of peace and harmony. Inevitably, the following session would be very stormy. The therapist pointed out this pattern and said, "As unpleasant as it may be, it seems as though you feel relatively comfortable and safe here when you are angry and dismiss me as useless and meaningless to you. Even so, moments emerge when you give in to what appears to be a natural tendency to relate to me in a positive way. But these moments are followed by reinforcement of your angry and devaluing attitude toward me. It seems as though that attitude serves a purpose [pointing out the defense] of protecting you from the positive, attached feelings that make you very uncomfortable [beginning to address the conflict]. A big part of our job here is to understand what it is about your positive feelings toward others, your longings, that makes you so uncomfortable that you replace them with the angry and violent feelings that are what people see and that guarantee that your underlying longings will not be satisfied."

The patient's initial response was "bullshit." However, after more cycles in which the therapist pointed out the pattern of the patient's relating to him positively and then becoming violently angry and rejecting, the patient said: "I've been thinking, and I think you're right. I really do want to be close to people, but that scares me so much I can't stand those feelings." This freed the patient to experience an important part of herself that she had previously kept out of consciousness and to explore why it was difficult for her to experience and express those feelings.

SUMMARY

Psychodynamic therapy has a long tradition of addressing our understanding of personality disorders and how to treat them. Psychodynamic models may differ in certain areas, such as the degree to which personality disorders are considered the result of intrapsychic conflict or of a deficit in psychic structure or self-structure. According to the model's position on this issue, the technical approach may put more emphasis on interpretation versus empathy. Nevertheless, it is important to keep in mind a common theme: the role of early development in combination with the individual's temperament in creating a psychic structure that does not adapt well to dealing with the complexities of the real world and the need to integrate or complete that psychic structure to help the individual replace failure and frustration in life with a realistic measure of satisfaction and achievement.

REFERENCES

Adler G: Borderline Psychopathology and Its Treatment. New York, Jason Aronson, 1985

American Psychiatric Association: Diagnostic and Statistical Manual of Mental Disorders, 3rd Edition. Washington, DC, American Psychiatric Association, 1980

American Psychiatric Association: Diagnostic and Statistical Manual of Mental Disorders, 4th Edition. Washington, DC, American Psychiatric Association, 1994

American Psychiatric Association: Diagnostic and Statistical Manual of Mental Disorders, 4th Edition, Text Revision. Washington, DC, American Psychiatric Association, 2000

American Psychiatric Association: Practice guidelines for the treatment of patients with borderline personality disorder. Am J Psychiatry 158 (suppl 10):1–52, 2001

Bateman AW, Fonagy P: The effectiveness of partial hospitalization in the treatment of borderline personality disorder: a randomized controlled trial. Am J Psychiatry 156:1563–1569, 1999

Bateman AW, Fonagy P: Treatment of borderline personality disorder with psychoanalytically oriented partial hospitalization: an 18-month follow-up. Am J Psychiatry 158:36–42, 2001

Bateman AW, Fonagy P: The development of an attachment-based treatment program for borderline personality disorder. Bull Menninger Clin 67:187–211, 2003

Bateman A, Fonagy P: Intensive Multi-Context Psychotherapy for Severe Personality Disorder: A Manualized Application of a Psychoanalytic Attachment Theory Based Model. Oxford, UK, Oxford University Press (in press)

Blatt SJ, Levy KN: Attachment theory, psychoanalysis, personality development, and psychopathology. Psychoanalytic Inquiry 23:102–150, 2003

Bowlby J: Attachment and Loss, Vol 1: Attachment. London, Hogarth Press and the Institute of Psycho-Analysis, 1969

Bowlby J: Attachment and Loss, Vol 2: Separation, Anxiety, and Anger. London, Hogarth Press and the Institute of Psycho-Analysis, 1973

Bowlby J: Attachment and Loss, Vol 3: Loss, Sadness, and Depression. London, Hogarth Press and the Institute of Psycho-Analysis, 1980

Bretherton I: New perspectives on attachment relations: security, communication, and internal working models, in Handbook of Infant Development, 2nd Edition. Edited by Osofsky JD. Oxford, England, Wiley, 1987, pp 1061–1100

Buie DH, Adler G: Definitive treatment of the borderline personality. Int J Psychoanal Psychother 9:51–87, 1982

Chessick RD: The Technique and Practice of Intensive Psychotherapy. New York, Jason Aronson, 1974

Clarkin JF, Yeomans FE, Kernberg OF: Psychotherapy for Borderline Personality. New York, Wiley, 1999

Clarkin JF, Foelsch PA, Levy KN, et al: The development of a psychodynamic treatment for borderline personality: a preliminary study of behavioral change. J Personal Disord 15:487–495, 2001

Clarkin JF, Levy KN, Lenzenweger MF, et al: The Personality Disorders Institute/Borderline Personality Disorder Research Foundation randomized control trial for borderline personality disorder. J Personal Disord 18:52–72, 2004

Diamond D, Clarkin J, Levine H, et al: Borderline conditions and attachment: a preliminary report. Psychoanalytic Inquiry 19:831, 1999

Fairbairn WRD: An Object-Relations Theory of the Personality. New York, Basic Books, 1954

First MB, Spitzer RL, Gibbon M, et al: The Structured Clinical Interview for DSM-III-R Personality Disorders (SCID-II), part I: description. J Personal Disord 9:2, 1995

Fonagy P, Target M: Mentalization and the changing aims of child psychoanalysis. Psychoanalytic Dialogues 8:87, 1998

Fonagy P, Leigh T, Kennedy R, et al: Attachment, borderline states and the representation of emotions and cognitions in self and other, in Emotion, Cognition, and Representation. Edited by Cicchetti DT, Sheree L. Rochester, NY, University of Rochester Press, 1995, pp 371–414

Fonagy P, Gergely G, Jurist E, et al: Affect Regulation, Mentalization, and the Development of the Self. New York, Other Press, 2003

Freud S: The ego and the id (1923), in The Standard Edition of the Complete Psychological Works of Sigmund Freud, Vol 14. Translated and edited by Strachey J. London, Hogarth Press, 1961, pp 1–66

Gabbard GO: Psychodynamic Psychiatry in Clinical Practice: The DSM-IV Edition. Washington DC, American Psychiatric Press, 2000

Gabbard GO: Psychoanalysis and psychoanalytic psychotherapy, in Handbook of Personality Disorders: Theory, Research, and Treatment. Edited by Livesley J. New York, Guilford, 2001, pp 359–376

Gunderson JG: Borderline Personality Disorder. Washington DC, American Psychiatric Press, 1984

Gunderson JG: Borderline patient's intolerance of aloneness: insecure attachments and therapist availability. Am J Psychiatry 153:752–758, 1996

Gunderson JG: Borderline Personality Disorder: A Clinical Guide. Washington DC, American Psychiatric Publishing, 2001

Jacobson E: The Self and the Object World. New York, International Universities Press, 1964

Kernberg OF: Borderline Conditions and Pathological Narcissism. New York, Jason Aronson, 1975

Kernberg OF: Internal World and External Reality: Object Relations Theory Applied. New York, Jason Aronson, 1980

Kernberg OF: Structural interviewing. Psychiatr Clin North Am 4:169–195, 1981

Kernberg OF: Severe Personality Disorders. New Haven, CT, Yale University Press, 1984

Kernberg OF: Psychoanalytic object relations theories, in Psychoanalysis: The Major Concepts. Edited by Moore B, Fine B. New Haven, CT, Yale University Press, 1995

Kernberg OF: A psychoanalytic theory of personality disorders, in Major Theories of Personality Disorder. Edited by Clarkin JF, Lenzenweger MF. New York, Guilford, 1996, pp 106–140

Kernberg OF, Selzer MA, Koenigsberg HW, et al: Psychodynamic Psychotherapy of Borderline Patients. New York, Basic Books, 1989

Klein M: Notes on some schizoid mechanisms (1946), in Envy and Gratitude and Other Works, 1946–1963. New York, Free Press, 1975, pp 1–24

Koenigsberg HW, Kernberg OF, Stone MH, et al: Borderline Patients: Extending the Limits of Treatability. New York, Basic Books, 2000

Kohut H: The Analysis of the Self: A Systematic Approach to the Psychoanalytic Treatment of Narcissistic Personality Disorders. New York, International Universities Press, 1971

Kohut H: The Restoration of the Self. New York, International Universities Press, 1977

Kohut H: How Does Analysis Cure? Chicago, IL, University of Chicago Press, 1984

Leichsenring F, Leibling E: The effectiveness of psychodynamic therapy and cognitive behavior therapy in the treatment of personality disorders: a meta-analysis. Am J Psychiatry 160:1223–1233, 2003

Lenzenweger MF, Clarkin JF: The personality disorders: history, classification, and research issues, in Major Theories of Personality Disorder. Edited by Clarkin JF, Lenzenweger MF. New York, Guilford, 1996, pp 1–35

Levy KN, Blatt SJ: Attachment theory and psychoanalysis: further differentiation within insecure attachment patterns. Psychoanalytic Inquiry 19:541–575, 1999

Loranger AW, Janca A, Sartorius N: Assessment and Diagnosis of Personality Disorders: The ICD-10 International Personality Disorder Examination (IPDE). Cambridge, England, Cambridge University Press, 1997

Luborsky L: Principles of Psychoanalytic Psychotherapy: A Manual for Supportive-Expressive Treatment. New York, Basic Books, 1984

Luborsky L, Mintz J, Auerbach A, et al: Predicting the outcome of psychotherapy: findings of the Penn Psychotherapy Project. Arch Gen Psychiatry 37:471–481, 1980

Meissner WW: Psychotherapeutic schema based on the paranoid process. Int J Psychoanal Psychother 5:87–114, 1976

Meissner WW: Psychotherapy and the Paranoid Process. Northvale, NJ, Jason Aronson, 1986

Ornstein PH: Psychoanalysis of patients with primary self-disorder: a self psychological perspective, in Disorders of Narcissism: Diagnostic, Clinical, and Empirical Implications. Edited by Ronningstam EF. Washington, DC, American Psychiatric Press, 1998, pp 147–169

Reich W: Character Analysis. New York, Farrar, Straus and Giroux, 1972

Rockland LH: Supportive Therapy: A Psychodynamic Approach. New York, Basic Books, 1989

Rockland LH: Supportive Therapy for Borderline Patients: A Psychodynamic Approach. New York, Guilford, 1992

Shaver PR, Collins N, Clark CL: Attachment styles and internal working models of self and relationship partners, in Knowledge Structures in Close Relationships: A Social Psychological Approach. Edited by Fletcher J. Hillsdale, England, Lawrence Erlbaum Associates, 1996, pp 25–61

Strupp HH, Binder JL: Psychotherapy in a New Key: A Guide to Time-Limited Dynamic Psychotherapy. New York, Basic Books, 1984

Valzelli L: Psychobiology of Aggression and Violence. New York, Raven, 1981

Waldinger RJ: Intensive psychodynamic therapy with borderline patients: an overview. Am J Psychiatry 144:267–274, 1987

Wallerstein RS: Forty-Two Lives in Treatment: A Study of Psychoanalysis and Psychotherapy. New York, Guilford, 1986

Westen D: Divergences between clinical and research methods for assessing personality disorders: implications for research and the evolution of Axis II. Am J Psychiatry 154:895–903, 1997

Yeomans FE, Selzer MA, Clarkin JF: Treating the Borderline Patient: A Contract-based Approach. New York, Basic Books, 1992

Yeomans FE, Clarkin JF, Kernberg OF: A Primer of Transference-Focused Psychotherapy for the Borderline Patient. Northvale, NJ, Jason Aronson, 2002

Zanarini MC, Gunderson JG, Frankenburg FR, et al: The revised Diagnostic Interview for Borderlines: discriminating BPD from other Axis II disorders. J Personal Disord 3:10–18, 1989

Zetzel ER: The so-called good hysteric. Int J Psychoanal 49:256–260, 1968

18

Schema Therapy

Jeffrey Young, Ph.D.
Janet Klosko, Ph.D.

Schema therapy is an integrative psychotherapy that blends elements from cognitive-behavioral, attachment, gestalt, object relations, constructivist, and psychoanalytic schools. Young and his colleagues have been developing schema therapy for the past 20 years (Young 1999; Young et al. 2003). Schema therapy is especially well-suited to patients with entrenched, chronic psychological disorders who are considered difficult to treat, including patients with personality disorders and those with significant characterological issues underlying their Axis I disorders.

Schema therapy evolved from Beck's cognitive therapy (Beck et al. 1979). Effective cognitive-behavioral treatments are available for many Axis I disorders, including mood, anxiety, sexual, eating, somatoform, and substance use disorders (Barlow 2001). These treatments traditionally have been short-term and have focused on reducing symptoms and building skills. However, although many patients are helped by cognitive-behavioral treatments, many others are not. For example, in depression, the success rate is more than 60% immediately after treatment, but with a relapse rate of about 30% after 1 year (Young et al. 2001). Often it is patients with underlying personality disorders who fail to

respond to traditional cognitive-behavioral therapy (CBT; Beck and Freeman 1990).

ASSUMPTIONS OF TRADITIONAL COGNITIVE-BEHAVIORAL THERAPY VIOLATED BY CHARACTEROLOGICAL PATIENTS

Traditional CBT makes several assumptions about patients that often prove untrue of those with characterological problems. One such assumption is that patients will comply with the treatment protocol. Standard CBT assumes that patients are single-mindedly motivated to reduce symptoms, build skills, and solve their current problems and that, therefore, they will be compliant. However, characterological patients tend to be more ambivalent. Their motivation is complicated, and they are often unwilling or unable to comply with CBT procedures.

Another such assumption in CBT is that, with brief training, patients can access their cognitions and emotions and report them to the therapist. Early in therapy, patients are expected to observe and record their thoughts and feelings. However, patients with characterological problems are frequently unable to do so. Many of these patients habitually engage in cognitive and affective avoidance.

CBT assumes that patients can change their problematic cognitions and behaviors through empirical analysis, logical discourse, experimentation, gradual steps, and repetition. However, for characterological patients, this outcome is often not the case. In our experience, their distorted thoughts and self-defeating behaviors are extremely resistant to modification solely through cognitive-behavioral techniques. Rigidity is a hallmark of personality disorders (American Psychiatric Association 2000). Characterological patients generally lack the psychological flexibility necessary for short-term change.

CBT also assumes that patients can engage in a collaborative relationship with the therapist within a few sessions. Difficulties in the therapeutic relationship are typically not a major focus of treatment. Rather, such difficulties are viewed as obstacles to be overcome in order to attain the patient's compliance. However, patients with characterological disorders often have difficulty forming a therapeutic alliance, reflecting their difficulties relating to others generally. Lifelong disturbances in relationships with significant others are another hallmark of personality disorders (Millon 1981). Some of these patients, such as those with borderline or dependent personality disorders, become so absorbed in trying to get the therapist to meet their emotional needs that they usually will not complete CBT self-help assignments. Others, such as those with narcissistic, paranoid, schizoid, or obsessive-compulsive personality disorders, are so disengaged or hostile that they are unable to collaborate with the therapist. Because interpersonal issues are often the core problem, the therapeutic relationship is a proper arena for assessment and treatment.

Finally, in CBT, the patient is presumed to have problems that are readily discernible as targets of treatment. In contrast, patients with characterological problems often have presenting problems that are vague, chronic, and pervasive. They are fundamentally dissatisfied in love, work, or play. These very broad life themes can be difficult to translate into concrete targets for standard CBT.

DEVELOPMENT OF SCHEMA THERAPY

Young developed schema therapy to treat patients with characterological problems (Young et al. 2003).

The model is based primarily on clinical experience and draws on techniques from many schools of therapy. Schema therapy is usually intermediate or longer term. It expands on traditional CBT by placing greater emphasis on exploring the childhood and adolescent origins of psychological problems, on emotive techniques, on the therapist–patient relationship, and on maladaptive coping styles.

Schema therapy is designed to treat the chronic, characterological aspects of disorders, not acute psychiatric symptoms (such as full-blown major depression or recurring panic attacks) and is often undertaken in conjunction with other modalities, including psychotropic medication. Our experience and that of other schema therapists around the world suggests that, in addition to the broad spectrum of personality disorders, schema therapy is especially useful in treating chronic depression and anxiety, eating disorders, couples problems, long-standing difficulties maintaining satisfying intimate relationships, and relapsing substance use disorders. There is ongoing research on the effectiveness of schema therapy in treating many of these disorders.

Schema therapy addresses the core psychological themes that are characteristic of patients with personality disorders. We call these core themes *early maladaptive schemas*. The model traces these schemas from early childhood to the present, with emphasis on the patient's interpersonal relationships. The therapist allies with patients in fighting their schemas using cognitive, affective, behavioral, and interpersonal strategies. When patients repeat dysfunctional patterns based on their schemas, the therapist empathically confronts them with the reasons for change. Through limited reparenting, the therapist supplies patients with a partial antidote to their unmet childhood needs.

There are three main constructs in our conceptual model: schemas, coping styles, and modes. Briefly, *schemas* are the core psychological themes; *coping styles* are characteristic behavioral responses to these schemas; and *modes* are the schemas and coping responses that are active at a given time.

Early Maladaptive Schemas

Young hypothesized that negative schemas, formed primarily as a result of toxic childhood experiences, were at the core of personality disorders (Young et al. 2003). He delineated a set of early maladaptive schemas, self-defeating patterns that begin early in development and repeat throughout the person's life. Our definition of an *early maladaptive schema* is a broad, pervasive theme or pattern composed of memories, emotions, cognitions, and bodily sensations regarding oneself and one's relationships with others that is developed during childhood or adolescence, elaborated throughout one's lifetime, and dysfunctional to a significant degree. Note that, according to this definition, an individual's behavior is not part of the schema itself; behaviors are driven by schemas but are not part of schemas. (From now on, we use the terms *schema* and *early maladaptive schema* interchangeably).

The most damaging schemas from our list of 18 usually involve childhood experiences of abandonment, abuse, neglect, or rejection. In adulthood, these schemas are triggered by life events that the person perceives as similar to the toxic childhood events. When a schema is triggered, the person experiences strong negative emotions, such as grief, shame, fear, or rage. However, not all schemas are based in childhood trauma. An individual can develop a Dependence/Incompetence schema without experiencing a single instance of childhood trauma. Rather, the individual might be completely sheltered and overprotected. However, although not all early maladaptive schemas have trauma as their origin, all of them are destructive, and most are caused by noxious experiences that are repeated throughout childhood and adolescence. The effects of all these related, harmful experiences are cumulative, and together they lead to the emergence of a schema.

Schemas fight for survival. This is the result of the human drive for consistency. The schema is what the individual knows. Although it causes suffering, it is comfortable and familiar. It feels right. Individuals feel drawn to people who trigger their schemas, a phenomenon we call *schema chemistry*. Schemas are regarded by patients as a priori truths and thus influence the processing of later experiences. They play a major role in how patients think, feel, act, and relate to others.

Schemas begin as reality-based representations of the child's environment. It has been our experience that individuals' schemas fairly accurately reflect the tone of their early environment. For example, if a patient tells us that his family was rejecting when he was young, he is usually correct, even though he may not understand why he was rejected. His attributions for their behavior may be wrong, but his basic sense of the emotional climate and how he was treated is almost always valid. The dysfunctional nature of schemas usually becomes most apparent later in life, when patients continue to perpetuate their schemas in their interactions with other people, even though their perceptions are no longer accurate.

The more severe the schema, the greater the number of situations that activate it. So, for example, if an individual experiences criticism that is early, frequent,

extreme, and carried out by both parents, then contact with almost anyone is likely to trigger a Defectiveness schema. If an individual experiences criticism that is later, occasional, milder, and carried out by only one parent, then fewer people later in life are likely to activate the schema; for example, the schema may only be triggered by demanding authority figures of the critical parent's gender. Furthermore, in general, the more severe the schema, the more intense the negative affect when the schema is triggered and the longer it lasts.

There are positive and negative schemas as well as early and later schemas. Our focus is on early maladaptive schemas, so we do not spell out these positive, later schemas in our theory. However, some writers have argued that for each of our early maladaptive schemas, there is a corresponding adaptive schema (see Elliott's polarity theory, Elliott and Lassen 1997). Similarly, there are healthy and unhealthy coping styles and modes. We do spell out some positive modes (mainly, the Healthy Adult).

Origins of Schemas

Our basic view is that schemas result from an interaction between unmet core emotional needs in childhood and the child's innate temperament. We have postulated five core emotional needs:

1. Secure attachments to others (includes safety, stability, nurturance, and acceptance)
2. Autonomy, competence, and sense of identity
3. Freedom to express valid needs and emotions
4. Spontaneity and play
5. Realistic limits and self-control

According to the schema model, a psychologically healthy individual is one who can adaptively get these core emotional needs met. The goal of schema therapy is to help patients find more adaptive ways to meet their core emotional needs.

Early Life Experiences

The schemas that develop earliest and have the most impact typically originate in the nuclear family. Other influences become increasingly important as the child matures, such as peers, school, groups in the community, and the surrounding culture, and may also lead to the development of schemas. However, schemas developed later are generally not as pervasive or as powerful. ("Social isolation" is an example of a schema that usually develops later and may not reflect the dynamics of the nuclear family.)

Table 18–1. Early maladaptive schemas with associated schema domains

Disconnection and Rejection

Expectation that one's needs for security, safety, stability, nurturance, empathy, sharing of feelings, acceptance, and respect will not be met in a predictable manner. Typical family origin is detached, cold, rejecting, withholding, lonely, explosive, unpredictable, or abusive.

1.	Abandonment/Instability	Perceived instability or unreliability of those available for support and connection. Involves the sense that significant others will not be able to continue providing emotional support, connection, strength, or practical protection because they are emotionally unstable and unpredictable (e.g., angry outbursts), unreliable, or erratically present; because they will die imminently; or because they will abandon the patient in favor of someone "better."
2.	Mistrust/Abuse	Expectation that others will hurt, abuse, humiliate, cheat, lie, manipulate, or take advantage. Usually involves the perception that the harm is intentional or the result of unjustified and extreme negligence. May include the sense that one always ends up being cheated relative to others or "getting the short end of the stick."
3.	Emotional deprivation	Expectation that one's desire for a normal degree of emotional support will not be adequately met by others. The three major forms of deprivation are A. Deprivation of nurturance: Absence of attention, affection, warmth, or companionship B. Deprivation of empathy: Absence of understanding, listening, self-disclosure, or mutual sharing of feelings from others C. Deprivation of protection: Absence of strength, direction, or guidance from others
4.	Defectiveness/Shame	Feeling that one is defective, bad, unwanted, inferior, or invalid in important respects or that one would be unlovable to significant others if exposed. May involve hypersensitivity to criticism, rejection, and blame; self-consciousness, comparisons, and insecurity around others; or a sense of shame regarding one's perceived flaws. These flaws may be private (e.g., selfishness, angry impulses, unacceptable sexual desires) or public (e.g., undesirable physical appearance, social awkwardness).
5.	Social isolation/Alienation	Feeling that one is isolated from the rest of the world, different from other people, and/or not part of any group or community.

Impaired Autonomy and Performance

Expectations about oneself and the environment that interfere with one's perceived ability to separate, survive, function independently, or perform successfully. Typical family origin is enmeshed, undermining of child's confidence, overprotective, or failing to reinforce child for performing competently outside the family.

6.	Dependence/Incompetence	Belief that one is unable to handle everyday responsibilities in a competent manner without considerable help from others (e.g., take care of oneself, solve daily problems, exercise good judgment, tackle new tasks, make good decisions). Often presents as helplessness.
7.	Vulnerability to harm or illness	Exaggerated fear that imminent catastrophe will strike at any time and that one will be unable to prevent it. Fears focus on one or more of the following: a) medical catastrophes (e.g., heart attacks, AIDS); b) emotional catastrophes (e.g., going crazy); c) external catastrophes (e.g., collapsing elevators, victimization by crime, airplane crashes, earthquakes).
8.	Enmeshment/Undeveloped self	Excessive emotional involvement and closeness with one or more significant others (often parents) at the expense of full individuation or normal social development. Often involves the belief that at least one of the enmeshed individuals cannot survive or be happy without the constant support of the other. May also include feelings of being smothered by, or fused with, others *or* insufficient individual identity. Often experienced as a feeling of emptiness and floundering, having no direction, or in extreme cases questioning one's existence.

Table 18–1.   Early maladaptive schemas with associated schema domains *(continued)*

9. Failure	Belief that one has failed, will inevitably fail, or is fundamentally inadequate relative to one's peers in areas of achievement (school, career, sports). Often involves beliefs that one is stupid, inept, untalented, ignorant, lower in status, or less successful than others.

Impaired Limits

Deficiency in internal limits, responsibility to others, or long-term goal-orientation. Leads to difficulty respecting the rights of others, cooperating with others, making commitments, or setting and meeting realistic personal goals. Typical family origin is characterized by permissiveness, overindulgence, lack of direction, or a sense of superiority rather than appropriate confrontation, discipline, and limits in relation to taking responsibility, cooperating in a reciprocal manner, and setting goals. In some cases, child may not have been pushed to tolerate normal levels of discomfort or may not have been given adequate supervision, direction, or guidance.

10. Entitlement/Grandiosity	Belief that one is superior to other people, entitled to special rights and privileges, or not bound by the rules of reciprocity that guide normal social interaction. Often involves insistence that one should be able to do or have whatever one wants, regardless of what is realistic, what others consider reasonable, or the cost to others; *or* an exaggerated focus on superiority (e.g., being among the most successful, famous, wealthy) to achieve power or control (not primarily for attention or approval). Sometimes includes excessive competitiveness toward, or domination of, others—asserting one's power, forcing one's point of view, or controlling the behavior of others in line with one's own desires—without empathy or concern for others' needs or feelings.
11. Insufficient self-control/ self-discipline	Pervasive difficulty or refusal to exercise sufficient self-control and frustration tolerance to achieve one's personal goals or to restrain the excessive expression of one's emotions and impulses. In its milder form, the patient presents with an exaggerated emphasis on discomfort avoidance: avoiding pain, conflict, confrontation, responsibility, or overexertion at the expense of personal fulfillment, commitment, or integrity.

Other-Directedness

Excessive focus on the desires, feelings, and responses of others at the expense of one's own needs to gain love and approval, maintain one's sense of connection, or avoid retaliation. Usually involves suppression and lack of awareness regarding one's own anger and natural inclinations. Typical family origin is based on conditional acceptance: children must suppress important aspects of themselves to gain love, attention, and approval. In many such families, the parents' emotional needs and desires—or social acceptance and status—are valued more than the unique needs and feelings of each child.

12. Subjugation	Excessive surrendering of control to others because one feels coerced—usually to avoid anger, retaliation, or abandonment. The two major forms of subjugation are

> A. Subjugation of needs: Suppression of one's preferences, decisions, and desires.
> B. Subjugation of emotions: Suppression of emotional expression, especially anger.

Usually involves the perception that one's own desires, opinions, and feelings are not valid or important to others. Frequently presents as excessive compliance, combined with hypersensitivity to feeling trapped. Generally leads to a build-up of anger, manifested in maladaptive symptoms (e.g., passive-aggressive behavior, uncontrolled outbursts of temper, psychosomatic symptoms, withdrawal of affection, "acting-out," substance abuse).

13. Self-sacrifice	Excessive focus on voluntarily meeting the needs of others in daily situations at the expense of one's own gratification. The most common reasons are to prevent causing pain to others, to avoid guilt from feeling selfish, or to maintain the connection with others perceived as needy. Often results from an acute sensitivity to the pain of others. Sometimes leads to a sense that one's own needs are not being adequately met and to resentment of those who are taken care of. (Overlaps with concept of codependency.)

Table 18–1.   Early maladaptive schemas with associated schema domains *(continued)*

Other-Directedness *(continued)*

14. Approval-seeking/ Recognition-seeking	Excessive emphasis on gaining approval, recognition, or attention from other people, or fitting in, at the expense of developing a secure and true sense of self. One's sense of esteem is dependent primarily on the reactions of others rather than on one's own natural inclinations. Sometimes includes an overemphasis on status, appearance, social acceptance, money, or achievement as means of gaining approval, admiration, or attention (not primarily for power or control). Frequently results in major life decisions that are inauthentic or unsatisfying or in hypersensitivity to rejection.

Overvigilance and Inhibition

Excessive emphasis on suppressing one's spontaneous feelings, impulses, and choices or on meeting rigid, internalized rules and expectations about performance and ethical behavior, often at the expense of happiness, self-expression, relaxation, close relationships, or health. Typical family origin is grim, demanding, and sometimes punitive: performance, duty, perfectionism, following rules, hiding emotions, and avoiding mistakes predominate over pleasure, joy, and relaxation. There is usually an undercurrent of pessimism and worry that things could fall apart if one fails to be vigilant and careful at all times.

15. Negativity/Pessimism	Pervasive, lifelong focus on the negative aspects of life (e.g., pain, death, loss, disappointment, conflict, guilt, resentment, unsolved problems, potential mistakes, betrayal, things that could go wrong) while minimizing or neglecting the positive or optimistic aspects. Usually includes an exaggerated expectation—in a wide range of work, financial, or interpersonal situations—that things will eventually go seriously wrong or that aspects of one's life that seem to be going well will ultimately fall apart. Usually involves an inordinate fear of making mistakes that might lead to financial collapse, loss, humiliation, or being trapped in a bad situation. Because potential negative outcomes are exaggerated, these patients are frequently characterized by chronic worry, vigilance, complaining, or indecision.
16. Emotional inhibition	Excessive inhibition of spontaneous action, feeling, or communication, usually to avoid disapproval by others, feelings of shame, or losing control of one's impulses. The most common areas of inhibition involve a) inhibition of anger and aggression; b) inhibition of positive impulses (e.g., joy, affection, sexual excitement, play); c) difficulty expressing vulnerability or communicating freely about one's feelings or needs; or d) excessive emphasis on rationality while disregarding emotions.
17. Unrelenting standards/ Hypercriticalness	Underlying belief that one must strive to meet very high internalized standards of behavior and performance, usually to avoid criticism. Typically results in feelings of pressure or difficulty slowing down and in hypercriticalness toward oneself and others. Must involve significant impairment in pleasure, relaxation, health, self-esteem, sense of accomplishment, or satisfying relationships. Unrelenting standards typically present as a) perfectionism, inordinate attention to detail, or an underestimate of how good one's own performance is relative to the norm; b) rigid rules and "shoulds" in many areas of life, including unrealistically high moral, ethical, cultural, or religious precepts; or c) preoccupation with time and efficiency so that more can be accomplished.
18. Punitiveness	Belief that people should be harshly punished for making mistakes. Involves the tendency to be angry, intolerant, punitive, and impatient with those people (including oneself) who do not meet one's expectations or standards. Usually includes difficulty forgiving mistakes in oneself or others because of a reluctance to consider extenuating circumstances, allow for human imperfection, or empathize with feelings.

We have observed four types of early life experiences that foster the acquisition of schemas. The first, *toxic frustration of needs* occurs when the child experiences "too little of a good thing" and acquires schemas such as Emotional deprivation or Abandonment/Instability through deficits in the early environment. The child's environment is missing something important, such as stability, understanding, or love. The second type of early life experience is *traumatization*. Here, the child is harmed, criticized, controlled, or victimized and develops schemas such as Mistrust/Abuse, Defectiveness, or Vulnerability to harm. In the third type, the child experiences *"too much of a good thing"*: the parents provide the child with too much of something that, in moderation, is healthy for a child. With schemas such as Dependence or Entitlement, for example, the child is coddled or indulged. The fourth type of life experience that creates schemas is *selective internalization* or identification with significant others. The child selectively identifies with, and internalizes, the parent's thoughts, feelings, and experiences. Basically, the child internalizes the parent's schema. This is a common origin for the Vulnerability schema. The child takes on the parent's fears and phobias. We believe that temperament largely determines whether a child identifies with and internalizes specific characteristics of a parent.

Emotional Temperament

In addition to early childhood experiences, the child's biological temperament plays an important role in the development of schemas. A great deal of research supports the importance of the biological underpinnings of personality. For example, Kagan et al. (1988) generated a body of research on temperamental traits present in infancy and found them to be remarkably stable over time. Figure 18–1 shows some dimensions of emotional temperament that we hypothesize might be largely inborn and relatively unchangeable through psychotherapy alone. One might think of temperament as the individual's unique mix of points on this set of dimensions (as well as other aspects of temperament that will undoubtedly be identified in the future).

Temperament interacts with childhood events in the formation of schemas. Different temperaments selectively expose children to different life circumstances. For example, an aggressive child might be more likely to elicit physical abuse from a violent parent than a passive, appeasing child. In addition, different temperaments render children differentially susceptible to similar life circumstances. Given the same treatment, two children might react very differently. For example, consider two boys who are both rejected by their mothers. The shy child hides from the world and becomes increasingly withdrawn and dependent on his mother, whereas the sociable child ventures forth and makes other, more positive connections. Indeed, sociability has been shown to be a prominent trait of resilient children who thrive despite abuse or neglect.

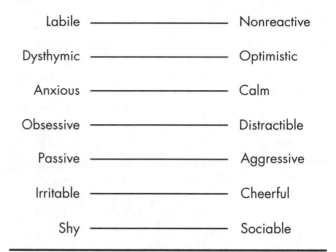

Figure 18–1. Dimensions of emotional temperament that may be inborn and relatively unchangeable through psychotherapy alone.

Schema Domains and Early Maladaptive Schemas

We group the 18 schemas into five broad categories of unmet emotional needs that we call schema domains. Table 18–1 lists the five domains and the 18 schemas that compose them.

Every thought, feeling, behavior, and life experience relevant to a schema can be said either to perpetuate the schema—elaborating and reinforcing it—or to heal the schema and thus weaken it. Schema perpetuation is everything the patient does (internally and behaviorally) that maintains the schema. For example, a female patient with a Mistrust/Abuse schema lends her boyfriend money, which he is slightly late in paying back. The patient thinks that her boyfriend deliberately misled her: "He's just using me. He doesn't really care." She feels humiliated and enraged and expresses herself accordingly, accusing her boyfriend of trying to "rip her off." Alarmed by her behavior, he breaks up with her. The patient's conclusion, that she "can't trust men," reinforces her schema. Her cognitive distortions, extreme emotional reactions, and self-defeating behaviors ultimately perpetuate, rather than heal, her mistrust schema.

Schema healing is the ultimate goal of schema therapy. With schema healing, all elements of a schema are diminished: the intensity of the memories connected to the schema, the schema's emotional charge, the strength of the bodily sensations, and the maladaptive cognitions. Schema healing also involves behavior change, as patients learn to replace maladaptive coping styles with adaptive patterns of behavior. Treatment thus includes cognitive, affective, and behavioral interventions. As schemas heal, they become more difficult to activate. When they are activated, the experience is less overwhelming, and the patient recovers more quickly. Patients increasingly respond to the triggering of their schemas in a healthy manner. They select more loving partners and friends, and they view themselves in more positive ways.

Schemas are hard to change. They are deeply entrenched beliefs about the self and the world, learned very early in life. They are often all the patient knows. Destructive as they are, schemas provide patients with feelings of security and predictability. Healing requires the willingness to face schemas and do battle with them. This process demands discipline and frequent practice. Patients must systematically observe the schema and work at it almost daily. Therapy is like waging war with the schema. The therapist and patient form an alliance to fight the schema.

THREE MALADAPTIVE COPING STYLES

As noted, our model differentiates between the schema itself and the strategies an individual uses to cope with the schema. The schema contains memories, emotions, bodily sensations, and cognitions, whereas behavior is part of the coping response. We differentiate schemas from coping styles because patients use different coping styles in different situations at different stages of their lives to cope with the same schema. Thus the coping styles for a given schema do not necessarily remain stable over time, whereas the schema itself usually does. Furthermore, different patients use widely varying, even opposite, behaviors to cope with the same schema. For example, three patients cope with their Vulnerability schemas through different mechanisms. Although all three feel threatened, one seeks out partners and friends for protection, one avoids leaving home, and one adopts a fearless attitude, facing the fear alone. The coping behavior is not intrinsic to the schema.

We have identified three basic maladaptive coping styles: surrender, avoidance, and overcompensation. Faced with a toxic frustration of needs, the child can respond with some combination of these three coping responses. In any given situation, the child will probably use only one of them, but the child can exhibit different coping styles in different situations or with different schemas. These coping styles are usually adaptive in childhood and can be viewed as healthy survival mechanisms. Yet they become maladaptive as the child grows older, because the coping styles continue to perpetuate the schema even when conditions change and the individual has more promising options.

Surrender

When patients surrender to a schema, they accept that is its true. They do not try to avoid it or fight it. They feel the emotional pain of the schema directly. They repeat schema-driven patterns so that, as adults, they continue to relive the childhood experiences that created the schema. For example, if as children they lived in an atmosphere of emotional deprivation, then as adults they seek out or remain in relationships with people who are emotionally cold. Patients who surrender to their schemas typically choose partners who are likely to treat them as the "offending parent" did. They then frequently relate to these partners in ways that exacerbate the situation. In the therapy relationship, these patients also may play out the schema with themselves in the child role and the therapist in the role of the offending parent.

Avoidance

When patients avoid as a coping style, they try to arrange their lives so that the schema is never activated. They avoid thoughts and feelings connected to the schema. They may withdraw socially, drink excessively, take drugs, have promiscuous sex, overeat, compulsively clean, seek stimulation, or become workaholics. They avoid situations that might trigger the schema, such as intimate relationships or work challenges. Many patients shun whole areas of life where they feel vulnerable. Often they avoid engaging in therapy: these patients might "forget" to complete homework assignments, refrain from expressing affect, raise only superficial issues, come late to sessions, or terminate prematurely.

Overcompensation

When patients overcompensate, they go to the opposite extreme in fighting the schema. They try to be as different as possible from the children they were when the schema was acquired. If they were treated as worthless as children, then as adults they try to be perfect. If they were subjugated as children, then as adults they control everyone. If abused, they abuse others. Faced with the schema, they counterattack. Overcompensation can be viewed as a partially healthy attempt to fight back against the schema that unfortunately overshoots the mark. Many "overcompensators" appear healthy. In fact, some of the most admired people in society—media stars, political leaders, business tycoons—are overcompensators. It is healthy to fight back against a schema as long as the behavior is proportionate to the situation, takes into account the feelings of others, and can reasonably be expected to lead to a desirable outcome. However, overcompensators typically get locked into counterattacking. Their behavior is usually excessive, insensitive, or unproductive. For example, it is beneficial for an emotionally deprived patient to ask others for emotional support, but an overcompensating patient with emotional deprivation goes too far and becomes demanding and feels overly entitled.

Overcompensation develops because it offers an alternative to the pain of the schema. It is a means of escape from the sense of helplessness and vulnerability that the patient felt growing up. Narcissistic overcompensations typically serve to help patients cope with core feelings of emotional deprivation and defectiveness. Rather than feeling ignored and inferior, these patients can feel special and superior. However, although they may be successful in the outside world, their overcompensations often isolate them and ultimately bring them unhappiness. They continue to overcompensate, no matter how much it drives away other people. In so doing, they lose the ability to connect deeply with others. They are so invested in appearing to be perfect that they forfeit true intimacy. Furthermore, no matter how perfect they try to be, they are bound to fail at something eventually, and they rarely know how to handle defeat constructively. They are unable to take responsibility for their failures or acknowledge their limitations, and therefore they have trouble learning from their mistakes. When narcissists experience sufficiently powerful setbacks, their ability to overcompensate collapses, and they often decompensate by becoming clinically depressed. When overcompensations fail, the underlying schemas reassert themselves with enormous emotional strength.

We hypothesize that temperament is one of the main factors in determining why individuals develop certain coping styles rather than others. In fact, temperament probably plays a greater role in determining patients' coping styles than it does in determining their schemas. Individuals who have passive temperaments are probably more likely to surrender or avoid, whereas individuals who have active or aggressive temperaments may be more likely to overcompensate.

Table 18–2 provides some examples of maladaptive coping responses for each schema. Most patients use a combination of coping responses and styles.

SCHEMA MODES

Schema modes are the schemas and coping responses—healthy or unhealthy—that are active at a given mo-

ment. A mode answers the question, "Right now, what schemas and coping responses is the patient manifesting?" A patient may shift from one mode into another, activating previously dormant schemas or coping styles. We are interested in working with both adaptive and maladaptive modes: we try to help patients switch from a dysfunctional mode to a healthy mode as part of the schema healing process.

Development of the Mode Concept

The concept of modes originated from our work with borderline patients, although now we apply it to many other diagnostic categories as well. One problem we were having applying the schema model to borderline patients was that they seemed to have an overwhelming number of schemas. For example, when we give borderline patients the Young Schema Questionnaire (YSQ; Young and Brown 2001), it is common for them to score high on almost all of the schemas. We found that we needed a different unit of analysis, one that would group schemas together and make them more manageable to treat.

Borderline patients were also problematic for the original schema model because they continually shift from one extreme affective state to another: one instant they are angry, then the next they are sad, robotic, terrified, impulsive, or filled with self-hatred. Our original model, because it focused primarily on trait constructs (schemas and coping styles), did not seem sufficient to account for the phenomenon of shifting states. We thus decided to move away from a trait model in treating borderline patients and toward a state model, with the mode as the primary construct.

Each patient exhibits certain characteristic modes, by which we mean characteristic groupings of schemas and coping styles. Similarly, some Axis II diagnoses can be described in terms of their typical modes. The borderline patient usually exhibits four schema modes, shifting rapidly from one to the other. One moment the borderline patient is in the Abandoned Child mode, experiencing the pain of her schemas; the next moment she may flip into the Angry Child mode, expressing rage about her unmet needs; she may then shift into the Punitive Parent mode, punishing herself for expressing anger; and finally, she may retreat into the Detached Protector mode, blocking her emotions and detaching from other people.

A difference between healthy and more impaired individuals lies in the effectiveness of the "Healthy Adult" mode. While we all have this mode, it is stronger and more frequently activated in psychologically

Table 18–2.   Examples of common coping responses for specific schemas

Early maladaptive schema	Surrender	Avoidance	Overcompensation
Abandonment/ Instability	Selects partners who cannot make a commitment and remains in the relationships	Avoids intimate relationships; drinks when alone	Clings to and "smothers" the partner to point of pushing partner away; vehemently attacks partner for even minor separations
Mistrust/Abuse	Selects abusive partners and permits abuse	Avoids becoming vulnerable and trusting anyone; keeps secrets	Uses and abuses others ("get others before they get you")
Emotional deprivation	Selects emotionally depriving partners and does not ask to get needs met	Avoids intimate relationships altogether	Acts emotionally demanding with partners and close friends
Defectiveness/ Shame	Selects critical and rejecting friends; puts self down	Avoids expressing true thoughts and feelings and letting others get close	Criticizes and rejects others while seeming to be perfect oneself
Social isolation	At social gatherings, focuses exclusively on one's differences from others rather than one's similarities	Avoids social situations and groups	Becomes a chameleon to fit into groups
Dependence/ Incompetence	Asks significant others (parents, spouse) to make all of one's financial decisions	Avoids taking on new challenges, such as learning to drive	Becomes so self-reliant that one does not ask anyone for anything ("counter-dependent")
Vulnerability to harm and illness	Obsessively reads about catastrophes in newspapers and anticipates them in everyday situations	Avoids going places that do not seem totally "safe"	Acts recklessly, without regard to danger ("counter-phobic")
Enmeshment/ Undeveloped self	Tells one's mother everything, even as an adult; lives through partner	Avoids intimacy; stays independent	Tries to become the opposite of significant others in all ways
Subjugation	Lets the other individual control situations and make choices	Avoids situations that might involve conflict with another individual	Rebels against authority
Failure	Does tasks in a half-hearted or haphazard manner	Avoids work challenges completely; procrastinates tasks	Becomes an "overachiever" by ceaselessly driving oneself
Self-sacrifice	Gives a lot to others and asks for nothing in return	Avoids situations involving giving or taking	Gives as little to others as possible
Approval-seeking/ Recognition-seeking	Acts to impress others	Avoids interacting with those whose approval is coveted	Goes out of one's way to provoke the disapproval of others; stays in the background
Punitiveness	Treats self and others in harsh, punitive manner	Avoids others for fear of punishment	Behaves in an overly forgiving way
Negativity/ Pessimism	Focuses on the negative, ignores the positive; worries constantly; goes to great lengths to avoid any possible negative outcome	Drinks to blot out pessimistic feelings and unhappiness	Is overly optimistic ("Pollyanna"-ish); denies unpleasant realities
Emotional inhibition	Maintains a calm, emotionally flat demeanor	Avoids situations where people discuss or express feelings	Awkwardly tries to be the "life of the party," even though it feels forced and unnatural

Table 18–2. Examples of common coping responses for specific schemas *(continued)*

Early maladaptive schema	Surrender	Avoidance	Overcompensation
Unrelenting standards	Spends inordinate amounts of time trying to be perfect	Avoids or procrastinates situations and tasks in which performance will be judged	Does not care about standards at all; does tasks in a hasty, careless manner
Entitlement/ Grandiosity	Bullies others into getting one's way, brags about one's accomplishments	Avoids situations in which one is average, not superior	Attends excessively to the needs of others
Insufficient self-control/ self-discipline	Gives up easily on routine tasks	Avoids employment or accepting responsibility	Becomes overly self-controlled or self-disciplined

healthy people. The Healthy Adult mode can moderate dysfunctional modes. For example, when psychologically healthy people become angry, they have a Healthy Adult mode that can usually keep angry emotions and behaviors from going out of control. In contrast, borderline patients typically have a very weak Healthy Adult mode, so that, when the Angry Child mode is triggered, there is no strong counterbalancing force. The anger almost completely takes over the borderline patient's personality. *In schema therapy, the therapist tries to strengthen the borderline patient's Healthy Adult mode to nurture the Abandoned Child, set limits on the Angry Child, defeat the Punitive Parent, and replace the Detached Protector with an authentic connection to life.*

In addition to borderline patients, we have found the mode approach to be useful for patients with narcissistic personality disorder, especially those whom we call "fragile narcissists." These patients typically display the narcissistic behaviors described in DSM-IV-TR (American Psychiatric Association 2000) in order to overcompensate for underlying Emotional Deprivation and Defectiveness schemas. We have identified three main modes in our narcissistic patients: the Self-Aggrandizer, the Detached Self-Soother, and the Lonely Child. We describe schema therapy for patients with borderline and narcissistic personality disorders more fully in *Schema Therapy: A Practitioner's Guide* (Young et al. 2003).

We are in the process of studying modes in patients with antisocial personality disorder. It is possible that, eventually, we will be able to apply the mode approach to many other DSM-IV-TR personality disorders. However, most personality disorders are best conceptualized in terms of our original model of schemas and coping styles. For example, paranoid personality disorder is explained by the schema of Mistrust/ Abuse; avoidant personality disorder is explained by the schema of Defectiveness, with avoidance as a coping style; obsessive-compulsive personality disorder is explained by the schema of Unrelenting Standards,

with compulsive behavior as the coping style; and dependent personality disorder is explained by the schema of Dependence/Incompetence. There is not a one-to-one correspondence between our model and the DSM-IV-TR personality disorders. Rather, we present an alternative system.

SCHEMA ASSESSMENT AND CHANGE

We briefly describe the steps in assessing and changing schemas.

Assessment and Education Phase

The therapist helps patients to identify their schemas and to understand the origins of their schemas in childhood and adolescence. The therapist educates the patient about the schema model. Our self-help book, *Reinventing Your Life* (Young and Klosko 1994), is helpful in this endeavor. Patients learn to recognize their maladaptive coping styles (surrender, escape, and counterattack) and to see how their coping styles perpetuate their schemas. We teach patients about their primary modes and help them observe how they move from one mode to another.

The assessment is multifaceted, including a life history interview, several schema questionnaires, self-monitoring assignments, and imagery exercises that trigger schemas emotionally and help patients make emotional links between current problems and related childhood experiences. By the end of this phase, the therapist and patient have developed a complete schema-focused case conceptualization.

Treatment Phase

The schema therapist does not adhere to a rigid protocol. Rather, the therapist blends cognitive, experiential, behavioral, and interpersonal strategies in a flexible manner, depending on the needs of the patient.

Cognitive Techniques

Patients learn to build a case against the schema. They disprove the validity of the schema on a rational level. As long as patients believe their schemas are valid, they will not be able to change. Patients list all the evidence supporting and refuting the schema throughout their lives, and the therapist and patient evaluate the evidence. In most cases, the evidence will show that the schema is false. The patient is not inherently defective, incompetent, or a failure. Rather, through a process of indoctrination, the schema was taught to the patient in childhood. However, sometimes the evidence is not sufficient to disprove the schema. For example, patients might in fact be failures at work. As a result of procrastination and avoidance, they have not developed the requisite skills. If there is not enough evidence to challenge the schema, then patients evaluate what they can do to change this aspect of their lives. For example, the patient might learn more effective work habits. The therapist and patient summarize the case against the schema on a "flashcard." Patients carry these flashcards with them and read them when they are facing schema triggers.

Experiential Techniques

Patients fight the schema on an emotional level. Using such experiential techniques as imagery and role-plays, they express anger and sadness about what happened to them as children and say what they needed but did not get. In imagery, they confront the parent and other significant childhood figures, and they protect and comfort the vulnerable child. Patients link childhood images with images of upsetting situations in their current lives. With the help of the therapist, they confront the schema and its message directly, opposing the schema and fighting back.

Behavioral Pattern Breaking

The therapist helps the patient design behavioral homework assignments in order to replace maladaptive coping responses with new, more adaptive patterns of behavior. The patient comes to see how certain partner choices or life decisions perpetuate the schema and begins to make healthier choices that break old self-defeating patterns. The therapist helps the patient prepare for homework assignments by rehearsing new behaviors in imagery and role-plays. The therapist uses flashcards to help the patient overcome obstacles to behavioral change.

Mode Work

Although we developed the concept of a mode as we focused the model on increasingly severe patients, we now use it with many of our higher-functioning patients as well. Mode work has become an integral part of schema therapy. We have identified four main types of modes: Child, Maladaptive Coping, Dysfunctional Parent, and Healthy Adult. Each mode is associated with certain schemas and coping styles.

The child modes are the Vulnerable Child, the Angry Child, the Impulsive/Undisciplined Child, and the Happy Child. We believe these child modes are innate and universal. We have identified three types of maladaptive coping modes: the Compliant Surrenderer, the Detached Protector, and the Overcompensator. They correspond, respectively, to the coping processes of surrender, avoidance, and overcompensation. We have identified two dysfunctional parent modes: the Punitive Parent and the Demanding Parent. These parent modes are especially prominent in borderline and narcissistic patients, respectively.

The Healthy Adult mode is the part of the self that serves an "executive" function relative to the other modes. Building the patient's Healthy Adult to work with the other modes more effectively is the overarching goal of mode work. Like a good parent, the Healthy Adult mode serves the following three basic functions: 1) nurtures, affirms, and protects the Vulnerable Child; 2) sets limits for the Angry Child and the Impulsive/Undisciplined Child, in accord with the principles of reciprocity and self-discipline; and 3) battles or moderates the Maladaptive Coping and Dysfunctional Parent modes. During the course of treatment, patients internalize the therapist's behavior as part of their own Healthy Adult mode. Initially, the therapist serves as the Healthy Adult whenever the patient is incapable of doing so. Gradually the patient takes over the Healthy Adult role.

We have developed seven general steps in mode work:

1. Identify and label the patient's modes
2. Explore the origin and (when relevant) adaptive value of the mode in childhood or adolescence
3. Link maladaptive modes to current problems and symptoms
4. Demonstrate the advantages of modifying or giving up one mode, if it is interfering with access to another mode
5. Access the Vulnerable Child through imagery
6. Conduct dialogues between the modes
7. Help the patient generalize mode work to life situations outside therapy sessions

Therapist–Patient Relationship

The therapist assesses and treats schemas, coping styles, and modes as they arise in the therapeutic relationship. The therapist–patient relationship serves as a partial antidote to the patient's schemas. The patient internalizes the therapist as a Healthy Adult who fights against schemas and pursues an emotionally fulfilling life.

Two features of the therapy relationship are especially important elements of schema therapy: the therapeutic stance of empathic confrontation and the use of limited reparenting. Empathic confrontation involves showing empathy for the patients' schemas and coping styles, while still highlighting the reasons for change. Limited reparenting involves supplying, within the appropriate bounds of the therapeutic relationship, what patients needed from their parents as children but did not get.

SCHEMAS, COPING STYLES, AND AXIS II DIAGNOSES

We have reviewed the limitations of the Axis II diagnostic system in DSM-IV elsewhere (Young and Gluhoski 1996), including low reliability and validity for many categories and the unacceptable level of overlap among the categories. Here, however, we want to emphasize what we see as more fundamental conceptual flaws in the Axis II system. We believe that in an attempt to be as "behavioral" as possible in establishing criteria, the developers have lost both the essence of what distinguishes Axis I from Axis II disorders and what makes chronic disorders hard to treat.

According to our model, schemas are at the core of personality disorders, whereas the behavioral patterns listed in DSM-IV-TR are primarily coping responses to the schemas. For most DSM-IV-TR categories, the coping behaviors *are* the personality disorders, in the sense that many diagnostic criteria are lists of coping behaviors. In contrast, the schema model accounts for chronic, pervasive characterological patterns in terms of both schemas and coping styles; relates the schemas and coping styles to their origins in early childhood; and provides direct and clear implications for treatment. Furthermore, each patient is viewed as having a unique profile, including several schemas and coping styles, each present at different levels of strength (dimensional), rather than as one single Axis II category.

As we have stressed, healing schemas should be the central goal in working with patients at a charac-terological level. Changing the behavioral responses, or coping styles, is almost impossible without changing the schemas that are driving them. Also, because the coping behaviors are not as stable as schemas—they change depending on the schema, the life situation, and the patient's stage of life—the patient's symptoms (and DSM-IV-TR diagnosis) might keep appearing to shift.

COMPARISON WITH LINEHAN'S DIALECTICAL BEHAVIOR THERAPY

Linehan (1993) viewed borderline personality disorder as reflecting a pattern of behavioral, emotional, and cognitive dysregulation. Dialectical behavior therapy (DBT) integrates concepts from Buddhism with a broad range of cognitive-behavioral strategies. The core treatment procedures are mindfulness meditation, problem solving, exposure techniques, skills training, contingency management, and cognitive modification. Whereas DBT is specifically tailored to treat patients with borderline personality disorder, schema therapy was developed to treat all of the personality disorders. However, if we focus on the treatment of borderline patients, we note similarities and differences between the two models.

Both schema therapy and DBT take an integrative, active, and practical approach to borderline patients. Linehan's concept of "dialectics" resembles schema therapy's concept of "empathic confrontation": in both, the therapist strives for the optimal balance between acceptance and confrontation. Schema therapy also shares Linehan's empathic response to the borderline patient's intense affect and behavior. Unlike clinicians who see the borderline patient's self-destructive and impulsive behaviors as rooted in aggression or as efforts to manipulate the therapist, both DBT and schema therapy view these behaviors as attempts to cope with extreme emotional pain.

Despite these similarities, there are significant differences between the two approaches. We believe that schema therapy's conceptual model more clearly delineates the borderline patient's psychological structure—in terms of the four primary modes of the Abandoned Child, the Angry Child, the Punitive Parent, and the Detached Protector—giving the therapist greater ease and depth in understanding the rapid and seemingly chaotic shifts in the borderline patient's affective states. Furthermore, although Linehan stresses the need for the therapist to validate borderline patients, hers is not a reparenting model: schema therapy focuses more directly on fulfilling the patient's unmet emotional needs. We find that partially meeting the patient's emotional needs leads to stable improvements in most borderline patients. Limited reparenting provides patients with leverage in the fight against their schemas and over time enhances their capacities to soothe and comfort themselves. The therapist provides a model patients gradually internalize as their own Healthy Adult mode.

Another difference between DBT and schema therapy is our greater focus on uncovering and expressing affect. When treating borderline personality disorder, the schema therapist first focuses on forming an attachment to the patient's youngest and most vulnerable mode—the Abandoned Child. The therapist encourages the patient to stay in the Abandoned Child mode and to express her feelings fully. The therapist concentrates on providing understanding and validation and only introduces cognitive-behavioral elements later, once the patient experiences the therapeutic relationship as stable. In schema therapy of borderline personality disorder, most cognitive-behavioral strategies are aimed at building the patient's Healthy Adult mode, modeled after the therapist.

Limit setting is a central element of both DBT and schema therapy for borderline patients. DBT uses contingency management to address suicidal and other acting-out behaviors. Schema therapy accomplishes this goal with increased reparenting, limit setting, mode work, and empathic confrontation. Schema therapists set limits more as circumstances call for them, as a parent would, rather than more formally in the form of contracts at the beginning of treatment.

Compared with DBT, schema therapy deals with deeper personality structures and overall well-being. This difference is reflected in the research. Treatment outcome studies of DBT focus primarily on acting-out behaviors, such as self-harm and suicidal gestures. In contrast, treatment outcome research on schema therapy assesses a broader range of borderline symptoms, such as mood and social functioning. As we described in the last section, research on the effectiveness of schema therapy in the treatment of borderline personality utilizes a more encompassing set of outcome measures.

Case Example

Melissa is a 37-year-old patient with borderline personality disorder. She enters treatment following a brief hospitalization for a suicidal gesture precipitated by a break-up with a boyfriend. This relationship was the latest in a string of disastrous relationships with men. Melissa explains this by saying, "I have a weakness for bad boys." When she was 7 years old, her father walked her to school, kissed her good-bye as on any other day, then unexpectedly left the family to live with another woman. Melissa did not see him again until she was 28 years old. He called occasionally, but if she expressed anger about his disappearance, he hung up on her. As a young teen she began engaging in promiscuous sex and underwent a number of traumatic experiences. For example, in junior high school she got drunk and was raped by two male students she thought were her friends. Melissa has a long history of drinking and engaging in reckless sexual behavior.

Treatment With Schema Therapy

David, Melissa's schema therapist, begins seeing her on an outpatient basis twice a week. Because she is a borderline patient in severe distress, David forgoes the usual questionnaires. (Borderline patients tend to score high on everything and then become overwhelmed.) Instead, David focuses on limited reparenting, limit setting, and mode work.

Limited Reparenting

Within the appropriate bounds of the therapeutic relationship, David begins to reparent Melissa's Abandoned Child mode. The purpose of this limited reparenting is to create an environment that is a partial antidote to the one she knew as a child. David focuses on meeting the core emotional needs that were not met for Melissa by her father. In sessions, David encourages Melissa to stay in the Abandoned Child mode, and he provides stability, nurturance, and protection. He encourages her to express her genuine needs and feelings, including anger. He helps her endure time between sessions by giving her flashcards that assure her he is still there. He lets her leave him a short phone message each night telling him how she is doing. He gives her advice about day-to-day matters.

Limit Setting

Because Melissa is entering treatment after a suicidal gesture, David makes limit setting an important part of the early phase of treatment. In the first session, he asks her to agree that she will not make a suicide attempt without contacting him first. Melissa views this requirement as caring and agrees to it readily. In addition, she agrees to follow the hierarchy of rules that the therapist sets for dealing with suicidal crises. (We give a detailed description of this hierarchy of rules in Young et al. [2003]). Applying the principle of "empathic confrontation," David validates her feelings but challenges her self-destructive behaviors. As we often see with our borderline patients, within a few weeks Melissa settles down in therapy, and her suicidal behaviors cease. David also sets limits on Melissa's drinking, with an escalating set of consequences on limits violations. Once she connects with David as a stable, nurturing base, then her impulsive, self-destructive behaviors reduce significantly.

Schema therapy provides extensive guidelines for limit setting with borderline patients, whose needs invariably exceed what most therapists are able to provide over the long run. Limits are based upon the patient's safety and the therapist's personal rights. If the patient is unsafe, the therapist sets whatever limits are necessary to provide safety. However, once the patient is safe, our rule of thumb is that therapists should not agree to do anything for the patient they are going to resent doing. This varies from therapist to therapist. Thus, David gives Melissa as much outside contact as he can without becoming angry. For example, at the start of treatment, Melissa asks if she and David could e-mail each other once a day, in addition to her leaving her daily phone message. David does not agree to this, knowing he would resent doing it over time. David is careful to think through his limits ahead of time and to adhere to them. He sets limits in a personal way, using self-disclosure of intentions and feelings whenever possible. He sets natural consequences for violating limits. For example, when Melissa calls him more often than agreed on, he sets a period when she cannot call.

Mode Work

Against the backdrop of limited reparenting and limit setting, David introduces mode work. To reiterate, we have identified four main modes that characterize the borderline patient: the Abandoned Child, the Angry Child, the Punitive Parent, and the Detached Protector. In a nutshell, treatment helps the patient build a Healthy Adult mode, modeled on the therapist, that can take care of the Abandoned Child, set limits on the Angry Child, defeat the Punitive Parent, and replace the Detached Protector with healthier coping behaviors. The patient gradually internalizes the therapist's reparenting as her own Healthy Adult mode.

The therapist tracks the patient's modes from moment to moment in sessions, selectively using the strategies that fit each one of the modes. When the patient is in the Abandoned Child mode, the therapist empathizes with her and protects her. When the patient is in the Angry Child mode, the therapist sets limits on behavior and helps the patient express emotions and needs appropriately. When the patient is in the Punitive Parent mode, the therapist joins with the patient in combating the punitive parent. When the patient is in the Detached Protector mode, the therapist reassures the patient that it is safe to be vulnerable with the therapist. When the patient is suicidal or parasuicidal, the therapist identifies the mode that is experiencing the urge and addresses the urge in accord with the mode that is generating it.

David introduces the concept of modes and helps Melissa identify her primary modes. Like most borderline patients, Melissa relates readily to the concept of modes. They begin with her Abandoned Child mode. David asks Melissa to read the chapter on abandonment in *Reinventing Your Life* (Young and Klosko 1994). Imagery exercises help Melissa connect her present difficulties with men to her childhood experiences with her father. David and Melissa identify her Angry Child mode. For example, discussing her past relationships with men, David and Melissa note her Angry Child, who berates her boyfriends when they are temporarily unavailable, accuses them of infidelity whether they are guilty or not, and punishes them for lapses in attention by flirting with other men. They identify her "Abandoning Father," Melissa's version of the Punitive Parent, who compares her unfavorably to other women, has many sexual affairs, and threatens imminent abandonment. Finally, they identify her Detached Protector, who engages in compulsive, anonymous sex or stays detached rather than risking true intimacy.

Once the patient's modes have been identified, the therapist conducts dialogues between the modes, usually in imagery or role-play exercises, to help the patient work through current problems. The dialogues are moderated by the Healthy Adult mode, at first played by the therapist and later by the patient. For example, in one session, Melissa role-plays a discussion between her Healthy Adult and Abandoned Child modes to find a way to stay emotionally connected rather than becoming detached during sex with her new boyfriend. Such dialogues lie at the heart of mode work.

Cognitive-behavioral and affective techniques are all part of mode work. In treating Melissa's Abandoned Child mode, David teaches her deep breathing and mindfulness exercises for affect regulation. He instructs her in assertiveness skills. He educates her about normal human needs, including the emotional needs of children, assigning her the first few chapters of *Reinventing Your Life* (Young and Klosko 1994). He helps her compose flashcards to read whenever she feels upset or abandoned. He helps her work through images of upsetting events from childhood, entering the images and reparenting her. Later in therapy, when she feels secure, he guides her through traumatic images of her rape in junior high school. David enters the image, confronts the perpetrators, and protects and comforts Melissa's teenage self.

In treating Melissa's Detached Protector mode, David uses cognitive techniques to highlight the advantages of experiencing emotions and connecting to other people. David and Melissa plan homework assignments in which she practices connecting to others rather than switching into the Detached Protector mode. Melissa rehearses for these homework assignments in imagery and role-plays during sessions. In experiential exercises, David conducts dialogues in which the Detached Protector becomes a character.

In fighting the Punitive Parent mode, the therapist allies with the patient against the Punitive Parent. The goal is to defeat and cast out the Punitive Parent. David uses cognitive techniques to demonstrate that punishment is not an effective strategy for self-improvement. When Melissa makes mistakes, he does not support the idea of punishment as a value. David sets up experiments to test Melissa's hypothesis that "all men leave." He works to reattribute her father's abandonment of her to her father's own issues rather than to some lack in herself. Her father did not leave because she was not "good enough." No matter how good she was, he would not have stayed. David helps Melissa fight the Punitive Parent in imagery. He enters the image and confronts the Punitive Parent. Melissa gradually learns to confront the Punitive Parent on her own.

In fighting the Angry Child mode, the therapist sets limits on rageful behavior, validates the patient's underlying needs, and teaches more effective ways of communicating. David educates Melissa about anger and teaches her anger management and assertiveness techniques. Melissa practices these techniques in imagery, role-plays, and homework assignments. Melissa comes to recognize the black-and-white thinking that fuels her anger to extremes. They write flashcards for her to read whenever her Angry Child mode is threatening to emerge in a self-defeating way. They negotiate compromises between the Angry Child and the Healthy Adult in which she is able to express her anger, but only in appropriate ways.

Treatment Progress

Schema therapy of borderline personality disorder generally proceeds through three stages: 1) bonding and emotional regulation, 2) the mode change phase, and 3) the autonomy stage. This is true for Melissa's course of therapy. In the early months of treatment, she becomes secure in the therapeutic relationship and stops many of her self-destructive behaviors. David gradually introduces mode work, and Melissa slowly develops a Healthy Adult mode that can moderate her other modes. By the third year of therapy, Melissa is ready to form relationships with men outside of therapy with whom she can appropriately express her genuine needs and feelings.

EMPIRICAL SUPPORT FOR SCHEMA THERAPY

Assessment Studies

Considerable research on Young's early maladaptive schemas has been done using the YSQ. The YSQ has been translated into many languages, including French, Spanish, Dutch, Turkish, Japanese, Finnish, and Norwegian. The first comprehensive investigation of its psychometric properties was conducted by Schmidt et al. (1995). The schemas demonstrated high test-retest reliability and internal consistency. The YSQ also demonstrated good convergent and discriminant validity in regard to measures of psychological distress, self-esteem, cognitive vulnerability to depression, and personality disorder symptomatology. A factor analy-

sis using both clinical and nonclinical samples revealed similar sets of primary factors that closely matched Young's clinically developed schemas. The investigators replicated these results in a second sample taken from the same population. This study was replicated by Lee et al. (1999) using an Australian clinical population. In accord with previous findings, 16 factors emerged as primary components, including 15 of the 16 originally proposed by Young. A higher-order factor analysis closely fit the schema domains proposed by Young.

Other studies have examined the validity of the individual schemas and how well they support Young's model. Freeman (1999) explored the use of Young's schema theory as an explanatory model for nonrational cognitive processing and found that endorsement of early maladaptive schemas was predictive of interpersonal maladjustment. Rittenmeyer (1997) looked at the convergent validity of Young's schema domains with the Maslach Burnout Inventory (Maslach and Jackson 1986) and found that two schema domains, "overconnection" and "exaggerated standards," correlated strongly with the "emotional exhaustion" scale of the Maslach Burnout Inventory.

Modes were studied in borderline patients by Arntz A, Klokman J, Sieswerda S ("An Experimental Test of the Schema Mode Model of Borderline Personality Disorder, unpublished data, 2004). Subjects completed the Schema Mode Questionnaire. Compared with normal subjects, borderline patients were significantly more likely to score high on all four borderline personality disorder modes (Abandoned Child, Detached Protector, Angry Child, Punitive Parent) and scored lowest on the Healthy Adult mode.

DSM-IV Studies

Carine (1997) investigated whether the presence of Young's schemas discriminated patients with DSM-IV Axis II psychopathology from patients with other types of psychopathology. Group membership in the Axis II cluster was predicted correctly 83% of the time. Carine also found that affect appears to be an intrinsic part of schemas.

Although the YSQ was not designed to measure specific DSM-IV personality disorders, there are significant associations between early maladaptive schemas and personality disorder symptoms (Schmidt et al. 1995). The total score highly correlates with the total score on the Personality Disorder Questionnaire–Revised (Hyler et al. 1987), a self-report measure of DSM-III-R (American Psychiatric Association 1987) personality pathology. The schemas of Insufficient

Self-Control and Defectiveness had the strongest associations with personality disorder symptoms. Individual schemas have been found to be significantly associated with theoretically relevant personality disorders. For example, Mistrust/Abuse is highly associated with paranoid personality disorder, Dependence is associated with dependent personality disorder, Insufficient Self-Control is associated with borderline personality disorder, and Unrelenting Standards is associated with obsessive-compulsive personality disorder (Schmidt et al. 1995).

Treatment Studies

As we write this chapter, a major multicenter outcome study of schema therapy has recently been completed in the Netherlands. We are able to report some preliminary results here. The study compares Young's schema therapy with Kernberg's transference-focused psychotherapy (Yeomans et al. 2002) in the treatment of borderline personality disorder. Preliminary results indicate that schema therapy is significantly more effective and has a dramatically lower dropout rate.

In the study, patients attended outpatient therapy sessions twice a week for up to 3 years, with regular assessments throughout. A wide range of psychometric instruments were used, including the Borderline Personality Disorder Severity Index (BPDSI), a psychometrically validated semistructured clinical interview based on DSM-IV diagnostic criteria for borderline personality disorder; self-report questionnaires measuring quality of life; and measures of general psychopathology, psychoanalytic constructs, schemas, and social functioning.

Researchers have analyzed data for 86 patients (80 females, 6 males). There was a large and significant difference in dropout rates for the two treatments. The dropout rate for schema therapy was 7% in the first year, 9% in the second year, and 11% in the third year. The dropout rate for transference-focused psychotherapy was 31% in the first year, 14% in the second year, and 5% in the third year. Thus, the total dropout rate was 27% for schema therapy and 50% for transference-focused psychotherapy over the 3 years.

The data show that approximately 45% of the schema therapy patients and 25% of the transference-focused psychotherapy patients qualified as "cured" on the BPDSI, the major measure used in the study. Based on the reliable change index for the BPDSI, 66% of schema therapy patients and 42% of transference-focused psychotherapy patients experienced "clinically significant improvement." On a composite factor score of all other measures of psychopathology, personality,

and the YSQ, schema therapy was significantly more effective than transference-focused psychotherapy. Both treatments showed significant improvement in quality of life measures and proved to be cost effective.

CONCLUSIONS

Schema therapy integrates cognitive-behavioral, attachment, gestalt, object relations, constructivist, and psychoanalytic schools into a unified conceptual model. Young developed schema therapy to treat patients with characterological problems who were not adequately helped by traditional treatments. Schema therapy can be brief, intermediate, or longer-term. There are three main constructs in the model: *schemas* are the core psychological themes, *coping styles* are characteristic behavioral responses to the schemas, and *modes* are the schemas and coping styles that are active at a given moment. Treatment weaves together cognitive, experiential, behavioral, and interpersonal techniques.

There is empirical support for schema therapy. The YSQ has been shown to have good reliability, internal validity, and convergent validity with other measures of personality disorder pathology. Borderline patients score higher than control subjects on the Schema Mode Questionnaire, which assesses the four modes we have hypothesized to underlie borderline personality disorder. Preliminary results of a Dutch study comparing schema therapy with Kernberg's transference-based psychotherapy for borderline patients indicate that schema therapy was significantly more effective in decreasing the severity and frequency of borderline personality disorder symptoms. Schema therapy had significantly fewer dropouts than transference-based psychotherapy.

REFERENCES

American Psychiatric Association: Diagnostic and Statistical Manual of Mental Disorders, 3rd Edition, Revised. Washington, DC, American Psychiatric Association, 1987

American Psychiatric Association: Diagnostic and Statistical Manual of Mental Disorders, 4th Edition. Washington, DC, American Psychiatric Association, 1994

American Psychiatric Association: Diagnostic and Statistical Manual of Mental Disorders, 4th Edition, Text Revision. Washington, DC, American Psychiatric Association, 2000

Barlow DH: Clinical Handbook of Psychological Disorders, 3rd Edition. New York, Guilford, 2001

Beck AT, Freeman A: Cognitive Therapy of Personality Disorders. New York, Guilford, 1990

Beck AT, Rush AJ, Shaw BF, et al: Cognitive Therapy of Depression. New York, Guilford, 1979

Carine BE: Assessing personal and interpersonal schemata associated with Axis II Cluster B personality disorders: an integrated perspective. Dissertation Abstracts International 58:1B, 1997

Elliott CH, Lassen MK: A schema polarity model for case conceptualization, intervention, and research. Clin Psychol Sci Pract 4:12–28, 1997

Freeman N: Constructive thinking and early maladaptive schemas as predictors of interpersonal adjustment and marital satisfaction. Dissertation Abstracts International 59:9B, 1999

Hyler S, Reider RO, Spitzer RL, et al: Personality Diagnostic Questionnaire–Revised. New York, New York State Psychiatric Institute, 1987

Kagan J, Reznick JS, Snidman N: Biological bases of childhood shyness. Science 240:167–171, 1988

Lee CW, Taylor G, Dunn J: Factor structures of The Schema Questionnaire in a large clinical sample. Cogn Ther Res 23:421–451, 1999

Linehan MM: Cognitive-behavioral treatment of borderline personality disorder. New York, Guilford, 1993

Maslach G, Jackson SE: Maslach Burnout Inventory Manual. Palo Alto, CA, Consulting Psychologists Press, 1986

Millon T: Disorders of Personality. New York, Wiley, 1981

Rittenmeyer GJ: The relationship between early maladaptive schemas and job burnout among public school teachers. Dissertations Abstracts International 58:5A, 1997

Schmidt NB, Joiner TE, Young JE, et al: The Schema Questionnaire: investigation of psychometric properties and the hierarchical structure of a measure of maladaptive schemata. Cogn Ther Res 19:295–321, 1995

Yeomans F, Kernberg O, Clarkin J: A Primer of Transference-Focused Psychotherapy for the Borderline Patient. Northvale, NJ, Jason Aronson, 2002

Young JE: Cognitive Therapy for Personality Disorders. Sarasota, FL, Professional Resources Press, 1999

Young JE, Brown G: Young Schema Questionnaire. New York, Schema Therapy Institute, 2001

Young JE, Gluhoski VL: Schema-focused diagnosis for personality disorders, in Handbook of Relational Diagnosis and Dysfunctional Family Patterns. Edited by Kaslow FW. New York, Wiley, 1996, pp 300–321

Young JE, Klosko J: Reinventing Your Life. New York, Plume, 1994

Young JE, Weinberger AD, Beck AT: Cognitive therapy for depression, in Clinical Handbook of Psychological Disorders, 3rd Edition. Edited by Barlow D. New York, Guilford, 2001, pp 264–308

Young JE, Klosko JS, Weishaar ME: Schema Therapy: A Practitioner's Guide. New York, Guilford, 2003

19

Dialectical Behavior Therapy

Barbara Stanley, Ph.D.
Beth S. Brodsky, Ph.D.

Dialectical behavior therapy (DBT) was developed 15 years ago by Marsha Linehan as a treatment specifically for suicidal and self-injuring individuals with borderline personality disorder (BPD) (Linehan 1993a), a population with a broad range of serious problems in addition to suicidality (Kehrer and Linehan 1996). A form of cognitive-behavioral psychotherapy, DBT can be adapted for use in other personality disorders, particularly those in which there is significant behavioral and emotional dyscontrol (Stanley et al. 2001). However, other than its use in BPD to date, most adaptations of DBT have been directed toward Axis I diagnoses, such as eating disorders (Telch et al. 2001), or special segments of the psychiatric population, such as adolescents (Rathus and Miller 2002) or geriatric patients (Lynch et al. 2003).

DBT has been evaluated in several efficacy studies, and it is currently undergoing a large-scale evaluation under our direction, funded by the National Institute of Mental Health (NIMH), at the New York State Psychiatric Institute/Columbia University Department of Psychiatry. In this chapter, we summarize DBT as described in the two published treatment manuals (Linehan 1993a, 1993b) and as we apply it in our efficacy study.

DBT was developed in response to the need for empirically supported psychotherapies for chronically suicidal individuals with BPD. Although originally developed for the self-injuring, it is also used in the segment of the BPD population that does not exhibit self-harm behaviors (Robins et al. 2001). Treatment retention of individuals with BPD is a well-known and significant problem, as is their lack of progress and dissatisfaction with their therapies. At the time when DBT was developed, empirical support for existing therapies, including supportive and psychodynamically oriented treatment, was lacking. Cognitive-behavioral therapy (CBT) showed efficacy in patients with de-

This work was supported in part by National Institute of Mental Health grant #R01 MH61079 to Dr. Stanley.

The authors would like to thank Alex Chapman, Ph.D., postdoctoral fellow in Behavior Research and Therapy Clinics, under the direction of Marsha Linehan, Ph.D., of the University of Washington, for his thoughtful comments on an earlier draft of this chapter.

pression and anxiety disorders, but individuals with BPD had trouble tolerating standard CBT (Dimeff and Linehan 2001). CBT places a strong emphasis on change strategies that, by themselves, are very difficult for individuals with BPD to accept and utilize. BPD patients tend to experience an almost exclusive focus on change as criticism and invalidation of their suffering rather than its intent as helpful. This approach, in turn, exacerbates their already harsh self-criticism and contributes to their poor retention rate in therapy.

In attempting to tackle this problem, DBT explicitly emphasizes the need to balance change strategies with acceptance and validation techniques. This balance is important for two primary reasons. First, acceptance and change, in and of themselves, are important ingredients in any successful psychotherapy. Many problems and issues confronted in psychotherapy cannot be changed. An obvious example is past history and childhood experiences. Patients are sometimes entrenched in a place of nonacceptance about their past and consequently are unable to move beyond a stance that it "should not have happened." Second, acceptance and change have a dynamic interplay that creates a *dialectic*. Increased acceptance enables greater change, whereas more change allows for increased tolerance and acceptance of what cannot be changed.

This chapter describes the theoretical underpinnings of DBT, provides an overview of the components of standard DBT treatment as developed for individuals with BPD who experience self-injurious and suicidal behavior, discusses basic DBT techniques and strategies, reviews the empirical findings of its efficacy, and provides case material demonstrating crucial aspects of the treatment. The intent of this chapter is to provide an overview of DBT and illustrate how it uniquely addresses the difficulties specific to the treatment and retention of individuals with BPD. For a comprehensive description of DBT, the treatment manuals (Linehan 1993a, 1993b) should be consulted.

THEORETICAL PERSPECTIVES

Biosocial Theory of Borderline Personality Disorder

DBT was developed from a particular theoretical perspective on the nature of BPD (Linehan 1987, 1993a). BPD is viewed as a disorder of *dysregulation*—dysregulation of behavior, affect, cognition, and interpersonal relationships. The chronic suicidal behavior characteristic of many individuals with BPD is seen as a consequence of these dysregulations. The biosocial theory (Linehan 1993a) on which DBT rests attributes the dysregulation to a transaction between an inborn emotional vulnerability and an emotionally invalidating childhood environment. The biologically based emotional vulnerability is characterized by an intense, quick reaction to emotionally evocative stimuli in the environment, along with a slow return to baseline after emotional arousal. The invalidating environment consists of caretakers who may punish, ignore, reject, and/or disregard the child's emotional experience and therefore do not provide conditions in which the individual can learn to regulate emotional experiences. A transaction between these two elements—in which 1) the emotional sensitivity leads to increased perception of threat in interpersonal situations and 2) the invalidating response from the environment exacerbates the emotional vulnerability—results in a propensity to dysregulation. Linehan (1993a) also applies learning theory to explain how the emotionally vulnerable individual develops self-destructive behaviors to obtain a nurturing response from the invalidating environment. As the behaviors escalate, they are intermittently reinforced, making them very difficult to unlearn.

The most egregious example of an invalidating environment would be one involving sexual abuse, physical abuse, or neglect. Besides being a clear example of invalidation of the child's needs, the experience of childhood abuse and neglect is often characterized by much inconsistency and conflict as the child experiences both nurturing and abuse/neglect from the same caretaker. Given the high prevalence of reported childhood abuse among individuals with BPD (Brodsky et al. 1995; Herman et al. 1989; Ogata et al. 1990), the biosocial theory maintains that abuse cannot be ignored as contributory to the etiology of BPD. Nor is abuse thought to have been present in all individuals who develop BPD. Less explicit forms of invalidation such as repeated dismissal or denial of a child's emotional experience and reinforcement of maladaptive coping mechanisms can also lead to severe impairment in self-regulation (Stanley and Brodsky 2005). For example, if children who cry in response to disappointments are repeatedly told "You have nothing to cry about," the result is often not what is intended—that is, to make them feel better. Instead, if it is a frequent occurrence, children begin to mistrust their inner states and become unable to read their own emotional cues. Children begin to question whether in fact there is something to cry about and become confused about their internal sense of upset and uncertain about what they are feeling. If carried forward into adulthood, their emotional experiences remain somewhat mysterious to them. Emotions are misperceived, misread, mistrusted, and experienced as an unidentifiable jumble of upset.

It is important to note that this theoretical stance does not ascribe "weights" to how much biological vulnerability and environmental invalidation is necessary to yield BPD. If an individual has a biological predisposition to emotional sensitivity, vulnerability, and reactivity, he or she is likely to be more easily hurt. Patients with preexisting vulnerability experience hurts more deeply, react more strongly, and have a greater propensity to feel invalidated. Thus, it can be challenging to provide a validating and supportive environment for the emotionally sensitive child. Finally, it is also important to underscore the fact that this theoretical perspective awaits empirical validation. Although some research has begun to examine this theory of BPD, at this point it remains a theoretical perspective, and it may be shown ultimately that either biological predispositions or environmental factors are the overriding determinants of BPD. Nevertheless, like other forms of psychotherapy, DBT was developed from a theoretical orientation, but its techniques and applicability are not dependent on it.

Treatment Theoretical Underpinnings

DBT is a theoretically and philosophically coherent treatment, with dialectical philosophy at its core, embedded within which is behavioral science (learning principles) and Zen mindfulness practice (Linehan 1993a). These perspectives have direct applicability in the treatment techniques and the understanding of patients and their problems.

LEARNING PRINCIPLES

The predominant theoretical approach of DBT is learning principles. An exhaustive review of learning principles is beyond the scope of this review, but in brief, behaviors are understood as maintained through either operant or classical conditioning. This distinction serves to shape the way in which behavior change should be approached. If a maladaptive behavior is understood as maintained through operant conditioning, removal of reinforcers is called for. Alternatively, positive reinforcement of adaptive behaviors can be implemented. If a maladaptive behavior is maintained through respondent (classical) conditioning, loosening

the connection between the conditioned and unconditioned stimuli is important.

Although learning principles are prominent in all forms of CBT, some forms of CBT emphasize the importance of, and therefore focus on, the role of cognitions. Other forms of CBT place an emphasis on behavior. For example, the CBT developed by Beck emphasizes the importance of distorted cognitions (Beck et al. 2003). Exposing and examining these faulty cognitions then becomes an important focus of the treatment. Correcting them is believed to be the pathway to change. Alternatively, DBT places a greater emphasis on emotion. Given the behavioral perspective, DBT defines cognition as behavior. DBT focuses on understanding that reinforcers maintain a maladaptive behavior and attempts to loosen the links that lead to the behavior through a variety of means. This focus does not imply that DBT never examines distorted cognitions nor that Beck's CBT never examines behavioral reinforcers. Instead, CBT varies in its approach to problems, as do the variety of psychodynamically oriented psychotherapies.

DBT aims to provide increased support for patients to remain safe on an outpatient basis as well as support for the therapist working with the chronically suicidal outpatient. This goal is achieved through applying learning principles toward capability and motivation enhancement of both patient and therapist. Patient capability is enhanced through the teaching of adaptive skillful behaviors, and motivation is enhanced through the reinforcement of progress and nonreinforcement of maladaptive behaviors. For the therapist, a DBT outpatient consultation team is a source of support and guidance as well as an aid to keep the therapist focused on the treatment goals and format.

MINDFULNESS ORIENTATION

Certain aspects of Eastern philosophy are integral to DBT (Robins 2002), particularly a focus on acceptance and the importance of mindfulness practice. Linehan (1997) observed that an exclusive focus on change in behavior therapy is experienced as invalidating by traumatized or rejection-sensitive individuals, and it can result in early dropout or resistance to change within the treatment. Therefore, the DBT strategy involves acceptance of whatever is valid about the individual's current behaviors, viewing these behaviors as the patient's best efforts to cope with unbearable pain. However, she also noted that ignoring the need for change is just as invalidating because it does not take the problems and negative consequences of the patient's behavior seriously. This can lead to hopelessness and suicidality. Thus, acceptance and validation are combined with change strategies. The balance of change with acceptance is one of the most unique aspects of the dialectical approach (described later) and is solidly based in the Zen mindfulness perspective. Change is achieved through the tension and resolution of this essential conflict between acceptance of individuals as they are right now and the demand that they change. Thus, the dialectical strategy encourages cognitive restructuring from an "either/or" to a "yes/and" perspective—directly addressing the dichotomous thinking that is characteristic of individuals with BPD and that often leads to maladaptive behaviors (Linehan 1997).

Mindfulness practice teaches controlling the mind to stay in the present moment without judgment. This practice is extremely useful in helping patients remain in the present rather than focusing on past worries or future fears. As patients fight urges to hurt themselves, mindfulness practice is useful in helping them distract themselves from urges, and it ultimately helps them to reduce the intensity of their urges.

DIALECTICAL APPROACH

DBT is based on a dialectical perspective representing a reconciliation of opposites by arriving at a synthesis of these opposites. A dialectical worldview is the overarching perspective in DBT and is manifest in the strategies and assumptions of the treatment. Therapists create a balance between accepting the patients' dysfunctions and helping patients modify their thinking and behavior. The dialectical philosophy leads to the following assumptions that underlie DBT. The first explicit assumption is that patients are doing the best they can. At the same time, patients want to improve, but they need to do better, try harder, and be more motivated to change. A second assumption is that patients may not have caused all of their own problems, but they have to solve them anyway. An additional assumption is that patients cannot fail in therapy; rather, if failure occurs, it is the treatment that fails (Linehan 1993a, 1997). These philosophical assumptions serve to enhance motivation and inform the therapeutic stance at all times (Cialdini et al. 1975; Freedman and Fraser 1966). For example, the first assumption encourages a nonjudgmental approach and discourages negative thinking on the therapist's part in the face of ongoing difficult patient behavior. The second assumption validates the need for change, without blame or judgment,

and promotes effective problem solving. Furthermore, it also underscores the belief that the therapist cannot save the patient—the patient must do most of the work with the help of the therapist. The therapist's role is to encourage self-care rather than to take care of the patient. If the patient does not make progress, gets worse, or drops out of treatment, the burden of the failure is assumed by the therapy—that is, that the therapy was not successful in enhancing motivation, and it removes blame from the patient regarding lack of motivation. This approach is particularly helpful to patients who experience tremendous, crippling self-blame that can inhibit taking chances and extending themselves in both therapy and life generally.

TREATMENT COMPONENTS: A TWO-PRONGED APPROACH

DBT consists of two components in which patients participate: individual psychotherapy and group skills training (Figure 19–1). This approach derives from a point of view that individuals need not only to understand their maladaptive patterns of behavior as they occur in individual psychotherapy, but they also have certain deficits that can best be overcome by developing a means of compensation and skills. These patients often report that they know *why* they "do what they do" but they "do not know what to do instead" or how to get themselves to do what they know they should do. Although the first half of this statement may be only partially correct, the second half is almost always true. A two-pronged approach to treatment acknowledges this problem by adopting a stance that patients may need to be taught coping strategies and skills in a more explicit manner than is typically done with patients who have personality disorders. Thus, this approach suggests that both an understanding of maladaptive patterns of thinking and behavior and skill development are useful in treating patients with personality disorders. Personality disorders are seen, in part, as deficits in certain skill areas that prevent the person from behaving in an effective manner. In addition to these two forms of patient contact, a consultation team for DBT therapists is considered an integral aspect of the treatment.

Individual Therapy

Patients attend at least one, sometimes two, individual therapy sessions of 50–60 minutes each week. Double sessions of 90–110 minutes can be utilized (Linehan 1993a). Although not always possible, it is desirable to

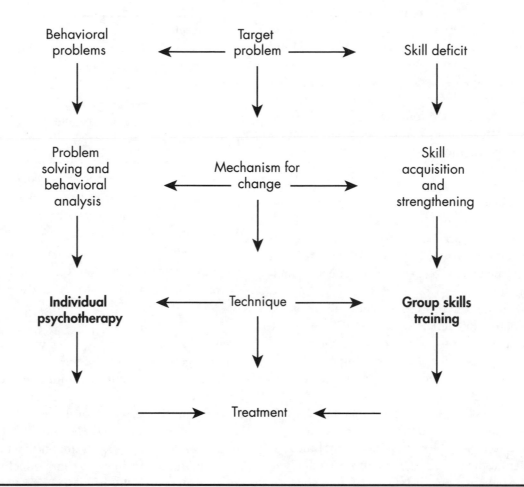

Figure 19–1. Two-pronged approach.

have the flexibility to alter session lengths depending on the patient's needs and the task at hand. For example, patients who have difficulty opening up or who have trouble closing up at the end of sessions may benefit from longer sessions for a period of time until they develop the capacity to transition in and out of sessions. Also, there are times when the type of treatment work benefits from longer sessions. When conducting trauma exposure sessions, longer session lengths are required. Alternatively, some patients have difficulty tolerating the intense closeness that can be experienced in individual treatment for more than brief periods of time. While this capacity to tolerate closeness is being worked on with the patient, allowing briefer sessions avoids premature termination.

The individual therapy session is structured by the treatment hierarchy and a number of behavioral techniques. Any life-threatening behaviors (target 1) are the top priority and must be addressed within an individual session if they have occurred. Therapy-interfering behaviors (target 2) are the second in priority and

are the first priority in the absence of life-threatening behaviors. As long as target 1 and 2 behaviors are either absent or addressed within a session, quality-of-life issues may also be targeted within any given session. The patient is required to keep a daily record of behaviors, level of misery, and suicidal ideation on what is called a *diary card* (Linehan 1993b) (described in more detail later). Therapist and patient review the diary card together and use it to create an agenda for the session. If the patient engaged in self-injury, a behavioral analysis (described later) is required.

Skills Training

Generally speaking, skills training is based on learning theory and utilizes behavioral principles such as shaping, modeling, repeated practice, behavioral rehearsal, homework, and reinforcement of socially appropriate behaviors. Behavior change is facilitated by the combination of the direct instruction of information, modeling of behaviors by role models, prompting of specific behaviors, and positive reinforcement of successive approximations toward the desired goal. The specific goal or behavior to be changed will differ depending on the patient's presenting problem. The teaching of skillful behaviors with which to replace the maladaptive ones is a major component of capacity enhancement in DBT. Attending a weekly skills training group in which skills are taught within a didactic framework, preferably by a therapist other than the individual therapist, is an essential component of the treatment. The group serves to introduce and teach the concepts of skills, and it provides an opportunity to interact with other patients who are also learning skills. A skills training manual (Linehan 1993b) describes the skills and how to teach them and contains worksheets and homework assignments to facilitate learning. In vivo skills coaching is conducted in such a way as to enhance patient capability and motivation.

The first step in the process of skills training is the assessment of the skill deficit, which in DBT takes place in the individual therapy session. Once the specific deficit has been identified, skills training may be implemented. Direct instruction on the skill to be learned begins the training. This instruction gives the patient the required knowledge to perform the skill. Next is modeling, by the therapist or skills trainer, of the skill behavior to be learned. Modeling has many functions for the patient (Spieglar and Guevremont 1998). First, it teaches the patient a new behavior through observation of a model. Second, the patient is prompted to perform a behavior after observing a model engage in the behavior. Third, the patient is motivated to engage in similar behavior after observing the favorable consequences it receives, which is the concept of *vicarious reinforcement*. Lastly, after observing a person who is serving as a model safely engaging in the anxiety-provoking behavior, the patient's anxiety is decreased.

After the skill has been modeled for the patient, it is the patient's turn to perform the behavior, often referred to as *behavior rehearsal*. The first step is prompting or reminding the patient to perform a behavior. Next is the process of shaping, which is the reinforcing of components of the target behavior that are successively closer approximations of the actual target behavior. Feedback is given to the patient regarding success, and reinforcement of the behavior results. After the skill has been rehearsed or practiced, the patient is then asked to participate in a role-play situation that requires use of the skill. Outside of skills training sessions, patients may be asked to complete homework assignments that will require more use of the skill.

Table 19–1.   Dialectical behavior therapy skills training modules

I.   Mindfulness
   A.   Focusing on the moment
   B.   Awareness without judgment

II.   Distress tolerance
   A.   Crisis survival strategies
   B.   Radical acceptance of reality

III.   Emotion regulation
   A.   Observe and identify emotional states
   B.   Validate and accept one's emotions
   C.   Decrease vulnerability to negative emotions
   D.   Increase experience of positive emotions

IV.   Interpersonal effectiveness
   A.   Assertiveness training
   B.   Cognitive restructuring
   C.   Balancing objectives with maintaining relationships and self-esteem

Eventually, this repeated practice will lead to mastery of the targeted skill or behavior.

Linehan (1993b) outlined four specific skills training modules that target the four areas of dysregulation of BPD: mindfulness skills address cognitive dysregulation, distress tolerance skills address behavioral dysregulation, emotion regulation skills address affect dysregulation, and interpersonal effectiveness skills address dysregulation of interpersonal relationships (Table 19–1).

Although the modules were developed for BPD, they have broad applicability to other problems and disorders, such as avoidant, dependent, and paranoid personality disorders (Stanley et al. 2001). The individual modules have been designed to remedy a specific dysfunction; however, they reinforce each other, thus creating a comprehensive treatment of the "whole patient."

The first module is *core mindfulness* skills training, which focuses on dysregulations of self and cognition. Mindfulness skills are based on Eastern Zen Buddhist principles. Patients are taught techniques for focusing their thoughts and attention on the present, establishing attentional control, and coupling awareness with nonjudgmental thinking. The goal is to help the patient establish a lifestyle of mental awareness and inner connectivity.

The second module is *distress tolerance* skills training, which focuses on teaching skills to help the patient tolerate and deal with problems such as impulsivity and suicidal ideation. The fundamental goal of this module is learning the skills of both distracting from a distressing situation as well as accepting situations when they cannot be changed. Distress tolerance skills focus on how to live through a crisis situation without engaging in destructive behaviors. Crisis survival strategies include distracting and self-soothing techniques, pro-and-con analyses, and strategies for accepting reality rather than fighting it.

The third skill module is *emotion regulation*, which teaches the necessary skills to control dysregulated experiences and expressions of anger, anxiety, fear, and depression as well as dysregulated positive emotions such as love and joy. Emotion regulation skills include observing and identifying emotional states and validating and accepting one's emotional reactions. There are also techniques for avoiding vulnerability to negative emotions and increasing the experience of positive emotions.

Finally, the fourth module is *interpersonal effectiveness* training, which exposes borderline patients to effective strategies for mending interpersonal conflict. Interpersonal effectiveness skills incorporate assertiveness training techniques with cognitive restructuring. Patients are encouraged and taught to challenge distorted cognitions related to interpersonal interactions and to identify and stay mindful of their goals within these interactions. They learn techniques for effectively making requests or saying no to unwanted demands and balancing their objectives with maintaining relationships and self-esteem.

Case Example

Ms. L is a highly intelligent 28-year-old woman working as a secretary and studying for her bachelor's degree. She lives with her boyfriend of 6 years; the two were in couples therapy seeking help in deciding whether to get married. Ms. L was referred by the couples therapist to individual therapy for the treatment of binge-eating disorder: the patient's obesity and out-of-control binge eating were interfering with the couple's sex life. During the course of individual psychotherapy, it became apparent that the patient was exhibiting symptoms of BPD that were contributing to the primary difficulties in her relationship with her boyfriend. Her binge eating was an impulsive behavior that was often triggered by fears of abandonment, feelings of emptiness, and identity diffusion, and the binge eating was a self-soothing mechanism for feelings of uncontrollable rage. The patient was also having difficulties in her relationships with supervisors at work due to a tendency to idealize, and then devalue, those in authority and to feel used and victimized and view the supervisors with suspicion when under stress. The individual therapist identified the need for the patient to develop more skillful cop-

ing mechanisms to replace the binge eating and impaired interpersonal functioning and referred her for adjunct DBT skills training. Although Ms. L was not initially interested in changing her interpersonal behaviors, because she viewed her difficulties with her supervisors as external to herself, she was highly motivated to gain control over her eating and agreed to undergo skills training.

Ms. L immediately took to the skills training. She found the mindfulness skills extremely helpful in allowing her to observe and describe urges to binge, which gave her increasing control over her eating behaviors. She learned distress tolerance skills that helped her distract from and also tolerate the feelings of anger and emptiness without resorting to binge eating. She was able to use the support of the other group members to observe her interpersonal patterns, and she became more willing to try new ways of interpreting the behaviors of others. She described it thus: "Mindfulness skills helped me more clearly distinguish between my thoughts and behaviors in an interpersonal interaction and what the contribution of the other person was."

STAGES OF TREATMENT AND TREATMENT HIERARCHY

DBT has four stages of treatment. Stage 1 specifically targets the reduction of life-threatening behavior and is therefore the most researched and of particular interest to clinicians who treat the chronic suicidality of BPD patients on an outpatient basis. Within the context of treating self-injury, other behavioral, interpersonal, cognitive, and emotional difficulties are also addressed. These include behaviors that interfere with the therapy and interpersonal difficulties. Once a patient has control over self-injurious behaviors, the patient enters into stage 2. Stage 2 in DBT helps patients increase emotional experiencing. Because many individuals with BPD have a history of childhood abuse (Brodsky et al. 1995; Herman et al. 1989), exposure-based procedures are used to treat the residue of childhood trauma (Foa 1997). Other quality-of-life issues, such as self-actualization in social and vocational arenas, become the target of treatment during stage 3. Finally, stage 4 treatment focuses on increasing joy and a sense of completeness and connectedness.

HIERARCHY OF TREATMENT GOALS

A standard hierarchy of goals is built into stage 1 DBT (Table 19–2). The primary goal is the reduction of life-threatening behaviors. The first task of the clinician is to establish a commitment from the patient to accept this hierarchy of goals, particularly the primary one of reducing self-injury. The sessions in which this commitment is negotiated are considered the pretreatment phase.

Table 19–2.   Hierarchy of dialectical behavior therapy goals in stage 1

1.   Reduction of life-threatening behaviors
2.   Reduction of therapy-interfering behaviors
3.   Reduction of quality-of-life-interfering behaviors

A second goal in stage 1 is the reduction of therapy-interfering behaviors. Such behaviors include lateness, missed sessions (of individual and/or skills groups), failure to keep a diary card (described later), and any other behavior on the part of the patient or therapist that interferes with the therapy. The third goal is the reduction of quality-of-life-interfering behaviors, such as interpersonal difficulties and personal and vocational functioning.

Case Example

Ms. M is a 28-year-old single white woman living with two roommates in a major metropolitan area. She was referred to DBT from a day program she had been attending for 3 months following hospitalization for a suicide attempt. The suicide attempt consisted of a serious overdose of her roommate's benzodiazepines, which Ms. M took impulsively after an argument with her boyfriend. She had lost consciousness, was found by her roommate, and was taken to the emergency department where she received gastric lavage. She regained consciousness after a few hours, and other vital signs were not affected.

At the time of the attempt, Ms. M was taking art courses and looking for a position as an office worker. In the past, after graduating from college, she had worked as an administrative assistant at a bank for about 2 years until she became depressed, somewhat paranoid, and angry. She would miss work frequently and get into altercations with coworkers when she was there. As she described it, "I stopped coming to work because I felt as if my boss was deliberately trying to give me a hard time." She was referred to DBT because she had been diagnosed with BPD and was intermittently suicidal. She experienced suicidal ideation, she occasionally engaged in self-injury consisting of cutting her inner arm without intent to die, her mood fluctuated from depression to anger to feelings of emptiness, and she had interpersonal difficulties due to increased guardedness and suspiciousness

when she was under stress. She reported a severe history of repeated sexual abuse at the hands of her stepfather between the ages of 8 and 12. When drunk he would enter her room at night and would frighten her into having intercourse and remaining quiet about it. This abuse ended when her mother and stepfather divorced. Ms. M suspected that her mother knew about the abuse but was uncertain that this was the case. She developed an inability to trust her own perceptions and had a very conflicted relationship with her mother, whom she perceived as weak and in need of protection. Ms. M had a treatment history of not regularly attending therapy and not remaining with one particular therapy treatment for more than a few months. She reported on intake that she had never found therapy very helpful and never felt that she could allow herself to trust a therapist to understand or help her.

Following the DBT hierarchy, the therapist identified treatment goals with Ms. M. Target 1 was the reduction of life-threatening behaviors. For Ms. M, these were suicide attempts in the form of overdoses, nonsuicidal self-cutting behaviors, and suicidal ideation. Target 2 was the correction of treatment-interfering behavior; Ms. M needed to attend therapy and skills training group sessions consistently and on time and with diary card and skills homework prepared. Target 3 would attend to quality-of-life issues—in this case, finding and maintaining employment.

The main challenge was to obtain Ms. M's commitment to the goal of reducing self-injury. From the patient's perspective, the self-injury was not problematic. She would vacillate between feeling that "having to live with the horrible feelings and memories is just too much to bear and suicide feels like the only way out" and "I don't think I will do something stupid like that (overdosing on pills) again; I'm not suicidal anymore." Her stated goal for treatment was to work through her childhood trauma, which was the main cause of her unhappiness and hopelessness.

Every time the therapist asked Ms. M to commit to the goal of reducing her self-injury, she would respond, "You just don't get it," start crying, and withdraw from interaction. Ms. M was experiencing the focus on change of her behavior as invalidation of her trauma history. Thus, the therapist implemented the "foot in the door" rather than the "door in the face" techniques. This intervention required a major focus on validation—of the pain, the hopelessness, and the horror of her childhood abuse.

The use of validation strategies over a number of sessions allowed Ms. M to feel that the therapist understood the disruption that her trauma history caused her in all areas of her life, despite the insistence on reducing her self-injury. The therapist explained that she was very interested in working with Ms. M on healing from the trauma. However, Ms. M needed first to be able to control the life-threatening behaviors and increase her adaptive coping strategies for dealing with the painful feelings surrounding the trauma. Ms. M and the therapist eventually made a commitment to work together to reduce her self-injury.

Consistent attendance to therapy was identified as a second goal of treatment. Finding employment would be a third, a quality-of-life goal that they would work toward in the absence of self-injury or therapy-interfering behavior. Although Ms. M agreed to focus on reduction of self-injury as the primary goal, the therapist agreed to balance this focus with understanding that the suicidal feelings and self-injury were validations of Ms. M's pain. Several times during the course of Ms. M's treatment she would miss a session only to return and insist that she needed to focus on the trauma and not on the reduction of her self-injury. Later analysis revealed that she had felt invalidated by too strong an emphasis on change in the previous session. At these times, the commitment needed to be revisited on both sides: Ms. M's commitment to reducing her behaviors, and the therapist's commitment to balancing change with validation.

This case demonstrates the DBT treatment hierarchy and how it is implemented when working with patients. In Ms. M's case, the patient was experiencing an overwhelming number of problems simultaneously. Having a treatment hierarchy provided both the patient and the therapist with a "road map" for the treatment and helped to prevent the continual "putting out of fires" that can characterize many treatments with BPD individuals. This latter approach often comes at the expense of working on longer-term goals and issues that will equip the individual for leading a more functional and independent life.

MAJOR TREATMENT TECHNIQUES AND STRATEGIES

A broad range of techniques is employed in DBT. An exhaustive review is beyond the scope of this chapter. Instead, in this section we give some examples of the major tools and techniques to give the reader a sense of how the treatment is conducted.

Behavioral Analysis

A major change technique used in the individual session is the step-by-step behavioral analysis of self-injurious or therapy-interfering behaviors. The dialectical approach to behavioral analysis is unique to DBT. This approach involves identifying the vulnerability the patient brings to the situation, the precipitating event, and the reinforcing consequences of the self-injurious behavior. The positive consequences for the patient, such as immediate relief from unbearable emotional pain, are highlighted and validated. The patient and therapist then collaborate in reconstructing the series of events (thoughts, feelings, actions, and environmental events) that led to the self-injury. The therapist asks for as much detail as possible and weaves solutions or alternative skillful behaviors the patient might have used into the thread of the analysis. Behavioral analysis is a useful tool for gaining understanding into the emotional and behavioral events that lead to an unwanted behavior and for generating specific solutions. It is also built into DBT as an aversive consequence of the maladaptive behavior. The expectation of spending a good portion of the next therapy session involved in a painstaking analysis of a self-injurious act often serves as a deterrent.

Crisis Management, Coaching, and Intersession Contact

Therapist availability between sessions is critical when treating suicidal patients. In DBT, in vivo skills coaching is conducted by the individual therapist to provide the necessary support for learning new behaviors "in the moment." Patients are encouraged to call or page individual therapists between sessions when they are fighting urges to self-injure and require help in implementing a substitute skillful behavior. During these phone contacts, the therapist and patient decide on a number of skillful ways of handling the current stressful situation. Skills coaching through phone consultation is also a strategy for encouraging the generalization of skillful behavior to other life situations.

Rather than resulting in constant calling by the patient, phone contacts are focused and limited to skills coaching and relationship repair. If the patient calls but is not really interested in problem solving, the therapist indicates availability when the patient is interested in skills coaching and quickly ends the contact. If skills coaching is agreed on, therapist and patient quickly review which skills the patient has already tried, and the therapist "cheerleads" and helps the patient generate a plan to try new skills. The therapist praises the patient for calling and validates the difficulty of tolerating the pain and trying a new behavior. These contacts are generally brief and goal directed, often result in the prevention of self-injury, and therefore are positively reinforcing for the therapist (if not the patient).

The 24-hour rule of DBT states that patients cannot call the therapist for 24 hours after they have engaged in self-injury. This rule does not apply to scheduled appointments. If a patient calls the therapist after the fact, the therapist, once ascertaining that the patient is safe from further self-harm, expresses regret that they cannot speak for the next 24 hours. The therapist wishes out loud that the patient had called sooner so he or she could have received skills coaching and support. The therapist then expresses the desire to hear from the patient as soon as the 24-hour period is past. Thus, patients are encouraged to call before they engage in self-injurious behavior, giving the therapist a chance to intervene. The rationale for this rule is to avoid reinforcement of life-threatening behavior and to provide the opportunity for reinforcement of appropriate help-seeking behavior.

If a patient uses between-session contact inappropriately and begins to burn out the therapist, it is addressed as a therapy-interfering behavior—addressed by conducting behavioral analyses, generating solutions, and applying skills to the reduction of the behavior. Thus, patients are encouraged to call before they engage in self-injurious behavior, giving the therapist a chance to intervene.

Case Example

Ms. N is a 24-year-old female with a history of more than 20 brief psychiatric hospitalizations for suicidality. In response to her distress, Ms. N often takes overdoses of available medications and then goes or is taken to the emergency department. These visits usually result in hospitalization, which Ms. N finds both helpful—because it gives her a rest from the troubles of her life—and disruptive because of the negative reactions of family and friends and because she misses work and other responsibilities. Ms. N expressed a desire not to be hospitalized anymore. The therapist suggested that developing a safety plan would help in the short term while skills and strategies were being developed to handle distress.

About 6 months into Ms. N's treatment, she paged her therapist on a Sunday morning because she had taken a "handful" (10–12) of pills to help her calm down after being very upset by an interaction with her boyfriend. The patient said she could not remember exactly which pills she took. It is important to note that although the "24-hour rule" emphasizes the importance of asking for help prior to engaging in a self-injurious behavior, the safety of the patient is evaluated and a safety plan is developed at any point that the patient contacts the therapist. Ms. N's boyfriend had called her at the last minute the previous evening to cancel their plans because he wanted to see a friend first and then meet later. She became very angry with him and told him not to bother coming at all. She then felt very lonely and guilty that she had yelled at him. She became agitated, lying awake all night thinking that he would leave her. She then took the pills to help her get to sleep.

The therapist reminded the patient that it might have been helpful to page the therapist before taking the pills, evaluated the patient's current safety, and determined with the patient that she should go to the emergency department to get a medical evaluation. Ms. N expressed a desire to be admitted to the hospital because she was tired and needed a rest. She stated that she did not really want to kill herself but was not sure she could prevent herself from taking pills again and that she wanted to go to the hospital to "get away from things" and have a rest. The therapist validated her feelings of wanting a rest but also reminded her of all that they had been working on and expressed the wish that Ms. N would stay out of the hospital so that they could have their outpatient appointment the next day. The therapist offered to do whatever she could to help the patient tolerate staying out of the hospital and not resort to taking another overdose. The therapist reminded Ms. N that it was her choice whether to present herself to the emergency department as in need of hospitalization. The therapist encouraged Ms. N to call from the emergency department so that the therapist could either coach her to stay out of the hospital or engage the hospital staff to make them aware of the treatment goals.

Ms. N called as requested—she had been medically cleared but still wanted to be hospitalized for a rest. The therapist spoke with emergency staff and asked them to evaluate her suicidality. The therapist also encouraged them to make their decision to hospitalize based on the current level of suicidality rather than the patient's desire to be hospitalized. The therapist indicated that she would be willing to see Ms. N the next day as an outpatient and work with her to keep her safe outside the hospital. Ms. N called later that day, complaining that the emergency staff had made her wait 10 hours and she just wanted to go home. The therapist let Ms. N know that she was looking forward to seeing her the next day for their appointment.

This case illustrates how a DBT approach works both to ensure the safety of a potentially suicidal patient in crisis and to encourage the patient to stay out of the hospital and continue building a life worth living. This vignette also describes the way in which DBT encourages managing the contingencies in the environment (working with the emergency department staff) in order not to reinforce less skillful behavior and to promote more skillful behavior (i.e., encouraging Ms. N to figure out a way to control her suicidal urges to stay out of the hospital and resume outpatient therapy).

Diary Cards

Patients keep track of all target 1 problems (life-threatening and self-injurious behaviors as well as behaviors that have an impact on target 1 problems) on a daily basis. Some examples of these problems might be overall mood, use of nonprescribed substances, urges to self-injure, and adherence to medication regimens. In addition, the therapist and patient decide together about any other important behaviors, urges, and feelings to track. These may include eating disorders, urges to physically hurt other people, and impulsive behaviors such as shoplifting.

The diary card serves as the means for setting the session agenda and is reviewed with the patient at the outset of each session. These cards are particularly useful for patients who experience frequent episodes of dissociation or who tend to remember only what happened in their current mood states. The cards are also helpful for patients who feel a great deal of shame about their behaviors. If the shameful behaviors are not recorded on the card, patients often feel too embarrassed to bring them up. Surprisingly, although some patients do not record all relevant behaviors and urges on the cards, it seems easier for patients to be truthful and record these items on the cards than to take the initiative of bringing up these behaviors and urges in a session. Diary cards jog the memory of patients and often result in having available information that would never have been brought up or recollected.

VALIDATION

Validation is a strategy that is used in many forms of psychotherapy including supportive, psychodynamic, and client-centered therapies. Linehan (1993a) presented the essence of validation in the context of DBT psychotherapy: "The therapist communicates to the client that her responses make sense and are understandable within her current life context or situation. Validation strategies require the therapist to search for, recognize, and reflect to the client the validity inherent in her response to events" (p. 223). Validation is at the core of the acceptance/change dialectic and is a crucial aspect of the therapeutic approach in DBT. Linehan therefore delineated five levels of validation: 1) listening and observing; 2) accurate reflection; 3) articulating the unverbalized; 4) validating in terms of sufficient, but not necessarily valid, causes; 5) validating as reasonable "in the moment." As mentioned earlier, validation is much less frequently utilized in CBT. In DBT, discussions of the patient's emotional experiences, suffering, and difficulty with changing are some of the occasions for using validation. The basic function of validation is to communicate to patients that their responses are understandable and make sense within their current life situation or context (Linehan 1993a).

Validation should never be patronizing, and it should never validate that which is invalid. Validation is composed of three steps: 1) active observing of what the patient is reporting; 2) reflection of the patient's feelings, thoughts, and behaviors in a nonjudgmental and nonauthoritarian manner, whereby the therapist phrases the reflection not as a pronouncement but more as a question; and 3) direct validation of the validity and "understandability" of the patient's response.

BALANCING CHANGE AND ACCEPTANCE

There is an ongoing focus on maintaining a balance between change and acceptance strategies within each intervention and over the course of the treatment. Validation and acceptance without a change focus can lead to demoralization that things will never be any different. An approach that focuses too intensely on change can make a patient feel poorly understood and criticized. This effect, in turn, can increase a patient's self-blame and lead to early treatment dropouts.

CONSULTATION TEAM

An assumption of DBT is that therapists treating suicidal individuals with BPD also need support. An integral aspect of DBT is the role of the consultation team to which therapists can bring any problems they are experiencing with their patients. The consultation team assumes a dialectic stance and provides both suggestions and support. In addition, the team provides a valuable function of helping therapists stay on track and follow the treatment hierarchy as prescribed. It is important to note that this consultation team is more similar to a supervision team than a patient's "treatment team." In the DBT model, team members in a day hospital or an inpatient setting tend not to have meetings jointly with the patient in order to avoid "splitting" or to avoid presenting a unified front to patients—which can be experienced as overwhelming and intimidating to patients. Instead, each staff member's experience with the patient is treated as valid and a synthesis of their experiences is sought. Furthermore, staff members are treated in the therapy as any other person in the patient's life. Therefore, instead of intervening and talking to the other staff member about a patient's complaint or upset, the therapist coaches a patient in how to handle the complaint directly with the staff member. For example, if a patient in DBT complains bitterly to the therapist that the psychiatrist is often late to appointments and the patient finds it enraging, the therapist's first approach is to help the patient express the feelings about the lateness directly to the psychiatrist rather than the therapist discussing it with the psychiatrist.

EFFICACY DATA

DBT was originally tested in a randomized, controlled clinical trial (Linehan et al. 1991, 1993, 1994; Shearin and Linehan 1992). The 1-year DBT treatment compared with treatment as usual showed significant effects in three areas: 1) suicidal behavior and self-mutilation, 2) maintenance in treatment, and 3) amount of inpatient treatment. DBT subjects engaged in significantly fewer self-injurious acts than treatment-as-usual subjects. This effect was most marked in the first 4 months of treatment. DBT patients also had significantly fewer severe self-injurious acts, in terms of medical consequences, than treatment-as-usual patients. Also, DBT patients had greater retention in individual therapy compared with treatment-as-usual patients (84% remaining in DBT treatment) and had significantly fewer days of hospitalization per person. In addition, DBT showed greater reduction in anger and improved functioning (Linehan et al. 1994). There were no group differences on measures of depression, hopelessness, suicidal ideation, or reasons for living. On 1-year follow-up, Linehan et al. (1993) found that DBT subjects had significantly fewer suicidal and self-mutilating behaviors, less anger, fewer psychiatric inpatient days, and better social adjustment than treatment-as-usual subjects.

DBT has also been tested as a 6-month treatment in two small sample studies (Koons et al. 2001; Stanley et al. 1998). Stanley et al. (1998), in a pilot study, found that individuals in DBT demonstrated decreased rates of self-injurious behavior and urges to self-injure and decreased hopelessness and subjective depression over the course of a 6-month treatment. Treatment retention was very high, with a 95% completion rate. Koons et al. (2001), in an outpatient study of female veterans with BPD, found that those in DBT had lower rates of self-injury, suicidal ideation, hopelessness, anger, and depression when compared with a treatment-as-usual group. In addition, Verheul et al. (2003) conducted a 12-month trial comparing DBT with treatment as usual in the Netherlands. This trial of 58 females with BPD found that DBT had a better retention rate and greater reductions in self-injury and other forms of self-damaging impulsive behavior. Suicide attempt rates were low in both groups and approached but did not reach significance, with 7% of the DBT group making suicide attempts compared with 26% of the treatment-as-usual group.

DBT has also been adapted for inpatient settings (Simpson et al. 1998; Swenson et al. 2001; Turner 2000). Barley et al. (1993) conducted a partial replication of DBT's efficacy in a pre/post design by showing a reduction in rates of suicidal behavior and self-mutilation incidents with DBT. Monthly rates of self-destructive behavior on an inpatient unit were compared before and after the introduction of DBT with rates on a similar general adult inpatient unit using a non-DBT treatment. Mean monthly rates of self-injurious behavior on the DBT unit were significantly lower after the introduction of DBT, whereas rates on the non-DBT unit were not significantly altered during the same time period. Therefore, DBT appears to be effective in treating the more serious behavioral aspects of BPD, namely suicidal behavior and self-mutilation. In addition, Bohus et al. (2000), in an uncontrolled inpatient trial of DBT, found that parasuicidal females with BPD showed decreased self-injury, depression, dissociation, and anxiety postdischarge. Although there are no trials of patients with other personality disorders, efficacy data have been shown for DBT with domestic violence partners (Fruzzetti and Levensky 2000) and in bulimia (Safer et al. 2001), binge-eating (Telch et al. 2001), hyperactivity (Hesslinger et al. 2002), and substance use disorders (Linehan et al. 1999, 2002; van den Bosch et al. 2002). Also, adaptations and efficacy in special populations have been explored, including forensic patients (McCann et al. 2000; Trupin et al. 2002), the elderly depressed (Lynch et al. 2003), and adolescents (Miller et al. 1997; Rathus and Miller 2002). Further treatment outcome studies comparing DBT with other forms of psychotherapy and/or psychopharmacological treatment are currently under way. See Scheel (2000) and Robins and Chapman (2004) for a comprehensive critical review of empirical findings regarding DBT for all disorders.

CONCLUSIONS

DBT is a cognitive-behavioral treatment that has demonstrated efficacy in BPD. It has also been adapted to other disorders and specialized populations. Although it has not yet been adapted to other personality disorders, it is likely to be useful in those disorders in which impulsivity and behavioral dyscontrol are prominent.

REFERENCES

Barley WD, Buie SE, Peterson EW, et al: Development of an inpatient cognitive-behavioral treatment program for borderline personality disorder. J Personal Disord 7:232–240, 1993

Beck A, Freeman A, Davis D: Cognitive Therapy of Personality Disorders, 2nd Edition. New York, Guilford, 2003

Bohus M, Haaf B, Stiglmayr C, et al: Evaluation of inpatient dialectical behavior therapy for borderline personality disorder: a prospective study. Behav Res Ther 38:875–888, 2000

Brodsky BS, Cloitre M, Dulit RA: Relationship of dissociation to self-mutilation and childhood abuse in borderline personality disorder. Am J Psychiatry 152:1788–1792, 1995

Cialdini RB, Vincent JE, Lewis SK, et al: Reciprocal concessions procedure for inducing compliance: the door-in-the-face technique. J Pers Soc Psychol 31:206–215, 1975

Dimeff L, Linehan M: Dialectical behavior therapy in a nutshell. The California Psychologist 34:10–13, 2001

Foa EB: Psychological processes related to recovery from a trauma and an effective treatment for PTSD. Ann NY Acad Sci 821:410–424, 1997

Freedman JL, Fraser SC: Compliance without pressure: the foot-in-the-door technique. J Pers Soc Psychol 4:195–202, 1966

Fruzzetti AE, Levensky ER: Dialectical behavior therapy for domestic violence: rationale and procedures. Cogn Behav Pract 7:435–447, 2000

Herman JL, Perry JC, van der Kolk BA: Childhood trauma in borderline personality disorder. Am J Psychiatry 146:490–495, 1989

Hesslinger B, Tebartz van Elst L, Nyberg E, et al: Psychotherapy of attention deficit hyperactivity disorder in adults: a pilot study using a structured skills training program. Eur Arch Psychiatry Clin Neurosci 252:117–184, 2002

Kehrer CA, Linehan MM: Interpersonal and emotional problem-solving skills and parasuicide among women with borderline personality disorder. J Personal Disord 10:153–163, 1996

Koons C, Robins CJ, Tweed JL, et al: Efficacy of dialectical behavior therapy in women veterans with borderline personality disorder. Behav Ther 32:371–390, 2001

Linehan MM: Dialectical behavior therapy: a cognitive-behavioral approach to parasuicide. J Personal Disord 1:328–333, 1987

Linehan MM: Cognitive-Behavioral Treatment of Borderline Personality Disorder. New York, Guilford, 1993a

Linehan MM: Skills Training Manual for Treating Borderline Personality Disorder. New York, Guilford, 1993b

Linehan MM: Dialectical behavior therapy for borderline personality disorder. J Calif Alliance Ment Ill 8:44–46, 1997

Linehan MM, Armstrong HE, Suarez A, et al: Cognitive-behavioral treatment of chronically parasuicidal borderline patients. Arch Gen Psychiatry 48:1060–1064, 1991

Linehan MM, Heard HL, Armstrong HE: Naturalistic follow-up of a behavioral treatment for chronically parasuicidal borderline patients. Arch Gen Psychiatry 50:971–975, 1993

Linehan MM, Tutek D, Heard HL, et al: Interpersonal outcome of cognitive-behavioral treatment for chronically suicidal borderline patients. Am J Psychiatry 5:1771–1776, 1994

Linehan MM, Schmidt HI, Dimeff LA, et al: Dialectical behavior therapy for patients with borderline personality disorder and drug-dependence. Am J Addict 8:279–292, 1999

Linehan MM, Dimeff LA, Reynolds SK, et al: Dialectical behavior therapy versus comprehensive validation therapy plus 12-step for the treatment of opioid dependent women meeting criteria for borderline personality disorder. Drug Alcohol Depend 67:13–26, 2002

Lynch TR, Morse JQ, Mendelson T, et al: Dialectical behavior therapy for depressed older adults: a randomized pilot study. Am J Geriatr Psychiatry 11:33–45, 2003

McCann RA, Ball EM, Ivanoff A: DBT with an inpatient forensic population: the CMHIP forensic model. Cogn Behav Pract 7:447–456, 2000

Miller AL, Rathus JH, Linehan MM, et al: Dialectical behavior therapy adapted for suicidal adolescents. Journal of Practical Psychiatry and Behavioral Health 3:78–86, 1997

Ogata SN, Silk KR, Goodrich S, et al: Childhood sexual and physical abuse in adult patients with borderline personality disorder. Am J Psychiatry 147:1008–1013, 1990

Rathus JH, Miller AL: Dialectical behavior therapy adapted for suicidal adolescents. Suicide Life Threat Behav 32:146–157, 2002

Robins CJ: Zen principles and mindfulness practice in dialectical behavior therapy. Cogn Behav Pract 9:50–57, 2002

Robins CJ, Chapman AL: Dialectical behavior therapy: current status, recent developments, and future directions. J Pers Disord 18:73–89, 2004

Robins CJ, Ivanoff AM, Linehan MM: Dialectical behavior therapy, in Handbook of Personality Disorders: Theory, Research, and Treatment. Edited by Livesley WJ. New York, Guilford, 2001, pp 117–139

Safer DL, Telch CF, Agras WS: Dialectical behavior therapy for bulimia nervosa. Am J Psychiatry 158:632–634, 2001

Scheel KR: The empirical basis of dialectical behavior therapy: summary, critique, and implications. Clin Psychol Sci Pract 7:68–86, 2000

Shearin EN, Linehan MM: Patient-therapist ratings and relationship to progress in dialectical behavior therapy for borderline personality disorder. Behav Ther 23:730–741, 1992

Simpson EB, Pistorello J, Begin A, et al: Use of dialectical behavior therapy in a partial hospital program for women with borderline personality disorder. Psychiatr Serv 49:669–673, 1998

Spieglar MD, Guevremont DC: Contemporary Behavior Therapy, 3rd Edition. Pacific Grove, CA, Brooks/Cole Publishing, 1998

Stanley B, Brodsky B: Suicidal and self-injurious behavior in borderline personality disorder: the self-regulation action model, in Understanding and Treating Borderline Personality Disorder: A Guide for Professionals and Families. Edited by Gunderson JG, Hoffman PD. Washington, DC, American Psychiatric Publishing, 2005, pp 43–63

Stanley B, Ivanoff A, Brodsky B, et al: Comparison of DBT and treatment as usual in suicidal and self-mutilating behavior. Paper presented at the Annual Meeting of the Association for the Advancement of Behavior Therapy, Washington, DC, November 1998

Stanley B, Bundy E, Beberman R: Skills training as an adjunctive treatment for personality disorders. J Psychiatr Pract 7:324–335, 2001

Swenson CR, Sanderson C, Dulit RA, et al: The application of dialectical behavior therapy for patients with borderline personality disorder on inpatient units. Psychiatr Q 72:307–324, 2001

Telch CF, Agras WS, Linehan MM: Dialectical behavior therapy for binge eating disorder. J Consult Clin Psychol 69:1061–1065, 2001

Trupin EW, Stewart DG, Beach B, et al: Effectiveness of dialectical behaviour therapy program for incarcerated female juvenile offenders. Child and Adolescent Mental Health 7:121–127, 2002

Turner RM: Naturalistic evaluation of dialectical behavior therapy-oriented treatment for borderline personality disorder. Cogn Behav Pract 7:413–419, 2000

van den Bosch LMC, Verheul R, Schippers GM, et al: Dialectical behavior therapy of borderline patients with and without substance abuse problems: implementation and long-term effects. Addict Behav 27:911–923, 2002

Verheul R, van den Bosch LMC, Koeter MWJ, et al: Dialectical behavior therapy for women with borderline personality disorder. Br J Psychiatry 182:135–140, 2003

20

Interpersonal Therapy

John C. Markowitz, M.D.

Literature exists on the interpersonal theory and assessment of personality disorders (e.g., Benjamin 2003a; Horowitz et al. 1988; Kiesler 1983, 1986). But treatment outcome research determines the utility of clinical theory, and as yet, few empirical studies have tested the application of these theories to treatment. To paraphrase T.H. Huxley (1870/1894), many a beautiful theory has been killed by nasty, ugly little data. Or, as stated by the late Gerald L. Klerman, M.D., who with Myrna M. Weissman, Ph.D., pioneered interpersonal psychotherapy (IPT): If the treatment doesn't work, who cares about the theory? This chapter focuses on treatment rather than theory and, hence, will be short. The chapter summarizes interpersonal issues related to personality disorders and focuses on IPT (Weissman et al. 2000) as a potential treatment for borderline personality disorder (BPD).

Interpersonal issues are ubiquitous in human experience, and they may sometimes provide an avenue for treatment. Some personality disorders may easily be conceptualized in interpersonal terms: BPD, for example, is defined by a number of interpersonally focused behaviors. Three of its nine DSM-IV-TR (American Psychiatric Association 2000) diagnostic criteria include

"frantic efforts to avoid...abandonment," "a pattern of unstable and intense interpersonal relationships characterized by alternating between extremes of idealization and devaluation," and "inappropriate, intense anger or difficulty controlling anger" as displayed in repeated confrontations with others (p. 710). Most of the criteria for avoidant personality disorder are also interpersonal, for example, "avoids occupational activities that involve significant interpersonal contact, because of fears of criticism, disapproval, or rejection" (American Psychiatric Association 2000, p. 721). By contrast, schizoid and schizotypal personality disorders are internally focused and may be considered interpersonal mainly in a negative sense, characterized by the absence of interpersonal involvement. Whether interpersonal approaches help patients anywhere along this continuum requires examination in—as yet undone—controlled clinical trials.

INTERPERSONAL THEORY

Some theorists have applied an interpersonal perspective to describe patients with personality disorders, of-

---

Supported in part by an Independent Investigator Award from the National Alliance for Research on Schizophrenia and Depression.

ten using the structure of an interpersonal grid. These grids may provide clinicians with helpful conceptualizations of interactions between individuals.

The Interpersonal Outlook

The interpersonal school of psychoanalysis arose in the 1940s as a response to the intrapsychic theories then predominant. Without challenging theories of unconscious drives and defenses, clinical theorists such as Sullivan (1953) emphasized man as a social animal and the importance of the social environment, beginning in childhood and continuing into the present. Sullivan shifted the role of the psychiatrist from observer of a patient's internal world to "participant observer," an active part of the patient's social field in the office. Sullivan and others noted the impact of current life events on patients' psychopathology. These observations seem commonplace today, but they were radical in their day. Sullivan defined *personality* as "the relatively enduring pattern of recurrent interpersonal situations which characterize a human life" (pp. 110–111) but had little to say about the (yet to be defined) personality disorders. He treated mainly inpatients with psychotic disorders.

Bowlby (1973, 1998) subsequently explored how children develop interpersonal attachments initially to their mothers and subsequently to other caregivers. Infants and children develop models for future relationships based on such prototypical experiences. Depending on the quality of early relationships, Bowlby theorized, children develop secure or insecure attachments and consequent ability or inability to tolerate intimacy and separation in relationships. A child's emotional attachment to his or her mother provides an initial experience of basic affects such as anger, fear, anxiety, security, love, and happiness.

If primary attachment figures are available and responsive, the individual develops a positive self-concept and an ability to form secure attachments, with open communication of positive and negative feelings. When faced with a crisis, the secure individual can respond by seeking appropriate social supports, reducing stress and anxiety. By contrast, a child with frightening, inconstant, or unavailable caregivers is likely to feel anxious and insecure, either overly dependent on or avoidant of relationships, with less comfort in social communication and less ability to utilize social supports when stressed (Bowlby 1988). Bowlby's attachment theory fits nicely into our understanding of the course of personality disorders. Whatever their genetic predisposition (Livesley et al. 1998; Maier et al. 1998; Torgersen 2000), individuals who de-

velop personality disorders do so early in life, and interactions with significant others in childhood provide a reasonable template for the patterns of interpersonal difficulties with which older patients with personality disorders present for treatment.

Other interpersonal factors also contribute to our understanding of psychopathology. Research on mood disorders long ago demonstrated that the availability of social supports protects against developing syndromal illness, whereas lack of perceived social support increases risk. Environmental life events have been shown to be both triggers and consequences of mood and anxiety symptoms, and those life events involving interpersonal agency have greater impact than impersonal ones (Janoff-Bulman 1992). These relationships between psychopathology and interpersonal interactions form much of the theoretical basis of IPT (Klerman et al. 1984).

The "Interpersonal Circle"

One way to describe the experience of individuals is to graph their interpersonal tendencies on a multiaxial grid. This grid usually consists of two axes, one of intimacy and the other of control. The first axis stretches on a continuum from affiliation or intimacy to avoidance or withdrawal, and the second axis stretches from dominance or aggression to submission or passivity. The first of these personality maps was developed during the 1950s (Freedman et al. 1951; Leary 1957), and they have been refined since that time. Examples include Kiesler's interpersonal circle (Kiesler 1983, 1986) and Horowitz's circumplex Inventory of Interpersonal Problems (Horowitz et al. 1988). The latter, for example, codes responses from a self-report questionnaire onto a graphic circle of factors such as assertiveness, sociability, intimacy, responsibility, submissiveness, and controllingness.

Benjamin (2003a, p. 24) has noted that these grids have not been widely used, perhaps in part because they fail to capture all of the DSM personality disorders. She has devised perhaps the most intricate such model, entitled Structural Analysis of Social Behavior (SASB). This approach, intended for patients with personality disorders, has three domains, each of which constitutes a two-dimensional grid: one focusing on an interpersonal other (orthogonal dimensions: attack vs. active love, emancipate vs. control); one focusing on oneself (recoil vs. reactive love, separate vs. submit); and one introjective (self-attack vs. active self-love, self-emancipate vs. self-control) (Benjamin 2003a). These axes reflect Sullivan's emphasis on love and power as central human needs. People in relationships tend to show complementarity in their interactions (Benjamin 2003a, pp. 47–48); for example, one person's "attack" elicits another's "recoil."

From these constructs, one can produce interpersonal profiles for each of the DSM-IV-TR personality disorders. For example, for BPD, Benjamin delineated the theme "My misery is your command" (Benjamin 2003a, p. 115) and posited pathogenic hypotheses of the patient's early life experience involving "a painful yet erotic incestual relationship" (p. 118), with associated family chaos, traumatic abandonment, self-punishment for autonomy, and a belief that significant others secretly like misery. The interpersonal behavior of borderline individuals can be mapped onto the SASB grids, and expected treatment developments follow. The patient with BPD starts out at "trust" and elicits "protect" from the therapist, to which the patient initially responds with "active love." Should, however, the patient feel "ignore[d]," to which he or she is acutely sensitive, "control," "blame," and "attack" come to the fore, seeking the therapist's return to "protect." Meanwhile, on the introjective grid, the patient moves to "self-attack" and "self-neglect." And so on (Benjamin 2003a).

These illustrative descriptions are recognizable from clinical practice, but whether they constitute a distinct psychotherapy can be debated. One might anticipate that the maladaptive interpersonal behavioral patterns described would improve with successful treatment, and indeed, studies have found that interpersonal problems do improve with various treatments. For example, pharmacotherapy of chronic depression (Markowitz et al. 1996), brief supportive group psychotherapy for Cluster C personality disorders (Rosenthal et al. 1999), and day treatment of patients with personality disorders (Wilberg et al. 1999) all yielded widespread improvement on the Inventory of Interpersonal Problems (Horowitz et al. 1988). It has not been shown that these interpersonal improvements resulted from specifically interpersonal interventions.

The SASB system diagnoses patients through their interpersonal patterns of behavior as an alternative to the standard DSM approach. It also suggests a treatment approach based on the idea of reciprocal and complementary relationships (e.g., "manage" evokes "obedience"). Benjamin's model seems to provide a basic structure for looking at interpersonal interactions in psychodynamic psychotherapy and anticipating transferential developments that may arise based on patients' prior patterns of behavior. The SASB model for treatment informs a "reconstructive" psychodynamic approach (Benjamin 2003b), lying at the interpersonal

end of the intrapsychic/interpersonal axis of the psychodynamic spectrum. It may share interpersonal emphases, for example, with supportive-expressive psychodynamic psychotherapy (Luborsky 1984), which in a different but related manner examines patients' wishes and responses in interpersonal situations. Treatment is open-ended and usually takes at least 1–2 years.

Benjamin's latest rendition of her psychotherapeutic approach incorporates both psychodynamic and cognitive techniques (Benjamin 2003b). Other interpersonal theorists have also developed psychotherapeutic approaches (e.g., Horowitz 2003). IPT is an eclectic sui generis treatment, neither psychodynamic nor cognitive, eschewing interpretation of transference and dreams, focusing on the patient's current interpersonal functioning outside the office rather than on the therapeutic dyad, assigning no formal homework and eschewing a focus on cognitions (Markowitz et al. 1998). Thus "interpersonal psychotherapies" is a loose rubric comprising a range of psychotherapeutic techniques.

CLINICAL ISSUES

The treatment of a personality disorder through IPT must focus on the interactions the patient has with others. Patients present for treatment with symptoms and maladaptive behavioral patterns of long standing. They are often discouraged about the prospect for improvement; because they have been this way for so long, they feel that their personality disorder is "who they are." The traditional approach to treating such patients has been open-ended, intensive (several times a week), lengthy (often for years) psychodynamic psychotherapy. This chapter focuses on BPD, because this is the area in which IPT has begun to be applied.

Borderline Personality Disorder

This chapter focuses on BPD both because it is a prevalent and difficult diagnosis of psychiatric patients and because we at New York State Psychiatric Institute have begun studying its treatment in a treatment trial. Part of what makes up BPD is the interpersonal chaos patients with this diagnosis provoke and respond to. Instability in interpersonal relationships has been shown to be an important component of BPD in factor analyses (Clarkin et al. 1993; Sanislow et al. 2002). Patients with BPD not only experience this chaos in everyday life but also bring it into the office as well. Therapists generally recognize patients with BPD as clinical challenges and frequently associate the diagnosis with poor treatment outcome. These are patients who scramble appointment schedules, call frequently and desperately for help or to threaten suicide, and frequently appear in emergency departments. BPD is often seen in clinical practice (Widiger and Weissman 1991); is highly comorbid with mood disorders, anxiety disorders, and substance abuse (Zanarini et al. 1998); and is associated with impaired social and occupational functioning (Skodol et al. 2002) and with impulsivity and suicide risk (Gardner and Cowdry 1985).

Recent research and clinical wisdom support the American Psychiatric Association treatment practice guideline for BPD (American Psychiatric Association 2001), which emphasizes the importance of psychotherapy as part of the treatment regimen. One psychotherapy that has demonstrated efficacy for patients with BPD is dialectical behavioral therapy (DBT; Linehan 1993), a variant of cognitive-behavioral therapy that has been shown in several studies to reduce impulsive behavior in self-harming patients with BPD (Linehan et al. 1991; Verheul et al. 2003). Although groundbreaking in establishing that psychotherapy could help control impulsive behaviors, DBT has shown less efficacy for the mood symptoms of borderline patients and has also shown some falloff of effect on follow-up.

Another approach involving treatment in an 18-month psychodynamic day hospital yielded improvement both in self-destructive behaviors and in depressed mood symptoms (Bateman and Fonagy 2001). This study left open the question of whether the day hospital setting or the specific psychotherapeutic interventions benefited patients. Other research suggests that patients with BPD may improve in and out of treatment: only 44% of a carefully diagnosed sample followed over time still met diagnostic criteria after 1 year (Shea et al. 2002). Thus, although the diagnosis of BPD has long evoked fear and therapeutic nihilism, there is hope for improvement.

INTERPERSONAL PSYCHOTHERAPY

IPT is a time-limited, diagnosis-focused, life-event-based treatment of demonstrated efficacy for major depression, mood disorders, bulimia, and likely for anxiety and other DSM-IV-TR Axis I disorders (Weissman et al. 2000). It is a simple, practical, optimistic treatment. Its central precepts are 1) a medical model, namely that the patient has a treatable illness that is not his or her fault; and 2) that symptoms and life events bear an important relationship. The first principle relieves the patient of

guilt and unnecessary self-blame for symptoms and labels the problem as an ego-alien illness rather than what the patient has generally perceived as a personal defect or flaw. The second principle, although not pretending to explain etiology—because we do not know the etiology of any psychiatric disorder—provides a conceptual understanding of illness based on factors that are at least partly within the patient's control, whether he or she feels in control or not. The IPT therapist offers the patient a chance to solve an interpersonal crisis in the course of a brief psychotherapy, with the expectation that the patient will both improve his or her life situation and relieve troublesome symptoms. Randomized, controlled trials have validated this approach particularly for major depressive episodes and increasingly for other DSM-IV-TR Axis I diagnoses as well. Indeed, reliance on outcome research to validate theory has been the approach of IPT researchers from the inception of the treatment. For personality disorders, however, the empirical literature for interpersonally targeted interventions of any kind is extremely limited.

IPT is based both on the theories of Sullivan, Bowlby, and others and on empirical research findings connecting mood and environment (Klerman et al. 1984). The theoretical background, then, may be seen as a common root for SASB and IPT, but is IPT for BPD a return to a Sullivanian developmental outlook? Not really. The IPT therapist reconstructs difficult and maladaptive interpersonal patterns from the past but focuses squarely on the present and future.

IPT has been delivered both as an acute and as a maintenance treatment (Frank et al. 1990; Reynolds et al. 1999) and in individual, couples, and group formats (Weissman et al. 2000). The acute treatment, which generally involves a predetermined 12–16 sessions in as many weeks, consists of three phases (Weissman et al. 2000).

Initial Phase

In the opening phase, which lasts no more than three sessions, the therapist takes a careful, interpersonally focused history with dual diagnostic aims. The first aim is to ascertain the target diagnosis (e.g., major depression) using DSM-IV-TR or ICD-10 (World Health Organization 1992) diagnostic criteria and rating scales (e.g., the Hamilton Rating Scale for Depression [Ham-D; Hamilton 1960]) to reify the illness as something other than the patient. This task is particularly important for patients with chronic illnesses such as dysthymic disorder (Markowitz et al. 1998), social phobia (Lipsitz et al. 1999), and personality disorders, in which the chronicity of the illness leads the patient to confuse it with who he or she is.

The second aim of the opening phase is to diagnose the "interpersonal inventory": the patient's interpersonal style, patterns of relationships with others, and social supports. The therapist elicits patterns of past relationships but is particularly interested in current relationships, both because they can provide needed social support to suffering patients and because interpersonal difficulties may have arisen either as a precipitant or a consequence of the patient's illness. The therapist seeks in this history recent life events, such as *complicated bereavement* (the death of a significant other), a *role dispute* (struggle with a significant other), or *role transition* (a life change such as a geographic move, end or start of a relationship or career, onset of a physical illness), that can be temporally linked to the onset of symptoms and around which the treatment might be focused. In the absence of any life events, the focus becomes *interpersonal deficits* (i.e., social isolation and an absence of life events).

Having raised alternative treatment options, the therapist proposes an IPT treatment with the following type of formulation:

> You've given me a lot of helpful information, and if it's okay with you, I'd like to give you some feedback. You have the symptoms of a major depressive episode, as your score of 24 on the Ham-D showed. Depression is a common and treatable illness, and it's not your fault. From what you've told me, it sounds as though your depressive symptoms began after you began to argue with your spouse over whether or not to have another baby. That's a very stressful situation, and we call that kind of struggle a *role dispute*. I propose that we spend the next 12 weeks helping you to solve that struggle at home. Even though you say you feel hopeless about it, there are probably things you could do. If you can resolve that problem, that should not only make your life situation better but improve your mood disorder as well. Does that make sense to you?

With the patient's agreement on this practical focus, treatment enters the second phase. The formulation explicitly links symptoms to life situation and provides a focus for the subsequent treatment. With the patient's agreement on this focus, the therapist can bring the patient back to key interpersonal themes in session after session.

Other aspects of the initial phase of IPT are developing a therapeutic alliance, based on the therapist's sympathetic, encouraging support of the patient; giving the patient the *sick role* (Parsons 1951), which defines the target psychiatric disorder as a medical illness and thus excuses the patient from blame but underscores the need to work toward remission and to gain or regain the healthy role; and providing psychoeducation about the diagnosis and its treatments. Serial assessment of symptoms using rating scales furthers the psychoeducational process while simultaneously informing both patient and therapist about the progress of treatment.

Middle Phase

In the middle phase of IPT, patient and therapist work on the treatment focus, with each focus employing a different set of strategies. Regardless of the focus, however, each session follows a pattern. The therapist's initial question, "How have things been since we last met?" elicits either an event or the patient's mood during the week's interval between sessions. The therapist's next question asks the patient to link the recent event to its effect on the patient's mood or, conversely, to link mood to recent events. After two questions, then, the therapist has identified a recent, affectively charged event, precisely the sort of incident that provides a good substrate for psychotherapy. Therapist and patient then explore this emotional event. If the incident has gone well, and the patient is feeling better, the therapist offers congratulations, reinforcing the patient's use of effective social skills. If it has gone poorly, the therapist expresses sympathy and pulls for painful affect but then helps the patient to explore alternative options: "What else could you try to do in that situation?" When patient and therapist have settled on an option, they role-play to help the patient rehearse these actions. The session frequently ends with a summary of what has just transpired.

The reader may grasp from this description that IPT focuses entirely on social encounters and their associated affects. It is little wonder, given this focus, that patients develop new social skills following IPT treatment. The IPT therapist normalizes emotions as signals of social encounters, which is useful to the patient to recognize what is occurring and how he or she may want to respond. No formal homework is assigned (meaning the patient cannot fail at doing homework), but the therapy's brief time limit and goal of resolving an interpersonal problem area provide an overarching task for the patient to complete. The concept of a medical syndrome excuses patients from self-blame for their symptoms but gives them the responsibility of working to change dysfunctional behavior so that they can interact with others more comfortably and effectively.

Final Phase

In the final sessions of IPT, the therapist remarks on termination as a bittersweet role transition—a life change with both positive and negative aspects. Sadness is normalized as an appropriate response to separation and is distinguished from the related feeling of depression. The therapist bolsters the patient's sense of independence and self-confidence by reviewing why the patient has gotten better. Given the treatment's emphasis on outside events rather than intraoffice process, it is evident that the reasons for improvement come from the patient's own actions: for example, finding an effective way to discuss and argue with the spouse at home about the baby issue and arriving at a reasonable compromise. The therapist may have been a helpful coach, but the patient receives the lion's share of credit for his or her own gains. If IPT has not been helpful, the therapist gives the patient credit for trying and points out that not all treatments work; pharmacotherapy provides a good analogy in these cases. The point is to excuse the patient from unnecessary self-blame and to explore other available treatment options. If IPT has helped, but the patient has a history of recurrent episodes or high levels of residual depressive symptoms, it may be appropriate to conclude the acute therapy but contract anew for a less intensive but more protracted maintenance course of IPT.

ADAPTING INTERPERSONAL PSYCHOTHERAPY FOR BORDERLINE PERSONALITY DISORDER

Working with Andrew Skodol, M.D., and colleagues at the New York State Psychiatric Institute, I obtained a grant from the National Alliance for Research on Schizophrenia and Depression to adapt IPT for BPD (IPT-BPD). IPT has worked well for relatively acute Axis I diagnoses such as major depressive disorder, but its adaptation to BPD presents difficulties. Among these are 1) the conceptualization of the disorder, 2) the chronicity of the disorder, 3) difficulties in forming and maintaining a treatment alliance, 4) the length of the intervention, 5) suicide risk, and 6) termination. In addition, preparing for a treatment study raised the question of 7) which patients with BPD to treat. The IPT-BPD manual developed for the study addresses these issues as follows.

Conceptualization of Borderline Personality Disorder

Researchers have noted the resemblance between and overlap of BPD and mood disorders. Many—in some

samples, nearly all—patients diagnosed with BPD meet criteria for major depression and/or dysthymic disorder (Akiskal et al. 1985; Zanarini et al. 1998). From a clinical perspective, patients seen in our protocol for BPD have shared interpersonal patterns with many chronically depressed patients. Like depressed individuals, they often feel depressed and guilty and see anger as a "bad" emotion, thus avoiding it when possible. Unlike most depressed patients, patients with BPD periodically explode, expressing anger in a manner that frightens themselves and others and has little benefit in solving interpersonal situations. This unhappy outcome convinces patients that anger is indeed "bad," and they thus to try to suppress it. Individuals with BPD are often inhibited in their behaviors, much as depressed individuals are, but they are sporadically impulsive in self-destructive ways.

For the purposes of this study, working with a spectrum of BPD patients who manage to have some interpersonal relationships, we characterized BPD as a mood-inflected chronic illness similar to dysthymic disorder but punctuated by sporadic, ineffective outbursts of anger and impulsivity. This medical model allows the patient to shift unneeded guilt from self to syndrome. Given the confusion and stigma attached to the borderline rubric, therapists provide psychoeducation about the name of the syndrome and what it does and does not mean. Our expectation is that IPT approaches similar to those for depressed patients will often be helpful.

Chronicity of the Disorder

The IPT model fits acute disorders nicely: symptoms arise in temporal association to life events, either preceding or postdating them. In either case, the therapist connects mood symptoms to life situations, a formulation that makes intuitive sense even to patients with poor concentration and sometimes concrete thinking. Chronic illness, however, fits less well. If you have been ill for decades, recent events seem less related to the illness, and indeed, you may not feel that you have an illness at all. To adapt IPT for chronic Axis I syndromes such as dysthymic disorder (Markowitz 1998) and social phobia (Lipsitz et al. 1999), we took advantage of the patient's perspective—that, precisely because of the duration of the illness, the patient would confuse symptoms with him- or herself. Therapy then became an *iatrogenic role transition* (Markowitz 1998): during the course of a relatively brief treatment, the patient would learn to distinguish a chronic illness (understandably confused with personality or self) from self. By taking healthy actions in interpersonal encounters, the patient would come to see how chronic illness had inhibited his or her interpersonal skills. Developing new (i.e., non-dysthymic) skills would then yield success experiences (Frank 1971), better interpersonal functioning, and better mood. The resolution of the iatrogenic role transition would be to shed the long-standing diagnosis.

In treating dysthymic disorder, therapists encourage patients that depression is *not* their personality, even if it feels as though it is. This intervention becomes more complicated in the instance of treating a personality disorder. The usual IPT approach is applied, nonetheless: BPD is diagnosed and deemed a chronic but treatable illness that affects interpersonal functioning. The goal of treatment is to develop better, more adaptive interpersonal skills so that the patient functions better and feels better. Treatment raises the exciting expectation that the patient may be able to shed this condition, which the patient has had throughout adulthood, in a relatively brief course of treatment.

Difficulties in Forming and Maintaining a Treatment Alliance

Depressed patients come to treatment in great pain and generally cooperate with treatment to relieve it. Working with patients with BPD is more complex; for this trial, we foresaw the need to form a therapeutic alliance with patients for whom such an alliance is potentially difficult. The IPT model is generally patient-friendly—that is, the therapist is an encouraging, therapeutically optimistic ally in the struggle against an illness. Because therapists' interpretations risk making patients feel criticized or threatened, and hence risk a therapeutic rupture, IPT focuses as much as possible on relationships external to the office. This focus minimizes the threat to the therapeutic alliance (Safran and Muran 2000). When conflict between patient and therapist does occur, it is addressed in here-and-now interpersonal terms, trying to understand and to optimize how the patient is feeling and handling current patterns and communications.

Patients with BPD notoriously tend to "split" (in psychodynamic terms) or think "dichotomously" (in cognitive terms). That is, they may feel strongly positive about a person or situation at one point and then abruptly reverse their polarity with seeming amnesia or at least lack of integration of their previous outlook. The goal of any helpful therapy for BPD patients must be to ultimately help patients integrate "mixed feelings," the positive and the negative aspects inherent in all relationships. In IPT, this integration is not done through

focusing on the therapeutic relationship but in exploring the range of feelings a patient has about significant relationships and the people in them. The therapist validates the patient's feelings but then probes for negative feelings in positively held relationships and vice versa. The therapist also explicitly normalizes the idea that mixed feelings are reasonable and tolerable: for example, that you can (and sooner or later may well) hate people you love, depending on what is happening in your relationship.

If a rupture should occur, the IPT therapist validates the patient's feelings wherever possible; encourages active communication of the disagreement in here-and-now interpersonal terms; and underscores the importance of continuing to work together, because this sort of interpersonal difficulty is precisely the kind of problem that arises with BPD. IPT therapists are free to apologize and to give the patient space as judged clinically appropriate.

> Mr. O, a 38-year-old single man, now abstinent following years of alcohol dependence, presented with BPD and paranoid personality disorder. His principal affect was rage, and he had run through seven sponsors at Alcoholics Anonymous. Despite the therapist's attempts to focus on his daily life outside the office, his hypersensitivity to their interaction led to frequent disruptions. He would notice and object if the tape recorder had been moved a few inches from one session to the next. He objected to the therapist's jewelry and the stylishness of her clothing. When he became angry, he would storm out of the office, slamming the door and announcing he would not return. Yet return he did, to repeat the scenario.
>
> The therapist had doubts about whether treatment could develop but did her best. She noted that anger was the problem that had brought Mr. O to treatment and that it was a key symptom (#8 on the DSM-IV-TR criteria list) of BPD. Anger was just what they needed to work on. She apologized for upsetting the patient but then explored with him what other options he had for expressing his feelings about relationships. As things were mended in the office, she tried to focus on anger difficulties in outside relationships. Although the pattern continued, it also changed over time. With the therapist's tolerance and support, the patient began to stay longer in sessions in which he felt enraged, at first fuming silently. Further into treatment, he was able not only to remain in the room but to voice his feelings. Treatment focus shifted back to outside relationships. He also began to discuss his related fear of abandonment and fear of dropping his guard lest others reject him.

Length of Treatment

Sixteen weeks, the usual maximal length of acute IPT, seemed inadequate to treat BPD. There are no published studies of IPT for Axis II disorders, although an earlier unpublished study by Gillies and colleagues (Angus and Gillies 1994) had attempted a 12-week trial. Without a clear precedent in IPT research, our research group arbitrarily decided to attempt a two-stage treatment. In the first, the acute phase, the patient receives eighteen 50-minute IPT sessions over 16 weeks. The goals of that initial phase are to establish a therapeutic alliance, limit self-destructive behaviors, and hopefully provide initial symptomatic relief. If the patient tolerates this first phase, a continuation phase of 16 sessions in as many weeks follows. Goals of continuation treatment involve building on initial gains, maintaining a strong therapeutic alliance as termination approaches, and developing more adaptive interpersonal skills.

Thus, patients with BPD can receive up to 34 IPT sessions over 8 months in this pilot study. In addition, patients are offered a 10-minute telephone contact once weekly, as needed, in order to handle crises and maintain therapeutic continuity. It should be noted that both the length and the intensity of treatment in this IPT protocol are considerably less than that in DBT, which comprises individual and group sessions weekly for a year (Linehan 1993), and less than that in the 18-month Bateman and Fonagy (2001) psychodynamic day hospital program.

The extended treatment framework, added to the reflection of patients' chaotic lives in the content of treatment, means that the focus of IPT-BPD was necessarily loosened somewhat. These patients present with no shortage of interpersonal life events, which is good from an IPT perspective, providing numerous opportunities for connecting affect to life situations. Although Angus and Gillies (1994), in adapting IPT for BPD patients, had created a fifth interpersonal problem area, *self-image*, and other adaptations of IPT have made equivalent additions (Weissman et al. 2000), our group has not seen the need to use this fifth category or to develop other new foci. We expected that most patients with BPD would have role disputes and role transitions.

Suicide Risk

Most outcome research trials of psychotherapy and pharmacotherapy have excluded patients at high suicide risk. (DBT has been a great exception in this regard.) This exclusion is understandable: clinicians hope to give patients at high risk the most complete treatment available, and research trials tend to restrict the treatments their subjects can receive. On the other hand, the exclusion of suicidal patients from research studies limits clinical knowledge about how best to treat them. In this study, we decided to allow patients who were already receiving stable dosages of medication to continue on their medication, assuming they still met DSM-IV (American Psychiatric Association 1994) criteria for BPD. We provide frequent assessments, telephone contacts, and weekly sessions to maintain patient contact and a therapist with a supportive, engaging stance to try to minimize the risk of therapeutic ruptures (Safran and Muran 2000).

Helping patients to avoid self-destructive behavior must be a key aspect of any treatment for BPD. In fact, our experience thus far has been that all patients have suicidal ideation, and some have impulses to act on it, but most have been willing to see such impulsive acts as avoidance of their feelings in relationship situations and thus willing to suspend the behaviors during the therapy. That suicidal behavior has not been more of a problem thus far may reflect the heterogeneity of the borderline diagnostic spectrum and the sample this study is selecting for treatment.

Termination

Given that issues of separation and abandonment are central for many individuals with BPD, termination poses a concern. In general, termination has not been as difficult a treatment phase in IPT as in open-ended psychodynamic psychotherapy, in part because of the de-emphasis of the therapeutic relationship and brief, clear time limit in IPT. Termination is announced well in advance, and the patient is reminded about it periodically. Treatment termination represents an opportunity to examine the patient's feelings about this difficult life event, to look at the positive and negative aspects of the relationship, and (it is hoped) to integrate them. As in standard IPT, the therapist helps bolster the patient's sense of independence by helping the patient to review the treatment to that point. Why has the patient been feeling better? It is because he or she has made strides in the treatment, learning to handle affects and relationships differently. The therapeutic relationship may be considered another such opportunity for dealing with interpersonally linked feelings in a here-and-now, nontransferential fashion.

Patient Selection

Patients with BPD constitute a highly heterogeneous group (Sanislow et al. 2002). Because the diagnosis requires five of nine DSM-IV-TR criteria, patients who carry the same diagnosis may differ markedly from one another. In this preliminary trial focusing on interpersonal problems, we decided to exclude patients with BPD characterized by predominant emptiness and isolation—in effect, those who met criteria for comorbid schizoid or schizotypal personality disorder. This exclusion ensured that patients would have the relationships and life events that IPT addresses and would obviate the need for the least developed, least useful IPT problem area, interpersonal deficits.

TREATMENT OUTCOMES OF INTERPERSONAL APPROACHES TO PERSONALITY DISORDERS

An IPT approach could potentially treat patients with at least some of the personality disorders. To date, there has been little treatment outcome research to establish whether such an approach is actually efficacious. In the realm of personality disorders, however, this paucity is not overly surprising. Several reasons may account for this.

Most outcome research since the publication of DSM-III in 1980 has focused on Axis I rather than Axis II disorders (American Psychiatric Association 1980). The model for and most common example of this research has been the randomized, controlled pharmacotherapy trial, comparing medication with placebo over the relatively short time course in which such medication is expected to work. Psychotherapy outcome research has tended to follow this model.

Most psychotherapy outcome trials have involved time-limited (usually 12–20 weeks, with once-weekly sessions), manualized psychotherapies such as cognitive-behavioral therapy and IPT. Their brief course fits the randomized, controlled "horse race" model. Therapies of such brevity might be expected to work better for episodes of illness, such as Axis I mood and anxiety disorders, than for lifelong personality disorders. Indeed, it might seem foolhardy to apply so brief a treatment to such a long-standing syndrome.

The longer treatment trials that Axis II personality disorders are anticipated to need make such research more expensive and complicated. The execution and funding of trials for Axis II disorders were, at least initially, probably a lesser priority for psychotherapy researchers and funding sources such as the National Institute of Mental Health than showing that psychotherapies efficaciously treat Axis I disorders.

There has not been a complete absence of outcome research for Axis II, as a meta-analysis by Leichsenring and Leibing (2003) shows. Yet much of the literature on interpersonally focused psychotherapies for personality disorders has been theoretical or descriptive, not based on outcome. Library- and Web-based literature searches for interpersonal outcome trials of personality disorders yield no results. Meanwhile, IPT, the interpersonal approach best tested in the outcome literature, has focused almost entirely on Axis I syndromes. Now that the worth of IPT has been established in treating Axis I disorders, it may be time to include personality disorders among diagnostic targets for IPT. At the same time, it would be useful to test in outcome research whether clinical descriptors such as SASB and interpersonal reconstructive therapy (Benjamin 2003b) have efficacy and advantages as treatment strategies.

Whereas IPT has been well studied as a treatment for various subpopulations of patients with Axis I mood disorders, eating disorders, and increasingly, anxiety disorders, there are no controlled data on its use with Axis II disorders. IPT might be expected to be more helpful for Cluster B or C personality disorders than Cluster A, given the interpersonal issues involved. BPD has appeared to two teams of investigators to be a good area to start on Axis II, given its overlap with mood disorders, for which IPT has shown efficacy; given its strong interpersonal features; and given its public health implications. By contrast, schizoid personality disorder is harder to find and less likely a good "fit."

In Toronto, Canada, Angus and Gillies (1994; also cited in Chapter 23 of Weissman et al. 2000) made an initial attempt to adapt IPT as a treatment for patients with BPD. They maintained the time-limited format, the usual IPT techniques, and the four interpersonal problem areas but added a fifth potential focus, *self-image* (Angus and Gillies 1994). They did so because identity disturbance specifically related to uncertain self-image is a prototypic feature of BPD. Relationship difficulties were viewed as being exacerbated by unstable affect—particularly with regard to anger regulation—and an uncertain and volatile sense of self.

Therapists offered reassurance and support, clarified cognitive/affective markers that triggered and often obscured interpersonal difficulties, helped patients to problem solve interpersonal dilemmas, and identified and addressed the patient's maladaptive interpersonal style in sessions. In the final sessions, the therapist attempted to integrate major interpersonal themes discussed in earlier sessions and to identify and maintain new interpersonal coping strategies. Recognizing the separation difficulties of borderline patients, therapists departed from traditional IPT in discussing termination throughout the course of therapy.

Gillies and colleagues began a pilot randomized treatment trial, treating 24 patients with BPD with either IPT or relationship management therapy (Dawson 1988; Marziali and Munroe-Blum 1994) in 12 weekly sessions and then following patients monthly for 6 months. Relationship management therapy strives to help patients cope with ambiguity and uncertainty. Its dropout rate, unfortunately, exceeded 75%, leading the investigators to abandon the randomized trial and treat the remaining subjects with IPT. Thirteen women age 18 years and older, recruited through mental health professionals and general practitioners, entered IPT. Patients with legal difficulties or current substance abuse were excluded. About a third of the patients studied took antidepressant or anxiolytic medication, which was maintained at stable dosages throughout the trial. Eight percent of subjects met criteria for a current major depressive episode.

Attrition in the IPT condition was low: 12 of the 13 (92%) patients completed the treatment course. Overall pathology and self-reported symptoms declined. Patients identified IPT therapists' engagement and high verbal activity as helpful factors. Gillies noted (personal communication, August 1998) that the study required three consecutive missed sessions as the criterion for dropout. Patients sometimes avoided sessions in periods of intense affect or anger. The investigators felt that permission to attend sporadically may have helped patients to continue and complete the course. Unfortunately, this study has never been published.

The current open trial for IPT-BPD at New York State Psychiatric Institute has thus far enrolled six subjects: one man and five women, mean age 39 years (range 29–52), two divorced and four never married, three working part-time and three unemployed. Two were maintained on stable pharmacotherapy. All met DSM-IV criteria for BPD, all had comorbid mood disorders, most had histories of substance abuse, and most met criteria for several personality disorders. Five of the six had made several suicide attempts. Subjects were rated monthly by self-report measures and by independent raters at 16-week intervals. There has been one dropout to date. Four subjects completed the acute phase of treatment, with three responding. The one nonresponder had comorbid anorexia nervosa and treatment-resistant chronic major depression, was admitted despite meeting study exclusion criteria, and made a suicide attempt during the trial. The three responders all entered the continuation phase and have completed it. As in the Toronto study, therapists had to be flexible about rescheduling sessions, but additional telephone contacts were not always necessary.

In the acute phase, Ham-D, Beck Depression Inventory (Beck 1978), Symptom Checklist–90—Revised (Derogatis et al. 1973), Social Adjustment Scale, and Clinical Global Impression Scale (Guy 1976) scores fell impressively for the responders. The three subjects who completed the continuation phase were not only no longer depressed but also no longer met DSM-IV criteria for BPD. They appeared to have gained understanding about their affective states and to have developed new strategies for handling relationships. The plan is to admit a total of 16 subjects to the protocol and, if the results remain encouraging, to follow it with a controlled trial.

Case Example

Ms. P, a 29-year-old single lesbian artist, met Diagnostic Interview for Personality Disorders–IV (Zanarini et al. 1987) criteria for borderline, paranoid, and avoidant personality disorders and Structured Clinical Interview for DSM-IV (First et al. 1995) criteria for dysthymic disorder and eating disorder not otherwise specified, with a history of past major depression and substance abuse/dependence. At baseline, she scored 280 on the Symptom Checklist–90, 21 on the Ham-D, and 24 on the Beck Depression Inventory and had a Clinical Global Impression Scale severity score of 4 (moderately ill). She was maintained on a serotonin reuptake inhibitor and had had years of prior psychotherapy, with apparently indifferent results. She had felt socially awkward, isolated, and "different" since childhood, the sole child of a failure father and overbearing mother. Teased mercilessly at school, she became a class clown. She said she had been depressed since age 11. She denied serious conflicts about lesbianism but reported relationships based on drug use and sexual contacts without emotional depth. On the rare occasion she did fall in love, she pursued shallow, self-absorbed women who mistreated and then abandoned her. She spent most of her time in the company of her depressed, obese male roommates, whose behavior evoked rage that she worked hard to suppress. She was conscious of trying to "put on an act" with people in social and work settings, trying to act nice and eager but feeling angry and mistrustful beneath this facade.

Ms. P accepted the diagnosis of BPD and read up on it. She liked the idea of blaming an illness rather than herself for her symptoms and interpersonal difficulties, although it took practice to actually do so. She also agreed that she was in a *role transition*: approaching 30, unsure what to do about her career and relationships, trying to avoid drug use and painful interpersonal rejections. She felt she had wasted her 20s in menial, part-time, museum-related jobs since graduating from an elite university.

She was cooperative but cautious and controlling in initial sessions. She took an intellectualized and affectively distanced stance, freely using psychoanalytic jargon (which the therapist ignored) and referring to a potential lover as "my mother." The therapist gently noted this distancing and pulled for affect in discussing Ms. P's encounters with coworkers, roommates, and dates. The patient said she was a perfectionist and believed that any exhibition of weakness would make her feel like a complete failure. She was tired of her "act" and wanted to have deeper relationships but feared rejection: not liking herself, how could she expect others to like her?

In focusing on seemingly minor interactions, such as Ms. P's smiling suppression of her irritation with others, the therapist validated her feelings (was it reasonable to feel annoyed when other people bothered her?) and explored options for expressing this. After a few sessions, she began to accept anger as a normal response to environmental annoyance, risked expressing how she felt rather than continuing her "act," and was delighted to find that others responded appropriately: they stopped the annoying behaviors and did not hate her for speaking up, as she had feared.

Dissatisfied with her patchy work history, which did not allow her to express her creativity, Ms. P decided to apply to fine arts graduate school. This step, however, led her to avoid pursuing a romantic relationship, because she did not want to have to break one off if she had to leave town for school. She did continue, however, to work on improving communication and the open expression of her feelings with those around her. Although her stance remained somewhat brittle and intellectualized, she tolerated her feelings increasingly openly.

At the end of 16 weeks, Ms. P's Symptom Checklist–90 score had dropped from 280 to 203, her Ham-D score had dropped to 9, and her Beck Depression Inventory score dropped to 17, showing an improvement in depressive symptoms. She was rated a 2 for improvement ("much improved") and 2 for severity ("borderline mentally ill") on the Clinical Global Impression Scale. During the continuation phase she was accepted at an out-of-town university for a graduate degree. This was addressed as a new, mostly positive role transition. She also survived and celebrated her 30th birthday. Treatment focused on her packing her belongings to move, on saying good-bye to those around her, and on a nascent romantic relationship that started despite her previous forswearing of that possibility. Termination of the treatment also received considerable discussion. As the patient reviewed her progress, she recognized her increasing comfort with expressing her emotions and thanked the therapist for his help. The therapist noted that she had done most of the work. They made plans for ongoing treatment in her new city. At termination, Ms. P no longer met criteria for depression or for BPD. Her Symptom Checklist–90 score was 141, her Beck Depression Inventory score was 10, and she received Clinical Global Impression Scale scores of 1 for improvement ("very much improved") and 1 for severity.

CONCLUSION

The treatment of BPD represents the first foray onto Axis II for IPT. It presents exciting but difficult challenges. Can a time-limited psychotherapy treat a personality disorder? What are the useful limits of an interpersonal approach to Axis II—that is, which personality disorders will prove treatable and to what degree? What are reasonable goals for brief therapy with such difficult and chronically ill patients? How brief should such therapy be? The exclusion criteria in the Toronto IPT study may have led to the selection of a relatively less severely ill subset of patients meeting the diagnosis of BPD, as evinced by the relative infrequency of mood disorders. The New York study has only fragmentary results, and it too is not attracting the most continually self-damaging patients. These patients appear somewhat less risky and suicidal than those on whom DBT focuses. Yet, precisely because the spectrum of BPD is so varied, a range of treatments may be useful for different types of patients and pathologies.

Interpersonal approaches seem potentially useful for the treatment of at least some personality disorders, likely more so for Axis II Cluster B ("dramatic") and C ("anxious") than for the paranoid Cluster A. As Table 20–1 illustrates, many of the Cluster B and C personality disorders are partly or largely defined in interpersonal terms. Having defining traits that are interpersonal does not mean that such patients are perforce treatable by interpersonal means. We might speculate that schizoid and antisocial patients would, for different reasons, be unwilling or unable to form a therapeutic alliance. Patients with histrionic personality, like those with BPD, might engage initially but find it hard to stay involved enough to seriously examine their interpersonal interactions. Those with dependent personality disorder could likely be engaged in treatment; the challenge would be to help them make independent decisions and take independent steps. Although one might imagine that patients with avoidant personality disorder might be more suitable for IPT than the rigidly defensive obsessive-compulsive personality types, research on depressed patients with these traits found that completers of the National Institute of Mental Health Treatment for Depression Collaborative Treatment study fared better in IPT if they had obsessive rather than avoidant traits (Barber and Muenz 1996).

Adapting IPT to other personality disorders would presumably follow the same general format, defining

Table 20–1.   Interpersonal aspects of personality disorders

Personality disorder	Interpersonal features[a]
Paranoid	1. Suspicious of others 2. Reluctant to confide 3. Bears grudges 4. Counterattacks for perceived slights
Schizoid	1. Lacks desire for relationships 2. Chooses solitude 3. Lacks confidants 4. Emotionally cold
Schizotypal	1. Suspicious of others 2. Odd speech (affecting communication) 3. Inappropriate or constricted affect (affecting relatedness) 4. Lacks confidants
Antisocial	1. Deceitful 2. Irritable and aggressive 3. Reckless disregard for others 4. Lacks remorse
Borderline	1. Fears abandonment 2. Unstable, intense relationships, alternating between extremes of idealization and devaluation 3. Inappropriately, intensely angry
Histrionic	1. Needs to garner attention 2. Seductive or provocative interactions 3. Rapidly shifting, shallow expression of emotions 4. Impressionistic style of speech (affecting communication) 5. Self-dramatizing 6. Suggestible 7. Misreads intimacy of relationships
Narcissistic	1. Requires excessive admiration 2. Sense of entitlement 3. Exploits others 4. Lacks empathy 5. Envies, or feels envied 6. Arrogant and haughty
Avoidant	1. Avoids interpersonal contacts, fearing rejection 2. Cautious to get involved with others 3. Restrained intimacy for fear of ridicule 4. Preoccupied with social criticism or rejection 5. Inhibited in new interpersonal situations 6. Reluctant to take social risks
Dependent	1. Requires reassurance to make decisions 2. Abdicates responsibility to others 3. Avoids disagreements 4. Self-abasing to obtain support from others 5. Urgently seeks new relationships for support when one ends
Obsessive-compulsive	1. Work devotion limits relationships 2. Inflexible 3. Unwilling to delegate to or collaborate with others 4. Rigid and stubborn

[a]Adapted from DSM-IV-TR symptom criteria (American Psychiatric Association 2000). Used with permission.

the personality disorder as a treatable illness characterized by maladaptive patterns of interpersonal function and helping the patient to understand and alter those interactions in day-to-day encounters. Thus a patient with dependent personality disorder, for example, would be encouraged to understand interpersonal conflicts as inevitable and confrontations as useful ways to resolve conflicts. Difficulties with taking risks would be explained as symptoms of dependent personality disorder, and the IPT therapist would help the patient prepare to take such risks, probably beginning first at the level of quotidian incidents and building up to more "dangerous" encounters. It is unclear whether new interpersonal problem areas would be needed as treatment foci.

Yet all remains speculation without treatment studies to test efficacy. BPD may be a good diagnosis with which to begin, given its prevalence, particularly in treatment settings; its associated debility; and its overlap with mood disorders for which IPT has shown efficacy. Definitive statements about the efficacy of interpersonal approaches to personality disorders lie far in the future. Establishing efficacy will require acute comparative trials with careful follow-up assessments and also likely will require ongoing continuation or maintenance therapy, but at least the initial steps in this process are under way.

REFERENCES

Akiskal HS, Yerevanian BI, Davis GC, et al: The nosologic status of borderline personality: clinical and polysomnographic study. Am J Psychiatry 142:192–198, 1985

American Psychiatric Association: Diagnostic and Statistical Manual of Mental Disorders, 3rd Edition. Washington, DC, American Psychiatric Association, 1980

American Psychiatric Association: Diagnostic and Statistical Manual of Mental Disorders, 4th Edition. Washington, DC, American Psychiatric Association, 1994

American Psychiatric Association: Diagnostic and Statistical Manual of Mental Disorders, 4th Edition, Text Revision. Washington, DC, American Psychiatric Association, 2000

American Psychiatric Association: Practice guideline for the treatment of patients with borderline personality disorder. Am J Psychiatry 158:1–52, 2001

Angus L, Gillies LA: Counseling the borderline client: an interpersonal approach. Canadian Journal of Counseling/Revue Canadienne de Counsel 28:69–82, 1994

Barber JP, Muenz LR: The role of avoidance and obsessiveness in matching patients to cognitive and interpersonal psychotherapy: empirical findings from the Treatment for Depression Collaborative Research Program. J Consult Clin Psychol 64:951–958, 1996

Bateman A, Fonagy P: Treatment of borderline personality disorder with psychoanalytically oriented partial hospitalization: an 18-month follow-up. Am J Psychiatry 158:36–42, 2001

Beck AT: Depression Inventory. Philadelphia, PA, Center for Cognitive Therapy, 1978

Benjamin LS: Interpersonal Diagnosis and Treatment of Personality Disorders, 2nd Edition. New York, Guilford, 2003a

Benjamin LS: Interpersonal Reconstructive Therapy: Promoting Change in Nonresponders. New York, Guilford, 2003b

Bowlby J: Attachment and Loss, Vol 1. Separation: Anxiety and Anger. New York, Basic Books, 1973

Bowlby J: A Secure Base: Parent–Child Attachment and Healthy Human Development. New York, Basic Books, 1988

Bowlby J: Developmental psychiatry comes of age. Am J Psychiatry 145:1–10, 1998

Clarkin JF, Hull JW, Hurt SW: Factor structure of borderline personality disorder criteria. J Personal Disord 7:137–143, 1993

Dawson DF: Treatment of the borderline patient, relationship management. Can J Psychiatry 33:370–374, 1988

Derogatis LR, Lipman RS, Covi L: The SCL-90: an outpatient psychiatric rating scale. Psychopharmacol Bull 9:13–28, 1973

First MB, Spitzer RL, Williams JBW, et al: Structured Clinical Interview for DSM-IV. New York, Biometrics Research Department, New York Psychiatric Institute, 1995

Frank E, Kupfer DJ, Perel JM, et al: Three-year outcomes for maintenance therapies in recurrent depression. Arch Gen Psychiatry 47:1093–1099, 1990

Frank J: Therapeutic factors in psychotherapy. Am J Psychother 25:350–361, 1971

Freedman MB, Leary TF, Ossorio AG, et al: The interpersonal dimension of personality. J Pers 20:143–161, 1951

Gardner DL, Cowdry RW: Suicidal and parasuicidal behavior in borderline personality disorder. Psychiatr Clin North Am 8:389–403, 1985

Guy W: ECDEU Assessment Manual for Psychopharmacology—Revised (DHEW Publ No ADM 76–338). Rockville, MD, U.S. Department of Health, Education, and Welfare, Public Health Service, Alcohol Drug Abuse, and Mental Health Administration, NIMH Psychopharmacology Research Branch, Division of Extramural Research Programs, 1976

Hamilton M: A rating scale for depression. J Neurol Neurosurg Psychiatry 25:56–62, 1960

Horowitz LM: Interpersonal Foundations of Psychopathology. Washington, DC, American Psychological Association, 2003

Horowitz LM, Rosenberg SE, Baer BA, et al: Inventory of interpersonal problems: psychometric properties and clinical applications. J Consult Clin Psychol 6:885–892, 1988

Huxley TH: Presidential address (1870) to the British Association for the Advancement of Science (1894). Biogenesis and Abiogenesis, Vol 8: Collected Essays.

Janoff-Bulman R: Shattered Assumptions: Toward a New Psychology of Trauma. New York, Free Press, 1992

Kiesler DJ: The 1982 interpersonal circle: a taxonomy for complementarity in human transactions. Psychol Rev 90:185–214, 1983

Kiesler DJ: The 1982 interpersonal circle: an analysis of DSM-III personality disorders, in Contemporary Directions in Psychopathology: Toward the DSM-IV. Edited by Millon T, Klerman GL. New York, Guilford, 1986

Klerman GL, Weissman MM, Rounsaville BJ, et al: Interpersonal Psychotherapy of Depression. New York, Basic Books, 1984

Leary T: Interpersonal Diagnosis of Personality: A Functional Theory and Methodology for Personality Evaluation. New York, Ronald Press, 1957

Leichsenring F, Leibing E: The effectiveness of psychodynamic psychotherapy and cognitive behavior therapy in the treatment of personality disorders: a meta-analysis. Am J Psychiatry 160:1223–1232, 2003

Linehan MM: Cognitive-Behavioral Therapy for Borderline Personality Disorder. New York, Guilford, 1993

Linehan MM, Armstrong HE, Suarez A, et al: Cognitive-behavioral treatment of chronically parasuicidal borderline patients. Arch Gen Psychiatry 48:1060–1064, 1991

Lipsitz JD, Fyer AJ, Markowitz JC, et al: An open trial of interpersonal psychotherapy for social phobia. Am J Psychiatry 156:1814–1816, 1999

Livesley WJ, Jang KL, Vernon PA: Phenotypic and genetic structure of traits delineating personality disorder. Arch Gen Psychiatry 55:941–948, 1998

Luborsky L: Principles of Psychoanalytic Psychotherapy: A Manual for Supportive/Expressive Treatment. New York, Basic Books, 1984

Maier W, Franke P, Hawellek B: Special feature: family genetic research strategies for personality disorders. J Personal Disord 12:262–276, 1998

Markowitz JC: Interpersonal Psychotherapy for Dysthymic Disorder. Washington, DC, American Psychiatric Press, 1998

Markowitz JC, Friedman RA, Miller N, et al: Interpersonal improvement in chronically depressed patients treated with desipramine. J Affect Disord 41:59–62, 1996

Markowitz JC, Svartberg M, Swartz HA: Is IPT time-limited psychodynamic psychotherapy? J Psychother Pract Res 7:185–195, 1998

Marziali E, Munroe-Blum H: Interpersonal Group Psychotherapy for Borderline Personality Disorder. New York, Basic Books, 1994

Parsons T: Illness and the role of the physician: a sociological perspective. Am J Orthopsychiatry 21:452–460, 1951

Reynolds CF III, Frank E, Perel JM, et al: Nortriptyline and interpersonal psychotherapy as maintenance therapies for recurrent major depression: a randomized controlled trial in patients older than fifty-nine years. JAMA 281:39–45, 1999

Rosenthal RN, Muran JC, Pinsker H, et al: Interpersonal change in brief supportive psychotherapy. J Psychother Pract Res 8:55–63, 1999

Safran JD, Muran JC: Negotiating the Therapeutic Alliance. New York, Guilford, 2000

Sanislow CA, Grilo CM, Morey LC, et al: Confirmatory factor analysis of DSM-IV criteria for borderline personality disorder: findings from the Collaborative Longitudinal Personality Disorders Study. Am J Psychiatry 159:284–290, 2002

Shea MT, Sout R, Gunderson J, et al: Short-term diagnostic stability of schizotypal, borderline, avoidant, and obsessive-compulsive personality disorders. Am J Psychiatry 159:2036–2041, 2002

Skodol AE, Gunderson JG, McGlashan TH, et al: Functional impairment in patients with schizotypal, borderline, avoidant, or obsessive-compulsive personality disorder. Am J Psychiatry 159:276–283, 2002

Sullivan HS: The Interpersonal Theory of Psychiatry. New York, WW Norton, 1953

Torgersen S: Genetics of patients with borderline personality disorder. Psychiatr Clin North Am 23:1–93, 2000

Verheul R, van den Bosch LMC, et al: Dialectical behaviour therapy for women with borderline personality disorder. Br J Psychiatry 182:135–140, 2003

Weissman MM, Markowitz JC, Klerman GL: Comprehensive Guide to Interpersonal Psychotherapy. New York, Basic Books, 2000

Widiger TA, Weissman MM: Epidemiology of borderline personality disorder. Hosp Community Psychiatry 42:1015–1021, 1991

Wilberg T, Urnes O, Friis S, et al: One-year follow-up of day treatment for poorly functioning patients with personality disorders. Psychiatr Serv 50:1326–1330, 1999

World Health Organization: International Statistical Classification of Diseases and Related Health Problems, 10th Revision. Geneva, World Health Organization, 1992

Zanarini MC, Frankenburg FR, Chauncey DL, et al: The Diagnostic Interview for Personality Disorders: interrater and test-retest reliability. Compr Psychiatry 28:467–480, 1987

Zanarini MC, Frankenburg FR, Dubo ED, et al: Axis I comorbidity of borderline personality disorder. Am J Psychiatry 155:1733–1739, 1998

21

Supportive Psychotherapy

Ann H. Appelbaum, M.D.

CONCEPTUAL BASIS

Anyone seeking to help a patient with psychotherapy must provide support of the kind and in the amount the patient needs. Failure to provide this support spells failure of the attempt at treatment. Basically healthy patients provide their own support by assuming the treater they have sought out is competent and has their best interests at heart. They can forgive the grossest rudeness (or at least accept it) by making excuses for the doctor ("He is so important and busy that he can't be expected to conform to ordinary courtesy"). Yet even the most mature people lose their ability to provide support from within when they are excessively scared or in pain, and the treater must assess the level of distress and respond to it appropriately. Psychoanalytically informed therapists provide reassurance, encouragement, active teaching, comforting, and a host of other interventions that they regard as "appropriate" on the basis of a dynamic understanding of the unconscious processes underlying the patient's distress and the therapist's reactions. The concepts that guide the therapist are those of current psychoanalytic theory as it has been enriched by theories of object relations, attachment, ego psychology, self psychology, and developmental observation.

Although patients may experience as supportive any measure that relieves anxiety, dynamic supportive psychotherapy is defined by psychoanalytic prin-

ciples and certain techniques employed to implement them. From the point of view of an outside observer (e.g., consultant, supervisor, researcher), a therapist is seen as providing supportive psychodynamic psychotherapy when he or she acts according to accepted practice principles by applying some specific techniques and avoiding others.

BASIC PRINCIPLES OF SUPPORTIVE THERAPY FOR PERSONALITY DISORDERS

Defining Supportive Psychotherapy

Psychoanalytically informed supportive therapy is defined by its goals, its method, and its techniques because these differentiate it from expressive therapy. Granting that in everyday practice the distinction between the two therapy approaches is less sharp than it is in theory and that skillful therapists typically mix the two methods as indicated, it may be helpful to sketch out the theoretical differences between the two approaches as they are applied to the treatment of patients with personality disorders.

The goals of supportive therapy can vary from restoration and maintenance of functioning to fulfillment of whatever may be the individual's capacities for happiness and healthy living. The latter is often referred to as "adaptation," a somewhat confusing term that often arouses the question, "adaptation to what?" The answer to this question is adaptation to whatever is irremediably limited by the patient's circumstances. In expressive therapy, the therapist's goal does not include maintenance of functioning, because patients referred for expressive treatment are usually seen as able to function on their own with only brief regressions during treatment. Verbalized insight, as well as adaptation, is a criterion of therapeutic success in expressive therapy, where the overall goal can be described as a general expansion of patients' awareness of their inner life and of its manifestations in current feelings and fantasies. Behavioral change for the better is seen as a consequence of developing such insight.

The methods of supportive and expressive psychotherapy differ consonant with their differing goals. The basic strategy of supportive therapy is to create an atmosphere of safety within which the patient can work with the therapist to overcome the internal and external obstacles that prevent achievement of the patient's goals. The basic strategy of expressive therapies is the creation of a treatment situation that highlights the patient's transference wishes and fears. As supportive and expressive psychotherapy goals and basic strategies differ, so too do their methods—with expressive therapy relying on techniques that facilitate the interpretation of transference—and supportive therapy relying on maintaining a reflective state in which identification with the reflectiveness of the therapist is most likely to occur.

Basic Strategy

In treating patients with personality disorders, it is well to keep in mind that disturbances in the management of feelings is almost always a fundamental problem. To do useful work in therapy, patients must be helped with affect regulation, learning to tune affect down or up to produce the state in which they can attend and think. Therapy is best carried out with the patient in the quiet, alert state most conducive to learning, a concept derived from developmental psychology. Peter Wolff (1966) discovered, by continuously observing neonates over a 24-hour period, that they had six emotional states ranging from deep sleep to hard crying. One state, observable only fleetingly at first, was a quiet, alert state in which the infant attended to the outside world. Over the ensuing months this state became more frequent and prolonged, and it was in this state that the baby could play with the parents and learn about the world around it.

Supportive therapy with adults seeks to bring about the adult counterpart of the "learning state" so that the

patient can learn to endure and ultimately enjoy interacting with the therapist in pursuit of the goals of therapy. These goals are determined in part by the amount of time the two participants have to work together: are they in a clinic where the treatment with any particular student must end in July? If so, there must be an initial discussion as to what goals can realistically be met in the time available. Initial goals are further determined by the patient's aspirations and by the strength available to work toward those aspirations.

Some examples may be useful. The following examples are drawn from psychoanalytically trained therapists in private practice who formed a study group to learn more about supportive psychotherapy.

Case Example

A 50-year-old dancer with narcissistic personality disorder came depressed to the therapist, lamenting the manifestations of aging that were limiting the parts she could play. At first she was full of self-contempt when she contemplated moving on to teaching, but with the help of the therapist she began to reminisce about all her own old teachers and how much they were respected by the dance aficionados of the time and idolized by their students. Over a period of 2 years she established herself as a teacher and regained her lofty charm.

The therapist's help consisted of listening with interest to the many stories the patient wanted to tell and empathizing with her hatred of the inroads of age. The therapist chose this route because the patient's self-centeredness, grandiosity, and inability to accept normal aging and its consequences seemed to be indications that the basic structure of her personality was too rigid and too delicate to sustain major change. The patient's indifference to everything other than the world of dance, her lack of any but the most shallow relationships, her easy rejection of anyone who failed to admire her, and her dependence on dance as the major support of her sense of self further convinced the therapist that an expressive therapy seeking to explore the meanings of her narcissistic pathology would either require an inordinate length of time or would fail. The supportive approach rapidly resolved the presenting "depression" (better described as a monumental sulk, for there were no vegetative symptoms) and restored the patient's legitimate pride in herself as a dancer.

Case Example

A business consultant with a history of suicide attempts and considered to have a borderline personality disorder with narcissistic features, came to therapy because of chronic anger. He saw all his bosses as fools and his peers as idiots. He was fired repeatedly, as a consequence of obstreperous behavior in which he showed up the limitations of his supervisors in public. He had run up massive debts and was forced to live with his parents because he could not afford a place of his own. The therapist focused on the patient's altercations with bosses, offering "lessons in hypocrisy." The patient drew himself up in righteous indignation, protesting, "Being a hypocrite is utterly against my principles!" "I didn't say I would help you *become* a hypocrite," replied the therapist, "only that I could help you *act* like one for purposes of survival."

On this basis the patient agreed to begin treatment, pledging to confine his diatribes to the sessions. He soon got an excellent job and was not only able to keep it during the treatment but was promoted several times. The treatment gradually took on the qualities of a partnership in which there was a high level of mutual respect, and both parties were equally invested in sorting out the feelings that tended to build up to episodes of rage or desperation. The therapist made no attempt to explore the unconscious elements in their relationship, remaining confident that this young man's partially formed identity would best be helped to solidify were he to become master of his intense affects.

The approach to this case is in contrast to how expressive therapy might approach this patient. Transference-focused therapy (Kernberg 1983), for example, would be alert to those moments when the patient's rage and contempt would be directed toward the therapist (as was starting to happen in the "hypocrisy lesson" episode). The therapist would not offer "lessons" in the first place but instead would focus on the rage being directed at the therapist and then offer an hypothesis such as, "It's as if the offer itself of help underlines the feelings of need that you are so ashamed of and makes you want to turn on your helper and make your therapist feel stupid and corrupt."

Methods

The following recommendations to therapists are about how to establish and maintain a "learning" state by keeping the patient's anxiety at an optimal level. To implement this basic strategy successfully, the therapist must think analytically while maintaining an attitude of kind objectivity.

Attending to the Patient's Physical Comfort

To establish the learning state in the first encounter, the therapist tries to make the patient comfortable. Throughout the treatment, the therapist sees to it that there are no interruptions (Havens 1989). The therapist's telephone and beeper are turned off, and if this is technically impossible the therapist explains in advance that the telephone might ring during the session but will not be answered unless, for instance, the therapist is expecting an emergency call. A "Do Not Disturb" sign is on the door.

Establishing and Maintaining Conditions of Emotional Safety

An atmosphere of emotional safety is fostered when the therapist lays out the conditions of treatment in clear and simple terms. The therapist must be explicit about what is needed from the patient to do his or her work effectively. He or she must unapologetically specify what can and cannot be done to make the patient feel better and what the patient must do to keep the treatment going (stay alive, avoid self-injury or actions like law-breaking that risk interrupting treatment, stop abusing mind-altering substances, and stay as fit as possible). The patient must try to be honest. Lies or withholding important information should be cleared up with the therapist as soon as possible. Both parties should be punctual and respectful of the constraints (e.g., time, money) that limit the other's choices.

Early in treatment, or even before formally beginning, it is often wise for the therapist to meet with the family and the patient to explain the therapist's understanding of the trouble, why supportive treatment is being prescribed, and how the family can help. Special psychological and neuropsychological testing is often indicated in these cases. The results and their implications for treatment should be shared with patient and family together, if possible.

The therapist maintains emotional safety by keeping a steady level of interest, while avoiding implicitly using his or her perceived superior power to influence the patient. Consider the following exchanges:

> Patient: Mind if I turn this lamp off?
> Therapist: Not at all.

Note that the therapist does not regard every interchange as intrinsic to therapy but at certain times treats the patient as a guest; he or she does not look for concealed meanings in everyday requests; attempt to "clarify" with statements such as "I wonder why the lamp is bothering you today?"; "confront" with "That light has been on for 6 months—there must be something different about today"; or interpret with "Perhaps too much light was shed on the subject of your anger at me last time." Why not? The "clarifying" intervention implicitly informs patients not to ask for consideration in the sessions, which can have the unintended consequence of stifling the expression of wishful fantasies later on. The "confrontational" intervention embarrasses the patient and stirs up defensiveness, which should be kept at a minimum in supportive therapy. The "interpretation" implies (correctly, perhaps, but inappropriately for supportive therapy) that without knowing it, the patient is hiding something from himself and the therapist can see it. All three types of intervention disturb the relationship between patient and therapist by implying a power discrepancy that the patient feels but usually cannot describe because it is covert, implicit, and not openly acknowledged by the therapist. These three staples of psychoanalytic technique are designed to shake up the defensive structure of neurotic patients whose symptoms are frozen in that structure and who can endure the temporary disruption of the relationship with the analyst in the interest of eventually feeling and functioning better. The treatment of choice for personality disorders is supportive therapy, in which the triad of clarification, confrontation, and interpretation is used sparingly, if at all. This approach is particularly true of the early diagnostic phase, when the therapist is developing a preliminary understanding of the case.

Throughout the treatment, the therapist is aware that emotional safety is jeopardized by change in the immediate environment of therapy. If, for example, flowers appear suddenly on the coffee table, a patient may wonder—from whom? why now? Furniture is rearranged—for whose comfort? Christmas cards are displayed in the waiting room and office, and the patient thinks, "Should I have sent one?" Enhancing the patient's awareness of the therapist's interest in other people can stir a sense of rivalry before the patient is ready to deal with it. By the same token, therapists should avoid unnecessary contributions to the envy and sense of deprivation that most patients with personality disorders struggle with.

Interacting With the Patient From the Beginning

Interact with the patient from the start of therapy unless the patient launches into his or her story at once. Most patients with personality disorders react to a silent therapist with escalating anxiety, especially at the beginning of sessions. They may deal with their anxiety by asking the therapist to ask them questions. Often patients have been interviewed many times and have well-rehearsed answers for the standard questions of the psychiatric examination. They feel at home in the well-learned role of patient and provide the kind of answers most likely to result in whatever action they hope the therapist will take. A therapist seeking to develop a relationship with a new patient by

asking questions may be in for an uncomfortable session of laconic responses or silence.

Avoiding Interrogation

A direct question arouses defensiveness, and defensiveness interferes with the learning state. Asking a question is almost always an implicit assertion of power. Any therapist who doubts this dictum has only to reflect on his own feelings when his patient walks in and says, "How was your holiday? Nice tan, where did you go?" Many therapists feel quite uncomfortable. Some feel somewhat indignant at the thought that the patient is "turning the tables." After all, the therapist is the one who is supposed to ask questions; the patient is supposed to answer them. The questioner has the power, the other is endangered, defensive, or submissive and obedient.

Discrepancies of power are already implicit in the therapy situation for a number of reasons. First is the status of the therapist as an authority, and this status is often conflated with power by patients and therapists alike. Second, the patient nearly always meets the therapist on the latter's turf. Third is the unequal flow of personal information from patient to therapist. Many patients with personality disorders resent and fear this power gradient because of the abuse of power they experienced in early life and because of the rage this experience filled them with, rage that feels as though it may spill over and destroy the relationship they need the most. To avoid adding to the humiliation and rage of the patient, wise therapists find ways of eliciting whatever information they need mostly without asking questions.

Case Example

A gifted resident complained to her supervisor about a patient who would not answer her questions and thus was preventing her from "taking" a history. (Note the connotation of extracting information from an unwilling informant.) When the supervisor told her she could learn all she needed to know without asking questions, the resident was silent for a while and then said, "I feel completely disarmed." Shocked at what she had just heard herself say, she realized that she had been using questions as weapons to maintain her advantage as the doctor without acknowledging to herself how important it was to her that she be respected and submitted to by her patients. Hers was a covert need for power, and questions are a covert expression of that need.

When she next interviewed the patient she began with a statement: "It must be rough on you to be cooped up on a hospital ward on such a lovely spring day." The patient replied, "Actually, it doesn't matter to me where I am or what the weather's like. It's like I'm crying inside all the time, and I don't even know why." The diagnostic interview was well advanced by that one poignant response. The doctor had prompted the learning state required for meaningful discourse.

The novelist Canetti, in his book *Crowds and Power*, showed how the primitive origin of questioning is the need to determine whether the other is suitable as prey (Canetti 1962). Hence the primitive and all but universal reaction of anxiety when a question is asked, and hence also the dislike aroused in others by the person whose major form of social interaction is the question. True, there are innocuous, playful, and pro forma questions, but they are now part of therapeutic technique.

Responding to the Patient's Questions

The latent aggression of a question is readily apparent to a therapist when the patient asks a question. The therapist may notice a feeling of discomfort, quickly dispelled by responding with "What brought that to mind just now?" Indeed, some therapists have been taught never to answer a patient's question but to respond with a question instead. The patient gets the message that the question was "inappropriate"; becomes flustered, upset, embarrassed, and angry; and learns not to ask any more questions. If the patient does not have a severe personality disorder, the worst outcome of this little episode is the permanent stifling of questions, which makes the therapist more comfortable but may deprive the treatment of important data. The best outcome is that the patient is able to analyze the reaction and see how incongruent the sensitivity to the "superior power" of the therapist is to the current reality of the relationship. Patients with severe personality disorders are not so capable of useful self-reflection. With deep, if not murderous resentment of the capacity of others to exert power over them, with searing shame at the discrepancy of power and privilege between others and themselves, they react to covert expressions of the other's power with rage, flight, or regression. "Responding" to questions does not necessarily mean answering them. The therapist may need to say at times something like, "I feel we don't know each other quite well enough for me to feel easy about answering that question. I'd rather put it on the back burner for now and return to it later if it remains an issue."

Avoiding Confrontation and Interpretation

Avoid confrontation and interpretation, at least in the early stages of therapy. Ever since Strachey's 1934 paper on the nature of the therapeutic action of psychoanalysis, psychoanalytically trained therapists have believed that analysis of transference is the intervention that brings about change. Without any scientific test of Strachey's assertion, they have believed that the structural changes that are the substrates of enduring improvements will not develop in the absence of systematic interpretation of transference. Currently, researchers are beginning to address the question of whether the success of interpretive therapies, such as psychoanalysis and transference-focused psychotherapy, derives primarily from the verbal interpretive interventions of the therapist. It remains to be shown whether the supportive elements of psychoanalysis are themselves mutative in that they facilitate an interpretive process in the patient, reinforced by the developing identification with the therapist's way of thinking about the patient's trouble (Holinger 1999). The patient's need to understand and integrate external and internal reality contributes to the motivation to pursue therapy. Yet that motive is impaired by anxiety, which is dealt with by the anti-integrative activity of *splitting*, the unconscious process that keeps bad, toxic, terrifying representations of self and other separate from good, rewarding, comforting ones.

Many psychoanalytic authors, including Appelbaum (1981, 1994), Dewald (1972), Gedo (1979), Holinger (1999), Loewald (1960), and Wallerstein (1986), have questioned whether interpretation is the only (or even the major) route to structural change. Changes referred to as "structural" when they come about in psychotherapy occur during normal development in the absence of interpretation but in the context of an environment that provides sufficient support to maturational processes. Children respond to the influence of their parents first by imitating them and gradually by internalizing aspects of the parents in the process of identification. Later they identify themselves with other important figures that come to stand for the parents. In health, as they establish these identifications, most children eventually develop a stable sense of self and ways of defending that effectively manage anxiety without sacrificing allegiance to reality; a firm yet benevolent conscience that produces signal guilt to prevent guilt-producing actions while permitting the reasonable pursuit of pleasure (change in the superego); and the capacity to love without fearing loss of the self in experiences of fusion and without excessive anxiety in the face of separations (reflecting change in both ego and superego). When such changes occur in the course of therapy the treatment is considered highly successful. As supportive elements cannot be entirely removed from transference-focused psychotherapy, a viable approach to the question of what brings about change in psychotherapy would be a treatment such as that described here that creates conditions facilitating the patient's own interpretive work by supplying the conditions favorable to self-reflection.

Verbal confrontation and interpretation tend to increase anxiety and defensiveness, producing in patients whose personality is fundamentally sound a momentary disturbance in the relationship with the analyst. In analysis and expressive therapy, the frequency of sessions facilitates the prompt examination and repair of such ruptures, along with the mutual study of the origin of the defensive reaction. Patients with personality disorders, however, tend to regress when sessions are more frequent than twice weekly, and their tendency to distort relationships is generally so great that repair of ruptures can be the major ongoing task of the participants. Techniques that increase defensiveness are contraindicated in these cases.

Fostering Verbal Expression of Thoughts and Feelings

Patients with severe personality disorders are often extremely limited in the use of language. They are likely to say, "I'm upset" or "I'm having a hard time" to cover the whole range of painful, hostile feelings. Once the patient feels safe and welcome in the therapist's presence, the therapist can begin helping the patient sort out and name her feelings. Pine (1985) has shown how moving from the "action mode" to the verbal mode of communication helps patients feel less alien.

Case Example

Therapist: Maybe the upset has something to do with last night when you phoned me and I wasn't there. That could be disappointing. Or it could be really scary.
Patient: No, I don't think I was disappointed or scared.
Therapist: Could you pause for a moment before you go on, because I want to call your attention to two things I think are quite important. One is that you have gotten the courage to disagree with me, and it sounded like it was easy. And the other is that it is just as important to identify what you don't feel as it is to get clear about what you do feel. We've been working so hard on naming your feelings that I think it's worth paying attention to it when that starts getting easy.
Patient: Well, I can't be too sure what I was feeling when I tried to reach you. But I know I was upset. My Mom had called…[she goes on to describe the disturbing phone call]. I guess it wasn't so bad, same old thing, really. But when I hung up I cried a little and then I found myself dialing your number. Like I thought talking to you would sort of erase how bad my Mom had made me feel…like guilty, I guess. And just hearing your voice on the answering machine was comforting enough.

Notice that the therapist hazarded a guess about the upset: Why that particular guess? The patient had given so little information that the therapist did well to listen to her own feelings of guilt stirred by having been unavailable. Noting the complementary identification of neglectful mother/self with patient/baby (Racker 1968) provided information that could be used for a response ("listening to the countertransference"). The therapist took a chance on being wrong. Why not pursue the matter further before making a guess?—"Did something happen that upset you? What was it? Why was your Mom's call so upsetting?"—but the therapist knew better and had no intention of derailing the interaction by questioning the patient, who clearly wanted to tell her story and would do so in her own time.

Finding Something About the Patient to Like and Respect

If finding something to like about the patient proves an impossible task, seek consultation and either discover what is of value at least potentially in the patient or arrange referral. Thomas Main (1960), who described the effect of borderline pathology among hospitalized patients on the hospital staff, observed the outward manifestations of splitting—each member of the nursing staff reacting to a different object relationship manifested in the patient's reactions to him or her. The result was chaos in the staff that matched that of the patient's mind. The remedy was for the staff to meet regularly to share impressions and develop a unified approach. This principle is valid today in the outpatient treatment of difficult cases. Forming a study group that meets regularly is a valuable protection against becoming exhausted and impatient in what can often seem a futile effort to help.

Keeping the End in Mind From the Beginning

Time-limited treatment is generally not good for patients with personality disorders. Current experience has shown that the most significant results of treatment (such as moving from disability status to full-time employment or finding a suitable partner instead of unstable, abusive ones) rarely show up before the third year of once- or twice-weekly sessions. This observation seems to reflect a response not so much to the number of sessions but rather the length of time the patient needs to have an ongoing relationship with the therapist before the therapist can become a stable internal object.

Case Example

A dramatic example was a young man who, terrified of the feelings aroused in the therapy situation, canceled all but 28 of the 120 sessions scheduled for him. When he did attend, his participation was desultory, yet in his life he made considerable progress. The steady, undemanding attitude of a fatherly therapist set the patient free to try to fulfill his own ambitions, bit by bit, confident both of the therapist's approval and the belief that his idealized therapist was absolutely dedicated to seeing the treatment through to its end. In point of fact, the therapist found it very difficult to sustain his undemanding position. He sometimes resented the patient's casual manner of canceling sessions, and he believed keenly that the patient would make much better progress if he would attend every session. The study group supported the therapist through each crisis of frustrated therapeutic zeal and helped him remain patient while keeping an eye on how the patient was doing.

When a time limit is set by external policies or by the therapist's life situation, it should be discussed with the patient before any commitment is made. Patient and therapist can then proceed to establish goals they can reasonably expect to meet in the time available. The therapist must keep these goals in mind. They may change, in which case a formal revision is in order.

At the halfway point of a time-limited therapy, patient and therapist should review their goals and adjust them, if need be, in light of how much time remains for them to be together. This review of what they have accomplished and what remains to be done is of immense importance given these patients' difficulty with endings and therapists' reluctance to inflict the pain of saying goodbye. It almost always comes as a shock to both parties to face the fact that ending will actually occur. Facing it early gives them time to express their feelings about it and to make plans as to whether and how and with whom therapy will continue.

Case Example

A therapist whose patient was making good progress in a 2-year research project was reminded by the study group that she was several months beyond the halfway point of the treatment. The study group asked her what the goals of the treatment were and she replied, "Well, I know what my goal is, to help her free herself from her hostile entanglement with her mother…I'm not sure what her goal is." The group pointed out that the therapist's goal was a very long-range one indeed; perhaps she and the patient could agree on a goal that had some chance of being reached in the 4 months that remained of the treatment. The therapist returned the next week to report that the patient's goal was to take driving lessons! Actually this was quite achievable and not unrelated to the therapist's ambitions for her.

In the training clinics of many teaching hospitals, patients are simply handed over from a graduating student to a beginner each July, an unfortunate practice that denigrates psychotherapy. "We're just here to teach the residents," one patient said. "I get a lot more help from the receptionist than from my therapists. After all, she's known all about me for years, and I know a lot about her, too. We talk about our grandchildren and about everything, I guess, and she never leaves." The practice of passing patients on deprives patients and therapists of the experience of ending as a serious matter. Furthermore, the strain on the therapist of ending all the cases at once is almost always excessive, resulting in emotional withdrawal and hasty planning just when patients most need a steady hand at the helm. It is much wiser to try to end cases when an ending of a phase of treatment comes about naturally.

Schlesinger (2005) described the "mini-endings" that occur in the course of treatment, not only in anticipation of weekends and vacations but also on the completion of a piece of work that leaves the patient feeling at loose ends for a while. The patient no longer knows what the treatment is all about, feels like canceling sessions, and in this mood is open to discussion of whether to go on or to take a break and decide whether to begin again. A fruitful discussion may ensue, leading to a real ending complete with an examination of the patient's attachment to the clinic itself, to the routines that may have been laid down over years of clinic attendance, to the clinic staff that may have become a second family, and to the therapist. Parting, after this sort of discussion, leaves patient and therapist with the mixed feelings of sadness and pride in their accomplishment that are the hallmark of a true "commencement." The resident who says good-bye to the patients one by one as appropriate in the months before leaving the service finds time freed up to do evaluations, consultations, and referrals, an important part of the training of future therapists.

Case Example

An example of an ending not attended to is that of a therapist who had the opportunity to work with a patient for 2 years in the clinic and thought they were making such excellent progress that they could continue in private practice after the resident's graduation. The therapist mentioned this to the patient not long before a month-long summer break. When sessions resumed at the end of August, the patient seemed quite different. He had little to say and appeared to have lost interest in the issues they had been working on before. In November the resident took the matter up with the supervisor. "I'd planned to invite this patient into my private practice, but he's turning out to be not nearly as intelligent and motivated as he seemed before. Actually, nothing has happened in the therapy since the end of August." "Nothing," said the supervisor, "doesn't quite describe what looks like some sort of major signal of distress. Could your patient be worrying about the end of his treatment with you?" The resident brought the matter up in the next session, whereupon the patient's eyes filled with tears. "When you didn't say any more about my continuing with you after next June, I thought you must have changed your mind, and I couldn't ask you because if you had changed your mind I wouldn't have been able to stand it. Now it feels like a ton of lead has just been lifted off my shoulders." The treatment immediately resumed its former characteristics of vividness and fruitful interchange.

INDICATIONS FOR SUPPORTIVE THERAPY FOR PATIENTS WITH PERSONALITY DISORDERS

For personality disorders, indeed for all patients, supportive therapy as described here is the treatment of choice during the initial diagnostic phase. If relinquishing interpretation is the hallmark of supportive therapy, it would follow that the diagnostic phase is a period of supportive therapy. It is not so rare an occurrence that a patient pronounces his presenting problem solved at the end of the diagnostic phase and takes leave of the therapist before "starting treatment." Unaware that a successful piece of supportive therapy has been accomplished by accident rather than by intent, the therapist sees the patient's leaving as "resistance" or a "flight into health" or the result of the therapist's incompetence. The therapist may pursue the patient in the attempt to get the "real" treatment started. Such pursuit is usually not only futile but also harmful: "Am I really that sick?" the patient wonders. A good experience of therapy is thus transformed into one that stirs self-doubts and lessens the likelihood of the patient returning for another course of therapy in the future.

When the diagnosis of personality disorder emerges from the diagnostic phase, it is likely one will be dealing with special vulnerabilities and sensitivities, cognitive difficulties, malignant introjects, defective affect regulation, and identity diffusion to one extent or another. Different diagnostic patterns call for different varieties of treatment, as follows.

Paranoid Personality Disorder

Paranoid patients need individual supportive therapy as described in detail by Gabbard (2000), whose treatment recommendations closely resemble those described here. If the patient presents with major depression in which paranoid features are often prominent, the depression must be successfully treated before it is possible to make a diagnosis of personality disorder.

Therapists who undertake to treat a patient with paranoid personality disorder must be prepared for a long and arduous task that puts considerable strain on the therapist's ability to contain and use his reactions to the patient's unflagging accusations and suspicions. A nondefensive response, with steady effort to understand the patient's point of view, may lead finally to identification with the therapist's thoughtful interest. If so, the patient begins to see how the truculent, vigilant search for the venality of others has served as protection against feelings of worthlessness and vulnerability. At this point, the patient may become deeply sad, arousing in the therapist the wish to comfort rather than help the patient understand his or her sadness. In the absence of clear-cut vegetative signs, treating the patient for "depression" with medication is both ineffectual and counterproductive. It is an unspoken vote of no confidence both in the treatment and in the patient's achievement of the ability to endure the sadness the patient has been defending against for years.

Paranoid patients have special vulnerabilities that must be taken into account. So great is their fear of others controlling them or seeing things that have escaped their own careful scanning that their defensive response to interpretation is particularly intense. They are prone to misunderstanding acts of kindness or words of encouragement as seductions.

Case Example

A young woman rejected her therapist's innocent offer to change the time of their appointments so that the patient could catch her bus, because it would require "payback." It later emerged that her father had bribed her for sexual favors.

Indeed, closeness in any form is intensely threatening to paranoid patients. An attitude of respectful reserve reassures them. Although one might start a session with a borderline patient with a warm greeting, such as "I'm glad to see you—I've been thinking a lot about our last session and wondering how it affected you," such a greeting would set a paranoid patient on edge: "What else has she been thinking? Why all the enthusiasm? What makes her think I was 'affected' by the session?" It is much wiser to greet the patient with a simple, "Good evening," offer a seat near the door, and await the barrage of reproaches.

Schizoid and Schizotypal Personality Disorder

Supportive therapy is indicated for schizoid and schizotypal patients who challenge the skills of the therapist not by combativeness and suspicion but rather by silence, dismissiveness, and apparent indifference.

Case Example

A young businessman, after several years of apparently superficial talking between long periods of silence, suddenly attempted suicide. Shaken, the therapist refused to resume the treatment after the patient's discharge from the hospital. The new therapist found it difficult to be with the patient. His description of his childhood as in a world of stone seemed to fit the stony indifference, polite but distant, with which he treated the therapist. After several months he mentioned that he had always had an interest in sculpture and would like to take lessons. The therapist did not hear this unprecedented remark, and it would have gone unnoticed had the session not been recorded on audiotape. The patient never mentioned it again. When the young doctor informed him that he was moving away, he declined the offer of a referral.

The therapist had been lulled into indifference by the patient's dismissive response to all his efforts to develop a relationship. The therapist never presented his uncharacteristic indifference as a problem to his study group, nor did he think about the patient much between sessions. The patient was succeeding in protecting his vulnerable feelings of worthlessness and longing with the façade of stony self-sufficiency. Just twice did he let down his guard, first with the suicide attempt and then with the risky remark about wanting to study sculpture. In supportive therapy, that remark would have stirred the alert therapist to respond (with care not to let too much enthusiasm frighten the patient away) that it might do the patient good to pursue that interest. Perhaps they could have a conversation about sculpture, he and this man imprisoned in a world of stone.

Borderline Personality Disorder

Borderline patients addicted to self-injury can benefit from a preliminary phase of education such as dialectical behavior therapy (Linehan 1993), which is of particular help in teaching patients that their illness is not their fault but is their responsibility, that they have to work to achieve what others develop naturally—namely, the ability to put their feelings into words rather than communicating in the language of action. Patients who come

for therapy without such preparatory treatment will need a period of education about their illness and how to manage their behavior as the introduction to therapy. Once they have gained control over self-destructive actions, supportive therapy is the treatment of choice until a solid identification with the therapist's reflective attitude has been achieved and along with it consolidation of a sense of self. At this point the termination phase of treatment can begin, a process that may lead to a decision to end treatment altogether or to referral for a more exploratory therapy.

Narcissistic Personality Disorder

Narcissistic patients can be exceptionally challenging, especially when their character includes paranoid and antisocial elements, the triad of malignant narcissism described by Kernberg (1989). Identification with the therapist may occur, if ever, very late in treatment, whereas superficial imitation that occurs early represents efforts to "have" what the therapist has, not to think or feel toward his or her own mind as the therapist does. Supportive therapy as described here may be effective with these patients, although an active exploratory therapy such as transference-focused therapy (Kernberg et al. 1989) is generally regarded as the treatment of choice.

Antisocial Personality Disorder

No psychoanalytically informed therapy has thus far been found effective for antisocial patients. It is therefore of special importance to make a careful, extensive diagnostic study of such cases to differentiate them from other personality disorders with antisocial features for which therapy may be effective if carried out in the hospital.

Histrionic Personality Disorder

Histrionic patients respond best to supportive therapy because, like borderline patients, they tend to communicate in the language of action (e.g., theatrical hyperemotionality, impulsiveness) and may require extensive supportive work before being able to express themselves in words. They are also given to the rapid development of erotized transference, responding poorly to attempts at interpretation (Blum 1973).

Hysterical Personality Disorder

Hysterical personality disorder was dropped from DSM-IV (American Psychiatric Association 1994), but these patients continue to present themselves for treatment nonetheless. They generally have symptoms related to the oedipal phase of development, tend to have strong interpersonal relationships, and tend to be thoughtful and introspective. Thus they respond well to expressive therapies, including psychoanalysis.

Obsessive-Compulsive Personality Disorder

In general, patients with obsessive-compulsive personality disorder need psychoanalysis or expressive psychotherapy. Special care is required, however, in establishing the diagnosis before making a referral for such therapy, because in some cases the obsessional and compulsive symptoms serve to manage the intolerable anxiety of an underlying psychosis.

In all these cases, an initial trial of therapy without explicit verbal interpretive interventions may prove to be so effective that referral for the more costly and time-consuming interpretive therapies may not be necessary.

Avoidant Personality Disorder

The term *avoidant personality disorder* seems to describe a category of people who are constitutionally excessively shy, while longing for normal relatedness and fun (Kagan et al. 1988). Little evidence is available that one form of treatment is more effective than another in helping these patients overcome their fear of making fools of themselves in social situations. Common sense and anecdotal evidence strongly suggest that the kind of therapeutic relationship offered by supportive therapy, with a generous dose of ingenious cognitive-behavioral interventions, would be the ideal introduction to psychotherapy for these patients. Having developed some confidence in their ability to overcome their symptoms, they might well move into psychoanalysis to clarify the events and fantasies of early life that set the constitutional-genetic predisposition on the path of symptom formation.

Dependent Personality Disorder

A diagnosis of dependent personality disorder may well account for more rejections of patients by therapists than any of the other disorders. Gabbard (2000) has written a sensitive account of the feelings stirred in therapists by these patients, who present nakedly the wishes for unconditional care that most people succeed in defending against. A supportive therapy that accepts those wishes and tries to help patient attain them without alienating others may succeed in easing the negative impact these patients have on others.

Case Example

Patient: I don't know if I can stand this treatment. I need contact. I was thrown out of dialectical behavior therapy for overuse of my therapist's beeper, and thrown out of treatment with a therapist I really loved because I called her up all the time.

Therapist: Well, here we are, anyway, assigned to try to work together. I don't have a beeper and sometimes don't get to answer phone messages until late in the evening. But you may have learned more than you realize from your previous treatment. I am willing to see what we can do. You can call me any time and leave a message, and I'll respond unless you tell me I don't need to.

The patient called several times a day at first, but rarely asked to be called back. Therapy was successfully terminated as initially planned at the end of a year.

SIGNIFICANCE OF ONGOING SUPERVISION

Most experienced, well-trained psychotherapists work for long stretches of time without seeking supervision or consultation. If they do so, it is all too often because a case has reached an impasse or is going badly. Therapists and their colleagues tend to connect supervision with failure, excessive dependency, or professional immaturity. Such derogation of supervision seems odd when one considers its honored place in other disciplines. Established actors continue to take acting lessons all their lives, as do accomplished dancers and musicians. In the medical profession a high value has somehow been placed on "going it alone," and this ethos seems to have infected the practice of many a psychotherapist.

Patients with personality disorders, and with identity diffusion and reliance on splitting as their major defense, present a therapist with challenges far beyond those to be expected when dealing with neurotic illnesses. Desperate suffering, anxiety that renders the patient almost unintelligible, importunate phone calls, self-injury, threats of suicide, dangerous behavior outside of sessions, even assaultiveness toward the therapist or—at the other extreme—withdrawnness, obscure communication, and lack of the expected feelings connected with horrendous stories are all behaviors that keep a therapist off-balance and uneasy, sometimes frightened and sometimes lulled into a state of indifference. The therapist can lose track of the goal of treatment and "go along" for months or even years with a conviction that the patient is a "lifer," needing endless contact with the therapist to stay out of trouble.

Working with some personality-disordered patients can be dangerous. Therapists must be prepared for threats of suicide, homicide, and assault. They may become the victims of stalking, lawsuits, or formal complaints of unethical behavior. In many if not most cases, such events are linked to therapists' failure to think ahead and bring their concerns into consultation (Gabbard and Lester 1995).

A patient's personality pathology can undermine the skills of an otherwise competent therapist. The therapists of these patients need a special form of supervision to avoid the pitfalls and impasses that the best of therapists can blunder into with patients with personality disorders. Although there is general agreement in the literature that individual supervision is necessary for therapists in danger of committing boundary violations, a case can be made for ongoing group supervision as the most effective way to keep the therapists of personality-disordered patients on track. In such groups different members respond to different facets of the patient, reflecting back to the therapist a more modulated and complex understanding of the case. A coherent theory of treatment with a well-articulated rationale is essential. It might be said that an effective study group is like an external representation of the internal integration we hope to help bring about in our patients.

RESEARCH DATA

Rockland's (1992) book on psychotherapy for borderline patients is the only recent major contribution emphasizing supportive treatment, but it is directed toward the treatment of borderline pathology rather than personality disorders in general. No one has recently undertaken a systematic reexamination of psychoanalytic supportive therapy with an eye to studying empirically its effectiveness in the treatment of our most challenging cases, those diagnosed as personality disorders. Two studies are relevant, however. One is the Psychotherapy Research Project of the Menninger Foundation (Kernberg et al. 1972) that sought to compare psychoanalysis and psychotherapy in a naturalistic study. Today, many of the subjects would be diagnosed as having various personality disorders. The findings have inspired a plethora of papers and books, Robert Wallerstein's *Forty-Two Lives in Treatment* foremost among them. Wallerstein (1986) pointed out that in some cases what is usually regarded as structural change came about in patients treated with supportive-expressive psychotherapy, whereas patients with severe personality disorders fared badly in psychoanalysis.

A current study being conducted by the Personality Disorders Institute at the Westchester division of New York Presbyterian Hospital seeks to compare the effectiveness of dialectical behavior therapy and transference-focused psychotherapy in a randomized 1-year treatment. A control group of patients in supportive therapy was offered in place of the "treatment as usual" control originally planned on the grounds that there is no treatment as usual for these patients. A manualized treatment was devised that was clearly distinguishable on videotape from the other two treatments. The results of this study will cast light on the question of whether treatment method or some other factor within the therapist–patient relationship is mutative for borderline patients. Unanswered questions will remain that demand empirical studies into the treatment of choice for the other personality disorders.

SUMMARY

Decades of clinical experience and hundreds of books and articles attest to the capability of supportive therapy to help patients in all diagnostic categories. Yet in contrast to transference-focused psychotherapy on the one hand and the various manualized cognitive-behavioral therapies on the other, psychoanalytically informed supportive therapy has not been rigorously defined in a way that has achieved general acceptance or lent itself to empirical study when applied to patients with severe character disorders. Traditionally, it was implicitly regarded as doing whatever was possible within a professional framework to help a patient use what strengths he or she has when the patient is too ill or too poor to engage in psychoanalysis or expressive psychotherapy. The present text is a step toward refining that definition, setting psychoanalytic supportive therapy apart from other therapies through its emphasis on maintaining a "learning" state in the patient so as to keep defensiveness at a minimum. Explicit verbal interpretations, asking questions, and confronting the patient can all be seen as covert expressions of the therapist's superior power, and many patients with severe character disorders do see them this way. Hence supportive therapy as conceived here avoids these indirect assertions of power by the therapist. (There may be times, usually in the early months of treatment, when direct assertions of power, such as forbidding some dangerous act, are necessary. These do not interfere with the treatment because the patient readily understands the need to be controlled at such times.) The basic assumption that change comes about through identification with the therapist's reflective attitude governs the therapist's overall conduct. The interpretive process goes on in the mind of the therapist and is transformed into interventions that foster that same process in the mind of the patient—who ultimately arrives, autonomously, at the mutative interpretations.

Case Example

A 12-year-old boy diagnosed as having borderline personality disorder finished his treatment with the following summary: "At first I knew I was crazy. My mind whirled like a merry-go-round and the only way I could get off was by yelling inside 'I'M IN THERAPY!' [The initial response to the "holding function" described by Winnicott (1960). Therapy was something he was "in."] Later, after I'd calmed down, I'd ask myself, 'What would Dr. T. say about this?' [Remembering an aspect of the identification figure.] Later still, I noticed I was talking to myself just like a therapist! [Imitation as an early stage of identification.] Now if I'm worried I go off by myself and meditate in my own way. I don't need you any more." [Identification complete. Identification figure has been absorbed into the self.]

REFERENCES

Appelbaum AH: Beyond interpretation: a response from beyond psychoanalysis. Psychoanal Inq 1:167–185, 1981

Appelbaum AH: Psychotherapeutic routes to structural change. Bull Menninger Clin 58:37–54, 1994

Blum H: The concept of erotized transference. J Am Psychoanal Assoc 21:61–76, 1973

Canetti E: Crowds and Power. New York, Continuum, 1962

Dewald P: Psychotherapy: A Dynamic Approach. New York, Basic Books, 1972

Gabbard GO: Psychodynamic Psychiatry in Clinical Practice. Washington, DC, American Psychiatric Press, 2000

Gabbard GO, Lester E: Boundaries and Boundary Violations in Psychoanalysis. New York, Basic Books, 1995

Gedo J: Beyond Interpretation. New York, International Universities Press, 1979

Havens L: A Safe Place. Cambridge, MA, Harvard University Press, 1989

Holinger P: Noninterpretive interventions in psychoanalysis and psychotherapy. Psychoanal Psychol 16:233–251, 1999

Kagan J, Reznick JS, Snidman N: Biological bases of childhood shyness. Science 240:167–171, 1988

Kernberg O: Object relations and character analysis. J Am Psychoanal Assoc 31(suppl):247–272, 1983

Kernberg OF: The narcissistic personality disorder and the differential diagnosis of antisocial behavior. Psychiatr Clin North Am 12:533–570, 1989

Kernberg O, Burstein ED, Coyne L, et al: Psychotherapy and psychoanalysis. Bull Menninger Clin 36:3–275, 1972

Kernberg O, Selzer MA, Koenigsberg HW, et al: Psychodynamic Psychotherapy of Borderline Patients. New York, Basic Books, 1989

Linehan MM: Cognitive-Behavioral Treatment for Borderline Personality Disorder. New York, Guilford, 1993

Loewald H: On the therapeutic action of psychoanalysis. International Journal of Psychoanalysis 41:16–33, 1960

Main T: The ailment. Br J Med Psychol 33:29–31, 1960

Pine F: Developmental Theory and Clinical Process. New Haven, CT, Yale University Press, 1985

Racker H: Transference and Countertransference. New York, International Universities Press, 1968

Rockland L: Supportive Therapy for Borderline Patients: A Psychodynamic Approach. New York, Guilford, 1992

Schlesinger H: Endings and Beginnings. Hillsdale, NJ, Analytic Press, 2005

Strachey J: The nature of the therapeutic action of psychoanalysis. International Journal of Psychoanalysis 15:127–159, 1934

Wallerstein RS: Forty-Two Lives in Treatment. New York, Guilford, 1986

Winnicott D: The theory of the parent–child relationship. International Journal of Psychoanalysis 41:585–595, 1960

Wolff P: The Causes, Controls and Organization of Behavior in the Neonate. Madison, CT, International Universities Press, 1966

22

Group Treatment

William E. Piper, Ph.D.
John S. Ogrodniczuk, Ph.D.

This chapter focuses on group treatment for personality disorders. Group treatment is a general type of therapy, similar to individual therapy or family therapy. Group therapies may take many different forms based on their theoretical and technical orientations. Because of the presence of multiple patients, group therapies have certain unique features that distinguish them from other general types of therapy. These unique features may facilitate or complicate the treatment of personality disorders. Similarly, personality disorders have certain features that may facilitate or complicate their treatment with group therapies.

Initially, this chapter considers these facilitating and complicating features of group therapies and personality disorders. Next, forms of group treatment that differ in format, intensity, and objectives are considered, followed by a discussion of research support for group treatments. The perceived usefulness of group treatment for each of the 10 DSM-IV-TR (American Psychiatric Association 2000) personality disorders is reviewed, and two case examples of patients treated with one of the most powerful forms of group treatment—day treatment—are presented. Finally, a number of conclusions are offered.

GROUP FEATURES THAT FACILITATE TREATMENT OF PERSONALITY DISORDERS

Because personality disorders are serious long-term conditions that are resistant to change, powerful treatments are needed. Group treatments are capable of mobilizing strong forces for change, such as peer pressure. The group, which is sometimes referred to as a *cohesive social microcosm*, can exert considerable pressure on patients to participate. It is capable of eliciting the typical maladaptive behaviors of each patient. The other patients can observe, provide feedback, and offer suggestions for change. The patient can subsequently practice adaptive behavior. This process is commonly referred to as *interpersonal learning*. Other patients may learn through observation and imitation. Simply recognizing that other patients share one's difficulties (*universality*) and helping other patients with their problems (*altruism*) can be therapeutic. These various processes (cohesion, interpersonal learning, imitation, universality, and altruism) are regarded as powerful unique therapeutic factors of group treatment (Yalom 1995).

There are other facilitative features of group treatment as well. Paralyzing negative transference toward the therapist is less likely to occur in group therapy compared with individual therapy because the situation is less intimate, and strong affects such as rage are diluted and expressed toward other patients. Similarly, feedback from the therapist in the individual therapy situation may be dismissed as biased, but this is much less likely to occur in response to feedback from several peers in a therapy group. In addition, because of the variety of affects expressed by different patients, integration of positive and negative affects is facilitated.

GROUP FEATURES THAT COMPLICATE TREATMENT OF PERSONALITY DISORDERS

Group features may also produce complications. Some patients with personality disorders resent sharing the therapist and feel neglected and deprived. In the group situation, regressive behavior such as emotional outbursts, aggressive actions, or suicidal threats are more difficult to manage and contain than in individual therapy. Groups are prone to scapegoating; patients with personality disorders provide many provocations. There are a number of concerns in the group situation, relative to individual therapy, that many patients with personality disorders find troublesome, including loss of control, individuality, understanding, privacy, and safety (Piper and Ogrodniczuk 2004). The therapist is subject to such concerns as well.

PERSONALITY DISORDER FEATURES THAT FACILITATE GROUP TREATMENT

The predominant feature of patients with personality disorders that facilitates group treatment is their strong tendency to openly demonstrate interpersonal psychopathology through behavior in the group. Compared with patients with many Axis I disorders, patients with personality disorders are more likely to demonstrate rather than describe their interpersonal problems. Although this also occurs in individual therapy, the stimuli from multiple patients precipitate pathological interpersonal behavior more intensely and quickly in group therapy. This behavior can be clearly recognized and dealt with immediately in the group. A second facilitative feature of patients with some personality disorders (e.g., dependent, histrionic, borderline) is that they are "other-seeking." They tend to value the connections in the group.

PERSONALITY DISORDER FEATURES THAT COMPLICATE GROUP TREATMENT

Many of the behaviors characteristic of those with personality disorders complicate group treatment. Because these behaviors are often offensive to members of the group, they tend to weaken cohesion and distract members from working. Usually, such patients challenge the guidelines and norms that have been established in the group. Examples of antitherapeutic behaviors include minimal disclosure, excessive disclosure, scapegoating, extra-group socializing, absenteeism, lateness, and premature termination.

When a patient's antitherapeutic behaviors persist in the group over time, the behaviors may be conceptualized as roles. The persons occupying the roles are commonly labeled as "difficult" patients in the group therapy literature (Bernard 1994; Rutan and Stone 2001). These difficult patients are often those with personality disorders. Examples of difficult roles and the DSM-IV-TR personality disorders often associated with them are the silent or withdrawn role (schizoid, schizotypal, paranoid, avoidant); the monopolizing role (histrionic, borderline, narcissistic); the boring role (narcissistic, obsessive-compulsive); the therapist helper role (histrionic, dependent); the challenger role (antisocial, borderline, obsessive-compulsive); and the help-rejecting complainer role (borderline, narcissistic, histrionic). Although these roles are occupied by individual persons, they frequently express something that other patients wish to have expressed and therefore are supported by others in the group. Among the personality disorders regularly seen in outpatient groups, patients with borderline and narcissistic personality disorders are usually viewed as the most difficult to treat and manage (Leszcz 1989; Tuttman 1990). For that reason, a combination of group therapy and individual therapy is often recommended.

DIFFERENT FORMS OF GROUP TREATMENT

Forms of group treatment differ in structure (format), intensity, and objectives. Four forms can be distinguished.

Short-Term Outpatient Group Therapy

Short-term outpatient group therapy often involves a single session per week for 20 or fewer weeks. Certain focal symptoms (e.g., depression) or behaviors (e.g., affect expression, social skills) are targeted for change. These groups are usually not intensive in nature. They do not attempt to change the basic personality traits or personality structure that characterize personality disorders. Many examples are described in the literature, including supportive groups for patients who experience complicated grief (Piper et al. 2001) or for patients who are undergoing organ transplantation (Abbey and Farrow 1998).

Long-Term Outpatient Group Therapy

Long-term outpatient group therapy consists of one or two sessions per week for at least 1–2 years. It focuses on the interpersonal world of the patient. It is intensive in nature and over time involves confrontation and interpretation of the patient's core conflicts, defensive style, and long-term maladaptive behaviors. It attempts to change the basic personality traits and personality structure that characterize personality disorders. Long-term outpatient group therapy is regarded as an appropriate and effective group treatment for personality disorders, especially when used in combination with long-term individual psychotherapy. The latter allows stabilization of the patient and an opportunity to disclose private and sensitive information that would be difficult to reveal in the group setting initially, although over time such revelation becomes possible. This group approach assumes that over time the group comes to represent a social microcosm in which the interpersonal difficulties of the patients become vividly illustrated by the interpersonal behavior of the patients in the group. Two well-known texts that focus on long-term group psychotherapy are those of Rutan and Stone (2001) and Yalom (1995).

Day Treatment

Day treatment is a form of partial hospitalization. It is designed for patients who do not require full-time hospitalization and who are unlikely to benefit a great deal from outpatient group therapy. Day treatment patients have often had an unsuccessful course of outpatient group therapy. Patients typically participate in a variety of therapy groups for several hours each day for 3–5 days per week. The therapy groups are often from different technical orientations. For example, behavioral and cognitive interventions can be used in structured, skills-oriented groups; whereas dynamic interventions are used in unstructured, insight-oriented groups. Family and couples interventions may also be employed. Day treatment is an intensive form

of therapy. Its goals include relief of symptoms, reduction of problematic behaviors, modification of maladaptive character traits, and facilitation of psychological maturation.

Several other features contribute to making day treatment a powerful treatment. First is the intensity of the group experience. Patients participate in a number of different groups each day. Second, the groups vary in size, structure, objectives, and processes. This variety provides a comprehensive approach. Third, the different groups are integrated and synergistic. Patients are encouraged to think about the entire system. Fourth, patients benefit from working with multiple staff members and a large number of other patients. Fifth, day treatment capitalizes on the traditional characteristics of a therapeutic community (democratization, permissiveness, communalism, reality confrontation). These features strengthen cohesion, which helps patients endure difficult periods of treatment. The structure of day treatment programs encourages patients to be responsible, engenders mutual respect between patients and staff, and facilitates patients' participation in the treatment of their peers. Well-known approaches to day treatment programs are described by Bateman and Fonagy (1999) and Piper et al. (1996).

Inpatient/Residential Treatment

Inpatient/residential treatment involves 24-hour care. Inpatient treatment is usually prompted by a crisis, such as a significant suicide attempt. The main objective is to provide support and observation in an effort to stabilize the patient until outpatient care can be resumed. It is intensive treatment. Although group treatment is usually a part of the ward regimen, it may represent only a small part of the program and is not likely to be aimed at modifying long-standing personality traits. In North America, the lengths of stay in hospitals have been decreasing significantly in response to escalating costs. Thus, inpatient treatment is often short-term treatment of 1 week or less. Two different approaches to inpatient treatment are described by Rosen et al. (2001).

Although once popular, residential treatment for severe personality disorders also has decreased due to high costs. In the past, such treatment has been intensive both in terms of structure and objectives. Treatment has included multiple sessions of group therapy and individual therapy aimed at modifying long-term maladaptive behavior and personality structure. Stays have involved months, sometimes years, of treatment. Another example of residential treatment is that which occurs in some prisons. Some institutions have treatment programs for inmates with antisocial personality disorder (ASPD) who have been convicted of crimes. Some experts have objected to residential care for personality disorders on the grounds that it promotes dependency. An approach to working with patients in residential treatment groups is described in a recent article by Kibel (2003).

RESEARCH SUPPORT FOR THE GROUP TREATMENT OF PERSONALITY DISORDERS

There is a striking absence of evaluative research on treatments for personality disorders. In the case of group treatments, the number of studies are few indeed. There are very few randomized clinical trials of psychosocial treatments. However, the trials that have been published provide encouraging findings. In this section, we summarize findings from several of the recent clinical trials. Outpatient group therapy studies are followed by partial hospitalization studies.

Randomized Clinical Trials

Cappe and Alden (1986) compared brief (8 weekly 2-hour sessions) behavioral group therapy with a waiting list control condition for a sample of 52 patients with avoidant personality disorder. The patients who were treated with a combination of graduated exposure training and interpersonal process training improved significantly more than patients who received only graduated exposure and patients on the waiting list. In a similar trial, Alden (1989) compared three variations of brief behavioral group therapy (10 weekly 2.5-hour sessions) with a waiting list control condition for a sample of 76 patients with avoidant personality disorder. All three treatment conditions demonstrated greater improvement than the waiting list control condition. However, the author noted that despite significant improvements, the patients did not achieve normal functioning.

Linehan et al. (1991) compared dialectical behavior therapy (DBT), which involved 2.5 hours of group skills training and 1 hour of individual therapy per week for 1 year, with regular community treatment (usually individual therapy) for a sample of 44 patients with borderline personality disorder. DBT resulted in greater reductions in symptoms and parasuicidal and dysfunctional behaviors, decreased dropouts, fewer and shorter inpatient admissions, and improved work status compared with regular treatment. However, no differences were evident on self-reported levels of depression, hopelessness, or suicidal ideation. Although useful, the authors argued that treatment of 1 year's duration was not sufficient.

Marziali and Munroe-Blum (1994) compared time-limited interpersonal group therapy, which consisted of weekly 90-minute sessions for 25 weeks and biweekly sessions for the next 10 weeks (30 sessions in total), with open-ended, weekly individual therapy for a sample of 79 patients with borderline personality disorder. All patients demonstrated significant improvement on outcome measures with no difference between the two treatment conditions. However, both conditions suffered high dropout rates.

Piper et al. (1993) compared time-limited day treatment, which consisted of group treatment in the form of a diverse set of daily group therapies for 7 hours per day, 5 days per week, for 18 weeks, with a waiting list control condition for a sample of 120 patients with affective and personality disorders. The most prevalent personality disorders were dependent and borderline. Day treatment patients demonstrated greater improvement on a comprehensive set of seven outcome variables that included symptoms, interpersonal behavior, self-esteem, and life satisfaction. The control condition patients evidenced little improvement—that is, minimal spontaneous remission. Improvements for the day treatment patients were maintained at 8-month follow-up.

Bateman and Fonagy (1999, 2001) compared psychoanalytically oriented day treatment, which consisted of a combination of group and individual therapies for 5 days a week for a maximum of 18 months, with a standard care control condition, which consisted of infrequent meetings with a psychiatrist but no formal therapy, for a sample of 44 patients with borderline personality disorder. Day treatment patients showed significant improvements that exceeded minimal change for standard care on a variety of outcome variables, including suicide attempts and acts of self-mutilation and self-reports of depression, anxiety, general symptoms, interpersonal functioning, and social adjustment. Day treatment patients maintained these gains and in some cases improved on them at 18-month follow-up.

Naturalistic Studies

Findings from a number of carefully conducted naturalistic outcome studies that focused on the group treatment of personality disorders also have been published. These tend to be pre-post, single-condition studies or studies with nonrandomly assigned conditions. These studies involved outpatient group therapy (Budman et al. 1996), day treatment (Hafner and Holme 1996; Tasca et al. 1999; Wilberg et al. 1998, 1999), and residential treatment (Chiesa et al. 2003). In general, the findings from these naturalistic studies were consistent with those of randomized clinical trials in providing evidence of favorable outcomes for patients with personality disorders, in particular those with borderline personality disorder. Most of the randomized clinical trials and naturalistic studies focused on group treatments from a psychodynamic or cognitive-behavioral orientation. A recent meta-analytic review that focused on both group and individual treatments of personality disorders from psychodynamic and cognitive-behavioral orientations concluded that both orientations were effective treatments (Leichsenring and Leibing 2003).

Clinical Reports

Clinical reports of successful group treatments of patients with personality disorders are the most prevalent type of evidence in the literature. They provide the basis for most recommendations about the suitability of specific personality disorders for group treatment. The following section reflects conclusions from a number of reviews that are based primarily on clinical reports (Azima 1993; Gunderson and Gabbard 2001; Robinson 1999; Sperry 1999). There is considerable consensus among these reviews.

FORMS OF GROUP TREATMENT FOR SPECIFIC PERSONALITY DISORDERS

Cluster A

Schizoid Personality Disorder

There is agreement that some schizoid patients can definitely benefit from group treatment, which involves social learning stemming from consistent exposure to other patients. Difficulties can involve passivity and silence, which may irritate other patients.

Schizotypal Personality Disorder

Group therapy may play an invaluable role in schizotypal patients, particularly in increasing socialization skills. Difficulties can arise if the patient's peculiarities are bizarre and difficult for other patients to tolerate. Prolonged silence can also be problematic. Preparation in individual therapy can be very helpful.

Paranoid Personality Disorder

Paranoid patients usually do not do well in a group because of their hypersensitivity, suspiciousness, and misinterpretation of others' comments. Feedback from other group members can be very powerful if the patient remains in the group and is receptive to feedback.

Cluster B

Borderline Personality Disorder

Group therapy can be extremely effective for borderline personality disorder patients and is often combined with individual therapy. In group therapy, both transference and countertransference are diffused, and thus it is more tolerable for both parties. As a result, interpretations may be better tolerated in group therapy. Nevertheless, the patient's tendency to express anger and other strong affects in an unpredictable manner can lead to rejection and scapegoating. Such patients are very challenging to treat.

Narcissistic Personality Disorder

Group therapy for narcissistic patients is usually regarded as problematic. Lack of empathy, a sense of entitlement, and hunger for admiration are not engaging characteristics of this disorder. Scapegoating is common. Dropout rates are high. If the patient can be convinced to stay, much useful learning can occur. Group therapy is often combined with individual therapy.

Histrionic Personality Disorder

For those with histrionic personality disorder, group therapy can definitely be helpful. Such patients can help energize the group. However, there is a better prognosis for those with less dramatic behavior. Difficulties follow if the patient slips into the role of monopolizer or help-rejecting complainer.

Antisocial Personality Disorder

Outpatient group therapy is not suitable for patients with ASPD, although some intensive residential programs and therapeutic community programs in prisons have reported successes (Dolan 1998; Warren and Dolan 1996).

Cluster C

Avoidant Personality Disorder

Group therapy can be extremely useful for those with avoidant personality disorder because such patients are usually well motivated. Often the therapy group follows a course of individual therapy.

Dependent Personality Disorder

For dependent patients, group therapy is regarded as an effective treatment, and some believe that it is the treatment of choice because the patients' dependent cravings can be gratified and their overclinging can be confronted (Azima 1993). Group therapy provides many opportunities for dependent patients to learn to be more independent and expressive.

Obsessive-Compulsive Personality Disorder

Group therapy can be helpful for some obsessive-compulsive patients. Difficulties involve the patient's tendencies to act as an additional therapist and to be stubborn and too work oriented. This behavior usually results in resentment from the other patients.

Summary

Thus, according to the clinical literature, schizoid, schizotypal, borderline, histrionic, avoidant, and dependent personality disorders are regarded as particularly suitable for group treatment. In contrast, paranoid, narcissistic, and obsessive-compulsive personality disorders are regarded as difficult to treat. Most group treatments are contraindicated for ASPD. Although single personality disorders, such as borderline, are often addressed in the clinical literature, it is quite common for patients to meet criteria for several personality disorders (Dolan et al. 1995), and this comorbidity complicates treatment. Research evidence from the individual therapy literature has shown that the number of personality disorders a patient is diagnosed with is inversely related to favorable outcome (Ogrodniczuk et al. 2001).

The following illustration summarizes the treatment of a patient with dependent personality disorder and narcissistic traits in an intensive (7 hours per day, 5 days per week), time-limited (18 weeks), group-oriented day treatment program with a daily census of approximately 35 patients. This powerful program is fully described in Piper et al. (1996).

Case Example

Mr. Q was a 50-year-old unemployed divorcé who lived with his 75-year-old widowed mother. His father had died 7 years previously. Mr. Q presented with feelings of discontent about his life. He had a pervasive feeling of having failed in his relationships and in the workplace. He was diagnosed as having a dependent personality disorder with significant narcissistic traits. He was experiencing a difficult phase of his life. At Mr. Q's admission, the therapist's etiological formulation read as follows:

Patient's hereditary factors may be indicated by his father's depression at age 50. In terms of psychosocial factors, his current distress seemed to have been triggered by recent negative criticism at work and a growing perception of failure. His feelings likely intensified through un-

successful attempts at farming, entrepreneurship, and sales. He experienced both feelings of inadequacy and rage because others were unable to recognize his special and unique qualities. The belief that he should be a strong role model seemed to start in his family of origin, where he was the eldest. His efforts to succeed were not acknowledged by either parent. There seemed to be a lack of support for expressing his opinions or making decisions. He felt controlled by his mother. Neither parent seemed receptive of his viewpoints. His unconscious life seemed dominated by negative self-images and experiences of rejection, devaluation, and control.

In relationships with women, Mr. Q tried to see himself as the strongest and most deserving of attention. He perceived himself as giving to women and being there for them but avoided thinking about how much he needed from them. He was drawn to women like his mother, whom he saw as emotional, controlling, and unable to meet his needs. He dealt with these relationships in the same way his father had dealt with his mother—by being submissive and by walking away from conflicts. In so doing, however, Mr. Q became resentful and furious toward women. He also acknowledged avoiding closeness with women. In his last serious relationship, 10 years earlier, he had hoped that he had found his idealized mother-figure. The woman was seen as caring, easygoing, and submissive. Mr. Q felt deeply betrayed when she suddenly left after 2 years. Following this break-up, he may have had a major depression. He avoided dealing with his emotions by becoming preoccupied with pastimes such as woodwork and music. He eventually returned to another woman, his mother, where he has continued to feel controlled and neglected but was unable to recognize his conflicting needs for closeness and independence. This conflict contributed to his feelings of frustration and inadequacy.

In summary, Mr. Q was described as a dependent man whose lack of self-assertion in relation to women had contributed to failure in intimate relationships. His craving for perfectly attuned attention and responsiveness to his physical and emotional needs also interfered with his relationships. The result was a growing sense of dissatisfaction with his life.

On admission to the day treatment program, Mr. Q received the following DSM-IV-TR diagnostic profile:

Axis I:	Phase-of-life problem
Axis II:	Dependent personality disorder with significant narcissistic traits
Axis III:	None
Axis IV:	Negative criticism at work
Axis V:	Global assessment of functioning Current: 60 Highest during past year: 70

Mr. Q formulated in his own words the following problem areas that he most wanted to work on in treatment: 1) Work problems: I have failed in the past and am afraid to try again, to get back into it. 2) Relationships: I am afraid to get involved; I need a wife and a family, but I have built up walls.

Mr. Q's paternalism and grandiosity emerged early in his treatment. He quickly assumed the role of giving advice to fellow patients and lending an ear to those in distress. At the same time, his difficulty identifying his own feelings and needs was evident. He frequently treated the female members of the group with a mixture of devaluation and condescension for their inability to respond to his needs in the group. He often sat next to the male psychiatrist in the large psychotherapy group but had difficulty elaborating on the possible reasons for his need to be near the male leader of the program.

The staff members and fellow patients consistently confronted him about his tendency to create distance by giving advice and by not elaborating on personal issues. He gradually became able to talk about the failures in his life and began to express feelings of hurt, anger, shame, and guilt. During the middle phase of the 18-week program, in an interview with his mother, he expressed his feelings of anger toward her for her controlling and neglectful ways. He explained his needs to separate emotionally and physically from her and for her to recognize his needs. In therapy groups, he was able to understand how his conflictual relationship with his mother had resembled his relationships with other women in his life. He began to see that his advice giving was part of a ploy to create dependency on him so that his needs and demands could be catered to. He was deeply conflicted about dependency in relation to women. Difficulty acknowledging his own dependency drove him to make women dependent on him while at the same time he resented his role in supporting them. His fear of independence interfered with his ability to assert himself with his mother and with other significant women.

During the final phase of treatment, loss issues became predominant. His youngest daughter confronted him about his emotional distance as a father. This confrontation enabled Mr. Q to begin exploration of unresolved grief in relation to his own father. Not only was he faced with the loss of his father through death but also through emotional distance during his early developmental years. In the therapy groups, Mr. Q began to see that his giving advice to fellow patients had been done partly in the hope that he would receive similar support and caring from the staff members and from the male psychiatrist in particular, who represented his father. He also began to recognize that his escalating and sometimes frantic demands, enacted especially with the female group members, reflected his needs for confirmation of his self-worth and the availability of someone to complete his fragmented self-image.

Outcome

At the time of his discharge, Mr. Q still was living with his mother but had definite plans to move out.

He did not elaborate on his intentions regarding his current girlfriend. He found a temporary job and intended to return to a career in sales. Mr. Q showed considerable improvement on measures of general symptomatic distress, mood level, self-esteem, and defensive functioning. He demonstrated moderate improvements in areas reflecting sexual, family, and social functioning as well as life satisfaction. He also made significant improvements in the two problem areas identified at the beginning of treatment.

We believe that the success of Mr. Q's treatment can, in part, be attributed to the basic therapeutic features of day treatment, which include exposure to multiple patients and multiple staff members in a variety of therapy groups for several hours each day over several months. The diversity of groups allows patients to begin to participate in one group in which they feel comfortable before actively participating in others. It also provides a comprehensive approach to treatment. The experience provides many opportunities for the unique features of group treatment (cohesion, interpersonal learning, imitation, universality, altruism) to have their effects. The time-limited program in which Mr. Q participated created pressure to work hard in a relatively short period of time in his life.

Case Example

Ms. R was a 26-year-old single nursing assistant who lived on her own. She presented for help because of repeated destructive relationships with men and an inability to tolerate male authority figures, especially at work. A recent confrontation with a male supervisor, in which she had become extremely angry, weepy, and confused, precipitated the crisis that prompted her to seek help. At admission, the therapist's etiological formulation read as follows:

Ms. R's family of origin was divided as a result of the emotional distance between her father and mother. Mother was seen as overinvolved, dependent, and verbally abusive toward Ms. R. Her father was seen as distant and emotionally unavailable to her. She tried hard to win his approval and acceptance through the pursuit of academics and sports, but her efforts went unnoticed. Ms. R's father abandoned the family for another woman when Ms. R was 13. She felt deserted and responsible for his leaving. She developed a persistent feeling of being a bad person. Unable to vent her anger and rage at her father for leaving and at her mother for letting him go, she instead became her mother's protector. At school, she was a protector of the underdog. This role continued into her adult life and into her work environment. As a result, she frequently came into considerable conflict with authority figures. There was evidence of triangulation in Ms. R's relationships in which she symbolically ended up fighting for her mother against her father. There was also a strong pre-oedipal pat-

tern to her history. *This pattern was manifested in the theme of destruction throughout her adult life: the self-abuse through bulimic behavior, alcohol abuse, and physical abuse by her boyfriends. Her desperation for a relationship with her father may have hidden a deep sense of emotional neglect at the hands of her inadequate mother.*

In summary, Ms. R was described as an emotionally labile woman whose pervasive sense of inadequacy culminated in frequent acts of self-destruction. Her oppositional disposition toward authority figures and fear of intimacy with men often interfered with her relationships. This disposition resulted in a growing sense of instability in her mood and her relationships.

On admission to the day treatment program, Ms. R received the following DSM-IV-TR diagnostic profile:

Axis I:	Bulimia nervosa, cyclothymia, alcohol dependence (in remission)
Axis II:	Borderline personality disorder with significant dependent traits
Axis III:	None
Axis IV:	Discord with boss, discord with parents and sibling
Axis V:	Global assessment of functioning Current: 52 Highest during past year: 65

Ms. R formulated the following problem areas in her own words that she most wanted to work on in treatment: 1) to be able to deal with my depression and mood swings; 2) to improve my relationships with others; and 3) to understand and stop my eating disorder.

Summary of Ms. R's Experience in the Day Treatment Program

Representative of Ms. R's functioning outside of the treatment setting, her passage through the day treatment program was stormy. Early in treatment, she demonstrated difficulty adhering to the limits defined by the therapists. She missed groups and spent considerable time counseling other patients during breaks. Within the groups, she would focus on other patients' problems rather than her own. She was openly scathing of the therapists' perceived failure to do the right thing for the patients. However, she would move in quickly to defend them when they were confronted by other patients.

Through consistent confrontation and limit-setting on the part of the therapists, Ms. R began to explore her feelings of rejection and of being uncared for by her family. Ms. R found herself becoming attached to two male patients. This attachment enabled her to explore her mixed feelings toward her father and brother. She also began to consider how she had assumed the role of the bad child in her family and had been scapegoated by her brother. How-

ever, she showed considerable reluctance to be open with her feelings toward her mother.

Ms. R experienced considerable stress as she entered the termination phase of treatment. Her symptoms returned with full force as she was confronted with losing the group, a deep reminder of the loss of her family when her father left. She once again began to test the limits of the therapists' tolerance through absenteeism and counseling fellow patients outside designated group hours. The other group members confronted Ms. R about her defiant behavior and helped her recognize it as a repetition of old maladaptive patterns: she loses important people in her life because she is a "bad" person. Contained by the group, she was able to talk about her painful feelings in relation to losing the two male patients to whom she had become attached. She was also able to confront her father to let him know for the first time of her feelings of rejection. Ms. R also began to recognize that her intolerance of authority and oppositional behavior were manifestations of the conflict between her wish to be accepted and cared for and her fear of being rejected.

Outcome

Upon her discharge from the day treatment program, Ms. R returned to work but continued to experience an uneasy relationship with her supervisor. She showed moderate improvements on measures of interpersonal functioning and general symptomatic distress. She also made modest improvements in two of the three problem areas that she identified at the beginning of treatment. Regarding her bulimia, there was little improvement. It was concluded that although the groups were helpful for Ms. R, the 18-week time limit was insufficient to deal effectively with her multiple, long-standing problems. Long-term group treatment was suggested.

CONCLUSIONS

Evidence of Efficacy and Effectiveness

The number of randomized clinical trials that have been conducted to evaluate the efficacy of group treatments for personality disorders is small, and they focus primarily on borderline, avoidant, and dependent personality disorders. However, although few in number, the findings of these studies definitely support the efficacy of group treatments. Randomized clinical trials represent a strong experimental design that provides confidence that the treatment was responsible for the outcome. However, they have been criticized for being artificial and not representing the way that treatment is conducted in everyday clinical situations. Studies that sacrifice experimental rigor but are conducted in everyday clinical situations are naturalistic and said to provide information about the effectiveness of treatment. Thus, it is important to know that the findings from the small number of carefully conducted naturalistic studies are consistent with efficacy studies in supporting the use of group treatment for patients with personality disorders. Clinical reports provide additional supportive conclusions, although the difficulties in treating personality disorders are widely acknowledged. It is well known that personality disorders are serious long-term conditions that are resistant to change. It would be a mistake to overemphasize the success of group treatments.

It is likely that the successes that group treatments have achieved are related to unique features arising from the presence of peers in groups. Group influence is a powerful agent. It becomes even more powerful in programs such as day treatment in which patients participate in a large number of groups that focus on different aspects of the patient's difficulties and capitalize on synergistic effects (Ogrodniczuk and Piper 2001).

Underutilization of Group Treatments for the Treatment of Personality Disorders

Given the positive nature of the efficacy and effectiveness findings and the high prevalence of patients with personality disorders, one would expect that group treatments for personality disorders would be much more prevalent in treatment settings and in research investigations. There is considerable evidence from reviews of the research literature that group and individual therapies produce similar results for a wide range of disorders (Fuhriman and Burlingame 1994; Piper and Joyce 1996; Smith et al. 1980).

Bender et al. (2001) conducted a treatment utilization study that focused on comparisons among four types of personality disorders and major depression. Although the study did not focus on differences between treatments for each personality disorder, the lifetime amounts of treatment, expressed as the mean number of months, indicated that the patients had received considerably more individual therapy than group therapy. The number of months for individual therapy and group therapy, respectively, were 43.7 versus 5.3 for schizotypal, 50.6 versus 8.0 for borderline, 31.7 versus 7.2 for avoidant, and 34.5 versus 3.7 for obsessive-compulsive personality disorders.

Resistance to conducting group therapy appears to stem from several sources. As indicated previously, issues related to perceived loss of control, individuality, understanding, privacy, and safety often lead to apprehension on the part of patients and therapists

about participating in group therapy. The therapist may collude with patient bias against group therapy as a "second-class" treatment because the patient does not receive as much individual attention as in individual therapy. In addition, from the perspective of the therapist, groups are perceived as more difficult to organize and as requiring greater administrative time. It is also true that many therapists have not received formal training in group therapy. This deficit is especially true for the more powerful forms of group treatment, such as day treatment programs, which are designed to treat large numbers of patients. Historically, there have also been financial and legal (liability) disincentives that have discouraged therapists from creating and conducting partial hospitalization programs in favor of maintaining full-time inpatient care (Piper et al. 1996). Unfortunately, the end result is underutilization of group therapy.

Future Research Topics and Directions

There are a number of worthwhile directions for future research. Particularly salient is the need for more randomized clinical trials that investigate the efficacy of different group therapies for personality disorders. Cluster A patients have been rarely studied, perhaps because they often do not seek treatment (Gabbard 2000). New approaches to the treatment of personality disorders, such as interpersonal reconstructive therapy (Benjamin 2002) and systems training for emotional predictability and problem solving (STEPPS; Blum et al. 2002), deserve study. Randomized trials that involve matching patients to treatment will be especially welcome, as well as effectiveness studies conducted at routine clinical sites.

Another important topic for future inquiry is that of combined treatments. With increasing frequency, clinicians are recommending that patients with certain personality disorders (e.g., borderline, narcissistic) receive a combination of treatments, such as group psychotherapy combined with individual psychotherapy or medication. Evaluations of the cost-effectiveness of group therapies are also needed. It is important to know whether group treatments result in lower future health care costs than other forms of treatment. Bateman and Fonagy (2003) provided preliminary evidence that intensive day treatment may be more cost-effective than treatment that is usually provided to patients with borderline personality disorder.

Studies of group composition (e.g., homogeneous vs. heterogeneous) would be welcome in order for clinicians to make more informed patient selection decisions. Some patients should not be in groups with certain other types of patients. Inappropriate group composition may lead to failure for some patients or for the whole group.

Premature termination is a significant problem in the treatment of patients with personality disorders. It not only means that the patient fails to receive the treatment that he or she needs, but it also affects the patients who remain in the group as well as the therapist. Studies that examine different approaches to improving patients' capacity to remain engaged in treatment are highly desirable.

Finally, future studies need to consider a broader range of outcomes. Symptom severity and current social functioning have been overrepresented. Clinicians treating patients with personality disorders are likely more concerned about whether they can effect change in the core personality traits and structures that characterize patients with personality disorders (Shea 1993). Clearly, there are many worthwhile research endeavors that can increase our understanding of the appropriate role of group treatments for patients with personality disorders.

REFERENCES

Abbey S, Farrow S: Group therapy and organ transplantation. Int J Group Psychother 48:163–185, 1998

Alden L: Short-term structured treatment for avoidant personality disorder. J Consult Clin Psychol 57:756–764, 1989

American Psychiatric Association: Diagnostic and Statistical Manual of Mental Disorders, 4th Edition, Text Revision. Washington, DC, American Psychiatric Association, 2000

Azima FJ: Group psychotherapy with personality disorders, in Comprehensive Group Psychotherapy. Edited by Kaplan HI, Sadock BJ. Baltimore, MD, Williams and Wilkins, 1993, pp 393–406

Bateman A, Fonagy P: Effectiveness of partial hospitalization in the treatment of borderline personality disorder: a randomized controlled trial. Am J Psychiatry 156:1563–1569, 1999

Bateman A, Fonagy P: Treatment of borderline personality disorder with psychoanalytically oriented partial hospitalization: an 18-month follow-up. Am J Psychiatry 158:36–42, 2001

Bateman A, Fonagy P: Health service utilization costs for borderline personality disorder patients treated with psychoanalytically oriented partial hospitalization versus general psychiatric care. Am J Psychiatry 160: 169–171, 2003

Bender DS, Dolan RT, Skodol AE, et al: Treatment utilization by patients with personality disorders. Am J Psychiatry 158:295–302, 2001

Benjamin LS: Personality disorders, in Psychotherapy Relationships that Work: Therapists' Relational Contributions to Effective Psychotherapy. Edited by Norcross J. Oxford, England, Oxford University Press, 2002, pp 423–438

Bernard HS: Difficult patients and challenging situations, in Basics of Group Psychotherapy. Edited by Bernard HS, MacKenzie KR. New York, Guilford, 1994, pp 123–156

Blum N, Pfohl B, St John D, et al: STEPPS: a cognitive-behavioral systems-based group treatment for outpatients with borderline personality disorder—a preliminary report. Compr Psychiatry 43:301–310, 2002

Budman SH, Demby A, Soldz S: Time-limited group psychotherapy for patients with personality disorders. Int J Group Psychother 46:357–377, 1996

Cappe RF, Alden LE: A comparison of treatment strategies for clients functionally impaired by extreme shyness and social avoidance. J Consult Clin Psychol 54:796–801, 1986

Chiesa M, Fonagy P, Holmes J: When less is more: an exploration of psychoanalytically oriented hospital-based treatment for severe personality disorder. Int J Psychoanal 84:637–650, 2003

Dolan B: Therapeutic community treatment for severe personality disorders, in Psychopathy: Antisocial, Criminal, and Violent Behavior. Edited by Millon T, Simonsen E. New York, Guilford, 1998, pp 407–430

Dolan B, Evans C, Norton K: Multiple Axis II diagnoses of personality disorder. Br J Psychiatry 166:107–112, 1995

Fuhriman A, Burlingame GM: Group psychotherapy: research and practice, in Handbook of Group Psychotherapy: An Empirical and Clinical Synthesis. Edited by Fuhriman A, Burlingame GM. New York, Wiley, 1994, pp 3–40

Gabbard GO: Psychotherapy of personality disorders. J Psychother Pract Res 9:1–6, 2000

Gunderson JG, Gabbard GO: Personality Disorders in Treatments of Psychiatric Disorders, 3rd Edition. Edited by Gabbard GO. Washington, DC, American Psychiatric Publishing, 2001, pp 2222–2368

Hafner RJ, Holme G: The influence of a therapeutic community on psychiatric disorder. J Clin Psychol 52:461–468, 1996

Kibel HD: Interpretive work in milieu groups. Int J Group Psychother 53:303–329, 2003

Leichsenring F, Leibing E: The effectiveness of psychodynamic therapy and cognitive behavior therapy in the treatment of personality disorders: a meta-analysis. Am J Psychiatry 160:1223–1232, 2003

Leszcz M: Group psychotherapy of the characterologically difficult patient. Int J Group Psychother 39:311–335, 1989

Linehan MM, Armstrong HE, Suarez A, et al: Cognitive-behavioral treatment of chronically parasuicidal borderline patients. Arch Gen Psychiatry 48:1060–1064, 1991

Marziali E, Munroe-Blum H: Interpersonal Group Psychotherapy for Borderline Personality Disorder. New York, Basic Books, 1994

Ogrodniczuk JS, Piper WE: Day treatment for personality disorders: a review of research findings. Harv Rev Psychiatry 9:105–117, 2001

Ogrodniczuk JS, Piper WE, Joyce AS, et al: Using DSM Axis II information to predict outcome in short-term individual psychotherapy. J Personal Disord 15:126–138, 2001

Piper WE, Joyce AS: A consideration of factors influencing the utilization of time-limited, short-term group therapy. Int J Group Psychother 46:311–328, 1996

Piper WE, Ogrodniczuk JS: Brief group therapy, in Handbook of Group Counseling and Psychotherapy. Edited by DeLucia-Waack J, Gerrity DA, Kalodner C, et al. Beverly Hills, CA, Sage, 2004, pp 641–650

Piper WE, Rosie JS, Azim HFA, et al: A randomized trial of psychiatric day treatment for patients with affective and personality disorders. Hosp Community Psychiatry 44:757–763, 1993

Piper WE, Rosie JS, Joyce AS, et al: Time Limited Day Treatment for Personality Disorders: Integration of Research and Practice in a Group Program. Washington, DC, American Psychological Association, 1996

Piper WE, McCallum M, Joyce AS: Patient personality and time-limited group psychotherapy for complicated grief. Int J Group Psychother 51:525–552, 2001

Robinson DJ: Field Guide to Personality Disorders. Port Huron, MI, Rapid Psychler, 1999

Rosen D, Stukenberg KW, Sacks S: The group-as-a-whole relations model of group psychotherapy. Bull Menn Clin 65:471–488, 2001

Rutan JS, Stone WN: Psychodynamic Group Psychotherapy, 3rd Edition. New York, Guilford, 2001

Shea MT: Psychosocial treatment of personality disorders. J Personal Disord 7 (suppl):167–180, 1993

Smith M, Glass G, Miller T: The Benefits of Psychotherapy. Baltimore, MD, Johns Hopkins University Press, 1980

Sperry L: Cognitive Behavior Therapy of DSM-IV Personality Disorders: Highly Effective Interventions for the Most Common Personality Disorder. Philadelphia, PA, Brunner/Mazel, 1999

Tasca GA, Balfour L, Bissada H, et al: Treatment completion and outcome in a partial hospitalization program: interactions among patient variables. Psychother Res 9:232–247, 1999

Tuttman S: Principles of psychoanalytic group therapy applied to the treatment of borderline and narcissistic disorders, in The Difficult Patient in Group: Group Psychotherapy With Borderline and Narcissistic Disorders. Edited by Roth BE, Stone WN, Kibel HD. Madison, CT, International Universities Press, 1990, pp 7–29

Warren F, Dolan B: Treating the "untreatable": therapeutic communities for personality disorders. Therapeutic Communities: International Journal for Therapeutic and Supportive Organizations 17:205–216, 1996

Wilberg T, Karterud S, Urnes O, et al: Outcomes of poorly functioning patients with personality disorders in a day treatment program. Psychiatr Serv 49:1462–1467, 1998

Wilberg T, Urnes O, Friis S, et al: One-year follow-up of day treatment for poorly functioning patients with personality disorders. Psychiatr Serv 50:1326–1330, 1999

Yalom ID: The Theory and Practice of Group Psychotherapy, 4th Edition. New York, Basic Books, 1995

23

Family Therapy

G. Pirooz Sholevar, M.D.

The rich literature in family and couples therapy is focused primarily on the examination of interactions and relationships among family members rather than on characteristics of individuals. Recently, however, there has been a renewed interest in the empirical exploration of family variables in major mental disorders particularly schizophrenia, depression, and alcoholism. The major findings in this area have enriched significantly our therapeutic knowledge and impact on major mental disorders. Personality disorders have not been a major beneficiary of empirical family investigations yet, for a variety of reasons that remain speculative. This omission is significant because many early pioneers in family therapy had a keen interest in personality disorders, partly due to their psychoanalytic orientation and training. A major reason for this omission has been the fear that by attending to the enduring character structure, traits, and disorders, one can easily lose the essential focus on the interactional and relational dimension in the family system, which is the fundamental principle in family systems theory. It is the goal of this chapter to examine the relational and interactional dimensions of the behavior of individuals with enduring character disorders within a family systems theoretical framework.

Early family experiences provide the context for the development of a healthy personality organization as well as one in which different disorders develop. The developmental trends established in childhood are further consolidated through continued interactions with parents and other family members. Subsequent social interactions with peers and experiences in the community are influential in the modification or redirection of personality traits, but they usually do not have the decisive impact of early family relationships.

Learned patterns of coping develop as a result of the interaction of the individual's biological constitution, including temperamental factors, with social reinforcement experiences to form personality traits or structure. Characteristics of family environment, such as a pattern of dealing with conflict and supportiveness, can determine the coping style of the individual (Head et al. 1991; Millon 1981).

Espy (1994) outlined characteristics of the character-disordered family system. He described a variety of methods used by the family to control its members, including threats, deception, betrayal, and physical punishment. The disordered family relationship becomes internalized in family members in the form of personality disorders. Other investigators, using a variety of investigative tools including the Family Environment Scale (Moos and Moos 1980, 1986), have described the failure of such families to achieve cohesiveness, empathic interactions, and reciprocity. As a result, communication is generally used as a method of control and power play to coerce other members to give in to the demands and will of others. Defensive affects are used as a way of intimidating and distancing others rather than providing a basis for meaningful communication and shared meaning in the service of satisfying the basic and developmental needs of family members.

Later-life experiences shape the formation of the individual's personality and provide the major tools of social development. In cases of personality constriction or disorders, premarital dating and marital choices are influenced substantially by a replication or rejection of former experiences with primary objects. A marital partner who is chosen based on replication can lead to a harmonious, although constricted, marital interaction with limited capacity for growth. The choice of a marital partner opposite of the early objects may hold the promise of personality expansion but can result in significant turmoil and the potential for marital breakup in cases in which the level of difference is significant.

A person with a healthy and resourceful personality establishes a relatively open and unrestricted interaction with a large number of diverse personalities in a broad range of situations, selects an equally healthy marital partner, and produces resourceful children. Such individuals adapt satisfactorily to most circumstances and may only develop transitory symptoms when encountering challenges. Restricted and disordered personalities can become symptomatic in minimally stressful circumstances. They can produce significant symptomatology, depression, or functional breakdown in challenging times. In cases of severe disorders, such as extreme degrees of schizotypal or antisocial personalities, the person may be unable to establish or sustain relationships, which can result in remaining single or divorcing after a short period of marriage or forming a highly pathological family unit.

Parenting factors were initially addressed by psychoanalytically oriented psychiatrists and mental health professionals in terms of parenting styles, such as overprotectiveness, neglect, and projection of childhood introjects of parents onto their children, resulting in projective identification. Such factors were described initially in terms of overprotectiveness (Levy 1943), parental moral deficits (Johnson and Szurek 1952), and especially by a host of more recent investigators examining the projections by the parents of their own pathogenic introjects formed in the parent's early childhood onto their children. In projective identification, parts of the self are split off and projected onto another person with consequent feelings of identification with that other person. Zinner (1976) emphasized the interactional component of this unconscious defense mechanism; this mechanism can be maintained only if there is willing unconscious collusion between the subject and object so that the object repeatedly manifests the qualities that the subject has projected onto him or her. The mechanism occurs frequently in the relationship between some couples and also between parents and their adolescent children. Projective identification serves as the basis for a dysfunctional or pathological identity formation in the child who forges a life course dictated by such introjects—rather than forming a flexible and multifaceted identity to negotiate different situations, seeking long-term success, and avoiding failure (Sholevar and Schwoeri 2003c).

PARENTING

Parental psychopathology and parenting styles have a decisive role in the genesis of personality disorders in the next generations. Both Axis I and Axis II disorders in parents, as well as parental ineffectiveness in addressing traumatic situations, play a significant role in the genesis of personality disorders in offspring. Some of the contributions of parents are direct, such as modeling dysfunctional patterns of coping and interpersonal relationships for their children. Parental influences can also be indirect, such as relative neglect of the children, which can expose them to traumatic situations such as sexual abuse inside and outside the family. Such traumatic incidents can become worse when parents discourage children from letting them know about the traumatic situations, disbelieve children when they reveal the trauma, or call them "liars" for the revelations.

Rutter and Quinton (1984) stated that parental personality disorder has more severe impact on the child than an Axis I disorder. This phenomenon is due to a variety of factors including the periodic and episodic nature of Axis I disorders, which can include periods of recovery and remission between clinical episodes. Some of the trauma of a parental emotional disorder may be addressed or resolved during symptom-free periods. Axis II disorders can have more of a detrimental impact due to their continuous nature as well as the lack of awareness and rationalization of parents of their maladaptive personality traits.

Personality disorders in previous generations can be less severe, and parents can exhibit only traits (or subsyndromal forms) of a personality disorder rather than a fully developed state or disorder. Generally, personality traits intensify across generations and lead to fully developed personality disorders in succeeding generations. This situation can become worse if a personality-disordered parent marries someone who shares the same personality disorder or has a complementary personality pattern. For example, the marriage of a person with borderline personality disorder (BPD) to a spouse with an antisocial or narcissistic personality disorder can lead both to intensification of symptoms in the offspring and to broadening of the range of symptoms by incorporating a larger number of dysfunctional behaviors from both parental personalities.

MARITAL CHOICE

Systematic investigation of assortative mating in people with personality disorders, or even mental illness in general, is lacking. In clinical practice, people with personality disorders frequently show a preference for selecting mates with certain personality disorders or Axis I diagnoses. However, this sample may be biased because the people who marry someone with a similar or pathologically complementary personality disorder may develop a more severe form of clinical disorder, which can make it more likely for them to consult a psychiatrist or other mental health professional. Furthermore, individuals with personality disorders who marry relatively symptom-free individuals may go through a corrective experience and gradually reduce their symptomatic and problematic personality traits and interpersonal dysfunctions.

Certain personality disorder combinations are frequently brought to the attention of psychiatrists and mental health professionals. The combination of a person with BPD and partner with narcissistic personality disorder has been frequently reported. A narcissistic man may be attracted to a woman with a borderline personality disorder because of her initial overidealization and lack of self-definition, which can accommodate his hunger for admiration; the intense dependency needs of persons with BPD may lead them to invest in narcissistic persons with the hope of eventual reward. Such a union can frequently lead to the intensification of personality pathology and precipitation of depression and suicidal behavior in the patient with BPD.

Another dysfunctional combination is the marriage of two people with BPD who may become attracted to each other initially based on the use of common defensive patterns and unconscious wishes but who soon find themselves in significant trouble due to the mutual impulsivity, explosiveness, intense defensive affects, poor capacity for problem solving, and limited ability to form intimate relationships.

The pairing of antisocial personality disorder with BPD is an ominous combination. The difficulties will be similar to those described for the narcissistic and borderline personalities but on a much more intense level due to the addition of active exploitation, total lack of regard for the needs of others, and legal complications.

It is the premise of family and couples therapy that personality and character constrictions are rooted in early developmental failures and lead to marital characteristics that are an extension of personality dysfunction. The interactional and marital disorder creates a relational and social context that perpetuates intrapsychic conflicts and hinders the forward movement of the couple and their children (Johnson and Lebow 2000; Sholevar and Schwoeri 2003b). Therefore, family and couples therapy provides an invaluable and unique therapeutic tool for the detection, exploration, and treatment of personality disorders; their roots in the families of origin; and their detrimental impact on the marriage through interlocking of personality disorders and interference with the development of the children.

THERAPEUTIC PRINCIPLES WITH PERSONALITY DISORDERS

The drama of the lives of character-disordered persons is played out in their interpersonal interactions with their spouses, children, and others in their social network. The person with a personality disorder observes, analyzes, and reports such data in a defensive, one-sided, and egocentric way. Family and couples therapy provides for a multilateral perspective on this drama, which can be uniquely helpful in many treatment resistant situations as is described here:

1. Delineation of personality traits and disorders can be made more accurately and completely within the context of family and couples therapy. Marital partners frequently witness the display of healthy or dysfunctional character traits by their spouse in different social or work situations. Spouses also can be the targets of the people with personality disorders, although they may contribute partially or substantially to undesirable events. Pathological personality traits can be reported readily—and frequently

without charity—by the spouse and other family members in family and couples sessions. At times, the spouse may act in a passive and compliant manner and collude with the person with the personality disorder to conceal his or her disruptive and pathological behavior. However, their adolescent children may reveal the parental personality disorder and the collusive compliance of the other parent in a disruptive situation.

2. Family and couples therapy allows the examination and understanding of the interplay of precipitating factors in situations in which a spouse displays pathological personality traits. The spouse can have the advantage of witnessing social events with their multiple circular contributors, negative escalations, and reinforcers. The therapist can arrive at a multifaceted, dynamic, and comprehensive picture of interpersonal interactions rather than a description of pathological personality traits devoid of context.

3. Pathological personality traits can be denied and rationalized, not only by the person with the psychopathology but also by his or her spouse. This *shared defensiveness* and rationalization can be detected in conjoint therapy.

4. Transference and enactment of early attitudes, feelings, and relationships onto the spouse can be a very valuable source of information. The intense "marital transference" (Sager 1976, 1986; Sholevar 2000; Sholevar and Schwoeri 2003c, 2003d; Sonne and Swirsky 1986) can compete with and at times undermine the development of a strong transference reaction and neurosis in individual therapy and in the psychoanalytic situation. The enactment and detection of marital transference in joint therapy allows the therapist to recognize early and unresolved conflicts that are enacted in the marital relationship and, therefore, to make these conflicts amenable to intervention and interpretation.

5. People with severe personality disorders can choose partners with complementary pathological traits and form highly pathological, disruptive, and destructive relationships. The interaction of powerful and destructive forces in the couple, frequently rooted in unresolved early conflicts, can create a stormy family atmosphere and be displayed in the treatment situation. The couples' observing egos can be submerged during the interpersonal conflicts. Conjoint therapy can allow the observing ego of the therapist to align with the functional observing ego of each family member in order to put in focus pathological elements, such as

projections, projective identifications, and enactments of unresolved past experiences.

6. Prevention of severe psychopathology in the next generation is a significant therapeutic goal with personality disorders due to their ominous impact on the developmental course of children. Family therapy allows the therapist to interrupt circular pathological interactions of the parents and point out the neglect of the children's basic, developmental, or future needs. For example, a couple who have engaged primarily in mutual blaming in the same manner for 20 years are reminded that they do not follow through with their wish for college educations for their adolescent children by helping them to prepare for SAT tests or by providing them with information about colleges and college selection processes. Repeated interventions based on the genetic roots of their behavior over 2–3 years helps the parents to set aside their narcissistic orientations and support their children in developing plans for college.

7. Family and couples therapy can reduce secondary gains from personality disorders or expected reparation from the partner for childhood traumas such as sexual abuse, physical abuse, or neglect. It can refocus the family on preventing the enactment of the traumatic situations at the expense of the spouse or children, and it can emphasize forging a more productive course for the family in the future.

8. Conjoint therapy allows for engagement and participation of a highly resistant character-disordered person in psychotherapy.

FAMILY INTERVENTIONS WITH PERSONALITY DISORDERS

The early pioneers in family and couples therapy paid keen attention to individuals with obsessive-compulsive personality disorder (OCPD) and those with histrionic personality disorder for their propensity to marry each other, with the underlying common fantasy that the person with OCPD will bring organization and intellectuality and the person with histrionic personality will contribute vitality to the union, which will enrich both spouses. The common failure of this fantasy leaves both partners feeling criticized, demeaned, and humiliated, which results in frequent early divorce. The union between persons with paranoid personality and depression prone people also has received some attention (Berman et al. 1986).

Currently, three of the Cluster B personality disorders have been the primary focus of family and couples therapy literature because they form the most dysfunctional family and marital relationships and are highly resistant to therapeutic interventions. Furthermore, the interlocking pathological and neurotic marriages of individuals with severe forms of personality disorder or unusually complementary needs leads to resistances that can exceed the therapeutic resourcefulness of most therapists and result in counterproductive/counter-therapeutic interventions and negative therapeutic outcomes.

Borderline Personality Disorder

BPD is characterized by an unstable image of self and others, poor impulse control, low frustration tolerance, affective instability, negative affects, and primitive defenses (Zanarini and Frankenburg 1997). Emotional decompensation occurs under the stress evoked in close interpersonal relationships. People with BPD harbor a pervasive fear of abandonment, sense of aloneness, and empty despair. There is a history of parental unavailability, insensitivity, and intrusiveness in early childhood that undermines the establishment of an autonomous sense of self in the child and exposes him or her to repeated traumas in early childhood (Lachkar 1992; Zinner 1976).

Gunderson (1984) emphasized the intense, unstable interpersonal relationships in patients with BPD, characterized by alteration between extremes of overidealization and devaluation. These relationships tend to fluctuate widely and do not persist through frustrations. There is a denial of separation and an inability to form wholesome relationships or mourn the loss of the failed ones. The inability to synthesize contradictory qualities of good and bad in a person results in devaluation of other people after a conflict and failure to solve problems and differences. It forces the individual with BPD to precipitously abandon one relationship and search and find another person who is idealized initially, only to be devalued after disappointment and frustration at a later time.

Goldstein (1990) described three common family types in BPD patients: overinvolved family, rejecting family, and idealizing or denying families. The *overinvolved* family is intense, overly hostile, and in open conflict with the person with BPD. One of the parents generally overprotects the person with BPD while the other one is devaluing, critical, and rejecting. *Rejecting* families view the person with BPD as an unwelcome and disruptive force and act as though the family would be better off without him or her. They deny any marital difficulties and form a tight marital bond to exclude the patient. In *idealizing or denying* families, the family members view each other as perfect. They minimize and deny the difficulties of the person with BPD, and they deny marital problems and present a superficial picture of complete harmony. Gunderson et al. (1980) described two major family patterns: 1) lifelong unavailability or neglect, and 2) one in which parents actively withdraw or are inconsistently present during critical periods of their children's lives. In a controlled study, Gunderson and Lyoo (1997) reported that individuals with BPD perceived their family environment and relationships more negatively in comparison with parents or individuals in normal families. Parents of patients with BPD agreed more with each other rather than with their offspring about the family environment; with both parents' perceptions often close to normative standards. Stone (1990) and Zanarini and Frankenburg (1997) described a high incidence of traumatic situations including sexual and physical abuse, witnessing parental/marital violence, fiery temper, parental divorce, even the suicide of the parents when the children were young. Herman et al. (1989) and Zanarini and Frankenburg (1997) also reported a high incidence of posttraumatic stress disorder and dissociative symptoms.

Severe dysfunction in the family system leads to impulsive attempts at problem solving based on defensive affects rather than on recognizing, analyzing, and negotiating differences. Feldman et al. (1995) demonstrated that families in which the mother has BPD are less cohesive than those of a control group as measured by the Family Environment Scale. They exhibit a higher level of psychopathology and significant difficulty with impulse control spectrum disorders. The children receive lower scores on the Global Assessment Scale.

Overidealization and excessive devaluation in BPD is based on family characteristics in which the attributes of "goodness" (providing, gratifying, loving) and "badness" (depriving, punishing, and hating) in a person are separated from each other and reinvested in different people so that each family member appears relatively unambivalent (Shapiro 1986). Dependence, in contrast to autonomy, is viewed as a "bad" quality, which impedes the expression and satisfaction of the dependency needs of the children. The denial of the need for dependency even on a temporary basis can result in significant defensiveness that will handicap future relationships of the person with BPD. This denial results in difficulties in a variety of familial, marital, and parental roles (Gunderson et al. 1980).

The marriage and family lives of patients with BPD are marked by impulsive actions such as violence, suicide attempts, substance abuse, a chronically conflictual and unsatisfactory marriage, and abrupt abandonment of the family at the height of friction (Lachkar 1992). Borderline patients tend to parentify their own children and excessively bind their children to themselves. In these families, adolescents can engage in highly pathological behaviors such as running away or attempting suicide to separate from parental control. Borderline patients exert extreme possessiveness of their children and demand absolute, unlimited control while threatening rejection. This rejection is usually rooted in the parents' unresolved grief over their own past losses. Painful affects are frequently dormant in the family and emerge disproportionately at the time of frustration and disappointment. The function of such painful affects is to reestablish ties with a frustrating, but psychologically important, early object (Kissen 1995; Sholevar 1997).

Families with a borderline member use projection and projective identification as interpersonal attempts to deal with loss (Schwoeri and Schwoeri 1981, 1982; Zinner 1976). The unconscious projection of feared separation or loss culminates in bitter, unexplained arguments and, often, in violent acting-out. Very often there is a replay of violent behavior resulting from the shared pathology in the family.

The lack of resolution of the separation-individuation stage of development, lack of attainment of object constancy, and the unstable internal image of the parent at times of separation lead to the instability of self-image, which is manifested by the feeling of vulnerability to abandonment and helplessness, lack of vitality, inability to control impulses, and self-destructive actions. Pain offers a false sense of aliveness and vitality to counter the feeling of being in a "black hole." Repeated traumatic experiences revive the feeling of attachment to early traumatic and disappointing objects (Kissen 1995; Sholevar 1997). A conflictual and violent marital relationship is a revival of such traumatic ties. Instability of the image of others is manifested by splitting of people into highly idealized or villainized images, which results in periods of extreme closeness and "falling in love" followed by "hatred" at the time of minor disappointment and threats of separation.

Breakups of relationships are often followed by flight into a relationship and marriage to someone of equally diffuse identity who is immediately idealized. For example, selection of a narcissistic partner and establishment of a narcissistic/borderline marriage facilitates idealization. This type of marriage is expected to directly *compensate* for one's early disappointments. The idealized stage of marriage soon breaks down. Partners react to marital disappointment by prematurely planning for a child in order to re-create an idealized stage of union. Once a child arrives on the scene, one or both of the spouses abandon each other in favor of the new child and the triangular stage of family development does not take place. Intense and inappropriate involvement with the child results in further weakening of the marital relationship. Separation and divorce at this stage is a likely outcome for BPD patients. Fearing abandonment, flight from the marriage frequently occurs by becoming impulsively involved with an inappropriate and emotionally unstable person who lacks self-definition and stability and is willing to become an unwitting partner to the continuation of this psychological drama.

The fight over control and autonomy is resumed between the borderline patient and her child once the child is of school age and into late adolescence. It is the intense fighting between the mother and child and the mother's wish to either control or put away her child that frequently brings the family to the clinician's office with a problem that has both an individual and a family dimension (Villenueve and Roux 1995).

Zinner (1976) stated that projection of disavowed elements of the self onto the spouse has the effect of charging a marital relationship with conflicts that have been transposed from an intrapsychic sphere to an interpersonal one. The operation of projective identification is more than a matter of externalization of disavowed traits. The contents of the projected material contain highly conflicted elements of the spouse's object relationships with his or her family of origin. This externalization of aspects of old conflicted relationships also has a *restorative* function: a need to bring back to life—in the form of the spouse—the individual's lost infantile objects, both good and bad.

One of Zinner's (1976) case examples is of a couple who perceived themselves as polar opposites. The husband was exceedingly rational, incapable of affectionate intimate ties, contemptuous of emotional display, and indifferent to sex. In contrast, the wife was viewed as volatile, impulsive, clinging, and erotic. Each of the partners could maintain such single-minded perceptions of him- or herself and the other through the projection of conflicting aspects of their personality onto their mate. When the projections failed periodically, the husband would fly into rages, which were experienced as dissociative lapses. Zinner asserted that intrapsychic conflicts that have been externalized through projective identification should be reinternalized through interpretation so the process of *working through* can be achieved at an intrapsychic level.

Zinner's formulation of projective identification is similar to the term *collusive marriages* coined by Dick (1967), in which interactions are largely determined by mutual projective identifications. Dick viewed such dyads as though they are a "joint personality" characterized by a kind of division of function by which each partner supplies a set of qualities, the sum of which creates a "complete dyadic unit." Dick emphasized that the psychological incompleteness of each partner is manifested by the lack of ambivalence: "the dyadic unit contains the ambivalence lacking in each individual" (p. 301).

Ringstrom (1998) proposed the concept of competing selfobject functions in the couple, a self psychology proposition position, in contrast to an object relations concept of projective identification (Dick 1967; Zinner 1976) or marital transference (Sager 1976, 1986; Sholevar 1996, 2000; Sonne and Swirsky 1986). He presented a dramatic session of a husband bullying his wife in a reenactment of his abusive family environment as a child when his subjective and inner feelings of reality were crushed by the collective abusive acts of his family. Selfobject functions are experienced by an individual as those persons, places, or things that restore one's sense of continuity, cohesion, and worth (Kohut 1971; Ringstrom 1998; Shane and Shane 1993; Sonne and Swirsky 1986). The selfobject needs of the wife, longing for the restoration of her feeling of depletion, competed with the selfobject needs of the husband for affirmation and validation of his success. The competing selfobject needs of the couple precipitated the marital crisis, which manifested itself by the husband bullying his wife for insensitivity, hostility, and spoiling his success. The therapist responded to the husband with his own selfobject need of standing up to the bully, which threatened the continuity of treatment. The sensitive interpretation of the selfobject needs of the partners (and the therapist) as an enactment of their early experiences in their families of origin resulted in insight into the longings of everyone involved and therapeutic gain.

Treatment

The ultimate goal of treatment is for family members to learn the value of meaningful and noncoercive communication of basic needs and to arrive at negotiated agreements. Disappointments are an integral part of human relationships, but they can be resolved through effective communication and the application of problem-solving methods. The accomplishment of these goals requires modification of highly pathological defenses such as projective identification, splitting, idealization, and denial. The psychodynamic family therapist searches for the genetic roots of marital and parent–child disturbances of the family in a multigenerational context. However, disturbances in the relationships of the borderline family can also be addressed by concentrating on diffuse boundaries that result in repetitive and conflictual communications and the absence of problem solving. The establishment of adequate, functional boundaries between the nuclear and extended families in borderline patients may be an essential task for maintaining the integrity of the nuclear family and its members.

A decrease in the intensity and immediacy of need expression in interpersonal relationships is necessary. It is helpful to reduce the level of intense affect and "affectation" in order to enhance cognitive processing and reveal underlying patterns in interpersonal conflicts. Frequently, the borderline person is caught in multiple ambiguous situations in which contextual and consequential factors are ignored and the poor outcome is blamed intensely on the partner. Such situations occur repeatedly over a long period of time and are stacked up on top of each other and treated as though they establish an unquestionable conclusion or fact. The therapist can slow down the intense blaming, affective storms, and the strong need for expressiveness and reveal the lack of listening capacity and overvaluation of expressing one's point of view repeatedly in a coercive fashion. By enhancing the listening function, the current situation can be sufficiently cooled off so one can investigate the patterns and the underlying needs and demonstrate to the couple that the same ambiguity has existed in a series of historical situations and has served as the basis for ongoing relational conflicts. The ultimate goal is to help the couple and the family to become open to alternative interpretations and solutions, respect their differences, and negotiate mutually acceptable solutions.

The therapeutic task is for the therapist to establish a bond with unsatisfied attachment feelings within the BPD person and her partner and help them to differentiate between the defensive affects of rage and anger and the basic feelings of helplessness, betrayal, insecurity, and neediness. Furthermore, the therapist needs to help the couple to recognize that being needy and expecting need satisfaction from one's partner is a fundamental function of the human relationship rather than something that should be a source of shame leading to rejection.

The Emotionally Focused Therapy approach of

Johnson (1996, 2002; Johnson and Lebow 2000) is particularly applicable to the treatment of patients with BPD in family and couples therapy. Johnson's distinction between the *defensive* and *attachment* affects sheds light on the defensive nature of stormy affective expressions of borderline persons that exaggerate and evade basic differences and conflicts in the relationship and lead to impulsive and destructive actions to the exclusion of cognitive processing. She recommends that the therapist help the couple to recognize that such affective storms are based on shared defensive moods, negative escalation, and failure to apply cognitive processing. The affective storms are the products of "emotional hypochondriasis" and "hyperbolic stance" described by Zanarini and Frankenburg (1994). *Emotional hypochondriasis* refers to the transformation of unbearable feelings such as rage into unremitting attempts to get others to recognize the enormity of one's emotional pain. The *hyperbolic stance* is to state one's views dramatically and repeatedly. Such communications are a coercive and destructive force against marital and family relationships as well as an individual's satisfactory adjustment and developmental progression. The therapist can help the couple and the family members to form a coalition against such affective storms and treat them as an extraneous factor that requires careful scrutiny and containment. This containment can result in the emergence of "soft" attachment feelings that help the couple recognize the need for closeness, intimacy, understanding, and support from each other, which can then be negotiated in a sensitive and reciprocal fashion. This intervention can lead to a higher recognition of the internal needs and establishment of relational reciprocity when both couple or all family members can participate in responding to and satisfying each other's basic and attachment needs. This process can create a contrast to the early family experiences of persons with personality disorder in which their attachment and dependency needs as growing children were denied, denigrated, and neglected by their parents.

Ringstrom (1994) alerted therapists to the common occurrence in many dysfunctional couples in which each partner acts as though he or she is the one who holds the more correct version of reality and attempts to "annihilate" the views of the partner to allow a single subjective view of reality to prevail. The therapist should assert that neither partner nor the therapist's view of the reality is "truer" than the other person's view and that the goal of treatment is to arrive at a shared vision of reality that recognizes everyone's perspective.

Persons with BPD, particularly women, have a high incidence of sexual (and physical) abuse in their childhood in comparison with control clinical groups (Zanarini and Frankenburg 1997). The traumatic impact of sexual abuse can manifest itself in a variety of forms in family and couples therapy, including the inability of the couple to share power and authority or negotiate a reciprocal intimate and sexual relationship. Sexual dysfunction in the marriage can result in sexual acting-out of the partner as well as the sexually abused person with BPD. A BPD patient can display fearfulness and avoidance of sexual encounters with the partner but be overly flirtatious with people outside of the marriage. Such behaviors will enhance the likelihood of the partner getting involved outside of the marriage, with the potential for relational breakup. The partner with BPD may enjoy admiration received from an idealized person outside of the marriage, which can help repair shaky self-esteem at the expense of marital stability.

The therapeutic intervention for the family therapist is to help the couple to forge a reciprocal and more functional intimate and sexual relationship. Facilitation of the expression and recollection of early traumatic situations, and modeling empathic listening by the therapist, can stand in contrast to the disbelief of the family of origin of the revelation of sexual abuse by the patient as a child. This initial step should be followed by equal attention to the pressing current issues most relevant to the BPD person and her partner. Characterological and interpersonal dimensions such as demanding, controlling, and coercion should be addressed in this context to avoid clinical deterioration (Sholevar and Schwoeri 2003a; Zanarini and Frankenburg 1997).

Protection of children against sexual abuse in the nuclear and extended family and by strangers is a goal that can be enhanced more readily in family and couples family than in other forms of treatment.

The person with BPD who is married to a narcissistic or antisocial spouse may require protection from constant blaming and attacking behavior of the partner, who will use coercive measures to force the BPD person to admire the spouse and submit to exploitation.

Narcissistic Personality Disorder

Narcissistic personality organization and disorder have received significant attention due to the investigations of Kohut (1971) and Kernberg (1975). The narcissistically vulnerable individual has a tendency to marry a spouse with a complementary narcissistic vulnerability in a collusive manner in order to conceal his or her narcissistic problems and underlying developmental conflicts. The marriages of narcissistically vulnerable people have been described extensively by Lansky (1981, 1986). Narcissistic couples are excessively sensitive to criticism due to their humiliation-prone personalities, which make them very sensitive to shame and criticism. They lack empathy for other people and each other's feelings and instead react to each other with blaming, attacking, and a lack of genuine empathy. They employ pathological distance regulation and avoid a mutually gratifying relationship out of the fear of experiencing emptiness and personality fragmentation. As children, narcissistic patients experienced neglect and emotional absence from one or both of their own parents. At times, they were parentified and forced to cater to the emotional needs of their siblings or parents. A history of sexual or physical abuse, neglect, or exploitation is common.

There are several common patterns in narcissistic marriages. The more common presenting picture is one of "blaming couples" who show surprising cohesiveness despite their chronic state of marital stress and symptomatology. Impulsive actions and a high level of reactivity are common. Such couples tend to be more treatable than other more severely disturbed ones whose disorders are treatment resistant. Demanding and blaming couples tend to alienate their families and to be very isolated. Psychotherapy can be difficult with such couples, particularly if there is a high level of manipulativeness and substance abuse. "Preoccupied couples" are usually high achievers and successful vocationally, socially, and in the community. The external obligation is frequently used as an excuse to avoid intimacy. Treatment can be difficult due to their external successes and rationalization.

Narcissistic interactions in couples generally conceal underlying developmental arrest marked by an inability to develop a nurturing and intimate relationship. Couples tend to see themselves as cheated, deficient, and in need of attention or recompense. Nurturance provokes feelings of shame and personality fragmentation. A propensity for personality disorganization is countered by pathological distance regulation. A high level of mutual reactivity is a common manifestation. In narcissistic marriages, ordinary disagreements can serve as opportunities to express infantile rage in the form of blame. One aspect of such disorders is to conceal inadequacy and project it onto a spouse or a child. In some narcissistically vulnerable marriages, conflicts may be covert and difficult to recognize, occurring particularly when there is a conflict of loyalty between one's job and family.

Individuals with narcissistic personality disorder have a strong need for appreciation, excessive feelings of entitlement, and expectation of special treatment. They attempt to search for a partner who will satisfy their needs based on her or his own vulnerability. As a result, in addition to marriages of mutually narcissistic partners, narcissistic individuals commonly choose a marital partner with BPD or depressive disorder. They use excessive blaming and attack on their partner as a way of coercing the partner to give in to their excessive demands. They use a variety of rationalizations in order to force the partner to satisfy their needs. When their expectations invariably are not met, they withdraw from the relationship and isolate themselves.

Treatment

In family and couples therapy for narcissistic disorders, the "narcissistic defenses" by which the couple tries to extract special concessions from each other should be explored and brought into the open. These defenses include preoccupation with themselves, excessive blaming, and attacking behavior on the partner in order to coerce him or her to give in to the other's excessive needs. Interpretations have to be made within a very empathic context to prevent further narcissistic injury and establish a bond with the healthier inner elements of the personality.

Such interventions and interpretations should enable narcissistic persons to recognize their repetitive self-defeating patterns that have resulted in multiple failures in relationships and in the workplace in spite of their tremendous talents and ability. The ultimate goal is to forge a modified relational contract with the partner in a way that would be more equitable and reciprocal based on the principle of give and take. Withdrawal from the interactions and relationships at times of disappointment should be interpreted within the context.

The goal of treatment with narcissistic couples is to reduce reactivity and collusive defenses, avoid humiliation, and enhance empathy in order to allow for growth and change. Lansky (1986) recommended a "conductor" type of therapeutic style (Bowen 1976, 1978; Sholevar and Schwoeri 2003d) by which the therapist takes command of the treatment situation to prevent overreactivity between the couple.

The therapist may choose to use the "funneling through the therapist" technique (Bowen 1976, 1978; Sholevar and Schwoeri 2003d) to undermine the defensive and pathological overreactivity and collusion. In this technique, the therapist asks that all transactions in the session go through him or her. The second goal of this technique is to enhance empathic listening, by which the therapist attempts to understand each spouse and help them to understand each other.

An important goal of treatment is to address the intergenerational aspects of narcissistic disorders. Intergenerational constructions are particularly helpful and necessary in dealing with humiliation. Narcissistic tendencies and disorders have a high propensity to repeat themselves in the next generations. Therefore, it is necessary to prevent such disorders in the younger generations by reducing blaming and collusion and enhancing empathy. The use of a genogram in the early phase of treatment is helpful. A common finding is that for each spouse, his or her childhood identification with the same-sex parent had been constantly criticized by the opposite-sex parent, thus weakening her or his gender identity. Another goal of intergenerational psychotherapy is the reconstruction and resolution of traumatic events in the early life of the couple, such as parental absences, neglect, and abuse.

Antisocial Personality Disorder

Parental factors in antisocial personality disorder, as in many other personality types, are usually the end result of multigenerational family dysfunction and deficit. Parents are unaware of their disruptive impact on the development of their children. The parental dimension has been studied recently by a number of investigators, particularly Patterson (1982) and Forehand and McMahon (1981a, 1981b), who have examined parent management practices. Parents can intervene with their children in an impulsive and punitive fashion based on their own poor frustration tolerance, impulsivity, and stressful life situations. They can become involved in coercive family processes (Patterson 1982) by which a parent interacts with the child in an impulsive and unstrategic fashion and escalates an argument when a child reacts with equally strong noncompliance and defiance. The parent may eventually back off, withdraw his or her efforts, and let the child win a particular episode. The repetition of this situation, known as a "coercive trap," can teach children that a display of aggression and explosive behavior can ensure winning their point of view, and they can adopt this method as a central organizing principle in forming their behavioral repertoire. This practice can lead to childhood oppositional defiant behavior and adolescent conduct disorder, with a high percentage ending with antisocial personality disorder as adults.

The antisocial person reaches adulthood after many years of practicing noncompliance, oppositionalism, defiance, and coerciveness and becomes proficient in using direct and indirect aggression efficiently. He or she has very little awareness of the perspectives or internal experiences of other people who are coerced or victimized (lack of "victim empathy"). Coercive measures are used consistently in social situations and with spouse and children. They succeed initially, but eventually disastrous outcomes ensue. The use of coercive interpersonal measures in a marriage can explain the frequency of marital breakup of antisocial persons. Furthermore, noncompliance and coercive interpersonal measures can explain frequent job loss by antisocial persons, resulting in financial hardship on the family.

Men with antisocial personality disorder marry and produce children at a high rate, although they do not always stay around to help with the upbringing of the children. In this way, the contribution of antisocial personality disorder to production of emotional disturbance in the next generation is maximized.

Treatment

The lifelong exploitative and self-defeating interactional patterns of the antisocial person should be brought into the open in the family by exploration of different situations. The collusive defenses of the spouse and the patient should be delineated to allow the antisocial acts to come into light. For example, a wife participates enthusiastically in spending the enormous sums of money brought home by her husband without questioning its source. Exploration of the issue reveals the husband's illegal business just before legal action is taken and the story breaks out in the newspaper.

Antisocial persons can arouse strong countertransference feelings in the therapist to "take him or her on" personally rather than to help the family take an active part and protect themselves against exploitations. It is usually more effective to enhance the family's ability to band together in self-protection against the antisocial person rather than to challenge the antisocial person, which can result in the family siding with the antisocial person and abrupt treatment termination.

Dependent Personality Disorder

Millon (1981) hypothesized that the experiential history of patients with dependent personality disorder consists of narrow sources of stimulation from the environment and a lack of emphasis and training in independent functioning, coupled with parental overprotection. Parents of a dependent person typically restrict ventures outside of the home and do things for the child rather than allow her or him to develop new skills. This hypothesis was confirmed by Head et al.

(1991), who demonstrated in a controlled study that a family environment characterized by low expressiveness and high control would lead to dependent personality disorder. The families of people with dependent personality disorder, in comparison with the families of a normal control group, were characterized by low cohesion, expressiveness, independence, and intellectual-cultural orientation. The family environment lacked intrafamilial support. In addition to a significantly lower level of expressiveness, there was a higher level of control.

The families of individuals with dependent personality disorder were similar to those of a normal control group in terms of achievement orientation and organization. They were similar to the control clinical group by exhibiting low cohesion, low independence, and low intellectual/cultural orientation in the family background. They were characterized by rigid rules governing family life, including a high level of family control and failure to encourage openness in action and expression of feelings. The environment was overprotective by fostering dependence on rigid rules to govern life and discouraging the ability to act and express oneself openly, which interfered with the development of autonomy in the offspring. The person grew up to be uncertain about making important decisions or solving problems without the advice of others and allowed the others to make his or her decisions.

Avoidant Personality Disorder

Avoidant personality disorder represents the exaggeration of the childhood trait of fearfulness. The family exhibits a clear characteristic of parental overprotection by not exposing their offspring to social situations in which they can learn to overcome anxiety. Personality constriction in avoidant personality disorder is usually much more extensive than in dependent personality disorder. People with avoidant personality disorder extract a heavy cost from spouses, children, and other family members. This burden results in weakening family bonds and cohesiveness and avoidance of family and social rituals that are essential to optimal family functioning and development (Wolin and Bennett 1984). People with avoidant personality disorder can also exaggerate pathological personality traits in their spouses and lead to deviant care for their children.

Treatment

People with dependent and avoidant personalities frequently choose partners who enjoy assuming a dominant position as a marital partner, and the couple can function in complementary and successful marital roles under normal circumstances; the dominant partner leads the family affairs and the dependent and avoidant person follows in a relatively cooperative fashion. Family roles are divided with a narrow band of functional overlap. The level of satisfaction of the partner of a dependent person is usually higher than that of the partner of an avoidant person because people with dependent personality disorder show a higher level of cooperation. Spouses or partners of people with avoidant personality disorder have a higher likelihood of feeling burdened by the limitations of the avoidant person and have to assume a higher level of responsibility and burden in family tasks.

Family or individual therapy with persons with dependent or avoidant personality is generally requested only when the burden on the spouse exceeds his or her level of tolerance and he or she feels unfairly constrained by an excessive portion of family tasks. Such couples may also enter family therapy when the developmental progression of their children is arrested or misfortunes affect the family. A person with avoidant personality disorder may enter family therapy due to failure of individual therapy, resulting from family or marital conflict or excessive secondary gain from the disorder.

The following principles can be used in family and couples therapy with dependent and avoidant personality disorders:

1. The pain of the spouse and other family members should be "actualized" (Minuchin 1974) by helping family members to express their feelings openly without fear of making the dependent or avoidant person worse. Broad-based expression of feelings can result in the emergence of a multidimensional and multilateral picture of the family and the enormous cost experienced by all family members. Secondary gain from the disorder then becomes relatively unimportant in comparison to its cost.

2. The model of the "overadequate-inadequate" couple as described by Bowen and others (Bowen 1976; Kerr 2003) is a useful model for exploring the intricacies of personality characteristics of dependent and avoidant persons and their partners. The clarification of the role of each partner and its embeddedness in their family of origin can bring the psychological picture in full view and undermine the adherence of the couple to their costly and dysfunctional marital roles, which limit their marital satisfaction and have detrimental impacts on the development of their children. The assumption of authority and initiative by the therapist to explore

marital and family roles and functions as described in the technique of "funneling through the therapist" (Bowen 1976; Kerr 1986, 2003; Sholevar and Schwoeri 2003d) can reduce the family resistance and enhance empathic listening and the impact of interventions.

3. Family interventions with persons with dependent and avoidant personality can become necessary when the spouse has a physical illness, such as a heart attack, and a realignment in family roles and functions becomes necessary.

Case Example

Ms. S, a 36-year-old married woman and mother of three children, including two teenagers, consulted a family therapist for treatment of multiple and severe "phobias" that had not responded to a wide range of psychotherapies and pharmacotherapy. Her family life had become severely constricted. She could not accompany her husband to his many professional meetings due to fear of flying. Her husband would engage in heavy drinking and smoking in her absence to the point that his health was seriously endangered. The teenage children had to accompany their mother frequently to the local convenience store because she could not tolerate the crowd or waiting in the store. Ms. S would sit in the car with the engine running while the teenage daughters ran in to buy milk and bread. They had to repeat the same routine one or more times on a daily basis to buy other items. The children referred to their mother as an emotional cripple, and her husband treated her as crazy and hopeless. The husband was initially threatened by Ms. S's good looks and enjoyed feeling superior to her due to her disorder. However, he felt increasingly burdened by the cost of her extensive and severe avoidant behavior.

The family exhibited a high level of cooperation and informativeness in the initial sessions, followed by a high level of collective resistance, blaming everything on Ms. S and insisting on the need for individual psychotherapy and medication for her. They had to be reminded of the failure of many previous therapies and the need for a new and broader approach.

The focus of family sessions was to help all family members to express their feelings and recognize the enormity of every family member's pain. The family eventually united when they recognized the extent of the disability that had pervaded everyone's life and kept them socially isolated and emotionally disengaged and unavailable to each other. The impact of parental dysfunction on the development of the children became painfully clear.

The first symptomatic improvement emerged when the husband, a man with a narcissistic character disorder, abruptly ceased smoking followed by parallel reduction in his excessive drinking. He tearfully remembered the sudden death of his alcoholic brother from acute pancreatitis and gastrointestinal bleeding, leaving his young wife to raise two children. The improvement in the husband was followed by an unexpected announcement by Ms. S that she would accompany her husband to Hawaii on short notice.

The teenage children exhibited a fair amount of resistance by exhibiting disruptive behavior when the parents began to assume parental authority. The children's rebellious behavior was addressed in the context of the family.

The following case example (Sholevar 1996, 2000) illustrates the use of couples therapy to recognize and interpret transference reactions of a couple toward each other—marital transference—a phenomenon that had not occurred in the course of simultaneous psychoanalysis of the couple, although each spouse had made considerable gains in personal, professional, and social functioning. Considering the common occurrence of strong transference reaction of many couples to each other, couples therapy can offer a powerful tool for detecting and interpreting marital transference. Strong transference reactions outside of the analytic situation can reduce the development of transference neurosis in the analytic situation and its amenability to interpretation in individual psychoanalytic treatment. The character traits of each spouse can also be better delineated in couples therapy because both partners will report it; the person with character disorder traits may be unaware or reluctant to reveal them. The two-dimensional description of events by the couple can reveal their conscious and unconscious motivations and can disclose the genetic roots of certain character traits.

Case Example

Mr. T and Ms. T entered treatment because Ms. T complained that Mr. T was nonresponsive to her needs and noncommunicative. Mr. T admitted to feelings of social and individual inadequacy on the surface but subtly accused his wife of being demanding and critical. The dissatisfaction had prevailed during their marriage of 23 years. Their sexual relationship had ceased for many years after a long period of unsatisfactory sexual practice. Mr. T felt inadequate because he "came too fast," while implying that Ms. T was hard to arouse. The couple had five children who had done very well educationally.

The couple had completed relatively successful individual psychoanalysis, simultaneously, for 6 years prior to seeking couples therapy. Both analysts felt that the psychoanalytic treatment was successful, but the couple felt less satisfied due to the persistence of marital problems. Mr. T remained aloof and intellectual in his psychoanalytic treatment, and

Ms. T felt that her analyst was cold, detached, and did not respond to her strong and relatively immediate needs for reinforcement.

The couple retained a very submissive and child-like position in relation to their fathers, who were both extremely successful and wealthy businessmen. The image of the couple's mothers remained in the background because they were not a source of conflict for the couple and were a less significant source of parenting. Mr. T's father was perceived as dominating toward Mr. T (and Ms. T), and Ms. T's father was perceived as demeaning and critical of her personality for being self-serving.

The long course of couples therapy focused on the following issues. Ms. T's major conflict was with her father; she felt he did not appreciate her and her many good qualities and was cold and subtly sadistic toward her. She had similar transference feelings toward her husband and her analyst. Mr. T felt put down and undermined by his father as a child and had become skilled in protecting himself from expected attacks by detaching from other people while appearing involved. This detached quality had characterized his relationships in general, had remained relatively unresolved during his psychoanalysis, and had limited his success in marriage and at work.

Marital transference was characterized by the constant attacks by Ms. T on her husband; he, on the other hand, acted oblivious or immune to her attacks. He attempted to appear engaged with Ms. T and the therapist but was covertly disengaged and frustrated. Marital transference of both spouses was further extended and displaced onto the marital therapist.

The therapeutic interventions were

- To delineate the character traits and structure of both spouses: Ample information was provided by each spouse in excess of what was provided in individual therapy;
- To interpret the marital transference and transference to the previous analysts and the marital therapist on different occasions based on which transference reaction was "less heated" and more amenable to interpretation;
- To interpret the hidden and unsatisfactory maternal transference that had remained dormant;
- To interpret the same transference reactions and phenomena, particularly the maternal ones, when they were displayed toward their children and close friends outside of the family.

It was the ability to interpret the transference reactions in multiple domains and levels that allowed for a more satisfactory therapeutic outcome than had been achieved in the analyses of the spouses. The marital relationship became more functional and satisfactory by the resolution of marital transference.

CONCLUSIONS

Healthy and disordered personalities are developed within the context of the family. Personality disorders are likely to develop in individuals at risk, if families are dysfunctional. Vulnerable people proceed to perpetuate psychological dysfunction by exhibiting a propensity to select marital partners who share their interpersonal dysfunctions on conscious and unconscious levels. The likely selection of a partner with a similar or complementary personality or Axis I disorder can lead to interlocking pathological and neurotic marriages (Sholevar and Schwoeri 2003c). This type of family or marital dysfunction is considered a midrange family dysfunction (Beavers 2003). The children reared in such a family environment are at a high risk for developmental, personality, and Axis I disorders.

Family systems theory provides for a systematic framework to obtain multilateral information about individuals with personality disorder and their historical and contemporary living contexts. The organization of the information on systemic and individual bases and their multiple feedback and homeostatic loops can provide for a rich picture, enabling the clinician to intervene effectively by balancing and unbalancing the family and couples' interactions. Psychoanalytically oriented therapists can perceive clearly the unconscious lives of the family members and their dormant intrapsychic contributions.

REFERENCES

Beavers WR: Functional and dysfunctional families, in Textbook of Family and Couples Therapy. Edited by Sholevar GP. Washington, DC, American Psychiatric Publishing, 2003, pp 317–341

Berman E, Lief H, Williams AM: A model of marital interaction, in Handbook of Marriage and Marital Therapy. Edited by Sholevar GP. Elmsford, New York, Pergamon, 1986, pp 3–34

Bowen M: Theory in the practice of psychotherapy, in Family Therapy: Theory and Practice. Edited by Guerin PJ. New York, Gardner, 1976, pp 76–104

Bowen M: Family Therapy in Clinical Practice. New York, Jason Aronson, 1978

Dick HV: Marital Tensions: Clinical Studies Towards a Psychological Theory of Interactions. New York, Basic Books, 1967

Espy J: The character disordered family system. Gestalt Journal 17:93–105, 1994

Feldman R, Zelkowitz P, Weiss M, et al: A comparison of the families of mothers with borderline personality disorder (BPD). Compr Psychiatry 36:157–163, 1995

Forehand R, McMahon R: Helping the Noncompliant Child: A Clinician's Guide to Parent Training. New York, Guilford, 1981a

Forehand R, McMahon RJ: Teaching parents to modify child behavioral problems: an examination of some follow-up data. J Pediatr Psychol 6:313–322, 1981b

Goldstein EG: Borderline Disorders: Clinical Models and Techniques. New York, Guilford, 1990

Gunderson JG: Borderline Personality Disorder. Washington, DC, American Psychiatric Press, 1984

Gunderson J, Lyoo IK: Family problems and relationships for adults with borderline personality disorder. Harv Rev Psychiatry 4:272–278, 1997

Gunderson JG, Kerr J, Englund DW: The families of borderlines: a comparative study. Arch Gen Psychiatry 37:27–33, 1980

Head S, Baker J, Williamson DA: Family characteristics of dependent personality disorder. J Personal Disord 5:256–263, 1991

Herman JL, Perry JC, van der Kolk B: Childhood trauma in borderline personality disorder. Am J Psychiatry 146:490–495, 1989

Johnson A, Szurek SA: The genesis of antisocial acting out in children and adults. Psychoanal Q 21:323–343, 1952

Johnson S: The Practice of Emotionally Focused Marital Therapy: Creating Connection. New York, Brunner/Mazel, 1996

Johnson S: Emotionally Focused Couple Therapy for Trauma Survivors: Strengthening Attachment Bonds. New York, Guilford, 2002

Johnson S, Lebow J: The "coming of age" of couple therapy: a decade review. J Marital Fam Ther 26:23–38, 2000

Kernberg OF: Borderline Conditions and Pathological Narcissism, New York, Jason Aronson, 1975

Kerr M: Multigenerational family systems theory of Bowen, in Textbook of Marriage and Marital Therapy. Edited by Sholevar GP. Elmsford, NY, Pergamon, 1986

Kerr M: Multigenerational family systems theory of Bowen and its application, in The Textbook of Family and Marital Therapy. Edited by Sholevar GP. Washington, DC, American Psychiatric Publishing, 2003, pp 103–126

Kissen M: Affect, Object, and Character Structure. Madison, CT, International University Press, 1995

Kohut H: The Analysis of the Self. New York International Universities Press, 1971

Lachkar J: The Narcissistic/Borderline Couple: A Psychoanalytic Perspective on Marital Treatment. New York, Brunner/Mazel, 1992

Lansky MR (ed): Family Therapy and Major Psychopathology. New York, Grune & Stratton, 1981

Lansky MR: Marital therapy for narcissistic disorders, in Clinical Handbook of Marital Therapy. Edited By Jacobson N, Gurman A. New York, Guilford, 1986

Levy D: Maternal Overprotection. New York, Columbia University Press, 1943

Millon T: Disorders of Personality: DSM-III, Axis II. New York, Wiley, 1981

Minuchin S: Families and Family Therapy. Cambridge, MA, Harvard University Press, 1974

Moos RH, Moos BS: Family Environment Scale. Palo Alto, CA, Consulting Psychologists Press, 1980

Moos RH, Moos BS: Family Environment Scale Manual, 2nd Edition. Palo Alto, CA, Consulting Psychologists Press, 1986

Patterson G: Coercive Family Process: A Social Learning Approach to Family Intervention, Vol 3. Eugene, OR, Castalia Publications, 1982

Ringstrom P: An intersubjective approach to conjoint therapy, in Progress in Self Psychology, Vol 10. Edited by Goldberg A. Hillsdale, NJ, Analytic Press, 1994, pp 159–182

Ringstrom P: Competing self-object functions: the bane of conjoint therapist. Bull Menninger Clin 62:314–325, 1998

Rutter M, Quinton D: Parental psychiatric disorders: effects on children. Psychol Med 14:853–880, 1984

Sager CJ: Marriage Contracts and Couple Therapy. New York, Brunner/Mazel, 1976

Sager CJ: Marital contracts, in Textbook of Marriage and Marital Therapy. Edited by Sholevar GP. Elmsford, NY, Pergamon, 1986, pp 35–76

Schwoeri L, Schwoeri F: Family therapy of borderline patients: diagnostic and treatment issues. International Journal of Family Psychiatry 2:237–250, 1981

Schwoeri L, Schwoeri F: Interactional and intrapsychic dynamics in a family with a borderline patient. Psychotherapy: Theory, Research, and Practice 19:198–204, 1982

Shane M, Shane E: Self psychology after Kohut: one theory or many? J Am Psychoanal Assoc 41:777–797, 1993

Shapiro R: Psychodynamic approaches to family therapy, in Treatment of Emotional Disorders in Children and Adolescents. Edited by Sholevar GP. Elmsford, NY, Pergamon, 1986

Sholevar GP: Psychoanalytic marital therapy: a case presentation. Grand Rounds, Robert Wood Johnson Medical School, University of Medicine and Dentistry–New Jersey, Camden, NJ, 1996

Sholevar GP: "Affect as process" and affect, object and character structure: an essay review. Int J Psychoanal 78:1239–1245, 1997

Sholevar GP: Marital therapy with character disorders. Presented at the meeting of Philadelphia Psychoanalytic Society and Association. Philadelphia, PA, February 2000

Sholevar GP, Schwoeri LD: Family therapy with incest, in Textbook of Family and Couples Therapy. Edited by Sholevar GP. Washington, DC, American Psychiatric Publishing, 2003a, pp 695–715

Sholevar GP, Schwoeri LD: Family therapy with personality disorders, in Textbook of Family and Couples Therapy. Edited by Sholevar GP. Washington, DC, American Psychiatric Publishing, 2003b, pp 715–723

Sholevar GP, Schwoeri LD: Psychodynamic family therapy, in Textbook of Family and Couples Therapy. Edited by Sholevar GP. Washington, DC, American Psychiatric Publishing, 2003c, pp 77–102

Sholevar GP, Schwoeri LD: Techniques of family therapy, in Textbook of Family and Couples Therapy. Edited by Sholevar GP. Washington, DC, American Psychiatric Publishing, 2003d, pp 225–250

Sonne JC, Swirsky D: Self-object considerations in marriage and martial therapy, in Handbook of Marriage and Marital Therapy. Edited by Sholevar GP. Elmsford, NY, Pergamon, 1986, pp 77–102

Stone MH: The Fate of Borderline Patients: Successful Outcome and Psychiatric Practice. New York, Guilford, 1990

Villenueve C, Roux N: Family therapy and some personality disorders in adolescence, in Adolescent Psychiatry, Vol 20. Edited by Marohn RC, Feinstein SC. New York, Jason Aronson, 1995, pp 365–380

Wolin S, Bennett L: Family rituals. Fam Process 23:401–420, 1984

Zanarini MC, Frankenburg FR: Emotional hypochondriasis, hyperbole, and the borderline patient. J Psychother Pract Res 3:25–36, 1994

Zanarini MC, Frankenburg FR: Pathways to the development borderline personality disorder. J Personal Disord 11:93–104, 1997

Zinner J: The implications of projective identification, in Contemporary Marriage for Marital Interaction in Structure, Dynamics and Therapy. Edited by Grunebaum H, Christ J. Boston, MA, Little, Brown, 1976, pp 293–308

24

Psychoeducation

Perry D. Hoffman, Ph.D.
Alan E. Fruzzetti, Ph.D.

Psychoeducation is a mode of intervention that has become a well-established treatment component for a considerable number of psychiatric disorders. It is particularly prevalent with Axis I disorders, such as schizophrenia and bipolar disorder, for which it has demonstrated benefits for patients and their families and has a low cost of delivery. However, despite the established efficacy of psychoeducation in the treatment of Axis I disorders, few psychoeducation programs for personality disorders have been developed.

The rationale for the development of the psychoeducation modality was based on the hypotheses that 1) an educational approach can be of benefit to people in their efforts to manage a particular illness and 2) a psychoeducation model can be directed toward the individual patient, her or his family member(s), or both. However, despite the increasing popularity of the concept and term *psychoeducation*, it lacks consistent definition. For example, in a literature review on psychoeducation and personality disorders, 11 journal and book articles were identified as having "psychoeducation" as their central topic. Most of these references, however, were not directed to any specific psychoeducation program but typically reiterated the importance of psychoeducation in treatment. In fact, in

many of the articles that use the term, psychoeducation appears to be interchangeable with education, and this latter word is perhaps the more appropriate term to define the treatment being suggested. In practice, the use of the term *psychoeducation* is varied.

So what *is* psychoeducation? One definition would posit it as a heterogeneous set of interventions that includes a range of approaches. However, when employed comprehensively, psychoeducation is a modality of treatment that provides 1) patient and/or family education, 2) coping skills, 3) family skills, and 4) training in problem-solving techniques. A set of guidelines for recovery and maintenance is sometimes offered as well. The focus of the components is to help patients and/or family members engage in behaviors that have been shown either to augment other treatment components to improve patient outcomes or to more generally facilitate patient and family well-being.

Psychoeducation is different from other multimodal treatments in that its primary focus is on education—information/facts and skill building. Unlike other interventions, a focus on family dynamics is not central. Rather, the ultimate goals of the modality are to increase coping abilities and promote behavioral change. As already noted, although the mode of psychoeducation is frequently employed with medical, developmental, or psychiatric disorders, psychoeducation as a meaningful aspect of treatment with personality disorders is still in its infancy. However, although research is limited, the existing data and clinical experience indicate that psychoeducation offers a viable and effective component in the treatment of specific aspects of personality disorders.

The purposes, therefore, of this chapter are to define and describe the range of psychoeducation programs, outline the different types of psychoeducation that have some bearing on personality disorders specifically, and review data that are relevant to the further development and implementation of psychoeducation with personality disorders. We begin by briefly reviewing the work done in the area of psychoeducation and schizophrenia. This review provides a brief overview of the relevant history and begins to explicate the prototypic paradigm that has served as the general model for psychoeducation across all psychiatric disorders.

THEORY AND RATIONALE

Historical Development

Over the past three-plus decades, there has been a major effort to develop and implement comprehensive, multicomponent treatment programs for those affected by mental illness either directly or indirectly. A major focus has been on programs for patients and their families. Several factors are the impetus for this focus.

Deinstitutionalization in the 1960s shifted the burden of care of those with severe and chronic disorders from institutional facilities to family settings. When the mandate to reduce the numbers of patients in institutions was effected, the rider to offer comprehensive outpatient services did not sufficiently materialize. Consequently, most individuals with psychiatric illnesses were returned to live in the community with their family members even though minimal outpatient ancillary psychiatric services were available.

Research on one psychosocial predictor of relapse, expressed emotion, documented that with certain psychiatric illnesses specific characteristics of the family environment were correlated with patient outcome (Anderson et al. 1980). Expressed emotion ratings, as assessed in the Camberwell Family Interview, a semi-structured audiotaped interview, indicated the number of critical comments and levels of hostility and emotional overinvolvement that family members ex-

pressed about their ill relatives. Research on most diagnoses has consistently demonstrated that modification of family attributes and behaviors, in particular certain family member attitudes and other behaviors associated with beliefs expressed about the patient, resulted in reduction of relapse rates.

Research on schizophrenia shifted the hypotheses of etiology from subjective and empirically unsupported observations (e.g., the "schizophrenogenic mother" as a causality factor) to more evidence-based factors based on medical/biological and social/family science. This critical change in the understanding of the etiology of schizophrenia also gave rise to an appreciation of the needs and experiences of family members. Constructs such as family member burden, grief, and depression were recognized (Greenberg et al. 1993; Maurin and Boyd 1990; Schene 1990), with a consequent change in perception of relatives from the strictly pathological model of family members as "patients" to family members as potential "providers" (Marsh 1992).

In the 1970s, psychoeducation programs for family members with a relative with schizophrenia were implemented, and the family treatment modality called *family psychoeducation* (a term apparently first used in print by Anderson et al. [1980]) began to be established. A substantial (and increasing) body of empirical research supports this treatment modality as perhaps the most successful family treatment component for schizophrenia (Falloon et al. 1984, 1985; Hogarty et al. 1986; Leff et al. 1982; McFarlane 1995, 2003). Subsequently, this family psychoeducation model has been adopted and adapted for other diagnoses, such as bipolar disorder (Miklowitz et al. 2003) and major depression (Anderson and Holder 1989; Keitner et al. 2003). The modality of family psychoeducation has been shown consistently to reduce relapse rates (Lam 1991), and family member levels of stress and feelings of burden have been shown to be significantly reduced (Cuijpers 1999).

Family Psychoeducation: Components and Definitions

Comprehensive patient psychoeducation and family psychoeducation models may include several key components or intervention targets: 1) educating patients and family members about a particular disorder and its etiologic factors, research findings, factors that ameliorate or exacerbate symptoms or severity, treatment options and expected outcomes, and community resources; 2) teaching coping skills and individual and family well-being skills to manage the disorder and its effects and minimize disability and maximize functioning; 3) offering a problem-solving forum in which participants learn to translate the knowledge and skills into changed attitudes, emotional reactions, and social behaviors toward the patients or other family members; and 4) providing ongoing support to the patient and to family members.

Not all programs that are designated "psychoeducation" or "family psychoeducation" include all four components listed above. Some programs have been developed for patients only and some for patients and family members, whereas others are directed just to family members of patients. In addition, there is abundant literature on skills training programs for both patients and families, and often these programs include one or more of the other components or targets. Such skills training programs, however, are rarely designated as "psychoeducation." Thus, the inconsistency of terms employed in labeling programs makes it difficult to evaluate psychoeducation objectively and comprehensively.

We now explore each of these four components to try to establish the "core" targets and approaches that allow for a less amorphous definition of psychoeducation.

Education

The educational component is predicated on the assumptions that "knowledge is power" and that offering information to families about their relative's disorder is helpful to them and, in turn, to the patient. Participants are given the most current information on etiology, treatment options, medications and pharmacological issues, and research findings. Issues regarding early trauma and environmental influences, developments in medications, and implications of research findings are usually of particular interest to participants. However, knowledge alone does not seem to suffice to improve outcomes (Hoffman et al. 2003; Posner et al. 1992); the educational facet of the program requires the additional and complementary component of skill acquisition.

Providing education to patients and family members presents many challenges clinically. For example, it is not uncommon for parents, partners, or children of patients with personality disorders to have various Axis I and Axis II disorders themselves. Consequently, although one member of the family may be designated as the patient, others in the family could benefit from skill building treatment as well. Although challenging, this program affords the clinician an opportunity to help other individuals consider behavioral change and to intervene directly into the family system (or refer to family therapy) to help the entire family. On occasion, family members may be so impaired themselves that enlisting them in a program primarily designed to help another family member may be impossible, but in our experience, even moderately impaired family members can benefit from psychoeducation. However, depending on their capacity for cooperative exchange, they may or may not be appropriate for group psychoeducation programs.

When discussing the etiology of personality disorders, it may at first glance seem callous or counterproductive to describe the putative role of family interactions because this information may lead to defensiveness in the parents of a patient. However, if done in a nonblaming way, family members may not become defensive at all; rather, they may identify factors in their own development that help them understand their own struggles, which in turn may help them blame the patient less. Thus, it is imperative that whoever leads the psychoeducation interventions has and promotes a well-grounded nonjudgmental perspective.

Family members bring varied levels of information. Accurate general knowledge about borderline personality disorder (BPD) is quite poor (Hoffman et al. 2003). The Internet is a frequent source of information, and it includes much that is contradictory. For example, resources range from patient sites that include a lot of vitriolic accusations toward parents to other sites for "caregivers" that complain bitterly and judgmentally about individuals with BPD. Consequently, many family members alternate between anger/defensiveness (being told that parents of those with BPD are always "abusers") and fear/guilt. It is important for clinicians to point out the variety of outcomes and causes associated with personality disorders.

Finally, it is crucially important to stress that we do not really know very much about specific etiologic pathways for any personality disorder. Thoughtful professionals may reasonably interpret myriad studies in a variety of ways. What is clear is the heterogeneity of factors, including family interaction and family functioning, which may be found in the developmental histories of our patients. Thus, being physically or sexually abused may be a risk factor for several personality disorders, yet the vast majority of survivors of physical and sexual abuse do not develop personality disorders. Similarly, having loving, attentive parents who do not have substance abuse or other mental health problems is a protective factor for most people. Yet some people with severe personality disorders have parents who fit this description. The current focus in the child development literature on transactional models (ongoing, reciprocal influence between individual psychological and biological factors and responses from parents and other caregivers) holds promise for more elucidation in the near future (Cummings et al. 2000; Eisenberg et al. 2003). However, at this time we can only speculate on the causes of any given case and must consider the impact of our hypotheses on patients and family members and their abilities to love and support each other, without blame, in the future. The best data we have suggest that current family functioning factors are very relevant to both short- and long-term patient outcomes.

Skills Training

Skills training enjoys abundant empirical proof as an effective program component in helping patients and family members. Patient skills training may include social skills, problem solving, assertion training, stress management, anger management, and relaxation techniques (O'Donohue and Krasner 1995). Family skills include communication (accurate expression, validation), parenting, collaborative problem solving, and other relationship and interpersonal skills (Fruzzetti AE, "Brief DBT Family Interventions to Augment Patient Outcomes," April 2004). However, skill acquisition is only one piece of effective skills training: skill application and skill generalization are also necessary components to help ensure skill transfer into daily life. In-session exercises may be introduced to implement the newly taught skill. Some programs, in addition, require weekly practice assignments for which tasks are completed outside of the group and then reviewed in the subsequent meeting.

For example, just about every adult "knows" that good communication involves accurate expression and accurate listening. However, most participants in psychoeducation do not distinguish between "description" and "blaming" when thinking about "accurate" expression. Family members often say things such as "Well, it is accurate to say he's lazy." Thus, it may take a lot of practice transforming the "knowledge" into effective practice (e.g., "I see him sitting around all day, and I know he's depressed; it makes me unhappy to see him this way, and sometimes I feel overwhelmed and frustrated, even resentful, that I do almost all the chores around the house").

Social Support

In addition to education and skill acquisition, family psychoeducation provides an opportunity for the development of an alliance and partnership among professional and family care providers and collaboration with the pa-

tient her- or himself. Such alliances and partnerships allow the possibility of greater continuity and consistency of care. Also, highly valued is the support system that develops among the participants (Hoffman et al. 1999). Group affiliation promotes a network among members who share similar struggles and experiences and who, all too often, feel isolated from friends and even other family members. These commonalities create mutual bonds of understanding and support that are seldom experienced in other life settings.

Family members and patients bring a lot of practical expertise to group psychoeducation because they often have learned how to cope with, or how to solve, certain problems with which other families currently struggle. Consequently, family members and patients can often provide not only specific suggestions for handling a situation but also the social and emotional support needed to implement a solution.

Problem Solving/Integrating Knowledge and Skills Into Changed Behaviors

The problem-solving component may be the one least consistently found in psychoeducation programs. It is also the closest to cognitive-behavioral family/group therapy. Specific problems as experienced by participants are brought to the group with the explicit purpose of having the group collectively work to apply their newly acquired skills and with the goal of effectively resolving or managing the given situation. A structured behavioral protocol is typically available. Such written protocols include guidelines that offer specific behavioral practices for participants to follow, with the objective that all individuals will recognize and accept the need for change.

The focus toward the end of a psychoeducation program on problem solving provides patients and families opportunities to put whole skill sets together to ameliorate current problems that could easily become crises. The ability to have seen good skills modeled by other members of the group (or group leaders), to have learned both individual coping skills and good relationship/family skills, and to have received support from peers all provide the ability and motivation to try new approaches or behaviors.

Despite the appealing rationale of these intervention components, and considerable positive data with Axis I disorders, again we must stress that application to personality disorders is nascent, and much research remains to be done.

We now turn to the programs currently available specifically for personality disorders.

PSYCHOEDUCATION FOR PERSONALITY DISORDERS

Although psychoeducation programs have not been developed for most personality disorders, there are several programs for BPD, and they will be reviewed in some detail. Perhaps because of its prevalence in clinical populations, BPD is better represented in the personality disorder literature compared with other Axis II diagnoses. Thus, perhaps there is some correspondence between this relative focus on BPD and the subsequent development of programs for the disorder. In addition, programs have been developed for avoidant personality disorder, and the several types of programs for domestic violence at least overlap the issues pertaining to antisocial personality disorder (ASPD; Dutton 1998; Fruzzetti and Levensky 2000), which is highlighted later.

Psychoeducation for Cluster A Disorders

No patient or family psychoeducation programs have been established for patients or their families with Cluster A diagnoses, but there are many successful programs for related Axis I disorders. Although the potential utility is obvious, and there are no data to contraindicate psychoeducation programs for any personality disorder, it is surprising that researchers have not adapted those programs for use with Axis II/ Cluster A problems.

Psychoeducation for Avoidant Personality Disorder

Avoidant personality disorder has several behavioral and theoretical connections to Axis I disorders. Although there is some evidence that it can be reliably discriminated from social phobias and schizoid personality disorder (Trull et al. 1987; Turner et al. 1986), the distinction between these Axis I and Axis II problems is often blurred. For example, several studies have shown positive outcomes using psychoeducation and graduated exposure techniques, which are the standard psychological interventions used in treating the related Axis I disorders. In one study employing social skills training and patient psychoeducation, Alden (1989) found significant improvement in most domains, and those treatment gains were maintained at follow-up 3 months later. Because these studies aggregate various interventions (psychoeducation plus other interventions), it is difficult to isolate the effect of psychoeducation per se.

Psychoeducation for Antisocial Personality Disorder

No studies have specifically evaluated psychoeducation for ASPD, although many studies have evaluated various psychoeducation and skills training programs for anger, aggression, or violent behaviors—symptoms that overlap to some extent with ASPD. The extent of this overlap is not clear, however, and the effectiveness of these treatments in reducing violence recidivism is controversial (Fruzzetti and Levensky 2000).

Although only a minority of men who batter their partners meet criteria for ASPD or other personality disorders, and only a minority of ASPD men batter (Dutton 1998), there has been a lot of research on treating male batterers. Thus, although it is not clear the extent to which these data generalize to ASPD in general, understanding the treatments may be instructive nevertheless.

Most batterer treatment programs utilize psychoeducation and cognitive-behavioral interventions. A typical curriculum includes instruction in anger management and violence interruption skills (e.g., anger recognition, time-out, self-talk, and relaxation), sex-role education, sex-role resocialization, and discussions of patriarchal and male power issues. Programs often include training in skills to improve relationship functioning, such as communication and conflict resolution skills, social skills, and assertion skills (Holtzworth-Munroe et al. 1995).

Dialectical behavior therapy (DBT), developed by Linehan and colleagues (1993a, 1993b), has recently begun to be applied to batterers (Fruzzetti and Levensky 2000) and to mixed ASPD/BPD inpatients in forensic settings (McCann et al. 2000). McCann and colleagues (2000) have shown promising results applying DBT, including reduced critical incidents, reduced aggression, and lower provider burnout.

Patient Psychoeducation for Borderline Personality Disorder

Although no isolated psychoeducation program for BPD patients has been shown to be effective, one treatment does have a substantial patient psychoeducation component: DBT (Linehan 1993a, 1993b). In more than a dozen controlled studies, DBT has been shown to be an effective treatment for BPD and its associated problems (e.g., parasuicide, substance abuse, eating disorders, anger, social adjustment, hospitalization; Bohus et al. 2000; Koons et al. 2001; Linehan et al. 1991; Turner 2000; Verheul et al. 2003). Successful outcomes have been demonstrated with borderline clients with severe substance abuse (Linehan et al. 1999), older patients with refractory depression (Lynch et al. 2002), adolescents with significant BPD features and high levels of suicidality (Rathus and Miller 2002), and adolescents remanded to the criminal justice system (Trupin et al. 2002). Although there have been no published studies that controlled specifically for follow-up treatment (e.g., randomized patients to no treatment, uncontrolled treatment, and specific follow-up treatment conditions after a fixed length of treatment), gains made during the treatment phase seem to be maintained during naturalistic follow-ups (Linehan et al. 1993; Verheul et al. 2003). Interestingly, the one study that looked at the use of DBT skills separately (Linehan et al. 1991) showed no benefit to adding skills training to treatment as usual, apparently because the modes of treatment (e.g., individual psychotherapy) are needed to highlight and reinforce the psychoeducation principles and psychological skills taught in the DBT skills training group.

DBT patient psychoeducation and skills training include four separate modules that have specific targets: 1) mindfulness, to increase attention control and awareness of self and others, decrease sense of emptiness, and reduce cognitive dysregulation; 2) emotion regulation, to understand the role of emotions in life, identify and label emotions accurately, reduce vulnerability and suffering associated with negative emotion, and tolerate and/or change negative emotions; 3) distress tolerance, to interrupt crises, counterbalance impulsiveness, and facilitate tolerating emotions and situations without engaging in dysfunctional behaviors that exacerbate the situation or negative emotion; and 4) interpersonal effectiveness, to achieve interpersonal objectives without damaging the relationship or the person's self-respect. In DBT these skills are typically taught in a group format, and patients also receive individual therapy in which the skills are reviewed, reinforced, and used as solutions to current treatment targets.

Family Psychoeducation for Borderline Personality Disorder

Family psychoeducation programs for BPD include 1) psychoeducational multifamily therapy groups (Gunderson and Berkowitz 2002); 2) DBT–family skills training groups (DBT-FST; Hoffman et al. 1999); 3) DBT with adolescents, designed by Alec Miller and colleagues (Rathus and Miller 2002); 4) DBT family skills groups for couples or for parents (Fruzzetti AE, "Brief DBT Family Interventions," April 2004; Fruzzetti and

Fruzzetti 2003); 5) systems training for emotional predictability and problem solving (Systems Training for Emotional Predictability and Problem Solving [STEPPS]; Blum et al. 2002); and 6) family connections (FC; Hoffman et al. 2004), a family education program for family members of persons with BPD. Each of these programs is discussed further below.

All family psychoeducation programs stress that involvement of families is central to patient outcomes and well-being. The research on BPD and the unique expressed emotion finding of Hooley and Hoffman (1999) very much support this concept. The results most pertinent from this study document that for BPD, contrary to all other diagnoses, the higher the family member's level of emotional overinvolvement, the better the patient did at 1-year outcome. Unlike with other mental illnesses where emotional overinvolvement is typically perceived as a pejorative characteristic and targeted for change, emotional overinvolvement with BPD patients seems to represent a positive attribute for the ill relative. The feelings and behaviors expressed by the family member are hypothesized by Hooley and Hoffman to perhaps be experienced as ones of caring and concern. Thus, removing the negative connotation of "over" in *over*involvement, which is misleading for the BPD population, these expressed emotion data well support the rationale for family member involvement in psychoeducation programs as a treatment component for BPD. Each one of the six interventions outlined in the following sections promotes family involvement and has as a central goal to educate family members on effective ways of being emotionally involved.

Multifamily Group Therapy

Gunderson and his colleagues at McLean Hospital in Belmont, Massachusetts, have been conducting family groups since the mid-1990s (Gunderson 2001). The format and structure, with additions and modifications specifically adapted to the needs of the BPD population, are based on the programs for schizophrenia pioneered and evaluated by William McFarlane. Gunderson's treatment follows McFarlane's three-phase format, which includes 1) joining, 2) half-day psychoeducation workshops, and 3) biweekly multifamily group meetings.

In the joining phase, the relatives from one family meet alone with the leaders, whose primary goal is to create an alliance and connection with the relatives. Information on the diagnosis of BPD is provided, and information and history of the family members' experiences and perspectives on their relative's difficulties are shared. Acknowledgment of the family members' anger and angst is crucial—allowing for the open expression of feelings, both positive and negative, and concerns. Although there is no time limit on this phase of the treatment, participants nearing completion of this joining phase are asked to commit, in general, to a 4-month period for the remainder of the modality.

The second phase in the psychoeducation multifamily group therapy format is the half-day psychoeducation workshop, in which participants are taught about BPD and offered an annotated list of guidelines with coping strategies. This component of the program is conducted with several families at one time and offers participants the experience of hearing from and sharing with others in similar situations. Families are given the opportunity to discuss *Family Guidelines*, a booklet that includes recommendations on a variety of important issues such as the "temperature" of the family environment, managing crisis, addressing problems, and limit setting (Gunderson and Berkowitz 2002).

The final and lengthiest phase of this modality is the multifamily group, in which families meet every other week for 90 minutes. This mode, which runs for approximately 1 year, includes an average of six families and focuses primarily on problem solving. Although the individual diagnosed with BPD is invited to participate, it is reported that typically few choose to do so and patient attendance is reported to be poor (Gunderson 2001).

Data available on this intervention show that 66.7% of family members reported decreased burden as well as an increased ability to modulate angry feelings. One hundred percent of participants felt supported by the group and indicated an improvement in communication with their family member. Seventy-five percent reported that the communication improvement was "great" (Gunderson 2001).

Dialectical Behavior Therapy–Family Skills Training

Hoffman and colleagues have designed DBT-FST, a manualized psychoeducation family treatment for BPD (Hoffman PD, "Dialectical Behavior Therapy–Family Skills Training [DBT-FST]," unpublished treatment manual, White Plains, NY, New York Presbyterian Hospital, January 1994). Based on Linehan's DBT (Linehan 1993a), the treatment is primarily based on acceptance and change strategies and includes both the DBT client and his or her family members. DBT-FST was intentionally created to offer participants an opportunity to learn about the disorder and to develop self and relationship skills with the ultimate goal of enhancing both individual and relationship needs. This treatment incorporates several of the structures of standard DBT, such as skill acquisition and skill generalization, directly into the family program. Skill attainment is through skill lecture and skill rehearsal, and skill generalization is promoted through problem-solving discussion and practice among family and group members.

DBT-FST adds another element called "structuring the environment," a component that offers a forum to put skill acquisition and skill generalization practice directly into the family environment. Whereas standard DBT has "coaching" to assist clients with an immediate environmental stressor, the family modality works from a broader base, coaching multiple players at the same time. The family forum, therefore, provides everyone the chance for self and relationship change both emotionally and behaviorally. All of this occurs in the context of a no-blame and nonjudgmental setting. Because the goal of DBT-FST is for mutual benefit to both client and relative, the dialectical target is a synthesis that balances the needs of both.

There are four primary goals of DBT-FST. The first goal is to educate family participants on two central aspects of BPD: 1) its definitions and presenting problems, and 2) the etiologic theory of BPD on which DBT is based. The second goal is to teach a new language of communication based on the DBT skills. Relatives and clients readily acknowledge a lack of commonality in words and terminology in their communications, so providing a common set of structures and labels is very useful. The third goal is to promote an attitude that is nonjudgmental. Frequently, there are family patterns of accusations and finger pointing. High-stress families such as those that attend DBT-FST are typically quicker to assess fault and blame toward each other than in other relationships in their lives. The fourth goal is to provide a safe forum where discussions and problem solving on family issues may occur so that new communication patterns are established and a new repertoire for problem solving is developed.

Experience has shown that the issues surrounding etiology and, in particular, the role of the environment are difficult for both family members and clients to discuss. However, a dialectical dialogue is particularly crucial for the well-being of each individual and of the relationship. The following excerpt, taken from the DBT-FST manual (Hoffman PD, "Dialectical Behavior Therapy–Family Skills Training," 1994), demonstrates the frame that has been used for this topic:

Why does a person develop the disorder? Considerable research has been done to understand how these problems evolve. There are several theories as to why, maybe, and we emphasize maybe, someone develops borderline personality disorder. Most theorists agree that there is a constitutional or biological predisposition to the disorder. What this specific predisposition is, however, remains unknown. Unlike schizophrenia and depression where researchers identified a problem with certain brain receptors, BPD research is still in its infancy in this area. Three factors, however, seem to occur consistently in BPD: 1) emotion dysregulation, 2) environmental factors, and 3) the transaction between the two. This transaction is called the biosocial theory.

The second component of the biosocial theory is the individual's experience of his or her environment. As was already identified, there is a biological factor that probably lays the foundation for the disorder, which is a high emotional sensitivity. Experiences are felt more intensely and the outside world is often experienced, seen, or felt as an unsafe place. In addition to this biological factor, there is also a social factor. There is something in the environment that plays a role in the development of these problems. That unknown something can range from extremes such as sexual or physical abuse, to other environmental factors that may seem insignificant or trivial— and to that another person without emotional vulnerability, they probably are. To put it in a more general way, the environment somehow became a mismatch with the child and his or her temperament. The environment could not meet the child's needs. Another way to think of this interaction is as a "goodness of fit" or "poorness of fit" between the child and the environment and in this case an incompatibility exists. Again, it is important to note that we are talking about this incompatibility from varying degrees; at the extreme end of the spectrum is the child who was sexually and physically abused, or at the other end is where the parent could not understand the child's needs or read the cues of the child. (pp. 15–16)

Although typically the family members who attend and participate in groups such as DBT-FST are not ones who have sexually abused their child, it is also important not to minimize those clients who have been abused by other relatives or nonfamilial persons. This presentation of abuse and the concept of an incompatibility in the parenting/family relationship have been generally well received and allow for validation and support of the experiences of both the clients and the family members.

Dialectical Behavior Therapy With Adolescents

DBT with adolescents, designed by Miller and colleagues (Miller 1999; Rathus and Miller 2002), is a multifamily group skills program for suicidal adolescent patients with BPD features and their families. This 16-week program includes both patients and family members and puts parents (or another adult in the patient's life) in the role of "skills coach" to facilitate the patient's mastering of DBT skills (Linehan 1993b). This treatment program (multifamily skills group plus individual DBT therapy for the adolescent patient) has been shown to be successful in reducing suicidality, hospitalizations, and depression while increasing treatment retention and global adjustment (Rathus and Miller 2002). However, no component analysis studies have attempted to determine the impact of the family psychoeducation component per se.

Dialectical Behavior Therapy Family Skills Groups

DBT family skills groups are a result of the work of Fruzzetti and colleagues (Fruzzetti and Fruzzetti 2003). It includes education materials and skill modules for families, with specific psychoeducation/skill programs and parenting psychoeducation/skill programs for couples, designed for families affected by BPD.

Couples.   Couple skills groups include the patient and her or his partner or spouse. This program in couple psychoeducation includes reducing dysfunctional interactions (especially those related in any way to individual target behaviors such as parasuicide, aggression, or substance abuse); understanding and improving couple communication (accurate expression and validation); and improving couple interaction patterns, problem management, and closeness and intimacy. Skills are taught in each of these areas and have been introduced in single-family formats (Fruzzetti AE, "Brief DBT Family Interventions," April 2004; Fruzzetti and Fruzzetti 2003) and in couple groups (Mosco and Fruzzetti 2003). These programs have demonstrated significant reductions in individual distress and depression for partners and significant improvements in validation and relationship satisfaction (Mosco and Fruzzetti 2003). Some evidence also suggests that these interventions may augment individual DBT treatment (Fruzzetti AE, "Brief DBT Family Interventions," April 2004). However, because no studies to date have employed comparison groups, caution must be used in interpreting these results.

Parents.   Groups for parents whose adolescent children have BPD (or significant BPD features) have recently been developed. Sometimes, of course, these groups include parents who are themselves BPD patients. The goals of these groups include education about parent and adolescent roles, effective self-management practices, and effective parenting practices (Fruzzetti AE, "Family Skill Training," unpublished treatment manual, Reno, NV, University of Nevada,

July 2002). This particular group is challenging both because of the inherent fear that parents of suicidal adolescents have and because many of these parents are themselves very distressed and lacking in skills. Thus, the dialectic of "taking care of yourself is taking care of your children; and taking care of your children is taking care of yourself" is embraced wholeheartedly. The basic idea is for parents to learn many of the same skills that their kids need—to manage their emotions and themselves, in addition to learning good parenting skills (e.g., limit setting, positive attention, listening and validation, fostering independence). Although preliminary data are promising for this multilevel intervention program, DBT parenting groups are currently being evaluated for their effectiveness.

Systems Training for Emotional Predictability and Problem Solving

Blum and colleagues (2002), researchers at the University of Iowa, have developed STEPPS, a program for patients and families that focuses on psychoeducation (Blum et al. 2002). STEPPS is a two-phase treatment that includes a 20-week basic skills group and a 1-year biweekly advanced program. It is formulated on two modalities: 1) cognitive-behavioral training and skills training and 2) a systems component that encompasses the patient's environment and the individuals that compose that environment. The patient system includes anyone with whom the patient has regular contact and who is deemed important to educate about the disorder. Family and significant others become an integral part of the treatment and are encouraged to attend education and skill sessions to learn ways to support the patient's treatment and to reinforce her or his newly acquired skills. The patient assumes the role of co-teacher to inform people important to them on the disorder and also to educate them on skills that are helpful to manage one's emotions more effectively. A preliminary study suggests that participation in STEPPS is associated with a moderate decrease in negative moods and impulsive behaviors (Blum et al. 2002).

Although family psychoeducation developed to improve patient outcomes has been highly valued, family advocacy groups have stated their concerns that the needs of family members beyond those related to improved patient outcomes are not always fully addressed within this modality. Some dissatisfaction, in part, was due to the expressed emotion rationale for family psychoeducation programs and its potential implication of "blaming the family." Another concern focused on the time requirements of some traditional psychoeducation programs, which require at least 9 months of weekly or biweekly participation. To overcome such concerns, another type of family psychoeducation, family education, has been developed (Solomon 1996). The primary focus of family education is on the needs of the family members. The modality is not based on the medical model that stressed family pathology; rather, this variant of psychoeducation draws on stress, coping, and support models and is directed to the needs of the nondiagnosed family member(s). Targets for change include the family member's well-being (e.g., levels of distress, burden, grief, and mastery).

Family Connections

FC, a family education program, is a variant of DBT-FST that includes only family members and not patients. We developed FC to provide all four functions of psychoeducation: education/knowledge, coping and family skills, social support, and problem solving. The groups are co-led by trained family members who volunteer their time in a mentoring capacity. FC is a 12-week multifamily group program that follows a standardized manual. The course content, adapted in consultation with family members and consumers, was taken from an existing curriculum used by several clinician/researchers over the past decade (Fruzzetti AE, "Brief DBT Family Interventions," April 2004; Hoffman et al. 1999). FC provides participants information and research, teaches skills to improve well-being, and offers an opportunity for attendees to acquire tools to help manage their own emotional states more effectively (Hoffman et al. 2003, in press). Using information and education modules as building blocks, the course centers on skill acquisition and skill application. Additionally, because families of persons with BPD typically express feelings of isolation and aloneness, FC provides the opportunity for them to work together as a group on skill building, to share experiences and hear that others are going through similar situations, and to develop a support network. In data to date, the participants have reported a sense of support and connection and a reduction in isolation (Hoffman et al., in press).

The goals of FC are 1) to reduce family member grief, 2) to lessen family member burden, 3) to lower family member levels of depression, and 4) to increase family empowerment. Data from an evaluation of FC documented a reduction in subjective and objective burden, relationship and role burden, and grief, along with an increase in family member level of empowerment (Hoffman et al. 2003). Changes were maintained at 3-month follow-up.

CONCLUSIONS

There are several well-established and empirically supported applications of psychoeducation for personality disorders in general and for BPD in particular (Hoffman and Fruzzetti in press). However, few examples reported in the literature demonstrate the specific effects of psychoeducation on patient outcomes. In contrast, good effects have been shown in programs using psychoeducation as part of a treatment package for BPD (e.g., DBT, STEPPS), and good outcomes have been shown for using family psychoeducation to improve family functioning and/or the well-being of nonpatient family members. Clearly, more research is needed to develop and apply psychoeducation to the variety of personality disorders currently under study and to understand the relative importance of psychoeducation to improve patient outcomes across all personality disorders.

REFERENCES

Alden L: Short-term structured treatment for avoidant personality disorder. J Consult Clin Psychol 57:756–764, 1989

Anderson CM, Holder DP: Family systems and behavioral disorders: schizophrenia, depression, and alcoholism, in Family Systems in Medicine. Edited by Ramsey CM. New York, Guilford, 1989

Anderson CM, Hogarty GE, Reiss DJ: Family treatment of adult schizophrenic patients: a psycho-educational approach. Schizophr Bull 6:490–505, 1980

Blum N, Pfohl B, John DS, et al: STEPPS: a cognitive-behavioral systems-based group treatment for outpatients with borderline personality disorder—a preliminary report. Compr Psychiatry 43:301–310, 2002

Bohus M, Haaf B, Stiglmayr C, et al: Evaluation of inpatient dialectical-behavioral therapy for borderline personality disorder: a prospective study. Behav Res Ther 38:875–887

Cuijpers P: The effects of family interventions on relatives' burden: a meta-analysis. Journal of Mental Health–U.K. 8:275–285, 1999

Cummings EM, Davies PT, Campbell SB: Developmental Psychopathology and Family Process: Theory, Research, and Clinical Implications. New York, Guilford, 2000

Dutton DG: The Abusive Personality: Violence and Control in Intimate Relationships. New York, Guilford, 1998

Eisenberg N, Valiente C, Morris AS, et al: Longitudinal relations among parental emotional expressivity, children's regulation, and quality of socioemotional functioning. Dev Psychol 39:3–19, 2003

Falloon IR, Boyd JL, McGill CW: Family Care of Schizophrenia: A Problem-Solving Approach to the Treatment of Mental Illness. New York, Guilford, 1984

Falloon IR, Boyd JL, McGill CW, et al: Family management in the prevention of morbidity of schizophrenia: clinical outcome of a two-year longitudinal study. Arch Gen Psychiatry 42:887–896, 1985

Fruzzetti AE, Fruzzetti AR: Borderline personality disorder, in Treating Difficult Couples: Helping Clients With Co-existing Mental and Relationship Disorders. Edited by Snyder D, Whisman MA. New York, Guilford, 2003, pp 235–260

Fruzzetti AE, Levensky ER: Dialectical behavior therapy with batterers: rationale and procedures. Cogn Behav Pract 7:435–447, 2000

Greenberg JS: Mothers caring for an adult child with schizophrenia: the effects of subjective burden on maternal health. Family Relations: Interdisciplinary Journal of Applied Family Studies 42:205–211, 1993

Gunderson JG: Borderline Personality Disorder: A Clinical Guide. Washington, DC, American Psychiatric Publishing, 2001

Gunderson JG, Berkowitz C: Family Guidelines. Belmont, MA, New England Personality Disorder Association, 2002

Hoffman PD, Fruzzetti AE: Family interventions for borderline personality disorder, in Borderline Personality Disorder. Edited by Zanarini MS. New York, Marcel Dekker (in press)

Hoffman PD, Fruzzetti AE, Swenson CR: Dialectical behavior therapy: family skills training. Fam Process 38:399–414, 1999

Hoffman PD, Buteau E, Hooley JM, et al: Family members' knowledge about borderline personality disorder: correspondence with their levels of depression, burden, distress, and expressed emotion. Fam Process 42:469–478, 2003

Hoffman PD, Fruzzetti AE, Buteau E, et al: Family connections: a program for relatives of persons with borderline personality disorder. Fam Process (in press)

Hogarty GE, Anderson CM, Reiss DL, et al: Family psycho-education, social skills training, and maintenance chemotherapy in the aftercare treatment of schizophrenia, I: one-year effects of a controlled study on relapse and expressed emotion. Arch Gen Psychiatry 43:633–642, 1986

Holtzworth-Munroe A, Markman H, O'Leary KD, et al: The need for marital violence prevention efforts: a behavioral-cognitive secondary prevention program for engaged and newly married couples. Appl Prev Psychol 4:77–88, 1995

Hooley JM, Hoffman PD: Expressed emotion and clinical outcome in borderline personality disorder. Am J Psychiatry 156:1557–1562, 1999

Keitner GI, Archambault R, Ryan CE, et al: Family therapy and chronic depression. J Clin Psychol 59:873–884, 2003

Koons CR, Robins CJ, Tweed JL, et al: Efficacy of dialectical behavior therapy in women veterans with borderline personality disorder. Behav Ther 32:371–390, 2001

Lam DH: Psychosocial family intervention in schizophrenia: a review of empirical studies. Psychol Med 21:423–441, 1991

Leff J, Kuipers L, Berkowitz R, et al: A controlled trial of social intervention in the families of schizophrenic patients. Br J Psychiatry 141:121–134, 1982

Linehan MM: Cognitive-Behavioral Treatment of Borderline Personality Disorder. New York, Guilford, 1993a

Linehan MM: Skill Training Manual for Treating Borderline Personality Disorder. New York, Guilford, 1993b

Linehan MM, Armstrong HE, Suarez A, et al: Cognitive-behavioral treatment of chronically parasuicidal borderline patients. Arch Gen Psychiatry 48:1060–1064, 1991

Linehan MM, Heard HL, Armstrong HE: Naturalistic follow-up of a behavioral treatment for chronically parasuicidal borderline patients. Arch Gen Psychiatry 50:971–974, 1993

Linehan MM, Schmidt H III, Dimeff LA, et al: DBT for patients with BPD and drug-dependence. Am J Addict 8:279–292, 1999

Lynch TR, Morse JQ, Mendelson T, et al: Dialectical behavior therapy for depressed older adults: a randomized pilot study. Am J Geriatr Psychiatry 11:33–45, 2002

Marsh DT: Families and Mental Illness: New Directions in Professional Practice. New York, Prager, 1992

Maurin JT, Boyd CB: Burden of mental illness on the family: a critical review. Arch Psychiatr Nurs 4:99–107, 1990

McCann RA, Ball EM, Ivanoff A: DBT with an inpatient forensic population: the CMHIP forensic model. Cogn Behav Pract 7:447–456, 2000

McFarlane WR, Link B, Dushay R, et al: Psychoeducational multiple family groups: four-year relapse outcome in schizophrenia. Fam Process 34:127–144, 1995

McFarlane WR, Dixon L, Lukens E, et al: Family psychoeducation and schizophrenia: a review of the literature. J Marital Fam Ther 29:223–245, 2003

Miklowitz DJ, George EL, Richards JA, et al: A randomized study of family focused psychoeducation and pharmacotherapy in the outpatient management of bipolar disorder. Arch Gen Psychiatry 60:904–912, 2003

Miller AE: Dialectical behavior therapy: a new treatment approach for suicidal adolescents. Am J Psychother 53:413–417, 1999

Mosco EA, Fruzzetti AE: The effects of emotion regulation and validation skill training: a test of validating and invalidating behaviors as mechanisms of change. Paper presented at the 37th annual convention of the Association for the Advancement of Behavior Therapy, Boston, MA, 2003

O'Donohue WT, Krasner L: Handbook of Psychological Skills Training. New York, Allyn and Bacon, 1995

Posner CM, Wilson KG, Kral MJ, et al: Family psychoeducational support groups in schizophrenia. Am J Orthopsychiatry 62:206–218, 1992

Rathus JH, Miller AL: DBT adapted for suicidal adolescents. Suicide Life Threat Behav 32:146–157, 2002

Schene AH: Objective and subjective dimensions of family burden: towards an integrative framework for research. Soc Psychiatry Psychiatr Epidemiol 25:289–297, 1990

Solomon P: Moving from psychoeducation to family education for families of adults with serious mental illness. Psychiatr Serv 47:1364–1370, 1996

Trull TJ, Widiger TA, Frances A: Covariation of criteria sets for avoidant, schizoid, and dependent personality disorders. Am J Psychiatry 144:767–771, 1987

Trupin EW, Stewart DG, Beach B, et al: Effectiveness of dialectical behaviour therapy program for incarcerated female juvenile offenders. Child and Adolescent Mental Health 7:121–127, 2002

Turner RM: Naturalistic evaluation of DBT-oriented treatment for borderline personality disorder. Cogn Behav Pract 7:413–419, 2000

Turner SA, Beidel DC, Dancu DV, et al: Psychopathology of social phobia and comparison to avoidant personality disorder. J Abnorm Psychol 95:389–394, 1986

Verheul R, Van Den Bosch LM, Koeter MW, et al: Dialectical behaviour therapy for women with borderline personality disorder: 12-month, randomised clinical trial in The Netherlands. Br J Psychiatry 182:135–140, 2003

25

Somatic Treatments

Paul H. Soloff, M.D.

Personality is a behavioral syndrome defined by the interaction of dimensional traits that arise from biological and learned influences on perception, cognition, affect, and behavior. A personality disorder is said to exist when a person's habitual style of seeing, thinking, feeling, and acting results in maladaptive behavior in the interpersonal world (Millon and Davis 1996). Personality dimensions believed to have a biological origin are traditionally referred to as *temperament*, whereas those acquired through social and cultural learning are termed *character*. This dichotomy between nature and nurture in the development of personality is both artificial and misleading. From the moment of birth, character is conditioned by the interaction of inborn temperament with the interpersonal environment. For example, a passive infant will experience an entirely different interpersonal world than a physically active one. A shy child will get different feedback from family, friends, and schoolmates than an impulsive-aggressive child, thus shaping each child's self-image, attitudes, and values.

Temperament may include behavioral traits influenced by experience as well as those that are genetically determined. Acquired traits of temperament may result from overt injury to the central nervous system or subtle changes in neurobiology after traumatic experiences. For example, childhood maltreatment, especially sexual abuse, results in persistent aberrations of the hypothalamic-pituitary-adrenal system, which modulates the stress response (DeBellis et al. 1999a), and in volume loss in hippocampus and amygdala, which are involved in memory and affect regulation (DeBellis et al. 1999b; Driessen et al. 2000). A history of childhood sexual abuse is associated with diminished central serotonergic regulation in adult women with borderline personality disorder (BPD; Rinne et al. 2000). Diminished central serotonergic regulation is implicated in behavioral syndromes of disinhibition—that is, impulsivity, impulsive aggression, and suicidal behavior. Temperament involves the biological regulation of cognition, perception, information processing, affect, and impulse, which are mediated by variations in neurotransmitter function in specific neural circuits of the brain (Siever and Davis 1991). A pharmacological approach to treatment of personality disorders is based on the ability of medication to modify neurotransmitter functions that mediate expression of state symptoms and trait vulnerabilities related to personality dimensions.

BASIC ASSUMPTIONS UNDERLYING PHARMACOTHERAPY IN THE PATIENT WITH PERSONALITY DISORDER

In terms of neurotransmitter function, the distinction between Axis I and Axis II disorders is arbitrary. Symptoms characteristic of patients with personality disorder may be mediated, in part, by the same neurotransmitter systems as similar symptoms in Axis I disorders. For example, ideas of reference, paranoid ideation, and mild thought disorder in patients with schizotypal personality disorder may be mediated in part by the same dopaminergic neurotransmitter systems as more severe forms of thought disorder. Both respond to dopaminergic blockade with neuroleptic agents. Symptom severity may be related to other disease-specific genetic or biological differences in these disorders. For example, schizotypal personality disorder is not the same as schizophrenia.

Pharmacotherapy in personality disorders is narrowly focused on those few dimensions that command the most clinical attention, such as affective dysregulation (e.g., labile, depressed, angry, or anxious moods), cognitive-perceptual symptoms ("psychoticism"), and impulsive aggression. These symptoms prompt urgent care because they mediate suicidal behavior, self-injury, or assault, and result in emergency department visits or hospitalization. As a result, most drug trials have been conducted in patients with borderline, schizotypal, and antisocial personality disorders.

Pharmacological interventions directed toward dimensions of personality disorders is a relatively new concept. The empirical literature, although growing, is still woefully inadequate. The work group that developed the practice guideline for treating BPD (American Psychiatric Association 2001) identified approximately 60 published reports on pharmacotherapy of BPD; half were randomized controlled trials and the rest were open label or small sample studies. Interpreting this literature requires an appreciation of the unique difficulties in conducting pharmacotherapy trials with personality disorder patients. Examples of these difficulties include the following:

1. Before the introduction of structured diagnostic interviews, clinician diagnoses of personality disorders were notoriously unreliable, raising questions about validity of diagnoses and generalizability of results. Some early reports used definitions of personality disorders no longer accepted in the modern nomenclature (e.g., emotionally unstable character disorder [Rifkin et al. 1972]). Structured interviews for personality disorder diagnoses, corresponding to DSM definitions, are now the accepted gold standard for randomized, controlled studies.

2. By definition, personality disorders are Axis II diagnoses. Comorbidity with Axis I disorders is common and must be controlled in any research design.

3. Overlapping symptoms in definitions of Axis I and II disorders often make differential diagnosis and determination of etiology of symptoms difficult (e.g., mood instability in BPD and bipolar II disorder). The relationship between depression and BPD has generated controversy, because it is often unclear whether the depressed patient with BPD has one disorder or two (Gunderson and Philips 1991; Koenigsberg et al. 1999; Soloff et al. 1991).

4. Comorbidity with Axis II "near neighbors" is often unavoidable.

5. Because personality disorder diagnoses are defined as syndromes, there is marked heterogeneity in the symptom presentations within any given personality disorder. Target symptoms for pharmacotherapy must be quantified by standardized assessment measures tailored to specific personality disorder symptoms. For example, the Affective Lability Scale may be more appropriate than the Hamilton Rating Scale for Depression (Ham-D) when antidepressants are being used to stabilize mood fluctuations rather than to treat a comorbid major depression.

6. Symptoms in the patient with personality disorder may be stress-related and transient, resolving with time alone or with crisis intervention therapy. A placebo condition is required to control for spontaneous remission of symptoms in drug trials. The need for placebo control raises additional problems, such as patient compliance and cooperation with an extended drug trial. Impulsive-aggressive patients assigned to placebo, for example, may not complete the study (Hollander et al. 2001).

7. Measurement of efficacy against trait vulnerabilities, such as impulsive aggression, must be done in appropriately long time frames, because the base rates of targeted behaviors (e.g., assaults, suicide gestures) may be low in a short time frame. Dropout rates are typically high (Kelly et al. 1992).

A pharmacological approach to treatment of personality disorders is symptom-specific and based on modifying neurotransmitter function in cognitive, affective, and impulsive-behavioral symptom domains. Both acute state symptoms (such as anger and anxiety) and trait vulnerabilities (such as impulsivity and dysregulated affect) are targets for treatment. Pharmacotherapy is not a primary treatment for problems of character or maladaptive interpersonal relationships, which are the focus of psychotherapy. However, appropriate use of medication may facilitate psychotherapy and stabilize a patient through the process of change. To underscore the empirical nature of this treatment, it is important to note that the U.S. Food and Drug Administration has not approved any medication for treatment of a personality disorder. All recommendations made in this chapter are based on review of empirical studies and are, by definition, off-label uses.

PHARMACOTHERAPIES

Neuroleptics

Neuroleptics have been studied more extensively than any other medication class used in the treatment of personality disorder. Randomized, controlled studies have included inpatients, outpatients, and adult and adolescent patients treated with a wide variety of first-generation and second-generation (atypical) antipsychotic agents. Most of these studies have been conducted in patients with borderline and/or schizotypal personality disorders. Neuroleptic medications, used in low doses, are the treatment of first choice for cognitive-perceptual symptoms, especially stress-related ideas of reference, transient paranoid ideas, and illusions. However, neuroleptics also have a broad spectrum of effects and reduce symptom severity in all symptom domains, including affective and impulsive-behavioral symptoms.

Brinkley et al. (1979) first described a series of patients with BPD who improved with open-label treatment on low doses of haloperidol, perphenazine, or thiothixene. Although cognitive disturbance was the rationale for treatment (following the original usage of the term "borderline"), affective symptoms such as mood, anxiety, and anger also improved, as well as somatic complaints. Hymnowitz et al. (1986) reported significant improvement in schizotypal symptoms among patients with schizotypal personality disorder treated in a single-blind design with haloperidol (mean, 3.6 mg) for 6 weeks. Both schizotypal and borderline traits (measured by structured interview) improved among study completers. Although 50% of

subjects dropped out, significant effects were noted by 2 weeks on medication among those who completed the study. In open-label trials, Teicher et al. (1989) found that low doses of thioridazine (mean daily dose 92 mg) produced marked improvement in overall borderline psychopathology, including impulsive-behavioral symptoms and global symptom severity. Similar findings were reported in open-label studies of adolescents with BPD treated with flupenthixol (3 mg/day; Kutcher et al. 1995). Impulsivity, depression, and global function were all significantly improved.

Random-assignment, parallel comparison studies comparing two neuroleptics without placebo controls also demonstrated a broad spectrum of efficacy. Leone (1982) found that loxapine succinate (mean daily dose 14.5 mg/day) or chlorpromazine (mean daily dose 110 mg/day) produced improvement in depressed mood, anxiety, anger-hostility, and suspiciousness. Serban and Siegel (1984) reported that thiothixene (mean daily dose ± SD, 9.4 mg ± 7.6 mg) or haloperidol (mean daily dose ± SD, 3.0 mg ± 0.8 mg) produced improvements in anxiety, depression, derealization, paranoia (ideas of reference), and general symptoms in borderline and schizotypal personality disorder patients. A global measure of borderline psychopathology also improved with thiothixene.

Placebo-controlled, randomized studies confirmed the broad spectrum of efficacy for low-dose neuroleptics, although efficacy against schizotypal symptoms and psychoticism, anger, and hostility were most consistently noted. Goldberg et al. (1986) studied outpatients with either borderline or schizotypal personality disorder; they required each patient to have at least one mild psychotic symptom, introducing a bias toward cognitive-perceptual symptoms. Patients received thiothixene (mean daily dose 8.67 mg) for up to 12 weeks and reported significant improvement over placebo in psychotic cluster symptoms—specifically, illusions and ideas of reference—and also in self-rated obsessive-compulsive and phobic anxiety symptoms. The more severely symptomatic the patient was at baseline, the better the patient responded to thiothixene.

Cowdry and Gardner (1988) conducted a complex, placebo-controlled, four-drug crossover study among outpatients with BPD using trifluoperazine (mean daily dose 7.8 mg) as the neuroleptic condition, with each trial lasting 6 weeks. Patients were also required to meet criteria for hysteroid dysphoria, an affective syndrome defined by histrionic traits, mood reactivity, rejection sensitivity, and atypical depressive symptoms, and to have a history of extensive behavioral dyscontrol, introducing a bias toward affective and impulsive-behavioral symptoms. Those patients who were able to stay on trifluoperazine for 3 weeks or longer (7 of 12 patients) were among the best mood responders in the study, with significant improvement over placebo on physician ratings of depression, anxiety, rejection sensitivity, and suicidality.

Soloff et al. (1986, 1989) studied acutely ill inpatients with BPD defined by the Diagnostic Interview for Borderline Patients and compared haloperidol with amitriptyline and placebo in a 5-week trial. Symptom severity was an inclusion criterion, defined by a Global Assessment Scale (GAS) score of less than 50 and either a Ham-D score of 17 or greater (measuring depression) or a score of 66 or greater on the Inpatient Multidimensional Psychiatric Scale (assessing psychoticism). Patients receiving haloperidol (mean daily dose 4.8 mg) showed significantly more improved symptom severity across all symptom domains than those receiving placebo. Severity of schizotypal symptoms was a predictor of favorable response. In the final analysis of this study (Soloff et al. 1989), haloperidol was significantly superior to placebo on global measures, self- and observer-rated depression, anger and hostility, schizotypal symptoms, psychoticism, and actual impulsive behaviors on the ward—in effect, a broad spectrum of symptom presentations. Haloperidol was equal to amitriptyline against depressive symptoms.

A second study by the same group, using the same design but comparing haloperidol with phenelzine and placebo, failed to replicate the broad spectrum efficacy of haloperidol (mean daily dose 3.93 mg). Borderline patients in the nonreplicating study, defined by the Diagnostic Interview for Borderline Patients as in the previous study, spent less time in the hospital and were significantly less impaired (Soloff et al. 1993). They had less schizotypal symptoms, psychoticism, and impulsive ward behavior than did patients in the first study (Soloff et al. 1989), suggesting less symptom severity at baseline. By chance, patients randomized to haloperidol in the nonreplicating study also were more depressed than those assigned to phenelzine and had more comorbid major depressive disorder (MDD) (Soloff et al. 1993). Efficacy for haloperidol was limited to hostile belligerence and impulsive-aggressive behaviors. Cornelius et al. (1993) followed this sample in a continuation study of responders maintained on their original medication assignments for 16 weeks following an initial 5 weeks of acute treatment. Intolerance of medication over time resulted in significant noncompliance and dropout. The 22-week attrition rates were 87.5% for haloperidol, 65.7% for phenelzine, and 58.1% for placebo. Analysis of endpoint data (all subjects carried forward) revealed significant continuing improvement on haloperidol compared with placebo only in the treatment of irritability, with a trend in total hostility. Patients on haloperidol reported significant worsening in depressive symptoms over time, which was attributed in part to the side effect of akinesia. Clinical improvement was modest and of limited clinical importance. This study illustrates the difficulties of continuation treatment with high-potency neuroleptics in the patient with personality disorder.

In a 6-month study, Montgomery and Montgomery (1982) controlled for noncompliance by using depot flupenthixol decanoate 20-mg injections once a month in a study of recurrently parasuicidal patients with borderline and histrionic personality disorders. Patients receiving flupenthixol demonstrated significant decreases in suicidal behaviors by 4 months compared with the placebo group.

The introduction of second-generation neuroleptics increases clinicians' options for treating the patient with personality disorder. In an open-label trial, Frankenburg and Zanarini (1993) reported that clozapine (mean daily dose ± SD, 253.3 mg ± 163.7 mg) improved positive and negative psychotic symptoms and global functioning in 15 patients with BPD and comorbid Axis I psychotic disorder not otherwise specified who had been intolerant of, or whose illness had been refractory to, other neuroleptic trials. Patients were recruited from a larger study of patients with treatment-resistant psychotic symptoms, raising the question of whether their symptoms were truly part of the Axis II disorder. Improvement was modest but statistically significant. These concerns were addressed by Benedetti et al. (1998), who excluded all Axis I psychotic disorders from a cohort of patients with treatment-refractory BPD. Target symptoms included "psychotic-like" paranoid ideation and referential thinking (which were transient and stress-related), visual illusions, hypnagogic phenomena, and odd beliefs (which "never reached a clear-cut delusional or hallucinatory quality"). Patients' symptoms had been refractory to 4 months of prior treatment with medication and psychotherapy. In a 4-month trial of 12 patients treated with clozapine and concurrent psychotherapy (mean daily dose 43.8 mg ± 18.8 mg), Benedetti et al. (1998) reported that low-dose clozapine improved symptoms in all domains—cognitive-perceptual, affective, and impulsive-behavioral. Clozapine may also have utility in treatment of self-mutilation and aggression in Axis I psychotic patients with comorbid Axis II BPD (Chengappa et al. 1995, 1999).

Newer second-generation neuroleptics (e.g., olanzapine, risperidone, quetiapine) are less difficult to use than clozapine and are better tolerated than first-generation agents. Clozapine, arguably the most effective of the atypical agents, is associated with lowered white blood cell counts, jeopardizing the body's immune response—a rare but dangerous side effect. Because of this risk, weekly white blood cell counts must be obtained for the first 6 months of treatment and biweekly thereafter for the duration of clozapine therapy. Koenigsberg et al. (2003) found that low doses of risperidone (to 2 mg/day), compared with placebo, produced significant improvement by 3 weeks of treatment in negative and positive symptoms of psychoticism in patients with schizotypal personality disorder, sustained through a 9-week trial. Open-label trials of olanzapine (mean dose 9.32 mg) in patients with schizotypal personality disorder have produced improvement in measures of psychoticism (Brief Psychiatric Rating Scale [BPRS]); depressed mood (Beck Depression Inventory [BDI], Ham-D); impulsive aggression (Overt Aggression Scale [OAS]); and overall global functioning (GAS) in much longer trials of 26 weeks' duration (although only 8 of 11 patients completed the full trial) (Keshavan et al. 2004). Rocca et al. (2000) reported that risperidone (mean dose 3.27 mg/day) produced improvement in aggression, hostility and suspicion, depressive symptoms, and overall global functioning in an open-label trial of 8 weeks' duration in patients with BPD. Schultz et al. (1999) conducted an 8-week open-label, dose-finding study of olanzapine in patients with BPD and comorbid dysthymia. Patients received an average daily dose (± SD) of 7.5 mg ± 2.61 mg daily, with a range of 2.5 mg to 10 mg. Significant improvement was reported in all global scales including general symptom severity (Hopkins Symptom Checklist–90 [SCL-90]); hostility (Buss-Durkee Hostility Inventory); impulsivity (Barratt Impulsiveness Scale); depression (BPRS, SCL-90-DEP); and in interpersonal sensitivity, psychoticism, anxiety, and anger/hostility (SCL-90). Zanarini and Frankenburg (2001) improved on this design in a 6-month placebo-controlled, randomized study of olanzapine in BPD (mean dose ± SD, 5.33 mg ± 3.43 mg/day). They reported significant improvement over placebo in the areas of interpersonal sensitivity, anxiety, anger and hostility, paranoia (all SCL-90), dissociation, positive symptoms of psychoticism (Positive and Negative Syndrome Scale for Schizophrenia), and global function (Global Assessment of Functioning Scale).

In these acute treatment studies, low-dose neuroleptics produced improvement in treatment trials extending from 5 weeks to 6 months. A role for low-dose neu-roleptics in continuation and maintenance therapies of the patient with personality disorder has yet to be established through multiple controlled-treatment trials.

Antidepressants

Selective Serotonin Reuptake Inhibitors and Related Medications

Selective serotonin reuptake inhibitor (SSRI) antidepressants are the drugs of first choice in the treatment of both affective dysregulation and impulsive-aggressive behavior in patients with personality disorder. Symptoms of affective dysregulation include marked lability of mood (intense, reactive, angry, depressive, or anxious feelings). In extreme expression, anger can be expressed behaviorally as temper tantrums, physical assaults, property destruction, or self-injury. Rejection sensitivity and depressive "mood crashes" result from a similar disinhibition of mood. (Impulsive aggression is discussed later in greater detail.)

BPD has been studied most intensively with antidepressants because of the prominence of affective dysregulation as a major component of temperament. Mood instability, "mood crashes," and "rejection-sensitive dysphoria" are familiar clinical terms describing this trait vulnerability. Some investigators view the affective dysregulation of the borderline patient as a subclinical manifestation of an affective disorder, evidence that some variants of BPD may be part of the broader affective disorders spectrum (Akiskal et al. 1985). Reviewing the antidepressant literature, one should keep in mind that studies in which there is a lack of control for comorbid Axis I depression would be expected to demonstrate a favorable response for antidepressant treatments but may not reflect the pharmacologic responsiveness of the Axis II syndrome.

Early case experience and small open-label trials with fluoxetine, sertraline, and venlafaxine (a mixed SSRI/norepinephrine uptake blocker) indicated efficacy against affective, impulsive-behavioral, and cognitive-perceptual symptoms in patients with BPD. Aggression and irritability, depressed mood, and self-mutilation responded to fluoxetine (up to 80 mg), venlafaxine (up to 400 mg), or sertraline (up to 200 mg) in treatment trials of 8–12 weeks' duration (Cornelius et al. 1990; Kavoussi et al. 1994; Markovitz and Wagner 1995; Markovitz et al. 1991; Norden 1989). An unexpected finding in these early open-label reports was that improvement in impulsive behavior appeared rapidly, often within the first week of treatment, and disappeared as quickly with discontinuation or non-compliance (Coccaro and Kavoussi 1997). Improvement in impulsive aggression appeared to be independent of effects on depression and anxiety and occurred regardless of whether the patient had comorbid MDD. Failure to respond to one SSRI did not predict poor response to all SSRIs. For example, some patients with illness that was refractory to fluoxetine (80 mg) have proven responsive to a subsequent trial of sertraline. Similarly, some patients whose illness failed to respond to sertraline, paroxetine, or fluoxetine in a first trial have proven responsive to venlafaxine (Markovitz 1995). In one study, higher doses (e.g., to the point of inducing tremor) and a longer trial (24 weeks) of sertraline converted half of sertraline nonresponders to responders (Markovitz 1995).

Following these open-label reports, placebo-controlled, randomized studies were reported in patients with BPD (Markovitz 1995; Salzman et al. 1995). Neither study is easily generalizable. Salzman et al. (1995) conducted a 12-week trial of fluoxetine (20–60 mg/day) in 27 highly functional subjects (not identified as patients) with BPD or borderline-trait disturbances. The subjects had a mean baseline GAS score of 74. One advantage of this mildly symptomatic sample was the absence of other Axis I or II comorbid diagnoses. Exclusion criteria also included recent suicidal behavior, self-mutilation, substance abuse, or current severe aggressive behavior—that is, behaviors typical of borderline patients seeking treatment. This strategy limits generalizability to more seriously ill patients, but it allows for a test of efficacy against symptoms unencumbered by comorbidity. For subjects who completed the study ($n=22$), significant improvements were reported for subjects receiving fluoxetine compared with those receiving placebo in self- and observer-rated anger, depression, and global function. A large placebo response was noted. Improvement in anger was found to be independent of changes in depressed mood. Improvement in this highly functional sample was modest, with no subject improving more than 20% on any measure.

Markovitz (1995) studied 17 patients (9 receiving fluoxetine, 8 receiving placebo) for 14 weeks; those receiving fluoxetine were given doses ranging from 20 mg to 80 mg daily. This sample was noteworthy for the high rate of comorbid Axis I affective disorders (10 with MDD, 6 with bipolar disorder), anxiety disorders, and somatic complaints (e.g., headaches, premenstrual syndrome, irritable bowel syndrome). Although this sample is more typical of an impaired borderline patient population, comorbidity with affec-

tive and anxiety disorders confounds interpretation of results, because SSRIs are effective for these disorders independent of BPD. Patients receiving fluoxetine improved significantly more than those receiving placebo on measures of depression and anxiety and on global measures. Measures of impulsive aggression were not included in this study. Anecdotally, some patients with premenstrual syndrome and headaches noted improvement in these somatic presentations with fluoxetine, whereas none improved with placebo.

A double-blind, placebo-controlled study by Coccaro and Kavoussi (1997) focused attention on impulsive aggression as a dimensional construct (i.e., a symptom domain found across personality disorder categories but especially characteristic of BPD and other Cluster B personality disorders). They recruited 40 male subjects, not identified as patients, with prominent impulsive aggression as a behavioral disturbance in the context of a DSM-III-R (American Psychiatric Association 1987) personality disorder. Personality disorder diagnoses included 11 (28%) eccentric cluster disorders, 19 (48%) dramatic cluster disorders, and 16 (40%) anxious cluster disorders. There was a high rate of comorbidity with dysthymic disorder or depression not otherwise specified, although MDD and bipolar disorder were excluded. Anxiety disorders and alcohol and drug abuse were also prominent. Following a 12-week double-blind, placebo-controlled trial of fluoxetine (20–60 mg), subjects receiving fluoxetine had significantly greater improvement than those receiving placebo on specific measures of verbal aggression and aggression against property. Improvement was significant by week 10, with first trends ($P=0.06$) appearing by week 4. Improvement in irritability appeared by week 6, again with an early trend apparent by week 4. Global improvement, favoring fluoxetine, was significant by week 4. As in the open-label trials and the Salzman et al. (1995) study, these investigators found that the effects on aggression and irritability did not appear due to improvement in mood or anxiety symptoms. More recently introduced SSRIs appear to have similar properties. A recent open-label, 8-week study using citalopram (mean daily dose 45.5 mg) in patients with Cluster B personality disorder or intermittent explosive disorder (but no MDD) also demonstrated significant decreases in irritable (impulsive) aggression (Reist et al. 2003).

Rinne et al. (2002) recently reported a double-blind, placebo-controlled trial of fluvoxamine in female patients with BPD treated for 6 weeks at 150 mg and then followed in a "half-crossover" design (all patients on active drug) for 6 weeks with a 12-week open-label continuation. Significant improvement was found only in a scale measuring rapid mood shifts, with the most improvement in the first 6 weeks. There were no significant changes in anger or impulsivity. The authors suggested that effects on anger and impulsivity may be related to gender—that is, more easily demonstrated in male patients (as in the Coccaro and Kavoussi [1997] study mentioned previously), who may respond preferentially to an SSRI.

In summary, these studies show efficacy for SSRI antidepressants against affective symptoms in the patient with personality disorder, specifically depressed mood (Markovitz 1995; Salzman et al. 1995), anger (Salzman et al. 1995), and anxiety (Coccaro and Kavoussi 1997; Markovitz 1995), and against impulsive-behavioral symptoms, specifically, verbal and indirect aggression (Coccaro and Kavoussi 1997). Global symptom severity also improves (Coccaro and Kavoussi 1997; Markovitz 1995; Salzman et al. 1995). Effects on impulsive aggression (Coccaro and Kavoussi 1997) and anger (Salzman et al. 1995) are independent of effects on affective symptoms, including depressed mood (Coccaro and Kavoussi 1997; Salzman et al. 1995) and anxiety (Coccaro and Kavoussi 1997), and may be relative to gender (Rinne et al. 2002).

Monoamine Oxidase Inhibitors

Monoamine oxidase inhibitor (MAOI) antidepressants (phenelzine, tranylcypromine) are second-line treatments for depressed mood in the patient with personality disorder, especially "atypical" depression so common in the patient with BPD. They may also be helpful in reducing social anxiety and hypersensitivity in patients with avoidant personality disorder in the context of social phobia (Liebowitz et al. 1986). Atypical depression is characterized by prominent mood reactivity, hypersomnia, hyperphagia, anergia ("leaden paralysis"), and rejection sensitivity. To have a diagnosis of atypical depression, the patient must also meet full criteria for a diagnosis of major depression, minor depression, or intermittent depression, facilitating the discrimination of atypical depression from the mood symptoms of the patient with BPD. MAOIs have also been shown to be useful in the treatment of hostility and impulsivity related to mood symptoms in the BPD patient (Cowdry and Gardner 1988; Soloff et al. 1993).

MAOI antidepressants have been studied in patients with BPD in three placebo-controlled, randomized studies. Phenelzine was compared with imipramine (Parsons et al. 1989) and haloperidol (Soloff et al. 1993) in parallel drug comparison studies, and tranylcypromine with trifluoperazine, alprazolam, and carbamazepine in a four-drug, placebo-controlled crossover study (Cowdry and Gardner 1988). Parsons et al. (1989) studied outpatients with atypical depression as a primary disorder and BPD as a secondary comorbid condition and reported global improvement in up to 92% of patients receiving 60 mg of phenelzine compared with a 35% responder rate for those receiving 200 mg of imipramine. Similarly, Kayser et al. (1985) found that phenelzine was superior to placebo in treating depressed patients with features of hysteroid dysphoria. Cowdry and Gardner (1988) studied outpatients with BPD as a primary diagnosis and comorbid hysteroid dysphoria using tranylcypromine (40 mg). The MAOI treatment was found to improve a broad spectrum of mood symptoms including depression, anger, rejection sensitivity, (increased) euphoria, and capacity for pleasure. Tranylcypromine also significantly decreased impulsivity and suicidality, with a near significant effect on behavioral dyscontrol. Cowdry and Gardner (1988) noted that "the MAOI proved to be the most effective psychopharmacologic agent overall, with clear effects on mood and less prominent effects on behavioral control" (p. 118). When BPD is a primary disorder, with no specific recruitment for atypical depression or hysteroid features, results are less favorable. Soloff et al. (1993) studied a clinical inpatient sample that had comorbidity for MDD (53%), hysteroid dysphoria (44%), and atypical depression (46%) but was not selected for a specific depressive disorder. An acute effect for phenelzine was reported on a self-rated measure of anger and hostility. No specific efficacy was found against measures of atypical depression or hysteroid dysphoria. These three randomized, controlled trials were of 5–6 weeks in duration. A 16-week continuation study of responding patients in the Soloff et al. (1993) study showed some continuing improvement over placebo beyond the acute 5-week trial in areas of depression and irritability (Cornelius et al. 1993). Phenelzine appeared to be activating, a change that was viewed as favorable in the clinical setting.

Soloff et al. (1993) found that the effects of phenelzine on BPD were independent of current comorbid affective diagnoses. Cowdry and Gardner (1988), excluding subjects with current major affective disorder, noted a nonsignificant trend for patients with past histories of major depression with or without melancholia or of bipolar II disorder to show more improvement on tranylcypromine ($P=0.08$). The response to tranylcypromine was not related to a family history of these affective disorders. A history consistent with attention deficit disorder was associated with a favorable response to tranylcypromine.

MAOI antidepressants (especially phenelzine) have demonstrated efficacy against social anxiety and interpersonal hypersensitivity in patients with Axis I social phobia and/or avoidant personality disorder, suggesting an overlap in neurotransmitter mediation of these symptoms regardless of Axis I or II designation (Deltito and Perugi 1986; Deltito and Stam 1989; Liebowitz et al. 1986). In patients treated for social phobia with the reversible, selective monoamine oxidase A (MAO-A) inhibitor brofaromine (150 mg/day), personality traits related to avoidant social behavior were significantly reduced after a 12-week double-blind, placebo-controlled trial (Fahlen 1995). The frequency of patients meeting full criteria for comorbid avoidant and dependent personality disorder diagnoses was significantly reduced by active treatment compared with placebo.

Although empirical support for MAOI antidepressants in the BPD patient is similar to that of the SSRI antidepressants, this class of medications is considered a second choice because of dietary restrictions, drug interactions, and safety concerns (e.g., risk of hypertensive crises). Patients must be willing to comply with the tyramine-free diet and abstain from certain classes of medication (e.g., many decongestants, meperidine, some older antihypertensives) and drugs of abuse (especially cocaine and amphetamines) or risk acute hypertensive crisis. Only cooperative and compliant patients should be considered for MAOI therapy. Many borderline patients do test the dietary limits through minor indiscretions as a manipulative gesture in the context of psychotherapy; however, few are willing to risk a heart attack or stroke in order to "test" the psychiatrist. (One sophisticated borderline patient of mine intentionally ate a large portion of quiche Lorraine, made with excellent aged cheeses, resulting in a hypertensive headache, a visit to the emergency department, and a late-night call to her psychiatrist. Her excuse: "It looked like a piece of pie!") With proper patient selection and instruction, hypertensive crisis is a rare occurrence, most frequently precipitated by the accidental use of over-the-counter decongestant medication (e.g., pseudoephedrine) or drugs of abuse (e.g., cocaine). Fear of these medications among inexperienced clinicians, especially psychiatrists trained after the advent of SSRIs, has greatly reduced their use, even in disorders for which they have clear advantages (e.g., atypical pattern depression, refractory depression).

Tricyclics or Heterocyclics

Double blind, placebo-controlled trials of tricyclic antidepressant (TCA) treatments in BPD have been conducted using amitriptyline, imipramine, and desipramine in both inpatient and outpatient settings. Mianserin, a tetracyclic antidepressant not available in the United States, has been used in patients with BPD and histrionic personality disorder in an outpatient setting in England (Montgomery et al. 1983). Most of these studies were parallel comparison studies with a second medication and placebo.

A 5-week inpatient study of BPD patients comparing amitriptyline (mean dose 149 mg/day) with haloperidol and placebo found that amitriptyline was more effective in decreasing depressive symptoms and indirect hostility and in enhancing attitudes about self-control compared with placebo (Soloff et al. 1986, 1989). Interestingly, it was not effective against the "core" neurovegetative symptoms of depression but rather the "associated" symptoms of diurnal variation, depersonalization, paranoia, obsessive-compulsiveness, helplessness, hopelessness, and worthlessness (measured on the 24-item Ham-D). With less than half of the patients meeting criteria for major depression in this sample, there was no relationship between response to amitriptyline and research diagnostic criteria diagnosis of Axis I major depression. Schizotypal symptoms and paranoia predicted poor outcomes for amitriptyline.

A small crossover study comparing desipramine (mean dose 162.5 mg/day) with lithium carbonate (985.7 mg/day) and placebo in BPD outpatients with minimal Axis I mood comorbidity found no significant differences between desipramine and placebo at 3 weeks and 6 weeks against affective symptoms, anger and suicidal symptoms, or in therapists' or patients' perception of improvement (Links et al. 1990).

A small open-label study comparing amoxapine, an antidepressant with neuroleptic properties, in BPD patients with or without comorbid schizotypal personality disorder found that amoxapine was not effective for patients with BPD as a sole diagnosis but was effective for those patients with comorbid schizotypal personality disorder who had more severe symptoms. This latter group had improvement in cognitive-perceptual, depressive, and global symptoms (Jensen 1989). In the context of BPD, schizotypal symptoms may represent a dimension of syndrome severity rather than a discrete separate disorder (e.g., schizotypal personality disorder). Psychoticism in BPD reflects a temperamental vulnerability to cognitive-perceptual distortion under affective stress, not a persistent thought disorder.

In the Parsons et al. (1989) study comparing imipramine 200 mg with phenelzine (60 mg) in outpatients with a primary diagnosis of atypical depression and secondary BPD, imipramine was significantly less effective than the MAOI. The presence of BPD symptoms predicted a negative global response to imipramine but a positive global response to phenelzine.

Montgomery et al. (1983) conducted a study of the efficacy of mianserin on recurrent suicidal behavior using patients with diagnoses of borderline or histrionic personality disorder. Patients were recruited from the hospital after a suicide attempt and had histories of at least two prior attempts. They did not have comorbid Axis I depression. In a 6-month double-blind, placebo-controlled trial, mianserin (30 mg/day) had no prophylactic efficacy compared with placebo for mood symptoms or recurrence of suicidal acts.

The utility of TCAs for the treatment of affective dysregulation or mood symptoms in BPD or other personality disorders is highly questionable. When a clear diagnosis of major depression can be made, therapy should be directed at the Axis I disorder. Where atypical depression is present, the MAOI antidepressants may be preferred. At best, the response to TCA (e.g., amitriptyline) appears modest in magnitude. Paradoxical behavioral toxicity to amitriptyline has been reported in some inpatients with BPD, consisting of increased suicide threats, paranoid ideation, demanding and assaultive behaviors, and an apparent disinhibition of impulsive behavior (Soloff et al. 1986, 1987). A choice of antidepressant for Axis I major depression comorbid with BPD should take this literature into consideration. The possibility of behavioral toxicity, and the known lethality of TCAs in overdose, supports the preferential use of an SSRI or related antidepressant as treatment of first choice for the affective dysregulation of the patient with personality disorder.

Anxiolytics

Anxiety is a common and chronic complaint among many patients with personality disorders and is a defining characteristic of the "anxious-fearful" Cluster C disorders (avoidant, dependent, and obsessive-compulsive personality disorders). Although anxiety is widely treated as a symptom independent of any Axis I diagnosis, there is a paucity of studies of anxiolytic use in patients ascertained specifically for personality disorder diagnoses. For example, studies of alprazolam efficacy for avoidant personality traits

(mean daily dose 2.9 mg × 8 weeks) are reported in the context of treating social phobia (Reich et al. 1989).

Cowdry and Gardner (1988) included alprazolam, a short-acting, high-potency benzodiazepine, in their double-blind, placebo-controlled crossover study of female BPD outpatients with comorbid hysteroid dysphoria and extensive histories of dyscontrol (self-mutilation, overdoses, rage episodes). Patients received an average daily dose of 4.7 mg of alprazolam for a 6-week trial. Use of alprazolam was associated with serious episodes of behavioral dyscontrol involving drug overdoses, self-mutilation, and throwing a chair at a child. Seven of 12 (58%) patients receiving alprazolam had episodes of serious behavioral dyscontrol compared with 1 of 13 patients receiving placebo (8%). Four alprazolam trials were stopped by the blind investigator, whereas none of the placebo trials required early termination (Gardner and Cowdry 1985). Alprazolam has been associated with emergence of extreme anger and hostile behavior, including physical assaultiveness, in patients with panic disorder, agoraphobia, obsessive-compulsive disorder, and major depression. These patients had histories of "chronic anger and resentment whose overt expression was well suppressed" (Rosenbaum et al. 1984). However, open-label case experience suggests that alprazolam may be helpful against anxiety in carefully selected patients with BPD (Faltus 1984).

Open-label case experience has also been reported in patients with BPD using clonazepam, a long-half-life (18–50 hours) benzodiazepine with anticonvulsant properties similar to carbamazepine and serotonin-enhancing properties similar to lithium carbonate (Freinhar and Alvarez 1985). Clonazepam is helpful as an adjunctive agent in the treatment of impulsivity, violent outbursts, and anxiety in a variety of disorders, including bipolar mania, schizoaffective disorder, schizophrenia, and BPD. Its efficacy may be related to an increase in serotonin levels and increased serotonin synthesis and function (Chouinard 1987).

Benzodiazepines in general warrant careful supervision because of the potential for abuse and the development of pharmacological tolerance with prolonged use. The use of benzodiazepine anxiolytics in patients with BPD should be limited to patients who fail to respond to other antianxiety treatments (e.g., SSRI antidepressants) and who are at low risk for abuse. Short-half-life benzodiazepine anxiolytics (e.g., alprazolam) should be used with great caution because of the risk of behavioral disinhibition or impulsive aggression. Patients with histories of behavioral disinhibition who are in need of anxiolytic treatment may be treated with clonazepam, a long-half-life benzodiazepine. There are no currently available studies of nonbenzodiazepine anxiolytics in patients with personality disorder diagnoses in the absence of Axis I anxiety disorders.

Lithium Carbonate and Anticonvulsant Mood Stabilizers

Lithium carbonate and the anticonvulsant mood stabilizers phenytoin, carbamazepine, divalproex sodium, and lamotrigine have all been studied in patients with personality disorders for the treatment of impulse dyscontrol. These studies have been conducted in patients with borderline and antisocial personality disorders in whom behavioral impulsivity and impulsive aggression were prominent characteristics. A separate literature, although relevant, describes the successful use of anticonvulsants (e.g., carbamazepine) in the treatment of intermittent explosive disorder and "rage outbursts" independent of personality diagnosis (Mattes 1990). Efficacy of anticonvulsants against aggression in patients with personality disorder (e.g., borderline or antisocial) may be independent of electroencephalographic abnormalities (Reeves et al. 2003).

An early hypothesis concerning the origin of impulse dyscontrol suggested that explosive anger and impulsive aggression were mediated by the same neural mechanisms involved in seizure disorders (Barratt 1972). This hypothesis led to trials of the anticonvulsant phenytoin as a treatment for impulsive aggression and nonepileptic rage in a variety of settings and populations. The results of many early studies were inconclusive, due in part to methodological problems involving diagnosis and assessment of aggression. Nonetheless, in some studies phenytoin has proven effective as an antiaggressive agent. Barratt et al. (1997) conducted a double-blind, placebo-controlled crossover study in a correctional facility using inmates with antisocial personality disorder but no Axis I comorbidity. Using structured interviews for diagnoses and standardized measures for aggression, these investigators demonstrated that phenytoin (in doses up to 300 mg/day) significantly reduced impulsive-aggressive behavior but not premeditated aggression.

The efficacy of lithium carbonate in bipolar disorders led to therapeutic trials in patients presumed to have personality disorders characterized by mood dysregulation and impulsive aggression. Rifkin et al. (1972) demonstrated improvement in mood swings in 21 patients with emotionally unstable character disorder, a diagnosis characterized by brief but nonreactive mood swings, both depressive and hypomanic, in the context of a chronically maladaptive personality resembling "hysterical character." The authors noted that emotionally unstable character disorder was "subsumed by hysterical or explosive character disorder in DSM-II, although more recent reviews suggest that these patients had cyclothymic or bipolar II disorder" (Kroll 1988, p. 73; American Psychiatric Association 1968). A double-blind, placebo-controlled crossover study of 6 weeks' duration resulted in decreased variation in mood from day to day (e.g., fewer "mood swings") and global improvement in 14 of 21 patients during the lithium treatment.

Lithium was also shown to have antiaggressive efficacy in chronically assaultive male prisoners in a placebo-controlled crossover study in which subjects received at least 1 month of lithium therapy (Sheard et al. 1976) and in longer-term open-label trials with incarcerated aggressive prisoners (Tupin et al. 1973) and aggressive delinquents followed both in institutional settings and as outpatients (Sheard 1975). Decreases in aggressive behaviors were documented through objective behavioral measures. Diagnoses of patients in these studies were not controlled and included patients with schizophrenia in the Tupin et al. (1973) study and diverse personality disorders among the adult and adolescent delinquent subjects in the Sheard study (Sheard 1971, 1975). Subsequently, case reports reported both mood-stabilizing and antiaggressive effects of lithium in individual patients defined as having BPD (LaWall and Wesselius 1982; Shader et al. 1974).

Links et al. (1990) compared lithium with desipramine in 17 outpatients with BPD in a double-blind, placebo-controlled crossover study. All patients received lithium for 6 weeks (with 4 weeks at constant dose) at an average daily dose of 985.7 mg and received concurrent psychotherapy. Among 10 patients completing both lithium and placebo treatments, therapists' blind ratings indicated greater improvement during the lithium trial, although patients' self-ratings did not reflect significant differences between lithium and placebo treatment. The authors noted that therapists were favorably impressed by decreases in impulsivity during the lithium trial. There was a trend for patients receiving lithium to report less anger and suicidal symptoms than patients receiving desipramine.

The anticonvulsant mood stabilizers carbamazepine and divalproex sodium have been used empirically in the treatment of affective instability and impulsive-aggressive behavior in BPD. Carbamazepine has been studied in two double-blind, placebo-controlled studies using very different patient samples and resulting in inconsistent findings.

In the first study, Gardner and Cowdry (1986a; Cowdry and Gardner 1988) studied female borderline outpatients who also had comorbid hysteroid dysphoria and extensive histories of behavioral dyscontrol. Patients received 6-week trials of medication, with 4 weeks at steady dose (mean daily dose 820 mg). Among the 11 patients who completed both a placebo and a carbamazepine trial, patients showed less behavioral dyscontrol and less severe types of behavioral dyscontrol during the carbamazepine trials. Comparing all patients, there were fewer suicide attempts or other major dyscontrol episodes during the carbamazepine trials (1 in 14 patients) compared with the placebo trials (7 of 11 patients, $P=0.005$). Patients receiving carbamazepine also showed improvement in anxiety, anger, and euphoria by physician's assessments, although patients did not report improved mood. There was a significant decrease in impulsivity and suicidality during the carbamazepine trials compared with the placebo trials. In an earlier report from the same study, Gardner and Cowdry (1986b) reported development of melancholia during carbamazepine treatment as an untoward effect in 3 of 17 (18%) patients.

In the second study, De la Fuente and Lotstra (1994) failed to replicate the findings of efficacy for carbamazepine in BPD that were noted in the Cowdry and Gardner studies (1988). De la Fuente and Lotstra (1994) conducted a double-blind, placebo-controlled trial of carbamazepine among inpatients in whom BPD was the main diagnosis. They rigorously excluded patients with any comorbid Axis I disorder, including a history of epilepsy or electroencephalographic abnormalities. Unlike the studies of Cowdry and Gardner (1988), patients were not selected for histories of behavioral dyscontrol. In the study by de la Fuente and Lotstra (1994), 20 patients (10 receiving carbamazepine and 10 receiving placebo) were studied in the hospital with medication trials of up to 32 days in duration. Carbamazepine doses were adjusted to yield plasma levels in the low therapeutic range. There were no significant differences between carbamazepine and placebo on measures of affective or cognitive-perceptual symptoms, impulsive-behavioral "acting-out," or global assessments. The two patients who failed to complete the study dropped out because of "acting-out" behaviors. Both were receiving carbamazepine.

Divalproex sodium has been used in open-label trials targeting the agitation and aggression of BPD patients in a state hospital setting (Wilcox 1995) and the mood instability and impulsivity of BPD patients in an outpatient clinic (Stein et al. 1995). Wilcox (1995) reported a 68% decrease in time in seclusion and improvement in anxiety, tension, and global symptom scores (BPRS) among 30 borderline patients receiving divalproex sodium for 6 weeks in a state hospital setting. Patients did not have "psychiatric comorbid conditions" (by clinical assessment), although five had abnormalities on the electroencephalogram (EEG) (with no seizure disorders). Patients received doses titrated to plasma levels of 100 µg/mL. Concurrent psychotropic medications were allowed. Both divalproex sodium and the abnormal EEG were predictive of improvement, although only the medication effect was significant. The author noted that anxiety played a role in the agitation of these patients and that both the antiaggressive and antianxiety effects of divalproex sodium were instrumental in decreasing agitation and time in seclusion.

An open-label study by Stein et al. (1995) enrolled 11 cooperative outpatients with BPD, allowing assessments by both self- and observer-based measures on a broad range of symptoms and control over psychiatric comorbidity (measured by structured interviews). All patients had been in psychotherapy a minimum of 8 weeks and were free of other medications prior to starting divalproex sodium, which was titrated to plasma levels of 50–100 µg/mL. Among eight patients completing the study, half were responders on a measure of global improvement. Improvement was noted in physicians' ratings of mood, anxiety, anger, impulsivity, and rejection sensitivity; in patients' ratings of global improvement (SCL-90); and in observed irritability (OAS-Modified [OAS-M]). There were no significant changes in measures specific for depression and anxiety (e.g., Ham-D, Hamilton Rating Scale for Anxiety); however, baseline depression and anxiety scores were low in this outpatient population.

Kavoussi and Coccaro (1998) also reported significant improvement in impulsive aggression and irritability after 4 weeks of divalproex sodium in 10 patients with impulsive aggression as a behavioral dimension in the context of a DSM-IV (American Psychiatric Association 1994) personality disorder. Eight patients completed the 8-week study. Five patients (four completers) met criteria for BPD, and seven (six completers) had a Cluster B personality disorder. Among eight patients completing the full 8-week trial, six had a 50% or greater reduction in aggression and irritability (OAS-M). All patients had previously failed a trial of fluoxetine (up to 60 mg for 8 weeks) prior to taking divalproex sodium.

Hollander et al. (2001) studied 16 outpatients with

BPD (and no Axis I depression or bipolar diagnoses) comparing divalproex sodium with placebo in a 10-week randomized, controlled study. Dropout rates were high: 50% of those receiving divalproex sodium and 100% of those receiving placebo due to lack of efficacy or impulsive decisions. No placebo patient was a responder. Patients receiving divalproex sodium improved significantly on global functioning (GAS, Clinical Global Impressions—Improvement of Illness), with nonsignificant trends for improvement in aggression and depressed mood. Hollander et al. (2003) also demonstrated significant treatment effects for divalproex sodium against irritability and aggression compared with placebo in Cluster B patients in a multisite trial of 12 weeks' duration that also included comparison groups with other impulse control disorders, intermittent explosive disorder, or posttraumatic stress disorder. Differences between Cluster B patients receiving divalproex and those receiving placebo were significant in the last 4 weeks of the trial. Improvements in impulsive aggression were greater for the Cluster B patients than for groups of patients with other impulsive disorders. Treatment effects were enhanced by excluding patients with premeditated aggression rather than impulsive aggression.

Frankenburg and Zanarini (2002) conducted a 6-month double-blind, placebo-controlled trial of divalproex sodium (average dose 850 mg ± 249 mg) in female patients meeting criteria for both BPD and bipolar II disorder. Analyses at 8 weeks and endpoint (using analysis of last observation carried forward) demonstrated divalproex to be superior to placebo on measures of interpersonal sensitivity, anger/hostility (SCL-90), and impulsive aggression (OAS-M). Comorbidity with bipolar II disorder makes this study difficult to generalize to personality disorder patients without bipolar spectrum illness. However, the similarity in symptoms between bipolar II disorder and BPD suggests clinical usefulness of divalproex sodium trials with either disorder.

Newer anticonvulsant agents such as lamotrigine may also have utility in treating affective dysregulation and impulsivity in patients with personality disorder, although at present only case reports are available (Pinto and Akiskal 1998; Rizvi 2002).

COMORBIDITY AND TREATMENT RESISTANCE

The presence of a personality disorder complicates somatic treatments of Axis I disorders. This problem has been studied most intensively in the context of major depression, for which comorbid personality disorders have long been considered a potential source of treatment resistance. Historically, patients with neurotic, hypochondriacal, or hysterical personality traits or comorbid categorical diagnoses of personality disorder tended to fare worse in trials of antidepressant medications and electroconvulsive therapy (ECT; see Mulder [2002] and DeBattista and Mueller [2001] for reviews). The etiology of this apparent treatment resistance has never been clearly defined. Does a personality disorder increase the severity of depression or alter the biology of depressive symptoms and their response to medication? Treatment resistance may be an unintended consequence of clinicians' decisions, because the presence of a prominent personality disorder may influence the choice of treatment, its intensity, or its duration. Conversely, treatment resistance may be a consequence of patient behavior, resulting from noncompliance with treatment recommendations. Recent literature reviews suggest that treatment-resistant depression in the patient with personality disorder may be more apparent than real, an artifact of poorly designed research studies (Brieger et al. 2002; DeBattista and Mueller 2001; Mulder 2002; Petersen et al. 2002). Mulder (2002) suggested that, given reliable diagnoses, standard treatment trials, and adequate durations of treatment, comorbid personality disorder "does not appear to worsen outcome for patients with major depression, provided that the patients receive good standard treatment for their mood disorder" (p. 369).

ELECTROCONVULSIVE THERAPY

ECT is indicated for the treatment of Axis I psychiatric disorders that have proven refractory to pharmacotherapy and are known to respond to ECT. The vast majority of patients referred for ECT have an affective spectrum disorder, although patients with schizoaffective disorder and schizophrenia may also benefit. On rare occasions, ECT may be a treatment of first choice for responsive Axis I disorders when clinical presentation requires urgency (e.g., catatonia), when pharmacotherapy poses unacceptable risk (e.g., neuroleptic malignant syndrome), or by patient preference (reinforced by past success). Depressed patients with prominent personality disorders are often not referred for ECT because of a widespread belief among practitioners that their illness is refractory to this somatic treatment. The literature on the efficacy of ECT for the depressed patient with personality disorder is remarkably inconclusive. Methodological differences between studies make generalization difficult.

The prejudice against the use of ECT treatment for depressed personality disorder patients may be traced back to early case reports and clinical series that described diminished responsiveness to ECT in patients with "neurotic" depression, a broadly defined construct of low diagnostic reliability incorporating many traits now attributed to comorbid personality disorder. Patients with "hysterical personality features" and BPD had poor outcomes with ECT (Kramer 1982; Lazare and Klerman 1968). Following the introduction of structured interviews for Axis I and II disorders and standardized outcome measures, empirical studies began to temper this view.

Pfohl et al. (1984) studied 41 inpatients with DSM-III (American Psychiatric Association 1980) MDD and comorbid Axis II personality disorder and compared them with 37 patients with MDD alone. Patients received somatic treatment by antidepressant medication or ECT, with all treatment decisions made by their attending physicians. Standard ratings of mood (Ham-D, BDI) and global functioning (GAS) were done before treatment and at discharge from the hospital. Depressed patients with comorbid personality disorder receiving antidepressant medications were less improved at discharge than patients with MDD alone; however, there was no difference between groups for patients receiving ECT.

This result was extended in a naturalistic study of outcomes in the treatment of 228 depressed inpatients. Black et al. (1988) reported that depressed patients with personality disorder receiving adequate antidepressant medication were less likely to recover than patients with MDD alone. However, there were no differences between groups in recovery after ECT. Depressed patients with personality disorder were less likely to be referred for ECT and generally received less aggressive treatment. In an expanded study involving 1,471 depressed inpatients, Black et al. (1991) found that the presence of a personality disorder diagnosis was a significant statistical predictor of poor outcome for hospital treatment in general (with antidepressant medication or ECT). Depressed patients with a personality disorder diagnosis were 50% less likely to be recovered at hospital discharge than patients with MDD without a personality disorder. (There was no analysis by separate treatment groups.)

Zimmerman et al. (1986) found no significant differences in immediate response to ECT treatment (on Ham-D, BDI, or GAS) between DSM-III MDD patients with and without a comorbid personality disorder. Patients had similar pretreatment symptom severity on Ham-D, BDI, and GAS and received similar (although uncontrolled) ECT treatments and pharmacotherapy. Follow-up at 6 months (by phone) indicated more episodes of rehospitalization and higher symptom scores in the personality disorder group. Although starting with similar improvement at hospital discharge, patients with personality disorder were less likely to maintain recovery compared with the depressed patients with no personality disorder.

Casey and Butler (1995) and Casey et al. (1996) studied ECT treatment in 40 inpatients with DSM-III-R MDD who were examined for personality disorder using Tyrer's Personality Assessment Schedule posttreatment. Patients were rated pretreatment, posttreatment, and every 6 weeks for 6 months and at 1 year at discharge using an outcome measure of mood (Ham-D-21) and social functioning (Social Functioning Schedule). A 12-month follow-up rated patients globally according to medication usage and patient status. ECT practice and concurrent antidepressant medication usage were uncontrolled, although patients in both groups had similar numbers of treatments (5 with personality disorder and 5.2 with no personality disorder) and days in the hospital. Depressed patients with personality disorder had acutely poorer outcomes on both the depression and social functioning scale following ECT treatment compared with depressed patients with no personality disorder. The presence or absence of a personality disorder was the strongest predictor of the Social Functioning Schedule outcome, explaining 31% of variance at discharge. Significant differences between groups on Ham-D disappeared by the first 6-week follow-up and for the Social Functioning Schedule by 12 weeks. There were no differences between groups in rehospitalizations in 6 or 12 months. The authors concluded that the presence of a personality disorder adversely affects early symptomatic recovery after ECT but not longer-term outcome.

Blais et al. (1998) obtained personality testing pre- and post-ECT in a small study sample ($N=16$) of depressed patients to determine changes in significant personality traits with ECT. Using the self-rated Millon Clinical Multiaxial Inventory–II, the investigators found significant changes (improvement) in four personality scales with ECT treatment: avoidant, histrionic, aggressive/sadistic, and schizotypal. Changes in passive-aggressive and borderline personality scale scores tended toward improvement but fell short of significance. Other personality scales appeared stable and did not change with ECT. Controlling for pretreatment depression scores, only a pretreatment diagnosis of BPD predicted posttreatment depression scores (on the BDI), with higher pretreatment BPD scores predicting poorer outcome.

Feske and colleagues (2004) recently reported that outcome differences following ECT for depressed patients with a comorbid personality disorder depended on the type of personality disorder. They divided 139 patients with a primary diagnosis of unipolar MDD into groups with comorbid BPD ($n=20$), other personality disorders ($n=42$), or no comorbid personality disorder ($n=77$). ECT methods and concurrent medication were controlled by a standard protocol. Patients with comorbid BPD showed a poorer acute response to ECT than the other two groups, who did not differ significantly.

In a review of this literature, DeBattista and Mueller (2001) concluded that 40%–75% of patients with MDD and comorbid personality disorder have a 50% decrease in depression scale scores with ECT, an efficacy equal to response rates among other patients with treatment-resistant depression without personality disorder comorbidity. However, increased relapse rates, rehospitalization, and psychosocial dysfunction (6 months to 1 year posttreatment) suggest that underlying personality disorder affects long-term outcome.

A major confounding factor in these studies is difficulty separating affective symptoms of the depressive disorder from those intrinsic to the personality disorder. For example, the affective dysregulation ("mood crashes"), low self-esteem, pessimism, chronic suicidality, and self-injurious behaviors of the patient with BPD are often misconstrued as Axis I affective pathology and assessed by outcome measures (e.g., BDI, Ham-D) that may correlate highly with diagnostic criteria. Not infrequently, a clinician will target these personality traits for ECT treatment, resulting in a predictably poor outcome. A recommendation for ECT in the personality disorder patient with comorbid MDD, especially the borderline patient, must be guided by the presence and severity of verifiable neurovegetative symptoms such as sleep disturbance, appetite disturbance, weight change, low energy, anhedonia, and loss of libido. These symptoms should be confirmed by outside observers because they provide an objective gauge of treatment response. Periodic use of an objective rating scale, such as the Ham-D, facilitates documentation of change over the course of treatment. The greatest challenge for the clinician is not when to institute a course of ECT in the depressed personality disorder patient but when to stop ECT. As the neurovegetative symptoms of MDD resolve, the patient may continue to report personality characteristics that reflect the Axis II

pathology and are not responsive to ECT. For example, low self-esteem can be an acute symptom of MDD or a chronic personality trait. Knowledge of the patient's personality functioning prior to the onset of MDD is critical to knowing when the "baseline" has been achieved. Many personality disorder patients with illness termed "refractory" to ECT for persistence of depressive complaint are, in fact, already in remission of their Axis I disorder and exhibiting their chronic characterological complaints and behaviors.

CONCLUSIONS

Pharmacotherapy is an important adjunctive treatment in the overall management of the patient with severe personality disorder. Symptoms of cognitive-perceptual disturbance, affective dysregulation, and impulsive-behavioral dyscontrol are appropriate targets for medication trials. Problems of character and of interpersonal dynamics are the domain of the psychotherapies and will not respond to medication. Because personality disorders are dimensional syndromes, a symptom-specific approach is warranted, potentially involving multiple medications. It is important to study the effects of each medication before adding a second or third agent. Ineffective medications should be discontinued. Expectations of efficacy should be modest and residual symptoms are the rule.

Pharmacotherapy of the personality disorders is still a relatively new and evolving practice. Current recommendations are based on a woefully small database of drug trials. The patient with personality disorder is best served by a comprehensive treatment approach involving psychotherapy, symptom-specific medication management, and psychoeducation for the patient and family.

REFERENCES

American Psychiatric Association: Diagnostic and Statistical Manual of Mental Disorders, 2nd Edition. Washington, DC, American Psychiatric Association, 1968

American Psychiatric Association: Diagnostic and Statistical Manual of Mental Disorders, 3rd Edition. Washington, DC, American Psychiatric Association, 1980

American Psychiatric Association: Diagnostic and Statistical Manual of Mental Disorders, 3rd Edition, Revised. Washington, DC, American Psychiatric Association, 1987

American Psychiatric Association: Diagnostic and Statistical Manual of Mental Disorders, 4th Edition. Washington, DC, American Psychiatric Association, 1994

American Psychiatric Association: Practice Guideline for the Treatment of Patients with Borderline Personality Disorder. Washington, DC, American Psychiatric Association, 2001

Akiskal HS, Chen SE, Davis GC, et al: Borderline: an adjective in search of a noun. J Clin Psychiatry 46:41–48, 1985

Barratt ES: Impulsiveness and anxiety: toward a neuropsychological model, in Anxiety: Current Trends in Theory and Research. Edited by Spielberger C. New York, Academic Press, 1972, pp 195–222,

Barratt ES, Stanford M, Felthous AR, et al: The effects of phenytoin on impulsive and premeditated aggression: a controlled study. J Clin Psychopharmacol 17:341–349, 1997

Benedetti F, Sforzini L, Colombo C, et al: Low dose clozapine in acute and continuation treatment of severe borderline personality disorder. J Clin Psychiatry 59:103–107, 1998

Black DW, Bell S, Hulbert J, et al: The importance of Axis II in patients with major depression: a controlled study. J Affect Disord 14:115–122, 1988

Black DW, Goldstein RB, Nasrallah A, et al: The prediction of recovery using a multivariate model in 1,471 depressed inpatients. Eur Arch Psychiatry Clin Neurosci 241:41–45, 1991

Blais MA, Matthews J, Schouten R, et al: Stability and predictive value of self-report personality traits pre- and post-electroconvulsive therapy: a preliminary study. Comp Psychiatry 39:231–235, 1998

Brieger P, Ehrt U, Bloeink R, et al: Consequences of comorbid personality disorders in major depression. J Nerv Ment Dis 190:304–309, 2002

Brinkley JR, Beitman BD, Friedel RO: Low dose neuroleptic regimes in the treatment of borderline patients. Arch Gen Psychiatry 36:319–326, 1979

Casey P, Butler E: The effects of personality on the response to ECT in major depression. J Personal Disord 9:134–142, 1995

Casey P, Meagher D, Butler E: Personality, functioning, and recovery from major depression. J Nerv Ment Dis 184:240–245, 1996

Chengappa KNR, Baker RW, Sirri C: The successful use of clozapine in ameliorating severe self mutilation in a patient with borderline personality disorder. J Personal Disorder 9:76–82, 1995

Chengappa KNR, Ebeling T, Kang JS, et al: Clozapine reduces severe self-mutilation and aggression in psychotic patients with borderline personality disorder. J Clin Psychiatry 60:477–484, 1999

Chouinard G: Clonazepam in acute and maintenance treatment of bipolar affective disorder. J Clin Psychiatry 48:29–36, 1987

Coccaro EF, Kavoussi RJ: Fluoxetine and impulsive-aggressive behavior in personality disordered subjects. Arch Gen Psychiatry 54:1081–1088, 1997

Cornelius JR, Soloff PH, Perel JM, et al: Fluoxetine trial in borderline personality disorder. Psychopharmacol Bull 26:151–154, 1990

Cornelius JR, Soloff PH, Perel JM, et al: Continuation pharmacotherapy of borderline personality disorder with haloperidol and phenelzine. Am J Psychiatry 150:1843–1848, 1993

Cowdry RW, Gardner DL: Pharmacotherapy of borderline personality disorder: alprazolam, carbamazepine, trifluoperazine and tranylcypromine. Arch Gen Psychiatry 45:111–119, 1988

de la Fuente JM, Lotstra F: A trial of carbamazepine in borderline personality disorder. Eur Neuropsychopharmacol 4:479–486, 1994

DeBattista C, Mueller K: Is electroconvulsive therapy effective for the depressed patient with comorbid borderline personality disorder. J ECT 17:91–98, 2001

DeBellis MD, Baum AS, Birmaher B, et al: Developmental traumatology part I: biological stress systems. Biol Psychiatry 45:1259–1270, 1999a

DeBellis MD, Keshavan MS, Clark DB, et al: Developmental traumatology part II: brain development. Biol Psychiatry 45:1271–1284, 1999b

Deltito JA, Perugi G: A case of social phobia with avoidant personality disorder treated with MAOI. Compr Psychiatry 27:255–258, 1986

Deltito JA, Stam M: Psychopharmacological treatment of avoidant personality disorder. Compr Psychiatry 30:498–504, 1989

Driessen M, Herrmann J, Stahl K, et al: Magnetic resonance imaging volumes of the hippocampus and the amygdala in women with borderline personality disorder and early traumatization. Arch Gen Psychiatry 57:1115–1122, 2000

Fahlen T: Personality traits in social phobia, II: changes during drug treatment. J Clin Psychiatry 56:569–573, 1995

Faltus FJ: The positive effect of alprazolam in the treatment of three patients with borderline personality disorder. Am J Psychiatry 141:802–803, 1984

Feske U, Mulsant BH, Pilkonis PA, et al: Clinical outcome of ECT in patients with major depression and comorbid borderline personality disorder. Am J Psychiatry 161:2073–2080, 2004

Frankenburg FR, Zanarini MC: Clozapine treatment of borderline patients: a preliminary study. Compr Psychiatry 34:402–405, 1993

Frankenburg FR, Zanarini MC: Divalproex sodium treatment of women with borderline personality disorder and bipolar II disorder: a double blind placebo controlled pilot study. J Clin Psychiatry 63:442–446, 2002

Freinhar JP, Alvarez WA: Clonazepam: a novel therapeutic adjunct. Int J Psychiatry Med 15:321–328, 1985

Gardner DL, Cowdry RW: Alprazolam-induced dyscontrol in borderline personality disorder. Am J Psychiatry 142:98–100, 1985

Gardner DL, Cowdry RW: Positive effects of carbamazepine on behavioral dyscontrol in borderline personality disorder. Am J Psychiatry 143:519–522, 1986a

Gardner DL, Cowdry RW: Development of melancholia during carbamazepine treatment in borderline personality disorder. J Clin Psychopharmacol 6:236–239, 1986b

Goldberg SC, Schulz SC, Schulz PM, et al: Borderline and schizotypal personality disorders treated with low dose thiothixene vs. placebo. Arch Gen Psychiatry 43:680–686, 1986

Gunderson JG, Philips KA: A current view of the interface between borderline personality disorder and depression. Am J Psychiatry 148:967–975, 1991

Hollander E, Allen A, Lopez RP, et al: A preliminary double blind, placebo-controlled trial of divalproex sodium in borderline personality disorder. J Clin Psychiatry 62:199–203, 2001

Hollander E, Tracy KA, Swann AC, et al: Divalproex in the treatment of impulsive aggression: efficacy in Cluster B personality disorders. Neuropsychopharmacology 28:1186–1197, 2003

Hymnowitz P, Frances A, Jacobsberg LB, et al: Neuroleptic treatment of schizotypal personality disorders. Compr Psychiatry 27:267–271, 1986

Jensen HV: An open noncomparative study of amoxapine in borderline disorders. Acta Psychiatr Scand 79:89–93, 1989

Kavoussi RJ, Coccaro EF: Divalproex sodium for impulsive aggressive behavior in patients with personality disorder. J Clin Psychiatry 59:676–680, 1998

Kavoussi RJ, Liu J, Coccaro EF: An open trial of sertraline in personality disordered patients with impulsive aggression. J Clin Psychiatry 55:137–141, 1994

Kayser A, Robinson DS, Nies A, et al: Response to phenelzine among depressed patients with features of hysteroid dysphoria. Am J Psychiatry 142:486–488, 1985

Kelly T, Soloff PH, Cornelius JR, et al: Can we study (treat) borderline patients: attrition from research and open treatment. J Personal Disord 6:417–433, 1992

Keshavan M, Shad M, Soloff PH, et al: Efficacy and tolerability of olanzapine in the treatment of schizotypal personality disorder. Schizophr Res 71:97–101, 2004

Koenigsberg HW, Anwunah I, New AS, et al: Relationship between depression and borderline personality disorder. Depress Anxiety 10:158–167, 1999

Koenigsberg HW, Reynolds D, Goodman M, et al: Risperidone in the treatment of schizotypal personality disorder. J Clin Psychiatry 64:628–634, 2003

Kramer BA: Poor response to electroconvulsive therapy in patients with a combined diagnosis of major depression and borderline personality disorder (letter). Lancet 2:1048, 1982

Kroll J: The Challenge of the Borderline Patient: Competency in Diagnosis and Treatment. New York, WW Norton, 1988

Kutcher S, Papatheodorou G, Reiter S, et al: The successful pharmacologic treatment of adolescents and young adults with borderline personality disorder: a preliminary open trial of fluopenthixol. J Psychiatry Neurosci 20:113–118, 1995

LaWall JS, Wesselius CL: The use of lithium carbonate in borderline patients. J Psychiatr Treat Eval 4:265–267, 1982

Lazare A, Klerman GL: Hysteria and depression: the frequency and significance of hysterical personality features in hospitalized depressed women. Am J Psychiatry 124 (suppl):48–56, 1968

Leone N: Response of borderline patients to loxapine and chlorpromazine. J Clin Psychiatry 43:148–150, 1982

Liebowitz MR, Fyer AJ, Gorman JM, et al: Phenelzine in social phobia. J Clin Psychopharmacol 6:93–98, 1986

Links P, Steuiner M, Boiago I, et al: Lithium therapy for borderline patients: preliminary findings. J Personal Disord 4:173–181, 1990

Markovitz PJ: Pharmacotherapy of impulsivity, aggression and related disorders, in Impulsivity and Aggression. Edited by Hollander E, Stein D. New York, Wiley, 1995, pp 263–287

Markovitz PJ, Wagner SL: Venlafaxine in the treatment of borderline personality disorder. Psychopharmacol Bull 31:773–777, 1995

Markovitz PJ, Calabrese JR, Schulz SC, et al: Fluoxetine in the treatment of borderline and schizotypal personality disorders. Am J Psychiatry 148:1064–1067, 1991

Mattes JA: Comparative effectiveness of carbamazepine and propranolol for rage outbursts. J Neuropsychiatry Clin Sci 2:159–164, 1990

Millon T, Davis RD: Disorders of Personality: DSM-IV and Beyond. New York, Wiley, 1996

Montgomery SA, Montgomery D: Pharmacologic prevention of suicidal behavior. J Affect Disord 4:291–298, 1982

Montgomery SA, Roy D, Montgomery DB: The prevention of recurrent suicidal acts. Br J Clin Pharmacol 15 (suppl 2):183S–188S, 1983

Mulder RT: Personality pathology and treatment outcome in major depression: a review. Am J Psychiatry 159:359–371, 2002

Norden MJ: Fluoxetine in borderline personality disorder. Prog Neuropsychopharmacol Biol Psychiatry 13:885–893, 1989

Parsons B, Quitkin FM, McGrath PJ, et al: Phenelzine, imipramine and placebo in borderline patients meeting criteria for atypical depression. Psychopharmacol Bull 25:524–534, 1989

Petersen T, Hughes M, Papakostas GI, et al: Treatment-resistant depression and Axis II comorbidity. Psychother Psychosom 71:269–274, 2002

Pfohl B, Stangl D, Zimmerman M: The implications of DSM-III personality disorders for patients with major depression. J Affect Disord 7:309–318, 1984

Pinto OC, Akiskal HS: Lamotrigine as a promising approach to borderline personality: an open case series without concurrent DSM-IV major mood disorder. J Affect Disord 51:333–343, 1998

Reeves RR, Struve FA, Patrick G: EEG does not predict response to valproate treatment of aggression in patients with borderline and antisocial personality disorders. Clin Electroencephalogr 34:84–86, 2003

Reich J, Noyes R, Yates W: Alprazolam treatment of avoidant personality traits in social phobic patients. J Clin Psychiatry 50:91–95, 1989

Reist C, Nakamura K, Sagart E, et al: Impulsive-aggressive behavior: open-label treatment with citalopram. J Clin Psychiatry 64:81–85, 2003

Rifkin A, Quitkin F, Carillo C, et al: Lithium carbonate in emotionally unstable character disorder. Arch Gen Psychiatry 27:519–523, 1972

Rinne T, Westenberg HGM, den Boer JA, et al: Serotonergic blunting to *meta*-chlorophenylpiperazine (m-CPP) highly correlates with sustained childhood abuse in impulsive and autoaggressive female borderline patients. Biol Psychiatry 47:548–556, 2000

Rinne T, van den Brink W, Wouters L, et al: SSRI treatment of borderline personality disorder: a randomized, placebo controlled clinical trial for female patients with borderline personality disorder. Am J Psychiatry 159:2048–2054, 2002

Rizvi ST: Lamotrigine and borderline personality disorder (letter). J Child Adolesc Psychopharmacol 12:365–366, 2002

Rocca P, Marchiaro L, Cocuzza E, et al: Treatment of borderline personality disorder with risperidone. J Clin Psychiatry 63:241–244, 2000

Rosenbaum JF, Woods SW, Groves JE, et al: Emergence of hostility during alprazolam treatment. Am J Psychiatry 141:792–793, 1984

Salzman C, Wolfson AN, Schatzberg A, et al: Effect of fluoxetine on anger in symptomatic volunteers with borderline personality disorder. J Clin Psychopharmacol 15:23–29, 1995

Schultz SC, Camlin KL, Berry SA, et al: Olanzapine safety and efficacy in patients with borderline personality disorder and comorbid dysthymia. Biol Psychiatry 46:1429–1435, 1999

Serban G, Siegel S: Response of borderline and schizotypal patients to small doses of thiothixene and haloperidol. Am J Psychiatry 141:1455–1458, 1984

Shader RI, Jackson AH, Dodes LM: The anti-aggressive effects of lithium in man. Psychopharmacologia (Berl) 40:17–24, 1974

Sheard MH: Effects of lithium on human aggression. Nature, March 12, 1971, pp 113–114

Sheard MH: Lithium in the treatment of aggression. J Nerv Ment Dis 160:108–118, 1975

Sheard MH, Marini JL, Bridges CI, et al: The effect of lithium on impulsive aggressive behavior in man. Am J Psychiatry 133:1409–1413, 1976

Siever LJ, Davis K: A psychobiological perspective on the personality disorders. Am J Psychiatry 148:1647–1658, 1991

Soloff PH, George A, Nathan S, et al: Progress in pharmacotherapy of borderline disorders. Arch Gen Psychiatry 43:691–697, 1986

Soloff PH, George A, Nathan RS, et al: Behavioral dyscontrol in borderline patients treated with amitriptyline. Psychopharmacol Bull 23:177–181, 1987

Soloff PH, George A, Nathan RS, et al: Amitriptyline vs haloperidol in borderlines: final outcomes and predictors of response. J Clin Psychopharmacol 9:238–246, 1989

Soloff PH, Cornelius J, George A: The depressed borderline: one disorder or two? Psychopharmacol Bull 27:23–30, 1991

Soloff PH, Cornelius J, George A, et al: Efficacy of phenelzine and haloperidol in borderline personality disorder. Arch Gen Psychiatry 50:377–385, 1993

Stein DJ, Simeon D, Frenkel M, et al: An open trial of valproate in borderline personality disorder. J Clin Psychiatry 56:506–510, 1995

Teicher MH, Glod CA, Aronson SJ, et al: Open assessment of the safety and efficacy of thioridazine in the treatment of patients with borderline personality disorder. Psychopharmacol Bull 25:535–549, 1989

Tupin JP, Smith DB, Clanion TL, et al: The long term use of lithium in aggressive prisoners. Compr Psychiatry 14:311–317, 1973

Wilcox JA: Divalproex sodium as a treatment for borderline personality disorder. Ann Clin Psychiatry 7:33–37, 1995

Zanarini MC, Frankenburg F: Olanzapine treatment of female borderline patients: a double-blind placebo controlled pilot study. J Clin Psychiatry 62:849–854, 2001

Zimmerman M, Coryell W, Pfohl B, et al: ECT response in depressed patients with and without a DSM-III personality disorder. Am J Psychiatry 143:1030–1032, 1986

26

Therapeutic Alliance

Donna S. Bender, Ph.D.

Any patient beginning treatment enters a relationship, whether it is for a short time during a hospital stay or over many years in long-term psychotherapy. This relationship with the clinician has the potential for improving the patient's quality of life, perhaps through the alleviation of symptoms or more profoundly through shifts in character structure. It is sometimes difficult to determine a priori who will benefit from what treatment with whom, but one factor has stood out in the research lexicon as the most robust predictor of outcome: therapeutic alliance (Horvath and Greenberg 1994; Horvath and Symonds 1991; Orlinsky et al. 1994).

Because establishing a productive alliance arises within the matrix of a relationship between patient and therapist, when considering personality disorders one must note that most such disorders are associated in some way with significant impairment in interpersonal relations. Speaking about the nature of relationships of individuals characterized by certain types of personality pathology, Masterson (1988) has stated the following:

> Each type of pathology produces its own confusion and its own distorted version of loving and giving. The borderline patient defines love as a relationship with a partner who will offer approval and support for regressive behavior.... The narcissist defines love as the ability of someone else to admire and adore him, and to provide perfect mirroring.... Psychopaths seek partners who respond to their manipulations and provide them with gratification. The schizoid...finds love in an internal, autistic fantasy. (pp. 110–111)

In fact, several studies have shown that rather than categorical diagnosis, it is the preexisting quality of the patient's relationships that most significantly affects the quality of the therapeutic alliance (Gibbons et al. 2003; Hersoug et al. 2002; Piper et al. 1991). Consequently, the clinician must consider an individual's characteristic way of relating so that appropriate interventions can be employed to effectively retain and involve the patient in the treatment, regardless of modality. Forming an alliance is often difficult, however, particularly in work with patients with severely narcissistic, borderline, or paranoid proclivities, because troubled interpersonal attitudes and behaviors will also infuse the patient's engagement with the therapist. For example, narcissistic patients may not be able to allow the therapist to act as a separate, thinking person for quite a long time, whereas someone with borderline issues may exhibit wildly fluctuating emotions, attitudes, and behaviors, thwarting the potential helpfulness of the clinician.

DEFINITION OF THERAPEUTIC ALLIANCE

The concept of the therapeutic alliance is often traced back to Freud, who observed very early in his work the need to convey interest and sympathy to the patient to engage her or him in a collaborative treatment endeavor (Meissner 1996; Safran and Muran 2000). Freud (1912/1946) also delineated an aspect of the transference—the unobjectionable positive transference—which is an attachment that should not be analyzed because it serves as the motivation for the patient to collaborate: "The conscious and unobjectionable component of [positive transference] remains, and brings about the successful result in psychoanalysis as in all other remedial methods" (p. 319). This statement is an early precursor to the modern empirical evidence showing that alliance is related to treatment outcome across modalities.

There are several contemporary definitions of alliance that we might consider to further our discussion of treating patients with personality disorders. One conceptualization, using psychoanalytic language, was posited by Gutheil and Havens (1979): The patient's ability to form a rational alliance arises from "the therapeutic split in the ego which allows the analyst to work with the healthier elements in the patient against resistance and pathology" (p. 479). This definition is useful vis-à-vis personality disorders in two regards: 1) the recognition that there will be pathological parts of the patient's personality functioning that may serve to thwart the attempted helpfulness of the clinician, and 2) the need for the clinician to be creative in enlisting whatever adaptive aspects of the patient's character may avail themselves for the work of the treatment.

Another definition that was developed in an attempt to transcend theoretical traditions is Bordin's (1979) identification of three interdependent components of the alliance: bond, tasks, and goals. The *bond* is the quality of the relationship formed in the treatment dyad that then mediates whether the patient will take up the *tasks* inherent in working toward the *goals* of a particular treatment approach. At the same time, the clinician's ability to negotiate the tasks and goals with the patient will also affect the nature of the therapeutic bond. This multifaceted view of the alliance underscores the complexity of the factors involved (Safran and Muran 2000).

Arguably, if the goal of treatment is fundamental character change, the Bordin definition of alliance specifies necessary, but not sufficient, elements. Adler (1980) observed that patients with borderline and narcissistic difficulties may not be able to establish a mature working alliance until much later in a successful treatment. Others who typically work with more disturbed patients have noted that establishing a therapeutic alliance may be one of the primary goals of the treatment and that there may be different phases of alliance development as treatment progresses. Gunderson (2000) observed the following alliance stages in the course of conducting long-term psychotherapy with patients with borderline personality disorder:

> 1) Contractual (behavioral): initial agreement between the patient and therapist on treatment goals and their roles in achieving them (Phase I); 2) Relational (affective/empathic): emphasized by Rogerian client-centered relationships; patient experiences the therapist as caring, understanding, genuine, and likable (Phase II); 3) Working (cognitive/motivational): psychoanalytic prototype; patient joins the therapist as a reliable collaborator to help the patient understand herself or himself; its development represents a significant improvement for borderline patients (Phases III–IV). (p. 41)

Progression through these stages, if successful, typically takes a number of years. The implication is that to reach a point at which work leading to substantive and enduring personality change can occur may require a lengthy initial alliance-building period. As Bach (1998) noted, "Perhaps the primary problem in engaging the difficult patient is to build and retain what Ellman (1991) has called analytic trust. These difficult patients have generally lost their faith not only in their caregivers, spouses, and other objects but also in the world itself as a place of expectable and manageable contingencies" (p. 185).

ALLIANCE STRAINS AND RUPTURES

Although a strong positive alliance can predict a successful treatment outcome, the converse is also true: problems in the treatment alliance may lead to premature termination if not handled in a sensitive and timely manner. Evidence has shown that strains and ruptures in the alliance are often related to unilateral termination (Samstag et al. 1998). Thus, negotiating ruptures in the alliance is another issue that has garnered increasing attention in the psychotherapy literature.

Disruptions in the alliance are inevitable and occur more frequently than may be readily apparent to the clinician (Safran and Muran 2000). One study (Hill et al. 1993) asked patients to report about thoughts and feelings that they were not expressing to their therapists. Most things that were not discussed were negative, and even the most experienced therapists were aware of uncommunicated negative material only 45% of the time. It has also been suggested, however, that therapist awareness of patients' negative feelings may actually create problems; therapists, rather than being open and flexible in response, may at times become defensive and negative or may become more rigid in applying treatment techniques (Safran et al. 2001).

Safran and Muran (2000) outlined a model specifying two subtypes of ruptures: withdrawal and confrontation. Withdrawals are sometimes fairly subtle. One example is a therapist who assumes the treatment is progressing but may be unaware that a patient is withholding important information from lack of trust or for fear of feeling humiliated. Other types of withdrawal behaviors include such things as intellectualizing, talking excessively about other people, or changing the subject. Withdrawal behaviors may be more common in patients who are overly compliant at times, such as those with dependent or obsessive-compulsive personality disorder or those who are uncomfortable about interpersonal relations, such as patients with avoidant personality disorder.

Confrontations, on the other hand, are usually more overt, such as complaining about various aspects of therapy or criticizing the therapist. Some may be rather dramatic, such as a patient who storms out of session in a rage or leaves an angry message on the therapist's answering machine. Confrontation ruptures are likely to be more frequently experienced with more brittle patients such as those with borderline, narcissistic, or paranoid personality disorder. In any event, clinicians are best served by being alert to ruptures and adopting the attitude that these are often excellent opportunities to engage the patient in a collaborative effort to observe and learn about that patient's own style (Horvath and Greenberg 1994).

ALLIANCE CONSIDERATIONS BY DSM CLUSTER

For ease of discussion, the following section is organized by DSM-IV-TR (American Psychiatric Association 2000) personality disorder diagnostic clusters to address particular alliance-relevant issues associated with each. However, there is increasing evidence that the DSM categories and clusters do not adequately capture the complexity of character pathology traits

and symptoms. For instance, patients often meet criteria for at least two personality disorders, perhaps spanning different clusters, such as the co-occurrence of schizotypal personality disorder with borderline personality disorder or borderline personality disorder with avoidant personality disorder (McGlashan et al. 2000), or a patient may not meet full criteria for any one disorder but could still have prominent features associated with one or several personality disorders.

Thus, in practical terms, a clinician considering salient elements of the therapeutic alliance should determine which aspects of a patient's personality pathology are dominant or in ascendance at intake and at various points over the course of treatment. That being said, it has been suggested that the nature of the alliance established early in the treatment is more powerfully predictive of outcome (Horvath and Luborsky 1993). One example of the relationship of early alliance and outcome regarding personality disorders was demonstrated in a study of long-term psychotherapy with a group of borderline patients: therapist ratings of the alliance at 6 weeks predicted subsequent dropouts (Gunderson et al. 1997). As Horvath and Greenberg (1994) noted: "It seems reasonable to think of alliance development in the first phase of therapy as a series of windows of opportunity, decreasing in size with each session" (p. 3). Thus, Table 26–1 summarizes by personality disorder the tendencies that may serve to challenge early collaboration-building as well as aspects that a clinician might use to engage the patient.

Cluster A

Cluster A—the so-called odd-eccentric cluster—comprises schizotypal, schizoid, and paranoid personality disorders. What is most relevant for alliance building is the profound impairment in interpersonal relationships associated with these disorders. Because there are often pronounced paranoid or alienated features, people with these characteristics often do not seek treatment unless dealing with acute Axis I problems such as substance abuse.

Schizotypal

Schizotypal phenomena are thought by some to exist on the schizophrenia spectrum, given the associated disordered cognitions and bizarre beliefs. Because it is almost always the case that such individuals have one or no significant others outside family members, it is often assumed that schizotypal individuals have no desire to become involved in relationships. However, in many cases, it is more a matter of being excruciatingly

Table 26–1.   Alliance-relevant aspects of each personality disorder style

Personality disorder trait cluster	Alliance challenges	Points of possible engagement in treatment
Schizotypal	Suspiciousness/paranoia Profound interpersonal discomfort Bizarre thinking	Possible motivation for human connection
Schizoid	Social detachment Emotional aloofness	Underlying neediness and sensitivity
Paranoid	Expectations of harm or exploitation Hypersensitivity to perceived criticism Inclination to withdraw or attack	Underlying need for affirmation
Borderline	Unstable emotional and cognitive states Extremely demanding Proneness to acting-out	Relationship-seeking Responds to warmth and support
Narcissistic	Need for constant positive regard Contempt for others Grandiose sense of entitlement	Responds over time to empathy and affirmation
Histrionic	Attempts to charm and entertain Emotionally labile Unfocused cognitive style	Relationship-seeking Responds to warmth and support
Antisocial	Controlling Tendency to lie and manipulate No empathy or regard for others Use of pseudoalliance to gain some advantage	May engage in treatment if in self-interest or if Axis I symptoms cause sufficient distress
Avoidant	Expectations of criticism or rejection Proneness to shame and humiliation Reluctance to disclose information	Responds to warmth/empathy Desire for relationships in spite of vulnerabilities
Dependent	No value placed on independence/ taking initiative Submission leading to pseudoalliance	Friendly and compliant Likely to stay in treatment
Obsessive-compulsive	Need for control Perfectionistic toward self and others Fear of criticism from therapist Restricted affect Stubbornness	Conscientious Use of intellectualization may be helpful at times Will try to be a "good patient"

uncomfortable around people rather than a lack of interest in connection. This discomfort may not be readily apparent, so establishing an alliance with such patients may require being attentive to clues about what is not being said. The therapist may be a player in some elaborated fantasy that is making it difficult for the patient to find some minimum level of comfort. A recent study by Bender et al. (2003) assessed various attributes of how patients with personality disorder think about their therapists. Interestingly, results showed that patients with schizotypal personality disorder had the highest level of mental involvement with therapy outside the session, missing their therapists and wishing for friendship while also feeling aggressive or negative. One man with schizotypal personality disorder (who

had also become attached to the female research assistant) revealed the following view of his therapist:

> Very beautiful and attractive in a sense that I yearn to have a sexual relationship with her. She's very smart and educated. She knows what she wants out of life and I wish I were working for I could take her out to the movies and dinner. She turns me on and I desperately want to make love to her eternally. She's my life and knowing she doesn't feel the same, I live in dreams. (p. 231)

Schizoid

Benjamin (1993) noted that schizoid personality is more consistently associated with a lack of desire for intimate human connection. She described that some people with schizoid character can be found living very conventional lives on the surface, having families, jobs, and so on. However, usually things are arranged such that people are kept at an emotional distance. There may also be a pronounced lack of conflict, with associated affective coldness or dullness such that a truly schizoid person is unlikely to become anxious or depressed and thus is usually totally lacking any motivation to seek treatment. However, Akhtar (1992) suggested that underlying all of this apparent detachment is an intense neediness for others and the capability of interpersonal responsiveness with a few carefully selected people. Patients who may have more access to these latter attributes have a greater likelihood of forming an alliance in therapy if they choose to seek treatment.

Paranoid

The "paranoid" label largely speaks for itself. Paranoid individuals are incessantly loaded for bear and see bears where others do not—that is, they are vigilantly on the lookout for perceived slights, finding offense in even the most benign of circumstances. Alliance-building challenges are obvious. However, it has also been noted that paranoid individuals are often acting in defense of an extremely fragile self-concept and may possibly be reached over time in treatment with an approach that includes unwavering affirmation and careful handling of the many possible ruptures (Benjamin 1993).

Cluster B

The "dramatic" cluster includes antisocial, borderline, histrionic, and narcissistic personality disorders. Each of these character styles is associated in some way with pushing the limits, and great care is needed by clinicians to avoid crossing inappropriate lines in a quest to build an alliance. Thus, many Cluster B patients present some of the most daunting treatment challenges.

Borderline

Kernberg (1967) described the borderline personality as being riddled with aggressive impulses that constantly threaten to destroy positive internal images of the self and others. According to this model, the borderline person does not undergo the normal developmental process of psychological integration but rather, as a defensive attempt to deal with aggression, creates "splits" in his or her mind to protect the good images from the bad. This splitting leads to a fractured self-concept and

the identity problems associated with this disorder. Thus, one can expect the alliance-building work to be rather rocky because these patients frequently exhibit pronounced emotional upheaval, self-destructive acting-out, and views of the therapist that alternate between idealization and denigration. Within relationships, such individuals are very needy and demanding, often straining the boundaries of the treatment relationship and exerting pressure on clinicians to behave in ways they normally would not. Research has demonstrated that such pressures can impair the clinician's ability to reflect on his or her mental states and those of the patient (Diamond et al. 2003). Furthermore, clinicians who work with such patients must be able to tolerate and productively discuss anger and aggression. However, because borderline patients are, in most cases, relationship-seeking, this is a positive indicator for engagement in treatment.

One treatment study of borderline patients (Waldinger and Gunderson 1984) examined alliance development over time. Psychodynamic psychotherapy was employed using largely noninterpretive interventions in the initial alliance-building period (the issue of intervention choice is discussed further later in the chapter). The authors observed that a strong alliance and good treatment outcome were linked to two factors: 1) a solid commitment by the participating therapist to remain engaged in the treatment until significant gains had been made by the patients; and 2) special emphasis on facilitating the patients' expression of aggression and rage without fear of retaliation. Horwitz et al. (1996), who studied the therapeutic alliance over the course of treatment of borderline patients, noted that "clinical observation of our cases revealed that the repair of moment-to-moment disruptions in the alliance often was the key factor in maintaining the viability of the psychotherapy" (p. 173).

Narcissistic

Narcissistic character traits have received considerable attention in the clinical literature. Kohut (1977) described individuals in whom there is a fundamental deficit in the ability to regulate self-esteem without resorting to omnipotent strategies of overcompensation or overreliance on admiration by others. Some people who are narcissistically vulnerable have difficulty maintaining a cohesive sense of self because of ubiquitous shame, resulting from a sense that they fundamentally fall short of some internal ideal. They look for constant reinforcement from others to bolster their fragile self-images. This combination of traits has been referred to alternatively as *vulnerable, deflated,* or *covert narcissism.*

On the other side of the narcissistic "coin"—what the DSM narcissistic personality disorder diagnosis captures—are people who are intensely grandiose, seeking to maintain self-esteem through omnipotent fantasies and defeating others. They defend against needing others by maintaining fusions of ideal self, ideal other, and actual self-images. Thus, there is an illusion maintained whereby this type of narcissistic person has a sense that because he or she is perfect, love and admiration will be received from other "ideal people," and thus there is no need to associate with inferiors. In its most extreme form, this manifestation of character pathology has been referred to as *malignant narcissism* (Kernberg 1984).

It is obvious that such personality traits pose significant challenges in alliance building. It is often the case that the patient will need to keep the therapist out of the room, so to speak, for quite a long time by not allowing him or her to voice anything that represents an alternative view to that of the patient's. For such patients, other people, including the therapist, do not exist as separate individuals but merely as objects for gratifying needs. The clinician must tolerate this state of affairs, sometimes for a lengthy period of time. Meissner (1996) observed, "Establishing any degree of trust with such patients may be extremely difficult, but not impossible, for a consistent respect for their vulnerability and a recognition of their need not to trust may in time undercut their defensive need" (p. 228).

Histrionic

A patient with histrionic personality needs to be the center of attention and may behave in seductive ways in an attempt to keep the clinician entertained and engaged. At the same time, emotional expressions are often shallow and greatly exaggerated, and the histrionic patient assumes a deep connection and dependence very quickly. Details are presented in vague and overgeneralized ways. There is very little tolerance for frustration, resulting in demands for immediate gratification. As opposed to the more well-integrated, higher-functioning, neurotic "hysterical personality" often written about in the psychoanalytic literature, the histrionic personality disorder organization more closely resembles the borderline. Particular borderline aspects include a tendency to utilize splitting defenses, rather than repression, and a marked degree of identity diffusion (Akhtar 1992). The attention-seeking attribute can be helpful in establishing a preliminary alliance. However, as with patients with borderline pathology, the clinician must be prepared to manage escalating demands and dramatic acting-out.

Antisocial

Antisocial personality is associated with ongoing violation of society's norms, manifested in such behaviors as theft, intimidation, violence, or making a living in an illegal fashion such as by fraud or selling drugs. Also narcissistic by definition, people with antisocial personality disorder have little or no regard for the welfare of others. Clearly, this personality disorder is found extensively among inmates within the prison system. Stone (1993) suggested that there are gradations of the antisocial style, with the milder forms being more amenable to treatment. However, within the broader label of *antisocial* is a subset of individuals who are considered to be psychopathic. Psychopaths are sadistic and manipulative pathological liars; show no empathy, compassion, or remorse for hurting others; and take no responsibility for their actions. The most dramatic form is manifested by individuals who torture or murder their victims. Those who perpetrate such violence reside on the extreme end of the spectrum of antisocial behavior and would be the most difficult to treat.

In keeping with the notion that there is a spectrum of antisocial psychopathology, empirical evidence shows that some antisocial patients are capable of forming a treatment alliance resulting in positive outcome (Gerstley et al. 1989). Consequently, it has been recommended by some that a trial treatment of several sessions be applied with antisocial patients who may typically be assumed to be untreatable. However, there is always the risk that such patients, particularly within an institutional context (e.g., a hospital or prison), may exhibit a pseudoalliance to gain certain advantages (Gabbard 2000). For example, there could be a disingenuous profession of enhanced self-understanding and movement toward reform as an attempt to manipulate the therapist into recommending inappropriate privileges.

There is some indication that depression serves as a moderator in the treatment of antisocial patients. One study demonstrated that depressed antisocial patients are more likely to benefit from treatment compared with nondepressed antisocial patients (Shea et al. 1992). Thus, the presence of depression may serve as motivation for these patients to seek and comply with treatment.

Sadomasochistic Character

Cases in which difficult patients take a prominent role in orchestrating situations to sabotage a potentially helpful treatment are ubiquitous in the clinical literature. This type of dynamic points to an additional element commonly overlooked in treatments in general but of particular relevance when trying to establish and maintain an alliance with patients with character pathology: sadomasochism. Most dramatically overt in patients with borderline, narcissistic, and/or antisocial issues, relational tendencies that are anywhere from tinged to saturated by sadomasochistic trends span the spectrum of personality disorder pathology. The presence of sadomasochistic patterns does not mean that overt sexual perversions will be present, although they may be, but that the patient has characteristic ways of engaging others in a struggle in which one party is suffering at the hands of the other. Although masochism is taken up in the psychoanalysis chapter of this book (see Chapter 16, "Psychoanalysis"), patients with a sadomasochistic approach to relationships make it very difficult for the clinician working in any modality to be a helpful agent of change. Furthermore, it is sometimes the case with such patients that at the foundation of the alliance is a very subtle, or not so subtle, sadomasochistic enactment.

For example, a patient may, on the surface, be agreeing with the therapist's observations but is actually experiencing them as verbal assaults while masochistically suffering in silence and showing no improvement in treatment. There is the patient who is highly provocative, attempting to bait the therapist into saying and doing things that may prove to be counterattacks. There are also patients who act out in apparently punishing ways, such as attempting suicide using a newly prescribed medication when it seemed as though the treatment was progressing.

Bach (1994) described a sadomasochistic way of relating as arising as "a defense against and an attempt to repair some traumatic loss that has not been adequately mourned" (p. 4). This trauma could have come in the form of an actual loss of a parent, loss of love as a result of abuse or neglect, or some experience of loss of the self due to such things as childhood illness or circumstances leading to overwhelming anxiety. From this perspective, the cruel behavior of the sadist may, for instance, be an attempt to punish the object for threatened abandonment. The masochistic stance involves a way of loving someone who gives ill treatment—the only way of maintaining a connection is through suffering (Berliner 1947). Early in development, this way of loving is self-preservative—the sadism of the love object is turned upon the self as a way of maintaining a needed relationship (Menaker 1953). However, in an adult, this masochistic solution, with its always-attendant aggressive-sadistic elements, serves to cause significant interpersonal dysfunction.

Case Example

A single woman in her forties, Ms. U, was referred for psychotherapy after she had gone to see four or five other therapists, staying for only several sessions maximum because she found them all to be incompetent in some way. An avid reader of self-help literature, she considered herself an expert on the helping professions. Highly intelligent and extremely articulate, Ms. U was aspiring to be a filmmaker. She had gone through a series of "day jobs" with corporations, reporting that her women supervisors were always untalented, unreasonable, and critical of her. Her interpersonal relations were always tumultuous, her moods very unstable, and it was apparent that she had been grappling with narcissistic and borderline personality disorder issues for decades.

Sadomasochistic trends became apparent very quickly. In the first meeting, Ms. U launched the first of many critiques, reporting that she had found the therapist's greeting to be too upbeat but then also criticizing the therapist for not reassuring her that she would have a successful treatment. She ultimately announced that the therapist was "gifted," so she would continue with this treatment, but there were many sessions in which she would find fault or deliver lectures on technique and theory. At the same time, she was extremely brittle and incapable of reflecting on this type of behavior, feeling as a victim if there was any vague hint that she might be doing something questionable. Thus, while attacking the therapist, she was doing it in the service of collecting grievances and, as Berliner (1947) observed about such patients, she "would rather be right than happy" (p. 46). Hence, both the sadistic and masochistic sides of the same coin were in evidence.

As stated previously, with patients such as this one, it is very important to be able to tolerate the expression of aggression. Consequently, to maintain an alliance with this very difficult woman, the therapist had to constantly assess whether the attacks represented a rupture in the alliance that had to be addressed or whether Ms. U simply needed to give voice to some of her tremendous anger at the world. In the instances it was judged that the alliance was in jeopardy, the therapist would discuss Ms. U's reaction to the therapist's interventions, acknowledging Ms. U's distress and telling Ms. U that the therapist would reflect on what had led her to make such comments. Ms. U usually found great relief in this approach, appreciating the therapist's willingness to reflect on the situation.

What is central is that the therapist withstood being portrayed as bad or incompetent in the patient's mind without retaliating as though it were true. If the therapist had had a different psychology, it would have been rather easy to take up the role of sadist in all of this, perhaps wrapped in the flag of "interpreting her aggression"; however, Ms. U and this therapist were a good match, because such retributive behavior would have been a sadomasochistic enactment and would have caused Ms. U to take a hasty departure.

Cluster C

The "anxious/fearful" cluster comprises avoidant, dependent, and obsessive-compulsive personality disorders. Patients who are most closely characterized by Cluster C disorders are emotionally inhibited and averse to interpersonal conflict and are often considered to be the treatable "neurotics" on the spectrum of personality disorders. These patients frequently feel very guilty and internalize blame for situations even when it is clear there is none. This latter tendency often facilitates alliance building, because the patient is willing to take some responsibility for his or her dilemma and will somewhat more readily engage in a dialogue with the therapist to sort it all out, compared with patients with more severe Cluster A or B diagnoses (Stone 1993).

Dependent

Fearing abandonment, dependent patients tend to be very passive, submissive, and needy of constant reassurance. They go to great lengths not to offend others, even at great emotional expense, agreeing with others' opinions when they really do not or volunteering to do unsavory chores to stay in someone's good graces. In the context of treatment, dependent patients are easily engaged, at least superficially, but often withhold a great deal of material for fear of alienating the therapist in some way. The following is an example of how this might play out (Benjamin 1993).

> A patient [with dependent personality disorder] was chronically depressed, and the doctor tried her on a new antidepressant. She did not improve and had a number of side effects, but did not mention them to the doctor. Fortunately, the doctor remembered to ask for the specific side effects. The patient acknowledged the signs, and the doctor wrote a prescription for a different antidepressant. The patient was willing to acknowledge the signs of problems…, but she did not offer the information spontaneously. The doctor asked her why she did not say anything. She explained, "I thought that maybe they were just part of the way the drug worked…. I figured you would know what was best." (p. 405)

Benjamin also observed that one difficulty in working in psychotherapy with such patients is the reinforcement gained by the patient's behavior. That is, because the passivity and submissiveness usually result in being taken care of, despite the associated cost, dependent patients are loath to see the value in asserting some independence. Furthermore, there is a deeply ingrained assumption by these patients that they are actually incapable of functioning more independently and that being

more assertive will be experienced by others as alienating aggressiveness. Thus, a therapist must be very alert to the withdrawal types of strains and ruptures, such as withholding information, as well as to the challenge to the alliance that may occur when the therapist attempts to encourage more independence.

Avoidant

The avoidant individual is extremely interpersonally sensitive, afraid of being criticized, and constantly concerned about saying or doing something foolish or humiliating. In spite of an intense desire to connect with others, an avoidant person does not let anyone get close unless absolutely sure the person likes him or her. Because of this acute sensitivity, there is some evidence that some avoidant patients are somewhat difficult to retain in treatment. One study showed that a group of avoidant patients was significantly more likely to drop out of a short-term supportive-expressive treatment compared with obsessive-compulsive personality disorder patients (Barber et al. 1997). Clinicians who work with avoidant patients need to be constantly mindful of the potentially shaming effects of certain comments but can also work with the patient's underlying hunger for attachment to enlist them in building an alliance.

Furthermore, there is preliminary evidence supporting the notion that at least some patients diagnosed with avoidant personality disorder are actually better characterized as vulnerable narcissists. These patients covertly crave admiration to bolster their fragile self-esteem and secretly or unconsciously feel entitled to it rather than simply being afraid of not being liked or accepted (Dickenson and Pincus 2003). Gabbard (2000) also referred to this style as *hypervigilant narcissism*, emphasizing extreme interpersonal sensitivity, other-directedness, and shame proneness aspects. An underlying unrecognized narcissism in avoidant personality disorder has significant treatment implications, changing the nature of the forces affecting the alliance as well as shaping the types of treatment interventions that are indicated.

Obsessive-Compulsive

The obsessive-compulsive character is associated with more stable interpersonal relationships than some other styles, but typical defenses are centered on repression, with patterns of highly regulated gratification and ongoing denial of interpersonal and intrapsychic conflicts (Shapiro 1965). Self-willed and obstinate, with a constant eye toward rules and regulations, people with obsessive-compulsive attributes guard against any meaningful consideration of their impulses toward others. Maintaining control over internal experience and the external world is a top priority, so rigidity is often a hallmark of this character type. Except in its most severe manifestations, obsessive-compulsive character pathology is less impairing than some of the others and more readily ameliorated by treatment. Although stubborn and controlling and averse to considering emotional content, obsessive-compulsive individuals also generally try to be "good patients" and so can be engaged in a constructive alliance that is less rocky compared with other types of personality disorder patients.

Case Example

Mr. V, a 25-year-old philosophy graduate student, began a twice-weekly psychotherapy. His presenting complaint was difficulty with completing work effectively, particularly writing tasks, due to excessive anxiety and obsessionality (he met criteria for obsessive-compulsive personality disorder and generalized anxiety disorder). When he came for treatment, he was struggling to make progress on his masters thesis. Although Mr. V socialized quite a bit, he reported that intimate relationships often felt "wooden." He was usually overcommitted, with an endless list of "shoulds" that he would constantly mentally review and remind himself how much he was failing to satisfy his obligations. A central theme throughout treatment was his tendency to be self-denigrating, loathing himself as a person deserving of punishment in some way yet being extremely provocative (sadomasochistic trends). He also held very strong political beliefs, sure that his way of viewing things was superior to others'.

Establishing a productive alliance with Mr. V was not easily accomplished at first. In the early phase of treatment, he was extremely controlling and challenging in sessions, talking constantly and tangentially, often losing the core point of his statements because of a need to present excessive details. Any statement the therapist made was experienced as an intrusion or interruption. For example, if the therapist attempted to be empathic using a word Mr. V had not used, such as saying, "That sounds difficult," he would respond, "Difficult? I don't know if I'd choose the word difficult. Challenging, maybe, or daunting, but not difficult." Thus, for a number of months in the initial phase of the treatment, the therapist chose her words carefully, which eventually paved the way for increased dialogue about his problems. Mr. V also began to tolerate a discussion of his emotional life, a topic that previously had been very threatening to him.

Passive-Aggressive

Some of the aspects of this latter case example may be described as passive-aggressive, particularly the patient's tendency to excessively procrastinate in doing his work. Passive-aggressive traits include argumentativeness, scorning authority, resistance to carrying out social and occupational responsibilities, angry pessimism, alternating between defiance and contrition, envy, and exaggerated complaints about personal misfortune. These attributes pose challenges to the formation of an effective therapeutic alliance because these patients are likely to expect that the treatment holds no promise of helping, and they behave in ways that contribute to that outcome. The passive-aggressive (negativistic) personality disorder diagnosis was included in Cluster C in DSM-III-R (American Psychiatric Association 1987) but was subsequently shifted to the appendix of disorders needing further study in DSM-IV (American Psychiatric Association 1994). Some experts on phenomenology argue that this diagnosis is clinically very useful and should be restored to the DSM list of personality disorders (e.g., Wetzler and Morey 1999).

ALLIANCE CONSIDERATIONS WITHIN DIFFERENT TREATMENT PARADIGMS

Clearly, no matter what treatment paradigm one adopts for working with personality disorder patients, attention to the alliance is of utmost importance. Thoughts and feelings on the part of the therapist must be monitored closely, because interactions with difficult patients may often be provocative, inducing reactions that must be carefully managed. (Refer to Chapter 27, "Boundary Issues," for a discussion of some of the most serious consequences of treatments gone awry.) Although this topic is usually discussed as countertransference in the psychoanalytic/psychodynamic tradition, it is also quite applicable across all treatments (Gabbard 1999).

Treatment approach and technique must be flexible so that interventions can be made appropriate to the individual patient's style. Otherwise, the alliance may be jeopardized and the patient will not benefit or may leave treatment altogether. Furthermore, it is likely that noticeable improvements in symptoms and functioning in such patients will likely require a significantly longer period of treatment than for patients with no character pathology. Although the application of specific treatment approaches is discussed at length in other chapters of this book, it is worth mentioning here a few alliance-relevant considerations pertaining to each broad treatment context.

Psychodynamic Psychotherapy/ Psychoanalysis

One long-standing issue within the psychodynamic psychotherapy tradition is the application of particular techniques. Interpretation of the transference was long considered the heart of the psychoanalytic approach. However, as the application of this treatment evolved and clinicians gained more experience with more disturbed patients—most notably those with borderline and narcissistic trends—it became apparent that, in many cases, transference interpretations with such patients were often counterproductive. Refraining from making deep, interpretive interventions early on is consistent with notions of writers such as Winnicott (1965) and Kohut (1984) who asserted that certain, more disturbed, patients cannot tolerate such interpretations in the initial phase of treatment.

Gabbard (2000) stressed the importance of understanding that there is usually a mixture of supportive and expressive (interpretive) elements in every analysis or psychodynamic psychotherapy. That is, the expressive, insight-oriented mode of assisting patients in uncovering unconscious conflicts, thoughts, or affects through interpretation or confrontation may be appropriate at times, whereas a more supportive approach of bolstering the patient's defenses and coping abilities is preferable in other circumstances.

For instance, it may be difficult to focus on more insight-oriented interventions with a patient with borderline impairments until that patient is assisted in achieving a safe, more stable alliance. Similarly, the severely narcissistically impaired patient may not be able to accept the analyst's interpretations of his or her unconscious motivations for quite a long time, so that supportive, empathic communications may be more effective interventions in building an alliance by helping the patient feel heard and understood. Conversely, some obsessional patients may benefit earlier in treatment by interpretations of the repressed conflicts that may underlie the symptoms.

The results of the Psychotherapy Research Project of The Menninger Foundation, which included patients with personality disorders, led Wallerstein (1986) to conclude that both expressive and supportive interventions can lead to character change. At the same time, there is empirical evidence supporting the notion that a fairly solid alliance must be present to effectively utilize transference interpretations per se. Bond et al. (1998) demonstrated with a group of personality disorder patients in long-term treatment that for those patients whose alliance was weak, transference interpretations caused further impairment to the alliance. Conversely, the alliance was strengthened by transference interpretations when already solidly established. At the same time, supportive interventions and discussions of defensive operations resulted in moving the therapeutic work forward with both the weak and strong alliance groups of patients.

These findings are consistent with a study conducted by Horwitz et al. (1996) exploring the effect of supportive and interpretive interventions on the therapeutic alliance with a group of patients with borderline personality disorder. The authors concluded that although many times therapists are eager to pursue transference interpretations, such interventions are "high-risk, high-gain" and need to be employed carefully. They may damage the alliance with patients who are vulnerable and prone to feelings of shame and humiliation. Therefore, there must be flexibility in adjusting technique according to the dynamics of a particular patient at a particular time given the patient's capacities and vulnerabilities, appropriately balancing both supportive and expressive interventions.

Case Example

Ms. W sought treatment when she was in her early 30s. She was referred for psychotherapy from her graduate school's counseling center. Ms. W presented in a major depressive episode and met eight out of a possible nine criteria for borderline personality disorder. The initial phase of the twice-weekly psychodynamic treatment focused on her depression and helping her to stabilize sometimes-devastating affective instability. She also reported intermittent, but not life-threatening, instances of cutting herself, particularly after some unsatisfactory encounter with a friend or colleague.

The patient's lack of object constancy, her affective instability, and a fragmented sense of self contributed to great variations in the nature of Ms. W's presence in sessions. At times she would be overwhelmed by fatigue, whereas other times she would be engaging, funny, and analytical. She would often defend against undesirable thoughts or emotions by spending the session recounting the details of her day-to-day life in great detail. The disjunctions in self-states made it difficult at times to maintain continuity in the process, because Ms. W did not remember what happened from session to session.

A Kernbergian formulation (Kernberg 1967) of this patient was theoretically informative in describing some of her dynamics (defensive splitting had been one prominent theme in the treatment). However, the technical implications of this particular approach, with its direct confrontation of aggression in the transference early in the treatment (Kernberg 1987) would have endangered the sometimes fragile working alliance being forged. In fact, a few times when transference interpretations were attempted in the first phase of treatment, Ms. W became confused and distressed, quickly changing the subject away from a discussion of her relationship with the therapist, talking about ending treatment, or becoming very sleepy and shut down for several sessions. On one occasion early on when an attempt was made by the therapist to address something in their relationship, Ms. W became very angry and said, "Why is any of this about here? These are my problems and I don't see what any of this has to do with you!" Clearly, in the beginning phase of treatment with some patients, one needs a different way of entering the patient's psychic world (Ellman 1998). On the other hand, Ms. W was responsive to gentle interpretations of her defenses, such as the therapist pointing out to her that her self-harm behaviors were a way of "being mean" to herself instead of channeling anger toward those who had upset her.

Thus, for most of the first 3–4 years of this treatment, the primary tasks were to develop a working alliance and establish a "holding environment" (Winnicott 1965) within which Ms. W could begin to feel safe to explore her history, her feelings, and her own mind. This approach paid off, because it eventually became possible to uncover, in ways that were meaningful and transformative to Ms. W, some of the split-off rage and despair underlying the identity instability and distorted cognitive functioning. Deeper experience and exploration of these feelings paved the way for further integration and less disjunctive experiences in her life and from session to session, and working with the transference increasingly became both possible and very productive. Ms. W has not been depressed for years and no longer meets any borderline criteria.

Cognitive-Behavioral Therapies

In recent years, work has been done to apply to personality disorders cognitive and cognitive-behavioral treatments that have typically been used to treat Axis I symptoms. However, Tyrer and Davidson (2000) observed that the approaches generally taken in these therapies for Axis I "mental state disorders" cannot be simply transferred to treating personality disorders without certain adjustments. Most cognitive and cognitive-behavioral therapies are based prominently on a therapist–patient collaboration that is assumed to be present from very early in the treatment. Such a collaboration, which revolves around the patient undertaking specific activities and assignments, depends on the establishment of a solid working alliance; however, it is sometimes very difficult to engage certain personality disorder patients in the therapeutic tasks. To facilitate this alliance when working with personality disorder patients—in addition to requiring lengthier periods to complete these treatments—work needs to directly address patient–therapist collaboration with clearly set boundaries and to focus on the therapeutic relationship itself when appropriate (Tyrer and Davidson 2000).

For example, in using the initial sessions of dialectical behavior therapy (DBT) (see Chapter 19, "Dialectical Behavior Therapy") to begin establishing a working relationship, Marsha Linehan (1993) observed: "These sessions offer an opportunity for both patient and therapist to explore problems that may arise in establishing and maintaining a therapeutic alliance" (p. 446). Even though DBT is a manualized treatment with clearly elaborated therapeutic tasks, it is quickly evident, particularly in working with borderline patients, that a great deal of flexibility must be maintained within this paradigm to achieve an alliance. More specifically, there may be frequent occurrences of therapy-interfering behaviors ranging from ambivalence causing missed sessions to multiple suicide attempts that prevent the treatment from progressing as the method outlines.

Case Example

Ms. X, a young woman with dependent personality disorder, was referred for behavioral treatment of a phobia of all forms of transportation (her other issues were already being addressed in an ongoing psychotherapy). The therapist spent several sessions with Ms. X outlining the exposure techniques recommended for treating her phobia, but she was resistant to beginning any of the activities described. At the same time, while trying to pursue a classically behavioral approach, the therapist realized that it was very important for Ms. X to spend some of the time talking about her life and the impact the phobia symptoms had for her. This approach helped Ms. X to feel a connection to the therapist. The therapist made this relationship-building aspect explicit with Ms. X by agreeing to take a part of each session to talk about her situation, but the therapist also made it clear that it was necessary to reserve enough time for the exposure activities. This approach fostered an alliance sufficiently to begin the behavioral tasks. By being flexible, while setting clear tasks and boundaries, the therapist was able to engage Ms. X in the treatment, and she began taking short rides with the therapist on the bus, eventually overcoming these fears completely.

Psychopharmacology Sessions

One large-scale depression study (Krupnick et al. 1996) comparing several different psychotherapies with medication and placebo showed that the quality of the alliance was significantly related to outcome for all of the study groups. This finding demonstrates the importance of considering the alliance not only in psychotherapies but in medication sessions as well. Gutheil (1982) suggested that there is a particular aspect of the therapeutic alliance—what he calls the *pharmacotherapeutic alliance*—that is relevant to the prescription of medications. In this formulation of the alliance, it is recommended that the physician adopt the stance of *participant prescribing*—that is, rather than adopting an authoritarian role, the clinician should make every effort to involve the patient as a collaborator who engages actively in goal-setting and observing and evaluating the experience of using specific medications. Such collaboration, like other therapeutic processes, may be affected by the patient's transference distortions of the clinician.

This latter notion can be more broadly applied in transtheoretical terms to personality disorders, where it is appropriate to consider how the patient's characteristic style may influence his or her attitudes and behaviors toward taking psychiatric medications. Some patients may become upset if medication is not prescribed, feeling slighted because they think their problems are not being taken seriously. Others with paranoid tendencies may think the physician is trying to put something over on them, or worse. Some patients who are prone to somaticizing, such as those with borderline or histrionic tendencies, might be hypersensitive to any possible side effects (real or imagined) and argue with the prescriber about his or her competence. The following is another example (Benjamin 1993) illustrating the importance of being mindful of how personality disorder patients might react around issues of medication:

> A patient [with avoidant personality disorder] overdosed one evening on the medicine her doctor had prescribed for her persistent depression. She liked and respected him a lot. She was discovered comatose by a neighbor who wondered why her cat would not stop meowing. The neighbor was the patient's only friend. It turned out that that morning her doctor had wondered aloud whether she had a personality disorder. The patient was deeply humiliated by that idea but secretly agreed with it. She felt extremely embarrassed and was convinced that her doctor now knew she was a completely foolish person.... Rather than endure the humiliation of facing him again, she decided to end it all. (p. 411)

Psychiatric Hospital Settings

Across the spectrum of personality disorders, psychiatric hospitalizations—both inpatient and day treatment programs—are most common for those with borderline personality disorder (Bender et al. 2001).

The central consideration regarding the alliance in this treatment context is that there is always a team of individuals responsible for the patient. With patients with borderline issues, splitting tendencies frequently are quite pronounced. That is, as a way of trying to cope with inner turmoil, the patient's mental world is often organized in black/white, good/bad polarities, and through complicated (see explanation of projective identification in Chapter 16, "Psychoanalysis") interaction patterns with various staff members, this internal world becomes replayed externally, dividing staff member against staff member.

Gabbard (1989) observed that this dynamic is often set up because the patient will present one self-representation to one or several team members and a very different representation to another. One of these staff factions may be viewed as the "good" one by the patient and the other as the "bad" one—although these designations can flip precipitously in the patient's mind—and this split becomes enacted among team members as they begin to work at cross purposes. It can be seen rather readily that trying to develop a constructive alliance with such a patient can be extremely precarious, particularly given the ever-decreasing length of hospital stays under managed care. That means that communication and close collaboration among the members of the team are vital during every phase of the hospital treatment.

Matters are complicated further at times by the need to find a productive way for hospital staff to collaborate with clinicians providing ongoing outpatient psychotherapy and/or psychopharmacology treatments. Although the hospitalization may represent a significant rupture in the outpatient treatment alliance, this rupture does not necessarily indicate that the outpatient treatment was ineffective and must be terminated but that work will be needed to reestablish the continuity of the treatment relationship. However, it is not uncommon for the hospital staff, seeing the patient's current condition, to conclude that the outpatient clinicians were somehow not doing a competent job (this conclusion may, of course, be fueled by further splitting on the part of the patient). Moreover, at times it may be obvious that the outpatient treatment was inadequate or inappropriate. In any event, it becomes rather dicey for all parties concerned to sort out the proper role of hospital staff versus outpatient staff over the course of the inpatient or day treatment program.

Case Example

A young woman, Ms. Y, with borderline personality disorder was admitted to a psychiatric inpatient unit

Table 26–2. Instruments for measuring alliance

Instrument	Type of measure	Attributes
Pennsylvania scales		
Helping Alliance Counting Signs (Alexander and Luborsky 1986)	Observers or therapists rate transcripts on occurrences of seven subtypes	All of the Pennsylvania scales have been designed to measure a psychodynamic conceptualization of two dimensions of the alliance:
Helping Alliance Rating Measure (Alexander and Luborsky 1986)	Observers or therapists rate brief samples of transcribed, videotaped, or live therapy on occurrences of 10 subtypes	1) The patient's experience of the clinician providing needed help (type 1 signs) 2) The patient's experience of working in collaboration with
Helping Alliance Questionnaire Method (Alexander and Luborsky 1986)	Patient self-report (11 items)	the therapist in working toward treatment goals (type 2 signs)
Vanderbilt scales		
Vanderbilt Psychotherapy Process Scale (Suh et al. 1986)	Observers rate videotaped therapy segments (80 items)	Measures positive and negative aspects of patient and therapist attitudes and behaviors, not simply alliance
Vanderbilt Therapeutic Alliance Scale (Hartley and Strupp 1983)	Observers rate videotaped therapy segments (44 items)	Alliance-specific version
Toronto scales		
Therapeutic Alliance Rating Scale (Marziali et al. 1981)	Observer-rated (42 items)	All Toronto scales are based on psychodynamic conceptualizations of the alliance along with Bordin's (1979)
Therapist Alliance Rating Scale–Therapist Version (Marziali 1984)	Therapist-rated (42 items)	integrative model; particular focus on affective elements of the alliance
Therapist Alliance Rating Scale–Patient Version (Marziali 1984)	Patient-rated (42 items)	
Working Alliance Inventory (Horvath and Greenberg 1986)	Therapist- and patient-rated versions each have 36 items	Designed for application to all models of therapy; measures Bordin's (1979) bond, tasks, goals dimensions of alliance; applicable to very early treatment sessions
California scales		
California Therapeutic Alliance Rating System (Marmar et al. 1989b)	Observer-rated audiotapes (41 items)	Includes four scales: 1) Therapist positive contribution 2) Therapist negative contribution 3) Patient positive contribution 4) Patient negative contribution
California Psychotherapy Alliance Scales (Marmar et al. 1989a)	Therapist- and patient-rated versions (31 items)	Adds: 1) Patient working capacity 2) Patient commitment 3) Therapist understanding and involvement 4) Working strategy consensus 5) Goal consensus
Therapeutic Bond Scales (Saunders et al. 1989)	Patient-rated (50 items)	Measures three dimensions: 1) Working alliance 2) Empathic resonance 3) Mutual affirmation

Source. Adapted from Martin et al. (2000)

after coming to the emergency department reporting acute suicidal ideation. This patient had been hospitalized several times previously, was in the mental health field, and "knew the ropes" quite well. She had been assigned a psychiatrist who was responsible for overall case management and a psychologist who was to provide short-term psychotherapy on the unit.

The initial psychotherapy session was extremely difficult, with Ms. Y refusing to speak very much and regarding the therapist with rageful contempt. However, after several more encounters, there was some softening by Ms. Y and she began to discuss the upsetting circumstances that led to her hospitalization. It appeared there might be the beginnings of a working alliance. Indeed, as she opened up more about her life, she reported feeling slightly more hopeful and less fragmented.

However, at the same time, she had created quite a bit of trouble with the rest of the staff by being very demanding and uncooperative and attempting to initiate discharge procedures even while refusing to deny that she would kill herself. Having reached a point of needing to take some action in the courts to keep Ms. Y hospitalized, the psychiatrist hastily called a meeting including himself, the psychologist, and the patient. Having had no opportunity to confer with other team members on the matter, the psychiatrist proceeded to tell Ms. Y that he was initiating legal proceedings to keep her in the hospital. Mindful of the splitting tendencies of such patients, the psychiatrist was careful to make it clear that he represented the viewpoint of the entire team, including the psychologist. However, he unwittingly created another split. Ms. Y, feeling betrayed, stared hatefully at the psychologist, the fragile working alliance was shattered, and she subsequently refused to participate in psychotherapy or any other therapeutic activities for the rest of the hospitalization. It is possible this rupture could have been ameliorated had there been adequate consultation among treatment team members so that a less alienating approach could be formulated.

STUDYING THE THERAPEUTIC ALLIANCE

There has not been a great deal of empirical inquiry, particularly across long-term treatments, about the nature and vicissitudes of the alliance when working specifically in treating character pathology. Thus, we are left to hope that this work will be taken up in the future by those who have some interest in pursuing this line of research. In this vein, utilizing a meta-analysis conducted by Martin et al. (2000), the major instruments for studying alliance are briefly summarized in Table 26–2.

CONCLUSION

Establishing an alliance in any treatment paradigm requires a great deal of empathy and attunement to a patient's way of seeing the world. Attention to alliance-building is even more important when working with patients with personality disorders, because these individuals often present with disturbed patterns of interpersonal relations. Research has shown not only the importance of building an alliance but also that this alliance is vital in the earliest phase of treatment. One cannot rigidly pursue the dictates of one's treatment paradigm without being prepared to make frequent adjustments to address the various ruptures that may occur. Gleaning clues from the patient's accounts of his or her relationships can serve to guide the clinician's general interpersonal stance. Furthermore, monitoring the therapeutic alliance in response to clinical interventions is a useful way to assess the effectiveness of one's approach and is informative in determining appropriate adjustments in the style and content of the therapist's interactions with the patient.

REFERENCES

Adler G: Transference, real relationship and alliance. Int J Psychoanal 61:547–558, 1980

Akhtar S: Broken Structures: Severe Personality Disorders and Their Treatment. Northvale, NJ, Jason Aronson, 1992

Alexander LB, Luborsky L: The Penn Helping Alliance Scales in The Psychotherapeutic Process: A Research Handbook. Edited by Greenberg LS, Pinsof WM. New York, Guilford, 1986, pp 325–366

American Psychiatric Association: Diagnostic and Statistical Manual of Mental Disorders, 3rd Edition, Revised. Washington, DC, American Psychiatric Association, 1987

American Psychiatric Association: Diagnostic and Statistical Manual of Mental Disorders, 4th Edition. Washington, DC, American Psychiatric Association, 1994

American Psychiatric Association: Diagnostic and Statistical Manual of Mental Disorders, 4th Edition, Text Revision. Washington, DC, American Psychiatric Association, 2000

Bach S: The Language of Perversion and the Language of Love. Northvale, NJ, Jason Aronson, 1994

Bach S: On treating the difficult patient, in The Modern Freudians. Edited by Ellman CS, Grand S, Silvan M, et al. Northvale, NJ, Jason Aronson, 1998, pp 185–195

Barber JP, Morse JQ, Krakauer ID, et al: Change in obsessive-compulsive and avoidant personality disorders following time-limited supportive-expressive therapy. Psychotherapy 34:133–143, 1997

Bender DS, Dolan RT, Skodol AE, et al: Treatment utilization by patients with personality disorders. Am J Psychiatry 158:295–302, 2001

Bender DS, Farber BA, Sanislow CA, et al: Representations of therapists by patients with personality disorders. Am J Psychother 57:219–236, 2003

Benjamin LS: Interpersonal Diagnosis and Treatment of Personality Disorders. New York, Guilford, 1993

Berliner B: The role of object relations in moral masochism. Psychoanal Q 27:38–56, 1947

Bond M, Banon E, Grenier M: Differential effects of interventions on the therapeutic alliance with patients with personality disorders. J Psychother Pract Res 7:301–318, 1998

Bordin ES: The generalizability of the psychoanalytic concept of the working alliance. Psychotherapy: Theory, Research and Practice 16:252–260, 1979

Diamond D, Stovall-McClough C, Clarkin JF, et al: Patient–therapist attachment in the treatment of borderline personality disorder. Bull Menninger Clin 67:227–259, 2003

Dickenson KA, Pincus AL: Interpersonal analysis of grandiose and vulnerable narcissism. J Personal Disord 17:188–207, 2003

Ellman SJ: Freud's Technique Papers: A Contemporary Perspective. Northvale, NJ, Jason Aronson, 1991

Ellman SJ: The unique contribution of the contemporary Freudian position, in The Modern Freudians. Edited by Ellman CS, Grand S, Silvan M, et al. Northvale, NJ, Jason Aronson, 1998, pp 237–268

Freud S: The dynamics of the transference (1912), in Collected Papers, Vol 2. Translated by Riviere J. London, Hogarth Press, 1946, pp 312–322

Gabbard GO: Splitting in hospital treatment. Am J Psychiatry 146:444–451, 1989

Gabbard GO: An overview of countertransference: theory and technique, in Countertransference Issues in Psychiatric Treatment. Edited by Gabbard GO (Review of Psychiatry Series, Vol 18; Oldham JM, Riba MB, series eds). Washington, DC, American Psychiatric Press, 1999, pp 1–25

Gabbard GO: Psychodynamic Psychiatry in Clinical Practice. Washington, DC, American Psychiatric Press, 2000

Gerstley L, McLellan AT, Alterman AI, et al: Ability to form an alliance with the therapist: a possible social marker of prognosis for patients with antisocial personality disorder. Am J Psychiatry 146:508–512, 1989

Gibbons MBC, Crits-Cristoph P, de la Cruz C, et al: Pretreatment expectations, interpersonal functioning, and symptoms in the prediction of the therapeutic alliance across supportive-expressive psychotherapy and cognitive therapy. Psychother Res 13:59–76, 2003

Gunderson JG: Psychodynamic psychotherapy for borderline personality disorder, in Psychotherapy for Personality Disorders. Edited by Gunderson JG, Gabbard GO (Review of Psychiatry, Vol 19; Oldham JM, Riba MB, series eds). Washington, DC, American Psychiatric Press, 2000, pp 33–64

Gunderson JG, Najavits LM, Leonhard C, et al: Ontogeny of the therapeutic alliance in borderline patients. Psychother Res 7:301–309, 1997

Gutheil TG: The psychology of psychopharmacology. Bull Menninger Clin 46:321–330, 1982

Gutheil TG, Havens LL: The therapeutic alliance: contemporary meanings and confusions. Int Rev Psychoanal 6:467–481, 1979

Hartley D, Strupp H: The therapeutic alliance: its relationship to outcome in brief psychotherapy in Empirical Studies of Psychoanalytic Theories. Edited by Masling J. Hillsdale, NJ, Erlbaum, 1983, pp 1–27

Hersoug AG, Monsen J, Havik OE, et al: Quality of working alliance in psychotherapy: diagnoses, relationship and intrapsychic variables as predictors. Psychother Psychosom 71:18–27, 2002

Hill CE, Thompson BJ, Cogar MC, et al: Beneath the surface of long-term therapy: therapist and client report of their own and each other's covert processes. J Couns Psychol 40:278–287, 1993

Horvath AO, Greenberg LS: The development of the working alliance inventory, in The Psychotherapeutic Process: A Research Handbook. Edited by Greenberg LS, Pinsof WM. New York, Guilford, 1986, pp 529–556

Horvath AO, Greenberg LS (eds): The Working Alliance: Theory, Research, and Practice. New York, Wiley, 1994

Horvath AO, Luborsky L: The role of therapeutic alliance in psychotherapy. J Consult Clin Psychol 61:561–573, 1993

Horvath AO, Symonds BD: Relation between working alliance and outcome in psychotherapy: a meta-analysis. J Couns Psychol 38:139–149, 1991

Horwitz L, Gabbard GO, Allen JG, et al: Borderline Personality Disorder: Tailoring the Psychotherapy to the Patient. Washington, DC, American Psychiatric Press, 1996

Kernberg OF: Borderline personality organization. J Am Psychoanal Assoc 15:641–685, 1967

Kernberg OF: Severe Personality Disorders: Psychotherapeutic Strategies. New Haven, CT, Yale University Press, 1984

Kernberg OF: An ego psychology–object relations theory approach to the transference. Psychoanal Q 56:197–221, 1987

Kohut H: The Restoration of the Self. New York, International Universities Press, 1977

Kohut H: How Does Analysis Cure? Chicago, IL, University of Chicago Press, 1984

Krupnick JL, Sotsky SM, Simmens S, et al: The role of the therapeutic alliance in psychotherapy and pharmacotherapy outcome: findings in the National Institute of Mental Health Treatment of Depression Collaborative Research Program. J Consult Clin Psychol 65:532–539, 1996

Linehan MM: Cognitive-Behavioral Treatment of Borderline Personality Disorder. New York, Guilford, 1993

Marmar CR, Gaston L, Gallagher D, et al: Alliance and outcome in late-life depression. J Nerv Ment Dis 177:464–472, 1989a

Marmar CR, Weiss DS, Gaston L: Towards the validation of the California Therapeutic Alliance Rating System. Psychol Assess 1:46–52, 1989b

Martin DJ, Garske JP, Davis MK: Relation of the therapeutic alliance with outcome and other variables: a meta-analytic review. J Consult Clin Psychol 68:438–450, 2000

Marziali E: Three viewpoints on the therapeutic alliance scales similarities, differences and associations with psychotherapy outcome. J Nerv Ment Dis 172:417–423, 1984

Marziali E, Marmar C, Krupnick J: Therapeutic alliance scales: development and relationship to psychotherapy outcome. Am J Psychiatry 138:361–364, 1981

Masterson JF: The Search for the Real Self: Unmasking the Personality Disorders of Our Age. New York, The Free Press, 1988

McGlashan TH, Grilo CM, Skodol AE, et al: The Collaborative Longitudinal Personality Disorders Study: baseline Axis I/II and II/II diagnostic co-occurrence. Acta Psychiatr Scand 102:256–264, 2000

Menaker E: Masochism: a defense reaction of the ego. Psychoanal Q 22:205–220, 1953

Meissner WW: The Therapeutic Alliance. New Haven, CT, Yale University Press, 1996

Orlinsky DA, Grawe K, Parks BK: Process and outcome in psychotherapy: Noch einmal, in Handbook of Psychotherapy and Behavior Change, 4th Edition. Edited by Bergin AE, Garfield SL. New York, Wiley, 1994, pp 270–376

Piper WE, Azim HFA, Joyce AS, et al: Quality of object relations versus interpersonal functioning as predictors of therapeutic alliance and psychotherapy outcome. J Nerv Ment Dis 179:432–438, 1991

Safran JD, Muran JC: Negotiating the Therapeutic Alliance. New York, Guilford, 2000

Safran JD, Muran JC, Samstag LW, et al: Repairing alliance ruptures. Psychotherapy 38:406–412, 2001

Samstag LW, Batchelder S, Muran JC, et al: Predicting treatment failure from in-session interpersonal variables. J Psychother Pract Res 5:126–143, 1998

Saunders SM, Howard KI, Orlinsky DE: The Therapeutic Bond Scales: psychometric characteristics and relationship to treatment effectiveness. Psychol Assess 1:323–330, 1989

Shapiro D: Neurotic Styles. New York, Basic Books, 1965

Shea MT, Widiger TA, Klein MH: Comorbidity of personality disorders and depressions: implications for treatment. J Consult Clin Psychol 60:857–868, 1992

Stone MH: Abnormalities of Personality. New York, WW Norton, 1993

Suh CS, Strupp HH, O'Malley SS: The Vanderbilt Process Measures: The Psychotherapy Process Scale (VPPS) and the Negative Indicators Scale (VNIS) Inventory, in The Psychotherapeutic Process: A Research Handbook. Edited by Greenberg LS, Pinsof WM. New York, Guilford, 1986, pp 285–323

Tyrer P, Davidson K: Cognitive therapy for personality disorders, in Psychotherapy for Personality Disorders. Edited by Gunderson JG, Gabbard GO (Review of Psychiatry, Vol 19; Oldham JM, Riba MB, series eds). Washington, DC, American Psychiatric Press, 2000, pp 131–149

Waldinger RJ, Gunderson JG: Completed psychotherapies with borderline patients. Am J Psychother 38:190–202, 1984

Wallerstein RS: Forty-Two Lives in Treatment: A Study of Psychoanalysis and Psychotherapy. New York, Guilford, 1986

Wetzler S, Morey LC: Passive-aggressive personality disorder: the demise of a syndrome. Psychiatry 62:49–59, 1999

Winnicott DW: The Maturational Processes and the Facilitating Environment. London, Hogarth Press, 1965

27

Boundary Issues

Thomas G. Gutheil, M.D.

Experience teaches us that any discussion of boundary issues—boundary crossings and violations—must begin with certain caveats, best delivered in the form of axioms. First, only the professional member of the treatment dyad has a professional code to honor or violate; thus only the professional is responsible for setting and maintaining professional boundaries. Second, patients, having no professional code, may transgress or attempt to transgress professional boundaries; if they are competent adults, they are responsible or accountable for their *behavior*. However, the professional must hold the line. Third, to explore the dynamics of interaction between therapist and patient is neither to "blame the victim" (i.e., the patient) nor to exonerate the professional from responsibility for the boundaries.

Boundary issues in the treatment of psychiatric patients are universal, as are concerns about these issues. Therefore, to discuss boundary issues in relation to patients with personality disorders is not to imply that *all* or *only* personality-disordered patients experience or pose boundary problems. Instead, this chapter examines a subset of the wider universe of boundary-related potential problem areas.

According to my own evidence, the above caveats do not indicate obsessive caution. In 1989, I pointed out that patients with borderline personality disorder (BPD) presented particular challenges with regard to boundaries (Gutheil 1989). That article was based on my forensic caseload and thus drawn from empirical reality. As discussed therein, the topic of boundaries for patients with BPD is fraught with tension, confusion, and political incorrectness.

The profession as a whole has had its consciousness raised by the careful study of trauma victims, many of whom had become highly sensitive to boundary transgressions in their treaters; indeed, boundary issues within the nuclear families of these individuals may have constituted, or been a component of, the trauma. The frequent association of boundary problems as precursors to actual sexual misconduct also focused attention on the subject.

It is critically important to retain nonjudgmental clarity in the important area of boundary issues, because the consequences of confusion about this topic may be serious. This chapter aims to alleviate possible confusion. Before turning our attention to personality disorders and their implications for boundary theory, the basic elements are summarized.

BASIC ELEMENTS OF BOUNDARY THEORY

Just what is a boundary? A working definition might be that a *boundary* is the edge of appropriate, professional conduct. The definition is highly context dependent. The relevant contexts may be the treater's ideology, the stage of the therapy, the patient's condition or diagnosis, the geographical setting, or the cultural milieu, among others. Although attorneys, boards of licensure, and young clinicians may long for a checklist of approved and disapproved behaviors, the matter is not that simple. Context is a critical and determinative factor.

Besides complaint procedures and their aftermath, data about boundary issues come from consultations, supervision and training settings, the literature, professional meetings, informal remarks by colleagues, and formal studies. These data permit empirical examination of the varieties of boundary phenomena, the criteria for boundary assessment, and the clinical contexts in which problems arise. An extensive literature has grown up around this subject in recent decades, and the reader is directed to this literature for additional discussion beyond the narrower focus of this chapter (Epstein and Simon 1990; Gabbard 1999; Gabbard and Lester 2002; Gutheil and Gabbard 1993, 1998; Gutheil and Simon 2002; Ingram 1991; Langs 1976; Simon 1989, 1992; Smith 1977; Spruiell 1983; Stone 1976). In summary, boundary problems may emerge from role issues, time, place and space, money, gifts and services, clothing, language, and physical or sexual contact as elsewhere addressed (Gutheil and Gabbard 1993).

BOUNDARY CROSSINGS AND BOUNDARY VIOLATIONS

In an earlier publication, Gabbard and I proposed a distinction that has proven important both in theory and in litigation related to boundaries: the difference between boundary crossings and boundary violations (Gutheil and Gabbard 1993).

Boundary crossings are defined as transient, nonexploitative deviations from classical therapeutic or general clinical practice in which the treater steps out to a minor degree from strict verbal psychotherapy. These crossings do not hurt the therapy and may even promote or facilitate it. Examples might include offering a crying patient a tissue, helping a fallen patient up from the floor, helping an elderly patient on with a coat, giving a fragile patient a home telephone number for emer-

gencies, giving a patient traveling on foot a lift in your car during a blizzard, writing cards to a patient during a long absence, visiting a patient at home based on his or her medical needs, answering selected personal questions, disclosing selected personal information, and so on. None of these actions is psychotherapy in its pure "talking" form; they constitute instead a mixture of manners, helpfulness, support, or social amity. No one could reasonably claim that these actions are exploitative of the patient or the patient's needs. Depending on the context, the appropriate response to such actions is for the therapist to explore their impact, maximize their therapeutic utility, and detect and neutralize any difficulties the patient may have as a result. Even the therapist's well-mannered gesture of putting out a hand for a handshake may be experienced as an attack or threat by a patient with a horrendous trauma history. An important point about boundary crossings is that when they occur, the therapist should review the matter with the patient on the next available occasion and fully document the rationale, the discussion with the patient, and the description of the patient's response.

Boundary violations, in contrast, constitute essentially harmful deviations from the normal parameters of treatment—deviations that *do* harm the patient, usually through some sort of exploitation that breaks the rule of "First, do no harm." Usually, the therapist's needs are gratified by taking advantage of the patient in some manner. The therapy is not advanced and may even be destroyed by such violations. Examples might include taking advantage of the patient financially, using the patient to gratify the therapist's narcissistic or dependency needs, using the patient for menial services (cleaning the office, getting lunch, running errands for the therapist), or engaging in sexual or sexualized relations or relationship with the patient. A useful test for distinguishing a boundary crossing from a violation is whether the event can be discussed in the therapy (Gutheil and Gabbard 1993). An even better test is whether the behavior in question can be discussed openly (hence, is admissible) with a colleague. Many violators have admitted that they did not seek consultations with a colleague because they knew the consultant would tell them to stop the behavior. In any case, the only proper response to boundary violations is not to do them in the first place.

As the next section illustrates, the difference between these two types of boundary issues is highly context dependent. However, forensic experience demonstrates that some agencies, such as the more punitive state boards of registration, tend to view all boundaries from a rigid "checklist" perspective that does violence to clinical flexibility and the essential relevance of context.

CONTEXT DEPENDENCE

In a conceptual vacuum, it may be impossible to distinguish clearly a boundary crossing from a boundary violation. A therapist who sends a dependent patient a reassuring postcard from his vacation is merely crossing the boundary; however, if the postcard is highly eroticized, contains inappropriate content, and is part of an extended sexual seduction, the same gesture carries entirely different weight.

Another element of context is the type and goal of the therapy. A favorite example is an analyst doing classical psychoanalysis, for whom no justification would exist for accompanying an adult patient into the bathroom; however, in the behaviorist treatment of paruresis (fear of urinating in public restrooms), the last step in a behavioral paradigm of treatment might well be the therapist accompanying the patient there. This example also implies that the context may be affected by issues such as informed consent to the type of therapy, the nature and content of the therapeutic contract, the patient's expectations, and so on.

POWER ASYMMETRY AND FIDUCIARY DUTY

The concepts of power asymmetry and fiduciary duty play an important theoretical role in analyzing boundary problems and are frequently used in discussing the consequences of boundary breaches. *Power asymmetry* refers to the unequal distribution of power between the two parties in the therapeutic dyad: the therapist has the greater social and legal power than the patient. With this power comes the greater responsibility for directing and containing the therapeutic envelope. The occasional protest of "it's not my fault, the patient seduced me" carries little weight under this formulation.

A *fiduciary duty* is a duty based on trust and obligation. The doctor, as a fiduciary, owes a duty to the patient to place the latter's interests first; primarily, the doctor does what the patient needs, not what the doctor wants to do. Exploitative boundary violations are thus viewed as breaches of the doctor's fiduciary duty to the patient: the treater has placed his or her own gratification ahead of the patient's needs.

CONSEQUENCES OF BOUNDARY PROBLEMS

The consequences of boundary problems may be divided into those *intrinsic* to the therapy and those *ex-*

trinsic to the therapy. As indicated earlier, a serious and exploitative boundary violation may doom the therapy and cause the patient accurately to feel betrayed and used. The clinical consequences of boundary violations, including sexual misconduct, may encompass the entire spectrum of emotional harms from mild and transient distress to suicide.

The extrinsic harms fall into three major categories: civil lawsuits (in some jurisdictions, criminal charges for overtly sexual activity); complaints to the board of registration, the licensing agency; and ethics complaints to the professional society (such as the district branch of the American Psychiatric Association), usually directed to the ethics committee of the relevant organization.

The above three types of complaints constitute the most common forms of negative consequence from boundary problems; alas for fairness, neither attorneys, boards, nor ethics committees may be sufficiently sophisticated to distinguish between boundary crossings and violations. Thus, any boundary issues should be clearly described in the records together with their rationales, readily discussed, and explored within the therapy itself. The major categories of extrinsic harms are discussed below.

Civil Litigation

A civil lawsuit for boundary problems is based on the concepts that the treater's deviation(s) from the appropriate standard of care were occasioned by negligence and that the patient consequently sustained some form of damages (Gutheil and Appelbaum 2000). This blunt legal analysis scants the commonly encountered clinical complexity of these claims. Although lawsuits for clinician sexual misconduct were a serious problem in past decades, observers have noted an increase in what might be termed "pure" boundary cases; that is, cases in which actual sexual intercourse has not occurred, but the patient is claiming harm from boundary violations short of that extreme.

Other factors may come into play in the litigation arena. The growing awareness of both boundary issues and their common precursor role in actual sexual misconduct has led some disgruntled patients to use a boundary claim as a means of taking revenge against a disliked clinician. A current joke holds that under the advent of managed care and the severe restrictions placed on length of treatment, no therapy will continue long enough for the patient to develop erotic transferences for the doctor.

On the one hand, a malpractice suit against the clinician will be defended and—in case of a loss—paid for by the malpractice insurer; on the other hand, many insurance policies contain exclusionary language that avoids coverage for the more sexualized forms of boundary violation.

Board of Registration/Licensure Complaint

A complaint to the board of registration challenges the physician's fitness to practice, as supposedly rendered questionable by the boundary problem in question. There are three serious problems with this form of complaint. First, boards in some areas are extremely punitive, seeking to meet quotas of de-licensed practitioners and ignoring both context and evidence. Second, unlike a malpractice case, a loss in these cases may cost the clinician his or her license and livelihood. Finally, because a complaint to the board is not a malpractice issue, insurers often will not fund the defense, leaving the legal expenses to be met out-of-pocket by the doctor. One implication of this grim scenario is that board complaints should be taken very seriously and must include legal assistance, no matter how bizarre, overreactive, and trivial the complaint may seem.

Ethics Complaints

The field of ethics has produced a vast wealth of philosophical opinion and literature as to what does and does not constitute ethical conduct, but an ethics complaint to one's professional society has an extremely concrete denotation: it asserts that a specific section of the American Psychiatric Association Code of Ethics (American Psychiatric Association 2001) has been violated by the boundary issue in question. What is ethical is what is in the "book." The outcome of a formal ethics complaint (informal complaints are not accepted) ranges from censure and warning (not reportable to the National Practitioner Data Bank) to suspension or expulsion from the professional society (both of which are reportable). Such reportage may plague every subsequent job application and usually also reaches the relevant board of registration.

SOME PERSONALITY TYPES ENCOUNTERED IN CLINICAL PRACTICE

We turn now to boundary issues that arise in relation to various personality disorders. As a reminder, the clinical correlation of boundary problems with patients with a personality disorder neither blames the victim nor exonerates the treater, nor does it remove from the latter the burdens of setting and maintaining boundaries. Indeed, it takes two to generate a true boundary

problem. Thus, the following discussion addresses the interactions between patients with personality disorders and the clinicians attempting to treat them.

As might be inferred from the earlier discussion, no particular therapist, patient, or personality disorder should be considered immune from actual or potential boundary problems (Norris and Gutheil 2003). Indeed, both members of the dyad may present risk factors increasing the likelihood of boundary problems. Therapist issues may include life crises; transitions in a career; illness; loneliness and the impulse to confide in someone; idealization of a "special patient"; pride, shame, and envy; problems with limit setting; denial; and issues peculiar to being in a small-town environment wherein interaction with patients outside the office is unavoidable. Patient issues increasing vulnerability to boundary problems may include enmeshment with the therapist; retraumatization from earlier childhood abuse and felt helplessness from that earlier event; the repetition compulsion; shame and self-blame; feelings that the transference is "true love"; dependency; narcissism; and masochism (Norris and Gutheil 2003).

Empirically, the Cluster A group, marked by a tendency toward detachment, is less likely to be involved in a boundary issue than the other two clusters; however, individuals in the group with very poor social skills and poor perspective-taking of others may cross boundaries more out of social ineptness than other dynamics.

Histrionic and Dependent Personality Disorders

Consultative experience demonstrates that two symptoms manifested by patients with histrionic or dependent personality disorder—drama and neediness—tend to play roles in boundary excursions. A patient's intense need for contact, self-esteem, approval, or relief from anxiety or tension may pressure clinicians into hasty actions that cross boundaries.

> A dependent patient who had been out drinking for an evening called her therapist in a panic and begged him to pick her up at the bar and drive her home. Feeling somewhat trapped and choiceless, the therapist did so. The situation, though presented by the patient as an emotional emergency, was clearly one merely of "urgency."

Although probably harmless, such an event may well be used by a board of registration as evidence of boundary problems in the treater. Appropriate responses may have included the therapists' calling a cab, recommending public transportation if available, or the therapists' call to family or friends.

Dramatic behavior may "trigger" a boundary problem because of the clinician's wish to "turn down the volume":

> A patient with histrionic personality disorder, distraught after a session in which the therapist announced vacation plans, seated herself on the floor just outside the therapist's door and moaned loudly for a prolonged interval. The therapist, embarrassed by this scene taking place in full view of the clinic waiting room in front of other patients and staff, brought the patient back into the office and conducted an impulsive, prolonged session, intruding into other patients' appointments.

Patients are free to cross boundaries—but the limits must be set by the clinician. The patient in this vignette might have been told that the behavior was inappropriate and should be discussed at the next appointment. If the patient refused to leave, security might have been called and the matter explored at the next session.

Although supervisory data were lacking in this vignette, it appears likely that the dynamic operating therein was the therapist's countertransference-based inability to deal with his own sadistic feelings both about planning a vacation (and thus causing abandonment feelings in the patient) and about being able to turn the patient away when the latter was behaving inappropriately. Conflicts about sadism are a common source of boundary difficulties, especially in younger therapists; the issue of countertransference is further addressed later in the chapter.

One of the earliest and most famous examples of histrionic (it would then have been called "hysterical") behavior was the hysterical pregnancy and pseudochildbirth of Anna O., who was in the throes of an erotic transference to Joseph Breuer, as described in the *Studies in Hysteria* (Breuer and Freud 1893–1895/1955). Although Breuer is not recorded as violating any boundaries, the point can be made that patient reactions in this disorder may operate independently of the clinician's actual behavior, a fact leading to confusion among decision-making bodies.

Antisocial Personality Disorder

Individuals with antisocial personality disorder may strain the boundary envelope with the intent of furthering manipulation of the therapist or, through the therapist, others in the environment. Examples might include getting the therapist to advocate for the patient at work, at school, and in other areas in which the therapist is induced to step out of the limits of the clinical role to abet the patient's purposes.

Another boundary issue seen with patients in this category is excessive familiarity and pseudocloseness designed to get the therapist to perform uncharacteristic actions that transgress boundaries:

> Doctor (on first meeting): How do you do, I am Dr. Thomas Gutheil.
> Patient (with warm handclasp): Very glad to meet you, Thomas.
> Doctor (slightly nonplussed): Um, well, Thomas *is* my given name, but I go by "Doctor Gutheil."
> Patient (affably): Whatever you say, Tommy.

As illustrated, the patient may shift on first acquaintance to a first-name or nickname basis to establish an artificial rapport designed to persuade the therapist to alter the rules of proper conduct. The therapist may feel silly or stuffy correcting this undue familiarity or even bringing it up at all, but the effort should probably be made in concert with attempts to explore the meaning of the behavior.

Some common goals of this tendency toward pseudocloseness are obtaining excusing or exculpatory letters sent to nonclinical recipients; obtaining prescriptions of inappropriate, or inappropriately large amounts of, controlled substances; and intervention in the patient's extratherapeutic reality ("I need you to meet with my parole officer to go easier on me; you know how ill I am").

From the patient's viewpoint, the boundaries, if even recognized, may be ignored in a goal-directed manner. From the clinician's viewpoint, the boundary transgressions may lead to trouble, especially if the patient's actions encompass illegal behavior (e.g., selling prescriptions) into which the doctor is drawn by association.

The following is an unfortunately common clinically observed constellation of boundary problems: a female psychotherapist is treating a male patient with antisocial personality disorder, but she misses the antisocial elements in the patient, seeing him as a needy infant who requires loving care to "get better." In the course of this rescue operation, boundary incursions occur and increase (Gabbard and Lester 2002).

Borderline Personality Disorder

As in the previous diagnostic category, patients with BPD may manifest conscious or unconscious manipulative tendencies for a number of reasons. Some scholars assert that these patients manipulate because their low self-esteem leaves them feeling unentitled to ask directly to have their needs met. It is a clinical truism that a sense of being unentitled may be masked by an overt attitude of entitlement; the patient operates from the position that he or she is special and deserving of extra attention. This demand for specialness can lead therapists to grant favors that transgress boundaries with these patients. (Because BPD empirically poses the greatest boundary difficulties, the reader may wish to review the axioms given at the outset of this chapter in order to maintain a properly nonjudgmental perspective.)

The surprising power of the manipulation to slip under the clinician's radar, as it were, is one of the more striking findings in the boundary realm. "I sensed that I was doing something that was outside my usual practice and, in fact, outside the pale," the therapist will lament to the consultant, "but somehow I just found myself making exceptions for this patient and doing it anyway."

In an earlier paper (Gutheil 1989), I described my experience with therapists seeking consultation who would begin their narratives with, "I don't ordinarily do this with my patients, but in *this* case I...[insert a broad spectrum of inappropriate behaviors here]." The patients' sense of entitlement and of being "special" may infect the therapist with the same view of their specialness, such that even inappropriate exceptions are made.

The patient's own boundary problems—both in the ego boundary sense (Gabbard and Lester 2002) and in the interpersonal space—may evoke comparable boundary blindness in the therapist:

> A therapist noted that a patient with very primitive BPD would sidle out of the office along the wall in a puzzling manner that seemed to convey a fearful state. On exploration the patient revealed that she was struggling with the fantasy that if she passed too close to the therapist she might accidentally fall forward and sink into the therapist's chest and be absorbed as though into quicksand. (D. Buie, personal communication, 1969)

We may be able to detect clinically the unconscious wishes for fusion hidden under this fear, but the point of the anecdote is that for some patients, the boundary even of the physical self may be extremely tenuous. Indeed, wishes for fusion in both patient and therapist may provide the stimulus to boundary transgressions.

The patient with BPD may manifest impulsivity that presses the therapist to act precipitously without forethought: "I need you to do this now, right now!" The patient may demand an immediate appointment, an immediate telephone contact, an immediate home visit, an immediate ride home, an extended session, a medication refill, or a fee adjustment. Note, of course, that any or all of these may be clinically indicated but may also constitute or lead to boundary problems.

> A patient with BPD in a subsequent psychotherapy commented out of the blue that she really felt her previous therapist should not have charged her a fee but should in fact have paid her, because her case was so interesting.

Research data indicate that patients with BPD often have a history of trauma; that is, they were at one time victims (Herman, cited in Gutheil and Gabbard 1993). Some of these patients adopt a posture of victimization (an element of entitlement distinguishable from narcissistic entitlement). This posture may mobilize rescue feelings, fantasies, or attempts in the therapist that lead the latter to "bend the rules" to achieve the rescue and thus transgress boundaries. Indeed, consultative experience leads to the conclusion that a number of cases of sexual misconduct spring from claimed attempts to rescue the patient, to prevent suicide, to elevate the patient's self-esteem, or to provide a "good" relationship to counter a string of bad ones that the patient has experienced.

"Borderline rage" is also a factor in leading to boundary problems, often through its power to intimidate:

> A 6-foot, 7-inch tall former college linebacker, now a therapist, was asked in consultation why he went along with a boundary violation that he knew was inappropriate but was demanded by the patient: why did he not simply refuse? Looking down from his height he stated, "I just didn't dare."

As noted elsewhere, borderline rage may leave therapists feeling pressured into inappropriate self-disclosure, conceding to inappropriate requests, and manifesting other signs of being "moved through fear" (Gutheil 1989, p. 598).

Disappointed in many past relationships, the patient with BPD may contrive to "test the therapist's care or devotion" in boundary-transgressing ways that often represent reenactments of earlier developmental stages. One source of this view is the patient's perception that therapy offers some form of promise, such as the inclusion in the therapist's idealized family (Gutheil 1989; Smith 1977). The patient may demand to sit on the therapist's lap or to be held or hugged, arguing that without this demonstration of caring, there can be no trust in the therapy. Herman (cited in Gutheil and Gabbard 1993) pointed out that because so many patients with BPD have histories of sexual abuse, they may have been conditioned to interact with significant others on whom they depend in eroticized or seductive ways.

Forensic experience reveals the sad truth of how often these primitive maneuvers actually succeed, to the detriment of the therapy and often to the censure of the therapist. As might well be expected, the well-spring of these deviations is commonly the countertransference in the dyad, our next topic.

COUNTERTRANSFERENCE ISSUES

The patient's need for help and the treater's membership in a helping profession ordinarily provide a salutary and symmetrical reciprocity, but it is not immune to distortion or miscarriage. The basic wish to help and heal, unfortunately, may inspire efforts that—no matter how well-intended—transgress professional boundaries in problematic ways. The patient's transferential neediness and dependency may evoke a countertransferential need in the therapist to rescue, save, or heal the patient at any cost. Wishes to save the patient from anxiety, depression, or suicide are common stimuli to boundary violations in the name of rescue.

An example of this problem is what I call the "brute force" attempt at cure. Frustrated by the difficulty of working with the patient and disappointed at the latter's lack of progress, the therapist sees the patient more and more often each week, for longer and longer session times; weekends, holidays, even vacations are no exception to this relentless crescendo. Therapists in this situation are being held hostage by the patient's insatiable need and are setting themselves the wholly unrealistic goal of meeting that need by "giving more."

In a related manner, such patients' suicidal risk may lead the therapist to try desperate measures to prevent this outcome at all costs, including violating boundaries to achieve this rescue. Gabbard (2003) described this phenomenon in detail under the heading of the therapist's masochistic surrender, a dynamic issue closely linked to boundary problems.

This frustration may rise to the level of overt anger, in which the therapist acts out countertransference hostility by violating boundaries such as confidentiality. The therapist who angrily and inappropriately calls the patient's partner at home and rails at him or her to protest some action involving the patient has lost the compass that would keep one in bounds.

In a useful discussion Smith (1977) defined the "golden fantasy" entertained by some patients with BPD and others, the belief that all needs—relational, supportive, nurturing, dependent, and therapeutic—will be met by the treater. As the patient loses track of what constitutes the therapeutic aspect of the work, the

therapist may begin to lose track of the actual parameters within which the treatment should take place.

The American Psychiatric Association (2003) practice guideline stresses four basic points relating to patients with BPD and boundaries. First, monitor countertransference carefully; second, be alert to deviations from usual practice ("red flags"); third, always avoid boundary violations; and fourth, obtain consultation for "striking deviations from the usual manner of practice." These points are fully congruent with the material in this chapter.

In summary—because of borderline patients' own difficulties with boundaries, their capacity to evoke powerful countertransference reactions, and the particular elements of their interpersonal style—patients with BPD pose some of the most noteworthy examples of boundary problems and challenges to clinicians to maintain proper limits.

SOME CROSS-CULTURAL OBSERVATIONS

One might expect that boundary issues are a uniquely American problem, what with our litigious and entitled population and our active attention in the professional literature to boundary issues. However, a recent cross-cultural study (Commons et al. in press) comparing boundary matters in the United States and Rio de Janeiro, Brazil, turned up some interesting findings.

The U.S. sample and the Brazilian sample agreed at the extremes—that is, in both countries overt sexual misconduct at one end of the spectrum was seen as proscribed, and trivial deviations at the other end were seen as harmless. In the middle ranges, however, divergence was revealed. For example, subjects in the U.S. sample believed hugging a patient was suspect and kissing was surely wrong, but it was fully acceptable to display licenses, certificates, and some honors on the walls of the office. The Brazilian cohort found kissing the cheek in greeting to be universally acceptable and an accepted manner of greeting patients, whereas display of certificates was considered a deviation.

It is likely that both cultural differences and personal data, such as trauma history, shape a patient's perception of boundary problems and the degree of their harmful effect, if any.

RISK MANAGEMENT PRINCIPLES AND RECOMMENDATIONS

Clearly, a rigid formalism and an icy demeanor are not the solution to boundary problems when dealing with patients with personality disorders; patients so treated will simply leave treatment. Rather, some basic guidelines may prove helpful to the clinician who desires to stay out of trouble while preserving the therapeutic effect of the work.

1. First, clinicians of any ideological stripe must obtain some basic understanding of the dynamic issues relating to transference and countertransference. Training programs that foolishly boast of having transcended "that Freudian stuff" do a serious disservice to their graduates. A patient with BPD in the idealizing phase of treatment may worship the therapist, but if the latter is untrained in the vagaries of transference, he or she is left to assume that his/her own natural gifts of person have evoked this reaction—a dangerous view, indeed.

2. Treaters of these patients must keep in mind the latter's capacity to distort or overreact. If you write to such a patient and sign the letter, "Love, Dr. Smith," you may intend agape (nonerotic love), but the patient may interpret eros and expect treatment consistent with that emotion. Even if the patient initially understands the meaning, the regulatory agencies may interpret that salutation as a sign that the clinician has lost objectivity and may assume that boundaries have been violated (note that this sequence of events is not speculative but empirical). Therapists should of course take responsibility for their actions, but these patients can evoke strong feelings of guilt that distort the clinician's perception of what happened and who is responsible.

   For example, in a Board of Registration complaint, the patient claimed to have been hurt by some action of the doctor. Instead of writing "I am sorry you feel hurt," the doctor wrote, "I am sorry I hurt you." This ill-chosen expression of inappropriate self-blame made it almost impossible to convince the board that the doctor had remained within proper boundaries.

   The learning point here: When in doubt, obtain forensic or legal consultation.

3. The therapist should develop a "red flag" warning response when finding him- or herself doing what "I do not usually do"—that is, making an exception to customary practice. The exception in question may be an act of laudatory creativity in treatment, but it may also be a boundary problem. Self-scrutiny and consultation may be most useful at such times.

4. Gutheil and Simon (1995) observed that the neutral space and time—when both parties rise from their chairs and move toward the door at the end of a session—represents an occasion when both parties may feel that the rules do not really apply anymore because the session is theoretically over. We recommended that therapists pay attention to their experiences and to the events and communications that occur during this "window"—because a tendency toward crossing or even violating boundaries may emerge in embryonic form during this period, allowing the therapist to open the subject for exploration in the following session and, one hopes, to deflate its problematic nature.

5. When in doubt, get consultation; doing so honors my favorite maxim: "Never worry alone." Although getting consultation before taking a step that might present boundary ambiguities is an excellent idea, the therapist should also begin presenting the case to a colleague or supervisor when boundary problems begin to appear on the horizon or when the transference becomes eroticized. Such consultation will aid in keeping perspective and in ensuring that the standard of care is being met.

6. Any potential boundary excursion of uncertain meaning should be marked by three critical steps: professional behavior; discussion with the patient; and documentation. Under some circumstances, a tactful apology to the patient for misreading a situation may be in order. Failure to perform these steps casts the therapist in the light of one who wants to conceal wrongdoing.

   For example, driving home from a late last appointment, a therapist sees his patient slogging wearily homeward on foot through the 2-foot high drifts that a recent blizzard had deposited on the area. To prevent the patient from dying of exposure in the subfreezing weather, he offers her a ride home in his jeep. In the car he continues to behave in a formal, professional manner, despite the odd circumstances. At the office the next day, he records a careful note outlining his reasoning and the risk-benefit analysis of the incident. At the patient's next appointment, he inquires how the patient felt about the incident, and its therapeutic significance is explored.

7. Finally, the majority of boundary difficulties may be averted by the following approach: "Explore before acting." Impulsive responses to patient demands are likely to go astray, and such responses may inappropriately model impulsivity.

REFERENCES

American Psychiatric Association: The Principles of Medical Ethics With Annotations Especially Applicable to Psychiatry, 2001 Edition. Washington, DC, American Psychiatric Association, 2001

American Psychiatric Association: Practice Guideline for the Treatment of Patients with Borderline Personality Disorder. Washington, DC, American Psychiatric Association, 2003

Breuer J, Freud S: Studies on hysteria (1893–1895), in Standard Edition of the Complete Psychological Works of Sigmund Freud, Vol 2. Translated and edited by Strachey J. London, Hogarth Press, 1955, pp 1–319

Commons ML, Miller PM, Gutheil TG: Cross-cultural aspects of boundaries: Brazil and the United States. J Am Acad Psychiatry Law (in press)

Epstein RS, Simon RI: The exploitation index: an early warning indicator of boundary violations in psychotherapy. Bull Menninger Clin 54:450–465, 1990

Gabbard GO: Boundary violations, in Psychiatric Ethics, 3rd Edition. Edited by Bloch S, Chodoff P, Green SA. Oxford, England, Oxford University Press, 1999, pp 141–160

Gabbard GO: Miscarriages of psychoanalytic treatment with suicidal patients. Int J Psychoanal 84:249–261, 2003

Gabbard GO, Lester EP: Boundaries and Boundary Violations in Psychoanalysis, 2nd Edition. Washington, DC, American Psychiatric Publishing, 2002

Gutheil TG: Borderline personality disorder, boundary violations and patient-therapist sex: medicolegal pitfalls. Am J Psychiatry 146:597–602, 1989

Gutheil TG, Appelbaum PS: Clinical Handbook of Psychiatry and the Law, 3rd Edition. Baltimore, MD, Lippincott, Williams and Wilkins, 2000

Gutheil TG, Gabbard GO: The concept of boundaries in clinical practice: theoretical and risk management dimensions. Am J Psychiatry 150:188–196, 1993

Gutheil, TG, Gabbard GO: Misuses and misunderstandings of boundary theory in clinical and regulatory settings. Am J Psychiatry 155:409–414, 1998

Gutheil TG, Simon RI: Between the chair and the door: boundary issues in the therapeutic "transition zone." Harv Rev Psychiatry 2:336–340, 1995

Gutheil TG, Simon RI: Non-sexual boundary crossings and boundary violations: the ethical dimension. Psychiatr Clin North Am 25:585–592, 2002

Ingram DH: Intimacy in the psychoanalytic relationship: a preliminary sketch. Am J Psychoanal 51:403–411, 1991

Langs R: The Bipersonal Field. New York, Jason Aronson, 1976

Norris DM, Gutheil TG, Strasburger LH: "This couldn't happen to me": boundary problems and sexual misconduct in the psychotherapeutic relationship. Psychiatr Serv 54:517–522, 2003

Simon RI: Sexual exploitation of patients: how it begins before it happens. Psychiatr Ann 19:104–122, 1989

Simon RI: Treatment boundary violations: clinical, legal and ethical considerations. J Am Acad Psychiatry Law 20:269–288, 1992

Smith S: The golden fantasy: a regressive reaction to separation anxiety. Int J Psychoanal 58:311–324, 1977

Spruiell V: The rules and frames of the psychoanalytic situation. Psychoanal Q 52:1–33, 1983

Stone MH: Boundary violations between therapist and patient. Psychiatr Ann 6:670–677, 1976

28

Collaborative Treatment

Abigail Schlesinger, M.D.
Kenneth R. Silk, M.D.

WHAT IS SPLIT OR COLLABORATIVE TREATMENT?

Collaborative treatment can mean different things in different clinical practice settings. In this chapter, *collaborative treatment* refers to the treatment relationship that occurs when two (or more) treatment modalities are provided by more than one mental health or medical professional. This type of treatment arrangement has had many names, such as *split treatment, joint* (or *conjoint*) *treatment,* or in certain specific circumstances, *medication backup* (Riba and Balon 1999). We reserve use of the term *split treatment* to circumstances in which there is disagreement among or between the collaborators. Collaborative treatment can be contrasted with integrative treatment, in which one mental health care provider—most frequently a psychiatrist—performs all mental health modalities for a patient.

In the most common form of collaborative treatment, one clinician prescribes psychotropic medication (or somatic treatments) and another performs psychotherapy. In psychiatry, collaborative treatment often involves a psychiatrist prescribing psychiatric medication and another clinician (e.g., psychiatrist, psychologist, social worker, therapist, case manager) performing the therapy. Increasingly, collaborative treatment has come to represent a situation in which a primary care physician (PCP) prescribes psychotropic medication while a nonpsychiatrist clinician conducts psychotherapy. In addition, treatment can be divided up in many ways among PCPs, psychoanalysts, specialty medical doctors, psychiatrists, specialty psychiatrists, therapists, clinical nurse therapists, visiting nurses, physician assistants, case managers, different people and disciplines on an inpatient unit or in a partial hospital program, and many others.

The term *collaborative* highlights the need for treating clinicians to communicate and work together, because there are many legal, ethical, and treatment issues and pitfalls that can arise when more than one provider is involved in a person's treatment. Patients with personality disorders, especially those with Cluster B traits, tend to "split" even without a "split" treatment relationship, and this propensity must be kept in mind when entering into a collaborative care model with another clinician for a patient with a personality disorder. *Splitting*, which is elaborated on more thoroughly elsewhere in this book, in its most formal psychoanalytic sense is a defensive process wherein a patient appears to attribute good characteristics almost exclusively to one person (or one provider of treatment) while attributing the other treater with all bad or negative feelings. The patient appears to take the natural ambivalence one feels about almost all people and divide it into two packages—a positive package bestowed upon one person and a negative package bestowed upon another. Each package almost exclusively contains either good or bad attributes, rarely contaminated by the opposite attribute. Defensive splitting can be accompanied by *projective identification*, in which the patient projects different aspects of himself onto different treaters. The different treaters, in turn, unconsciously identify with those projected characteristics and may experience pressure to respond accordingly (Gabbard 1989; Gabbard and Wilkinson 1994; Ogden 1982).

> Ms. Z, a young woman diagnosed with borderline personality disorder (BPD), was in psychotherapy with a psychologist and receiving medication from a psychiatrist. Ms. Z had an extensive history of self-mutilating behavior. The psychologist was, even in his everyday interactions, quite restrained.
>
> Ms. Z was acutely aware of rejection, and she would call the psychiatrist to complain vociferously about her psychotherapist's lack of feeling or empathy. Every 6 or 9 months of this 5-year treatment, she would try to convince the psychiatrist, whom she knew did psychodynamic psychotherapy, to take over all of the treatment. The psychiatrist always sent Ms. Z back to discuss these issues with her psychologist, even though the psychiatrist was aware that many of the accusations made about the therapist were, in some ways, not untrue.[1]
>
> As the therapy progressed, Ms. Z's self-destructive behavior diminished and then eventually ceased as her interpersonal relationships grew more stable. Longer periods elapsed between her complaints about her therapist, and eventually the complaints stopped. The treatment terminated successfully.

This chapter discusses collaborative treatment in general and then collaborative treatment of patients with personality disorders. Much of what is discussed applies to any collaborative treatment, regardless of the patient's diagnosis, but the issues of collaboration are heightened when the patient has a diagnosis of a personality disorder. Although the techniques, strategies, or issues presented are pertinent to many patients with personality disorders, they cannot be applied to all such patients because we often discuss treatments in which psychotherapy is conducted by one person and psychopharmacology is managed by another, and there are few data to support prescribing medications to patients with schizoid, antisocial, histrionic, narcissistic, and dependent personality disorders.

EVIDENCE FOR EFFECTIVENESS OF COLLABORATIVE CARE

Although collaborative treatment is increasingly common in mental health care, the effectiveness of collaborative versus integrative treatment has not been well studied. There are no head-to-head efficacy studies comparing collaborative with integrative treatment, although there are studies that examine one treatment modality versus another modality versus both modalities together (Greenblatt et al. 1965; Klerman 1990).

Many patients with personality disorders have complex biological and psychosocial issues and do not respond as well to medications as would patients whose primary diagnosis is from Axis I (except perhaps those with schizotypal personality disorder [Paris 2003; Soloff 1990, 1998]). Treatment modalities beyond psychopharmacological treatment are necessary, and often each modality is provided by a different mental health professional. Thus there are many clinical situations in which multimodal treatment implies and warrants collaboration between at least two mental health professionals.

Most current outcome studies in psychotherapy and psychopharmacology do not measure the effects of any treatment other than the one being studied. There are surprisingly few studies—and even fewer randomized, controlled trials—comparing psychotherapy alone, medication alone, and psychotherapy and medicine in combination to determine the differential efficacy or effectiveness (Browne et al. 2002). Studies of cognitive-behavioral therapy and nefazodone for depression (Keller et al. 2000) and cognitive-behavioral therapy and tricyclic antidepressants for panic disorder (Barlow et al. 2000) have interesting findings about the course and continuation of response to specific interventions (Manber et al. 2003). Often patients with personality disorders are excluded from these studies, or personality disorders are not assessed. Thus, for patients with personality disorders, no clear conclusions can be made concerning the effectiveness of a medication versus psychotherapy; furthermore, no conclusions about effectiveness or efficacy can be made if these treatments are combined and performed by one provider versus being divided between two (or more) providers with

---

[1] This situation may occur frequently in collaborative treatment. The patient presents an observation about the collaborating psychotherapist that may be an astute and accurate perception of the psychotherapist. Despite the face validity of the observation, the psychiatrist must refrain from agreeing or disagreeing with the patient. Each patient brings his or her unique history and transference into play when making such observations, and a comment at this point might undermine that particular transferential process occurring in the psychotherapy.

one providing psychotherapy and the other prescribing medications. The exception may be the study by Kool et al. (2003), which found that patients with personality pathology and depression responded best to a combined approach of both psychopharmacology and psychotherapy, although personality pathology of patients with Cluster C diagnoses responded better than that of patients with Cluster B diagnoses.

IMPORTANCE OF COLLABORATIVE TREATMENT IN CURRENT PERSONALITY DISORDERS CARE

General Issues

A large proportion of antidepressants being prescribed in the United States is prescribed by PCPs (Lecrubier 2001). Serotonin reuptake inhibitors are less complicated to prescribe, with fewer general side effects and less lethality, than tricyclic antidepressants (Healy 1997). PCPs appear ready to provide the ongoing management of psychopharmacological medication in consultation with a psychiatrist. Although they do not always prescribe concurrent psychotherapy, a number of PCPs are collaborating with therapists of varying levels of training. An interesting triangular relationship can develop: a therapist, a PCP writing the prescriptions for psychotropic medication, and a psychiatrist for referral or collaboration. Smith (1989) wrote, "In contemporary treatment situations that include a patient, a therapist, a pharmacotherapist, and a pill, the transference issues can become more complex than the landing patterns of airplanes at an overcrowded airport" (p. 80). Add a managed care utilization reviewer to the picture, and things really get complicated.

Managed care companies often believe that patients with personality disorders use too much or at least more than their share of treatment. One of the challenges associated with providing collaborative care for these patients is convincing utilization reviewers that more than one modality of care is needed. To avoid divergent reports that negatively affect the reimbursed care for the patient, it is best to designate one member of the team to report the progress of treatment and the treatment plan to the reviewer. In general, this designated "reporter" should be the psychiatrist.

Increasing Prescription of Antidepressants

Despite the lack of hard evidence for the benefits of psychopharmacology in personality disorders, the practice of prescribing antidepressants for a wide array of symptom complexes suggestive of depression continues to increase (Healy 1997). Although depression is prevalent among patients with personality disorders (Skodol et al. 1999), quite often the nature of the depression, especially among patients with Cluster B disorders, is not the classic psychophysiological presentation frequently seen in a major depressive episode (Westen et al. 1992). There has been much debate about the type and nature of depression in patients with personality disorders. The effectiveness of antidepressants in treating depression in such patients is moderate at best, even as their prescriptions are increasing (Paris 2003). Many patients who may have been treated by psychotherapy alone in the past are now receiving psychopharmacological treatment as well. An emerging literature suggests that antidepressants can be helpful in the treatment of specific symptom complexes such as employing selective serotonin reuptake inhibitors or mood stabilizers for impulsivity, affect lability, and aggression in patients with BPD (Coccaro and Kavoussi 1997; Coccaro et al. 1989; Cowdry and Gardner 1988; Hollander et al. 2001; Markowitz 2001, 2004; Rinne et al. 2002; Salzman et al. 1995; Sheard et al. 1976; Soloff 1998; Soloff et al. 1993). The American Psychiatric Association practice guidelines recommend treatment with selective serotonin reuptake inhibitors in a symptom-specific manner for patients with BPD; this recommendation is based on evidence from several double-blind, placebo-controlled studies; a number of open studies; and clinical experience in conjunction with a relatively benign side-effect profile and risk of overdose (American Psychiatric Association 2001). Also, some strong evidence suggests that neuroleptics and atypical antipsychotics (Goldberg et al. 1986; Koenigsberg et al. 2003; Markowitz 2001, 2004; Schulz and Camlin 1999; Soloff et al. 1986b, 1993; Zanarini and Frankenburg 2001) can be effective for patients with schizotypal personality disorder and BPD.

Patients with personality disorders present with a complex admixture of symptoms and problems, some of which appear to arise from psychosocial issues and interpersonal events, whereas others appear more related to expressions of underlying traits such as baseline anxiety, emotional lability, and impulsivity (Livesley 2000; Livesley et al. 1998). When treatment is divided among two providers, the psychotherapist may believe that all problems arise from psychosocial issues and subtly demean, undermine, or dismiss the psychopharmacological treatment. Conversely, the psychopharmacologist may think that difficulties are primarily due to "trait expression" and that once the right combination of medications is discovered, all symptoms will be alleviated

STRENGTHS AND WEAKNESSES OF COLLABORATIVE TREATMENT

There are many positives to a collaborative treatment. Some of these positives have direct reference to patients with personality disorders.

1. Collaborative treatment can provide the patient with both a clinician to idealize and a clinician to denigrate within one treatment relationship. Although this situation might at first appear to be problematic, it can be useful if both providers confer with each other and work to have the patient develop a more balanced view of each of them. For example, both treaters may have an opportunity to model more appropriate coping mechanisms for the patient, or the idealized therapist might be able to work with the patient to modify or mollify the patient's denigration of the other treater and thus help keep the patient in treatment with the therapist being denigrated. The classic example is the patient with BPD, but patients with narcissistic personality disorder also contemptuously devalue and criticize treaters who do not treat them in the way in which they believe they are entitled. Feeling devalued can occur when faced with the moralistic, judgmental, and somewhat contemptuous attitude of the patient with obsessive-compulsive personality disorder. In all these instances, the "good" therapist may be able to provide support to the criticized, or "bad," therapist. One way this support may occur is by the "good" therapist providing examples of other situations in which he or she had the misfortune of owning and bearing the "bad" therapist label and how difficult it was to bear at the time but how useful it was to the eventual outcome of the treatment. The "good" therapist may also try to minimize the negative countertransferential feelings the "bad" therapist is experiencing and may be able to ward off the "bad" therapist's wish to end treatment with the patient.
2. Collaborative treatment provides a basis for ongoing consultation between providers. It also provides the potential for multiple perspectives on complicated clinical and diagnostic situations.

Such complex situations are not uncommon in patients with personality disorders, whose symptoms, behaviors, and interpersonal interactions can be so entwined that it is difficult to unravel the trait biological functioning from the interpersonally and experientially learned behaviors and maneuvers (Cloninger et al. 1993; Livesley et al. 1998).
3. When collaboration is with a PCP, the mental health professional can confer with someone who may have a longitudinal relationship with and understanding of the patient. The PCP often is viewed as fairly neutral by the patient and may be more impervious to the distortions of transference that appear frequently among patients with personality disorders. The PCP may be able to assist the patient in remaining medication compliant.
4. Patients with personality disorders can be very draining to treat. Patients with BPD can be demanding and threatening. Constant demands for attention from histrionic or narcissistic patient can become exhausting. The complaints of histrionic patients can be very difficult to listen to and to take seriously. Patients with dependent personality disorder can be draining and pulling, whereas the chronic anger and distrustfulness of patients with paranoid personality disorder can be quite difficult to tolerate. Therefore, a group of therapists and psychiatrists working as a team to provide overall patient management can support and confer with one another to reduce burnout.

Collaborative treatment can readily turn into a split treatment when the collaborators fail to collaborate. There can be many causes for this failure. Some patients with personality disorders have a tendency, as explained earlier, to split by attributing all good to one person and all bad to another. Although this splitting is most blatant among patients with BPD, it occurs in more subtle forms among patients with schizotypal, narcissistic, antisocial, and obsessive-compulsive personality disorders. Failure to collaborate in the treatment of these patients can lead to serious problems in the treatment. Table 28–1 presents specific issues that need to be considered in a collaborative treatment for each of the personality disorders.

Failure to collaborate or the end of collaboration can develop when the treaters identify with the projections of the patient. In this situation, each of the treaters begins to lose respect for the other treater as each begins to identify and psychologically own some of the negative projections of the patient (Gabbard 1989; Ogden 1982). Such events or situations are not uncommon on inpatient units where the split is often between the attending or resident psychiatrist and a member or members of the nursing staff, although they can occur between nurses as well (see Gabbard 1989; Gunderson 1984; Main 1957; Stanton and Schwartz 1954).

> A ward staff member suddenly accuses another staff member of deliberately trying to jeopardize the treatment of a specific patient, while each staff member believes that she or he alone really knows best. The director of the ward, who has frequently encountered such sudden disagreements, decides to deal with these types of difficulties by bringing together the "warring parties" and wondering out loud with them why each has suddenly begun to despise his or her other colleague on the unit. The director emphasizes that prior to the disagreement, each person appeared to have great respect for and to enjoy working with the other person. The director moves to a discussion of the patient and tries to show the parties how each is really only seeing a part of the patient, upon which they have each constructed the idea that they alone know how best to treat the patient.

Collaboration in divided treatment is essential but does not always occur easily or frequently; a concerted effort must be made. Regularly scheduled phone calls or e-mail exchanges may be the best way to sustain the collaboration even when there is skepticism as to its value or a belief that another provider is causing difficulty.

COLLABORATIVE TREATMENT AND PERSONALITY DISORDERS

Treatment with psychopharmacology and psychotherapy is more common now in the treatment of all personality disorders than it has ever been. This probably is due to a number of factors:

1. Use of psychopharmacological agents among all psychiatric patients has increased, reflecting the general ascendancy of biological psychiatry (Siever and Davis 1991; Siever et al. 2002; Silk 1998; Skodol et al. 2002).
2. Since the early 1990s, there has been an expansion in specific types of psychotherapy for patients with personality disorders, such as dialectical behavior therapy (Linehan et al. 1993), transference-focused psychotherapy (Clarkin et al. 1999; Kernberg et al. 2000), dynamic therapy (Bateman and Fonagy 1999, 2001), interpersonal reconstructive psycho-

therapy (Benjamin 2003), and schema-focused cognitive-behavioral therapy (Young et al. 2003). None of these therapies opposes the concurrent use of psychopharmacological agents.
3. Psychopharmacological agents are in more common use in psychiatric treatment today, and the medications used are generally safer and have more tolerable side-effect profiles (Healy 2002). Safety is important among a group of patients, particularly patients with BPD, who have very high suicide rates (Paris 2002; Stone 1990).
4. Managed care companies play a significant role. They are reluctant to approve treatment sessions with seriously ill patients (including a significant number of patients with personality disorders) who are not receiving medication.
5. There is a growing appreciation of the role of biological and constitutional factors in the etiology of personality disorder symptoms. The nature-nurture dichotomy has been replaced by consideration of the subtle interplay of biological predisposition, resulting in traits that are expressed through behavior that is affected by experiential and environmental factors (both shared and nonshared) (Rutter 2002). Such a theory of interaction between biological predispositions and life experience supports a multimodal treatment approach (Paris 1994).
6. The comorbidity of both Axis I and Axis II disorders has received increased consideration. If one prefers to treat Axis II problems with psychotherapy, Axis I comorbidity still must be considered and treated, or it will likely worsen the clinical manifestation of the Axis II disorder (Yen at al. 2003; Zanarini et al. 1998). Axis I comorbid diagnoses may respond to pharmacological agents, and even in the absence of a clear Axis I comorbid diagnoses, the patient may have pharmacologically responsive symptom clusters that are reminiscent of Axis I and should be treated as such.

SITUATIONS OF COLLABORATIVE TREATMENT

Although *collaborative treatment* usually refers to the arrangement in which a nonmedical psychotherapist performs the psychotherapy and a psychiatrist or other medical doctor prescribes medication, variations on that arrangement still qualify as collaborative treatment. Some such variations occur regardless of the diagnosis, but others are more prone to occur in the treatment of patients with personality disorders.

Table 28–1. Specific issues to address in collaborative treatment with specific personality disorders

Personality disorder	Classic features	Tips for providers of collaborative treatment
Paranoid	Distrust, suspiciousness	Be clear about frequency of contact among providers and be sure to inform patient whenever a contact between any of the providers has occurred. Regularly remind patient about sources of specific information and be sure that each treater knows whether the information he or she has about the patient comes from the patient or other sources (providers).
Schizoid	Detachment from emotional relationships	Work among providers to minimize redundancy of visits so that patient can come as infrequently as possible. Coordinate treatment visits so patient can visit all providers on the same day.
Schizotypal	Discomfort with close relationships, cognitive or perceptual distortions, eccentricities of behavior	Be prepared to contact other providers when increased distortions arise in sessions. Work together to minimize redundancy of visits (see schizoid above).
Antisocial	Disregard for rights of others	Convey clearly that all members of the treatment team will communicate regularly. Be prepared for misrepresentations of facts. Be prepared to verify information with providers. If different providers are getting very different facts from the patient, a designated provider needs to discuss the discrepancies with the patient.
Borderline	Instability in mood and interpersonal relationships, impulsivity	Provide support for the patient without becoming caught up in splitting among providers. Discuss strong countertransference feelings with other providers. Have a clear plan about roles and responses of all providers to emotional outbursts, threats, increased suicidality, other crises, and medication changes. Be careful that repeated crises or turmoil are not reinforced by increased attention from providers.
Histrionic	Excessive emotionality, attention seeking	Have a clear plan among providers as to how to handle emotional outbursts. Be prepared to contact other providers at periods of increasing physical symptoms and/or increasing attention-seeking behavior.
Narcissistic	Grandiosity, lack of empathy	Be prepared to contact other providers when overt or covert signs of increasing contempt toward one of the treaters occurs. Have a clear plan among providers regarding how to handle contemptuous behavior so that one of the providers addresses the issue even if the patient is expressing contempt toward only one of them.

Table 28–1. Specific issues to address in collaborative treatment with specific personality disorders (*continued*)

Personality disorder	Classic features	Tips for providers of collaborative treatment
Avoidant	Social inhibition, feelings of inadequacy, hypersensitivity to negative evaluation	Work among each other to encourage consistent treatment relationships and attitudes in all treatments involved in the collaboration. Be prepared to communicate with other providers whenever missed appointments with any provider occur. Coordinate treatment visits so patient can visit all providers on the same day.
Dependent	Submissive behavior, a need to be taken care of	Work with patient to minimize appointments and avoid overutilization of services. Work together to anticipate how to handle patient needs during vacations. Plan to ensure that increasing distress does not lead to increasing number of appointments.
Obsessive-compulsive	Preoccupation with order, cleanliness, control	Ensure that consistent recommendations are made by each provider. Be prepared to communicate with other providers when patient is having difficulty adhering to recommendations. Have a clear plan regarding how to confront a patient who constantly obsesses and complains about the lack of consistency or thoroughness of the treatment when the particular obsessing is a sign of disdain toward other people.

Note. In many personality disorders, in which there is no clear indication or no data to support the use of medications, collaborative treatment might arise because there is psychopharmacological treatment of a comorbid Axis I disorder. This table provides tips with respect to how the patient's personality disorder might be dealt with in a collaborative treatment even if the medication is being administered for reasons other than the patient's personality disorder diagnosis.

Comorbid Substance Abuse Treatment

Collaboration should occur when the patient is in both substance abuse treatment and treatment with a psychiatrist for personality disorder issues. Continuous use of substances can exacerbate personality disorder psychopathology, and in these instances it is very important that the substance abuse counselor and/or psychotherapist and the treating psychiatrist immediately confer (Casillas and Clark 2002; de Groot et al. 2003). If an increase in or a resumption of substance use after a period of abstinence should occur, the counselor/psychotherapist needs to initiate contact with the psychiatrist. Sometimes a patient will feel embarrassed about resuming use of substances after a period of sobriety and may ask the counselor/psychotherapist not to inform the psychiatrist. Obviously this wish cannot be granted, because there would be 1) collusion between the counselor/psychotherapist and the patient to keep the psychiatrist in the dark and 2) a splitting between the counselor/psychotherapist and the psychiatrist.

> An engineer in his mid-50s, Mr. BB was referred for substance abuse treatment after his second citation for driving while intoxicated. The substance abuse counselor referred Mr. BB to a psychiatrist for treatment of narcissistic personality disorder. Whenever Mr. BB increased his alcohol use, he would miss his appointments with the psychiatrist because he was embarrassed, although he *would* attend his substance abuse sessions. The psychiatrist called the substance abuse counselor whenever Mr. BB missed an appointment, and the counselor always convinced Mr. BB to return to and continue with the psychiatrist. The psychiatrist eventually concluded that Mr. BB's shame about his substance abuse behavior related more to avoidance than narcissism in interpersonal functioning, and this information allowed the substance abuse counselor to modify his approach to Mr. BB.

Somatic Complaints, the Primary Care Physician, and the Psychiatrist

Patients with personality disorders, particularly those with Cluster B and Cluster C personality disorders, have a tendency to be somatically preoccupied (Benjamin et al. 1989). Although the treating psychiatrist may suspect mere somatic preoccupation, one cannot make the mistake of not taking the complaint seriously. If complaints persist or if different somatic concerns frequently appear, it is important for the psychiatrist to share his concern with the physician working up the somatic issues. Together, the two physicians can decide how much physical exploration of

somatic concerns should occur and coordinate a consistent therapeutic response to persisting somatic issues (Williams and Silk 1997).

SEVEN PRINCIPLES TO FOLLOW IN COLLABORATIVE TREATMENT

A number of principles can apply to any collaborative treatment, but they have special application in personality disorders. Adherence to these principles can lead to a smoother and more synergistic approach to collaborative treatment (Silk 1995).

Understanding and Clarifying the Relationship Between the Therapist and the Prescriber

The relationship between a psychotherapist and a pharmacotherapist, or "prescriber," has been described as the "pharmacotherapy-psychotherapy triangle" (Beitman et al. 1984). In managed care, psychiatrists may be expected to provide medical backup for therapists whose work they do not know, whose approach they may not agree with, or whom they do not respect (Goldberg et al. 1991). Conversely, the psychotherapist may have to deal with a psychiatrist whom he or she does not know or agree with. In the best of worlds, neither the psychiatrist nor the psychotherapist would feel obligated to collaborate with a treater whom he or she does not respect.

Patients with personality disorders are quite sensitive to disagreements among members of the treatment team (Main 1957; Stanton and Schwartz 1954). Without communication and knowledge about what other professionals involved in the case are doing, the patient can become caught in the middle of disagreement (Stanton and Schwartz 1954). Each treater should respect what the other is trying to accomplish. This respect for treatment modality should be separated from personal feelings (although it is always easier if there is mutual liking). Each provider should be free to conduct an open communication with the other so that treatment collaboration and coordination can occur (Koenigsberg 1993).

Ideally, the prescriber and the therapist will know each other or at least know something about each other's practice and practice reputation. The prescriber should have an appreciation for the basic psychological issues involved in treatment and a general understanding of how they may manifest in psychopharmacological treatment. The prescribing psychiatrist needs to be clear with the therapist as to his or her beliefs in the putative efficacy of psychotherapy in the personality disorder in general as well as for each patient specifically. Psychotherapy will not proceed constructively if the prescriber does not believe in the usefulness of psychotherapy, particularly with personality-disordered patients (especially those belonging to Cluster B). Maintenance of therapeutic boundaries between treaters is crucial in patients with personality disorders and must be clarified (Woodward et al. 1993). Some questions to ask are: Should between-session phone calls be permitted in the pharmacological treatment if they are not permitted or are frowned upon in the psychotherapy? In what quantities will pills be prescribed, and what course should the therapist take if there is a sudden increase in the suicidality of the patient? When the patient requests a change or an increase in dosage, will the prescriber contact the therapist beforehand to understand better what issues might be coming up in the psychotherapy? How frequently will discussions between the prescriber and the therapist take place? How will issues that belong primarily in the psychotherapy be dealt with if they are brought up in the psychopharmacological treatment? Will the psychopharmacologist notify the psychotherapist that he or she has directed some issue back to the psychotherapist?

The psychotherapist, in a similar manner, needs to have respect for the prescriber and for the intervention of psychopharmacology (Koenigsberg 1993). Although there is probably little need for nonmedical therapists to be experts in psychotropic drug usage, nonmedical psychotherapists should understand the general indications for pharmacotherapy and be aware of the specificity as well as the limitations of the psychopharmacological treatment. The therapist should have some rudimentary knowledge of both the expected therapeutic effects as well as the possible side effects of at least the broader classes of psychotropic medications. In the course of the psychotherapy, the therapist should be willing to discuss, albeit on a limited basis, the patient's experience (both positive and negative) of taking the medication. Additionally, the therapist needs to have some knowledge of medications so that he or she can have some appreciation of what might be subjective versus objective reactions of the patient to taking the medication.

As stated earlier, no psychotherapist or psychopharmacologist should feel obligated to work with a collaborative partner with whom they do not agree or respect. They each must respect the roles and competence of their co-treater. In this atmosphere of mutual respect, both the prescriber and the therapist need to appreciate the perceived efficacy as well as limitations of each of the interventions. Both need to be able to tolerate treatment situations where progress is often slow, punctuated by periods of improvement and regression, and where the long-range prognosis is often guarded but not necessarily negative. Appreciating each other's difficulties and those of the patient in the treatment may help each treater avoid blaming the other (or the patient) during difficult periods.

Appelbaum suggested that, to address both clarity of treatment and treatment expectations, as well as medicolegal issues, the therapist and prescriber draw up a formal contract that delineates their respective roles as well as the expected frequency and range of, or limitations on, their communication (Appelbaum 1991; Chiles et al. 1991). Such a contract works well when the two people share responsibility for a number of patients (Smith 1989). These ideas about contracts are merely suggestions and certainly may not be necessary or useful when the two collaborators work in the same clinic or the same health system.

Much of what we diagnose as personality disorder reflects a group of patients who have chronic maladaptive interpersonal functioning across a wide range of settings. Interpersonal dysfunction cannot and should not be ignored, dismissed, or denied, and whenever and wherever it occurs in the therapeutic endeavor, it should be discussed not only between the two therapists but among the treaters *and* the patient. Transference is not solely reserved for transference-oriented psychotherapy (Beck and Freeman 1990; Goldhamer 1984), and "pharmacotherapy is [also] an interpersonal transaction" (Beitman 1993, p. 538).

Understanding What the Medication Means to Both Therapist and Prescriber

Medications may play both a positive and a negative role in treatment. The therapist and the prescriber need to be attuned to what the initiation of medication means to each of them.

Although DSM-IV-TR (American Psychiatric Association 2000) lists 10 personality disorders, in clinical practice patients with personality disorders defy easy classification and do not always fit neatly into any of these DSM categories (Westen and Arkowitz-Westen 1998). In addition, no medications have yet been indicated for any specific personality disorder. Although there are algorithms with respect to the pharmacological treatment of personality disorders (particularly BPD [American Psychiatric Association

2001; Soloff 1998]), there are no clear-cut rules as to when or what medication should be used in any given Axis II diagnosis. In circumstances with prescriber self-doubt, ambivalence, and uncertainty about either the diagnosis or, more probably, the chosen pharmacological agent, a defensive and authoritarian posture might be assumed by the prescriber in an attempt to assure that the pharmacological decision was correct. The prescriber and/or the therapist may deny ambivalence about the medication, become intolerant of the patient's (or the other provider's) questions and concerns, and present the possible therapeutic effects of the medications in a more positive light than the evidence would imply. This idealization of the medication, similar to the patient's periodic idealization of the treatment, will usually be short-lived.

Pessimism about progress in the therapy was given as a reason to consider prescribing medications by 65% of the respondent psychotherapists in a study by Waldinger and Frank (1989). Given that some patients with personality disorders, particularly BPD, seem especially attuned to feelings, a treater's pessimism or frustration with the course of therapy may be inadvertently and unconsciously conveyed to the patient. Conversely, a referral to a psychopharmacologist could be viewed as an opportunity for consultation and second opinion (Chiles et al. 1991).

It is easy for treaters to develop anger and rage at patients with personality disorders, particularly with patients with substantial borderline, narcissistic, and paranoid personality disorder characteristics, when there is little apparent therapeutic progress (Gabbard and Wilkinson 1994). At these times, one treater may try to pull back from the treatment or, conversely, try to take over control of the entire treatment. The best way to handle these feelings is not to isolate oneself but to approach the other provider and be willing to share one's frustrations. More often than not, the first provider will discover that the other provider shares similar frustrations. This shared frustration not only will lead to less tension in each provider and in the therapy but also, at times, to a discussion and a review of the treatment.

When medication is being considered in a collaborative treatment, the following questions may be asked: Where is the impetus for the medication coming from? Does the therapist think the medication will affect or change the therapeutic relationship? In turn, the prescriber should be able to let the therapist know if he or she feels that the therapist's expectations for the medication are unrealistic and what might be a reasonable expected response.

Understanding What the Medication Means to the Patient

Beginning pharmacotherapy or changing medication may not always be seen as favorable by patients, and a negative reaction to the idea of medication needs to be anticipated. A propensity to put the most negative spin on interpersonal encounters or perceived intentions may cause patients with personality disorders to experience the introduction of medication as a failure of their role in treatment or as the psychotherapist giving up on them. Patients might also, albeit rarely, experience the introduction of medication as a hopeful sign, as an additional modality that might help speed the progress of the treatment (Gunderson 1984, 2001; Waldinger and Frank 1989). Whatever the patient's reaction, understanding what the medication means to the patient and how the patient understands the use of medication within the context of the therapy as well as in the context of his or her own life experience is crucial (Metzl and Riba 2003).

Understanding the patient's reaction to the introduction of medication can be important not only for the patient's cooperation and compliance but also for transferential issues. The patient may take medication in a spirit of collaboration with the therapist and the prescriber. The patient may disagree with the decision, but cooperate out of a strong need to please. A patient's reactions will depend on whether the therapist and prescriber are truly collaborating or at odds.

The introduction of medication into any therapy, even if by a conferring psychiatrist, has repercussions on the transference (Goldhamer 1984). If the idea of medication is introduced early in the treatment process, the potential negative transferential reaction to the introduction of medications later may be minimized. It is important that the therapist and the prescriber be on the same page as to "how" medication will be chosen, introduced, continued, discontinued, and so on. Discussions at the beginning of treatment can model the ethos of an open forum for exchange of information about medications and other feelings.

> Mr. CC, a 50-year-old man with histrionic personality disorder and panic disorder, was referred to an anxiety disorder clinic after several emergency department visits because of uncomfortable arousal symptoms precipitated by an antidepressant (Soloff et al. 1986a). He received cognitive-behavioral therapy and responded well, although he had trouble starting an antidepressant without having his panic symptom increase. He did tolerate a low-dose benzodiazepine but was fearful of becoming "addicted" to the benzodiazepine and would intermittently reduce his dosage despite his

therapist's attempts to discourage it. When Mr. CC's insurance ran out, he stopped seeing his therapist because he was "doing so well," and he also stopped his medication. He began to have emotional outbursts and increased panic attacks and called the psychiatric emergency room inquiring about rehabilitation for drug abuse. Therapy was reinitiated after both the therapist and psychiatrist discussed Mr. CC's concerns about medication and how these concerns were affecting his life. The providers developed clear plans as to whom Mr. CC would call for "medication questions," whom for "exposure questions," and how they would respond to emotional upheavals.

Both therapist and prescriber should be aware that patients may use medications as transitional objects (particularly patients with borderline, histrionic, and perhaps severely dependent personality disorder [Cardasis et al. 1997; Gunderson et al. 1985; Winnicott 1953]). In this context, the patient's attachment and/or resistance to changing or altering medications may seem out of proportion to the actual therapeutic benefit derived from the medication (Adelman 1985). It may also explain why the patient who has repeatedly complained about the medications is unwilling to change them even when there has been little clear evidence that the medications have been effective.

Understanding That the Medication Will Probably Have Limited Effectiveness

Therapists and prescribers need to appreciate the therapeutic benefits and limitations of medication. Therapists should inquire about their patient's medications at moments of calm, not during periods of crisis. Perhaps the most instructive and useful time for (ex)change is when things are actually going well and treatment does not seem bleak or hopeless.

The prescriber should describe what features of a specific medication may or may not be useful in this particular patient at this particular time. The prescriber should tell the therapist what unusual idiosyncratic reactions to the medication might occur (Gardner and Cowdry 1985; Soloff et al. 1986a), especially because these paradoxical reactions or tendencies toward dependency may not always be listed in the package insert or in the *Physician's Desk Reference*.

With effective collaboration, medication decisions will not be solely in the hands of the prescriber. A dialogue between therapist and prescriber should take place as to how each particular type or category of medication with the particular patient might work.

Ms. DD was referred by a psychiatrist from out of town for treatment of anxiety and depression.

Ms. DD had a long history of major depressive episodes. At the time of the evaluation, she was taking five medications: two mood stabilizers, a low-dose atypical antipsychotic, an antidepressant, and a benzodiazepine. She insisted that this combination was the correct regimen for her and that the new psychiatrist not tamper with her medications. She said it took many months and finally a referral to the most prominent psychopharmacologist in her region before the right combination was found. She also stated that she was going to remain in psychotherapy with her old therapist through weekly long-distance phone contacts.

The new psychiatrist, after seeing Ms. DD five or six times, began to feel that Ms. DD primarily had a narcissistic personality disorder and that her depressions were brought about by her extreme sensitivity to anything that could remotely represent a narcissistic injury. The psychiatrist called Ms. DD's therapist, who acknowledged that although Ms. DD did have some narcissistic issues, she really had experienced a number of major depressive episodes during their treatment together.

After a few months, Ms. DD grew more depressed, but her depression was marked primarily by lethargy, absenteeism from work, and an inability to concentrate. She was, however, able to date and had no loss of libido or appetite. Instead of feelings of guilt or worthlessness, she had feelings of grandiosity and entitlement. Ms. DD requested a psychostimulant to help with her concentration and lethargy. The psychiatrist balked and tried to address some of the ways in which he felt her depression was atypical. He pointed out that she seemed more invested in wanting the psychiatrist to figure out what pills would make her better rather than in exploring events in her life that might be leading to what she thought was depression. She stormed out of the office. Later that week, Ms. DD called the psychiatrist to say that her therapist also believed that she could benefit from a psychostimulant, and she was going to find a psychiatrist who was an expert in depression and more up-to-date about treatment. Calls the psychiatrist made to Ms. DD's long-distance therapist went unanswered.

Understanding How the Medication Fits Into the Overall Treatment and Treatment Plan for the Patient

If a psychotherapist considers using medications at some time during the course of treatment, it is hoped that he or she will have an ongoing arrangement with a prescriber or know ahead of time who the prescriber might be. It is never wise to begin searching for a prescriber during a time of pressing need for medications.

The goal of treatment for a patient with personality disorder cannot be cure. Deciding to use medications or changing medications should not imply that one is "going for the cure." The goal of treatment should be to try to improve the ways in which our patients cope, to help them develop increased awareness of their cognitive rigidity and distortions, to assist them in becoming somewhat less impulsive and less affectively labile, and to try to increase the distance between, while reducing the amplitude of, their interpersonal crises (Koenigsberg 1993). These goals are attributable to both the psychotherapy and psychopharmacology and need to be appreciated by both the therapist and the prescriber. A prescriber who conveys a powerful belief in finding the "right" medication will promote an unrealistic and difficult situation.

Any therapy for patients with character disorders must have realistic and limited goals set early in the therapy, lest any of the players begin to idealize another player or another modality. Such idealization can only lead to disappointment and the multiple repercussions that occur in the treatment as a result.

Understanding the Potential and Actual Lethality of the Medication

Many psychotropic medications can be lethal, particularly tricyclic antidepressants, lithium, and the mood stabilizers/anticonvulsants. The monoamine oxidase inhibitors and the benzodiazepines also have a significant morbidity and mortality associated with overdose, especially when combined with other agents. Suicide potential needs to be continually assessed, and when it increases, a plan should be enacted that takes into account when the therapist will contact the prescriber, whether the prescriber is going to limit the size of the prescription, which of the treating professionals might hold onto the medications if a decision is made to limit their administration, and so on. At a minimum, if the therapist believes there is an increase in suicide potential, then the prescriber should be notified. If the therapist is fearful that the patient may overdose, this issue should be discussed openly with the prescriber.

Patients with personality disorders, particularly BPD, are potentially volatile and can act out when they feel that relationships are threatened (Gunderson 1984). The therapist–patient relationship is one that, when complicated by transference, can increase the possibility of acting-out in ways that include suicidal and other self-destructive behaviors; the prescriber–patient relationship is another that also holds the potential for these types of dangers. Mutual respect and communication between the therapist and the prescriber are indispensable to ensuring that a crisis is defused.

Understanding That Interpersonal Crises and Affective Storms Cannot Be Relieved Simply Through Initiation or Modification of the Medication

Introducing medication into the treatment of a patient with personality disorder should not be a spur-of-the-moment decision. It should be done in a controlled manner with forethought and not in the midst of an interpersonal or transferential crisis. Our patients' lives and affects do not follow well-designed courses or even respond to well-designed plans. Even if careful plans are made, the interpersonal crises and affective storms that occur in treatment, combined with the interpersonal demandingness and/or helplessness and passivity of the patient, put enormous pressure on the therapist to do something, to change something, to make the pain go away. There is a tendency to promise much more than can be accomplished, ultimately leading to idealization, disappointment, and subsequent devaluation. If there is a collaborative relationship, and it is very good and mutually supportive, then neither treater should deal with the patient's attacks and demands alone. Each can use the opportunity to think through and resolve the crisis.

In a crisis, all of the six points just described come into play. How well has there been open collaboration between the psychotherapist and the prescriber? How well do they work together, and can they trust each other and each other's judgment? How do they each, as well as the patient, understand the role of medication in the treatment and the medication's benefits and symbolic meaning? How well does each person understand the limits of the medication, and is one of the treaters overreacting, merely prescribing or wanting a prescription written for medication in order to feel that a crisis is being defused? What has been said about medications in the treatment in the past, and how and when have medications been used in the treatment? Have medications been employed successfully, and have they been used safely by the patient?

CONTRAINDICATIONS TO COLLABORATIVE TREATMENT

Before concluding, we need to make mention of situations in which collaborative treatment may be contraindicated. First, however, we must point out that when a patient needs both medication and psychotherapeutic treatment, it is very common that both treatments are provided by a single psychiatrist. We continue to urge treatment by one individual psychiatrist whenever possible if the psychiatrist feels capable of and competent in providing both the medication and the specific form of psychotherapy most useful to the patient.

There may be situations in which collaborative treatment is contraindicated. The first situation would be when the patient is extremely paranoid or psychotic. These types of patients may not agree to having people "talk about them" and thus would not sign a release of information for such exchanges to occur. Also, paranoid people often think that all or most other people are talking about them, and the therapist may not wish to reinforce this idea by means of an arrangement wherein people *are* talking about the patient.

There may also be instances in which patients have an admixture of serious medical and psychiatric problems. The medical problems may directly affect the patient's psychological problems and presentation as well as the patient's cognitive processes and ability to comprehend. A physician who understands the impact of medical conditions on psychological presentation and functioning and who can conduct the psychotherapy as well as manage the medications would be most helpful in these cases, especially if the medical condition or related psychological problems wax and wane. In this instance, drug–drug interactions may have a direct impact on psychological and medical well-being, and changes in medical condition may warrant repeated reevaluation of psychotropic drug regimens.

In other instances, practical reality issues may lead to treatment by a single provider rather than collaborative treatment. If a patient has a severe limit on the number of sessions of psychological or psychiatric treatment because of third-party payer restrictions, then the psychiatrist must consider how to use those sessions most efficiently and cost-effectively for the patient. In this instance, being able to manage medications and conduct psychotherapy in a single session may be important. A similar situation can occur when the patient has severely restricted financial resources or lives so far away that a trip to the psychotherapist and/or psychiatrist involves a significant expenditure of time or money. In this case, if both psychotherapy and psychopharmacology can be accomplished in a single trip or visit, then this approach should be seriously considered.

CONCLUSION

Collaborative treatment is increasing because of a number of factors, some economic, some because of advances in neuroscience and pharmacology, and some because of managed care and the way health care in the United States is delivered. The various combinations and permutations of collaborative treatment are growing beyond the standard combination of one person writing prescriptions for psychiatric medications while another person provides the psychotherapy. Psychiatrists, psychologists, PCPs, social workers, case managers, physician assistants, and visiting nurses are just some of the players involved in a collaborative treatment.

Advances in neuroscience and trends toward using psychotropic medications more regularly for patients with personality disorders have led to more such patients receiving collaborative treatment. Managed care puts pressure on psychiatrists to use medications for a "quicker" response, and patients, bolstered by direct-to-consumer advertising, assume a medication is available for every ailment. Given the co-occurrence of many Axis I disorders with personality disorders, it is not uncommon to find one provider managing medications while another directs or conducts psychodynamic, cognitive-behavioral, or interpersonal psychotherapy.

Patients with personality disorders have major difficulties in interpersonal relationships, and every visit with a psychopharmacologist or a psychotherapist is an interpersonal encounter. These interpersonal encounters must be managed carefully, and when there are two or more providers of treatment, the providers must communicate with each other on a regular basis. This communication is not only a hallmark of good psychiatric care but is also a method whereby two or more providers can coordinate their treatment approach and collaborate on decision making so that the experience can be a synergistic rather than a divisive one.

Collaborative treatment at its best occurs in an atmosphere of respect and results in open and free communication with fellow providers. An opportunity for collaborators to consult and learn from one another exists, and this collaboration has the potential to result in more comprehensive and thoughtful care for difficult-to-treat groups of patients.

REFERENCES

Adelman SA: Pills as transitional objects: a dynamic understanding of the use of medication in psychotherapy. Psychiatry 48:246–253, 1985

American Psychiatric Association: Diagnostic and Statistical Manual of Mental Disorders, 4th Edition, Text Revision. Washington, DC, American Psychiatric Association, 2000

American Psychiatric Association: Practice guideline for the treatment of patients with borderline personality disorder. Am J Psychiatry 158 (10 suppl):1–52, 2001

Appelbaum PS: General guidelines for psychiatrists who prescribe medications for patients treated by nonmedical psychotherapists. Hosp Community Psychiatry 42:281–282, 1991

Barlow DH, Gorman JM, Shear MK, et al: Cognitive behavioral therapy, imipramine, or their combination for panic disorder: a randomized controlled trial. JAMA 28:2529–2539, 2000

Bateman A, Fonagy P: Effectiveness of partial hospitalization in the treatment of borderline personality disorder: a randomized controlled trial. Am J Psychiatry 156:1563–1569, 1999

Bateman A, Fonagy P: Treatment of borderline personality disorder with psychoanalytically oriented partial hospitalization: an 18-month follow-up. Am J Psychiatry 158:36–42, 2001

Beck AT, Freeman A: Cognitive Therapy of Personality Disorders. New York, Guilford, 1990

Beitman BD: Pharmacotherapy and the stages of psychotherapeutic change, in American Psychiatric Press Review of Psychiatry, Vol 12. Edited by Oldham JM, Riba MB, Tasman A. Washington, DC, American Psychiatric Press, 1993, pp 521–539

Beitman BD, Chiles J, Carlin A: The pharmacotherapy-psychotherapy triangle: psychiatrist, non-medical psychotherapist, and patient. J Clin Psychiatry 45:458–459, 1984

Benjamin J, Silk KR, Lohr NE, et al: The relationship between borderline personality disorder and anxiety disorders. Am J Orthopsychiatry 59:461–467, 1989

Benjamin LS: Interpersonal Reconstructive Therapy. New York, Guilford, 2003

Browne G, Steiner M, Roberts J, et al: Sertraline and/or interpersonal psychotherapy for patients with dysthymic disorder in primary care: 6-month comparison with longitudinal 2-year follow-up of effectiveness and costs. J Affect Disord 68:317–330, 2002

Cardasis W, Hochman JA, Silk KR: Transitional objects and borderline personality disorder. Am J Psychiatry 154:250–255, 1997

Casillas A, Clark LA: Dependency, impulsivity, and self-harm: traits hypothesized to underlie the association between cluster B personality and substance use disorders. J Personal Disord 16:424–436, 2002

Chiles JA, Carlin AS, Benjamin GAH, et al: A physician, a nonmedical psychotherapist, and a patient: the pharmacotherapy-psychotherapy triangle, in Integrating Pharmacotherapy and Psychotherapy. Edited by Beitman BD, Klerman GL. Washington DC, American Psychiatric Press, 1991, pp 105–118

Clarkin JF, Yeomans FE, Kernberg OF: Psychotherapy for borderline personality. New York, Wiley, 1999

Cloninger CR, Svrakic DM, Przybeck TR: A psychobiological model of temperament and character. Arch Gen Psychiatry 50:975–990, 1993

Coccaro EF, Kavoussi RJ: Fluoxetine and impulsive aggressive behavior in personality-disordered subjects. Arch Gen Psychiatry 54:1081–1088, 1997

Coccaro EF, Siever L, Klar HM, et al: Serotonergic studies in patients with affective and personality disorders. Arch Gen Psychiatry 46:587–599, 1989

Cowdry RW, Gardner DL: Pharmacotherapy of borderline personality disorder: alprazolam, carbamazepine, trifluoperazine, and tranylcypromine. Arch Gen Psychiatry 45:111–119, 1988

de Groot MH, Franken IH, van der Meer CW, et al: Stability and change in dimensional ratings of personality disorders in drug abuse patients during treatment. J Subst Abuse Treat 24:115–120, 2003

Gabbard GO: Splitting in hospital treatment. Am J Psychiatry 146:444–451, 1989

Gabbard GO, Wilkinson SM: Management of Countertransference with Borderline Patients. Washington, DC, American Psychiatric Press, 1994

Gardner DL, Cowdry RW: Alprazolam induced dyscontrol in borderline personality disorder. Am J Psychiatry 142:98–100, 1985

Goldberg RS, Riba M, Tasman A: Psychiatrists' attitudes toward prescribing medication for patients treated by nonmedical psychotherapists. Hosp Community Psychiatry 42:276–280, 1991

Goldberg SC, Schulz SC, Schulz PM, et al: Borderline and schizotypal personality disorders treated with low-dose thiothixene vs. placebo. Arch Gen Psychiatry 43:680–686, 1986

Goldhamer PM: Psychotherapy and pharmacotherapy: the challenge of integration. Can J Psychiatry 38:173–177, 1984

Greenblatt M, Solomon MH, Evans A, et al (eds): Drug and Social Therapy in Chronic Schizophrenia. Springfield, IL, Charles C Thomas, 1965

Gunderson JG: Borderline Personality Disorder. Washington, DC, American Psychiatric Press, 1984

Gunderson JG: Borderline Personality Disorder: A Clinical Guide. Washington DC, American Psychiatric Publishing, 2001

Gunderson JG, Morris H, Zanarini MC: Transitional objects and borderline patients, in The Borderline: Current Empirical Research. Edited by McGlashan TH. Washington, DC, American Psychiatric Association, 1985, pp 43–60

Healy D: The Anti-Depressant Era. Cambridge, MA, Harvard University Press, 1997

Healy D: The Creation of Psychopharmacology. Cambridge, MA, Harvard University Press, 2002

Hollander E, Allen, A, Lopez, RP, et al: A preliminary double-blind, placebo-controlled trial of divalproex sodium in borderline personality disorder. J Clin Psychiatry 62:199–203, 2001

Keller MB, McCullough JP, Klein DN, et al: A comparison of nefazodone, the cognitive behavioral-analysis system of psychotherapy, and their combination for the treatment of chronic depression. N Engl J Med 342:1642–1670, 2000

Kernberg O, Koenigsberg H, Stone M, et al: Borderline Patients: Extending the Limits of Treatability. New York, Basic Books, 2000

Klerman GL: The psychiatric patient's right to effective treatment: implications of Osheroff vs. Chestnut Lodge. Am J Psychiatry 147:409–418, 1990

Koenigsberg HW: Combining psychotherapy and pharmacotherapy in the treatment of borderline patients, in American Psychiatric Press Review of Psychiatry, Vol 12. Edited by Oldham JM, Riba MB, Tasman A. Washington, DC, American Psychiatric Press, 1993, pp 541–563

Koenigsberg HW, Reynolds D, Goodman M, et al: Risperidone in the treatment of schizotypal personality disorder. J Clin Psychiatry 64:628–634, 2003

Kool S, Dekker J, Duijsens IJ, et al: Changes in personality pathology after pharmacotherapy and combined therapy for depressed patients. J Personal Disord 17:60–72, 2003

Lecrubier Y: Prescribing patterns for depression and anxiety worldwide. J Clin Psychiatry 62 (suppl 13):31–36, 2001

Linehan MM, Heard HL, Armstrong HE: Naturalistic follow-up of a behavioral treatment for chronically parasuicidal borderline patients. Arch Gen Psychiatry 50:971–974, 1993

Livesley WJ: A practical approach to the treatment of patients with borderline personality disorder. Psychiatr Clin North Am 23:211–232, 2000

Livesley WJ, Jang KL, Vernon PA: Phenotypic and genetic structure of traits delineating personality disorder. Arch Gen Psychiatry 55:941–948, 1998

Main TF: The ailment. Br J Med Psychol 30:129–145, 1957

Manber R, Arnow B, Blasey C, et al: Patient's therapeutic skill acquisition and response to psychotherapy, alone or in combination with medication. Psychol Med 33:693–702, 2003

Markowitz P: Pharmacotherapy, in Handbook of Personality Disorders, Theory, Research and Treatment. Edited by Livesley WJ. New York, Guilford, 2001, pp 475–493

Markowitz PJ: Recent trends in the pharmacotherapy of personality disorders. J Personal Disord 18:90–101, 2004

Metzl JM, Riba M: Understanding the symbolic value of medications: a brief review. Primary Psychiatry 10:1–4, 2003

Ogden TH: Projective Identification and Psychotherapeutic Technique. New York, Jason Aronson, 1982

Paris J: Borderline Personality Disorder: A Multidimensional Approach. Washington, DC, American Psychiatric Press, 1994

Paris J: Chronic suicidality among patients with borderline personality disorder. Psychiatr Serv 53:738–742, 2002

Paris J: Personality Disorders Over Time: Precursors, Course, and Outcome. Washington, DC, American Psychiatric Publishing, 2003

Riba M, Balon R (eds): Psychopharmacology and Psychotherapy: A Collaborative Approach. Washington, DC, American Psychiatric Press, 1999

Rinne T, van de Brink W, Wouters I, et al: SSRI treatment of borderline personality disorder: a randomized, placebo-controlled clinical trial for female patients with borderline personality disorder. Am J Psychiatry 159:2048–2054, 2002

Rutter M: The interplay of nature, nurture, and developmental influences: the challenge ahead for mental health. Arch Gen Psychiatry 59:996–1000, 2002

Salzman C, Wolfson AN, Schatzberg A, et al: Effect of fluoxetine on anger in symptomatic volunteers with borderline personality disorder. J Clin Psychopharmacol 15:23–29, 1995

Schulz SC, Camlin KL: Treatment of borderline personality disorder: potential of the new antipsychotic medications. Journal of Practical Psychiatry and Behavioral Health 5:247–255, 1999

Sheard M, Marini J, Bridges C, et al: The effect of lithium on impulsive aggressive behavior in man. Am J Psychiatry 133:1409–1413, 1976

Siever LJ, Davis KL: A psychobiological perspective on the personality disorders. Am J Psychiatry 148:1647–1658, 1991

Siever LJ, Torgersen S, Gunderson JG, et al: The borderline diagnosis III: identifying endophenotypes for genetic studies. Biol Psychiatry 51:964–968, 2002

Silk KR: Rational pharmacotherapy for patients with personality disorders, in Clinical Assessment and Management of Severe Personality Disorders. Edited by Links P. Washington, DC, American Psychiatric Press, 1995, pp 109–142

Silk KR (ed): Biology of Personality Disorders. Washington, DC, American Psychiatric Press, 1998

Skodol AE, Stout RL, McGlashan TH, et al: Co-occurrence of mood and personality disorders: a report from the Collaborative Longitudinal Personality Disorders Study (CLPS). Depress Anxiety 10:175–182, 1999

Skodol AE, Siever LJ, Livesley WJ, et al: The borderline diagnosis II: biology, genetics, and clinical course. Biol Psychiatry 51:951–963, 2002

Smith JM: Some dimensions of transference in combined treatment, in The Psychotherapist's Guide to Pharmacotherapy. Edited by Ellison JM. Chicago, IL, Year Book Medical, 1989, pp 79–94

Soloff PH: What's new in personality disorders? An update on pharmacologic treatment. J Personal Disord 4:233–243, 1990

Soloff PH: Algorithms for pharmacological treatment of personality dimensions: symptom-specific treatments for cognitive-perceptual, affective, and impulsive-behavioral dysregulation. Bull Menninger Clin 62:195–214, 1998

Soloff PH, George A, Nathan RS, et al: Paradoxical effects of amitriptyline in borderline patients. Am J Psychiatry 143:1603–1605, 1986a

Soloff PH, George A, Nathan RS, et al: Progress in pharmacotherapy of borderline disorders: a double-blind study of amitriptyline, haloperidol, and placebo. Arch Gen Psychiatry 43:691–697, 1986b

Soloff PH, Cornelius J, George A, et al: Efficacy of phenelzine and haloperidol in borderline personality disorder. Arch Gen Psychiatry 50:377–385, 1993

Stanton AH, Schwartz MS: The Mental Hospital: A Study of Institutional Participation in Psychiatric Illness and Treatment. London, England, Tavistock, 1954

Stone MH: The Fate of Borderline Patients: Successful Outcome and Psychiatric. New York, Guilford, 1990

Waldinger RS, Frank AF: Clinicians' experiences in combining medication and psychotherapy in the treatment of borderline patients. Hosp Community Psychiatry 40:712–718, 1989

Westen D, Arkowitz-Westen L: Limitations of Axis II in diagnosing personality pathology in clinical practice. Am J Psychiatry 155:1767–1771, 1998

Westen D, Moses M, Silk KR, et al: Quality of depressive experience in borderline personality disorder and major depression: when depression is not just depression. J Personal Disord 6:382–393, 1992

Williams BC, Silk KR: "Difficult" patients, in Primary Care Psychiatry. Edited by Knesper DJ, Riba MB, Schwenk TL. Philadelphia, PA, W.B. Saunders, 1997, pp 61–75

Winnicott D: Transitional objects and transitional phenomena. Int J Psychoanal 34:89–97, 1953

Woodward B, Duckworth KS, Gutheil TG: The pharmacotherapist-psychotherapist collaboration, in American Psychiatric Press Review of Psychiatry, Vol 12. Edited by Oldham JM, Riba MB, Tasman A. Washington, DC, American Psychiatric Press, 1993, pp 631–649

Yen S, Shea MT, Pagano M, et al: Axis I and Axis II disorders as predictors of prospective suicide attempts: findings from the collaborative longitudinal personality disorders study. J Abnorm Psychol 112:375–381, 2003

Young JE, Klosko JS, Weishaar ME: Schema Therapy: A Practitioner's Guide. New York, Guilford, 2003

Zanarini MC, Frankenburg FR: Olanzapine treatment of female borderline personality disorder patients: a double-blind, placebo-controlled pilot study. J Clin Psychiatry 62:849–854, 2001

Zanarini MC, Frankenburg FR, Dubo ED, et al: Axis I comorbidity of borderline personality disorder. Am J Psychiatry 155:1733–1739, 1998

Part V

Special Problems and Populations

29

Assessing and Managing Suicide Risk

Paul S. Links, M.D., F.R.C.P.C.

Nathan Kolla

Robins and colleagues in 1959 demonstrated the strong association between mental disorders and suicide, but the relationship between suicidal behavior and personality disorders (Axis II disorders) has only been systematically studied since the mid-1980s. The purpose of this chapter is threefold. First, the epidemiological evidence for the association between suicidal behavior and suicide in individuals diagnosed with personality disorders is reviewed. Second, we examine whether any potentially modifiable risk factors are associated with these diagnoses, based on existing empirical evidence. Last, clinical approaches to the assessment of the uncommunicative patient and patients with antisocial, borderline, and narcissistic personality disorder presenting at risk for suicide are discussed.

DEFINITION OF TERMS AND METHODOLOGY

For purposes of this review, *suicidal behavior* is defined through three components: suicide, suicide attempts, and self-injurious behaviors. The definitions of O'Carroll et al. (1996) have been adopted. They defined *suicide* as self-injurious behavior with a fatal outcome for which there is evidence (either explicit or implicit) that the individual intended at some (nonzero) level to kill him- or herself. A *suicide attempt* is defined as self-injurious behavior with a nonfatal outcome for which there is evidence (either explicit or implicit) that the individual intended at some (nonzero) level to kill

This chapter is adapted with permission from Links PS, Gould G, Ratnayake R: "Assessing Suicidal Youth With Antisocial, Borderline, or Narcissistic Personality Disorder." *Canadian Journal of Psychiatry* 48:301–310, 2003.

him- or herself. A definition of *self-injurious behavior* not intended to be fatal has also been utilized. Simeon and Favazza (2001) defined *self-injurious behavior* as all behaviors that involve deliberate infliction of direct physical harm to one's body with zero intent to die as a consequence of this behavior.

Our discussion of suicide risk focuses on the clinical entities known as personality disorders. Primarily, the diagnoses from DSM-III, DSM-III-R, DSM-IV, and DSM-IV-TR (American Psychiatric Association 1980, 1987, 1994, 2000) are discussed; however, we also include studies employing ICD-9 and ICD-10 diagnoses (World Health Organization 1977, 1992) for completeness. Personality or personality traits are often discussed from a dimensional approach. These dimensions have inherent advantages for measurement and statistical purposes, describing cases at categorical borders and connecting with the large body of normal personality research. A diagnostic or categorical approach has certain advantages for the practicing clinician, because a considerable body of research related to risk assessment exists based on psychiatric and personality disorder diagnoses. As discussed later, there is a lesser body of clinical research and little consensus related to personality dimensions and suicide risk assessment.

This review is based on the English-language literature from 1991 to 2003 using the search terms of all personality disorders and suicide and for suicidal behavior. In particular, this chapter focuses on research that examined potential risk factors for these diagnoses compared with those for other psychiatric disorders. The final section of this chapter describes clinical approaches to patients at risk for suicidal behavior who are uncommunicative and for those with antisocial, borderline, and/or narcissistic personality disorder. These observations are based on clinical experience and not on empirical evidence. The observations would not replace the need for doing a comprehensive suicide risk assessment based on formats such as those described by Jacobs et al. (1999), Rudd and Joiner (1998), and the American Psychiatric Association's (2003) practice guideline for assessing and treating patients with suicidal behavior. The difficult decisions that arise during a suicide risk assessment—such as whether the patient should be admitted to hospital, whether such admission should be involuntary, or whether the person's risk of suicide should be communicated to the family—are most soundly based on careful clinical assessment, because there is no measurement scale that can replace clinical expertise.

PERSONALITY, PERSONALITY DISORDERS, AND SUICIDE RISK ASSESSMENT

Goldsmith et al. (1990) articulated modern conceptualizations of the causal relationship between personality and/or personality disorder and suicidal behavior, but most importantly, they asked whether personality disorders directly predispose to suicidal behavior independent of other risk factors. Although the causal relationship between personality and/or personality disorders and suicidal behavior is likely complex, research since 1990 has suggested that certain personality features and/or disorders are related to suicidal behavior and are independent of other known risk factors.

Conner et al. (2001) thoroughly reviewed the empirical literature to determine whether psychological vulnerability was a risk factor for completed suicide. The authors argued that *personality traits* was too narrow a concept and that psychological vulnerabilities encompassed dysfunctional cognitions, behavior, and emotions. For example, hopelessness was examined as a form of psychological vulnerability, although it remains unclear whether hopelessness is best considered a personality trait, an affect, or a part of a psychiatric illness.

Reviewing databases from January 1966 to February 2000 and including only constructs found to be associated with suicide by at least two independent teams, Conner et al. (2001) identified five dimensions: impulsivity/aggression, depression, hopelessness, anxiety, and self-consciousness/social disengagement. The proportion of significant findings out of the studies testing the constructs did not differ significantly across the five dimensions: impulsivity/aggression (14/20, 70%); hopelessness (11/16, 69%); depression (13/22, 59%); anxiety (13/22, 59%); and self-consciousness/social disengagement (18/24, 75%). Given the breadth of concepts identified by their review, the authors concluded that "no single conceptual or empirically derived model of personality constructs" (p. 371) was sufficient to explain the relationship of psychological vulnerabilities to suicide. No such comprehensive review was found relating personality traits and suicide attempts.

Johnson et al. (1999) reviewed the empirical literature to determine the value of objective personality inventories for predicting assessment of "long-term" suicide risk. The authors searched PsychLit journal databases from January 1974 to March 1996 and restricted their inquiry to self-reported inventories and reports on entire measures rather than focusing on subscales. The measures reviewed included the California Personality Inventory; Edwards Personal Preference Schedule; Eysenck Personality Tests; Millon Clinical Multiaxial Inventories I–III; Minnesota Multiphasic Personality Inventories (MMPI) 1 and 2; Myers-Briggs Type Indicator; 16 Personality Factor Test; Neuroticism, Extroversion, Openness Personality Inventory; and the Personality Diagnostic Questionnaire.

Based on the review, the MMPI was considered the most empirically investigated objective personality measure; however, the authors found no "support of the notion that any MMPI item(s), scale or configural profile consistently differentiates suicidal from nonsuicidal patients" (p. 178). Overall, Johnson et al. (1999) concluded there was little indication of the utility for any single inventory, scale, or item in the prediction of long-term suicide risk.

These two authoritative reviews expose the limits of our current understanding of the relationship between personality and suicide. However, research continues, and three personality characteristics are highlighted as uniquely related to suicidal behavior and as principal areas for further study. Impulsive aggressiveness has been shown to have a unique relationship to a history of suicidal behavior, and Mann et al. (1999) demonstrated that impulsive aggressiveness was more strongly associated with a history of suicide attempts than was the strength of psychiatric symptomatology. In addition, various biological research strategies have demonstrated that low serotonergic function was specifically related to impulsive aggressiveness, providing evidence for the biological bridge between suicide and personality traits (Mann et al. 1999).

At the other extreme, the individual who appears perfectionistic and vulnerable to narcissistic injury might be at risk for suicidal behavior. Hewitt et al. (1998) demonstrated that perfectionism was significantly related to suicide risk even after controlling for the level of hopelessness and depression. In particular, perceiving oneself as not meeting others' expectations was significantly related to increased suicide risk. Finally, emotional dysregulation, characterized as rapidly shifting mood states, has been theoretically and empirically linked to suicidal behavior. Linehan (1993) hypothesized that emotional dysregulation in conjunction with an invalidating environment explained the suicidal behavior characteristic of individuals with borderline personality disorder (BPD). Fawcett et al. (1990) found that *depressive turmoil*, defined as rapid shifts from one dysphoric state to another without persistence of one affect, was significantly predictive

of suicide in their cohort of individuals with major affective disorders. Although emotional dysregulation should be a primary focus of research, the precise definition of this characteristic requires further refinement. Emotional dysregulation is often subsumed within the concept of neuroticism; however, we have suggested that emotional dysregulation or affective lability might encompass four elements: cyclicity, intensity, variability, or hyperreactivity of mood to external stimuli. Because suicidal behavior is undoubtedly multidetermined, complex modeling of various personality characteristics with other distal and proximal risk factors and utilizing multilevel analyses will be required to explain suicide or suicidal behavior as the outcome.

EPIDEMIOLOGICAL EVIDENCE

Most of the evidence points to the relationship between antisocial and borderline personality disorders and suicidal behavior. Therefore, we begin by reviewing the epidemiological evidence for each of the Cluster B personality disorders. The more limited literature related to Clusters A and C and suicidal behavior are reviewed according to the respective clusters rather than the individual personality disorders. To organize the literature, we discuss the rates of the various personality disorders in individuals who completed suicide or made suicide attempts. Then we present the rates of suicide and suicide attempts in samples of individuals with the various personality disorders.

Cluster B

Studies have been done of the rates of personality disorders in adolescents who died by suicide. Marttunen et al. (1991), from the Comprehensive Psychological Autopsy Study in Finland, estimated that 17% of adolescents ages 13–19 who died by suicide met criteria for conduct disorder or antisocial personality disorder (ASPD). When Marttunen et al. (1994) examined adolescents with nonfatal suicidal behavior, approximately 45% of males and one-third of females were characterized by antisocial behavior. In other research, suicidal behavior was found to be higher among adolescents with conduct disorders than in the comparison groups even after controlling for major depression (Brent et al. 1993b). Beautrais et al. (1996) studied individuals who had made medically serious suicide attempts and compared them with community comparison subjects. After controlling for the intercorrelations between mental disorders, these researchers found the risk of a serious suicide attempt was 3.7 times higher for individuals with ASPD than for those without. When they examined men under age 30, the risk of a serious suicide attempt was almost 9 times more likely among antisocial individuals than among those without the disorder; for women, the risk of a serious suicide attempt was 2.3 times higher.

A few studies have documented the lifetime risk of suicide in samples of individuals with ASPD. Maddocks (1970), in a 5-year follow-up of a small sample of 59 persons with the disorder, estimated a 5% lifetime risk of suicide. Laub and Vaillant (2000) examined causes of death of 1,000 delinquent and nondelinquent boys followed up from ages 14 to 65 years. Deaths due to violent causes (accident, suicide, or homicide) were significantly more common in delinquent compared with nondelinquent boys; however, equal proportions of both groups died by suicide.

Patients with BPD represent 9%–33% of all suicides (Kullgren et al. 1986; Runeson and Beskow 1991). Bongar et al. (1990) studied chronically suicidal patients with four or more visits in a year to a psychiatric emergency department, and most often these patients met criteria for BPD. These patients accounted for over 12% of all psychiatric emergency department visits during the year studied. Crumley (1979) has shown a high incidence of BPD in adolescents and young adults ages 15–24 who engage in suicidal behavior. Paris and Zweig-Frank (2001) indicated that this diagnosis significantly increases the risk of eventual suicide. Depending on the study, the lifetime risk of suicide among patients with BPD patients is between 3% and 10% (Paris and Zweig-Frank 2001). Those at highest risk appeared to be young, ranging from adolescence into the third decade (Berman 1985; Friedman and Corn 1987; Stone 1990), which likely reflects a decrease in severity of symptoms later in adulthood in the majority of patients (Crumley 1979; Stone 1990). The high rates of suicidal behavior in patients with BPD are reflected by, or some would say result from, the inclusion of recurrent suicidal behavior, gestures, threats, or self-mutilating behavior as a diagnostic criterion in DSM-IV-TR. A history of suicidal behavior is found in 55%–70% of individuals with a personality disorder (Casey 1989; Clarkin et al. 1984; Gomez et al. 1992) and in 60%–78% of individuals with BPD (Gunderson 1984; Kjellander et al. 1998).

Narcissistic personality disorder is an uncommon diagnosis in community samples compared with ASPD and BPD, and few data exist regarding the risk of suicide in individuals with this disorder. In samples of suicide victims studied with the psychological autopsy method, narcissistic personality is infrequently identified. However, Apter et al. (1993) studied 43 consecutive suicides by Israeli males ages 18–21 that occurred during their compulsory military service. Psychological autopsies were carried out using preinduction assessment information, service records, and extensive postmortem interviews. Based on this methodology, the most common Axis II personality disorders were schizoid personality in 16 of 43 (37.2%) and narcissistic personality in 10 of 43 (23.3%). Stone's (1990) extensive follow-up study of 550 patients admitted to the general clinical service of the New York State Psychiatric Institute provided some information on this outcome for individuals hospitalized with the diagnosis of narcissistic personality disorder. According to the 15-year follow-up, patients with the disorder or narcissistic traits were significantly more likely to have died by suicide compared with patients without the disorder or traits (14% versus 5%; $P < 0.02$).

Few studies have reported on the risk of suicide or suicide attempts in individuals with histrionic personality disorder, and studies that do comment on the relationship between this diagnosis and suicidal behavior have rarely controlled for the presence of BPD. Although histrionic personality disorder has been diagnosed in 1%–17% of all adult suicide attempters being assessed at hospital emergency departments (Braun-Scharm 1996; Dirks 1998; Ferreira de Castro et al. 1998; Gupta and Trzepacz 1997; Markar et al. 1991; Soderberg 2001) as well as in 16% of individuals forming a sample of adolescent inpatient suicide attempters (Brent et al. 1993a), Ferreira de Castro et al. (1998) noted that histrionic personality disorder was the most common personality disorder diagnosis (22% of all subjects) in their sample, comprising individuals who engaged in self-injurious behavior but whose intention was not death. Other studies examining the connection between histrionic personality disorder and completed suicide include Harwood et al.'s (2001) observation that 4% of their sample of individuals over the age of 60 had the disorder. The prevalence of suicidal tendencies in a sample of patients diagnosed with hysterical personality disorder, the ICD-9 equivalent of histrionic personality disorder, has been found to be approximately 39% (Ahrens and Haug 1996).

Clusters A and C

Epidemiological evidence for the risk of suicide or suicide attempts among individuals with either Cluster

A or Cluster C personality disorders is relatively scarce. Again, most studies do not control for the possibility of coexisting BPD mediating the observed suicidal behavior in the subjects examined. Depending on the study, the prevalence of Cluster A or C personality disorders in adults presenting to an emergency department following a suicide attempt or self-injury ranges from 3% to 5% for schizoid personality disorder (Braun-Scharm 1996; Dirks 1998; Ferreira de Castro et al. 1998), 9% for schizotypal personality disorder (Markar et al. 1991), 8%–10% for paranoid personality disorder (Persson et al. 1999; Soderberg 2001), 6%–20% for avoidant personality disorder (Persson et al. 1999; Soderberg 2001), 30% for anxious personality disorder (Dirks 1998), 1%–9% for dependent personality disorder (Braun-Scharm 1996; Dirks 1998; Gupta and Trzepacz 1997), 6% for obsessive-compulsive personality disorder (Soderberg 2001), and 13% for anankastic personality disorder (Dirks 1998). In their study of inpatient suicide attempters between the ages of 13 and 19, Brent et al. (1993a) reported that 27% fulfilled criteria for any Cluster A personality disorder and 70% for any Cluster C personality disorder. However, only a diagnosis of borderline or any personality disorder was significant in this sample of adolescent suicide attempters when compared with a group of psychiatric nonsuicidal control subjects.

Similar to the studies just cited, Haw et al. (2001) reported on the prevalence of ICD-10 personality disorders among individuals admitted to a British hospital following an episode of deliberate self-harm and diagnosed on follow-up approximately 12–16 months later. These researchers found that 5% of their sample fulfilled criteria for schizoid personality disorder, 15% for paranoid personality disorder, 21% for anxious personality disorder, 13% for dependent personality disorder, and 20% for anankastic personality disorder.

Several studies have employed the psychological autopsy method of retrospectively diagnosing personality disorders in completed suicides. Among individuals older than 23 whose deaths received a verdict of suicide or unknown cause, Houston et al. (2001) reported that 4% of the victims had a primary paranoid personality disorder, 4% a primary anxious personality disorder, and 7% a primary anankastic personality disorder, whereas 4% had secondary paranoid, anxious, and anankastic personality disorders. Analyzing data from the National Suicide Prevention Project in Finland, Isometsa et al. (1996) determined that 1% of their sample fulfilled criteria for paranoid personality disorder, 6% for avoidant personality disorder, 7% for dependent personality disorder, 3% for obsessive-

compulsive personality disorder, and 18% for Cluster C personality disorders not otherwise specified. Harwood et al. (2001) examined individuals over the age of 60 whose deaths received a verdict of suicide and found that 4% of their sample had had anankastic personality disorder during their lifetimes.

Studies have also reported on rates of attempted and completed suicides among individuals diagnosed with personality disorders. Fenton et al. (1997) located patients from the Chestnut Lodge Follow-Up Study who were originally diagnosed with schizotypal personality disorder and found that 3% had committed suicide, 24% had attempted suicide, and 45% had expressed suicidal ideation at some point during the previous 19 years. Among patients admitted to the psychiatric department of a German hospital between 1981 and 1994 who were assigned a primary diagnosis of personality disorder upon admission, Ahrens and Haug (1996) found that 44% of individuals diagnosed with schizoid personality disorder displayed suicidal tendencies, as did 47% of the patients with paranoid personality disorder or anankastic personality disorder.

Summary

Modestin et al. (1997) noted that suicidal behavior in women is independently correlated with each of the three personality disorder clusters, whereas suicidal behavior in men only correlates with the clusters as a group. Thus, although evidence suggests that Cluster A and C personality disorders are associated with the risk of suicide or suicide attempts, the relationship between Cluster B personality disorders and suicidal behavior has been well documented and appears to be more robust.

RISK FACTORS FOR SUICIDE AND SUICIDAL BEHAVIOR

Many studies have identified factors at a population level that alone or in combination increase the risk of suicide. Although extrapolating these risk factors to an individual allows for categorization of risk, it does little to predict which individual will suicide and when. "The goal of a suicide assessment is not to predict suicide, but rather to place a person along a putative risk continuum, to appreciate the bases of suicidality, and to allow for a more informed intervention" (Jacobs et al. 1999; p. 4). Many risk factors are fixed (age, race, gender), providing little opportunity to intervene. However, several of the most significant risk factors are modifiable. Forster and Wu (2002) captured the concept eloquently in the following statement, "Suicide is almost always the catastrophic result of inadequately treated psychiatric illness" (p. 105). Forster and Wu suggested concentrating on modifiable risk factors. Therefore, the purpose of this review is to discuss risk factors that place patients with personality disorders at a higher risk relative to other individuals with like disorders or place them at higher risk relative to other times in the course of their illness. In addition, purportedly modifiable risk factors are discussed because they might present opportunities for interventions. By far, the majority of the studies have focused on subjects with BPD, with little or no research on patients with other personality disorders. This chapter reviews each of the major risk factors and discusses, in some detail, findings from key studies—those employing carefully characterized comparison groups and controlling for potential confounding factors.

Comorbid Disorders

The presence of two or more psychiatric disorders appears to substantially increase the suicide attempt rate compared with the presence of a single disorder, and comorbidity is found to be higher in adolescents than in adults (Lewinsohn et al. 1995). Most of the research has been done with regard to BPD, and the following studies indicate that certain specific comorbidities may increase the risk for suicidal behavior in patients with BPD.

Major Depressive Episode

Several studies have documented that the existence of depression plus BPD may confer an increased risk for suicidal behavior. In adolescents, coexistence of disruptive behavior plus depression is felt to be a particularly "dangerous" combination (McCracken et al. 1993). The most careful study of this combination was completed by Soloff et al. (2000). They examined a well-characterized group of patients with BPD comorbid with major depressive episodes and compared them with subjects with BPD without a major depressive episode and with subjects with current major depressive episode only. The number of lifetime suicide attempts significantly differentiated the comorbid patients from the other two comparison groups, with a mean of 3.0 lifetime attempts among the comorbid group versus 1.9 lifetime attempts for subjects with pure BPD and 0.8 lifetime attempts for subjects with major depressive episodes only. Comorbid patients reported significantly higher levels of objective plan-

ning based on the most serious lifetime attempt than the other comparison groups. Using regression analysis, the researchers demonstrated that the number of lifetime attempts was predicted by BPD diagnosis and comorbidity, history of aggression, and the level of hopelessness. Overall, the patients with comorbidity demonstrated an increased risk for suicidal behavior, particularly with a higher number of lifetime attempts and evidence for more objective planning. The authors concluded that suicidal behavior in inpatients with BPD should not be considered "less serious" than the suicidal behavior of inpatients with a major depressive episode.

Substance Abuse Disorder

Comorbidity of substance abuse disorder with BPD has also been found to be related to increased suicidal behavior (Runeson and Beskow 1991; Soloff et al. 1994). Links et al. (1995) examined the prognostic significance of comorbid substance abuse in BPD patients. These patients were followed prospectively over a 7-year period. The researchers found that patients comorbid for substance abuse and BPD perceived themselves at significantly more risk for the likelihood of killing themselves than the comparison groups of BPD patients without comorbidity, patients with substance abuse without BPD, and patients with borderline traits only. The comorbid patients also demonstrated a more frequent pattern of self-mutilative behavior and reported a more frequent pattern of suicide threats and attempts than the noncomorbid patients. Yen et al. (2003) prospectively studied the diagnostic predictors of suicide attempts using the Collaborative Longitudinal Personality Disorders sample made up of four personality-disordered groups—schizotypal, borderline, avoidant, and obsessive-compulsive—and a group with major depressive disorder without personality disorder. The baseline diagnosis of a drug use disorder and BPD was predictive of suicide attempts during the follow-up interval; however, alcohol use disorder did not significantly add to the model once the BPD diagnosis was entered. Evidence also indicates that comorbidity between substance abuse disorder and conduct disorder increases the risk for suicidal behavior in youth (Kelly et al. 2002; Marttunen et al. 1991).

Recent Life Events

Adverse life events may push high-risk patients into actual suicidal crises. Kelly et al. (2000) studied the impact of recent life events and the level of social adjustment in patients with major depression, patients with

BPD, and patients comorbid for major depression and BPD. Kelly et al. (2000) found that the suicide attempters within this sample had experienced more adverse life events recently, particularly in the area of stressful events at home, either family or financially related. In addition, the total number of life events was related to increased risk of suicidal behavior. When the authors did a regression analysis to predict suicide attempter status, the diagnosis of BPD was predictive, as was the level of social adjustment in the family unit. However, once these variables were accounted for in the model, the level of recent life events was not predictive. Patients characterized by the presence of low social adjustment and the borderline diagnosis were found to be 16 times more likely to be classified as suicide attempters than the patients with major depressive episodes. Heikkinen et al. (1997) similarly reported that life events such as job problems, family discord, financial trouble, unemployment, and interpersonal loss were more common among suicide victims with personality disorders than among suicide victims without personality disorders. Interestingly, these researchers also concluded that interpersonal and job-related or financial problems most closely preceded suicide among individuals with personality disorders. On the other hand, rates of financial trouble and unemployment among individuals with Cluster C personality disorders were found to be no different from rates for suicide victims without a diagnosis of personality disorder. Runeson and Beskow (1991) also found the number of stressful life situations was related to death by suicide for adolescents with BPD versus others without BPD. These situations included such things as unstable employment, financial problems, lack of a permanent residence, and a sentence by a court of law.

Discharge from hospital should be considered a stressful event. Kullgren (1988) found that patients with BPD were at somewhat increased risk for suicide around the time of imminent discharge from hospital and that suicides of such patients occurred during the period of inpatient care and in the weeks following discharge. Kjelsberg et al. (1991) noted that patients with BPD who died by suicide during or following hospitalization were more frequently discharged after violating an in-hospital contract than were the surviving borderline patients.

History of Childhood Abuse

A history of childhood abuse needs to be mentioned because its association with suicidal behavior has been documented by several investigators (Dubo et al. 1997; Runeson and Beskow 1991; Stone 1990); however, it is debatable whether childhood abuse is a modifiable risk factor. Soloff et al. (2002) completed a key study examining the relationship between childhood abuse and suicidal behavior in a sample of borderline patients. They found that suicidal behavior, in terms of the number of attempts, was predicted by a history of childhood sexual abuse, by the severity of BPD, and by the level of hopelessness. In fact, childhood sexual abuse continued to predict the number of attempts independently, even after entering a number of other selected risk factors into the analysis. The severity of childhood sexual abuse was associated with the severity of comorbid depression in these patients, the presence of antisocial traits, and a trend toward greater hopelessness. Childhood sexual abuse as a risk factor for suicidal behavior may be mediated by these factors. Soloff et al. (2002) indicated that patients with a history of childhood sexual abuse had a 10-fold greater risk of suicidal behavior versus those patients without such a history.

Case Example

Ms. EE, a 28-year-old single female, presented herself to the emergency department complaining that she felt terrible. "I am close to overdosing," she explained. For the last 2 days, she had medicated herself by binging on cocaine and alcohol. The patient was clear about her distress. Two days prior to presentation, her gynecologist had informed Ms. EE that she needed a hysterectomy and that the surgery could not be put off any longer. Although the precipitating events were plain, a more complete picture emerged after the patient was hospitalized. She and her colleagues at work reported a 2-month history of declining work performance, increasing depression with suicidal ideation, and heightened irritability. Ms. EE had not been under psychiatric care for several years; however, she had a history of three previous suicide attempts, very stormy relationships, impulsivity including periodic binging on alcohol and cocaine, and chronic feelings of dysphoria. Her previous therapist had given her a diagnosis of BPD. During her worst bout of depression, Ms. EE carefully planned her first suicide attempt. She acquired several months' worth of prescription tricyclic antidepressants and made arrangements to be unavailable to her family for the weekend. While taking a hot bath, she ingested all of the pills and waited for her outcome. Fortunately, her stomach was the first organ affected, and she became violently ill and unable to keep her death potion down.

This case demonstrates the association between major depression and BPD and how it can lead to heightened risk for suicide. The underlying depression could have been missed if the time had not been taken to elicit a careful history of the last few weeks and months leading to Ms. EE's presentation. Collateral sources of information were extremely beneficial in confirming the patient's deteriorating mood. One should always look for the effects on functioning that comorbid depression most often has on borderline patients. Although anger is part of the borderline diagnosis, for this woman anger was an indication of her comorbid depression.

In summary, patients with ASPD or BPD are likely to be at increased risk when they demonstrate the risk factors described. In particular, patients with these disorders are likely to be at increased risk when they demonstrate a confluence of risk factors. The presence of comorbidity, particularly when it is acutely evident, may lead high-risk patients into episodes of acute suicidal behavior. The accumulation of recent life events and/or the lack of intimate or family support also indicates times of high risk for these patients. If factors such as a history of childhood sexual abuse and the associated psychopathological deficits, the level of hopelessness, or a history of impulsivity are modifiable based on clinical interventions, then potentially these interventions could reduce the ongoing risk in these patients.

CLINICAL APPROACH TO THE UNCOMMUNICATIVE PATIENT AND PATIENTS WITH ANTISOCIAL, BORDERLINE, AND NARCISSISTIC PERSONALITY DISORDER

Uncommunicative Patients

Uncommunicative patients are among the most difficult to assess for the risk of suicide. The presence or absence of suicidal ideation should be elicited if possible. However, the denial of suicidal ideation does not negate the risk of suicide. Duberstein and colleagues (Conner et al. 2001) found that individuals who suicided lacked an openness to experience, and the authors connected this personality feature to the interpersonal process of individuals who, when assessed, are less likely to feel and report feeling suicidal. Fawcett et al. (1990) found that suicidal ideation was not predictive of suicide in the short term, within 1 year of the assessment, but was related to suicide in the longer term. When questions related to suicidal ide-

ation are denied or not responded to, the clinician must judge the level of risk based on the inference of all available risk and protective factors.

In assessing the uncommunicative patient, the clinician has to pay particular attention to the interview process. What is the patient communicating through his or her lack of verbal communication? For many uncommunicative patients, their failure to respond expresses the lack of personal safety they feel during the assessment encounter. Creating some sense of safety may facilitate more verbal communication. For suicidal men, in particular, the clinician must attend to the process of the assessment interview. Suicidal men may enter a clinical encounter with the expectation that no help is available. Therefore, from a single question or comment the patient may interpret the clinician as being uninterested or dismissive, and the patient will terminate his willingness to be frank and truthful. The clinician must carefully attend to such lapses in cooperation. Finally, the clinician should remember that uncooperativeness is a patient characteristic that is predictive of the need for hospitalization, and sometimes this is the necessary outcome for such patients.

Case Example

Mr. FF, an 18-year-old man called "the Street Kid" by the emergency staff, presented himself to hospital stating "I'm suicidal. I don't feel safe." After uttering those few words, the patient remained mute and huddled in the corner of the examination room. When I entered the room, the patient was sitting cross-legged on the stretcher with his jacket hood covering almost all of his face. In spite of the winter jacket, scars from previous self-attacks were apparent on his wrists, hands, and neck.

"I'm the doctor with the Crisis Team. They asked me to speak with you. You are feeling suicidal?" No response. No acknowledgement at all.

"Can you tell me your name and where you're living?" No response.

"Have you ever been to this hospital before?" No response. Several questions later, I stated the following:

"You're obviously not feeling safe and not safe enough to speak with someone that you have never met before. Is there something I could do to make you feel safer while you're here in the hospital?" He made no response, although he moved his hooded head up as if to catch a glance of my face.

"Is there someone I could talk with who knows about your problems and can help me understand why you've come to the hospital today?"

"Angela, at Streetview, knows why I'm here," the patient abruptly responded.

"Is Angela a counselor at Streetview?"

"Yea. She told me to get lost…so I came here."

"That sounds pretty hurtful. Can you tell me more about what happened?"

For Mr. FF, identifying his hurt feelings allowed the interview to progress. The patient gave permission for the psychiatrist to speak with his counselors and the staff at "Streetview."

For the immediate management of individuals at risk for suicide, involvement of significant others including family members is crucial. The patient's primary care physician or family doctor should be another resource included in the aftercare plan. The family members or significant others need to understand the likelihood of future suicidal behavior to be able to monitor the risk effectively. They need to be involved in encouraging the patient to attend follow-up appointments. Family members or significant others need to be educated to take action and remove the patient's access to means of suicide; for example, disposing of firearms or large quantities of pills. Evidence has established that simple educational interventions significantly increase the chances that families will remove access to means (Brent et al. 2000; Kruesi et al. 1999).

In most cases when the patient is deemed a risk to him- or herself and will not provide consent to speak to family or significant others, the psychiatrist is well advised to attenuate confidentiality to the extent needed to address the safety of the patient (see American Psychiatric Association 2003). In the case of Mr. FF, we were able to resolve some of the miscommunication between himself and "Angela," which helped lessen his risk of suicide. He became more cooperative and agreed to a referral to a safe house. The safe house was able to offer Mr. FF a nonmedical community crisis bed for a few days to help resolve the situation.

Patients With Antisocial Personality Disorder

Patients with ASPD or conduct disorder present a unique challenge to the clinician. When these patients present in crisis, the clinician is faced with the risk of assessing the potential for violence in addition to the risk of suicide or suicidal behavior. For example, Marttunen et al. (1994) reported that 10 of 23 patients with antisocial behavior had a history of violence against others. In fact, all of the patients that met criteria for conduct disorder or ASPD had had a history of violence. Clinicians need to carefully consider interventions, such as hospitalization, based on the potential risk to the patient versus the risk this individual might represent to other patients.

Besides the usual factors involved in a risk assessment, when the clinician is trying to balance the risks to the patient versus others, the psychopathy concept can be clinically of value. Cleckley's (1976) classic description of *psychopathic personality disorder* described that these patients had a "disinclination" toward suicide. Clinically, he observed that among ward patients, suicidal behavior was much rarer among psychopathic patients than other patients. Cleckley wrote "instead of a predilection for ending their own lives, psychopaths, on the contrary, show much more evidence of a specific and characteristic immunity for such an act" (p. 359).

Cleckley's clinical observation has had some support from empirical research. Hare (1991) developed the Psychopathy Checklist–Revised to capture the aspects of Cleckley's psychopathic concept. Research has shown that the concept is composed of two underlying dimensions. The first dimension, called Factor 1 or "emotional detachment," includes the affective component of psychopathy: the glibness, superficial charm, grandiose sense of self-worth, pathological lying, cunning and manipulativeness, lack of remorse or guilt, shallow affect, callousness, lack of empathy, and failure to accept responsibility. Factor 2 relates to antisocial behavior; in this factor, items such as a proneness to boredom, poor behavioral controls, early problematic behavior, lack of realistic long-term goals, impulsivity, irresponsibility, juvenile delinquency, and revocation of conditional release were found (Hare 1991). In a direct examination of the relationship between the factors of psychopathy, ASPD, and suicide risk, Verona et al. (2001) attempted to determine whether a suicidal history was differently related to Factors 1 and 2. The authors found that suicidal history was significantly related to Factor 2. However, Factor 1 was negatively related to a history of suicidal behavior, although this relationship was not statistically significant.

The mechanism by which Factor 1 might work to lessen the risk of suicide seems related to the emotional deficit found in some psychopaths. Physiological studies have demonstrated that psychopathic individuals have reduced startle response when processing adverse stimuli (Herpertz et al. 2001; Patrick 1994). This deficit may indicate a temperamental difficulty in their capacity to reflect negative affect or to experience depression or dysphoric states (Lovelace and Gannon 1999). Therefore, the psychopathic Factor 1 might assist the clinician deciding on the relative risk a patient presents for himself or herself versus others. It appears that patients demonstrating elements of the Factor 1 "emotional detachment" are more likely to be a risk to others rather than themselves. In making particular decisions to admit such patients to an inpatient psychiatric environment, one must be careful to weigh the risks to vulnerable others versus the risk to the patient him- or herself.

Patients With Borderline Personality Disorder

The clinical assessment of the borderline patient in crisis is complicated. Often these patients have made multiple suicide attempts, and it is unclear whether a short-term admission will have any impact on the ongoing risk of suicidal behavior. Figure 29–1 demonstrates a way of assessing and communicating in the medical record the suicidal risk of patients with BPD and a history of repeated suicide attempts. These patients typically are at a chronically elevated risk of suicide much above that of the general population. This risk exists because of a history of multiple attempts; in addition, these patients' history of self-injurious behavior also increases the risk for suicide (Linehan 1993; Stanley et al. 2001). Stanley et al. (2001) found that patients with self-injurious behavior were at risk for suicide attempts because of their high level of depression, hopelessness, and impulsivity and also because they misperceive and underestimate the lethality of their suicidal behaviors. The patient's level of chronic risk can be estimated by taking a careful history of the previous suicidal behavior and focusing on the times when the patient may have demonstrated attempts with the greatest intent and medical lethality. By documenting the patient's most serious suicide attempt, one can estimate the severity of the patient's ongoing chronic risk for suicide.

In patients with BPD, the acute-on-chronic level of risk (i.e., the acute risk that occurs over and above the ongoing chronic risk; Figure 29–1) is related to several factors. An acute-on-chronic risk will be present if the patient has comorbid major depression or if the patient is demonstrating high levels of hopelessness or depressive symptoms, as reviewed earlier. The study by Yen et al. (2003) supported the need to look for an acute-on-chronic change in status; the authors demonstrated that a worsening of depression or substance use occurred in the month preceding a suicide attempt relative to the general levels of change in all other months. In addition, patients with BPD are known to be at risk for suicide around times of hospitalization and discharge. The clinical scenario of a patient presenting in crisis shortly after discharge from an inpatient setting illustrates a time when the risk assessment must be very carefully completed to ensure that a proper disposition is made. This patient is potentially at an acute-on-chronic risk and the assessment cannot be truncated because of the recent discharge from hospital. Proximal substance abuse can increase the suicide risk in a patient with BPD. Of course, the existence of a diagnosis of substance abuse increases the chronic risk for suicidal behavior. The risk is acutely elevated in patients who have less immediate family support or who have lost or perceive the loss of an important relationship.

Gunderson (1984) made the distinction that the borderline patient who is attempting to manipulate the environment is at less risk than the borderline patient who presents in a highly regressed dissociative state. At these times, interventions frequently have to be put in place acutely to reduce the risk of suicide attempts or self-harm. Using the acute-on-chronic model can be very effective for communicating in the medical record the decisions regarding interventions. For example, if a patient is felt to be at a chronic but not acute-on-chronic risk for suicide, one can document and communicate that a short-term hospital admission will have little or no impact on a chronic risk that has been present for months and years. However, an inpatient admission of a patient demonstrating an acute-on-chronic risk (Figure 29–1) might well be indicated. In this circumstance, a short-term admission may allow the level of risk to return to chronic preadmission levels. Managing the chronic level of suicide risk in patients with BPD often involves strategic outpatient management such as dialectical behavior therapy, which has been shown to be effective in reducing suicidal behavior (Koerner and Linehan 2000; Linehan 1993).

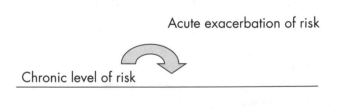

Figure 29–1. Acute-on-chronic suicide risk in a patient with borderline personality disorder.
Source. This figure is adapted with permission from Links PS, Gould G, Ratnayake R: "Assessing Suicidal Youth With Antisocial, Borderline, or Narcissistic Personality Disorder." *Canadian Journal of Psychiatry* 48:301–310, 2003

Patients With Narcissistic Personality Disorder

Assessing patients with narcissistic personality disorder for suicidal risk presents a unique clinical challenge. Ronningstam and Maltsberger (1998) thought-provokingly described how narcissistic patients can be at risk for suicide at times when they are not depressed. Certainly, narcissistic patients will be at increased risk during episodes of comorbid depression (Perry 1990). However, these patients present a unique clinical challenge because they can become acutely suicidal outside of episodes of clinical depression. Suicide attempts in narcissistic patients can arise because of their very fragile self-esteem and in response to perceived narcissistic injury. Ronningstam and Maltsberger (1998) described that suicidal behavior can have several meanings in these patients, including an attempt to raise self-esteem through a sense of mastery; as a way to protect themselves against anticipated narcissistic threats—"death before dishonor"; as a revengeful act against a narcissistic trauma; the false belief of indestructibility; and the expression of a wish to destroy or attack an imperfect self. Narcissistic individuals, therefore, can demonstrate a "Richard Corey" suicide—that is, like the title character in the poem by Edwin Arlington Robinson, they are individuals who take their lives in spite of seeming to have every happiness and good fortune.

The clinician can take four steps to monitor the risk of suicide and suicidal behavior in patients with narcissistic personality disorder. First, the patient should be routinely monitored for evidence of coexisting major depression or for an acute episode of lowered self-esteem resulting from a felt narcissistic injury. Because suicide attempts in narcissistic individuals tend to arise abruptly, the risk can be lessened by preventing the patient from having access to a means of suicide. Therefore, attention should be paid to ensure the patient has no access to highly lethal means of suicide such as guns or large quantities of pills. The patient's family and other significant supports should be aware of the potential for an acute onset of suicidal feelings and the need to avoid access to lethal means. Finally, Kohut (1972) suggested that narcissistic patients may be at less risk of acting out suicidal behavior once they have established a stable transference within a therapeutic relationship and the therapist has established some empathic closeness to the patient's fragmented self. The creation of a stable therapeutic relationship seems to be an important factor that can lessen the risk of suicide in patients with narcissistic personality disorder and should be a consideration in their ongoing outpatient management.

SUMMARY

The uncommunicative patient and patients with antisocial, borderline, and narcissistic personality disorder present unique challenges to clinicians. First, these diagnoses clearly identify individuals at increased risk for suicidal behavior and death by suicide. Second, the assessment of their risk of suicide is problematic. When patients deny or refuse to respond to questions regarding suicidal ideation or intent, the assessment needs to be carefully based on the balance of other risk and protective factors. For the antisocial patient, the risk of violence has to be judged in addition to the risk of suicide or self-harm. For borderline patients, one has to differentiate an acute from chronic risk and determine interventions based on this approach. Finally, narcissistic patients can be at high risk of suicide outside of times of clinical depression. These episodes can seem to arise in an unpredictable fashion. This chapter provides some clinical approaches to the assessment of these patients. However, in the future we hope that empirical evidence will provide a more sound footing for assessing and managing suicide risk in patients with antisocial, borderline, narcissistic, and other personality disorders.

REFERENCES

Ahrens B, Haug HJ: Suicidality in hospitalized patients with a primary diagnosis of personality disorder. Crisis 17:59–63, 1996

American Psychiatric Association: Diagnostic and Statistical Manual of Mental Disorders, 3rd Edition. Washington, DC, American Psychiatric Association, 1980

American Psychiatric Association: Diagnostic and Statistical Manual of Mental Disorders, 3rd Edition, Revised. Washington, DC, American Psychiatric Association, 1987

American Psychiatric Association: Diagnostic and Statistical Manual of Mental Disorders, 4th Edition. Washington, DC, American Psychiatric Association, 1994

American Psychiatric Association: Diagnostic and Statistical Manual of Mental Disorders, 4th Edition, Text Revision. Washington, DC, American Psychiatric Association, 2000

American Psychiatric Association: Practice Guideline for the Assessment and Treatment of Patients with Suicidal Behavior. Washington, DC, American Psychiatric Association, 2003

Apter A, Bleich A, King RA, et al: Death without warning? a clinical postmortem study of suicide in 43 Israeli adolescent males. Arch Gen Psychiatry 50:138–142, 1993

Beautrais AL, Joyce PR, Mulder RT, et al: Prevalence and co-morbidity of mental disorders in persons making serious suicide attempts: a case-control study. Am J Psychiatry 153:1009–1014, 1996

Berman AL: The teenager at risk for suicide. Med Aspects Hum Sex 19:123–129, 1985

Bongar B, Peterson LG, Golann S, et al: Self-mutilation and the chronically "suicidal" emergency room patient. Ann Clin Psychiatry 2:217–222, 1990

Braun-Scharm H: Suicidality and personality disorders in adolescence. Crisis 17:64–68, 1996

Brent DA, Johnson B, Bartle S, et al: Personality disorder, tendency to impulsive violence and suicidal behavior in adolescents. J Am Acad Child Adolesc Psychiatry 32:69–75, 1993a

Brent DA, Perper JA, Moritz G, et al: Psychiatric risk factors for adolescent suicide: a case-control study. J Am Acad Child Adolesc Psychiatry 32:521–529, 1993b

Brent DA, Baugher M, Birmaher B, et al: Compliance with recommendations to remove firearms in families participating in a clinical trial for adolescent depression. J Am Acad Child Adolesc Psychiatry 39:1220–1226, 2000

Casey PR: Personality disorder and suicide intent. Acta Psychiatr Scand 79:290–295, 1989

Clarkin JF, Friedman RC, Hurt SW, et al: Affective and character pathology of suicidal adolescent and young adult inpatients. J Clin Psychiatry 45:19–22, 1984

Cleckley H: The Mask of Sanity. St. Louis, MO, Mosby, 1976

Conner KR, Duberstein PR, Conwell Y, et al: Psychological vulnerability to completed suicide: a review of empirical studies. Suicide Life Threat Behav 31:367–385, 2001

Crumley FE: Adolescent suicide attempts. JAMA 241:2404–2407, 1979

Dirks BL: Repetition of parasuicide: ICD-10 personality disorders and adversity. Acta Psychiatr Scand 98:208–213, 1998

Dubo ED, Zanarini MC, Lewis RE, et al: Childhood antecedents of self-destructiveness in borderline personality disorder. Can J Psychiatry 42:63–69, 1997

Fawcett J, Scheftner WA, Fogg L, et al: Time-related predictors of suicide in major affective disorder. Am J Psychiatry 148:1189–1194, 1990

Fenton WS, McGlashan TH, Victor BJ, et al: Symptoms, subtype, and suicidality in patients with schizophrenia spectrum disorders. Am J Psychiatry 154:199–204, 1997

Ferreira de Castro E, Cunha MA, Pimenta F, et al: Parasuicide and mental disorders. Acta Psychiatr Scand 97:25–31, 1998

Forster PL, Wu LH: Assessment and treatment of suicidal patients in an emergency setting, in Emergency Psychiatry (Review of Psychiatry series, Vol 21; Oldham JM, Riba MB, series eds). Edited by Allen MH. Washington, DC, American Psychiatric Publishing, 2002, pp 75–113

Friedman RC, Corn R: Suicide and the borderline depressed adolescent and young adult. J Am Acad Psychoanal 15:429–448, 1987

Goldsmith SJ, Fyer M, Frances A: Personality and suicide, in Suicide Over the Life Cycle: Risk Factors, Assessment, and Treatment of Suicidal Patients. Edited by Blumenthal SJ, Kupfer DJ. Washington, DC, American Psychiatric Press, 1990, pp 155–176

Gomez A, Lolas F, Martin M, et al: The influence of personality on suicidal behavior. Actas Luso Esp Neurol Psiquiatr Cienc Afines 20:250–256, 1992

Gunderson JG: Borderline Personality Disorder. Washington, DC, American Psychiatric Press, 1984

Gupta B, Trzepacz PT: Serious overdosers admitted to a general hospital: comparison with nonoverdose self-injuries and medically ill patients with suicidal ideation. Gen Hosp Psychiatry 19:209–215, 1997

Hare RD: The Hare Psychopathy Checklist–Revised. Toronto, Canada, Multi-Health Systems, 1991

Harwood D, Hawton K, Hope T, et al: Psychiatric disorder and personality factors associated with suicide in older people: a descriptive and case-control study. Int J Geriatr Psychiatry 16:155–165, 2001

Haw C, Hawton K, Houston K, et al: Psychiatric and personality disorders in deliberate self-harm patients. Br J Psychiatry 178:48–54, 2001

Heikkinen ME, Henriksson MM, Isometsa ET, et al: Recent life events and suicide in personality disorders. J Nerv Ment Dis 185:373–381, 1997

Herpertz SC, Werth U, Lukas G, et al: Emotion in criminal offenders with psychopathy and borderline personality disorder. Arch Gen Psychiatry 58:737–745, 2001

Hewitt PL, Norton GR, Flett GL, et al: Dimensions of perfectionism, hopelessness, and attempted suicide in a sample of alcoholics. Suicide Life Threat Behav 28:395–406, 1998

Houston K, Hawton K, Shepperd R: Suicide in young people aged 15–24: a psychological autopsy study. J Affect Disord 63:159–170, 2001

Isometsa ET, Henriksson MM, Heikkinen ME, et al: Suicide among subjects with personality disorders. Am J Psychiatry 153:667–673, 1996

Jacobs DG, Brewer M, Klein-Benheim M: Suicide assessment: an overview and recommended protocol, in The Harvard Medical School Guide to Suicide Assessment and Intervention. Edited by Jacobs DG. San Francisco, CA, Jossey-Bass, 1999, pp 3–39

Johnson WB, Lall R, Bongar B, et al: The role of objective personality inventories in suicide risk assessment: an evaluation and proposal. Suicide Life Threat Behav 29:165–185, 1999

Kelly TM, Soloff PH, Lynch KG, et al: Recent life events, social adjustment, and suicide attempts in patients with major depression and borderline personality disorder. J Personal Disord 14:316–326, 2000

Kelly TM, Cornelius JR, Lynch KG: Psychiatric and substance use disorders as risk factors for attempted suicide among adolescents: a case control study. Suicide Life Threat Behav 32:301–312, 2002

Kjellander C, Bongar B, King A: Suicidality in borderline personality disorder. Crisis 19:125–135, 1998

Kjelsberg E, Eikeseth PH, Dahl AA: Suicide in borderline patients: predictive factors. Acta Psychiatr Scand 84:283–287, 1991

Koerner K, Linehan MM: Research on dialectical behavior therapy for patients with borderline personality disorder. Psychiatr Clin North Am 23:151–167, 2000

Kohut H: Thoughts on narcissism and narcissistic rage. Psychoanal Study Child 27:360–400, 1972

Kruesi MJP, Grossman J, Pennington JM, et al: Suicide and violence prevention: parent education in the emergency department. J Am Acad Child Adolesc Psychiatry 38:250–255, 1999

Kullgren G: Factors associated with completed suicide in borderline personality disorder. J Nerv Ment Dis 176:40–44, 1988

Kullgren G, Renberg E, Jacobsson L: An empirical study of borderline personality disorder and psychiatric suicides. J Nerv Ment Dis 174:328–331, 1986

Laub JH, Vaillant GE: Delinquency and mortality: a 50-year follow-up study of 1,000 delinquent and nondelinquent boys. Am J Psychiatry 157:96–102, 2000

Lewinsohn PM, Rohde P, Seeley JR: Adolescent psychopathology, III: the clinical consequences of comorbidity. J Am Acad Child Adolesc Psychiatry 34:510–519, 1995

Linehan M: Cognitive Behavioral Treatment of Borderline Personality Disorder. New York, Guilford, 1993

Links PS, Heslegrave RJ, Mitton JE, et al: Borderline personality disorder and substance abuse: consequences of comorbidity. Can J Psychiatry 40:9–14, 1995

Lovelace L, Gannon L: Psychopathy and depression: mutually exclusive constructs? J Behav Ther Exp Psychiatry 30:169–176, 1999

Maddocks PD: A five year follow-up of untreated psychopaths. Br J Psychiatry 116:511–515, 1970

Mann JJ, Waternaux C, Haas G, et al: Toward a clinical model of suicidal behavior in psychiatric patients. Am J Psychiatry 156:181–189, 1999

Markar HR, Williams JM, Wells J, et al: Occurrence of schizotypal and borderline symptoms in parasuicide patients: comparison between subjective and objective indices. Psychol Med 21:385–392, 1991

Marttunen MJ, Aro HM, Henriksson MM, et al: Mental disorders in adolescent suicides: DSM-III-R axes I and II diagnoses in suicides among 13- to 19-year-olds in Finland. Arch Gen Psychiatry 48:834–839, 1991

Marttunen MJ, Aro HM, Henriksson MM, et al: Antisocial behaviour in adolescent suicide. Acta Psychiatr Scand 89:167–173, 1994

McCracken JT, Cantwell DP, Hanna GL: Conduct disorder and depression, in Monographs in Clinical Pediatrics, Vol 6: Depression in Children and Adolescents. Edited by Koplewicz HS, Klass E. New York, Harwood Academic, 1993, pp 121–132

Modestin J, Oberson B, Erni T: Possible correlates of DSM-III-R personality disorders. Acta Psychiatr Scand 96:424–430, 1997

O'Carroll PW, Berman AL, Maris RW, et al: Beyond the Tower of Babel: a nomenclature for suicidology. Suicide Life Threat Behav 26:237–252, 1996

Paris J, Zweig-Frank H: A 27-year follow-up of patients with borderline personality disorder. Compr Psychiatry 42:482–487, 2001

Patrick CJ: Emotion and psychopathy: startling new insights. Psychophysiology 31:319–330, 1994

Perry CJ: Personality disorders, suicide and self-destructive behavior, in Suicide: Understanding and Responding. Edited by Jacobs D, Brown H. Madison, CT, International Universities Press, 1990, pp 157–169

Persson ML, Runeson BS, Wasserman D: Diagnoses, psychosocial stressors and adaptive functioning in attempted suicide. Ann Clin Psychiatry 11:119–128, 1999

Robins E, Murphy GE, Wilkinson RH, et al: Some clinical considerations in the prevention of suicide based on a study of 134 successful suicides. Am J Public Health 49:888–899, 1959

Ronningstam EF, Maltsberger JT: Pathological narcissism and sudden suicide-related collapse. Suicide Life Threat Behav 28:261–271, 1998

Rudd MD, Joiner T: The assessment, management, and treatment of suicidality: toward clinically informed and balanced standards of care. Clin Psychol Sci Pract 5:135–150, 1998

Runeson B, Beskow J: Borderline personality disorder in young Swedish suicides. J Nerv Ment Dis 179:153–156, 1991

Simeon D, Favazza AR: Self-injurious behaviors: phenomenology and assessment, in Self-Injurious Behaviors: Assessment and Treatment. Edited by Simeon D, Hollander E. Washington, DC, American Psychiatric Publishing, 2001, pp 1–28

Soderberg S: Personality disorders in parasuicide. Nord J Psychiatry 55:163–167, 2001

Soloff PH, Lis JA, Kelly T, et al: Risk factors for suicidal behavior in borderline personality disorder. Am J Psychiatry 151:1316–1323, 1994

Soloff PH, Lynch KG, Kelly TM, et al: Characteristics of suicide attempts of patients with major depressive episode and borderline personality disorder: a comparative study. Am J Psychiatry 157:601–608, 2000

Soloff PH, Lynch KG, Kelly TM: Childhood abuse as a risk factor for suicidal behavior in borderline personality disorder. J Personal Disord 16:201–214, 2002

Stanley B, Gameroff MJ, Michalsen V, et al: Are suicide attempters who self-mutilate a unique population? Am J Psychiatry 158:427–432, 2001

Stone MH: The Fate of Borderline Patients. New York, Guilford, 1990

Verona E, Patrick CJ, Joiner TE: Psychopathy, antisocial personality and suicide risk. J Abnorm Psychol 110:462–470, 2001

World Health Organization: International Classification of Diseases, 9th Revision. Geneva, World Health Organization, 1977

World Health Organization: International Statistical Classification of Diseases and Related Health Problems, 10th Revision. Geneva, World Health Organization, 1992

Yen S, Shea TM, Pagano M, et al: Axis I and Axis II disorders as predictors of prospective suicide attempts: findings from the Collaborative Longitudinal Personality Disorders Study. J Abnorm Psychol 112:375–381, 2003

30

Substance Abuse

Roel Verheul, Ph.D.
Louisa M.C. van den Bosch, Ph.D.
Samuel A. Ball, Ph.D.

Since the introduction of DSM-III in 1980, there has been a growing interest in the study of Axis II comorbidity among patients with substance use disorders (American Psychiatric Association 1980). The driving force behind this interest has been and still is the difficult clinical management of these dual-diagnosis patients as well as their high comorbidity. Although the evaluation of co-occurring personality disorders has been the subject of countless studies by addiction researchers, very little attention is paid by personality disorder researchers to the co-occurrence of substance abuse. This state of affairs is difficult to understand when one considers that substance abuse and personality disorders are far and away the most common form of dual diagnosis. In most personality disorder books, the topic of substance abuse is rarely given any coverage. Several reasons might account for this. First, the field of personality disorder research started relatively recently in the 1980s, whereas the field of addiction has long recognized the interconnection with personality dysfunction—if for no other reason than because the first two editions of DSM embedded alcohol and drug

addiction under sociopathy. Second, institutes and therapists specializing in the treatment of personality disorder, particularly out of a psychodynamic tradition, traditionally excluded patients with comorbid substance abuse from programs because they were considered to have little potential for change, could not be analyzed, and were at high risk for dropout. Finally, funding possibilities for Axis II research has been limited, at least when compared with funding for research on Axis I. Thus, the major part of Axis II studies have actually been conducted in samples of patients referred for treatment of Axis I disorders such as substance abuse.

An inevitable consequence of this situation is that this chapter is mostly based on studies focusing on the occurrence and implications of personality disorder in patients with substance use disorder. In addition, evidence from the literature on (normal) personality traits will be "borrowed" whenever informative. The primary focus in this chapter is on causal pathways and treatment issues, supplemented by some attention to epidemiology and diagnostic issues.

EPIDEMIOLOGY

Substance abuse is highly prevalent among individuals with Axis II disorders. For example, in a nonpatient sample, the lifetime prevalence of alcohol use disorders was found to range from 43% to 77% among patients with various personality disorders (Zimmerman and Coryell 1989). In a sample of more than 500 patients, Zanarini et al. (1998) reported substance use disorder to be prevalent in 64% of patients with borderline personality disorder (BPD) and in 54% of patients with other personality disorders.

A much larger number of studies has investigated the Axis II prevalence among patients with substance use disorder. Verheul et al. (1995, 1998a) have provided the most comprehensive overview to date. The best estimate of Axis II prevalence ranged from 44% among alcoholic patients to 79% among opiate abusers. The two most prevalent personality disorders among patients with substance use disorder are antisocial personality disorder (ASPD) and BPD, with reported best estimates of 22% for ASPD and 18% for BPD. Other personality disorders are usually prevalent among patients with substance use disorder in the range of 1%–10%. Thus high joint comorbidity is evident for ASPD and BPD and perhaps paranoid and avoidant personality disorders.

Reported prevalence rates of personality disorders in nonpatient samples of individuals with substance use disorder are at least three times higher than in normal individuals (i.e., those without mental disorders including substance use disorder) (Verheul et al. 1998a). The interpretation of these comorbidity figures is hampered because little knowledge is available about the extent to which a high Axis II prevalence among individuals with substance use disorder is attributable to conceptually overlapping diagnostic criteria and measurement issues such as trait-state artifacts. Clearly overlapping criteria seem to be restricted to only a few of the criteria for ASPD and BPD. The possibility of trait-state artifacts in patients with substance use disorder is discussed later.

ASSESSMENT AND DIAGNOSIS

Semistructured interviews and self-report questionnaires for the assessment of DSM-IV (American Psychiatric Association 1994) personality disorders provide diagnoses with reliability that is comparable with diagnoses of Axis I disorders obtained using standardized procedures (Ball et al. 2001). There is some consensus that self-reports overdiagnose personality disorders. This tendency might be especially relevant in patients with substance use disorder, because these instruments do not ask respondents to differentiate personality traits from the effects of substance abuse or other prolonged changes in mental status. Thus, diagnostic interviews may have greater specificity because questions and answers can be clarified to tease out whether a symptom is chronic and pervasive, more situation-specific, or related to substance abuse. Further clinical inquiry can also determine whether other behavioral examples of the trait exist that are not specifically related to substance abuse. An interview also provides important behavioral observations of the patient's interpersonal style that may inform clinical judgment (Zimmerman 1994). Some recent studies have shown promising findings in favor of the validity of Axis II diagnoses in substance abusers obtained using a semistructured interview schedule. First, Skodol et al. (1999) reported similar prevalence rates of personality disorders among patients with a current substance use disorder and patients with a lifetime substance use disorder. Second, in a sample of 273 patients with substance use disorder, remission of the disorder was not significantly associated with remission of personality pathology, suggesting that the two conditions follow an independent course (Verheul et al. 2000).

Part of the reliability and validity issue for personality disorder diagnosis in patients with substance use disorder centers on whether to include or exclude Axis II symptoms that seem to be substance related (i.e., behaviors directly related to intoxication and/or withdrawal or other behaviors required to maintain an addiction). The magnitude of the effect of exclusion on the prevalence estimate seems partly attributable to the strategy used for exclusion. Measures with more stringent criteria exclude any symptom that has ever been linked to substance abuse and yield significantly reduced rates. Measures that exclude symptoms only if they were completely absent before substance abuse or during periods of extended abstinence show minimal effects on rates. It is important to realize that the more stringent strategy will probably exclude all secondary personality pathology and may even exclude primary personality pathology. The less stringent strategy is meant to exclude behaviors and/or symptoms that do not persist beyond periods of abuse and do not qualify for a personality disorder diagnosis. Consequently, the less stringent approach will probably not exclude primary personality pathology and will have only a limited impact on secondary personality disorder.

Intuitively, one might suggest that excluding substance-related symptoms (at least following the less stringent strategy) would result in more valid diagnoses. Diagnosing personality disorders independent of substance use disorder is consistent with guidelines suggested by DSM-IV-TR (American Psychiatric Association 2000). However, the task of differentiating substance-related symptoms from personality traits is not easy for patients or clinical interviewers and thus may not be reliable. This task becomes almost impossible when the patient's entire adolescent and adult life is characterized by chronic abuse of substances. Furthermore, although most patients with substance use disorder can distinguish behaviors that are only related to substance intoxication or withdrawal, they have greater difficulty making the same distinction for other activities, such as lying or breaking the law, that may be related to obtaining substances. Such a distinction requires a high level of introspection and cognitive competence in making the judgment necessary to differentiate a trait from a situation or state. It also requires an empathic awareness of the impact of one's behavior on self and others and a willingness to accept responsibility for one's actions (Zimmerman 1994).

Patients with substance use disorder may be particularly impaired in the skills necessary to make these distinctions. Consistent with this view, Rounsaville et al. (1998) found that excluding substance-related symptoms reduced the reliability of ASPD diagnoses (but not of BPD diagnoses). Furthermore, they found that patients with independent diagnoses had a rather similar clinical profile compared with patients with substance-related diagnoses, thereby questioning the feasibility and clinical utility of exclusion. If one chooses to exclude substance-related symptoms from the measurement of any personality disorder, several considerations are in order:

- It is probably more reliable to determine whether a symptom should be eliminated as substance related on an item-by-item basis and not wait until the end of the interview or until all items relating to a specific disorder are administered.
- Criteria in which substance dependence is an inherent part should be scored as due to substance abuse unless nonsubstance-related behavioral indicators of the trait (e.g., impulsivity, unlawful behaviors) are also present.
- The interviewer should periodically remind patients that questions refer to the way the patients usually are—that is, when they are not symptomatic with either substance abuse or another Axis I disorder.

CAUSAL PATHWAYS

High (joint) comorbidity that cannot be explained by conceptual or measurement artifacts strongly suggests that the co-occurrence of substance use disorder and personality disorders is not due solely to random or coincidental factors. It seems reasonable to explore the assertion that substance use and personality disorders are in some way causally linked. Evidence for causal relationships between substance use and personality disorders can be derived from long-term longitudinal studies, epidemiological findings, genetic epidemiology, and retrospective studies that account for the order of onset of each disorder. Three superordinate meta-models of comorbidity can be distinguished: the primary substance use disorder model, the primary personality disorder model, and the common factor model.

Primary Substance Use Disorder Model

The primary substance use disorder model postulates that substance abuse contributes to the development of personality pathology. This pathway has received relatively little empirical attention. Bernstein and Handelsman (1995) tentatively proposed three mechanisms: 1) substance abuse often occurs within the context of a deviant peer group, and antisocial behaviors might be shaped and reinforced by social group norms (social learning hypothesis); 2) some Cluster A traits (e.g., suspiciousness, eccentric behaviors, ideas of reference, magical thinking), Cluster B traits (e.g., exploitativeness, egocentrism, manipulativeness), and Cluster C traits (e.g., passivity, social avoidance) may be shaped and maintained by the reinforcing and conditioning properties of psychoactive substances (behavioristic learning hypothesis); and 3) chronic substance abuse or withdrawal may alter personality through neuroadaptive changes or a direct effect on brain chemistry (neuropharmacological hypothesis).

As Bernstein and Handelsman (1995) pointed out, it is unclear to what extent these effects can "overwrite" or interact with preexisting personality patterns to form new personality configurations. Considering the primary substance use disorder model, it is important to distinguish new enduring personality patterns from temporary behavior patterns that disappear with reductions of substance use. The latter should not be taken into account for an Axis II diagnosis. According to DSM-IV-TR, it is only when the consequences of substance abuse persist beyond the period of alcohol and/or drug consumption that these features constitute personality pathology. To the best of our knowledge, there are currently no studies yielding substantive evidence in favor of the primary substance use disorder model; on the contrary, some indirect evidence refutes the model. For example, Axis II diagnoses in adults with alcoholism have been found to be associated with maladjustment in childhood, even after partialling out the current and cumulative effects of substance use (Bernstein et al. 1998; Morgenstern et al. 1997).

In summary, there is currently no direct evidence supporting the primary substance use disorder model, and there is some indirect evidence against the model. However, it would be premature to fully preclude the possibility that some symptoms in some individual patients with substance use disorder are shaped and maintained by the reinforcing and conditioning properties of psychoactive substances.

Primary Personality Disorder Model

The primary personality disorder model describes comorbid relationships in which (pathological) personality traits contribute to the development of substance use disorder. Since the 1990s, many studies have yielded empirical support for this model. Recently, it was proposed that the available evidence suggests at least two or three different developmental pathways from personality to addiction (Finn et al. 2000; Verheul and van den Brink 2000). These pathways were defined as the behavioral disinhibition pathway, the stress reduction pathway, and the reward sensitivity pathway.

Behavioral Disinhibition Pathway

The behavioral disinhibition pathway to substance abuse predicts that individuals scoring high on traits such as antisociality and impulsivity and low on constraint or conscientiousness have lower thresholds for deviant behaviors such as alcohol and drug abuse. This pathway might account for the association of ASPD and, to some extent, BPD with substance abuse. Of the three proposed pathways, this one is the best documented. First, high relative comorbidity is observed between substance use disorder and Axis I and Axis II disorders from the impulse control spectrum. For example, in a large sample recruited from the general population, individuals with substance use disorder were 17.2 times more likely to have ASPD than those without (Zimmerman and Coryell 1989). Second, several longitudinal studies have shown that teachers' ratings of low constraint, low harm avoidance, lack of social conformity, unconventionality, an-

tisociality, and aggression in children, particularly boys, predicted alcohol and drug abuse in adolescence and young adulthood (Caspi et al. 1997; Cloninger et al. 1988; Krueger et al. 1996; Masse and Tremblay 1997). The same pattern was observed in university students (Sher et al. 2000). Third, a recent study found that the onset of ASPD characteristics preceded that of alcohol dependence by approximately 4 years (Bahlman et al. 2002). The relationship between behavioral disinhibition and early onset addictive behaviors is probably mediated through deficient socialization, school failure, and affiliation with deviant peers (Sher and Trull 1994; Tarter and Vanyukov 1994; Wills et al. 1998). The behavioral disinhibition pathway is associated with an early onset of drinking, a more rapid development of alcohol dependence once drinking begins, and more severe symptoms than nonantisocial subjects (Verheul et al. 1998a).

Stress Reduction Pathway

The stress reduction pathway to substance abuse predicts that individuals scoring high on traits such as stress reactivity, anxiety sensitivity, and neuroticism are vulnerable to stressful life events. This pathway might account for the comorbidity of BPD, avoidant, dependent, and schizotypal personality disorder. These individuals typically respond to stress with anxiety and mood instability, which in turn can become a motive for substance use as self-medication. Longitudinal studies have shown that teachers' ratings of negative emotionality, stress reactivity, and low harm avoidance in children predicted substance abuse in adolescence and young adulthood (Caspi et al. 1997; Cloninger et al. 1988; Wills et al. 1998). Furthermore, Conrod et al. (1998) showed that coping motives for drinking as well as the fear-dampening properties of alcohol were far more pronounced among men scoring high on anxiety-sensitivity than among their low-scoring counterparts. The self-medication pathway, which has most frequently been investigated for alcoholism, typically accounts for late-onset alcohol use disorders and is more prevalent among women than among men.

Reward Sensitivity Pathway

The reward sensitivity pathway predicts that individuals scoring high on traits such as novelty seeking, reward seeking, extraversion, and gregariousness will be motivated to substance use for its positive reinforcing properties. This pathway might account for the comorbidity of antisocial, histrionic, and narcissistic personality disorder. Consistent with this hypothesis, some longitudinal studies (Cloninger et al. 1988; Masse and Tremblay 1997; Wills et al. 1998) have shown that novelty seeking as a temperamental trait in childhood predicts later substance use problems. Furthermore, some evidence suggests that students' scores of extraversion, at least among those without a family history of alcoholism, predict alcohol dependence at age 30 (Schuckit et al. 1994). As observed in animal studies, hyperresponsiveness to the positive reinforcing or rewarding effects of substances is partly accounted for by the sensitization processes initiated by the repetitive use of the substances themselves (Robinson and Berridge 1993) and to that extent is not precipitated by premorbid personality factors. However, this hyperresponsiveness or hypersensitivity might develop most strongly among individuals characterized by a more general sensitivity to positive reinforcements (Zuckerman 1999). A recent study showed that men with multigenerational family histories of alcoholism demonstrated elevated resting heart rates (index of psychostimulation) in response to alcohol intake, suggesting that this pathway partly mediates the role of genetic vulnerability in the etiology of alcoholism (Conrod et al. 1998).

Common Factor Model

The common factor model assumes that both personality pathology and substance abuse are linked to an independent third factor that contributes to the development of both disorders. This model is more likely for personality disorders that show relatively high joint comorbidity, such as ASPD and BPD. This hypothesis is consistent with a psychobiological perspective on personality disorders suggesting that BPD and ASPD are phenomenologically, genetically, and/or biologically related to Axis I impulse disorders such as substance abuse (Siever and Davis 1991; Zanarini 1993).

Family, twin, and adoption studies are generally considered most appropriate to evaluate whether a common risk factor is transmitted genetically or otherwise. Evidence from several adoption studies suggests that alcoholism and ASPD are genetically separate disorders (Cadoret et al. 1985). Furthermore, Loranger and Tulis (1985) reported that family members of patients with BPD were at greater risk for alcoholism than those of schizophrenic or bipolar-affective patients, but when patients were further subdivided based on their own level of alcohol consumption, family risk differences for alcoholism almost disappeared. A recent study reported that the shared genetic risk between major depression and alcohol and marijuana dependence was largely explained by genetic effects

on ASPD, which in turn was associated with increased risk of each of the other disorders (Fu et al. 2002). These data presented no evidence for cross-transmission of pure forms and no support for the shared-etiology model. However, the available studies do not preclude the possibility of common factors that, for example, are less specific to ASPD. For example, Slutske et al. (2002) reported that genetic influences contributing to variation in behavioral undercontrol accounted for about 40% of the genetic variation in alcohol dependence and conduct disorder risk and about 90% of the common genetic risk for alcohol dependence and conduct disorder. This and other studies (e.g., Krueger et al. 2002) suggest that genetic factors contributing to variation in dimensions of personality, particularly behavioral undercontrol or impulsivity, account for a substantial proportion of the genetic diathesis for alcohol dependence and most of the common genetic diathesis for alcohol dependence and conduct disorder among men and women.

Another approach in the search for common factors has relied on high-risk strategies, with the aim of identifying markers of biological vulnerability for both conditions. A recent study revealed that a reduced amplitude of the P300 component of the scalp-recorded event-related brain potential in men is strongly associated with a general tendency toward antisocial, defiant, and impulsive traits, which in turn increase the risk for alcohol abuse (Justus et al. 2001). Furthermore, some reviewers (Bernstein and Handelsman 1995; Siever and Davis 1991) have concluded that abnormalities in serotonergic function may form a biological substrate underlying both substance abuse and impulsive/aggressive behavior.

Comment

It is important to note that the different meta-models are not necessarily mutually exclusive. In any individual case, more than one model may have explanatory value. Furthermore, it is possible that one model best describes the initiation of a comorbid disorder, whereas another describes long-term maintenance of the same comorbid association. For example, a borderline patient may use stimulants to reduce feelings of boredom and use alcohol to regulate affective instability. After a while, the patient becomes addicted to both substances, which in turn aggravates the impulsivity and sets the conditions for aggressive suicide attempts. Simultaneously, the patient may get entangled with a deviant peer group, leading to both increased antisocial behavior and additional substance abuse.

TREATMENT OUTCOME

Outcomes of Treatments Focusing on Substance Abuse

Personality pathology has been found to be significantly related to poor treatment response and outcome in patients with affective and anxiety disorders (Reich and Vasile 1993). In the early 1990s it was generally believed that the same applied to patients with substance abuse. However, the available studies at the time had many methodological and interpretative problems, making it difficult to draw conclusions. Consequently, it was often unclear whether the reported effects on outcome were attributable to a poor treatment response of comorbid patients or to differences in pretreatment characteristics. Several studies published later on showed convincingly that personality pathology is associated with pre- and posttreatment problem severity but is not a robust predictor of the amount of improvement (e.g., Cacciola et al. 1995, 1996; Verheul et al. 1999). Furthermore, some studies showed that Axis II comorbidity is not associated with premature drop-out or a shorter time-in-program (Kokkevi et al. 1998; Marlowe et al. 1997; Verheul et al. 1998b), nor with less motivation to change (Verheul et al. 1998b). In the late 1990s, some authors concluded that the available studies did not allow any firm conclusions about the prognosis of patients with both substance use disorder and personality disorders. This conclusion from empirical studies was in sharp contrast with clinical experiences and knowledge.

A number of more recent studies have yielded results that provide somewhat more clarity. For example, two studies showed that Axis II disorders predict a shorter time to relapse after discharge (Thomas et al. 1999), even when controlling for the baseline severity of alcohol problems (Verheul et al. 1998b). Thus it seems that "an equal amount of improvement" does not resemble a similar risk of relapse. A possible explanation for this apparent discrepancy is that patients without personality pathology improve to a level of problem severity that no longer leaves them at risk for relapse, whereas patients with personality pathology are at risk for relapse despite their improvement. Other studies focused on "normal" personality traits and reported that low persistence (Cannon et al. 1997; Janowsky et al. 1999; Sellman et al. 1997) and high novelty seeking (Meszaros et al. 1999) are strong predictors of time to relapse. Finally, it was found that high neuroticism and low conscientiousness predicted the time to relapse after discharge and that the combination of these two features was associated with the highest odds of relapse (Fischer et al. 1998).

Early studies typically examined the impact of personality pathology separately from other patient characteristics, although this approach might have failed to identify possible interactions with other important characteristics. For example, one study examined motivation for change and time-in-program as potential moderators and mediators of the relationship between personality disorders and relapse (Verheul et al. 1998b). It appeared that although motivation for change was unrelated to personality pathology, it moderated the relationship between Axis II and relapse so that personality pathology was a strong predictor of relapse among less motivated individuals but not among their more motivated counterparts. In addition, two studies suggest that personality pathology interferes with the patient–therapist working alliance, thereby resulting in poorer outcomes or a higher risk for relapse (Gerstley et al. 1989; Verheul et al. 1998b). Finally, Pettinati et al. (1999) found that the combination of Axis I and Axis II psychopathology was the best predictor of a return to substance use at 1 year posttreatment compared with those factors alone.

An alternative explanation of the available data that seems to refute common clinical knowledge with respect to the prognosis of ASPD is that the disorder's criteria set identifies a heterogeneous group of patients that includes both individuals with only antisocial behaviors and individuals with both antisocial and psychopathic personality traits, such as shallow affect, grandiosity, and lack of empathy and remorse. The latter group might be particularly at risk of poor treatment response and outcome. Consistent with this view, Woody et al. (1985) have shown that opiate addicts with ASPD and a lifetime diagnosis of major depression were able to benefit about as much from individual psychotherapy as patients without ASPD. This finding is in comparison with "pure" ASPD subjects, who experienced very little benefit from psychotherapy. Another interesting study found that antisocial patients who were able to form a working alliance with their therapists had better treatment response and outcome at follow-up than did antisocial patients who lacked this ability (Gerstley et al. 1989).

Outcomes of Treatments Focusing on Personality Disorder

Little is known about the impact of substance abuse on outcome for patients in treatment for personality problems noted earlier, this neglect in literature might be accounted for by the exclusion of dual diagnosis patients from the treatment system. A similar phenomenon can also be observed in research. For example, patients with substance use disorder are often excluded from studies examining the efficacy of treatments designed to target borderline symptoms. The exclusion from research is often justified as a strategy to preserve the homogeneity in cohorts. This differential approach illustrates the limitations specific to a mental health system and a research policy oriented toward the treatment of single rather than multiple disorders (Ridgely et al. 1990).

To the best of our knowledge, only one study has investigated the impact of substance abuse on the outcome of a treatment focusing on Axis II. In their randomized trial of dialectical behavior therapy (DBT) among Dutch women with BPD, Verheul et al. (2003) found no differences in effectiveness for patients with versus those without substance use problems. This finding is in obvious contrast with the tradition described earlier.

Outcomes of Dual Focus Treatments

Two psychotherapies developed for the treatment of personality disorders—schema focused therapy and DBT—have been modified to meet the specific needs of dual-diagnosis patients.

Dual Focus Schema Therapy

The only documented integrated dual focus treatment for the broad range of Axis II is dual focus schema therapy (DFST), developed by Ball and Young (Ball 1998; Ball and Young 2000). DFST is a 24-week, manual-guided individual therapy including both symptom-focused relapse prevention and coping skills techniques and schema-focused techniques for maladaptive schemas and coping styles. Some preliminary empirical support can be derived from a randomized pilot study among 30 methadone maintenance patients comparing DFST with 12-step facilitation therapy (Ball et al. 1999). Patients met criteria for an average of 3.3 personality disorders, with ASPD present in over 70% and BPD and avoidant personality disorder present in over 50% of the cases. Patients assigned to DFST reduced substance use frequency more rapidly over the 24-week treatment than did patients assigned to 12-step facilitation therapy. Further inspection of the data suggested that a difference began to emerge at month 3, which corresponds to a point in the manual at which the treatment shifts from an assessment and education focus to an active change focus. Furthermore, DFST patients reported an increase from a good early therapeutic alliance to a very

strong alliance over the subsequent months of treatment, whereas the 12-step facilitation patients demonstrated no such increase. Consistent with this finding, DFST therapists reported feeling as though they had a stronger working alliance with patients than did 12-step facilitation therapists.

Case Example

Mr. GG was a 36-year-old divorced male whose primary Axis II diagnosis was obsessive-compulsive personality disorder. In addition to symptoms of depression, obsessive thoughts, compulsive behavior, and paranoid ideation, he had interpersonal problems related to being both exploitable and domineering as well as vindictive. He began using substances at the age of 14, had several prior substance abuse treatments, and had been on methadone for 1 year before starting individual therapy. His heroin dependence was in remission (on agonist medication), and his primary drug abuse problem was cocaine, with more sporadic use of a high-potency solvent to which his part-time job gave him ready accessibility. Mr. GG also met criteria for ASPD. This diagnosis does not frequently co-occur with obsessive-compulsive personality disorder; however, it was difficult to determine whether the ASPD diagnosis was independent of substance abuse given the very early age of onset and persistent use of multiple substances during adolescence and adulthood. In addition, Mr. GG met diagnostic criteria for depressive personality disorder, a category mentioned in the appendix of DSM-IV as needing further study.

Mr. GG was treated for 6 months as part of a research protocol evaluating DFST. His core early maladaptive schema was unrelenting standards/hypercriticalness (i.e., perfectionism, rigid rules, and preoccupation with time and efficiency), which appeared to originate from the seemingly contradictory combination of parental perfectionism (with physical or emotional abuse for Mr. GG's "failures" as child) and defeat secondary to both parents being torture survivors who escaped to the United States from another country. Mr. GG put a great deal of pressure on himself, and any minor deviation in his striving for perfection triggered a massive substance relapse, irresponsible giving up, and antisocial acting-out. He engaged in a number of maladaptive coping behaviors that perpetuated this schema, including expecting too much of himself and others and being a perfectionistic workaholic. At other times, he sought relief from the pressures of these standards and would avoid occupational or social commitments, develop somatic symptoms, procrastinate, or give up on himself and use drugs when he could not get things to be perfect. These avoidance strategies actually reinforced his high standards even more because he would subsequently have to redouble his efforts to get desired outcomes.

Mr. GG began therapy in a loud, challenging manner, wanting to know for sure that therapy was going to help him and that he was going to get as much out of it as we got out of him as a research participant. Because he continued to abuse cocaine and inhalants for the first 3 months, therapy necessarily remained more relapse-prevention focused while he struggled to grasp cognitively any of the schema-focused psychoeducational material. By month 4, he had achieved complete abstinence from solvents and was using cocaine much less frequently. This had a significant positive effect on his personality (more agreeable and sociable, less depressed and agitated); however, his unrelenting standards/hypercriticalness schema was expressed even more strongly. Cognitively oriented interventions included cost-benefit analyses of his unrelenting standards and reducing the perceived risks of imperfection in his relationships. A core cognitive distortion targeted for dispute was "When I don't accomplish or get what I want, I should get enraged, give up, use drugs, and be dejected." Experiential techniques involved imagery dialogues with his parents about how they always made mistakes seem like catastrophes. Behavioral techniques included learning to accept "good enough" work from himself and others, accepting directions from people he did not respect, and redeveloping old leisure interests. Therapeutic relationship interventions included the therapist modeling acceptance of his own mistakes, processing homework noncompliance due to self-imposed rigid standards, and confronting his dichotomous views of the therapist. Much of the work in Mr. GG's outside relationships and in therapy involved helping him change his dichotomous view of other people as well as his own recovery (i.e., all good/sober vs. all bad/relapsed). Despite a rather turbulent course of treatment, Mr. GG appeared genuinely interested in improving himself and made some significant changes. In addition to his reduced substance abuse, he also experienced significant reductions in psychiatric symptoms and negative affect.

Dialectical Behavior Therapy

The second dual focus treatment involves a modified version of DBT known as DBT-S. This program includes all of the components of standard DBT (i.e., weekly individual cognitive-behavioral psychotherapy sessions with the primary therapist, weekly skills training groups lasting 2–2.5 hours per session, weekly supervision and consultation meetings for the therapists, and phone consultation) plus application of dialectics to abstinence issues, application of a specific pharmacotherapy module, a treatment target hierarchy relevant to substance abuse, new strategies to keep difficult-to-engage and easily lost patients, the addition of six new and modified skills, an individual skills consultation mode, and increased emphasis on using natural and arbitrary reinforcers for maintenance of abstinence. There is some evidence from a randomized controlled trial that DBT-S is effective in reducing substance abuse in borderline patients with substance use disorder (Linehan et al. 1999). Subjects assigned to DBT-S had significantly lower dropout rates and showed significantly greater reductions in drug abuse throughout the treatment year and at 16-month follow-up compared with control subjects. However, no differences were reported in the medical or psychiatric inpatient treatment received by DBT-S and control subjects or in rates of parasuicidal behavior.

Case Example

Ms. HH was a 27-year-old patient with BPD. Her first suicide attempt was at the age of 12; alcohol abuse began at 16, followed by cocaine and heroin. Her first admission into a psychiatric hospital was at age 12, and she had had a criminal record since age 16. In addition to interpersonal problems, anger outbursts, parasuicidal behaviors, and aggressive impulsiveness, she abused heroin, cocaine, cannabis, and alcohol. Previously, she had been in psychiatric and addiction treatments on both an outpatient and an inpatient basis. Among her typical therapy-interfering behaviors was attempting to invite the therapist into a very special and sometimes intimate relationship. She usually dropped out each time she failed to seduce a therapist. At the time of admission to the DBT program, she was in an addiction-oriented day hospital program.

Soon after the start of therapy, a basic behavior pattern became clear: after work on Friday evening, she would start to feel lonely. The thought "I need to comfort myself" would pop up. She would close the curtains, drink a glass of wine, and smoke cannabis while listening to "good old days" music. Around 10 P.M. she would become restless, followed by feeling angry because she also deserved "some company." Then she would dress up in sexy clothes and go out for a drink. In the pub, she would often meet familiar drug dealers. After having had a few drinks together, the drug dealers would offer her cocaine. Because she could not afford to buy it, she would agree to have sex with them. Feelings of guilt would lead to more substance abuse, and finally she would lose contact with reality. The next morning, she would awake next to a stranger and would become self-destructive.

The behavior pattern described was targeted for treatment. Because of its threshold-lowering capacities for impulsive and self-destructive behavior, the alcohol abuse was given high priority early in treatment. Telephone consultation was of utmost importance in this stage. After 3 months, Ms. HH succeeded for the first time in not acting on the impulse to go to the bars late at night. Her contact with her father, mother, and sisters was restored. Because communication improved, reinforcement contingencies were changed. She resumed contact with a network of old friends who were not involved in drug abuse, and she accepted a new, more challenging job.

The cannabis use appeared to be the most change-resistant behavior. Reminding her of her own commitment (no hard or soft drugs), the therapist insisted that she practice her mindfulness skills every time she was tempted to use again. After 8 months she was clean and was able to "surf the craving." Then, finally, her attachment problems were targeted in treatment. Efforts to become more intimate with the therapist failed, as well as all efforts to make the therapist reject her (e.g., stalking by telephone, anger outbursts). The therapist was able to validate her behavior as fear of abandonment, and she finally recognized that she was more afraid of saying goodbye than of being rejected. After 54 sessions she left the program and the therapist by mutual agreement; she left a bouquet of flowers, combined with the words "this relationship is the most horrible thing that has ever happened to me in my life. Thanks so much."

Comment on Treatment Outcome

In summary, we have seen that 1) personality pathology has a strong impact on the course of addictive problems after discharge from addiction treatment, 2) individuals with substance use disorder are usually—without a proper theoretical or empirical basis—excluded from Axis II treatments, and 3) some preliminary data are supportive of treatments with a dual focus. Together, these data provide strong support for the current movement toward treatment approaches that pay simultaneous attention to both addictive and personality problems, such as DFST and DBT-S. However, we need more empirical evidence that these treatments really have improved effectiveness over existing approaches. Attention to the feasibility of these treatments is also required. As currently developed, DFST and DBT-S require additional or separate clinical training beyond the standard programs from which they are derived. The focus on one target behavior seems to be a common characteristic of the different DBT programs. The question is to what extent this approach is useful for common clinical practice, which includes patients who have multiple symptoms. It would therefore be worthwhile to examine the possibility of integrated, multitargeted treatment programs, rather than separate symptom-specific programs. This might imply that therapists are trained to address a range of symptomatic manifestations of personality pathology in the impulse control spectrum, including suicidal and self-damaging behavior, binge eating, and substance abuse.

TREATMENT GUIDELINES

In general, clinical guidelines for the treatment of personality disorders recommend psychotherapy whenever possible, complemented by symptom-targeted pharmacotherapy whenever necessary or useful. We see no reason to substantially deviate from this recommendation in dual-diagnosis patients, although effective treatment of these patients often requires modifications to traditional programs and methods. In the remainder of this chapter, some clinical recommendations for psychotherapy and pharmacotherapy, respectively, are formulated.

Psychotherapy

Dual Focus

Dual focus does not necessarily mean that attention to both foci should always take place simultaneously but rather that the program should consist of an integrated package of these elements. During the earlier sessions, it is often best to place the greatest emphasis on the establishment and maintenance of abstinence but with a secondary focus on identification of and psychoeducation about maladaptive personality traits. During later sessions, a greater emphasis can be placed on confronting and changing maladaptive traits.

Clinical Setting

Psychotherapy with patients with both substance use disorder and personality disorder probably should not be provided as a stand-alone treatment. Psychotherapy is likely to have greater success if it is provided in the context of a relatively long-term treatment program that provides sufficient structure and safety (e.g., day hospital, residential treatment, or methadone maintenance program).

Duration and Treatment Goals

The treatment of individuals with personality disorders can be a long-term process. The added problems of limited treatment retention and compliance associated with substance abuse raise questions of what the appropriate treatment goals are for this group. In most cases, the goal will not be to accomplish deep and permanent change in personality structure within a relatively short term. If facilities or resources are limited, a more practical aim may be to improve substance abuse treatment outcome by teaching patients how to cope with or modulate maladaptive personality traits.

Required Therapist Training

Patients with substance use disorder and severe personality disorders are commonly seen in treatment programs and consume a disproportionate amount of staff time. They tend to be admitted into treatment repeatedly and exhaust the resources of one counselor after another. Therapists treating these dual-disorder patients probably should be professional or highly skilled therapists with extensive education and training in psychotherapy, psychopathology, personality disorders, and addiction. Drug counselors with limited training and supervision are not capable of dealing properly with these patients. Given the challenges of treating this population, all therapists should have some forum for supervision.

Essential Ingredients

Effective treatment of patients with both substance use disorder and personality disorders requires special and professional attention from the very beginning. Particular emphasis on motivational interviewing (Martino et al. 2002) during the admission phase and throughout the entire treatment process may be necessary with these dual-diagnosis patients. In addition to the regular program modules, intensive individual counseling is recommended to establish a working alliance and to prevent these patients from leaving treatment early. Direct therapeutic attention to maladaptive personality traits may increase cognitive and coping skills, which in turn may improve symptomatology and reduce the risk for relapse. Finally, participation in an appropriate aftercare program is highly recommended.

Pharmacotherapy

Pharmacotherapy may have an important role in the treatment of dual-diagnosis patients. Medications may ameliorate some personality disorder symptoms while simultaneously improving the outcome of substance use disorder. It should be noted, however, that the co-occurrence of these disorders is also associated with high rates of noncompliance and an increased risk of lethal overdose as well as the potential for dependence on the medication.

Neuroleptics

Low doses of neuroleptics have been reported to be associated with a range of beneficial effects in patients with borderline, schizotypal, or paranoid personality disorders (Rocca et al. 2002; Soloff 1998) as well as with a decrease in craving in cocaine abusers (Gawin et al. 1989). However, recent trials do not support the anticraving or abstinence-promoting effect of neuroleptics (e.g., Dackis and O'Brien 2002).

Selective Serotonin Reuptake Inhibitors

Selective serotonin reuptake inhibitors have been shown to reduce aggression/impulsivity in patients with BPD and ASPD (Coccaro and Kavoussi 1997; Soloff 1998) and may have some positive effect on substance abuse in alcohol- and cocaine-dependent patients (Cornelius et al. 1997). However, a recent study showed that fluvoxamine, as compared with placebo, produced a robust and long-lasting reduction in rapid mood shifts in female borderline patients but had no effect on impulsivity or aggression (Rinne et al. 2002).

Mood Stabilizers

Lithium and other mood stabilizers (e.g., carbamazepine, divalproex sodium) have been reported to reduce aggressive and violent behaviors in antisocial prison inmates and to decrease "within-day mood fluctuations" in borderline patients (Cowdry and Gardner 1988; Stein 1992). Early anecdotal reports and a small double-blind, placebo-controlled study also suggested that lithium may be efficacious in the treatment of alcohol dependence. However, a large Veterans Administration study showed no benefits of lithium over placebo for alcohol-dependent patients with or without depressive symptoms (Dorus et al. 1989). Similar negative findings are now available for the treatment of cocaine dependence with mood stabilizers (Silva de Lima et al. 2002).

Benzodiazepines

Benzodiazepines are generally contraindicated for this group because of the risk of addiction and of paradoxical reactions involving behavioral disinhibition (Cowdry and Gardner 1988).

Buspirone

The partial serotonin agonist buspirone seems to combine a lack of abuse potential with a positive effect on social phobia and avoidant personality disorder (Zwier and Rao 1994) and a delay in the return to heavy alcohol consumption in anxious alcohol-dependent patients (Kranzler et al. 1994).

Stimulants

Various stimulants, including methylphenidate, pemoline, dexamphetamine, and levodopa, have been reported to reduce impulsivity in BPD and ASPD patients with a history of attention-deficit/hyperactivity disorder. It has been claimed that childhood hyperactivity and a history of drug abuse are predictors of a favorable response to both psychostimulants and monoamine oxidase inhibitors among patients with personality disorders (Stein 1992). However, stimulants are known for their addictive and abuse potential, and restraint should be used in prescribing these drugs.

Naltrexone

It has been reported that the opioid antagonist naltrexone is effective in the treatment of alcohol and opiate dependence as well as in the prevention of self-mutilation in a borderline patient (Griengl et al. 2001; Soloff 1993).

CONCLUSIONS

Substance abuse is highly prevalent among patients with personality disorder, irrespective of type, with prevalences of 50% and beyond. Among patients with substance use disorder, ASPD and BPD are the predominant Axis II diagnoses, with prevalences of approximately 20%. Thus high joint comorbidity is evident for ASPD/BPD and substance use disorder.

Personality disorders can be reliably and validly measured in patients with substance use disorder, but assessment and diagnosis require careful attention to disentangling substance-related and independent personality pathology.

With respect to causal pathways, the primary personality disorder model and common factor model have received the strongest empirical support. These models describe comorbid relationships in which personality traits contribute to the development of substance use disorder and in which both conditions are linked to an independent factor, respectively. Within the primary personality disorder model, the evidence supports multiple pathways from personality to substance use disorder—that is, the behavioral disinhibition, stress reduction, and reward sensitivity pathways. With respect to the common factor model, recent evidence suggests that genetic factors contributing to variation in personality dimensions, particularly behavioral undercontrol, might account for a substantial proportion of the comorbidity of ASPD and substance use disorder.

Contrary to expectations, recent evidence has convincingly shown that comorbid patients usually benefit from addiction treatments. However, they often only improve to a level of problem severity that leaves them at considerable risk for relapse. In addition, the maladaptive personality traits remain untreated and also contribute to higher odds of relapse. Also contrary to expectations, some evidence suggests that comorbid patients benefit from treatments focusing on the personality disorder as much as do those without substance use disorder. Yet the current clinical consensus is that, if possible, so-called dual focus treatments consisting of an integrated package of elements targeting both the substance use disorder and the maladaptive traits are preferable over strategies with a single focus. Some preliminary data are supportive of dual focus treatments.

Clinical guidelines for the treatment of personality disorder recommend psychotherapy whenever possible, complemented by symptom-targeted pharmacotherapy whenever necessary or useful. We see no reason to substantially deviate from this recommendation in dual-diagnosis patients, although effective treatment of these patients often requires modifications to traditional programs and methods.

REFERENCES

American Psychiatric Association: Diagnostic and Statistical Manual of Mental Disorders, 3rd Edition. Washington, DC, American Psychiatric Association, 1980

American Psychiatric Association: Diagnostic and Statistical Manual of Mental Disorders, 4th Edition. Washington, DC, American Psychiatric Association, 1994

American Psychiatric Association: Diagnostic and Statistical Manual of Mental Disorders, 4th Edition, Text Revision. Washington, DC, American Psychiatric Association, 2000

Bahlman M, Preuss UW, Soyka M: Chronological relationship between antisocial personality disorder and alcohol dependence. Eur Addict Res 8:195–200, 2002

Ball SA: Manualized treatment for substance abusers with personality disorders: dual focus schema therapy. Addict Behav 23:883–891, 1998

Ball SA, Young JE: Dual focus schema therapy for personality disorders and substance dependence: case study results. Cogn Behav Pract 7:270–281, 2000

Ball SA, Young JE, Rounsaville BJ, et al: Dual focus schema therapy vs. 12-step drug counseling for personality disorders and addiction: randomized pilot study. Paper presented at the ISSPD 6th International Congress of the Disorders of Personality, Geneva, Switzerland, September 1999

Ball SA, Rounsaville BJ, Tennen H, et al: Reliability of personality disorder symptoms and personality traits in substance-dependent inpatients. J Abnorm Psychol 110:341–352, 2001

Bernstein DP, Handelsman L: The neurobiology of substance abuse and personality disorders, in Neuropsychiatry of Personality Disorders. Edited by Ratey J. Cambridge, England, Blackwell Science, 1995

Bernstein DP, Stein JA, Handelsman L: Predicting personality pathology among adult patients with substance use disorders: effects of childhood maltreatment. Addict Behav 23:855–868, 1998

Cacciola JS, Alterman AI, Rutherford MJ, et al: Treatment response of antisocial substance abusers. J Nerv Ment Dis 183:166–171, 1995

Cacciola JS, Alterman AI, Rutherford MJ, et al: Personality disorders and treatment outcome in methadone maintenance patients. J Nerv Ment Dis 184:234–239, 1996

Cadoret RJ, O'Gorman TW, Troughton E, et al: Alcoholism and antisocial personality: interrelationships, genetic and environmental factors. Arch Gen Psychiatry 42:161–167, 1985

Cannon DS, Keefe CK, Clark LA: Persistence predicts latency to relapse following inpatient treatment for alcohol dependence. Addict Behav 22:535–543, 1997

Caspi A, Begg D, Dickson N, et al: Personality differences predict health-risk behaviors in young adulthood: evidence from a longitudinal study. J Pers Soc Psychol 73:1052–1063, 1997

Cloninger CR, Sigvardsson S, Bohman M: Childhood personality predicts alcohol abuse in young adults. Alcohol Clin Exp Res 12:494–505, 1988

Coccaro EF, Kavoussi RJ : Fluoxetine and impulsive aggressive behavior in personality-disordered subjects. Arch Gen Psychiatry 54:1081–1088, 1997

Conrod PJ, Pihl RO, Vassileva J: Differential sensitivity to alcohol reinforcement in groups of men at risk for distinct alcoholism subtypes. Alcohol Clin Exp Res 22:585–597, 1998

Cornelius JR, Salloum IM, Ehler JG, et al: Fluoxetine in depressed alcoholics: a double-blind, placebo-controlled trial. Arch Gen Psychiatry 54:691–694, 1997

Cowdry RW, Gardner DL: Pharmacotherapy of borderline personality disorder: alprazolam, carbamazepine, trifluoperazine and tranylcypromine. Arch Gen Psychiatry 45:111–119, 1988

Dackis CA, O'Brien CP: Cocaine dependence: the challenge for pharmacotherapy. Curr Opin Psychiatry 15:261–267, 2002

Dorus W, Ostrow D, Anton R, et al: Lithium treatment of depressed and non-depressed alcoholics. JAMA 262:1646–1652, 1989

Finn PR, Sharkansky EJ, Brandt KM, et al: The effects of familial risk, personality, and expectancies on alcohol use and abuse. J Abnorm Psychol 109:122–133, 2000

Fischer LA, Elias JW, Ritz K: Predicting relapse to substance abuse as a function of personality dimensions. Alcohol Clin Exp Res 22:1041–1047, 1998

Fu Q, Heath AC, Bucholz KK, et al: Shared genetic risk of major depression, alcohol dependence, and marijuana dependence: contribution of antisocial personality disorder in men. Arch Gen Psychiatry 59:1125–1132, 2002

Gawin FH, Allen D, Humblestone B: Outpatient treatment of crack cocaine smoking with flupenthixol decanoate: a preliminary report. Arch Gen Psychiatry 46:322–325, 1989

Gerstley L, McLellan AT, Alterman AI, et al: Ability to form an alliance with the therapist: a possible marker of prognosis for patients with antisocial personality disorder. Am J Psychiatry 146:508–512, 1989

Griengl H, Sendera A, Dantendorfer K: Naltrexone as a treatment of self-injurious behavior: a case report. Acta Psychiatr Scand 103:234–236, 2001

Janowsky DS, Boone A, Morter S, et al: Personality and alcohol/substance-use disorder patient relapse and attendance at self-help group meetings. Alcohol Alcohol 34:359–369, 1999

Justus AN, Finn PR, Steinmetz JE: P300, disinhibited personality, and early-onset alcohol problems. Clin Exp Res 25:1457–1466, 2001

Kokkevi A, Stefanis N, Anastasopoulou E, et al: Personality disorders in drug abusers: prevalence and their association with Axis I disorders as predictors of treatment retention. Addict Behav 23:841–853, 1998

Kranzler HR, Burleson JA, Del Boca FK, et al: Buspirone treatment of anxious alcoholics: a placebo-controlled trial. Arch Gen Psychiatry 51:720–731, 1994

Krueger RF, Caspi A, Moffit TE, et al: Personality traits are differentially linked to mental disorders: a multitrait-multidiagnosis study of an adolescent birth cohort. J Abnorm Psychol 105:299–312, 1996

Krueger RF, Hicks BM, Patrick CJ, et al: Etiologic connections among substance dependence, antisocial behavior, and personality: modeling the externalizing spectrum. J Abnorm Psychol 111:411–424, 2002

Linehan MM, Schmidt H, Dimeff LA, et al: Dialectical behaviour therapy for patients with borderline personality disorder and drug-dependence. Am J Addict 8:279–292, 1999

Loranger AW, Tulis EH: Family history of alcoholism in borderline personality disorder. Arch Gen Psychiatry 42:153–157, 1985

Marlowe DB, Kirby KC, Festinger DS, et al: Impact of comorbid personality disorders and personality disorder symptoms on outcomes of behavioral treatment for cocaine dependence. J Nerv Ment Dis 185:483–490, 1997

Martino S, Carroll K, Kostas D, et al: Dual Diagnosis Motivational Interviewing: a modification of Motivational Interviewing for substance-abusing patients with psychotic disorders. J Subst Abuse Treat 23:297–308, 2002

Masse LC, Tremblay RE: Behavior of boys in kindergarten and the onset of substance use during adolescence. Arch Gen Psychiatry 54:62–68, 1997

Meszaros K, Lenzinger E, Hornik K, et al: The Tridimensional Personality Questionnaire as a predictor of relapse in detoxified alcohol dependents. Alcohol Clin Exp Res 23:483–486, 1999

Morgenstern J, Langenbucher J, Labouvie E, et al: The comorbidity of alcoholism and personality disorders in a clinical population: prevalence rates and relation to alcohol typology variables. J Abnorm Psychol 106:74–84, 1997

Pettinati HM, Pierce JD, Belden PP, et al: The relationship of Axis II personality disorders to other known predictors of addiction treatment outcome. Am J Addict 8:136–147, 1999

Reich JH, Vasile RG: Effect of personality disorders on the treatment outcome of Axis I conditions: an update. J Nerv Ment Dis 181:475–484, 1993

Ridgely MS, Goldman HH, Willenbring M: Barriers to the care of persons with dual diagnoses: organizational and financing issues. Schizophr Bull 16:123–132, 1990

Rinne T, van den Brink W, Wouters L, et al: SSRI treatment of borderline personality disorder: a randomized, placebo-controlled clinical trial for female patients with borderline personality disorder. Am J Psychiatry 159:2048–2054, 2002

Robinson TE, Berridge KC: The neural basis of craving: an incentive-sensitization theory of addiction. Brain Res Rev 18:247–291, 1993

Rocca P, Marchiaro L, Cocuzza E, et al: Treatment of borderline personality disorder with risperidone. J Clin Psychiatry 63:241–244, 2002

Rounsaville BJ, Kranzler HR, Ball S, et al: Personality disorders in substance abusers: relation to substance use. J Nerv Ment Dis 186:87–95, 1998

Schuckit MA, Klein J, Twitchell G, et al: Personality test scores as predictors of alcoholism almost a decade later. Am J Psychiatry 151:1038–1043, 1994

Sellman JD, Muldert RT, Sullivan PF, et al: Low persistence predicts relapse in alcohol dependence following treatment. J Stud Alcohol 58:257–263, 1997

Sher KJ, Trull TJ: Personality and disinhibitory psychopathology: alcoholism and antisocial personality disorder. J Abnorm Psychol 103:92–102, 1994

Sher KJ, Bartholow BD, Wood MD: Personality and substance use disorders: a prospective study. J Consult Clin Psychol 68:818–829, 2000

Siever LJ, Davis KL: A psychological perspective on the personality disorders. Am J Psychiatry 148:1647–1658, 1991

Silva de Lima M, Garcia de Oliveira Soares B, Alves Pereira Reisser A, et al: Pharmacological treatment of cocaine dependence: a systematic review. Addiction 97:931–949, 2002

Skodol AE, Oldham JM, Gallaher PE: Axis II comorbidity of substance use disorders among patients referred for treatment of personality disorders. Am J Psychiatry 156:733–738, 1999

Slutske WS, Heath AC, Madden PA, et al: Personality and the genetic risk for alcohol dependence. J Abnorm Psychol 111:124–133, 2002

Soloff PH: Pharmacological therapies in borderline personality disorder, in Borderline Personality Disorder: Etiology and Treatment. Edited by Paris J. Washington, DC, American Psychiatric Press, 1993, pp 319–348

Soloff PH: Algorithms for pharmacological treatment of personality dimensions: symptom-specific treatments for cognitive-perceptual, affective, and impulsive-behavioral dysregulation. Bull Menninger Clin 62:195–214, 1998

Stein G: Drug treatment of the personality disorders. Br J Psychiatry 161:167–184, 1992

Tarter RE, Vanyukov M: Alcoholism: a developmental disorder. J Consult Clin Psychol 62:1096–1107, 1994

Thomas VH, Melchert TP, Banken JA: Substance dependence and personality disorders: comorbidity and treatment outcome in an inpatient treatment population. J Stud Alcohol 60:271–277, 1999

Verheul R, van den Brink W: The role of personality pathology in the etiology and treatment of substance use disorders. Curr Opin Psychiatry 13:163–169, 2000

Verheul R, van den Brink W, Hartgers C: Prevalence of personality disorders among alcoholics and drug addicts: an overview. Eur Addict Res 1:166–177, 1995

Verheul R, Ball SA, van den Brink W: Substance abuse and personality disorders, in Dual Diagnosis and Treatment: Substance Abuse and Comorbid Medical and Psychiatric Disorders. Edited by Kranzler HR, Rounsaville BJ. New York, Marcel Dekker, 1998a, pp 317–363

Verheul R, van den Brink W, Hartgers C: Personality disorders predict relapse in alcoholic patients. Addict Behav 23:869–882, 1998b

Verheul R, van den Brink W, Koeter MWJ, et al: Antisocial alcoholics show as much improvement at 14-month follow-up as non-antisocial alcoholics. Am J Addict 8:24–33, 1999

Verheul R, Kranzler HR, Poling J, et al: Axis I and Axis II disorders in substance abusers: fact or artifact? J Stud Alcohol 61:101–110, 2000

Verheul R, van den Bosch LMC, Koeter MWJ, et al: Efficacy of dialectical behavior therapy: a Dutch randomized controlled trial. Br J Psychiatry 182:135–140, 2003

Wills TA, Windle M, Cleary SD: Temperament and novelty seeking in adolescent substance use: convergence of dimensions of temperament with constructs from Cloninger's theory. J Pers Soc Psychol 74:387–406, 1998

Woody ME, McLellan T, Luborsky L, et al: Sociopathy and psychotherapy outcome. Arch Gen Psychiatry 42:1081–1086, 1985

Zanarini MC: Borderline personality disorder as an impulse spectrum disorder, in Borderline Personality Disorder: Etiology and Treatment. Edited by Paris J. Washington, DC, American Psychiatric Press, 1993, pp 67–86

Zanarini MC, Frankenburg FR, Dubo ED, et al: Axis I comorbidity of borderline personality disorder. Am J Psychiatry 155:1733–1739, 1998

Zimmerman M: Diagnosing personality disorders: a review of issues and research methods. Arch Gen Psychiatry 51:225–245, 1994

Zimmerman M, Coryell WH: DSM-III personality disorder diagnoses in a nonpatient sample: demographic correlates and comorbidity. Arch Gen Psychiatry 46:682–689, 1989

Zuckerman M: Vulnerability to psychopathology: a biosocial model. Washington, DC, American Psychological Association, 1999, pp 255–317

Zwier KJ, Rao U: Buspirone use in an adolescent with social phobia and mixed personality disorder (cluster A type). J Am Acad Child Adolesc Psychiatry 33:1007–1011, 1994

31

Violence

Michael H. Stone, M.D.

We are all passengers aboard one ship called Earth,
and we must not allow it to be wrecked by acts of violence;
there will be no second Noah's Ark.

Mikhail Gorbachev

The concept of violence is, semantically speaking, confined to the human domain. According to one definition, *violence* is a bodily response with the intended infliction of bodily harm on another person or persons (Glasser 1998). The term relates to destructive forms of interpersonal behavior and contrasts with the broader concept of aggression (De Zulueta 1993), which pertains to the animal kingdom in general. *Aggression* involves the use of force, not necessarily accompanied by physical injury, for the purpose of gaining some advantage (Hollin and Howells 1989). In the animal kingdom the advantage may concern the acquisition of food, the warding off of a predator, or the establishment of rank among social animals. There are biological substrates and specialized brain regions in animals (including humans) that subserve aggression as a way of warding off various threats and dangers (Perelberg 1999). Violence is invoked when the method of reducing or eliminating

the danger is effected through bodily harm, whether fatal or nonfatal, and is restricted to the human community. Many factors contribute to violence; here we concentrate on those relevant to personality and its disorders. Because the other factors often interact with and are mediated by personality, they also have an important place in our discussion. Several useful lists of such factors have been published, such as those of Hart (1998) and Monahan and Steadman (1994).

Among the important interacting factors are the biological (hormonal, neurotransmitter-related, and brain-injury related such as intoxication and head injury); psychological (personality disorder, psychosis, and cognitive impairment such as low intelligence); and social (cultural and job-related) (Hart 1998). The factors outlined in the MacArthur Risk Assessment Study were chosen as a result of research begun in 1988 by members of the Research Network group, headed by John Monahan (Steadman et al. 1994). In addition to those factors mentioned by Hart, the MacArthur group cited demographic factors (age, gender, race, socioeconomic status); history of crime and violence (arrests, self-reported violence); and social history (child rearing, child abuse within the family, family deviance)—factors often subsumed under the heading of environmental factors.

EVOLUTIONARY ASPECTS OF AGGRESSION AND VIOLENCE

In his monograph on aggression and violence, Valzelli (1981) cataloged the varieties of aggression in the animal kingdom: predatory, competitive, defensive, irritative, territorial, maternal-protective, and instrumental. All of these play a role in enhancing the survival of the individual, either by killing or immobilizing an attacker or by maintaining or augmenting social rank and thus mating potential. The latter is central to the evolutionary genetics concept of fitness, which is a measure of how many offspring an individual leaves in the next generation. Fitness also relates to the gains an animal makes as a result of its behavior, compared with the behavior of others in competition with it (Cartwright 2000). Fitness is unrelated to longevity, because an animal (or person) can live a long time yet produce no offspring, thus demonstrating low fitness; another, more aggressive individual may have casual sex with many partners, sire many children, invest little in their upbringing, and die in a barroom brawl at age 30 yet still demonstrate remarkable fitness.

The two types of aggression most relevant to our discussion are predatory and irritative (the latter sometimes called "affective," "reactive," or "impulsive"). In the animal kingdom, predatory aggression is evoked by hunger and the presence of an appropriate object of prey and may be regulated by (among other centers) the lateral hypothalamus (Valzelli 1981). Irritative aggression is evoked by a variety of stimuli and is commonly observed in anger or rage reactions. Aversive stimuli, such as a blow to the body, may elicit irritative aggression in animals as well as in man.

Violence, representing the translation in humans of aggression into outright physical attack, may be either lawful or unlawful. Here we are concerned with unlawful violence, although it is worth noting that the lawful forms relate to defense, as when one subdues a dangerous intruder or kills an acquaintance or relative who threatens bodily harm. A parent who kills someone attacking the parent's child is guilty of justifiable homicide and therefore not of murder (which implies unlawful killing). Even the reverse situation, in which a child kills someone attacking the parent, may be a justifiable homicide, such as in the 1957 case of Cheryl Crane, the 14-year-old daughter of actress Lana Turner. Crane stabbed to death Johnny Stompanato, who had been menacing her mother and herself (Rhodes 1999). Defensive (including maternal-protective) violence of this sort is part of the innate human behavioral repertoire and is not necessarily related to a disorder of personality.

In *predatory* violence one finds only minimal autonomic arousal, along with premeditation, absence of threat, and motives such as power, sex, revenge, or dominance. This violence is in contrast to *irritative* or *affective* violence, in which there is heightened sympathetic arousal, anger, or fear and an absence of planning but the presence (or assumption, even if false) of imminent threat (Meloy 2003). The purpose of affective violence is the enhancement of survival by warding off threat. Some would reserve the term irritative, on the human plane, for affective violence that significantly exceeds in destructiveness the minimum force needed to overcome an adversary.

In times of war or intergroup conflict, one may see irritative aggression and violence meted out even against innocent parties who have the misfortune to symbolize the "enemy" to the aggressor. Examples are legion: the twentieth century witnessed genocidal attacks of the utmost violence against Armenians, Russian kulaks, Jews, Chinese intelligentsia, Cambodians, Bosnians, Tutsis, and others who had not provoked their killers. Because wars are often begun as a premeditated attack against a nonprovoking enemy who is then slaughtered with grossly unnecessary force, including torture, predatory and irritative violence are often combined in the actions of the aggressors. The gain, in evolutionary terms, is the survival of the aggressor group (and its loyal population) and the extinction of the enemy group (and their population). One has only to think of Hitler's quest for lebensraum for the German people, as he incited them to war against the Slavic peoples to the east. The personalities of the aggressors in these situations can vary over a wide range from the fanatical, sadistic, and narcissistic to the quite ordinary.

We mention here the evolutionary aspects of violence to emphasize that, however pathological violent behavior may appear when viewed from a psychiatric perspective, there is always a reason for it, viewed as a phenomenon in nature—no matter how ignoble and grotesque that reason may seem to us. Quinsey et al.

(1998) made the argument that aggression and belligerence conferred adaptive advantages in the ancestral environment, with deceitfulness and dishonesty as elements added on later in our phylogenetic development. They cited the "fearless and fierce" Vikings of the ninth and tenth centuries as examples—men who pursued short-term mating tactics and an aggressive and risky approach to achieving social dominance. However, these qualities are precisely the same in what we now call the psychopath. The fact that the genes contributing to this pattern of dominance through violence—although less adaptive in current society—are still adaptive enough to persist generation after generation suggests that what we now consider a disorder (i.e., psychopathy) was, and to an extent remains, a "life-history strategy" (Mealey 1995).

A less controversial aspect of violence, in relation to human society, is that of *instrumental aggression*, which is limited to threatening behavior meant to intimidate those who might, through their own aggression, disrupt the body social. Leaders use this type of aggression through the laws they make to govern us, which can be backed up with actual violence if necessary—physical punishment or death meted out to those who violate social rules (Valzelli 1981). German sociologist Wolfgang Sofsky (1996), in his brilliant treatise on the use of violence as a tool in the formation of societies, put it this way: "The fear of pain is what compels men to the ratification of social contract" (p. 12).

PERSONALITY CONFIGURATIONS COMMONLY ASSOCIATED WITH VIOLENCE

A full accounting of all the personality configurations that may be associated with the pathological (i.e., not merely defensive) forms of violence requires that we widen our search beyond the personality disorders mentioned in DSM-IV-TR (American Psychiatric Association 2000). Violence may be seen in any of the 10 disorders in Axis II of DSM-IV-TR, but evidence suggests that the connection is strongest in the Cluster B disorders (especially antisocial and borderline personality disorders), less strong in the Cluster A disorders (predominantly in paranoid personality disorder), and weakest in the Cluster C disorders (predominantly in obsessive-compulsive personality disorder). Violent persons often meet criteria for more than one DSM disorder. In one study (based on DSM-III; American Psychiatric Association 1980), for example, 164 violent offenders in a British maximum security hospital and special units in prison showed six diagnostic pat-

terns: antisocial-narcissistic, paranoid-antisocial, borderline-antisocial–passive-aggressive, borderline, compulsive-borderline, and schizoid (Blackburn and Coid 1999). Offenders in the first three categories had more extensive criminal careers and often met criteria for psychopathy (Hare 1991). Data from Blackburn and Coid (1999) underline the point that violent offenders are, viewed from the prism of personality, a heterogeneous group. The common thread running through the first three patterns—those most predictive of violent behavior—is antisocial personality disorder (ASPD).

DSM-IV-TR Personality Disorders

Antisocial Personality Disorder

The current DSM-IV-TR definition of *antisocial personality disorder* is composed of three items that can be assigned to personality in the strictest sense: 1) deceitfulness, 2) impulsivity, and 3) lack of remorse, and four items that pertain to behavior: 1) repeated acts that are grounds for arrest, 2) reckless disregard for the safety of others (although this item could be conflated with the personality trait of contemptuousness), 3) failure to sustain work of financial obligations, and 4) aggressiveness (with frequent fights or assaults). One can thus view ASPD as a construct made up of two factors, analogous to the personality and behavioral components of psychopathy. Because only three of these seven items are necessary for the diagnosis in DSM's polythetic system, a person could conceivably demonstrate just the personality items (which also happen to represent an extreme form of narcissism), or just the behavioral items (which answer to a kind of wanton aggressiveness). We must keep these distinctions in mind when examining data in the following section dealing with which particular factors are most predictive of future violence. As with other DSM-IV-TR personality categories, ASPD seldom occurs in the absence of other personality disorders: the most common comorbid disorders are borderline and histrionic and, to a lesser extent, passive aggressive, paranoid, and narcissistic personality disorders (Widiger and Corbitt 1997).

Narcissistic Personality Disorder

Of the nine criteria for narcissistic personality disorder in DSM-IV-TR, at least three represent personality traits that overlap conceptually with those of ASPD (and psychopathy); namely, exploitativeness, arrogance, and lack of empathy. A sense of entitlement might be construed as another, because this trait points to the one-sidedness of the narcissist's relations with others and is suggestive of the contemptuousness also common in this disorder. More importantly, it can be said that almost all antisocial and habitually violent people show marked narcissistic traits, because they put their own needs and wants far ahead of the needs and rights of others. At the crossroads between narcissistic personality disorder and ASPD is the *malignant narcissism* described by Kernberg (1992), in which some capacity for loyalty and concern for others is retained (unlike what one sees in ASPD) despite the presence of narcissism, antisocial behaviors, paranoid traits, and ego-syntonic sadism (often including violent interactions with intimates and subordinates in the workplace).

Borderline Personality Disorder

The items of borderline personality disorder (BPD) conducive to violence are inordinate anger and impulsivity. These in turn contribute to a third item: unstable and intense interpersonal relationships. BPD is predominantly encountered in women, whereas those with ASPD (as well as psychopathy and sadism) are predominantly men. Women are much less aggressive than men in general, but among those women who are aggressive, BPD is overrepresented (Dougherty et al. 1999). BPD rarely occurs unaccompanied by other personality configurations, and these influence the propensity to violent behavior. Persons meeting criteria for both BPD and ASPD, for example, are more violence prone than those with BPD plus avoidant personality disorder.

Paranoid Personality Disorder

The characteristics of paranoid personality disorder pertinent to violence are quickness to react angrily or to counterattack (having misperceived the intent of others), grudge bearing, and unjustified suspiciousness about being harmed or exploited.

Obsessive-Compulsive Personality Disorder

The remaining personality disorders of DSM-IV-TR contribute less to violence than those already mentioned. Some men with obsessive-compulsive personality disorder are rigid, out of touch with feelings (whether their own or other people's), and hostile. Certain men with this configuration become highly intolerant of criticism or demands and end up battering their spouses or children or showing other forms of violence. Batterers have also been spoken of as demonstrating abusive personality (Dutton 1998), which focuses on the inordinate anger (rage) of BPD—the exercise of

control through violence. The description of abusive personality overlaps considerably with that of BPD.

Other Personality Types

Several personality configurations that figure importantly in the analysis of violent behavior are not included in the "official" diagnostic categories of DSM-IV-TR. These include psychopathy, passive-aggressive personality (included in DSM-III), hypomanic personality, and sadistic personality (the latter is described in the appendixes of DSM-III-R [American Psychiatric Association 1987] and DSM-IV-TR). Of these, psychopathy and sadistic personality are of special importance. In addition, several other disorders, defined partly by symptoms and partly by personality traits, also predispose to violent behavior: intermittent explosive disorder (IED), with its episodic outbursts of aggressive or violent behavior and attention-deficit/hyperactivity disorder (ADHD), with its intrusiveness and sometimes assaultiveness in adolescents. It is estimated that one-fourth of adolescents with ADHD go on to develop ASPD (Barkley 1990). Another example is stalking, which is not mentioned in DSM and is called "aggravated harassment" in the legal domain. Stalkers may pursue intimates (especially after a romantic rejection) or strangers (usually celebrities); may be psychotic (as in the case of Mark David Chapman, who killed John Lennon) or "borderline" in function; are more apt to be men than women, by a factor of 3:1 (Meloy 1996); and 3%–36% may show violent (assaultive, only rarely murderous) behavior (depending on the sample). Many different personality configurations may be present in stalkers: depressive-masochistic (in women who have been rejected by a lover), obsessional (in men rejected by a lover), paranoid, grandiose/narcissistic (in certain celebrity stalkers), or even schizoid. These lonely "psychotic" persons form pathological attachments to anyone (including mental health professionals) who extends them some measure of kindness or who represents some idealized figure (as in the case of Arthur Jackson, the paranoid schizophrenic who tried to kill actress Teresa Suldana in the hope that they would then be joined in heaven [Markman and Labreque 1994]).

Psychopathy

As for psychopathy, the diagnostic criteria most commonly used at present are those of the Psychopathy Checklist–Revised (PCL-R; Hare 1991), which includes 20 items, each of which can be scored a 0, 1, or 2, for a maximum score of 40. To diagnose psychopathy in categorical terms, a score of 30 or higher is used in the United States and Canada (25 or more in many European countries). Intermediate scores in the 15–29 range are viewed in dimensional terms as consistent with psychopathic traits. The PCL-R is seen as composed of two main factors (Harpur et al. 1988): 1) an interpersonal/affective factor (containing such traits as superficial charm, grandiosity, deceitfulness, absence of remorse, callousness and inability to take responsibility for one's actions, and manipulativeness); and 2) an impulsive behavior/social deviance factor (with such characteristics as impulsivity, lack of long-term goals, parasitic lifestyle, juvenile delinquency, early behavioral problems, and need for stimulation) (Hart et al. 1994).

Recently, a reexamination of the PCL-R by Cooke and Michie (2001) suggested that a three-factor solution, consisting of a cognitive, an affective, and a behavioral component, is preferable. Cooke's model is based on 13 items and omits the "criminological" items from the PCL-R, such as "failure of conditional release" and "criminal versatility" (relating to the number of different kinds of crime for which a subject had been arrested). Each approach has its advantages. The PCL-R may be more useful in estimating the risk of recidivism for violent and nonviolent offenses in a known forensic or prison population. Cooke's modification is more useful in work with first-time offenders and with those from more favorable socioeconomic backgrounds, who may have committed crimes for which they were never formally arrested, let alone incarcerated. From the perspective of *personality* in its purest sense, defined only in terms of traits, psychopathy represents the extreme of narcissism—that is, apart from shallow affect and irresponsible behavior, the psychopath is an egocentric and aggressive narcissist, indifferent to and contemptuous of the feelings of others.

According to Hare (1998), the psychopath is a "remorseless predator…who, lacking in conscience, finds it easy to use charm, manipulation, intimidation, and violence to control others and to satisfy their own selfish needs" (p. 128). If this constellation is present, therefore, the risk for criminal and particularly for violent behavior may be greatly elevated. In the example of rape, Groth and Birnbaum (1979) identified two main types: anger-rape (approximately one-third of cases) and power-rape (approximately two-thirds of cases). Anger-rape is motivated by revenge and retaliation; power-rape, which is usually premeditated, is motivated by the pleasure derived from the woman's helplessness and by the fantasy that she will "enjoy" the experience. Power-rape is the rape committed by the

psychopath. We would thus expect PCL-R scores to be higher in the power-rape than in the anger-rape cases.

In the next section, I examine the efficacy of the PCL-R and other rating scales in the prediction of violent recidivism for sexual and nonsexual offenses.

Sadistic Personality Disorder

Although no longer included in DSM-IV-TR, sadistic personality disorder remains a valid personality configuration, distinct enough from ASPD and psychopathy to warrant a separate place in the taxonomy. The key or prototypical attribute, from among the eight items for sadistic personality disorder described in the appendix to DSM-III-R, is taking pleasure in hurting others. Not all persons who demonstrate sadistic personality disorder, ASPD, or psychopathy are violent, but the presence of any of these three elevates the risk of violence; the acts committed by the sadist are more apt to involve torture and tend to be more gruesome or depraved than are those committed by individuals with ASPD or psychopathy in the absence of sadistic personality disorder.

FACTORS PREDISPOSING TO VIOLENCE AND THEIR ASSESSMENT

The number of factors known to affect the risk for violence, whether one is evaluating a person who has not yet been violent or one with a history of violence, is very large, rendering the task of assessing this risk complex and fraught with uncertainties. The efforts of Monahan and Steadman (1994) led to improvements since the mid-1980s (Monahan 1996), reducing the guesswork to a level at which the use of the newer risk-assessment instruments permits estimates that are usually more accurate than those derived from clinical judgment alone. Even so, clinical judgment may have been underestimated to some extent: a recent study by Lidz et al. (1993) of patients seen in an acute psychiatric clinic showed that patients who raised initial concern when first evaluated by psychiatrists and nurses proved more likely to have been violent in a 6-month follow-up period (53%) than those patients who did not raise such concern (36%). The investigators relied not only on official records and informants but also on self-reports by the patients—which, as Klassen and O'Connor (1987) demonstrated earlier, increased predictive accuracy by some 28%.

Before examining the risk factors in detail, with their varying "weights" and complex interactions, we should note that the most important predictor of violence is a previous record of violence (Monahan 1981). Beyond this, the many factors can be compartmentalized, as alluded to earlier, into the biological, psychological (including personality-related), and social—or, to use Monahan's schema, into the demographic, historical, contextual, and clinical.

Genetic/Constitutional Factors

The risk for violence in patients with schizophrenia or manic-depressive illness, both of which show strong genetic underpinnings, is about four to six times greater than the prevalence of either psychosis in the general population (Hodgins 1993). These odds ratios jump to 8.5 in males with major mental illness who abused substances as adults and to 15 if they abused substances before age 18. This ratio is relevant because many patients with schizophrenia also manifest paranoid or other Cluster A disorders. Those with manic depression may show hypomanic, paranoid, borderline, or passive-aggressive personalities. ASPD can occur in either group. Psychopathy may be less common in schizophrenia than in manic depression. Yet in a study by Côté and Hodgins (1990) of prison inmates with schizophrenia, 63% were comorbid for ASPD, a proportion of whom could also be considered psychopathic. Similar findings emerged from the forensic-hospital study of Rasmussen and Levander (1996), in which 22 of the 29 male schizophrenic patients who met criteria for ASPD also had PCL-R scores of more than 29 and were also psychopathic.

Certain interactions are more strongly associated with violence than others. Patients in whom schizophrenia is combined with marked paranoid traits are more vulnerable to command hallucinations and threat/control-override phenomena. In the latter instance, patients may feel (unrealistically) threatened by others or may have their personal controls "overridden" by their feelings—predisposing in either case to violent behaviors (Blumenthal and Levander 2000; Link and Stueve 1995).

Another condition with a strong genetic component is Asperger's syndrome, which resembles autism with its social isolation ("schizoidness") and eccentricity but has less intellectual impairment or language delay. Males are affected more than females. Males with Asperger's syndrome show a heightened risk for conduct disorder, with physical aggressiveness or threats of violence in adolescence, although this propensity seldom continues into adulthood (Maughn 1993).

Recent neuroimaging studies suggest that violent and impulsive behavior is associated with inferior frontal and medial temporal lobe dysfunction in the brain, with disruption in frontotemporolimbic circuits (Hoptman 2003).

Personality Factors

Personality is an amalgam of hereditary and environmental factors, each contributing to about half the variance. The inevitable interactions between temperament (the hereditary component) and character (the postnatal environmental component) make neat divisions between the two spurious, but twin and adoption studies do underscore that genes influence personality. Six of seven recent twin studies and six of each recent adoption studies summarized by Carey and Goldman (1997) showed significant heritability estimates for ASPD. Several studies suggest a modest genetic predisposition for the narrower construct of *psychopathy* (Raine 1993). As for violent—as opposed to property—crime, there are data on both sides of the issue. The Danish adoption study of Mednick et al. (1984) found a significant increase in property crime among adoptees in relation to the number of criminal convictions among their biological parents, but they found no significant correlation for violent crime. However, this study was based on the Danish population, where the base rate for violent crime is lower than in the United States, thus making it harder to detect a correlation if one existed. The twin study of Cloninger and Gottesman (1987) suggested a heritability quotient of 0.50 for violent crime (as against 0.78 for property crime). In Raine's (1993) view, it is when both genetic and environmental factors occur together that an individual is most likely to show criminal behavior, and the interaction between these two factors accounts for more of the variance than either factor alone.

The heightened risk of violence in the major psychoses, as noted earlier, is partly attributable to the personality traits that tend to accompany each condition. Paranoid traits are common in both schizophrenia and bipolar depression and contribute to risk because the suspiciousness and irritability can cause interpersonally stressful situations to boil over into violence. In a study of 250 nonpsychotic female prison inmates, paranoid and schizoid personality disorders were found to be associated with violent crime (Warren et al. 2002). In the study by Warren et al. (2002), Cluster B personality disorders were predominant (ASPD, 43%; BPD, 24%), but the Cluster A personality disorders were linked to the most extreme types of violence—perhaps, as the authors speculated, because of the social isolation, suspiciousness, and bizarre forms of thinking seen in schizoid/paranoid persons.

Paranoid personality can arise from factors independent of genes for psychosis, as can the related personality type called "fanatic" in Kurt Schneider's (1932) classification. The limitless violence of which religious and political fanatics are capable is well known; the same applies to fanatics who operate within narrower confines, such as racially motivated bigots or fanatics identified with a "cause" who feel justified in lynching or otherwise killing the targets of their hatred. In some instances, fanatical persons are severely disturbed in all spheres of social interaction and appear as misfits. In other instances, their hatred is compartmentalized in such a way that they remain able to relate amicably to family members and like-minded acquaintances, to whom they appear perfectly normal. It is their victims who see the other side.

Schizoid personality disorder in general is not nearly as high a risk factor for violent crime as are ASPD, paranoid personality disorder, and psychopathy, yet it may on occasion contribute to the commission of unusually grotesque violence, which is all the more striking when the schizoid offender has not also been the victim of childhood abuse or other negative environmental factors.

The key here may be the indifference to and lack of feeling for other people, as though they are mere inanimate objects. In my study of serial killers, the most unexpected finding was the high percentage who showed schizoid personality disorder: 47.4%, or 47 of 99 men (Stone 2001)—a striking ratio given that schizoid personality disorder is noted only in about 1% of the population.

In bipolar persons committing violent crimes, paranoid traits are as common as among those with schizophrenia; however, apart from that, one sees different personality constellations. One trait-cluster seen in the admittedly small number of bipolar men who have actually murdered a spouse or a lover consists of hypomanic, narcissistic, arrogant, insensitive, grandiose, pathologically jealous, and physically abusive traits. These men can also be understood as psychopaths (their PCL-R scores [Hare 1991] are often above 30) who use their enormous charm to win the affections of various women whom they subsequently terrorize, brutalize, and may eventually kill—either out of jealousy or out of the desire to be with another woman without the fuss of alimony or custody disputes.

Violence is one of the defining features (although not a necessary feature) of ASPD and is a typical but not invariable attribute of the psychopath. Males outnumber females in both disorders by a factor in the range of 5:1 to 10:1, depending on the sample.

ASPD is common in most groups of violent persons (Coid 2002). An important example is the subgroup of wife batterers who are also violent outside the marriage. These men are generally belligerent, verbally aggressive, controlling, sadistic, jealous, and prone to alcohol abuse, in contrast to the men who are violent only within the family (LaTaillade and Jacobson 1997). The latter group is more concerned with abandonment by their wives, is less often antisocial, and is apt to use low-level forms of violence.

Violence in persons with BPD, most of whom are women, is more often self-directed, in the form of self-mutilation or suicidal acts, and less often appears as the outwardly directed violence we are concerned with here. Assaultive behavior in borderline persons is precipitated usually by (actual or perceived) rejection (Tardiff and Koenigsberg 1985). The reaction may be impulsive and immediate or, in the case of the rejected borderline person who begins to stalk a former lover, more calculated and slower to reach the boiling point. Total strangers are rarely the targets of assaultiveness by those with BPD. In forensic settings, they may in their ragefulness and impulsivity strike out against staff members or other patients who annoy them in some way. Only in a few instances does the violence go all the way to murder, and then the victims are almost always intimates, such as lovers, mates, or the patient's children. With regard to potential for violence, BPD combined with ASPD is clearly a more dangerous combination than BPD with other personality types.

The inhibited/anxious personalities of DSM-IV-TR Cluster C show much less risk for violence than do the other disorders. In the annals of crime, there are the occasional examples of men with obsessive-compulsive personality disorder and sadistic traits who commit murder, more often of intimates than of strangers. Depressive personality, although not in DSM-IV-TR, belongs to this inhibited/anxious domain and is occasionally associated with violence (including murder) toward intimates (Malmquist 1995). Examples are men frightened of the responsibilities of parenthood; depressed, infanticidal women; and men who have lost their jobs. Murderous violence in the workplace usually occurs when a man has been fired from his job and becomes depressed and rageful. Many such men showed paranoid personalities to begin with and were hard to get along with, which is likely why they were dismissed in the first place.

If one can include murder by poisoning as an example of violence—albeit committed at a distance and without physical assault—then we can include certain passive-aggressive traits, usually in combination with schizoid aloofness, in our roster of personality configurations associated with violence. Persons with these trait configurations, when they become vengeful, typically eschew violence involving eye contact or physical contact (e.g., shooting or stabbing) in favor of methods that are more secretive and less visible.

IED, although a symptom (Axis I) disorder in DSM-IV-TR, has some attributes of personality disorder. Persons manifesting the sudden and unpredictable outbursts of violence characteristic of IED have been shown to have even lower concentrations of serotonin than offenders who commit premeditated acts of violence (Linnoila et al. 1983). In a related phenomenon called episodic dyscontrol, abnormal electrophysiological activity in the brain may underlie the sudden outbursts of irrational thinking and violence (Elliott 1982). These biological factors, in turn, exert an influence on the emerging personality.

Less obscure as to etiology than IED is another, more common, contributor to violent behavior—namely, head injury. Head injury often affects the frontal lobe areas, especially the orbitofrontal region that mediates social decision making (Volavka 1995). This region, and the nearby cingulated gyri, are the same areas implicated in psychopathy, whether *primary* (on a largely constitutional basis) or *secondary*. In *secondary psychopathy*, environmental factors involving severe childhood neglect and abuse are critical (Porter 1996); in *primary psychopathy*, genetic predisposition presumably provides the template upon which negative environmental experiences are often (although not always) engrafted. Severely traumatized persons may, as Porter (1996) asserted, learn over time to "turn off" their emotions to cope with horrific circumstances, thus emerging in adulthood as psychopathic personalities. With regard to postnatal head injury and its effects, 52% of wife batterers were noted in one study to have a history of head injury, as opposed to 22% of control subjects (Rosenbaum 1991); in another study, 61% of 62 habitually violent male prisoners had experienced severe head injuries (Bach-y-Rita and Veno 1974). Head injury appears to predispose to violent but not to nonviolent antisocial behavior (Brennan and Mednick 1997). Frontal-lobe impairment is considered an important factor in certain schizophrenic patients with marked proclivities to violence and antisocial traits (Krakowski et al. 1997).

Environmental/Psychological Factors

In the complex calculus of factors contributing to violence, seriously adverse family environment, abuse of substances in the teen years and beyond, and brain damage are important predictors. Brain damage may be either constitutional (i.e., in utero), reflecting the earliest "environment," or environmental in the more common sense of postnatal circumstances. Among the most robust predictors of future violence are juvenile criminal offenses, convictions for violent offenses, number of previous arrests, and severity of the original offense (Blumenthal and Levander 2000).

For reasons of simplicity and space, significant factors not already mentioned are set forth in Table 31–1, derived mainly from the schema suggested by Steadman et al. (1994). Steadman et al. (1994) outlines demographic and other dispositional factors, along with historical, contextual, and clinical factors.

Intergenerational factors are implicit in the table; abused children, for example, are at significantly increased risk for abusing their own children or their mates, especially if they witnessed their own parents behaving violently toward one another. In persons who behave violently there are usually a multiplicity of factors operating: personality disorder, adverse childhood experience, social and economic handicaps, cultural sanctions, and so on. Thus the instruments designed to predict future violence address this complexity by including a large number of items.

Assessment Instruments

The instruments used most widely at present for assessing the risk of criminality (against property as well as persons), violence, or both are the PCL-R (Hare 1991) mentioned earlier; the Violence Risk Assessment Guide (VRAG; Quinsey et al. 1998); and the "HCR-20"—a 20-item questionnaire containing 10 history items, 5 clinical management items, and 5 risk management items (Webster et al. 1997). These instruments are of particular use in evaluating known offenders, unlike the Cooke revision of the PCL-R, also described earlier, which does not carry the criminological items.

The PCL-R score is included as one of the items in both the VRAG and the HCR-20, and each of the newer instruments adds items not covered in the PCL-R: 11 extra items in the VRAG, 19 in the HCR-20. Not all the descriptors are of equal significance in forecasting violence. The most important additions in the VRAG are early age at index offense, history of alcohol abuse, and presence of a DSM-IV-TR personality disorder. The HCR-20 incorporates these and adds previous violence, unresponsiveness to treatment, and exposure to destabilizing events (such as being released, after stays in the hospital or in prison, back into a community dominated by antisocial gangs). As a predictor

Table 31–1. Additional factors and their influence on violence risk

Factor	Influence on violence risk	Reference
A. Dispositional		
Age	Risk maximal in age range 18–30 years	Blumenthal and Levander 2000
Sex	Males at higher risk, especially in homicides by youthful offenders	Snyder and Sickmund 1995; Swanson 1994
Social class	Risk elevated in lower and lower-middle classes	Straus and Gelles 1992; Swanson 1994
Race	Risk greater in African American and Hispanic male youths, but difference related mainly to socioeconomic factors	Young and Hammond 1997
IQ	Low IQ associated with conduct disorder and adult criminality; left-hemisphere deficits common in criminal psychopaths	Raine 1993; Wilson and Herrnstein 1985
B. Historical		
Parental involvement	Poor parental nurturance (neglect) and early loss of parents heightens risk	Klassen and O'Connor 1994; Widom 1989
Child abuse	Physically abused children (especially males) much more likely to engage in violence as adults; sexually abused children more likely to commit sexual crimes	Dutton and Hart 1992
Witnessing abuse	Marital aggression correlates with having seen one's parents hit one another	Kalmuss 1984
Employment	Low income or loss of job are risk factors for violence, as is unemployment	Hall 1978; Sviridoff and Thompson 1979
Job perception	Persons with antisocial personality disorder are often dissatisfied with work; work dissatisfaction in general a risk factor	Robins and Regier 1991
Arrest record	Previous record of arrests for violence associated with increased risk for future violence, especially in those with high Psychopathy Checklist scores	Blumenthal and Levander 2000; Hemphill et al. 1998
Self-reported violence	Self-reported violence added to the rates of violence as recorded only from records and informants	Swanson et al. 1990
Violence to self	Poor impulse control (as in borderline personality disorder) and suspiciousness (as in paranoid personality disorder) correlate with both suicidality and violence to others	Plutchik et al. 1989
C. Contextual		
Living arrangement	Being single is a risk factor; persons with antisocial personality disorder are less likely to marry than those with other personality disorders	Cloninger et al. 1997
Perceived support	Inadequate social support a factor for heightened risk (mentioned also in the HCR-20; Webster et al. 1997)	Steadman et al. 1994
Social network	Living in "inner-city" ghetto or living among delinquent peers heightens risk	Reid and Eddy 1997
D. Substance abuse		
Alcohol	Alcohol abuse heightens violence risk across all personality disorders, especially antisocial personality disorder and psychopathy	Klassen and O'Connor 1994
Other substances	Risk increased with psychoactive stimulants (cocaine, phencyclidine, amphetamines)	White 1997
E. Cultural	Cultural factors (e.g., "machismo" in Latin American culture) may heighten risk	Cooke 1998

of future violence, the social deviance factor (Factor 2) of the PCL-R gives a more accurate estimate than the interpersonal/affective factor (Factor 1), because the former highlights behavior rather than attitude. However, a high score on the PCL-R, whatever the item mix, points more robustly than does the diagnosis of ASPD to violent recidivism in those who have previously committed violent offenses. There are many ways this correlation has been demonstrated. In one 13-year follow-up study, for example, the percentage of offenders, after release from prison, who had still not been rearrested for a violent offense varied in accordance with their PCL-R scores. By the end of the follow-up period, 36% of those with low scores (0 to 19) had offended again, but 65% of those with scores greater than 29 had reoffended. The psychopaths (those with scores above 29) also reoffended earlier during the follow-up interval (Hemphill et al. 1998). The PCL-R was also found the best predictor of violence in the MacArthur Risk Assessment Study (Blumenthal and Levander 2000). Similarly, among adult sex offenders, those who used violence had significantly higher PCL-R scores than did nonviolent sex offenders (Hart and Hare 1997).

The next section provides some brief clinical vignettes illustrating a few of the varieties of violent personality-disordered offenders, some of whom were encountered in forensic hospitals.

CLINICAL EXAMPLES OF VIOLENT BEHAVIORS IN PERSONS WITH PERSONALITY DISORDER

Cluster A Disorders

George Trepal, a schizoid chemist with psychopathic traits, was annoyed by a neighboring family. He sneaked Coca-Cola bottles laced with thallium into their kitchen, poisoning the mother of the family to death and almost killing the children. (Good and Goreck 1995)

Sultan Abdul Hamid, who instigated the Armenian genocide of 1894–1895, had a paranoid/fanatical personality disorder. He had himself ensconced in a fortress with a miles-wide maze and staffed a private army to prevent intruders. Distrustful of his own troops, he insisted that the ships moored in the nearby Bosporus carry no ammunition. He carried a pistol with him at all times and shot anyone who startled him. (Balakian 2003)

Michael Ryan, a 27-year-old paranoid/schizoid man raised in a nonabusive family, grew up awkward and was bullied because he was a "misfit." He lived at home and had no friends. He became a "survivalist," wearing combat gear and eventually murdering 16 people (including his mother) in Hungerford, England, using an AK-47 he had purchased and with which he later killed himself when cornered by the police. (Joseph 1993) (This paranoid/schizoid constellation is typical of men committing mass murder.)

Cluster B Disorders

Pathologically jealous 17-year-old Melinda Loveless stabbed and burned to death a 12-year-old "rival" who had had sex with Melinda's homosexual lover. Melinda developed borderline personality in the aftermath of an extremely abusive and incestuous relationship with her father, also pathologically jealous, who stuck guns up the vaginas of her and her two sisters in order to intimidate them. (Jones 1994)

Saddam Hussein, narcissistic former tyrant of Iraq, has features of malignant narcissism and psychopathy. A violent bully in his teens, he rose to power by murder, torture, and intimidation of rivals. Grandiose, he had oversize posters and monuments of himself placed throughout the country and fostered by way of his reign of terror a kind of worship of his person. (Coughlin 2002)

Cluster C Disorders

Len Fagot, an ex-marine and New Orleans attorney, was obsessive-compulsive and rigid. Perfectionistic and parsimonious, he flew into rages if his will was not carried out. He became increasingly possessive and controlling of his four daughters and eventually staged the murders of two of his sons-in-law for insurance money. (Donahue and Hall 1991)

Primary Psychopathy

Randall Woodfield came from an upper-middle-class nonabusive family in Oregon. An exhibitionist in his teens, he raped several women and became a serial killer in his 20s. (Rule 1984)

Head Injury–Induced Psychopathy

Richard Starett was from an affluent, nonabusive family in Georgia. He suffered a severe head injury with a long period of unconsciousness after a fall at age 7 from a jungle-gym. He underwent a personality change afterward and became intrigued with sadistic magazines and voyeurism. He developed headaches, blackouts, and memory lapses. In his late 20s, he raped and killed ten women. The murders occurred in a setting of headaches with auras accompanied by an urge to kill and fueled by alcohol. (Naifeh and Smith 1995)

Secondary Psychopathy

A 30-year-old man diagnosed as schizophrenic was remanded to a forensic hospital after shooting three workmen while under the influence of hallucinogens (phencyclidine, cocaine). In his youth, his father repeatedly sodomized him after subduing him by choking him to near-unconsciousness. His mother would frequently whip him with an electric cord for minor acts of misbehavior. He had become emotionally numb, had engaged in armed robbery and theft during adolescence, and got into fights while in the army—from which he was discharged after abandoning his baby to go off drinking.

Sadistic Personality in a Psychopath

Gerald Schaefer was raised in a well-to-do Southern family of stern fundamentalist religious leanings. Not abused himself, he witnessed repeated beatings of his mother by his alcoholic father (who would also call her a "whore"). Torn by opposite feelings about sex, he was voyeuristic but would revile a woman who sunbathed, calling her a "slut." Working as a policeman, he would arrest women on fake charges, tie them up, rape them, subject them to prolonged and humiliating tortures, and then kill them. He may have killed 80 or more women before being arrested. (London 1997)

Hypomanic Personality

Richard Minns, a married health-spa tycoon in his late 40s, abandoned his family for a 21-year-old beauty queen. Described as arrogant, egotistical, paranoid, flashy, grandiose, jealous, vengeful, violent, and sensation seeking, he became obsessed with his mistress and later both pathologically jealous and physically abusive. She moved out, whereupon he hired hitmen to kill her (they managed only to render her paraplegic). He fled the United States for Europe and has never been located. (Finstad 1991)

A company executive with bipolar depression and a distinctly hypomanic personality had a lifelong history of aggressiveness and assaultiveness toward relatives (including all three of his wives) and subordinates. He oscillated between feelings of entitlement and contempt for the victims of his abusiveness and (especially in the case of his third wife) extreme remorse and self-mortification. On the behavioral side, he oscillated between serious assaultiveness (breaking his wife's jaw at one point) and suicidal gestures. The amplitude of his mood swings and destructiveness diminished over a 2-year period of largely supportive psychotherapy and mood stabilizers, although a week's hospitalization proved necessary as a cooling-off period following an incident in which he fractured his wife's jaw.

Depressive Personality

Dr. Bruce Rowan, who had a lifelong pessimistic, depressive disposition, made suicidal gestures in medical school but later married and adopted a child. However, he began to resent his wife's attention to the baby. He killed his wife with an axe, put her in a car, and pushed it down a hill to make it appear accidental. He stabbed himself then, although not fatally. He was acquitted on an insanity plea and remanded to a forensic hospital. (Smith 2000)

THERAPEUTIC INTERVENTIONS USED IN DEALING WITH VIOLENT PATIENTS

Most violent persons do not make themselves available to psychiatrists for treatment. What familiarity psychiatrists have with violent persons stems more from evaluation in emergency departments or in forensic settings. Focusing just on murder for the moment, it can be estimated that some 15 million persons fell victim to murder—apart from armed conflict between groups or nations—throughout the twentieth century, using an estimate of 5 homicides per 100,000 per year, with an average world population of 3 billion. This figure is less than one-tenth of the killings brought about by wars, engineered for the most part by leaders whose personalities bore decidedly narcissistic, psychopathic, sadistic, or paranoid/fanatical traits. Such men lie far beyond the circle within which the psychotherapy of violence has demonstrated any measure of effectiveness.

It is with the comparatively minor and nonrepetitive or at least not-too-ingrained forms of violence that we do our best work. Success is sometimes achieved, for example, with children and adolescents who show conduct disorders, ADHD, and the like, as well as with men who batter their mates, with mothers who are physically abusive toward their children, or with patients whose impulsive aggression (e.g., in the form of IED) leads to occasional assaultiveness toward nonfamily members.

Dynamic psychotherapy has limited utility with violent or with highly impulsive persons (Kay and Kay 1997). It may have some effectiveness in those who have a capacity for remorse and whose physical abusiveness has not been life threatening. Guidelines for this treatment have been provided by Tardiff (1996). For the remainder of those violent patients who are still amenable to verbal psychotherapy, cognitive and behavioral methods have proven superior. Such work is often carried out in groups, especially in the case of incarcerated (forensic or prison) patients. In ambulatory work, there are groups for spouses who

Table 31–2. Medications used in the treatment of violent patients

Type of medication	Conditions for which medication is useful
Antidepressants	Irritable aggression; disruptive children and adolescents with conduct disorder; SSRIs in personality disorders characterized by impulsivity
Lithium	Aggressiveness and violence in antisocial and other diverse groups; impulsive/combative women with BPD Episodic dyscontrol (often noted in those with BPD)
Beta-blockers (e.g., propranolol, nadolol)	Intermittent explosive disorder and other personality configurations stemming from neurological impairment; organic brain syndrome–related irritable/paranoid disorders
Stimulants (e.g., amphetamine, methylphenidate)	Conduct disorder with antisocial features; attention-deficit/hyperactivity disorder with antisocial/aggressive features
Neuroleptics	Psychotic patients with paranoid, schizoid, or manic/irritable personality configurations
Benzodiazepines	Violent/aggressive patients (often with paranoid features) seen in emergency departments; persons with episodic temper outbursts (impulsive/aggressive)
Anticonvulsants	Intermittent explosive disorder and a broad range of impulsive/aggressive and violent antisocial persons (especially in secure settings)
Libido-lowering drugs (e.g., medroxyprogesterone, triptorelin)	Male sexual offenders, such as child molesters who use minimal violence (rapists with psychopathic or marked antisocial personalities can seldom be relied on to take these medications except in secure settings)

Note. BPD=borderline personality disorder; SSRI=selective serotonin reuptake inhibitor.
Source. Adapted from Eichelman and Tardiff 1999.

batter their partners, but these are useful only where there is motivation, perseverance, and remorse on the part of the violent partner(s).

Because the large majority of violent persons abuse alcohol or other substances, often to prime themselves for the violence they are about to commit (in a kind of "willed dyscontrol"), joining and staying in a 12-step program (e.g., Alcoholics Anonymous, Narcotics Anonymous) is the first order of business, without which other therapeutic interventions are doomed to fail.

Therapy aside, clinicians should not overlook the effects of time and maturation. Many an antisocial, violent (though nonpsychopathic) adolescent ceases his violent ways, even without treatment, by age 40, as Robins and Regier (1991) have shown. However, despite the superiority of time to most other measures, it still requires—in passing from the violence of youth to the comparative calmness of middle age—a good 20 years.

The main task in any of the verbal approaches is to help the violent patient break the habit of violence through expansion of his hitherto extremely narrow range of behavioral "options." A paranoid/jealous wife batterer, for example, must come to understand that his assumptions of his spouse's supposed "infidelity" may be quite incorrect, or that if she had been unfaithful, he may have driven her to it by his hostile controllingness. If the two cannot resolve their differences and divorce is necessary, he must understand that there are other women in the world with whom a more gratifying relationship may be quite possible. This "gray area" where most of us live is foreign territory to the all-or-none thinking of the violence-prone partner.

As a rule, we will be more successful with battering spouses who restrict their violence to the marital relationship (and who may show borderline or depressive personality features more than antisocial ones) than with those who are violent in all spheres (where the antisocial features predominate and augur more poorly for improvement). Cultural issues need to be addressed in dealing with male batterers, many of whom have been steeped in the culture of machismo, where keeping a woman "in line" through physical intimidation seems normal and ego-syntonic (Holtzworth-Munroe and Meehan 2002). Because of cultural reinforcement, the related habits are all the harder to supplant with more adaptive ones.

PSYCHOPHARMACOLOGIC INTERVENTIONS

Provided the patients themselves are willing to take medications, there are now pharmacological measures for aiding in the control of many forms of violent behavior in personality disorders. The various drugs and the conditions for which they have been found useful have been summarized by Eichelman and Tardiff (1999). One of the first agents that proved effective in a general way with violent patients was lithium, whose utility was thus shown to extend beyond bipolar disorders (Sheard et al. 1976). The array of medications in current use in violence-prone patients with personality and other disorders is outlined in Table 31–2.

We are then left with a residue of scarcely treatable to altogether untreatable persons with violence embedded in their personality disorders. The latter includes psychopathy proper (i.e., with PCL-R scores in the high range of 30 or more); malignant narcissism (particularly in persons occupying positions of great power); sadistic personality, especially when occurring within the context of sexual sadism; antisocial or psychopathic personalities in which the violent offenses are repetitive rapes; and highly impulsive/aggressive personalities with "secondary" psychopathy brought about by what Lonnie Athens (1992) has called "virulency." *Virulency* is the final stage in his schema, in which certain persons pass through stages of extreme brutalization in their youth, followed by belligerency, "violent performances," and finally virulency, where all regard for human feelings has been expunged, leaving only a vengeful, implacable predator.

One of the key features of the persons (and they will mostly be males) in these last categories is lack of empathy or compassion for their victims (Ward et al. 1997). These are deficiencies not affected by medication and scarcely amenable to therapy of any sort. In general, when dealing with violent, personality-disordered persons it is important to know not only our capabilities but also our limitations.

REFERENCES

American Psychiatric Association: Diagnostic and Statistical Manual of Mental Disorders, 3rd Edition. Washington, DC, American Psychiatric Association, 1980

American Psychiatric Association: Diagnostic and Statistical Manual of Mental Disorders, 3rd Edition, Revised. Washington, DC, American Psychiatric Association, 1987

American Psychiatric Association: Diagnostic and Statistical Manual of Mental Disorders, 4th Edition, Text Revision. Washington, DC, American Psychiatric Association, 2000

Athens L: The Creation of Dangerous Violent Criminals. Chicago, IL, University of Chicago Press, 1992

Bach-y-Rita G, Veno A: Habitual violence: A profile of 62 men. Am J Psychiatry 131:1015–1017, 1974

Balakian P: The Burning Tigris. New York, HarperCollins, 2003

Barkley RA: Attention Deficit Hyperactivity Disorder: A Handbook for Diagnosis and Treatment. New York, Guilford, 1990

Blackburn R, Coid JW: Empirical clusters of DSM-III personality disorders in violent offenders. J Personal Disord 13:18–34, 1999

Blumenthal S, Levander T: Violence and Mental Disorder: A Critical Aid to the Assessment and Management of Risk. London, England, Jessica Kingsley, 2000

Brennan PA, Mednick SA: Medical histories of antisocial individuals, in Handbook of Antisocial Behavior. Edited by Stoff DM, J Breiling J, Maser JD. New York, Wiley, 1997, pp 269–279

Carey G, Goldman D: The genetics of antisocial behavior, in Handbook of Antisocial Behavior. Edited by Stoff DM, Breiling J, Maser JD. New York, Wiley, 1997, pp 243–254

Cartwright J: Evolution and Human Behavior. Cambridge, MA, MIT Press, 2000

Cloninger CR, Gottesman II: Genetic and environmental factors in antisocial behavior disorders, in The Causes of Crime: New Biological Approaches. Edited by Mednick SA, Moffitt TE, Stack SA. Cambridge, England, Cambridge University Press, 1987, pp 92–109

Cloninger CR, Bayon C, Przybeck TR: Epidemiology and Axis I comorbidity of antisocial personality, in Handbook of Antisocial Behavior. Edited by Stoff DM, Breiling J, Maser JD. New York, Wiley, 1997, pp 12–21

Coid JW: Personality disorders in prisoners and their motivation for dangerous and disruptive behavior. Crim Behav Ment Health 12:209–226, 2002

Cooke DJ: Psychopathy across cultures, in Psychopathy: Theory, Research and Implications for Society. Edited by Cooke DJ, Forth AE, Hare RD. Dordrecht, The Netherlands, Kluwer, 1998, pp 13–45

Cooke DJ, Michie C: Refining the construct of psychopathy: towards a hierarchical model. Psychol Assess 13:171–188, 2001

Côté G, Hodgins S: Co-occurring mental disorders among criminal offenders. Bull Am Acad Psychiatry Law 18:271–281, 1990

Coughlin C: King of Terror. New York, HarperCollins, 2002

De Zulueta F: From Pain to Violence: The Traumatic Roots of Destructiveness. London, England, Whurr, 1993

Donahue C, Hall S: Deadly Relations. New York, Bantam, 1991

Dougherty DM, Bjork JM, Huckabee HC, et al: Laboratory measures of aggression and impulsivity in women with borderline personality disorder. Psychiatry Res 85:315–326, 1999

Dutton DG: The Abusive Personality: Violence and Control in Intimate Relationships. New York, Guilford, 1998

Dutton DG, Hart SD: Evidence for long-term, specific effects of childhood and neglect on criminal behavior in men. International Journal of Offender Therapy and Comparative Criminology 36:129–137, 1992

Eichelman BS, Tardiff K: Long-term medications for violent patients, in Medical Management of the Violent Patient. Edited by Tardiff K. New York, Marcel Dekker, 1999, pp 255–275

Elliott FA: Neurological findings in adult minimal brain dysfunction and the dyscontrol syndrome. J Nerv Ment Dis 170:680–687, 1982

Finstad S: Sleeping with the Devil. New York, William Morrow, 1991

Glasser M: On violence: a preliminary communication. Int J Psychoanal 79:887–902, 1998

Good J, Goreck S: Poison Mind. New York, William Morrow, 1995

Groth AN, Birnbaum HJ: Men Who Rape: The Psychology of the Offender. New York, Plenum, 1979

Hall HV: Violence Prediction: Guidelines for the Forensic Practitioner. Springfield, IL, Charles C Thomas, 1978

Hare RD: The Hare Psychopathy Checklist Revised [PCL-R]. Toronto, Canada, Multi-Health Systems, 1991

Hare RD: Psychopathy, affect and behavior, in Psychopathy: Theory, Research and Implications for Society. Edited by Cooke DJ, Forth AE, Hare RD. Dordrecht, The Netherlands, Kluwer, 1998, pp 105–137

Harpur TJ, Hakstian AR, Hare RD: Factor structure of the Psychopathy Checklist. J Consult Clin Psychol 56:741–747, 1988

Hart SD: Psychopathy and risk for violence, in Psychopathy: Theory, Research and Implications for Society. Edited by Cooke DJ, Forth AE, Hare RD. Dordrecht, The Netherlands, Kluwer, 1998, pp 355–373

Hart SD, Hare RD: Psychopathy: assessment and association with criminal conduct, in Handbook of Antisocial Behavior. Edited by Stoff DM, Breiling J, Maser JD. New York, Wiley, 1997, pp 22–35

Hart SD, Hare RD, Forth AE: Psychopathy as a risk marker for violence: development and validation of a screening version of the Revised Psychopathy Checklist, in Violence and Mental Disorder: Development in Risk Assessment. Edited by Monahan J, Steadman HJ. Chicago, IL, University of Chicago Press, 1994, pp 81–98

Hemphill JF, Templeman R, Wong S, et al: Psychopathy and crime: recidivism and criminal careers, in Psychopathy: Theory, Research and Implications for Society. Edited by Cooke DJ, Forth AE, Hare RD. Dordrecht, The Netherlands, Kluwer, 1998, pp 375–399

Hodgins S: The criminality of mentally disordered persons, in Mental Disorder and Crime. Edited by Hodgins S. Newbury Park, CA, Sage, 1993, pp 3–21

Hollin CR, Howells K: An introduction to concepts, models and techniques, in Clinical Approaches to Violence. Edited by Howells K, Hollin CR. Chichester, England, Wiley, 1989

Holtzworth-Munroe A, Meehan JC: Husband violence: personality disorders among male batterers. Curr Psychiatry Rep 4:13–17, 2002

Hoptman MJ: Neuroimaging studies of violence and antisocial behavior. J Psychiatr Pract 9:265–278, 2003

Jones A: Cruel Sacrifice. New York, Pinnacle, 1994

Joseph J: Hungerford: One Man's Massacre. London, England, Gryphon, 1993

Kalmuss D: The intergenerational transmission of marital aggression. J Marriage Fam 46:11–19, 1984

Kay J, Kay RL: Individual psychoanalytic psychotherapy, in Psychiatry, Vol 2. Edited by Tasman A, Aky J, Lieberman JA. Philadelphia, PA, W.B. Saunders, 1997, pp 1373–1390

Kernberg OF: Aggression in Personality Disorders and Perversions. New Haven, CT, Yale University Press, 1992

Klassen D, O'Connor WA: Predicting violence in mental patients: cross validation of an actuarial scale. Presented at the Annual Meeting of the American Society of Criminology, Quebec City, Canada, November 1987

Klassen D, O'Connor WA: Demographic and case-history variables in risk assessment, in Violence and Mental Disorder: Development in Risk Assessment. Edited by Monahan J, Steadman HJ. Chicago, IL, University of Chicago Press, 1994, pp 229–257

Krakowski M, Czobor P, Libiger J, et al: Violence in schizophrenic patients: the role of positive psychotic symptoms and frontal love impairment. Am J Forensic Psychiatry 18:39–50, 1997

LaTaillade JJ, Jacobson NS: Domestic violence: antisocial behavior in the family, in Handbook of Antisocial Behavior. Edited by Stoff DM, Breiling J, Maser JD. New York, Wiley, 1997, pp 534–550

Lidz C, Mulvey E, Gardner W: The accuracy of prediction of violence to others. JAMA 269:1007–1011, 1993

Link BG, Stueve A: Evidence bearing on mental illness as a possible cause of violent behavior. Epidemiol Rev 17: 172–181, 1995

Linnoila M, Virkkunen M, Scheinin M, et al: Low cerebrospinal 5-hydroxyindoleacetic acid concentrations differentiates impulsive from nonimpulsive violent behavior. Life Sci 33:2609–2614, 1983

London S: Killer Fiction. Venice, CA, Feral House, 1997

Malmquist C: Depression and homicidal violence. Int J Law Psychiatry 18:145–162, 1995

Markman R, Labreque R: Obsessed: The Stalking of Teresa Suldana. New York, William Morrow, 1994

Maughn B: Childhood precursors of aggressive offending in personality-disordered adults, in Mental Disorder and Crime. Edited by Hodgins S. Newbury Park, CA, Sage, 1993, pp 119–139

Mealey L: The sociobiology of sociopathy: an integrated evolutionary model. Behav Brain Sci 18:523–599, 1995

Mednick SA, Gabrielli WH, Hutchings B: Genetic influences in criminal convictions: evidence from an adoption cohort. Science 224:891–894, 1984

Meloy JR: Stalking (obsessional following): a review of some preliminary studies. Aggress Violent Behav 1:147–162, 1996

Meloy JR: When stalkers become violent: the threat to public figures and private lives. Psychiatr Ann 33:659–665, 2003

Monahan J: Predicting Violent Behavior. Newbury, CA, Sage, 1981

Monahan J: Violence prediction: the past twenty years and the next twenty years. Crim Justice Behav 23:107–120, 1996

Monahan J, Steadman HJ (eds): Violence and Mental Disorder: Development in Risk Assessment. Chicago, IL, University of Chicago Press, 1994

Naifeh S, Smith G: A Stranger in the Family. New York, Dutton, 1995

Perelberg RJ: Psychoanalytic Understanding of Violence and Suicide. London, England, Routledge, 1999

Plutchik R, van Praag HM, Conte HR: Correlates of suicide and violence risk. Psychiatry Res 28:215–225, 1989

Porter S: Without conscience or without active conscience? The etiology of psychopathy revisited. Aggress Violent Behav 1:179–189, 1996

Quinsey VL, Harris GT, Rice ME, et al: Violent Offenders: Appraising and Managing Risk. Washington, DC, American Psychological Association, 1998

Raine A: The Psychopathology of Crime: Criminal Behavior as a Clinical Disorder. New York, Academic Press, 1993

Rasmussen K, Levander S: Symptoms and personality characteristics of patients in a maximum security psychiatric unit. Int J Law Psychiatry 19:27–37, 1996

Reid JB, Eddy JM: The prevention of antisocial behavior: some considerations in the search for effective interventions, in Handbook of Antisocial Behavior. Edited by Stoff DM, Breiling J, Maser JD. New York, Wiley, 1997, pp 343–356

Rhodes R: Why They Kill: The Discoveries of a Maverick Criminologist. New York, Knopf, 1999

Robins LN, Regier DA: Psychiatric Disorders in America: The Epidemiological Catchment Area Study. New York, Free Press, 1991

Rosenbaum A: The neuropsychology of marital aggression, in Neuropsychology of Aggression. Edited by Milner JS. Boston, MA, Kluwer, 1991, pp 167–180

Rule A: The I-5 Killer. New York, Signet, 1984

Schneider K: Psychopatische Persoenlichkeiten. Leipzig, Germany, F Deuticke, 1923

Sheard MH, Marini JL, Bridges CI, et al: The effects of lithium on impulsive aggressive behavior in man. Am J Psychiatry 133:1409–1413, 1976

Smith C: Bitter Medicine. New York, St Martin's, 2000

Snyder HN, Sickmund M: Juvenile Offenders and Victims. Washington, DC, Office of Juvenile Justice and Delinquency Prevention, U.S. Department of Justice, 1995

Sofsky W: Traktat über die Gewalt. Frankfurt am. Main, Verlag Fischer, 1996

Steadman HJ, Monahan J, Appelbaum PS, et al: Designing a new generation of risk assessment research, in Violence and Mental Disorder: Development in Risk Assessment. Edited by Monahan J, Steadman HJ. Chicago, IL, University of Chicago Press, 1994, pp 297–318

Stone MH: Serial sexual homicide: biological, psychological and sociological aspects. J Personal Disord 15:1–18, 2001

Straus MA, Gelles RJ: Physical Violence in American Families: Risk Factors and Adaptations to Violence in 8,145 Families. New Brunswick, NJ: Transaction, 1992

Sviridoff M, Thompson JW: Linkage between Employment and Crime: A Qualitative Study of Rikers Releases. New York, Vera Institute of Justice, 1979

Swanson JW: Mental disorder, substance abuse, and community violence: an epidemiological approach, in Violence and Mental Disorder: Development in Risk Assessment. Edited by Monahan J, Steadman HJ. Chicago, IL, University of Chicago Press, 1994, pp 101–136

Swanson JW, Holzer C, Gunju V, et al: Violence and psychiatric disorder in the community: evidence from the Epidemiological Catchment area surveys. Hosp Community Psychiatry 41:761–770, 1990

Tardiff K: Assessment and Management of Violent Patients, 2nd Edition. Washington, DC, American Psychiatric Press, 1996

Tardiff K, Koenigsberg HW: Assaultive behavior among psychiatric outpatients. Am J Psychiatry 142:960–963, 1985

Valzelli L: Psychobiology of Aggression and Violence. New York, Raven, 1981

Volavka J: Neurobiology of Violence. Washington, DC, American Psychiatric Press, 1995

Ward Y, McCormack J, Hudson SM, et al: Rape: assessment and treatment, in Sexual Deviance: Theory, Assessment and Treatment. Edited by Laws DR, O'Donohue W. New York, Guilford, 1997, pp 356–393

Warren JI, Burnette M, South SC, et al: Personality disorders and violence among female prison inmates. J Am Acad Psychiatry Law 30:502–512, 2002

Webster CD, Douglas KS, Eaves D, et al: HCR-20: Assessing Risk of Violence to Others, Version 2. Burnaby, British Columbia, Mental Health Law and Policy Unit, Simon Fraser University, 1997

White HR: Alcohol, illicit drugs and violence, in Handbook of Antisocial Behavior. Edited by Stoff DM, Breiling J, Maser JD. New York, Wiley, 1997, pp 511–523

Widiger TA, Corbitt EM: Comorbidity of antisocial personality disorder with other personality disorders, in Handbook of Antisocial Behavior. Edited by Stoff DM, Breiling J, Maser JD. New York, Wiley, 1997, pp 75–82,

Widom CS: The cycle of violence. Science 244:160–166, 1989

Wilson JQ, Herrnstein R: Crime and Human Nature. New York, Simon and Schuster, 1985

Yung BR, Hammond R: Antisocial behavior in minority groups: epidemiological and cultural perspectives, in Handbook of Antisocial Behavior. Edited by Stoff DM, Breiling J, Maser JD. New York, Wiley, 1997, pp 474–495

32

Dissociative States

José R. Maldonado, M.D.
David Spiegel, M.D.

THE NATURE OF DISSOCIATION

Definition

According to the Random House Webster's Dictionary, the word *dissociation* is defined as the act of dissociating or the state of being dissociated; or the splitting off of a group of mental process from the main body of consciousness (1999). In psychiatry, the term is used to describe the reversible separation of elements of "identity, memory, or consciousness" (American Psychiatric Association 2000) from the mainstream of consciousness or of behavior, as in dissociative amnesia, fugue, depersonalization, or dissociative identity disorder (DID). The word comes from the Latin verb *dissociare*, meaning to separate or to disunite: *dis* meaning asunder, *sociare* meaning to unite.

Phenomenology of Dissociation

Dissociation can be understood as a mechanism through which we are able to separate mental processes and contents. Under normal conditions, the (nonpathological) mechanism of dissociation allows us to carry on more than one complex task or action simultaneously by keeping out of consciousness routine experiences or tasks, for example the operation of implicit memory systems which allow us to perform complex physical activities with little conscious thought (Schacter 1992). Dissociation can also be triggered, not always voluntarily, as an attempt to preserve a sense of control, safety, and identity while exposed to overwhelming stress or trauma (Bremner et al. 1992; Maldonado and Spiegel 1998; Spiegel 1997; Spiegel and Cardena 1991). Pathological dissociation may be elicited as a response to traumatic events that threaten personal physical integrity or the safety of a loved one, or it may be elicited in response to extreme isolation and abandonment. The use of dissociative defenses can be so effective at allowing victims of trauma to separate themselves from the awareness of danger that some trauma survivors may act as if they were unaware of threats. In extreme cases, victims may act as if the traumatic experience had never happened.

The types of trauma leading to the use and development of dissociative defenses may vary widely, ranging from natural disasters, such as floods, nature fires, earthquakes (Koopman et al. 1995); to man-made accidental disasters, such as war and nuclear plant explosions (Marmar et al. 1998; Noyes and Kletti 1977; Spiegel 1997); to large scale intentional man-made disasters, such as ethnic cleansing, school shootings, acts of terrorism, the September 11, 2001, attack on New York City (Yehuda et al. 1996); to more personal traumas, such as car accidents, medical procedures, imprisonment (Maercker and Schutzwohl 1997), and

493

the most publicized of all forms of trauma: abandonment, neglect, and childhood physical and sexual abuse (Banyard 2001; Kluft 1985; Spiegel 1986, 1997).

Dissociation as a psychiatric disorder was initially described by the French philosopher and psychologist Pierre Janet. Janet utilized the French term désagrégation which carries with it a different and more accurate nuance than its English translation, dissociation. Désagrégation implies a separation of mental contents despite their general tendency to aggregate or be processed together. Thus, according to Janet, the problem experienced by these patients is a difficulty in integration of psychic processes, rather than a proliferation of components of consciousness, memory, identity, or perception. Janet (1889) viewed désagrégation (or its translation dissociation) as a purely pathological process, "a malady of the personal synthesis" (p. 332). Janet was also the first to study psychological trauma as a principal cause of dissociative phenomena.

During the twentieth century, Janet's work and theories of dissociation as a pathological process were eclipsed by the emerging psychoanalytic theories proposed by Sigmund Freud. Psychoanalysis emphasized the mechanism of repression, rather than dissociation. Despite their later divergence, early writings by Freud and Breuer explored unconscious phenomena through an examination of seemingly similar "dissociative phenomena." Taking from the theories on hysteria of their predecessor, Jean Marie Charcot, Breuer and Freud suggested that the dissociative symptoms exhibited by their patients were attributed to the patient's capacity to enter spontaneous and uncontrolled hypnoid states (Breuer and Freud 1893–1895/1955).

After Janet, there was little, if any, discussion about dissociation and its relation to trauma until the Second World War. During the postwar period, clinicians noted a high incidence of dissociative symptoms such as fugue states and amnesic syndromes among combatants. Traumatic neurosis was recognized among ex-inmates of concentration camps. Based on these observations, Hilgard (1977) developed a "neodissociation" theory that revived interest in Janetian psychology and psychopathology. The neodissociation model by Hilgard (1986) conceived of a mental structure with divisions that were horizontal rather than vertical, differing from the topographic model by Freud (1915/1963), which was composed of deepening layers of unconscious mental processing. Unlike Freud's system, Hilgard's allowed for immediate access to consciousness of any of a variety of warded-off memories. In Hilgard's model, amnesia is the crucial mediating mechanism that provides the barriers which divide one set of mental contents from another. Thus, the flexible and reversible use of amnesia is a key defensive tool. Therefore, a method that allows for controlled reversal of amnesic content would be an important therapeutic tool.

Historically, most research on dissociative disorders had been concerned with between-personalities amnesia, and little attention has been paid to within-personality memory function. In 1989, Schacter and colleagues examined the autobiographical memory of a patient with DID and her response to cuing procedures that were proven useful in previous studies of normal and abnormal memory. They found that the subject was able to retrieve autobiographical episodes from the recent past, although her performance differed in several respects from that of matched controls. They also found a striking deficit in the subject's childhood autobiographical memory: she was unable to recall a single episode from before age 10 in response to various retrieval cues, whereas control subjects had no difficulty recalling numerous childhood episodes. These findings add to published data and clinical experience that suggest significant memory problems, particularly in regard to autobiographical data, affecting subjects with clinical dissociation, including those with primary personality disorders.

Noll (1989) reviewed and outlined Jung's contributions to the study of dissociation. Jung was unique in recognizing that the "dissociability of the psyche" is a fundamental process that extends along the continuum from normal mental functioning to abnormal states. Thus, dissociation was recognized by Jung as a universal and necessary psychic activity for the development of personality through the differentiation of functions. However, when the cohesion of consciousness is shattered by extreme traumatic experiences (e.g., childhood physical or sexual abuse) this natural differentiation of function is intensified and the dissociative splits between autonomous forces in the psyche become more extreme, as in the case of borderline personality disorder (BPD) or DID.

Throughout the years, researchers and scientists have debated whether dissociation is a subtype of repression or vice versa. Current psychological testing techniques may never be able to clearly resolve this dilemma. Nevertheless, given the complexity of human cognitive processing mechanisms, what is remarkable is not that dissociative disorders occur at all, but rather that they do not occur more often (Baars 1988; Cohen and Servain-Schreiber 1992a, 1992b; Rumelhart and McClelland 1986; Spiegel 1991a, 1991b). We believe that as a general model for keeping information out of

Table 32–1. Differences between dissociation and repression

	Dissociation	Repression
Organizational structure	Horizontal	Vertical
Barriers	Amnesia	Dynamic conflict
Etiology	Trauma	Developmental conflict over unacceptable wishes
Contents	Untransformed: traumatic memories	Disguised, primary process: dreams, slips
Means of access	Hypnosis	Interpretation
Psychotherapy	Access, control, and working through traumatic memories	Interpretation, transference

conscious awareness repression differs from dissociation in six important ways (Maldonado and Spiegel 2002): organizational structure, functional barriers to prevent access to information, etiological causes, amnesic content, preferred means to access that content, and effective psychotherapeutic techniques to achieve symptom resolution (Table 32–1).

Putnam (1997) suggested the "discrete behavioral states" model of DID. Forrest (2001) described a possible biological mechanism to support this model by proposing the involvement of the orbital frontal cortex in the development of DID and suggesting a potential neurodevelopmental mechanism responsible for the development of multiple representations of the self. The proposed "orbital frontal" model integrates and elaborates on theory and research from four domains: the neurobiology of the orbital frontal cortex and its protective inhibitory role in the temporal organization of behavior, the development of emotion regulation, the development of the self, and experience-dependent reorganizing of neocortical processes. The hypothesis proposed by Forrest establishes that the experience-dependent maturation of the orbital frontal cortex in early abusive environments, characterized by discontinuity in dyadic socioaffective interactions between the infant and the caregiver, may be responsible for a pattern of lateral inhibition (i.e., dissociation or inhibition of conflicting subsets of self-representations that are normally integrated into a unified self). His basic idea is that the discontinuity in the early caretaking environment is manifested in the discontinuity in the organization of the developing child's self.

Depending on each therapist's clinical experience, level of skepticism, and appreciation of the history of hysteria and dissociation, DID may be interpreted as 1) the psychological "missing link" that realizes Freud's goal of uniting the psychology of dreams with psychopathology; 2) a fraudulent condition that is wittingly or unwittingly manufactured in the therapist's office; or 3) a population of disturbed and disturbing patients, once the subject of great scientific interest, who are now back in the fold of legitimacy as renewed attention has been paid to the long-term effects of traumatic stressors (Brenner 1999). Brenner has suggested that dissociation may be seen as a complex defense based on his extensive clinical experience with psychic trauma and his treatment of subjects with DID. Furthermore, he believes that DID may be considered a "lower level dissociative character" and that a unique psychic structure, which he calls the "dissociative self," creates alter personalities out of disowned affects, memories, fantasies, and drives. As many other experts on dissociation have suggested, Brenner believes that this "dissociative self" must be dissolved during the therapeutic process in order for integration of "alter personalities" to occur.

According to DSM-IV-TR, memory dysfunction is a central feature of dissociative disorders. Following the memory anomalies seen in subjects with DID outlined by Putnam (1994, 1995), the data seem to suggest that as a whole, amnesic barriers between alter personalities are typically impervious to explicit stimuli, as well as to conceptually driven implicit stimuli. The same research suggests that autobiographical memory deficits are also evident in DID. Although no experimental studies have addressed the issue of source amnesia (i.e., recall of mental content without recollection of the source of the information) or pseudomemories, some evidence (Dorahy 2001) shows that pseudomemories are an infrequent but real phenomenon in DID patients.

Dell (2002) conducted a study to investigate the dissociative phenomenology in patients with DID. In order to determine the use of dissociation as a psychological mechanism, he administered the Multidimensional Inventory of Dissociation to four different population groups: patients with DID, patients with dissociative disorder not otherwise specified (DDNOS), patients with mixed psychiatric disorders, and normal (control) individuals. Dell found that DID patients obtain significantly higher scores than the other three groups on 27 dissociation-related variables. These findings are virtually identical to the large body of published data on the dissociative phenomenology of DID. His findings suggest that dissociation is a unifactorial taxon or natural type that has different presentation aspects or epiphenomena (e.g., amnesia, depersonalization, voices, trance, etc.).

The literature has focused on the characterological features of DID, thus extending the "state versus trait" debate to the realm of the dissociative disorders. A number of different theories are presented describing DID as a variant of, on a continuum with, or being comorbid with the diagnoses of narcissistic personality disorder and BPD. Brenner (1996) suggested that DID would be best considered a distinct characterological entity. He presented two theories, which described DID as a personality disorder whose predominant defense is dissociation. The more developed model which possibly has more explanatory value is the "dissociative character." In this schema, DID would be considered a lower-level dissociative character, utilizing primitive forms of dissociation in which splitting is enhanced by an autohypnotic defensive altered state of consciousness. These patients experience altered states, which originate in response to the overstimulation stemming from external trauma, but get reactivated in response to here-and-now intrapsychic conflicts. Recognition of this dual quality of dissociation seems helpful in psychodynamic treatment, which allows for separate analysis of the traumatic content and the defenses facilitating these states. The nature of the content of what is "in dissociation" appears to have a dreamlike quality to it that may correspond to previous trauma but also be subject to some secondary revision. According to Brenner, the second organizing influence which contributes to seemingly separate identities is that of perverse sexuality. Thus, it appears that a number of dissociated sexual pathways may be followed in the same individual, which encapsulates aggression, childhood trauma, anxiety, and a sense of self. When this exceedingly complex psychic structure is successful, it may then free up some ego to proceed with aspects of healthy development.

Dissociative disorders represent a failure of integration of various aspects of identity, memory, and consciousness. Thus various components of identity in a dissociative disorder patient may be analogous to one

or more personality disorder syndromes. In fact, Ellason et al. (1995) administered the Millon Clinical Multiaxial Inventory-II to patients with DID and found that the most elevated personality disorder scales were avoidant, self-defeating, borderline, and passive-aggressive personality disorders. The diagnosis of a personality disorder in a patient with dissociative disorders should be made on the basis of the assessment of the "whole" human being—that is, on the presence of a pervasive and relatively inflexible pattern of behaviors that reflects the individual predominant mode of being—and not on the basis of personality traits contained within any single alternate personality or groups of personalities.

The personality disorders as defined by DSM-IV-TR (American Psychiatric Association 2000) are a heterogeneous group of conditions whose individual etiologies reflect a complex array of constitutional, genetic, environmental, interpersonal, and psychodynamic factors. The interplay of various etiological factors is variable and diverse among these determinants of the personality disorders and the traumatic forces that result in the development of a dissociative disorder. Nevertheless, some confluence of factors, namely abandonment and abuse, may be common among some dissociative and personality disorders (Fink 1991). For the Cluster A personality disorders (schizoid, schizotypal, paranoid), evidence supports a relationship between dissociative disorders and specific psychotic illnesses. The combination of dissociative pathology with these personality disorders commonly results in a greater impairment of reality testing than in either condition alone. The Cluster B personality disorders (histrionic, narcissistic, borderline, and antisocial) and Cluster C personality disorders (avoidant, obsessive-compulsive, dependent) are believed to be primarily developmental disturbances (Fink 1991). In general, many DID patients present with an apparent mixed personality profile consisting of an array of avoidant, compulsive, borderline, narcissistic, dependent, and passive-aggressive features.

A close review of similarities between personality disorders and dissociative disorders have suggested the common use of immature defense. Vaillant and Drake (1985) conducted a study of 307 inner-city men looking at different dimensions of psychosocial dysfunction by way of three assessment tools: the Health-Sickness Rating Scale (HSRS), Axis II of DSM-III, and dominant choice of ego mechanisms of defense. They found that the majority of subjects with personality disorders and low HSRS scores had a tendency to use primarily immature defense mechanisms (i.e., projection, schizoid fantasy, passive aggression, dissociation, hypochondriasis, and acting-out). Conversely, only a slim minority of subjects without personality disorders and of those with HSRS scores of over 70 were noted to favor such defenses. Their results confirm the notion that personality disorder subjects use a preponderance of immature defenses but do not clarify if this finding is a cause or effect; that is, are patients with personality disorder somehow developmentally arrested at the time of trauma and continue to use immature defenses, or do they revert to the use of immature defenses over time as an adaptation to traumatic events?

Prevalence of Dissociative Phenomena

Unfortunately few good epidemiological studies have been performed on dissociative disorders and phenomena. Some authors estimate the prevalence of dissociative disorders at only 1 per 10,000 in the general population (Coons 1984; Kluft 1991) with far higher proportions reported among psychiatric populations. Not surprisingly, the prevalence of dissociative symptoms seems to be associated with the specific population under study. Recent data suggest that the prevalence in the general population may be as high as 1% (Ross et al. 1991a, 1991b; Vanderlinden et al. 1991), whereas data from specialized inpatient populations suggest the prevalence may be as high as 3% (Kluft 1991; Ross et al. 1991a). Dissociative symptoms have also been reported in virtually every major psychiatric disorder and, in less severe forms, even in nonpatient ("normal") populations (Giese-Davis et al. 1997). In the general population, 6.3% of adults have reported three to four dissociative symptoms (Mulder et al. 1998). Looking at the acute and subacute psychiatric population of a day hospital, Lussier et al. (1997) found a 9% prevalence of a dissociative disorder. Coons (1998) reported that dissociative disorders might comprise 5%–10% of psychiatric populations.

Draijer and Langeland (1999) administered the Dissociative Experiences Scale (DES) and the Structured Trauma Interview (STI) to 160 inpatients consecutively admitted to a general psychiatric hospital. They found that 18% of the patients obtained a DES score greater than 30, which is usually considered the cutoff for dissociative disorders. In their sample, early separation was reported by 26.4% of the patients; 30.1% had witnessed violence amongst their parents; 23.6% reported physical abuse; 34.6% reported sexual abuse; 11.7% reported rape before age 16; and 42.1% reported combined sexual and physical abuse. In the studied population, the level of dissociation was pri-

marily related to reports of overwhelming childhood experiences (e.g., sexual and physical abuse). Furthermore, the severity of dissociative symptoms increased with the severity of the sexual abuse (e.g., involving penetration, multiple perpetrators, or abuse lasting more than 1 year). The highest dissociation levels were found in patients reporting cumulative sexual trauma (e.g., intrafamilial and extrafamilial) or both sexual and physical abuse. Of note, the degree of maternal dysfunction was directly related to the level of dissociation.

These findings were similar to those reported by Nijenhuis and colleagues (1998). They found that dissociative disorder patients had experienced more severe and multifaceted traumatization. In their sample, physical and sexual trauma predicted somatoform dissociation, while sexual trauma alone predicted psychological dissociation.

All available studies suggest that pathological dissociation is best predicted by early onset of reported intense, chronic, and multiple traumatization. Thus, physical trauma seems to elicit dissociation or compartmentalization of experience and may often become the matrix for later posttraumatic symptomatology, such as dissociative amnesia for the traumatic episode. Indeed, some trauma researchers (Kluft 1984b, 1984c, 1991; Spiegel 1984, 1986) have described patients with more extreme dissociative disorders, such as DID, as patients with a "chronic form of posttraumatic stress disorder (PTSD)." In these subjects, recollection of traumatic experiences tends to have an "on-off" quality involving either intrusion or avoidance memories (Horowitz 1976), in which victims (Spiegel 1984) either intensively relive the trauma as though it were recurring (i.e., flashbacks) or have difficulty remembering it (i.e., amnesia and psychic numbing) (Cardena and Spiegel 1993; Christianson and Loftus 1987; Madakasira and O'Brien 1987).

The apparent rise in reported cases of dissociative disorders may be a reflection of a greater awareness of the phenomena among mental health professionals, the availability of specific diagnostic criteria, and previous misdiagnosis of dissociative disorders as bipolar affective disorder, mood disorder with psychotic features, schizophrenia, or BPD. Critics of the diagnosis suggest a more controversial theory for the increase in reported cases. They suggest that dissociative disorders do not exist as spontaneous phenomena, but that they are the result of hypnotic suggestion and inadequate handling by overzealous therapists (Brenner 1994, 1996; Frankel 1990; Ganaway 1989, 1995; McHugh 1995a, 1995b; Spanos 1986; Spanos et al. 1985). Although those individuals who are most likely to have the disorder are highly hypnotizable and therefore relatively suggestible, this trait may not account for all cases, particularly those diagnosed without the use of hypnosis or by "skeptical" psychiatrists.

Dissociative disorders have been described in many cultures and settings (Maldonado and Spiegel 2002). Women make up the majority of cases, accounting for 90% or more of the reported cases in some studies (Coons et al. 1988; Putnam et al. 1986; Schultz et al. 1989). Of interest, the most common dissociative disorder diagnosis is the DDNOS category, both in the United States and in non-Western countries, where dissociative trance and possession trance are the most common dissociative disorder diagnoses (Adityanjee et al. 1989; Saxena and Prasad 1989). Of note, dissociative trance and possession trance are in an appendix of DSM-IV (American Psychiatric Association 1994) as exploratory diagnostic categories. Thus, when a subject meets diagnostic criteria for one of these phenomena, the patient should be diagnosed with DDNOS according to the current dissociative disorder nosology of the DSM-IV-TR.

Abuse and Trauma as Etiological Factors in Dissociative Symptoms

Clinical and empirical evidence suggests that dissociation may occur as a defense during trauma—as an attempt to maintain mental control at the very moment when physical control has been lost (Bremner and Brett 1997; Butler et al. 1996; Eriksson and Lundin 1996; Kluft 1984a, 1984c, 1985; Koopman et al. 1995; Putnam 1985; Spiegel 1984; Spiegel et al. 1988). In fact, the growing literature suggests a connection between a history of physical and sexual abuse in childhood and the development of dissociative symptoms (Anderson et al. 1993; Brown et al. 1999; Chu et al. 1999; Coons 1994; Coons and Milstein 1986; Ellason et al. 1996; Farley and Keaney 1997; Irwin 1999; Kluft 1984c; Mulder et al. 1998; Roesler and McKenzie 1994; Sar et al. 1996; Saxe et al. 1993; Scroppo et al. 1998; Spiegel 1984). Similarly, evidence is accumulating that dissociative symptoms are more prevalent in patients with Axis II disorders, such as BPD, when the patient has a history of childhood abuse (Brenner 1996; Brodsky et al. 1995; Chu and Dill 1990; Darves-Bornoz 1997; Herman et al. 1989; Zweig-Frank et al. 1994a, 1994b). When Mulder and colleagues (1998) examined the relationship between childhood sexual abuse, childhood physical abuse, current psychiatric illness, and measures of dissociation in an adult population, they found that 6.3% of the abused population suffered from three or more frequently occurring dissociative symptoms. Among these individuals, the rate of childhood sexual abuse was two and one-half times as high, the rate of physical abuse was five times as high, and the rate of current psychiatric disorder was four times as high as the respective rates for the other subjects.

Researchers have observed that numbing (i.e., loss of responsiveness in the wake of trauma) is a predictor of future use of dissociative defenses, such as in PTSD. Research on war veterans, hostages, and survivors of other life-threatening events indicates that more than half have experienced feelings of unreality, automatic movements, lack of emotion, hyperalertness, and a sense of detachment/depersonalization (Madakasira and O'Brien 1987; Noyes and Kletti 1977; Noyes and Slymen 1978; Sloan 1988; Solomon et al. 1988, 1989). Depersonalization, numbing, loss of interest, and an inability to feel deeply about anything were reported in about a third of the survivors of man-made and natural disasters (Cardeña and Spiegel 1993; Holen 1993).

Timmerman and Emmelkamp (2001) studied the relationship between traumatic experiences, dissociation, and BPD pathology among a group of male forensic patients ($n=39$) and male prisoners ($n=192$). Findings suggest that a history of sexual and emotional abuse were significantly more common among forensic patients than among prisoners. Forensic subjects also reported a broader range of traumas. Of interest, prisoners reported significantly higher dissociative symptoms. Analyses of the relationship of type of trauma on the one hand and dissociation and borderline personality pathology on the other showed that sexual abuse was significantly correlated with borderline personality pathology but not with dissociation among forensic subjects. Meanwhile, in the prison sample these associations were found only for familial, but not extrafamilial, sexual abuse. The results of this study support the hypothesis that sexual abuse is related to the presence of borderline personality psychopathology, although it does not support the same for the presence of dissociative symptoms. It also suggests, that at least in this particular population, dissociative symptoms are related to borderline personality pathology but not to the experience of traumatic events per se.

Golynkina and Ryle (1999) postulated that partial dissociation provoked by trauma and deprivation in childhood may result in the persistence of separate self-states. The characteristics of these self-states and alternations between them were suggested to account for the main features of BPD. Similarly, Figueroa and colleagues (1997) reported that a history of childhood sexual abuse (CSA) was correlated with general measures of psychopathology on the SCL-90-R in a sample of inpatients with BPD.

Thus, a good clinical research base outlines the links between reported sexual abuse and psychological symptoms and disorders. Nevertheless, there is less understanding of the psychological processes mediating that relationship. Ross-Gower and colleagues (1998) conducted a study to asses the role of dissociation as a mediator between reported sexual abuse and a range of psychopathological characteristics. They randomly obtained a sample of 45 women attending clinical psychology services. Each woman was interviewed regarding a reported history of sexual abuse and was asked to complete standardized measures of general psychopathology, BPD characteristics, and symptoms of dissociation. The results of the study suggest that sexual abuse (per se) was associated with the patient's extent of depression, somatization, compulsive behavior, phobic symptoms, and BPD characteristics. In each case, dissociation served as a complete mediator in that link. The study findings suggest that the effectiveness of clinical work with patients suffering these psychopathological features would be enhanced if the symptoms of dissociation were directly addressed in women with a reported history of sexual abuse. However, the same mediating relationship was not found when attempting to explain the greater psychopathological impact of other forms of abuse (such as traumatic childhood experiences and intrafamilial abuse).

Shearer (1994) administered published scales and structured interviews to 62 female inpatients meeting DSM-III-R criteria for BPD, 14 of whom also had a concomitant dissociative disorder diagnosis. The goal of the study was to determine whether trauma variables and certain behavioral correlates are differentially prevalent in BPD patients with high and low dissociative experiences. Shearer discovered that high dissociative experiences in patients with BPD were characterized by more self-reported traumatic experiences, posttraumatic symptoms, behavioral dyscontrol, self-injurious behavior, and alcohol abuse. Furthermore, multivariate analyses suggested that scores on the DES were predicted by several factors, particularly adult sexual assault, behavioral dyscontrol, and both sexual and physical abuse in childhood.

Young (1992) summarized the findings of many researchers, suggesting that trauma and sexual abuse may lead to long-term psychological effects, particularly the possible embodiment of trauma-related conflicts and the formation of personal identity and other problems of psychological integrity. Young was trying to identify the effect of severe sexual abuse on a child's sense of living in his or her body and, by extension, living in the world, thus raising the idea that trauma and dissociation are linked to the development and maintenance of a "posttraumatic" sense of personal identity. If so, then, several disorders or symptoms associated with sexual abuse—dissociation, DID, eating disorders, somatization disorder, self-mutilation, suicide, borderline personality organization, and self-injurious behaviors (i.e., suicide attempts and cutting)—could be explained in terms of their phenomenological coherence and relation to the problem of embodiment.

Sanders and Giolas (1991) assessed dissociative tendencies in a heterogeneous group of 47 disturbed adolescents (ages 13–17 years old, 35 girls, 12 boys) and examined the relationship between the degree of dissociation and the degree of reported childhood stress, abuse, or trauma. Subjects completed the DES and a child abuse and trauma questionnaire. The researchers also had access to the subject's hospital records. They found that scores on the DES correlated significantly with self-reported physical abuse or punishment, sexual abuse, psychological abuse, neglect, and negative home atmosphere, but not with abuse ratings made from hospital records. They concluded that dissociation represents a reaction to early negative experience and places dissociative disorders at the extreme end of a continuum of dissociative sequelae of childhood trauma.

Patients with a history of trauma and abuse are likely to develop both dissociative symptoms and those associated with personality disorders. Ross and Norton (1989) collected a series of 236 cases of multiple personality disorder (MPD) reported to them by 203 psychiatrists, clinical psychologists, and other health care professionals. MPD patients experienced extensive sexual (79.2%) and physical (74.9%) abuse as children. They had been in the health care system for an average of 6.7 years before being diagnosed with MPD and had an average of 15.7 personalities at the time of reporting. The most common alter personalities were a child personality (86.0%), a personality of a different age (84.5%), a protector personality (84.0%), and a persecutor personality (84.0%). MPD patients were highly suicidal, with 72% attempting suicide and 2.1% being successful. The patients frequently received diagnoses of other mental disorders. The most common previous diagnoses were for affective disorders (63.7%), personality disorders (57.4%), anxiety disorders (44.3%), and schizophrenia (40.8%).

Diagnostic Assessment of Dissociative States

Gleaves and colleagues (2001) reviewed the empirical evidence for the validity of the DID diagnosis, the vast majority of which has come from research conducted within the preceding 10 years. After reviewing three different guidelines to establish diagnostic validity, Gleaves et al. concluded that despite criticism regarding the considerable convergent validity of dissociative disorders as a "real psychiatric disorder," evidence supported the inclusion of DID in DSM-IV-TR. Gleaves et al. reached this conclusion as diagnoses such as DID appear to meet all of the guidelines for inclusion and none of the exclusion guidelines proposed by Blashfield and colleagues (1990). Of interest, DID is one of the few disorders currently supported by taxometric research. A review of the literature on trauma and dissociation reveals that dissociation phenomena and disorders have been diagnosed in all cultures and countries (Maldonado and Spiegel 2002).

Another useful differential diagnostic characteristic of patients with dissociative disorders, as compared with other psychiatric disorders, is that dissociative disorder patients score far higher than healthy individuals and psychotic patients on standard measures of hypnotizability (Lavoie and Sabourin 1973; Pettinati 1982; Pettinati et al. 1990; Spiegel and Fink 1979; Spiegel et al. 1982; van der Hart and Spiegel 1993).

New scales of trait dissociation have been developed in which patients with dissociative disorders score extremely high compared to healthy populations and other psychiatric patient groups (Ross et al. 1990; Steinberg et al. 1990). These include the DES (Bernstein and Putnam 1986; Carlson et al. 1993), the Somatoform Dissociation Questionnaires (SDQ-20 and SDQ-5; Nijenhuis et al. 1996 and 1997, respectively), the Clinician-Administered Dissociative States Scale (CADSS; Bremner et al. 1998), Structured Clinical Interview for DSM-IV Dissociative Disorder—Revised (SCID-D-R; Steinberg 2000), and the Adolescent Dissociative Experiences Scale (A-DES; Armstrong et al. 1997).

The issue of amnesia and memory distortion has been raised at times to explain, but often to discredit, the phenomenon of dissociation and the presence of dissociative disorders. DSM-IV-TR lists amnesia as one of the features of dissociative disorders. Unfortunately, the assessment of amnesia in DID must rely on self-report. Many authors criticize even the existence of the diagnosis as the veracity of amnesic episodes often cannot be independently verified. Allen and Mov-

ius (2000) assessed the memory of four subjects diagnosed with DID using an objective method involving the use of event-related potentials (ERPs), as well as indirect behavioral measures of memory, and that provided statistically supported assessments for each participant. Subjects meeting DSM-IV criteria for DID participated in an ERP memory assessment task, in which words learned by one identity (Identity A) were then presented to a second identity (Identity B). All participants—tested as Identity B—produced ERPs and behavioral evidence consistent with recognition of the material learned by Identity A. This study used a very small sample of subjects and its findings have not been replicated. Even though the authors suggested that these findings may raise questions regarding the veracity of reported memories of abuse by a patient claiming DID, a possible explanation for this finding includes the phenomenon of co-consciousness (i.e., partial awareness across concurrent dissociated mental states), the fact that no defense is perfect and thus repression or dissociation may be imperfect, and the nature of the studied memories. Many have reported that traumatic memories are processed differently than nontraumatic memories, thus this experiment may not reflect the true nature of repressed traumatic memories.

Jones and colleagues (1999) studied whether individuals with BPD had a higher tendency to be over general in their autobiographical recall and whether the extent of their over general recall covaries with their susceptibilities to dissociative experiences by comparing 23 patients with BPD and 23 matched controls. All subjects completed the Autobiographical Memory Test and self-report measures of depression, anxiety, trait anger, and dissociative experiences. They found that subjects with BPD scored significantly higher than the control group on the measures of depression, anxiety, trait anger, and dissociative experiences and also retrieved significantly more general memories on the Autobiographical Memory Test. The number of general memories retrieved by the BPD group correlated significantly with their dissociation scores but not with their scores on mood measures. They concluded that patients with BPD have significant difficulties in recalling specific autobiographical memories and that these difficulties may be related to their tendency to dissociate in order to help them avoid episodic information that would evoke acutely negative affect.

As described by Loewenstein (1991a), in searching for the diagnostic evidence of dissociation it is most useful to begin with inquiry about amnesia, autohypnotic, posttraumatic, pseudopsychotic, and passive-influence symptoms. It also helps to inquire about the possibility of a history of childhood abuse or traumatization. The interview should look for the more overt signs of dissociation, including spontaneous trances, age-regression, blending or overlap of states, or frank switching which may increase the level of confidence in making the diagnosis. Other diagnostic methods may include the use of ideomotor signals, formal induction of trance states (i.e., hypnosis), and even pharmacologically (i.e., barbiturate or benzodiazepine) facilitated interviews. Combined with diagnostic tools, such as the DES, the Dissociative Disorders Interview Schedule, and the Structured Clinical Interview for DSM-IV Dissociative Disorders, the clinical interview can help the clinician make the diagnosis of dissociative states with a much greater level of confidence.

Armstrong (1991) suggested that clinicians and researchers familiar with the BPD literature may see a correspondence between certain of his dissociative disorder Rorschach results and typical borderline characteristics. Most notably, in his sample, both groups (i.e., persons with dissociative disorders and persons with BPD) reason and view others in unusual but not psychotic ways and demonstrate certain difficulties in affect integration. On the other hand, the dissociative disorders group exhibited many attributes that contradict predictions one would make from a borderline perspective and which support Kluft's (1991) assertion that the majority of these patients have a more complex and structured personality system. Rather than holding oversimplified attitudes, they are attuned to the subtleties of experience. Their generally introversive personality style reflects a capacity for internalization, for ideational organization of anxiety, for taking analytic distance from themselves, and for viewing and relating to others in a complex and empathic fashion.

Despite the similarities, the borderline personality concept does not provide adequate description of dissociative disorder symptomatology. It lacks the specificity needed to describe the test phenomena that appear on the Rorschach test results of patients with dissociative disorders. Armstrong (1991) remarked that special test instructions, behavior ratings of extra-test dissociative phenomena, and the posttest process questions enable the investigator to see that although at a gross level certain vulnerabilities resemble borderline characteristics, the processes underlying these phenomena are quite distinct. Moreover, unexpected areas of strength and maturity also exist. These findings suggest that we are not viewing a developmental arrest, but rather, are seeing the signs of what developmental psychologists call a "strange" development (i.e., an atypical developmental pathway created by unusual interactions with the world). It may well be that much of the difficulty in establishing the validity of BPD test criteria has been due to the unwitting inclusion of dissociative disorder patients within these studies. If so, the distinction between borderline and dissociative test characteristics will lead to more accurate and refined studies of both groups.

Coons and Fine (1990) blindly rated the Minnesota Multiphasic Personality Inventory of 63 subjects, identifying each person as a dissociative disorder patient or not. The overall rate of correct identification for the entire sample was 71.4%, with a 68% rate of correct identification of patients with dissociative disorders. These rates suggest that the Minnesota Multiphasic Personality Inventory may be clinically useful in confirming the diagnosis of dissociative disorders.

COMORBIDITY: DISSOCIATION AND PERSONALITY DISORDERS

The major comorbid psychiatric diagnoses associated with dissociative disorders are depressive disorders (Putnam et al. 1986; Ross and Norton 1989; Ross et al. 1989; Yargic et al. 1998), substance use disorders (Anderson et al. 1993; Coons 1984; Dunn et al. 1995; Ellason et al. 1996; Putnam et al. 1986), and BPD (Anderson et al. 1993; Brodsky et al. 1995; Horevitz and Braun 1984; Shearer 1994; Yargic et al. 1998). Patients with dissociative disorders, particularly DID, frequently display self-mutilative behavior (Bliss 1980, 1984a, 1984b; Coons 1984; Gainer and Torem 1993; Greaves 1980; Putnam et al. 1986; Ross and Norton 1989; Zweig-Frank et al. 1994a, 1994b), impulsiveness, and overvaluing and devaluing of relationships, contributing to the fact that approximately a third of DID patients fit the criteria for BPD as well. Also present, but at a much lesser extent are sexual (Brenner 1996; van der Kolk and Fisler 1994), eating (Valdiserri and Kihlstrom 1995), somatoform (Spitzer et al. 1999; Yargic et al. 1998), and sleep disorders (Putnam et al. 1986). Conversely, recent research shows dissociative symptoms in many patients with BPD, especially those who report histories of physical and sexual abuse (Chu and Dill 1990; Ogata et al. 1990).

Zanarini and colleagues (2000) identified four risk factors associated with dissociative symptomatology in BPD patients, including inconsistent treatment by a caretaker, sexual abuse by a caretaker, witnessing sexual violence as a child, and adult rape history. Thus, both sexual trauma and some other factor(s) intrinsic to the borderline diagnosis itself predispose borderline patients to suffer from dissociative phenomena. Some have suggested that the single factor mediating the main differences between BPD and other personality disorders is the presence of dissociation (Wildgoose et al. 2000). Compared to control groups, BPD patients have much higher levels of dissociation (26% in BPD group vs. 3% in controls), as measured by the DES (Zanarini et al. 2000). Golynkina and Ryle (1999) described how the partial dissociation provoked by trauma and deprivation in childhood results in the persistence of separate self-states in patients with BPD. A study of patients engaging in deliberate self-injurious behavior demonstrated that the frequency of this behavior was primarily related to increased dissociation (Low et al. 2000). A secondary component is mediated by low self-esteem, anger, impulsivity, and a history of sexual and physical abuse (Low et al. 2000).

Ng and colleagues (2002) studied the personality traits of 58 individuals who suffered from dissociative trance disorder using the Eysenck Personality Questionnaire (EPQ) and clinical interviews and examined whether the personality profiles could predict the individual's frequency of trance states. The subjects were reassessed 1 year later to obtain the frequency of trance states. Compared to a control population, subjects with dissociative trance states scored lower in extraversion scores and had higher psychoticism, neuroticism, and lie scores. The total episodes of trances that occurred over the 1-year follow-up period were positively correlated with neuroticism and negatively with extraversion scores. The researchers suggested that the high lie scores in individuals with dissociative trance disorder could be a reflection of their concern of how others perceive them (Ng et al. 2002).

Waldo and Merritt (2000) administered the Inventory of Childhood Memories and Imaginings (Barber and Wilson 1978), the Structured Interview for DSM-IV Personality (SIDP-IV; Pfohl et al. 1997) and the DES (Bernstein and Putnam 1986) to a group of subjects identified as "high fantasizers" (i.e., having high imaginative and dissociative tendencies) and a matched control group. The authors found that "fantasizers" had increased rates of Cluster A and B personality disorders but were equivalent to controls in Cluster C diagnoses. For both Clusters A and B, 55% of the "fantasizers" received clinical diagnoses, obtaining significantly higher scores in the DES (Waller et al. 1996), DES-Taxon (DES-T; Waller et al. 1996, 2001), and Normal Dissociative Index scores. Although nearly one half of the fanta-

sizers' DES-T patterns were classified within the pathological dissociative taxon (Waller and Ross 1997), none of the controls and only 10.03% of the original screening sample received this disorder. In summary, the study found that both Axis II pathology and pathological dissociation were associated with fantasy proneness.

Dell (1998) administered the Millon Clinical Multiaxial Inventory-II (MCMI-II), the Minnesota Multiphasic Personality Inventory-2 (MMPI-2), and the DES to 42 patients with DID and 16 patients with dissociative disorder not otherwise specified. His results indicated that DID patients manifested severe personality pathology on a mean of four MCMI-II scales: avoidant (76%), self-defeating (68%), borderline (53%), and passive-aggressive (45%). DDNOS subjects exhibited even more severe personality pathology on fewer MCMI-II scales: avoidant (50%) and self-defeating (31%). Of interest, DID and DDNOS subjects differed in their scores on the DES, the PK-PTSD scale of the MMPI-2, and in the incidence of severe borderline pathology (53% vs. 6%). These patients exhibit increased personality pathology on the avoidant, self-defeating, borderline, and passive-aggressive scales. The robust convergence of findings among DID and PTSD subjects supports the construct validity of DID as a form of posttraumatic disorder and suggests a quite predictable "personality core" to the clinical picture of severely traumatized individuals.

In an attempt to determine the extent of dissociative experiences and the prevalence of dissociative disorders in a series of acute psychiatric inpatients and to correlate these experiences and disorders with some sociodemographic, clinical, and historical variables, Modestin and colleagues (1996) studied 207 consecutively admitted psychiatric inpatients. All subjects were examined with the DES, Structured Clinical Interview for DSM-III-R Personality Questionnaire (SCID-II PQ), Parental Bonding Instrument (PBI), and Frankfurter Self-Concept Scales (FS). In addition, patients scoring greater than 20 on the DES were also examined with the Dissociative Disorders Interview Schedule. They found that 20% of patients scored greater than 20 on the DES. Of the patients, 5% were subsequently diagnosed with a dissociative disorder. Significant positive correlations were found between DES scores and SCID-II PQ items' frequency with regard to all personality disorder types, especially borderline, antisocial, schizotypal, and dependent personality types. Less pronounced correlations were found between DES and PBI scores and between DES score and age. In their study, Axis I diagnoses did not seem to have any pronounced influence on the DES score. In contrast, patients with greater proneness to dissociation scored lower on most FS scales. As in other studies, there was a tendency for patients with dissociative disorders to report childhood abuse more frequently. Similarly, subjects with dissociative disorders had a significantly greater number of somatic symptoms.

Clinical data into the nature of dissociative states and disorders suggest that most patients with dissociation spend most of their lives not manifesting their dissociative tendencies in a "classic clinical manner" (Kluft 1991). Dissociation is a pathological process that involves the maintenance of memories associated with trauma hidden and out of consciousness. Thus, most patients with dissociative states do not show typical Axis II signs of restricted interpersonal development and childish behavior, sometimes referred to as the "teddy-bear sign." This by no means suggests that subjects with dissociation may not behave in a regressed manner, but that it is not the classic pattern of their presentation. Thus clinicians are asked to keep an eye on extremely overt childlike presentation as it may reflect either other Axis II pathology or an attempt to confabulate a dissociative disorder, either for secondary gain or other reasons.

Cluster A (Paranoid, Schizoid, Schizotypal)

Irwin (2001) administered the DES, the Schizotypal Personality Questionnaire-Brief, and the Childhood Trauma Questionnaire to a group of adults (n=116) without psychiatric diagnosis. Hierarchical regression analysis revealed that both pathological and nonpathological dissociative tendencies were predicted by the dimensions of schizotypy, even after the contribution of childhood trauma had been removed. He concluded that the relationship between dissociative tendencies and schizotypy is not an artifact of childhood abuse, but the clinical significance of this relationship remains to be established.

Pope and Kwapil (2000) studied the relationship between dissociative experiences and psychosis proneness in a sample of 523 college undergraduates. Subjects were administered the DES, the Perceptual Aberration Scale, the Magical Ideation Scale, the Social Anhedonia Scale, and the Physical Anhedonia Scale. Researchers found that the Perceptual Aberration and Magical Ideation Scales were positively correlated with DES scores. While the Social Anhedonia Scale had only a modest correlation with the DES, this relationship was largely mediated by the Perceptual Aberration and Magical Ideation Scales. On the other hand, the Physical Anhedonia Scale had no correlation with DES scores. Exploratory factor analysis of the psychosis-proneness

scales and the DES subscales resulted in a three-factor solution: dissociative experiences, positive schizotypy, and negative schizotypy. This result suggests that the DES depersonalization subscale is high on both the dissociation and positive schizotypy factors.

Previous research has noted a robust correlation between dissociation and schizophrenia-like symptoms. One way to interpret the relationship between dissociation and schizotypy is to assume that it is an artifact of fantasy proneness. In a study by Merckelbach and colleagues (2000), the authors studied 152 undergraduate students, using measures of dissociation, schizotypy, and fantasy proneness. They found that dissociative tendencies were related to the full range of schizotypal features. The results argue that the close connection between dissociation and schizotypy cannot be interpreted in terms of an artifact produced by fantasy proneness.

Of interest, while exploring the relationship between dissociative symptoms and other Axis I and Axis II symptoms among a sample of women diagnosed with eating disorders, Gleaves and Eberenz (1995) found that, in their sample, dissociative symptoms were most highly correlated with schizotypal symptomatology (r=0.59), uncorrelated with borderline or antisocial symptomatology, and slightly negatively correlated with histrionic symptomatology.

We have already discussed the relationship between traumatic experiences and dissociative tendencies, especially when the trauma occurs in early childhood. Berenbaum and colleagues (2003) studied a sample of 75 community women, looking for a history of trauma and/or maltreatment and the presence of symptoms of schizotypal personality disorder, using both questionnaire and interview measures. The study found that individuals with histories of trauma/maltreatment had elevated levels of schizotypal symptoms. Among types of trauma, a reported history of childhood neglect was especially strongly associated with schizotypal symptoms (Berenbaum et al. 2003). Unfortunately, the authors did not report on these subjects' dissociative tendencies.

Watson (2001) examined the associations among sleep-related experiences (e.g., hypnagogic hallucinations, nightmares, waking dreams, and lucid dreams), dissociation, schizotypy, and personality traits in two large student samples. Factor analyses indicated that dissociation and schizotypy are strongly correlated yet distinguishable constructs. Furthermore, he postulated that the differentiation between dissociation and schizotypy can be enhanced by eliminating detachment/depersonalization items from the dissociation scales. His findings also suggest that measures of dissociation, schizotypy, and sleep-related experiences all define a common domain characterized by unusual cognitions and perceptions.

Cluster B (Antisocial, Borderline, Histrionic, Narcissistic)

Schmahl and colleagues (2002) reviewed the published neurobiological data integrating the biological, psychological, and clinical findings of subjects with BPD. Their conclusions suggest that four core elements may play a major role in the development of BPD: interpersonal stress, affective instability, impulsivity, and dissociation and self-injurious behavior. The available neurobiological data suggest that genetic and environmental factors actually lead to brain alterations that form the basis for the specific presentations of the disorder, particularly the self-injurious and impulsive-aggressive behavior.

Stiglmayr and colleagues (2001) studied the relationship among aversive tension, affective dysregulation, and the dissociative features in female patients with BPD, compared with a healthy control group. The researchers found substantial and highly significant differences with regard to the duration and intensity of the subjectively perceived states of aversive tension among the two groups. Among patients with BPD there was a strong correlation between duration and intensity of tension, and experience of dissociative features, both somatoform and psychological. These findings underline the clinical importance of states of aversive tension in BPD suggesting the stress-related induction of dissociative features.

Wildgoose and colleagues (2000) studied a group of personality disordered subjects divided into two groups: subjects with BPD and subjects with all other types of personality disorders. Participants completed measures of dissociation, personality fragmentation, and psychiatric disturbance. The authors found that subjects in the BPD group had higher levels of a number of aspects of psychiatric symptomatology, most of which were mediated by aspects of dissociation. The phenomenology of personality fragmentation differentiated the two groups, with greater fragmentation observed in BPD subjects. Nevertheless, this fragmentation was not related to the higher levels of other aspects of psychiatric disturbance observed in subjects with BPD.

In order to study the severity and quality of dissociative experiences reported by borderline patients, Zanarini and colleagues (2000) compared BPD pa-

tients to Axis II controls. All subjects completed the DES. They found that the majority of BPD patients experience higher levels of dissociation, often similar to that reported by patients meeting criteria for PTSD or dissociative disorders. On the other hand, control subjects had a significantly low distribution of their overall DES scores. Not only did BPD patients had a significantly higher score than the controls on the DES item scores and a significantly higher overall DES score, but they had significantly higher scores on the three factors that have been found to underlie the DES: absorption, amnesia, and depersonalization. The authors suggested that the severity of dissociation experienced by BPD patients is more heterogeneous than previously reported. They also suggested that borderline patients have a wider range of dissociative experiences than are commonly recognized, including experiences of absorption and amnesia, as well as experiences of depersonalization.

The incidence of completed suicides in borderline patients has been estimated to range from 3% to 9% (Paris 2002; Yen et al. 2003). Suicidality as a presenting symptom is present in nearly 70% of patients with dissociative disorders (Putnam et al. 1986), with 2.1% of patients being successful (Ross et al. 1989). Thus as reported by Yen and colleagues (2003), among individuals diagnosed with personality disorders, exacerbation of comorbid Axis I conditions (including MDD, substance use, and dissociation) heightens the risk for a suicide attempt.

Yet others (Clary et al. 1984) have proposed that dissociative disorders represent a "special instance" of BPD, where the introjects are composed of a representation of the self, a representation of the object, and an affective bond. Similarly, Benner and Joscelyne (1984) concurred in this opinion when they suggested that MPD should not be viewed as a hysterical (i.e., dissociative) disorder but rather a borderline disorder. They based their opinion on the role of the defense mechanism they perceived to underlie the manifestations in both disorders (i.e., splitting), the process of object-relations formation, and the symptomatology in both disorders. As in the case of BPD, they suggest that DID subjects benefit from the role of limit setting, confrontation, and management of negative transference.

There is a general uncertainty as to what comprises the essence of histrionic personality disorder. Using phenomenological methodology, Sigmund and colleagues (1998) analyzed phenomena observable in the 'classic' hysterical personality, and classified it according to the basic functions of human experience and behavior. Their study suggested that the phenomenon of dissociation of the mental processes served as the basis for the various basic functions observed in these patients. They further suggested that a specific feature of histrionic personality disorder is that dissociation of mental contents of the personality permeates along a conscious-preconscious-unconscious continuum. They concluded that in patients with histrionic personality disorder, dissociation was, in the final analysis, the prerequisite for a compromised and partial acting-out of prohibited nonintegrated elements (e.g., aggression, as a coping strategy).

Cluster C (Avoidant, Dependent, Obsessive-Compulsive)

There are no published data regarding an association between dissociation and Cluster C personality disorders. Similarly, our clinical experience suggests that dissociative symptoms are not prevalent in this cluster of personality disorders.

RELATIONSHIP AMONG PERSONALITY DISORDERS, DISSOCIATION, AND OTHER AXIS I DISORDERS

Eating Disorders

Molinari (2001) reviewed the published literature on the role that sexual and physical abuse may play in predisposing women to eating disorders. He establishes that despite some discordant opinions, there is general consensus concerning the complex genesis of the eating disorders of some women. Some of the common symptoms of patients with eating disorders are strikingly similar to those of patients with some forms of dissociative disorders and include trancelike states during episodes of pathological eating behavior (Pettinati et al. 1985), reliving of the trauma, dissociation, personality disorders (particularly Cluster-B symptoms), pathological relationship with food, distortion of body image, suicide attempts, and self-inflicted punishment.

Co-occurrence of bulimia nervosa and BPD has been attributed to shared factors. As in the case of dissociative disorders, childhood abuse is one of those factors. Others have suggested a disturbance in central serotonin (5-hydroxytryptamine; 5-HT) mechanisms. To explore the neurotransmitter theory, Steiger and colleagues (2000) conducted a controlled assessment of the relationship between childhood abuse and 5-HT function in bulimics with and without BPD. The sample consisted of patients with bulimia nervosa, whose diagnosis had been confirmed with the use of the Eating Disorders Examination interview. In this sample, 35% of subjects had a concomitant diagnosis of BPD. Subjects were then compared to a sample of normal-eater controls. All subjects were assessed for clinical symptoms (e.g., eating disturbances, mood lability, impulsivity, and dissociation) and a possible history of childhood sexual and physical abuse. Platelet tritiated-paroxetine binding was studied in bulimics (about half of the sample had a diagnosis of BPD) and controls. Steiger et al. found that relative to normal eaters, bulimic subjects exhibited greater affective instability, overall impulsivity, and a history of physical abuse. BPD-bulimics showed elevated motor impulsivity, dissociation, and rates of sexual abuse. Paroxetine-binding tests indicated no differences attributable to comorbid BPD, instead linking bulimia nervosa with or without BPD to substantially reduced 5-HT transporter density. These results suggest that these pathologic entities are rather autonomous. In this sample, subjects with bulimia nervosa were found to have abnormal 5-HT transporter function and affective instability, but these findings were relatively independent of a history of childhood sexual abuse. On the other hand, those subjects diagnosed with BPD were found to have histories of sexual abuse, and to experience dissociative symptoms and behavioral impulsivity.

Impulse Control Disorders: Suicidal and Parasuicidal Behaviors

To investigate possible neurophysiologic underpinnings of self-injurious behavior in women with BPD, Russ and colleagues (1999) compared subjects among four groups of women; female inpatients with BPD who do (BPD-P group) and do not (BPD-NP group) report pain during self-injury, female inpatients with major depression, and normal-control women. To assess their pain experience, pain report and EEG power spectrum density were recorded during a laboratory pain procedure (i.e., the cold pressor test). Results show that the BPD-NP group reported less pain intensity during the cold pressor test compared to the other groups. Electroencephalographic data (i.e., total absolute theta power) was significantly higher in the BPD-NP group compared to the depressed and normal groups, suggesting possible neurological differences among the groups. EEG recordings suggested that theta activity was significantly correlated with pain rating and dissociative experiences. DES scores were significantly higher in the BPD-NP group compared to the depressed and normal groups and were significantly higher in the BPD-P group compared to the normal group. Measures of anxiety and depression were significantly lower in the normal group compared to all patient groups.

Zlotnick and colleagues (1999) looked at the relationship between Axis I and Axis II psychiatric disorders characterized by impulsive aggression and self-mutilative behavior. They administered diagnostic interviews for Axis I and Axis II disorders and questionnaires that measured a history of dissociation and childhood abuse, as well as self-mutilative acts within the last 3 months, to 256 outpatients. They found that Axis I disorders of substance abuse, posttraumatic stress disorder, and intermittent explosive disorder were significantly related to self-mutilative behavior, independent of the presence of the diagnosis of BPD and/or antisocial personality disorder. They also found that a higher level of dissociation was related to self-mutilation, after controlling for BPD and childhood abuse. Outpatients with certain Axis I disorders and those who dissociate may represent a sizable group of patients who are at risk for self-mutilative behavior.

In DSM-IV, it is suggested that the affective instability experienced by BPD patients is due to the subjects' marked reactions to environmental events. In an attempt to investigate affective responsiveness of abnormal personalities with self-harming impulsive behaviors, Herpertz and colleagues (1998) conducted a series of two affect-stimulation design experiments. The first one consisted of the presentation of a short story that allowed affective responses to various stimuli to be assessed in regard to quality, intensity, and alterations over time. The second one presented a typical frustration design, which provoked specific feelings of anger and disappointment. Impulsive personalities showed an affective hyperreactivity characterized by a decreased threshold for affective responses and by intensive, rapidly changing affects. Furthermore, affect experiences turned out to be qualitatively diffuse and undifferentiated. These results support the notion that the affective instability observed in patients with BPD should be differentiated from the autonomous deviations of mood typical of affective disorders and that the affective hyperreactivity is a crucial part of impulsive personality functioning, leading to interpersonal problems and impulse dyscontrol behaviors (i.e., self-injurious behaviors).

Similarly, Kemperman and colleagues (1997b) looked at the mood regulatory function of self-injurious behavior in patients with BPD. They studied a variety of mood and affective states in female inpatients with an Axis II diagnosis of BPD and a history of self-injurious behavior, using visual analog scales. Subjects were additionally divided into two groups according to whether they typically experience pain during self-injurious behavior (BPD-P group) or did not (BPD-NP group). For both groups, the visual analog scale ratings revealed significant mood elevation and decreased dissociation following self-injury, with a peak in dissociative symptoms during self-injury. The ratings of dissociative symptoms were found to be higher in the BPD-NP group when compared to the BPD-P group across all stages of self-injurious behavior.

To explore the relationship between dissociation, self-mutilation, and childhood abuse history, Brodsky and colleagues (1995) administered the DES, the Sexual Experiences Questionnaire, and the Hamilton Rating Scale for Depression, along with a comprehensive treatment history questionnaire to consecutively admitted female inpatients with BPD as diagnosed by the Structured Clinical Interview for DSM-III-R Personality Disorders. Brodsky et al. discovered that 50% of the subjects had a score of 15 or more on the DES, indicating pathological levels of dissociation; 52% reported a history of self-mutilation, and 60% reported a history of childhood physical and/or sexual abuse. The subjects who dissociated were more likely than those who did not to self-mutilate and to report childhood abuse. The same subjects had higher levels of depressive symptoms at the time of admission and higher frequency of seeking psychiatric treatment. Multiple regression analysis demonstrated that each of these variables predicted dissociation when each of the others was controlled for and that self-mutilation was the most powerful predictor of dissociation. Thus, they concluded that female inpatients with BPD who dissociate may represent a sizable subgroup of patients with the disorder who are at especially high risk for self-mutilation, childhood abuse, depression, and utilization of psychiatric treatment. The strong correlation found between dissociation and self-mutilation independent of childhood abuse history was significant and should encourage clinicians treating patients with BPD to address symptoms of dissociation first, while exercising caution in attributing them to a history of abuse.

Russ and colleagues (1996) studied a group of women with BPD who do not experience pain during self-injury. These subjects were found to discriminate more poorly between imaginary painful and mildly painful situations, to reinterpret painful sensations (a pain-coping strategy related to dissociation), and to have higher scores on the DES than similar female patients who experienced pain during self-injury and a sample of age-matched normal women. They postulated that the "analgesia" during self-injury by borderline patients may be associated with a cognitive impairment in the ability to distinguish between painful and mildly painful situations, as well as to dissociative mechanisms.

In a separate study, Kemperman and colleagues (1997a) attempted to examine whether differences in reported pain experienced during self-injurious behavior in female patients with BPD could be explained by neurosensory factors and/or attitudinal factors (response bias). After studying subjects for their thermal responsivity, they found that patients with BPD who do not experience pain during self-injury (BPD-NP group) had a difficult time discriminating between noxious thermal stimuli of similar intensity than female patients with BPD who do experience pain during self-injury (BPD-P group), than female patients with BPD who do not have a history of self-injury (BPD-C group), and than age-matched normal women. Patients in the BPD-NP group also had a higher response criterion (i.e., were more stoic) than subjects in the BPD-C group. These findings suggest that the apparent "analgesia" experienced by BPD subjects during self-injury may be related to both neurosensory, as well as attitudinal/psychological abnormalities.

Multiple previously published studies have reported that self-mutilation in patients with personality disorders were related to the presence of other psychological risk factors, primarily dissociation. Zweig-Frank and colleagues (1994a, 1994b) conducted a study to determine whether or not self-mutilation in patients with personality disorders was indeed related to other psychological risk factors, dissociation, or comorbid diagnoses. They compared patients diagnosed with BPD to subjects diagnosed with a personality disorder other than BPD. Of note, about half of the subject sample with BPD reported a history of self-mutilation. In all subjects, psychological risk factors were measured through histories of childhood sexual abuse, physical abuse, and separation or loss, as well as through scores on the Parental Bonding Index. Dissociation was measured by the DES. In this population of male subjects, researchers found no relationships between any of the psychological risk factors and self-mutilation. Subjects who mutilated themselves had higher scores on the DES in univariate analysis, but the scores in multivariate analyses dissociation did not discriminate between subjects who mutilated themselves and those who did not.

Psychosis

Many patients with personality disorders exhibit "psychotic" phenomena from time to time. In fact, some researchers have eloquently argued that paranoid schizophrenia and DID should be in the differential diagnosis of patients with certain types of personality disorders (Stubner et al. 1998). This relationship appears to be particularly true in patients with BPD who are described as experiencing "micropsychotic episodes," which can be defined as a range of specified "altered experiences of reality." Dowson and colleagues (2000) conducted a study of the associations between self-reported past psychotic phenomena and features of DSM-III-R personality disorders in 57 inpatients without a previous diagnosis of the main disorders that involve delusions and hallucinations. They found associations between past psychotic phenomena and features of BPD, between repeated self-harm and a report that "thoughts seemed put into the head," and between psychotic phenomena and features of other personality disorders, particularly schizotypal personality disorder. They found a particularly high prevalence of BPD in their study sample. Finally, these authors concluded that dissociation, in the context of the features of BPD, may be a causal factor for the development of some of the psychotic phenomena presented by patients with personality disorder.

Substance Abuse

Several studies have looked into the issue of substance abuse and personality disorders. As with other comorbid complications in patients with Axis II disorders, there seems to be a convergence with substance abuse, dissociation, and history of childhood trauma. Ellason and colleagues (1996) studied 106 patients admitted to a chemical dependency treatment unit and found that 65% of subjects reported a history of physical and/or sexual abuse during childhood and 26.4% met criteria for posttraumatic stress disorder. Not surprisingly, those subjects who reported a history of childhood abuse showed more symptoms of depression, dissociation, and BPD than those who denied childhood trauma. These findings seem to suggest that dissociative, mood, anxiety, and personality disorders may be common in patients with chemical dependency disorders who have histories of childhood trauma.

Conclusions

In summary, dissociative symptoms occur in many Axis I and II disorders, and comorbidity of dissociative and other disorders is common, especially when there is a history of trauma.

TREATMENT OPTIONS

We must begin this section with a warning. There is no systematic research conducted in the treatment of dissociative defenses of patients with personality disorders. Most of what we will discuss therefore is an extrapolation of data available in subjects with dissociative disorders in general.

Psychopharmacology

To date, no good evidence shows that medication of any type has a direct therapeutic effect on the dissociative process manifested by DID patients (Markowitz and Gill 1996). In fact, most dissociative symptoms seem relatively resistant to pharmacological intervention (Loewenstein 1991a, 1991b). Thus, pharmacological treatment has been limited to the control of signs and symptoms afflicting DID patients or comorbid conditions rather than the treatment of dissociation per se.

Evidence suggests that alterations of the endogenous opiate system contribute to dissociative symptoms in patients with BPD and PTSD. To test this theory, Bohus and colleagues (1999) treated two groups of female BPD patients (all met the diagnostic criteria of DSM-IV and the revised Diagnostic Interview for Borderline Patients) who experienced prominent dissociative phenomena including flashbacks with the nonselective opiate receptor antagonist naltrexone, 25–100 mg qid, for at least 2 weeks. Subjects completed a self-rated questionnaire measuring dissociation, analgesia, tonic immobility, and tension, before and during treatment with naltrexone. Some of the subjects completed a flashback protocol. They found that self-reported scores reflected a highly significant reduction of the duration and the intensity of dissociative phenomena and tonic immobility as well as a marked reduction in analgesia during treatment with naltrexone. Two-thirds of the subjects reported a decrease in the mean number of flashbacks per day. These findings suggest that, in subjects with BPD, an increased activity of the opioid system may contribute to dissociative symptoms, including the presence of flashbacks, and suggest that these symptoms may respond to treatment with opiate antagonists.

Overall, antipsychotics are rarely useful in reducing dissociative symptoms (Maldonado and Spiegel

2002). Nevertheless, Soloff (1987) suggested that a low-dose neuroleptic strategy may be indicated in BPD patients as an acute treatment for symptoms of anger, hostility, suspiciousness, ideas of reference, paranoid ideation, overwhelming anxiety, dissociative episodes, and related behavioral dyscontrol. Medication effects may be clinically significant, although modest in magnitude. He recommended a short duration of treatment (i.e., 3–12 weeks), although he acknowledged that continued pharmacotherapy may be warranted in selected cases. The risks of treatment include the well-recognized side effects of all atypical neuroleptics, the possibility of overdose, and interactions with alcohol and street drugs. As others have noted, he recognized that pharmacotherapy is only an adjunct to supportive psychosocial intervention.

Quetiapine, initially introduced in the United States as an atypical antipsychotic drug for the treatment of schizophrenia and other psychotic states, has been used in a variety of disease states, including mood and anxiety disorders, obsessive-compulsive disorder, aggression, hostility, posttraumatic stress disorder, delirium, and BPD. Unfortunately, there are no double-blind, placebo controlled studies to determine its usefulness or safety in patients with personality disorders or its effects on dissociation. Thus, as is the case with all of the atypical antipsychotic agents, more studies are needed (Adityanjee and Schulz 2002). When it comes to the use of neuroleptics, most researchers have reported an extremely high incidence of adverse side effects in patients suffering dissociative symptoms (Kluft 1984a, 1988).

As in the case of many other psychiatric disorders manifesting with episodic violence, subjects with dissociation-related agitation or violent outburst may benefit from the use of anticonvulsant agents. Coons (1992) has reported on the use of carbamazepine in such inpatients; unfortunately, the data published so far are limited to case reports.

Antidepressants are reported to have some possible indications for patients with dissociative disorders. Similar to patients with dissociative disorder, BPD subjects suffer from high levels of depression and/or dysthymia. The successful use of antidepressant medications in this patient population has been reported (Kluft 1984a). The use of antidepressant agents should be limited to the treatment of patients who exhibit clear symptoms of depression. The newer selective serotonin reuptake inhibitors (SSRIs) are preferred given their lower lethality in overdose compared with tricyclics and monoamine oxidase inhibitors (MAOIs). Unfortunately, medication side effects, particularly akathisia could prove difficult to differentiate from the worsening of symptoms (i.e., increased anxiety, dissociation, or acting-out). Medication compliance is a problem with these patients because dissociated personality states may interfere with the taking of medication by the patients' "hiding" or hoarding of pills, or patients may overdose.

Nonpharmacological Treatments

It is possible to help personality disorder patients gain control over their dissociative symptoms in several ways. The fundamental psychotherapeutic stance should involve acknowledging that they experience themselves as fragmented, yet the reality is that the fundamental problem is a failure of integration of memories and aspects of the self. Therefore, the goal in therapy is to facilitate integration of disparate elements (Maldonado and Spiegel 2002).

Wildgoose and colleagues (2000) suggested that treating patients with BPD may require psychotherapy, which must address both the experiences of dissociation, as well as personality fragmentation. On the other hand, Adler (1993) suggested that an effective psychodynamic formulation of borderline psychopathology must include an understanding of the borderline patient's aloneness problems, need-fear dilemma issues, and difficulties with primitive guilt. According to Adler, the aloneness problem is at the core of the disorder and contributes to the inability of BPD patients to maintain an evocative memory (e.g., to hold soothing introjects of significant people when under the stress of separation). Thus, Adler believes that a good psychodynamic formulation may provide the necessary framework to deal with difficult issues in cases of personality disorders, while helping the therapist process and effectively utilize countertransference. The ability to recognize projective identification is important, as it helps explain the complex transference/countertransference experiences elicited during the treatment of these patients and may be used in defining the resolution of the aloneness problems of borderline patients. He also recommends the use of limit-setting and transitional objects as needed. Utilizing a variety of intervention techniques, the overall structure of the psychotherapy of dissociative symptoms in the context of BPD can be summarized as in Table 32–2.

Regardless of the therapeutic approach or technique used in the treatment of dissociative symptoms, Kluft (1989) warned of the need to "pace the therapy, lest the already beleaguered patient become both acutely and chronically overwhelmed" (p. 91). The

Table 32–2. Summary of treatment options for patients with dissociative symptoms

1. Explore the extent of dissociative symptomatology
2. Explore current issues that may lead to dissociative episodes
3. Clarify and discuss the symptoms with the patient and possibly the family
4. Teach the patient how to access and learn to control dissociation, including the possible use of hypnosis in patients with full dissociative disorder
5. Work through any possible posttraumatic symptoms associated with the dissociative symptoms
6. Facilitate integration of dissociated identities or personality states and integrating amnesic episodes
7. Work through transference issues related to trauma and feelings about controlling dissociative symptoms
8. Consolidate and stabilizing gains
9. Support the patient in case of relapse

Source. Adapted from American Psychiatric Association: "Practice Guidelines for the Treatment of Patients With Borderline Personality Disorder." *American Journal of Psychiatry* 158 (10 suppl):1–52, 2001. Used with permission. Copyright 2001 American Psychiatric Association.

majority of the existent literature on the use of hypnosis for the treatment of dissociation comes from our experience with DID in particular and dissociative disorders in general. When hypnosis is used with DID, it may help address the processes of accessing alters or dissociated states, abreact traumatic memories, arrange or mediate reconciliations among alter states, and facilitates integration. Kluft (1989) discussed the use of several hypnotherapeutic techniques (to be used in or out of trance), which may offer temporary respite for overwhelmed patients. These techniques include alter substitution, the creation of safe places, distancing maneuvers, bypassing time, bypassing affect and/or memory, attenuating affect and/or memory retrieval, and rearranging the configuration of the alters by bartering or "shuffling the deck."

Cognitive Restructuring

Similar to the findings of studies addressing the treatment of dissociative disorders, recent studies (Wildgoose et al. 2001) suggest that personality fragmentation (e.g., dissociative tendencies) may be a core component of BPD. Wildgoose et al. suggested that successful treatment of BPD may depend on the extent to which dissociation is addressed. They demonstrated that a relative short course (16 sessions) of cognitive analytic therapy can increase personality integration by strengthening awareness, and hence control, of the dissociative processes that maintain fragmentation. During treatment, all BPD subjects experienced a reduction in the severity of the BPD. The findings of Wildgoose et al. generally support the suggestion that integration of dissociative tendencies should be enhanced in patients with BPD and that cognitive analytic therapy may be a useful method to achieve this goal.

Hypnosis

When it comes to the problem of dissociation, hypnosis can be helpful in diagnosis as well as therapy (Braun 1984; Maldonado and Spiegel 1995, 1998; Maldonado et al. 1997; Smith 1993; Smith et al. 1993; Spiegel and Spiegel 1978). The administration of objective measures of hypnotizability, such as the hypnotic induction profile (HIP; Spiegel and Spiegel 2004) may help determine if symptoms exhibited by the patient are, in fact, dissociative phenomena. If it is objectively determined that the patient possesses clinically usable hypnotic ability, he or she may be taught to enter a "controlled trance state," thus preventing or minimizing spontaneous dissociative phenomena. Hypnosis may also be used to allow for controlled access and processing of traumatic memories. The use of these techniques may help make the traumatic memories more bearable by placing them in a broader perspective, one in which the trauma victim also can identify adaptive aspects of his or her response to the trauma. This technique and similar approaches can help these individuals work through traumatic memories, enabling them to bear the memories in consciousness and therefore reducing the need for dissociation as a means of keeping such memories out of consciousness. Although these techniques can be helpful and often result in reduced fragmentation and enhanced integration (Maldonado and Spiegel 1995, 1998; Spiegel 1984), a number of complications can occur in the psychotherapy of these patients as well.

As previously described by Kluft (1992) and others, many dissociative symptoms are unresponsive or incompletely responsive to medications. This poses a unique challenge to physicians and staff treating personality disorder patients with dissociative disorders or symptoms. As described by Fine and Berkowitz (2001), "therapists skilled in the treatment of DID are typically fluent in the uses of hypnosis for stabilization, affect management, building a safe place and grounding…" (p. 275), taking advantage of the high hypnotizability of patients with dissociation. The implementation of these techniques greatly facilitates

acute crisis resolution, leading to a greater sense of safety on the part of patients. The ability to manage crises can in turn enhance the inpatient treatment staff's sense of mastery and minimize the need for emergency medication administration and restraints.

Not only does Kluft (1992) recommend the use of hypnotic techniques for the management of acute dissociative crises in patients with dissociative disorders, but he suggests that hypnosis treatment may very well be the treatment of choice for dissociative symptoms in general. Given that some personality disorder patients (e.g., those with BPD) may experience spontaneous and self-generated dissociative states and phenomena, sharing much in common with hypnotically induced states, formal hypnotic inductions may help facilitate control of spontaneous dissociative episodes and help reestablish a functional continuity of memory and identity. This ability can be especially useful in the context of comorbid dissociative disorders and borderline or other personality disorders, in that teaching enhanced control over dissociative symptoms may strengthen the therapeutic alliance and change the perspective on some symptoms previously seen as hostile acting-out rather than poorly controlled dissociation. Bowers (1991) proposed a neodissociative model, which views hypnotic behavior as capable of being both purposeful (in the sense that the suggested state of affairs is achieved) and nonvolitional (in the sense that the suggested state of affairs is not achieved by high level executive initiative and ongoing effort). The use of hypnosis for the treatment of dissociative states has been widely advocated and is part of the BPD treatment guidelines for comorbid dissociation, although critics of its use fear contamination or "creation of alters."

In a study of the effects of hypnosis on the features of dissociation, Ross and Norton (1989) compared 57 patients with DID who had been hypnotized both before and after diagnosis to 38 patients who had not been hypnotized during assessment or treatment. They found that the two groups did not differ on the diagnostic criteria or in the number of personalities, suggesting that hypnosis did not have a gross distorting effect on the features of dissociation in general, or DID in particular. They do warn that hypnosis may, however, affect the recall of sexual and physical abuse and the manifestation of certain types of dissociative personality states. This lack of distortion may indicate that the hypnotized group benefited from the use of hypnosis to help access more traumatic memories associated with child identities. Thus hypnosis can be helpful in identifying dissociative phenomena, explaining them to the patient, and teaching them a means of accessing, working through, and controlling dissociative symptoms.

Relaxation Techniques

Glantz and Goisman (1990) reported on a behavioral intervention specifically designed to merge split self-representations to be used as an adjunct to the psychotherapy of personality-disordered patients. The method, which is introduced only after signs of split self-representation have been identified through exploratory psychotherapy, consists of a series of steps. Patients are first taught a relaxation technique and are asked to practice at home. Once they are able to relax in the session, they are asked for visual images of first one and then another of the conflicting self-representations. After clear images have been elicited and discussed, they are encouraged to merge them. Finally, they are asked "Who's watching" or some similar question designed to elicit a statement about a unified self. They tested this technique in 27 patients meeting criteria for personality disorders in Clusters B and C of DSM-III-R. They reported that 24 of the subjects responded with greater compliance, reduced resistance, and improved relationships at work and elsewhere.

Group Psychotherapy

Similar to the use of group psychotherapy with dissociative disorder patients, Coons and Bradley (1985) remarked on the benefits and potential pitfalls of this treatment strategy in subjects with BPD with comorbid dissociative symptoms. Nevertheless, it is important to have a homogeneous group composed solely of one or the other diagnostic group and not to combine patients with personality and dissociative disorders. Given the complexity of the BPD patient and adding the factor of dissociation, issues such as group process, interpersonal dynamics, transference, countertransference, safety, and termination need to be clearly delineated from the beginning of the group experience and maintained throughout. This approach is particularly important when dealing with boundaries and the manifestation of "altered states." Given etiological issues discussed above, therapy at some point will focus and deal with past neglect and abuse.

Eye Movement Desensitization and Reprocessing

Beginning in the 1990s, there has been an increased interest in the use of eye movement desensitization and reprocessing (EMDR) for the treatment of PTSD, DID, and other psychiatric consequences of abuse. As Fine

and Berkowitz (2001) pointed out, "the technique seems aptly suited for the treatment of trauma, but can be destabilizing" (p. 275). Instead, they propose a treatment protocol, which combines the use of EMDR and hypnosis in the treatment of not only DID but also DDNOS and chronic PTSD. According to Fine and Berkowitz, this treatment method may be useful in helping clinicians—with advanced training, experience, and skill in both modalities independently—to achieve more stable results. Despite many studies of EMDR, no evidence shows that the specific use of eye or other movements contributes specifically to therapeutic outcome, and what works best is likely classical psychotherapeutic exploration of traumatic memories.

Dialectical Behavior Therapy

Dialectical behavior therapy (DBT) for BPD developed by M. Linehan was specifically designed for the outpatient treatment of chronically suicidal patients with BPD. Most of the research on DBT has focused on treatment in an outpatient setting. Hypothesizing that the course of therapy could be accelerated and improved by an inpatient setting at the beginning of outpatient DBT, Bohus and colleagues (2000) developed a treatment program of inpatient therapy for this patient group according to classic DBT guidelines. The program consisted of a 3-month inpatient treatment, followed by long-term outpatient therapy. The researchers conducted a pilot study involving 24 female patients and compared levels of psychopathology and frequency of self-injurious behavior at the beginning of treatment (i.e., prior to admission to the hospital) and at one month after discharge. They reported significant improvements in ratings of depression, dissociation, anxiety, and global stress. They also reported a highly significant decrease in the number of parasuicidal acts.

Ego-State Therapy

Ego-state therapy is a psychodynamic approach in which techniques of group and family therapy are employed to resolve conflicts between the various ego states that constitute a "family of self" within a single individual (Watkins 1993). Ego states may be hypnotically activated and made accessible for contact and communication by the therapist. Once contact is established, any behavioral, cognitive, or psychoanalytic technique may then be employed by a therapist skilled in this technique. As in the case of hypnosis, practitioners who advocate the use of ego-state therapy suggest that this approach has demonstrated that complex psychodynamic problems (i.e., dissociative symptoms) can often be resolved in a relatively short time compared to more traditional analytic therapies.

Similarly, Gainer and Torem (1993) described the use of ego-state therapy for the treatment of self-injurious behavior. They based their recommendations on the theory that in some patients, particularly those with DID, PTSD, and BPD, self-injurious behavior results from conflict among dissociated ego states. Their treatment strategy consists of identifying an ego state in which self-injurious behavior has occurred, activating the patient's ego strengths using inner-adviser techniques, and facilitating the integration of these resources within the ego state responsible for the behavior.

FORENSIC CONSIDERATIONS

Dealing With Transference

The issue of transference is important in every therapy situation, but it is particularly important in patients who have been physically and sexually abused. These patients have experienced the betrayal of someone they trusted (a caretaker) who, instead of providing care, comfort, and security, behaved in an exploitative and sometimes sadistic way. These patients may approach the therapeutic relationship with a sense of mistrust and apprehension. They may project their fears and past experiences onto the therapists, leading to problems with the transferential relationship (i.e., traumatic transference). Although their reality testing is good enough that they can perceive genuine caring, they expect their therapist either to exploit them (e.g., as the patients viewing the working through of traumatic memories as a reinflicting of the trauma and the therapists' taking sadistic pleasure in the patients' suffering), or to be excessively passive (e.g., with the patients identifying the therapist with some uncaring family figure who knew abuse was occurring but did little or nothing to stop it).

To avoid these kinds of problems, it is important to keep these transference issues in mind and address them early in the course of therapy. Attention to these issues can diffuse, but may not eliminate, the occurrence of such traumatic transference distortions of the therapeutic relationship (Maldonado and Spiegel 1995, 1998).

Dilution of Responsibility

In 1993, Steinberg and colleagues conducted an extensive literature review and suggested that several features characteristic of MPD (including amnesia, emo-

tional instability, and alterations in consciousness and personality) may cause varying degrees of influence over the criminal behavior of an individual with MPD. Thus, Steinberg et al. suggested that every case must be examined individually to assess the degree to which dissociative behavior may influence an individual's competence to stand trial and even possible insanity defense. They stressed the need and advantages of using formal diagnostic tools, such as the Structured Clinical Interview for DSM-IV Dissociative Disorders, in the forensic assessment of suspects manifesting dissociative symptoms and disorders.

Bray (2003) conducted a literature review looking at the issues of free will and moral responsibility in patients with BPD. He found that impulsivity, acting-out, and to some extent, less severe forms of dissociation do not vitiate responsibility. On the other hand, his findings suggest that more severe dissociative symptoms, like psychosis, may well render people with BPD less morally responsible for their actions. This view is not universally accepted by all researchers and therapists in the field of trauma and dissociation. In fact, some (Maldonado and Spiegel 2002) have suggested that even patients with significant dissociation should be held accountable and responsible for their actions, at least in the context of psychotherapy. It is unclear how the courts would deal with those issues, but it may be expected that comorbid conditions in BPD may affect the ability to act responsibly.

Criminal Responsibility

The controversy over the issue of dissociation as a diagnostic entity and a defense or symptom that may alter responsibility or culpability has added to the general discussion regarding dissociation in general. Many researchers have made attempts to find objective measures of dissociation to be applied in the field of forensic evaluations to try to rule out simulation, such as in cases of factitious dissociation, or malingering. Overall, a judicial review of the issues reflects a trend to disallow the concept of dissociative disorders as a criminal defense (Perr 1991).

There has been significant controversy regarding how the different identities (i.e., alters) typical for dissociative disorders should be interpreted. It is difficult to know whether alters are just metaphors for different emotional states or whether they represent truly autonomous entities that are capable of willful action. This issue becomes particularly important due to its legal implications and ramifications as it will dictate the way in which courts may handle cases that involve dissociation as a defense. Due to studies suggesting that alters of dissociative disorder patients differ in their memory performance or physiological profile, some researchers have suggested that alters are more than just metaphors.

The skepticism regarding the existence of dissociation in general may even be compounded in the case of criminals because of issues of suspected malingering. To assess the issue of veracity, Lewis and Bard (1991) reviewed the clinical records of 12 murderers who had been diagnosed with DID. Lewis and Bard were able to independently corroborate the presence of signs and symptoms diagnostic of DID in childhood and adulthood from several sources in all cases. Furthermore, objective evidence of a history of abuse was obtained in 11 cases. As reported by others, many subjects had amnesia for most of the abuse and had a tendency to underreport it.

Nevertheless, Merckelbach and colleagues (2002) pointed out that there is little consensus among dissociation experts about the degree to which various types of memory information (implicit, explicit, procedural) may leak from one alter to the another (i.e., coconsciousness). They further suggested that without such theoretical accord, any given outcome of memory studies on dissociative disorder subjects may be taken as support for the assumption that alters are in some sense "real." Because most psychophysiological studies on alter activity have lacked proper control conditions, most studies are inconclusive as to the status of alters. They thus conclude that the results of these studies are open to multiple interpretations and in no way refute an interpretation of alters in terms of metaphors for different emotional states (Merckelbach et al. 2002).

Similarly, many contemporary bioethicists claim that the possession of certain psychological properties is sufficient for having what is known as "full moral status." Bayne (2002) argued that there is tension between the psychological approach and a widely held model of DID. According to this model, the individual personalities or alters that belong to someone with DID possess those properties that proponents of the psychological approach claim suffice for full moral status. If this account of DID is true, then the psychological approach to full moral status seems to entail that the two standard therapies for treating DID might, on occasion, be seriously immoral, for they may well involve the (involuntary) elimination of an entity with full moral status. On the other hand, this argument seems to be repeatedly challenged every time a psychiatric patient is involuntarily treated, as often the refusal of treatment is in itself

a sign or symptom of their psychological disorder. As far as we have been able to find there has been no case law against a therapist for "eliminating" or "fusing" personality states.

It is our belief that patients with dissociative disorders do have enough implicit memory to be able to fully understand the issue of treatment nuances and goals, thus conferring patients enough mental capacity as to be considered competent to consent to treatment. In fact, our clinical experience suggests even personality states seem to have enough "co-consciousness" as to understand what happens in the therapy process.

There has been at least one reported case of a patient with a mixed (borderline-histrionic) personality disorder with dissociative features who was wrongfully diagnosed with DID. After the diagnosis, the case became the object of legal action as part of a malpractice suit. At trial, the court decided in favor of the patient leading to action against the diagnosing psychiatrist. This case raised serious and valid questions, in this case, about the possibility of auto-suggestion in mimicking dissociative disorders. The case also highlighted the suspicions with which courts look at the diagnosis. Legally, only carefully evaluated independent data about incongruent past patterns, or behavior suggesting alternate personality, can be considered reliable reference for the diagnosis (Serban 1992).

Other case reports have focused on cases of BPD or psychopathic character subjects factitiously presenting with features of "MPD." This finding has led to the recommendation (Bruce-Jones and Coid 1992) that subjects fulfilling diagnostic criteria for BPD or the psychodynamic features of borderline personality organization and presenting with dissociative features should be suspected of possible factitious behavior.

Coons (1991) warned about the fragmentary nature of the history presented by a group of 19 individuals who were charged with homicide. He warned of how it is usually impossible to state definitively who had genuine dissociation and who did not, thus raising the possibility of iatrogenesis and/or malingering. Even though he believed that most cases were associated with malingering, he also conceded that data from other sources suggested that the use of hypnosis in some of the individuals accused of homicide may iatrogenically produce DID-like phenomena when coupled with the defendant's desire to escape criminal responsibility. As stated by others, the risk of contamination may be decreased if practitioners use clear guidelines for the forensic evaluation of defendants in whom dissociative disorders are suspected.

Similarly, Lewis and Bard (1991) remarked that violence and dissociative disorders have very similar origins in early extraordinary physical and sexual abuse. Thus, they warn that as offenders become more knowledgeable about the possibility of diminished capacity associated with dissociative states, we can also expect to encounter more and better malingering among violent offenders related to dissociative episodes. Still, they fear that at present, we are far more likely to overlook the problem of dissociation (i.e., dissociative disorders) than we are to overdiagnose it. The main reason dissociation may be misdiagnosed in criminal offenders is probably because many of the characteristics of dissociative disorders are similar to the symptoms associated with some personality disorders, particularly antisocial personality. For example, the reported amnesia for a given behavior may be dismissed as lying. Fugue states may appear as attempts to evade justice. A patient inexplicably finding things in his or her possession may appear to be stealing. Episodes of self-mutilation and suicide attempts may look like attempts at manipulation. Finally, the use of different names at different times and under different circumstances may be interpreted as the conscious use of aliases in order to deceive and evade the law. Most often, the diagnosis of dissociative states is missed because the clinician does not even consider it a possibility.

As eloquently expressed by Halleck (1990), the controversies about issues of culpability in cases in which dissociation is raised as a defense can be clarified by considering the manner in which clinicians attribute responsibility for undesirable conduct associated with a psychiatric disorder. In treating patients with dissociative tendencies, clinicians must decide whether their therapeutic approach will emphasize the patient's responsibility for undesirable conduct or will minimize it. Certainly, practical and theoretical arguments can be made for both approaches. Clinically, using either approach has important consequences to patients, and inconsistent approaches have particularly harmful consequences. Halleck suggested that, until more objective data are available, the preferred method of dealing with patients with dissociation should continue to focus on maximizing their responsibility for any type of undesirable conduct.

Of interest, Silberman et al. (1985) conducted a study to assess the issue of learning and potential memory differences in subjects claiming to experience dissociated states. Subjects with dissociative disorders were not found to differ from controls in overall level of memory, and information learned by dissociative disorder subjects in disparate personality states did not result in greater compartmentalization than that of which control subjects were capable. However, there were qualitative differences between the cognitive performance of dissociative disorder patients and that of controls attempting to role-play alter personalities. Silberman et al. concluded that simple confabulation is not an adequate model for dissociative disorders and suggest a possible role for state-dependent learning in the phenomenology of dissociative states.

In a sample of men charged with a variety of offenses, Taylor and Kopelman (1984) found that nearly 10% of the men claimed amnesia for the offense leading to their conviction. Amnesia was found only among inmates who had committed violence and was most frequently associated with homicide. All of the inmates claiming amnesia had a comorbid psychiatric disorder. Of the sample, four fulfilled criteria for a primary depressive illness, the remainder being almost equally divided between schizophrenia and alcohol abuse. In this sample, the amnesic events had no direct legal implications, in that amnesia was not used as a defense. A variety of mechanisms were proposed by Taylor and Kopelman to account for the amnesia, including repression, dissociation, and alcoholic blackouts.

CONCLUSIONS

Dissociative symptoms and disorders commonly interact with other disorders such as BPD, especially in the context of a history of childhood trauma. Dissociation may underlie a variety of serious symptoms, including impulsiveness, self-harm, and revictimization. Adequate assessment and treatment of dissociation and working through of trauma-related symptomatology is crucial to the successful psychotherapeutic management of these complex disorders. These disorders share a common etiology that occurs early in life and that is likely to affect the development of personality structure, the lifelong pattern of interpersonal relationships, development of personal identity, management of impulsiveness, and affective instability. The presence of dissociative symptoms further complicates the management of BPD and other personality disorders, so recognition and treatment of dissociative symptoms can improve overall management of personality disorders. The fact that dissociative symptoms occur at the edge of conscious control makes their recognition and treatment crucial to better patient management and the working through of negative transference. Limits are better set when therapist and patient are clear on the patient's understanding and ability to control behavior, understand relationships, and manage affect. The sudden, unbidden, and rapid state shifting seen in dissociation can exacerbate problems in personality disorder patients, while understanding and management of such symptoms can stabilize the patient and facilitate treatment. It has been said that the problem with dissociative disorder patients is not that they have more than one personality but, rather, less than one personality. Their problem is difficulty with integration, and the damaged personality seen in personality disorder patients can be understood as another variant of the problems that accompany lifelong dissociation.

The following case example illustrates the ways in which untreated dissociative symptoms can complicate transference problems in psychotherapy—and how the use of hypnosis, working through of trauma-related memories, and emphasis on integration of dissociated elements of personality structure can be helpful in treatment.

Case Example

Ms. II was a 55-year-old mother with a history of sexual abuse by her father and grandfather and physical abuse by her mother. She was initially seen for a psychotic transference to a psychotherapist who had been encouraging regression by sitting Ms. II on her lap and hugging Ms. II when child alters emerged. Removing the patient from this harmful therapy was complicated by the typical borderline fear of abandonment. Indeed, Ms. II's dissociation fueled this fear because various personality states formed little connection with the new therapist and felt abandoned during the therapy, while other components felt allied with the prior therapist. Management of the dissociation with hypnosis helped to clarify which personality states were active, reasons for fears of abandonment, Ms. II's belief that she had to care for her new therapist rather than be cared for by him based on pathological early interactions with her parents, and selective amnesia for positive elements of her new therapeutic relationship. In this case, the dissociative elements amplified problematic aspects of the psychotherapy, and identification and control of them helped, initially by eliminating Ms. II's psychotic belief that her first therapist was her mother, and then by helping Ms. II to recognize and deal with ambivalent feelings toward both her earlier and current therapist and toward her parents.

An approach that acknowledges the patient's experience of fragmentation—but utilizes the controlled dissociation of hypnosis to establish connections across identity states—can help the patient to work through traumatic experiences that stimulate dissociation, enhance control over dissociated states, help the patient clarify transference fears and distortions, and reduce dissociative and associated depressive symptoms.

REFERENCES

Adityanjee, Raju GSP, Khandelwal SK: Current status of multiple personality disorder in India. Am J Psychiatry 146:1607–1610, 1989

Adityanjee, Schulz SC: Clinical use of quetiapine in disease states other than schizophrenia. J Clin Psychiatry 63 (suppl)13:32–38, 2002

Adler G: The psychotherapy of core borderline psychopathology. Am J Psychother 47:194–205, 1993

Allen JJ, Movius HL II: The objective assessment of amnesia in dissociative identity disorder using event-related potentials. Int J Psychophysiol 38:21–41, 2000

American Psychiatric Association: Diagnostic and Statistical Manual of Mental Disorders, Fourth Edition. Washington, DC, American Psychiatric Association, 1994

American Psychiatric Association: Diagnostic and Statistical Manual of Mental Disorders, Fourth Edition, Text Revision. Washington, DC, American Psychiatric Association, 2000

Anderson G, Yasenik L, Ross CA: Dissociative experiences and disorders among women who identify themselves as sexual abuse survivors. Child Abuse Negl 17:677–686, 1993

Armstrong J: The psychological organization of multiple personality disordered patients as revealed in psychological testing. Psychiatr Clin North Am 14:533–546, 1991

Armstrong JG, Putnam FW, Carlson EB, et al: Development and validation of a measure of adolescent dissociation: the Adolescent Dissociative Experiences Scale. J Nerv Ment Dis 185:491–497, 1997

Baars B: A Cognitive Theory of Consciousness. New York, Cambridge University Press, 1988

Banyard VL: Understanding links among childhood trauma, dissociation, and women's mental health. Am J Orthopsychiatry 71:311–321, 2001

Barber TX, Wilson SC: The Barber Suggestibility Scale and the Creative Imagination Scale: experimental and clinical applications. Am J Clin Hypn 21:84–108, 1978

Bayne TJ: Moral status and the treatment of Dissociative Identity Disorder. J Med Philos 27:87–105, 2002

Benner DG, Joscelyne B: Multiple personality as a borderline disorder. J Nerv Ment Dis 172:98–104, 1984

Berenbaum H, Valera EM, Kerns JG: Psychological trauma and schizotypal symptoms. Schizophr Bull 29:143–152, 2003

Bernstein EM, Putnam FW: Development, reliability, and validity of a dissociation scale. J Nerv Ment Dis 174:727–735, 1986

Blashfield RK, Sprock J, Fuller AK: Suggested guidelines for including or excluding categories in the DSM-IV. Compr Psychiatry 31:15–19, 1990

Bliss EL: Multiple personalities: A report of 14 cases with implications for schizophrenia and hysteria. Arch Gen Psychiatry 37:1388–1397, 1980

Bliss EL: Spontaneous self-hypnosis in multiple personality disorder. Psychiatr Clin North Am 7:135–148, 1984a

Bliss EL: A symptom profile of patients with multiple personalities, including MMPI results. J Nerv Ment Dis 172:197–202, 1984b

Bohus MJ, Landwehrmeyer GB, Stiglmayr CE, et al: Naltrexone in the treatment of dissociative symptoms in patients with borderline personality disorder: an open-label trial. J Clin Psychiatry 60:598–603, 1999

Bohus M, Haaf B, Stiglmayr C, et al: Evaluation of inpatient dialectical-behavioral therapy for borderline personality disorder: a prospective study. Behav Res Ther 38:875–887, 2000

Bowers KS: Dissociation in hypnosis and multiple personality disorder. Int J Clin Exp Hypn 39:155–176, 1991

Braun BG: Uses of hypnosis with multiple personality. Psychiatr Ann 14:34–40, 1984

Bray A: Moral responsibility and borderline personality disorder. Aust N Z J Psychiatry 37:270–276, 2003

Bremner JD, Brett E: Trauma-related dissociative states and long-term psychopathology in posttraumatic stress disorder. J Trauma Stress 10:37–49, 1997

Bremner JD, Southwick S, Brett E, et al: Dissociation and posttraumatic stress disorder in Vietnam combat veterans. Am J Psychiatry 149:328–332, 1992

Bremner JD, Krystal JH, Putnam FW, et al: Measurement of dissociative states with the Clinician-Administered Dissociative States Scale (CADSS). J Trauma Stress 11:125–136, 1998

Brenner I: The dissociative character: a reconsideration of "multiple personality." J Am Psychoanal Assoc 42:819–846, 1994

Brenner I: The characterological basis of multiple personality. Am J Psychotherapy 50:154–166, 1996

Brenner I: Deconstructing DID. Am J Psychother 53:344–360, 1999

Breuer J, Freud S: Studies on Hysteria (1893–1895). London, Hogarth Press, 1955

Brodsky BS, Cloitre M, Dulit RA: Relationship of dissociation to self-mutilation and childhood abuse in borderline personality disorder. Am J Psychiatry 152:1788–1792, 1995

Brown L, Russell J, Thornton C, et al: Dissociation, abuse and the eating disorders: evidence from an Australian population. Aust N Z J Psychiatry 33:521–528, 1999

Bruce-Jones W, Coid J: Identity diffusion presenting as multiple personality disorder in a female psychopath. Br J Psychiatry 160:541–544, 1992

Butler LD, Duran RE, Jasiukaitis P, et al: Hypnotizability and traumatic experience: a diathesis-stress model of dissociative symptomatology. Am J Psychiatry 153 (suppl 7):42–63, 1996

Cardeña E, Spiegel D: Dissociative reactions to the San Francisco Bay Area earthquake of 1989. Am J Psychiatry 150:474–478, 1993

Carlson EB, Putnam FW, Ross CA, et al: Validity of the Dissociative Experiences Scale in screening for multiple personality disorder: a multicenter study [see comments]. Am J Psychiatry 150:1030–1036, 1993

Christianson S, Loftus E: Memory for traumatic events. Appl Cogn Psychol 1:225–239, 1987

Chu JA, Dill DL: Dissociative symptoms in relation to childhood physical and sexual abuse [see comments]. Am J Psychiatry 147:887–892, 1990

Chu JA, Frey LM, Ganzel BL, et al: Memories of childhood abuse: dissociation, amnesia, and corroboration. Am J Psychiatry 156:749–755, 1999

Clary WF, Burstin KJ, Carpenter JS: Multiple personality and borderline personality disorder. Psychiatr Clin North Am 7:89–99, 1984

Cohen J, Servain-Schreiber D: Introduction to neural network mode in psychiatry. Psychiatr Ann 22:113–118, 1992a

Cohen J, Servain-Schreiber D: A neural network model of disturbance in the processing of context in schizophrenia. Psychiatr Ann 22:131–136, 1992b

Coons PM: The differential diagnosis of multiple personality. Psychiatr Clin North Am 12:51–67, 1984

Coons PM: Iatrogenesis and malingering of multiple personality disorder in the forensic evaluation of homicide defendants. Psychiatr Clin North Am 14:757–768, 1991

Coons PM: The use of carbamazepine for episodic violence in multiple personality disorder and dissociative disorder not otherwise specified: two additional cases. Biol Psychiatry 32:717–720, 1992

Coons PM: Child abuse and multiple personality disorder (letter). Am J Psychiatry 151:948, 1994

Coons PM: The dissociative disorders: rarely considered and underdiagnosed. Psychiatr Clin North Am 21:637–648, 1998

Coons PM, Bradley K: Group psychotherapy with multiple personality patients. J Nerv Ment Dis 173:515–521, 1985

Coons PM, Fine CG: Accuracy of the MMPI in identifying multiple personality disorder. Psychol Rep 66 (3 Pt 1):831–834, 1990

Coons PM, Milstein V: Psychosexual disturbances in multiple personality: characteristics, etiology, and treatment. J Clin Psychiatry 47:106–110, 1986

Coons PM, Bowman ES, Milstein V: Multiple personality disorder. A clinical investigation of 50 cases. J Nerv Ment Dis 176:519–527, 1988

Darves-Bornoz JM: Rape-related psychotraumatic syndromes. Eur J Obstet Gynecol Reprod Biol 71:59–65, 1997

Dell PF: Axis II pathology in outpatients with dissociative identity disorder. J Nerv Ment Dis 186:352–356, 1998

Dell PF: Dissociative phenomenology of dissociative identity disorder. J Nerv Ment Dis 190:10–15, 2002

Dorahy MJ: Dissociative identity disorder and memory dysfunction: the current state of experimental research and its future directions. Clin Psychol Rev 21:771–795, 2001

Dowson JH, Sussams P, Grounds AT, et al: Associations of self-reported past "psychotic" phenomena with features of personality disorders. Compr Psychiatry 41:42–48, 2000

Draijer N, Langeland W: Childhood trauma and perceived parental dysfunction in the etiology of dissociative symptoms in psychiatric inpatients. Am J Psychiatry 156:379–385, 1999

Dunn GE, Ryan JJ, Paolo AM, et al: Comorbidity of dissociative disorders among patients with substance use disorders. Psychiatr Serv 46:153–156, 1995

Ellason JW, Ross CA, Fuchs DL: Assessment of dissociative identity disorder with the Millon Clinical Multiaxial Inventory-II. Psychol Rep 76 (3 Pt 1):895–905, 1995

Ellason JW, Ross CA, Sainton K, et al: Axis I and II comorbidity and childhood trauma history in chemical dependency. Bull Menninger Clin 60:39–51, 1996

Eriksson N-G, Lundin T: Early traumatic stress reactions among Swedish survivors of the m/s Estonia disaster. Br J Psychiatry 169:713–716, 1996

Farley M, Keaney JC: Physical symptoms, somatization, and dissociation in women survivors of childhood sexual assault. Women Health 25:33–45, 1997

Figueroa EF, Silk KR, Huth A, et al: History of childhood sexual abuse and general psychopathology. Compr Psychiatry 38:23–30, 1997

Fine CG, Berkowitz AS: The wreathing protocol: the imbrication of hypnosis and EMDR in the treatment of dissociative identity disorder and other dissociative responses. Eye Movement Desensitization Reprocessing. Am J Clin Hypn 43:275–290, 2001

Fink D: The comorbidity of multiple personality disorder and DSM-III-R Axis II disorders. Psychiatr Clin North Am 14:547–566, 1991

Forrest KA: Toward an etiology of dissociative identity disorder: a neurodevelopmental approach. Conscious Cogn 10:259–293, 2001

Frankel FH: Hypnotizability and dissociation [see comments]. Am J Psychiatry 147:823–829, 1990

Freud S: Papers on Metapsychology (1915). London, Hogarth Press, 1963

Gainer MJ, Torem MS: Ego-state therapy for self-injurious behavior. Am J Clin Hypn 35:257–266, 1993

Ganaway GK: Historical versus narrative truth: clarifying the role of exogenous trauma in the etiology of MPD and its variants. Dissociation: Progress in the Dissociative Disorders 2:205–220, 1989

Ganaway GK: Hypnosis, childhood trauma, and dissociative identity disorder: toward an integrative theory. Int J Clin Exp Hypn 43:127–144, 1995

Giese-Davis J, Koopman C, Butler LD, et al: The Stanford Self-Efficacy Scale for serious illness: reliability, validity, and generalizability. Paper presented at the annual meeting of the American Psychological Society, Washington, DC, May 27, 1997

Glantz K, Goisman RM: Relaxation and merging in the treatment of personality disorders. Am J Psychother 44:405–413, 1990

Gleaves DH, Eberenz KP: Correlates of dissociative symptoms among women with eating disorders. J Psychiatr Res 29:417–426, 1995

Gleaves DH, May MC, Cardena E: An examination of the diagnostic validity of dissociative identity disorder. Clin Psychol Rev 21:577–608, 2001

Golynkina K, Ryle A: The identification and characteristics of the partially dissociated states of patients with borderline personality disorder. Br J Med Psychol 72 (Pt 4):429–445, 1999

Greaves GB: Multiple Personality. 165 years after Mary Reynolds. J Nerv Ment Dis 168:577–596, 1980

Halleck SL: Dissociative phenomena and the question of responsibility. Int J Clin Exp Hypn 38:298–314, 1990

Herman JL, Perry JC, van der Kolk BA, et al: Childhood trauma in borderline personality disorder [see comments]. Am J Psychiatry 146:490–495, 1989

Herpertz S, Gretzer A, Muhlbauer V, et al: Experimental detection of inadequate affect regulation in patients with self-mutilating behavior. Nervenarzt 69:410–418, 1998

Hilgard ER: Divided Consciousness: Multiple Controls in Human Thought and Action. New York, Wiley-Interscience, 1977

Hilgard ER: Divided Consciousness: Multiple Controls in Human Thought and Action. New York, Wiley-Interscience, 1986

Holen A: The North Sea Oil Rig Disaster. New York, Plenum, 1993

Horevitz RP, Braun BG: Are multiple personalities borderline? An analysis of 33 cases. Psychiatr Clin North Am 7:69–87, 1984

Horowitz M: Stress Response Syndromes. New York, Jason Aronson, 1976

Irwin HJ: Pathological and nonpathological dissociation: the relevance of childhood trauma. J Psychol 133:157–164, 1999

Irwin HJ: The relationship between dissociative tendencies and schizotypy: an artifact of childhood trauma? J Clin Psychol 57:331–342, 2001

Janet P: L'Automatisme Psychologique. Doctoral dissertation. Paris, Felix Alcan, 1889

Jones B, Heard H, Startup M, et al: Autobiographical memory and dissociation in borderline personality disorder. Psychol Med 29:1397–1404, 1999

Kemperman I, Russ MJ, Clark WC, et al: Pain assessment in self-injurious patients with borderline personality disorder using signal detection theory. Psychiatry Res 70:175–183, 1997a

Kemperman I, Russ MJ, Shearin E: Self-injurious behavior and mood regulation in borderline patients. J Personal Disord 11:146–157, 1997b

Kluft RP: An introduction to multiple personality disorder. Psychiatr Ann 14:19–24, 1984a

Kluft RP: Multiple personality in childhood. Psychiatr Clin North Am 7:121–134, 1984b

Kluft RP: Treatment of multiple personality disorder: a study of 33 cases. Psychiatr Clin North Am 7:9–29, 1984c

Kluft RP: Dissociation as a response to extreme trauma, in Childhood Antecedents of Multiple Personality. Edited by Kluft RP. Washington, DC, American Psychiatric Press, 66-97, 1985

Kluft RP: The postunification treatment of multiple personality disorder: first findings. Am J Psychother 42:212–228, 1988

Kluft RP: Playing for time: temporizing techniques in the treatment of multiple personality disorder. Am J Clin Hypn 32:90–98, 1989

Kluft RP: Multiple personality disorder, in American Psychiatric Press Review of Psychiatry, Vol 10. Edited by Tasman A, Goldfinger SM. Washington, DC, American Psychiatric Press, 1991, pp 161–188

Kluft RP: Enhancing the hospital treatment of dissociative disorder patients by developing nursing expertise in the application of hypnotic techniques without formal trance induction. Am J Clin Hypn 34:158–167, 1992

Koopman C, Classen C, Cardena E, et al: When disaster strikes, acute stress disorders may follow. J Trauma Stress 8:29–46, 1995

Lavoie G, Sabourin M: Hypnotic susceptibility, amnesia, and IQ in chronic schizophrenia. Int J Clin Exp Hypn 21:157–168, 1973

Lewis DO, Bard JS: Multiple personality and forensic issues. Psychiatr Clin North Am 14:741–756, 1991

Loewenstein RJ: An office mental status examination for complex chronic dissociative symptoms and multiple personality disorder. Psychiatr Clin North Am 4:567–604, 1991a

Loewenstein RJ: Psychogenic amnesia and psychogenic fugue: a comprehensive review, in American Psychiatric Press Review of Psychiatry, Vol 10. Edited by Tasman A, Goldfinger SM. Washington DC, American Psychiatric Press, 1991b, pp 189–222

Low G, Jones D, MacLeod A, et al: Childhood trauma, dissociation, and self-harming behaviour: a pilot study. Br J Med Psychol 73 (Pt 2):269–278, 2000

Lussier RG, Steiner J, Grey A, et al: Prevalence of dissociative disorders in an acute care day hospital population. Psychiatr Serv 48:244–246, 1997

Madakasira S, O'Brien KF: Acute posttraumatic stress disorder in victims of a natural disaster. J Nerv Ment Dis 175:286–290, 1987

Maercker A, Schutzwohl M: Long-term effects of political imprisonment: a group comparison study. Soc Psychiatry Psychiatr Epidemiol 32:435–442, 1997

Maldonado JR, Spiegel D: Using hypnosis, in Treating Women Molested in Childhood. Edited by Classen C. San Francisco, Jossey-Bass, Inc., 1995, pp 163–186

Maldonado JR, Spiegel D: Trauma, dissociation, and hypnotizability, in Trauma, Memory, and Dissociation. Edited by Bremner JD, Marmar CR. Washington, DC, American Psychiatric Press, 1998, pp 57–106

Maldonado JR, Spiegel D: Dissociative disorders, in The American Psychiatric Publishing Textbook of Clinical Psychiatry, Fourth Edition. Edited by Hales RE, Yudofsky SC. Washington, DC, American Psychiatric Publishing, 2002, pp 709–742

Maldonado JR, Butler L, Spiegel D, et al: Treatment of dissociative disorders, in A Guide to Treatments that Work. Edited by Nathan PE, Gorman JM. New York, Oxford University Press, 1997, 423–446

Markowitz JS, Gill HS: Pharmacotherapy of dissociative identity disorder. Ann Pharmacother 30:1498–1499, 1996

Marmar CR, Weiss DS, Metzler T: Peritraumatic dissociation and posttraumatic stress disorder, in Trauma, Memory, and Dissociation. Edited by Bremner JD, Marmar DR. Washington, DC, American Psychiatric Press, 1998, pp 229–252

McHugh PR: Dissociative identity disorder as a socially constructed artifact. Journal of Practical Psychiatry and Behavioral Health 1:158–166, 1995a

McHugh PR: Witches, multiple personalities, and other psychiatric artifacts. Nat Med 1:110–114, 1995b

Merckelbach H, Rassin E, Muris P: Dissociation, schizotypy, and fantasy proneness in undergraduate students. J Nerv Ment Dis 188:428–431, 2000

Merckelbach H, Devilly GJ, Rassin E: Alters in dissociative identity disorder: metaphors or genuine entities? Clin Psychol Rev 22:481–497, 2002

Modestin J, Ebner G, Junghan M, Erni T: Dissociative experiences and dissociative disorders in acute psychiatric inpatients. Compr Psychiatry 37:355–361, 1996

Molinari E: Eating disorders and sexual abuse. Eat Weight Disord 6:68–80, 2001

Mulder RT, Beautrais AL, Joyce PR, et al: Relationship between dissociation, childhood sexual abuse, childhood physical abuse, and mental illness in a general population sample. Am J Psychiatry 155:806–811, 1998

Ng BY, Yap AK, Su A, et al: Personality profiles of patients with dissociative trance disorder in Singapore. Compr Psychiatry 43:121–126, 2002

Nijenhuis ER, Spinhoven P, Van Dyck R, et al: The development and psychometric characteristics of the Somatoform Dissociation Questionnaire (SDQ-20). J Nerv Ment Dis 184:688-694, 1996

Nijenhuis ER, Spinhoven P, van Dyck R, et al: The development of the somatoform dissociation questionnaire (SDQ-5) as a screening instrument for dissociative disorders. Acta Psychiatr Scand 96:311-318, 1997

Nijenhuis ER, Spinhoven P, van Dyck R, et al: Degree of somatoform and psychological dissociation in dissociative disorder is correlated with reported trauma. J Trauma Stress 11:711–730, 1998

Noll R: Multiple personality, dissociation, and C.G. Jung's complex theory. J Anal Psychol 34:353–370, 1989

Noyes R Jr, Kletti R: Depersonalization in response to life-threatening danger. Compr Psychiatry 18:375–384, 1977

Noyes R Jr, Slymen DJ: The subjective response to life-threatening danger. Omega 9:313–321, 1978

Ogata SN, Silk KR, Goodrich S, et al: Childhood sexual and physical abuse in adult patients with borderline personality disorder [see comments]. Am J Psychiatry 147:1008–1013, 1990

Paris J: Chronic suicidality among patients with borderline personality disorder. Psychiatric Services 53:738–742, 2002

Perr IN: Crime and multiple personality disorder: a case history and discussion. Bull Am Acad Psychiatry Law 19:203–214, 1991

Pettinati HM: Measuring hypnotizability in psychotic patients. Int J Clin Exp Hypn 30:404–416, 1982

Pettinati HM, Horne RL, Staats JM: Hypnotizability in patients with anorexia nervosa and bulimia. Arch Gen Psychiatry 42:1014–1016, 1985

Pettinati HM, Kogan LG, Evans FJ, et al: Hypnotizability of psychiatric inpatients according to two different scales. Am J Psychiatry 147:69–75, 1990

Pfohl B, Blum N, Zimmerman M: Structured Interview for DSM-IV Personality. Washington, DC, American Psychiatric Press, 1997

Pope CA, Kwapil TR: Dissociative experience in hypothetically psychosis-prone college students. J Nerv Ment Dis 188:530–536, 2000

Putnam FW Jr: Dissociation as a response to extreme trauma, in Childhood Antecedents of Multiple Personality. Edited by Kluft RP. Washington, DC, American Psychiatric Press, 1985, pp 66–97

Putnam FW: Dissociation and disturbances of self, in Disorders and Dysfunctions of the Self, Vol 5. Edited by Cicchetti D, Toth SL. Rochester, NY, University of Rochester Press, 1994, pp 251–265

Putnam FW: Development of dissociative disorders, in Developmental Psychopathology, Vol 2. Edited by Cicchetti D, Cohen DJ. New York, Wiley, 1995, pp 581–608

Putnam FW: Dissociation in Children and Adolescents: A Developmental Perspective. New York, Guilford Press, 1997

Putnam FW, Guroff JJ, Silberman EK, et al: The clinical phenomenology of multiple personality disorder: review of 100 recent cases. J Clin Psychiatry 47:285–293, 1986

Roesler TA, McKenzie N: Effects of childhood trauma on psychological functioning in adults sexually abused as children. J Nerv Ment Dis 182:145–150, 1994

Ross CA, Norton GR: Effects of hypnosis on the features of multiple personality disorder. Am J Clin Hypn 32:99–106, 1989

Ross CA, Norton GR, Wozney K: Multiple personality disorder: an analysis of 236 cases. Can J Psychiatry 34:413–418, 1989

Ross CA, Joshi S, Currie R: Dissociative experiences in the general population. Am J Psychiatry 147:1547–1552, 1990

Ross CA, Anderson G, Fleisher WP: The frequency of multiple personality disorder among psychiatric inpatients. Am J Psychiatry 148:1717–1720, 1991a

Ross CA, Joshie S, Currie R: Dissociative experiences in the general population: a factor analysis. Hosp Community Psychiatry 42:297–301, 1991b

Ross-Gower J, Waller G, Tyson M, et al: Reported sexual abuse and subsequent psychopathology among women attending psychology clinics: the mediating role of dissociation. Br J Clin Psychol 37 (Pt 3):313–326, 1998

Rumelhart D, McClelland J: Parallel Distributed Processing: Explorations in the Microstructure of Cognition. Cambridge, The MIT Press, 1986

Russ MJ, Clark WC, Cross LW, et al: Pain and self-injury in borderline patients: sensory decision theory, coping strategies, and locus of control. Psychiatry Res 63:57–65, 1996

Russ MJ, Campbell SS, Kakuma T, et al: EEG theta activity and pain insensitivity in self-injurious borderline patients. Psychiatry Res 89:201–214, 1999

Sanders B, Giolas MH: Dissociation and childhood trauma in psychologically disturbed adolescents. Am J Psychiatry 148:50–54, 1991

Sar V, Yargic LI, Tutkun H: Structured interview data on 35 cases of dissociative identity disorder in Turkey. Am J Psychiatry 153:1329–1333, 1996

Saxe G, van der Kolk BA, Berkowitz R, et al: Dissociative disorders in psychiatric patients. Am J Psychiatry 150:1037–1042, 1993

Saxena S, Prasad K: DSM-III subclassification of dissociative disorders applied to psychiatric outpatients in India. Am J Psychiatry 146:261–262, 1989

Schacter DL: Understanding implicit memory: a cognitive neuroscience approach. Am Psychol 47:559–569, 1992

Schacter DL, Kihlstrom JF, Kihlstrom LC, et al: Autobiographical memory in a case of multiple personality disorder. J Abnorm Psychol 98:508–514, 1989

Schmahl CG, McGlashan TH, Bremner JD: Neurobiological correlates of borderline personality disorder. Psychopharmacol Bull 36:69–87, 2002

Schultz R, Braun BG, Kluft RP: Multiple personality disorder: phenomenology of selected variables in comparison to major depression. Dissociation 2:45–51, 1989

Scroppo JC, Drob SL, Weinberger JL, et al: Identifying dissociative identity disorder: a self-report and projective study. J Abnorm Psychol 107:272–284, 1998

Serban G: Multiple personality: an issue for forensic psychiatry. Am J Psychother 46:269–280, 1992

Shearer SL: Dissociative phenomena in women with borderline personality disorder. Am J Psychiatry 151:1324–1328, 1994

Sigmund D, Barnett W, Mundt C: The hysterical personality disorder: a phenomenological approach. Psychopathology 31:318–330, 1998

Silberman EK, Putnam FW, Weingartner H, et al: Dissociative states in multiple personality disorder: a quantitative study. Psychiatry Res 15:253–260, 1985

Sloan P: Post-traumatic stress in survivors of an airplane crash-landing: a clinical and exploratory research intervention. J Trauma Stress 1:211–229, 1988

Smith ED, Stefanek ME, Joseph MV, et al: Spiritual awareness, personal perspective on death, and psychosocial distress among cancer patients: an initial investigation. Journal of Psychosocial Oncology 11:89–103, 1993

Smith WH: Incorporating hypnosis into the psychotherapy of patients with multiple personality disorder. Bull Menninger Clin 57:344–354, 1993

Soloff PH: Neuroleptic treatment in the borderline patient: advantages and techniques. J Clin Psychiatry 48 (suppl):26–31, 1987

Solomon Z, Mikulincer M, Bleich A: Characteristic expressions of combat-related posttraumatic stress disorder among Israeli soldiers in the 1982 Lebanon War. Behav Med 14:171–178, 1988

Solomon Z, Mikulincer M, Benbenishty R: Combat stress reaction: clinical manifestations and correlates. Mil Psychol 1:35–47, 1989

Spanos NP: Hypnotic behavior: a social-psychological interpretation of amnesia, analgesia, and "trance logic." Behav Brain Sci 9:449–502, 1986

Spanos NP, Weekes JR, Bertrand LD: Multiple personality: a social psychological perspective. J Abnorm Psychol 94:362–376, 1985

Spiegel D: Multiple personality as a post-traumatic stress disorder. Psychiatr Clin North Am 7:101–110, 1984

Spiegel D: Dissociation, double binds, and posttraumatic stress in multiple personality disorder, in Treatment of Multiple Personality Disorder. Edited by Braun BG. Washington, DC, American Psychiatric Press, 1986, pp 61–77

Spiegel D: Dissociating Consciousness from Cognition. Behav Brain Sci 14:695–696, 1991a

Spiegel D: Foreword to dissociative disorders, in American Psychiatric Press Review of Psychiatry, Vol 10. Edited by Tasman A, Goldfinger SM. Washington, DC, American Psychiatric Press, 1991b, pp 143–144

Spiegel D: Trauma, dissociation, and memory, in Psychobiology of Posttraumatic Stress Disorder. Edited by Yehuda R, McFarlane A. New York, The New York Academy of Sciences, 1997, pp 225–237

Spiegel D, Cardena E: Disintegrated experience: the dissociative disorders revisited. J Abnorm Psychol 100:366–378, 1991

Spiegel D, Fink R: Hysterical psychosis and hypnotizability. Am J Psychiatry 136:777–781, 1979

Spiegel D, Detrick D, Frischholz E: Hypnotizability and psychopathology. Am J Psychiatry 139:431–437, 1982

Spiegel D, Hunt T, Dondershine HEl: Dissociation and hypnotizability in posttraumatic stress disorder. Am J Psychiatry 145:301–305, 1988

Spiegel H, Spiegel D: Trance and treatment: Clinical Uses of Hypnosis. Washington, DC, American Psychiatric Press, 1978

Spiegel H, Spiegel D: Trance and Treatment: Clinical Uses of Hypnosis. Washington, DC, American Psychiatric Press, 2004

Spitzer C, Spelsberg B, Grabe HJ, et al: Dissociative experiences and psychopathology in conversion disorders. J Psychosom Res 46:291–294, 1999

Steiger H, Leonard S, Kin NY, et al: Childhood abuse and platelet tritiated-paroxetine binding in bulimia nervosa: implications of borderline personality disorder. J Clin Psychiatry 61:428–435, 2000

Steinberg M: Advances in the clinical assessment of dissociation: the SCID-D-R. Bull Menninger Clin 64:146–163, 2000

Steinberg M, Rounsaville B, Cicchetti DV: The Structured Clinical Interview for DSM-III-R Dissociative Disorders: preliminary report on a new diagnostic instrument. Am J Psychiatry 147:76–82, 1990

Steinberg M, Bancroft J, Buchanan J: Multiple personality disorder in criminal law. Bull Am Acad Psychiatry Law 21:345-56, 1993

Stiglmayr CE, Shapiro DA, Stieglitz RD, et al: Experience of aversive tension and dissociation in female patients with borderline personality disorder—a controlled study. J Psychiatr Res 35:111–118, 2001

Stubner S, Volkl G, Soyka M: Differential diagnosis of dissociative identity disorder (multiple personality disorder). Nervenarzt 69:440–445, 1998

Taylor PJ, Kopelman MD: Amnesia for criminal offences. Psychol Med 14:581–588, 1984

Timmerman IG, Emmelkamp PM: The relationship between traumatic experiences, dissociation, and borderline personality pathology among male forensic patients and prisoners. J Personal Disord 15:136–149, 2001

Vaillant GE, Drake RE: Maturity of ego defenses in relation to DSM-III Axis II personality disorder. Arch Gen Psychiatry 42:597–601, 1985

Valdiserri S, Kihlstrom JF: Abnormal eating and dissociative experiences: a further study of college women. Int J Eat Disord 18:145–150, 1995

van der Hart O, Spiegel D: Hypnotic assessment and treatment of trauma-induced psychoses. Int J Clin Exp Hypn 41:191–209, 1993

van der Kolk BA, Fisler RE: Childhood abuse and neglect and loss of self-regulation. Bull Menninger Clin 58:145–168, 1994

Vanderlinden J, van Dyck R, Vandereycken W, et al: Dissociative experiences in the general population of the Netherlands and Belgium: a study with the Dissociative Questionnaire (DIS-Q). Dissociation 4:180–184, 1991

Waldo TG, Merritt RD: Fantasy proneness, dissociation, and DSM-IV Axis II symptomatology. J Abnorm Psychol 109:555–558, 2000

Waller G, Ohanian V, Meyer C, et al: The utility of dimensional and categorical approaches to understanding dissociation in the eating disorders. Br J Clin Psychol 40 (Pt 4):387–397, 2001

Waller NG, Ross CA: The prevalence and biometric structure of pathological dissociation in the general population: taxometric and behavior genetic findings. J Abnorm Psychol 106:499–510, 1997

Waller NG, Putnam FW, Carlson EB: Types of dissociation and dissociative types: a taxometric analysis of dissociative experiences. Psychological Methods 1:300–321, 1996

Watkins HH: Ego-state therapy: an overview. Am J Clin Hypn 35:232–240, 1993

Watson D: Dissociations of the night: individual differences in sleep-related experiences and their relation to dissociation and schizotypy. J Abnorm Psychol 110:526–535, 2001

Wildgoose A, Waller G, Clarke S, et al: Psychiatric symptomatology in borderline and other personality disorders: dissociation and fragmentation as mediators. J Nerv Ment Dis 188:757–763, 2000

Wildgoose A, Clarke S, Waller G: Treating personality fragmentation and dissociation in borderline personality disorder: a pilot study of the impact of cognitive analytic therapy. Br J Med Psychol 74 (Pt 1):47–55, 2001

Yargic LI, Sar V, Tutkun H, et al: Comparison of dissociative identity disorder with other diagnostic groups using a structured interview in Turkey. Compr Psychiatry 39: 345–351, 1998

Yehuda R, Elkin A, Binder-Brynes K, et al: Dissociation in aging Holocaust survivors. Am J Psychiatry 153:935–940, 1996

Yen S, Shea MT, Pagano M, et al: Axis I and axis II disorders as predictors of prospective suicide attempts: findings from the collaborative longitudinal personality disorders study. J Abnorm Psychol 112:375–381, 2003

Young L: Sexual abuse and the problem of embodiment. Child Abuse Negl 16:89–100, 1992

Zanarini MC, Ruser T, Frankenburg FR, et al: The dissociative experiences of borderline patients. Compr Psychiatry 41:223–227, 2000

Zlotnick C, Mattia JI, Zimmerman M: Clinical correlates of self-mutilation in a sample of general psychiatric patients. J Nerv Ment Dis 187:296–301, 1999

Zweig-Frank H, Paris J, Guzder J: Psychological risk factors and self-mutilation in female patients with BPD. Can J Psychiatry 39:259–264, 1994a

Zweig-Frank H, Paris J, Guzder J: Psychological risk factors and self-mutilation in male patients with BPD. Can J Psychiatry 39:266–268, 1994b

33

Defensive Functioning

J. Christopher Perry, M.P.H., M.D.

Michael Bond, M.D.

Clinicians who interview or treat individuals with personality disorders confront defenses and their behavioral correlates at many points. Even those who do not use a psychodynamic perspective to understand psychopathology find terms, phrases, or epithets such as the following very apt:

> resistant, lacks awareness, acts out a lot, complains but does not do anything about it, avoids doing the homework, acts very dependent, demanding, denial, blames others rather than himself or herself, lies to himself or herself, sees things only in black or white, does not listen, very regressed, sensitive to criticism, puts others down, sarcastic, unrealistic idolizing or relying on others when they are not going to help, does not talk about the important things, seems to forget a lot, cannot make up his or her mind, only talks in generalities, cannot seem to feel anything

This chapter reflects the point of view that the situations in which these terms might apply can perhaps be construed more scientifically and productively as relating to the patient's defensive functioning at the

time. This chapter briefly reviews some aspects about the theory and measurement of defenses and specific research relevant to personality disorders. The remainder of the text then discusses how the management and interpretation of defenses can help further the aims of psychotherapy. The chapter ends with some examples of defenses in specific therapeutic interactions. It is our experience that even therapists who use nondynamic treatments such as cognitive-behavioral therapy will find knowledge of defenses helpful in judging with what material the patient is able to work.

BACKGROUND

Current Views and Assumptions About Defenses

Although many aspects of psychodynamic theory have eluded scientific examination, researchers have focused on defense mechanisms for decades. Earlier efforts were thwarted by problems with definition and assessment issues, but recent work has proved more fortunate. Researchers have provided clear, non-overlapping definitions, sometimes including prototypical examples, to aid in making the low-inference clinical judgments necessary to identify each specific defense (see Table 33–2 later in this chapter for a glossary of defense mechanisms included in DSM-IV-TR). These developments have resulted in acceptable measurement reliability, which has allowed defense research to enter the scientific arena (see review in Perry and Ianni 1998). We suggest that there is an approximate consensus among researchers on the following aspects of the defense mechanism construct (Perry 1993; Perry and Ianni 1998; Vaillant 1993):

1. An overall definition of a defense is that it is the individual's automatic psychological response to internal or external stressors or emotional conflict (see Defensive Functioning Scale in DSM-IV-TR [American Psychiatric Association 2000, pp. 807–813]). Defenses are triggered by the occurrence of what Freud (1926/1959) called *signal anxiety*, arising whenever internal wishes or drives conflict with internalized prohibitions or external reality constraints.

2. Defenses generally act automatically, without conscious effort. Often, the individual is completely unaware of the defensive operation, although in some instances he or she may have partial awareness. A common usage of displacement exemplifies this phenomenon: an individual suddenly becomes irritated at a small annoyance and then realizes that this response has been misdirected away from a more significant source of annoyance that remains unresolved. A well-worn example is the individual who, upon coming home after an argument with the boss, becomes irritated at the spouse over an issue that usually would not evoke as much emotion.

3. Character traits are in part made up of specific defenses that individuals tend to use repetitively in diverse situations. Individuals tend to specialize, using a set or repertoire of defenses across a variety of stressors depending on the motives or conflicts active at the time. This observation suggests that defenses can be viewed as underlying dispositions that manifest under certain stressful states. Therefore, the defenses an individual shows at any point in time may vary in degree or specificity with the stressor, making some state effects expectable (Perry 2001). Whether there is specificity between the type of stressor and individual defense is an empirical question.

4. A past review tallied 42 different individual defense mechanisms described by various authors (Perry and Cooper 1986). Although there is no clear rationale for selecting a definitive list of defenses (Vaillant 1976), a process of consensus has favored those defenses with clear, nonoverlapping definitions, reliable application, and demonstrated empirical findings. This process is advanced but hardly completed.

5. Defenses affect adaptation (Vaillant 1976, 1993). Each defense presumably is highly adaptive in certain situations. In dangerous situations, such as battle, projection may help the individual resolve ambiguous situations by assuming that a threat is present and thus minimizing immediate personal harm. Similarly, the abused child's use of splitting of others' images allows him or her to coexist with the abusive caretaker on whom he or she is highly dependent for survival needs. Due to intense fear, the child temporarily splits off rage and experiences all problems as due to him- or herself (being all-bad), whereas the abusive caretaker is all-powerful and good. Later, in different circumstances, the child may experience the self and another with the meanings reversed. Despite the reality that each defense may be highly adaptive in certain situations, there is a clear hierarchy of defenses in relation to the overall adaptiveness of each one. Defenses at the lower end are usually maladaptive, save in a few situations, whereas those defenses at the higher end are adaptive in a broader array of circumstances.

6. When defenses are least adaptive, they protect the individual from awareness of the stressors, anxiety, or associated conflicts at the price of constricting awareness, a sense of freedom to choose, and flexibility to maximize positive outcomes. When defenses are most adaptive, they maximize awareness of internal and external motives, stressors, and constraints and thereby maximize the expression and gratification of wishes and needs, minimize negative consequences, and provide a sense of freedom to choose. Some individuals label the most adaptive defenses with the special term *coping mechanisms*, whereas many in the dynamic tradition retain the defense designation because the so-called coping mechanisms share many characteristics with other defenses. This question of terminology—defense versus coping—may mix questions of preference with science.

7. Whether defenses emerge in a certain developmental sequence is an empirically open issue, despite the use of developmental terms to describe groups of defenses, such as immature or mature. These developmental terms are used for reasons of history and convenience only. In fact, even preverbal toddlers may preferentially use so-called mature or high adaptive level defenses (Bader and Perry 2001), which suggests that much more is needed to understand why some adults come to use the lower-level defenses associated with personality disorders. However, in development during adulthood there appear to be sequences in which certain lower-level defenses progress to higher-level defenses on the continuum of adaptiveness (Vaillant 1993). For instance, acting-out in early life (e.g., rebelling against authority) may evolve later to reaction formation (taking the side of authority) and eventually to altruism (helping the unfortunate obtain fairness from authority). These sequences deserve study because they may hold important implications for patterns of therapeutic change in personality disorders both as a patient "trades up" within a therapy session and as he or she develops over time.

8. Defenses aid in understanding the problems and therapeutic challenges in treating personality disorders. Defenses in the lower half of the defense hierarchy mediate many of the most maladaptive ways of handling stress and conflict in personality disorders. Specific defense levels may be associated with certain individual disorders or clusters that relate to core psychopathology, such as splitting and projective identification in borderline personality disorder (BPD; Kernberg 1975; Perry and Cooper 1986) or omnipotence and devaluation in antisocial and narcissistic personality disorders (Perry and Perry 2004). Whenever used, these same defenses serve as instantaneous markers alerting the clinician that a core issue for a given personality disorder type is operating.

Hierarchy of Defenses

Defenses have been hierarchically ordered based on the empirical relationship to general measures of adaptiveness. A number of authors have contributed to this finding (Bond et al. 1983; Perry 1993; Perry and Cooper 1989; Vaillant 1976, 1993), culminating in a generally accepted hierarchy. Examples include the Defensive Functioning Scale in DSM-IV-TR (American Psychiatric Association 2000; Skodol and Perry 1993) and the Defense Mechanism Rating Scales (DMRS) hierarchy (see Table 33–1). Defenses that have common aims are grouped together in one of eight levels (more if sublevels are included). For instance, among the so-called immature defenses, the disavowal level includes three defenses: denial, rationalization, and projection. These have a common function of disavowing certain affects, actions, ideas, or motives that others can identify in the person using them. However, each defense differs in how the disavowed material is handled—whether actively avoiding it altogether (denial), covering it up with something more socially acceptable (rationalization), or misattributing it to others and thereby maintaining an interest in it but at a distance (projection). The defense levels range from the lowest level of defensive dysregulation (psychotic defenses) to the high adaptive level (mature defenses). Healthier individuals use a larger proportion of highly adaptive defenses and a lower proportion of defenses at the low end of the hierarchy.

MEASURING DEFENSIVE FUNCTIONING

This chapter focuses on clinical observer-rated and self-report methods, although other methods, such as projective tests, also are in use (see review by Perry and Ianni 1998).

Observer Ratings of Defenses

There are several observer-rated methods for identifying defenses (see review in Perry and Ianni 1998), but only some of the clinically based methods have been applied to the study of personality disorders.

Vaillant's Life Vignette Method

Vaillant (1976) defined 18 defense mechanisms to rate life vignettes obtained from patient interviews. The interviews elicited vignettes about the patients' responses to important events in their lives. The method qualitatively identifies an individual's three most prominent defenses used in the vignettes and has acceptable reliability (*mean r*=0.73). Defense maturity is also separately rated on a nine-point scale. Vaillant subsequently developed a Q-sort of 51 statements representing 15 defenses with three to six cards per defense (Roston et al. 1992), which is easier to use by less experienced raters. Interrater reliability is a bit lower than the clinical method (*median r*=0.55) but correlates moderately with it (*median r*=0.57).

Defense Mechanism Rating Scales

The fifth edition of the DMRS (Perry 1990a) was devised for rating the qualitative presence of a defense in a 50-minute dynamic interview. This qualitative scoring can be employed in clinical work without recordings or transcripts. Qualitative assessment yields information for the current time period, specifying which defenses the patient uses. This assessment can be used for a "defense diagnosis" informing clinical work but does not yield data on the actual frequency of usage of individual mechanisms. Relevant clinical data include events occurring in the interview itself, such as dialogue, actions by the patient, silences, and slips of the tongue, or vignettes reported from outside the interview. Additional clinical advice for accurate defense identification is available (Perry and Henry 2004). Published translations are available in French (Perry 2004), Italian (Perry 1994), Danish (Perry 2002), or directly from the author in German, Spanish, and Portuguese (Brazilian).

The DMRS can be used for quantitative assessment when interview recordings and transcripts are available. Using this scoring method, the rater identifies each defense as it occurs. The individual defenses are grouped into defense levels noted in Table 33–1. All of the defense scores can be summarized by an overall defensive functioning score (see Table 33–1). This overall score is calculated by multiplying each defense by a weight according to its place in the overall zero- to seven-point hierarchy of defenses and taking the weighted average of all the defenses rated in the session. The defense levels and overall defensive functioning score correlate in predicted directions with symptoms and functioning, with the lower level defenses predicting higher distress and impairment (Perry 1990b, 1996; Perry and Cooper 1989). Interestingly, disavowal defenses diverge slightly from this pattern. They did not predict self-report measures of distress over follow-up because they guard against recognition of it, but they did predict observer-rated measures of alcohol abuse and antisocial behavior and, to a lesser extent, anxiety and depression (Perry and Cooper 1989).

Defensive Functioning Scale

The Defensive Functioning Scale in DSM-IV-TR is very similar to the DMRS system and consists of a glossary of defense terms and definitions (see Table 33–2). The rater makes a clinical rating of the five most prominent defenses and three most prominent defense levels. The Defensive Functioning Scale has been shown to be reliable and have both convergent and discriminant validity compared with Axes I through V of DSM-III-R (American Psychiatric Association 1987; Perry and Hoglend 1998) and DSM-IV (American Psychiatric Association 1994; Blais et al. 1996; Hilsenroth et al. 2003). This scale is probably the most convenient method for the clinician to use in practice.

Self-Report Measurement of Defenses

Defense Style Questionnaire

The Defense Style Questionnaire (Bond and Wesley 1996; Bond et al. 1983) is the main self-report measure used in studying personality disorders. It has a short (40-question) and a longer (88-question) version and has been translated and validated in many languages including French, Spanish, Italian, Portuguese, German, Dutch, Norwegian, Chinese, and Japanese. The questionnaire items are designed to assess conscious derivatives of defense mechanisms, which are conscious or unconscious mental processes dealing with internal or external stressors. The premise underlying the Defense Style Questionnaire is that people are sufficiently aware of these characteristic styles to provide useful information for assessing defense styles.

Factor analysis of patients' responses yielded four factors of presumed defense mechanisms, which are referred to as *defense styles*. The styles are ranked on a continuum of adaptiveness from lowest to highest: 1) maladaptive action, 2) image-distorting, 3) self-sacrificing, and 4) adaptive. An overall defensive functioning score can be calculated, with a higher score indicating greater adaptiveness or maturity. Based on empirical study (Bond et al. 1983), patients are deemed to score high on styles 1, 2, and 3 if their score is 0.5 standard deviations above the mean for the normative nonpatient group and low on style 4 if their score is 0.5 standard deviations below the mean on that style. The maladaptive defense style—most associated with personality disorders—includes passive aggression and acting-out, whereas the image-distorting style includes splitting and omnipotence/devaluation, the self-sacrificing style includes reaction formation, and the adaptive style includes suppression.

DEFENSES ASSOCIATED WITH PERSONALITY DISORDERS

General Findings

Studies using the Defensive Functioning Scale have found that the diagnosis of any personality disorder (a mixture of types) was associated with significantly

Table 33–1. Defense Mechanism Rating Scales hierarchy of defense levels and individual defense mechanisms

7	High adaptive level (mature)	Affiliation, altruism, anticipation, humor, self-assertion, self-observation, sublimation, suppression
6	Obsessional level	Intellectualization, isolation of affect, undoing
5	Other neurotic level	a) Repression, dissociation; b) Reaction formation, displacement
4	Minor image-distorting level (narcissistic)	Devaluation of self or object images, idealization of self or object images, omnipotence
3	Disavowal level	Denial, projection, rationalization; although not a disavowal defense, autistic fantasy is scored at this level
2	Major image-distorting level (borderline)	Splitting of others' images, splitting of self-images, projective identification
1	Action level	Acting-out, help-rejecting complaining (hypochondriasis), passive aggression
0	Defensive dysregulation level (psychotic)	Distortion, psychotic denial, delusional projection, psychotic dissociation

Note. **Overall Defense Maturity:** This 0–7 scale summarizes defensive functioning by taking the mean score of all the defenses, each weighted according to the above 0–7 scheme.

lower defensive functioning ($r=-0.29$ in Perry and Hoglend 1998; $r=-0.31$ in Hilsenroth et al. 2003). Both studies also found that the Defensive Functioning Scale was factorially largely independent of most measures, except for some association with the presence of personality disorder pathology. Blais et al. (1996) found that total scores of each of the DSM personality disorders mostly correlated significantly with various lower defense levels: action, major image-distorting, disavowal, and minor image-distorting.

Rating early psychotherapy sessions using the DMRS quantitative method, Perry (2001) found that patients with personality disorders had an overall defensive functioning score of 4.32 (range of 3.31 to 4.97). All scores were below the lower threshold of 5.00 for neurotic patients. According to Vaillant's (1976) tripartite classification hierarchy, 49.3% of defensive functioning was attributable to the lower defenses (levels 1–4), 40.8% to neurotic defenses (levels 5–6), and 9.9% to the high adaptive defenses (level 7). Using the qualitative scoring method, Lingiardi et al. (1999) also found that personality disorders were associated with lower- and midlevel defenses. In particular, Cluster B disorders were associated with the action level, whereas Cluster C disorders were associated with midlevel defenses.

The level of stability of defenses across five weekly sessions indicated both state and trait characteristics (median value for the defense levels, intraclass $R=0.47$; overall defensive functioning score, intraclass $R=0.48$), whereas the number of defenses used (intraclass $R=0.14$) appeared more related to state characteristics

such as stress (Perry 2001). When corrected for the reliability of overall defensive functioning, the ratio of variance for patient to occasion (1.3:1.0) indicated that patient trait contributes about 30% more variance for overall defensive functioning than does state or occasion week to week. In particular, the high adaptive defenses were the least stable (intraclass $R=0.08$), indicating inconsistent use by personality disorders early in therapy.

In a follow-along study of borderline, antisocial, and schizotypal personality disorders and bipolar II disorder, Perry (1996) found that action and major image-distorting defenses and overall defensive functioning predicted self-destructive symptoms, such as recurrent suicidal ideation, suicide attempts, and self-cutting as well as symptoms (Perry and Cooper 1989) and exacerbations of episodes of depression (Perry 1988, 1990b). Action and disavowal defenses predicted alcohol and drug use, antisocial symptoms (Perry and Cooper 1989), and, along with minor image-distorting defenses, risk taking. Minor image-distorting defenses predicted dysthymic symptoms (Perry 1990b). Hysterical defenses were also associated with suicide attempts and self-cutting as well as anorexia. By contrast, obsessional defenses clearly showed a protective role against both impulsive and depressive symptoms (Perry 1988, 1990b, 1996; Perry and Cooper 1989). The robust patterns of prediction are consistent with the theoretical assumption that defenses are fundamental mechanisms of personality functioning that underlie a wide variety of symptoms and problematic behaviors.

Specific Personality Disorders

Observer-Based Findings

Vaillant and Drake (1985) examined a follow-up sample of inner-city men at age 47 for the presence of a personality disorder and for defenses rated from life vignettes gathered about the past decade. Of those with any Axis II diagnosis, 66% used mostly immature defenses (projection, fantasy, hypochondriasis, passive aggression, acting-out, and dissociation/denial) as opposed to 10% of those without an Axis II disorder. Conversely, the use of mature defenses such as humor, sublimation, and suppression correlated negatively with the presence of a personality disorder. The following specific personality disorders were highly associated with certain defenses:

> *Paranoid:* projection 100%, acting-out 75%
> *Schizoid:* autistic fantasy 33%
> *Antisocial:* acting-out 75%,
>   dissociation/denial 63%
> *Narcissistic:* dissociation/denial 83%,
>   acting-out 61%, projection 39%
> *Dependent:* dissociation/denial 56%
> *Passive-aggressive:* passive aggression 64%,
>   dissociation/denial 43%
> *Avoidant:* passive aggression 25%,
>   dissociation/denial 25%

BPD was not found in this middle-aged male sample. Unlike the other disorders, avoidant personality disorder did not demonstrate an association with particular defenses, suggesting that it may be dynamically more heterogeneous than the others. Conversely, narcissistic personality disorder demonstrated a defense profile similar to that of antisocial personality, although the former scored far lower on a sociopathic symptom scale than the latter. This finding suggested that both disorders may be dynamically related, as Perry and Perry (2004) later confirmed. Limitations in the data (i.e., dictated interview summaries) and rating method (qualitative) may have led to underidentification of defenses and thus diminished the above associations, when a strong association might have been expected.

In a study of personality and mood disorders using qualitative DMRS ratings only, Perry and Cooper (1986) found that borderline psychopathology was significantly associated with the major image-distorting defenses (splitting and projective identification; $r=0.36$) and the action defenses (acting-out, hypochondriasis, passive aggression; $r=0.26$). Antisocial psychopathol-

ogy correlated with minor image-distorting defenses (omnipotence, idealization, devaluation; $r=0.23$) and with disavowal defenses (denial, projection, and rationalization; $r=0.22$). By contrast, the mood disorder bipolar type II was associated with the higher-level obsessional defenses (isolation, intellectualization, and undoing; $r=0.37$). However, qualitative ratings of defenses were not able to discriminate the three study diagnoses from one another. Perry and Perry (2004) examined narcissistic personality disorder features in the same sample and found that the disorder was positively associated with four defenses: omnipotence, devaluation, autistic fantasy, and projection—and negatively associated with one: repression. These findings held up even when controlling for the association between narcissistic personality disorder and antisocial personality disorder in the sample. Together with other data on conflicts, these findings support the idea that narcissistic features are adaptations to underlying problems in regulating self-esteem and affect and are not synonymous with antisocial behavior.

Dahl (1984) examined hospitalized patients using the Bellak Ego Function Assessment. The borderline diagnostic group had overall defensive functioning that was significantly higher than a schizophrenic group but not different from a group with affective psychoses. Borderline patients scored lower than those with other personality disorders and neuroses, a finding in keeping with Kernberg's (1975) assertion that borderline personality organization is less healthy than neurotic personality organization. Also using the same instrument, Goldsmith et al. (1984) found that defensive functioning and level of object relations were the two ego functions that best differentiated borderline from neurotic patients.

In comparing patients with personality disorders with and without BPD, Perry (2001) found that the BPD group had a significantly lower overall defensive functioning score (4.07 versus 4.62), principally due to greater reliance on action and major image-distorting defenses. This finding confirmed the qualitative findings of earlier authors (e.g., Kernberg 1975). Interestingly, BPD patients often had a wide range of defenses in their repertoire, but their reliance on high adaptive, low action, and major image-distorting levels was not stable, varying greatly from week to week. In some sessions they functioned at a neurotic level, even displaying some high adaptive level defenses, whereas in other sessions their defensive functioning regressed considerably. This instability in defensive functioning mirrored affective, interpersonal, and other areas of instability.

Self-Report Findings

In a study of 78 patients with and 72 patients without BPD, Bond et al. (1994) compared the Defense Style Questionnaire scores of the two groups. The BPD group reported using maladaptive and image-distorting defense styles more often and adaptive defense styles less often than the non-BPD group. Although the BPD group used more splitting and acting-out, they used the adaptive defenses of suppression, sublimation, and humor less than others. This finding suggests that borderline patients' deficit in mastering anxiety, painful emotion, and threatening impulse is related to an underutilization of adaptive defenses and not only an overreliance on the characteristic image-distorting and maladaptive action defenses.

In a study of defense styles as predictors of personality disorder symptoms, Johnson et al. (1992) compared the Defense Style Questionnaire defense styles and the Personality Diagnostic Questionnaire–Revised (PDQ-R) assessing personality disorder. The Defense Style Questionnaire maladaptive and image-distorting defense styles were significantly and positively associated with the PDQ-R composite index (regression model R^2=0.27 and 0.34, respectively) as well as with a total of 11 and 7 of the personality disorder subscales, respectively. The image-distorting defense style was the sole predictor of narcissistic and antisocial personality disorder subscales. The adaptive and image-distorting defense styles both predicted scores on the histrionic personality disorder subscale. The adaptive (negative direction) and image-distorting styles both predicted sadistic personality disorder. The Defense Style Questionnaire adaptive style was significantly negatively associated with the PDQ-R composite index (regression model R^2=0.23).

In a study examining personality dimensions associated with depressive personality disorder, Lyoo et al. (1998) used the Defense Style Questionnaire in a sample of 26 patients with depressive personality disorder and 20 depressed patients without depressive personality disorder. Individuals with depressive personality disorder used the adaptive defense style less than did the depressed control subjects. They scored lower on the maladaptive defense style than Bond's patient group but higher than his nonpatient group.

A Finnish study (Sammallahti et al. 1994) found that omnipotence, devaluation, splitting, denial, isolation, and projective identification loaded on a factor that consisted of typical "borderline" defenses (Cronbach's alpha=0.72). A group of 31 patients with personality disorders had higher scores on this factor than did 42 neurotic patients or 353 community control subjects.

Five studies have found that the maladaptive style was significantly associated with personality disorder, especially with Cluster B disorders (Devens and Erickson 1998; Genden 1995; Mulder et al. 1999; Sinha and Watson 1999; Sun 2000). The adaptive style was negatively associated with Cluster B disorders.

Although certain specific defense mechanisms and defense styles are both significantly correlated empirically and associated theoretically with specific personality disorders, one cannot safely diagnose a personality disorder simply by identifying a characteristic defense. People use a wide range of defenses, and the defenses used vary somewhat with the person's external circumstances as well as with his or her state of mind. We can say that once a particular diagnosis is made based on the usual set of criteria, there is a high likelihood that the individual will use that disorder's characteristic defenses.

PSYCHOTHERAPY AND CHANGE IN DEFENSIVE FUNCTIONING

In personality disorders, defenses can be somewhat volatile from session to session, which represents state, not stable, trait change (Perry 2001). Table 33–3 presents the results of four naturalistic treatment studies that examined change using the DMRS overall defensive functioning. In a four-session dynamic intake, Drapeau et al. (2003) found that as distress diminished, patients used fewer defenses and overall defensive functioning increased somewhat, with an effect size of 0.46. Patients relied on fewer minor image-distorting and more obsessional defenses, indicating a decrease in protecting self-esteem in favor of greater reliance on minimizing distressing affect. These changes were modest and most likely represented a return to usual level of functioning, because overall defensive functioning and the proportion of high adaptive defenses were still low.

Some research on short-term psychotherapy demonstrates modest improvement in defensive functioning alongside other measures of symptoms and functioning. Examination of defenses in two samples, in which more than 60% had personality disorders, found that after about 6 months of treatment, overall defensive functioning improved about 0.4, which due to differences in heterogeneity yielded medium effect sizes of 0.41 (Perry et al. 1999) and 0.82 (Hersoug et al. 2002). In neither sample did overall defensive functioning reach the healthy-neurotic range. By contrast, a sample in which more than 80% of subjects had personality disorders (40% with

Table 33–2. Glossary of specific defense mechanisms and coping styles

acting out The individual deals with emotional conflict or internal or external stressors by actions rather than reflections or feelings. This definition is broader than the original concept of the acting out of transference feelings or wishes during psychotherapy and is intended to include behavior arising both within and outside the transference relationship. Defensive acting out is not synonymous with "bad behavior" because it requires evidence that the behavior is related to emotional conflicts.

affiliation The individual deals with emotional conflict or internal or external stressors by turning to others for help or support. This involves sharing problems with others but does not imply trying to make someone else responsible for them.

altruism The individual deals with emotional conflict or internal or external stressors by dedication to meeting the needs of others. Unlike the self-sacrifice sometimes characteristic of reaction formation, the individual receives gratification either vicariously or from the response of others.

anticipation The individual deals with emotional conflict or internal or external stressors by experiencing emotional reactions in advance of, or anticipating consequences of, possible future events and considering realistic, alternative responses or solutions.

autistic fantasy The individual deals with emotional conflict or internal or external stressors by excessive daydreaming as a substitute for human relationships, more effective action, or problem solving.

denial The individual deals with emotional conflict or internal or external stressors by refusing to acknowledge some painful aspect of external reality or subjective experience that would be apparent to others. The term *psychotic denial* is used when there is gross impairment in reality testing.

devaluation The individual deals with emotional conflict or internal or external stressors by attributing exaggerated negative qualities to self or others.

displacement The individual deals with emotional conflict or internal or external stressors by transferring a feeling about, or a response to, one object onto another (usually less threatening) substitute object.

dissociation The individual deals with emotional conflict or internal or external stressors with a breakdown in the usually integrated functions of consciousness, memory, perception of self or the environment, or sensory/motor behavior.

help-rejecting complaining The individual deals with emotional conflict or internal or external stressors by complaining or making repetitive requests for help that disguise covert feelings of hostility or reproach toward others, which are then expressed by rejecting the suggestions, advice, or help that others offer. The complaints or requests may involve physical or psychological symptoms or life problems.

humor The individual deals with emotional conflict or external stressors by emphasizing the amusing or ironic aspects of the conflict or stressor.

idealization The individual deals with emotional conflict or internal or external stressors by attributing exaggerated positive qualities to others.

intellectualization The individual deals with emotional conflict or internal or external stressors by the excessive use of abstract thinking or the making of generalizations to control or minimize disturbing feelings.

isolation of affect The individual deals with emotional conflict or internal or external stressors by the separation of ideas from the feelings originally associated with them. The individual loses touch with the feelings associated with a given idea (e.g., a traumatic event) while remaining aware of the cognitive elements of it (e.g., descriptive details).

omnipotence The individual deals with emotional conflict or internal or external stressors by feeling or acting as if he or she possesses special powers or abilities and is superior to others.

passive aggression The individual deals with emotional conflict or internal or external stressors by indirectly and unassertively expressing aggression toward others. There is a facade of overt compliance masking covert resistance, resentment, or hostility. Passive aggression often occurs in response to demands for independent action or performance or the lack of gratification of dependent wishes but may be adaptive for individuals in subordinate positions who have no other way to express assertiveness more overtly.

projection The individual deals with emotional conflict or internal or external stressors by falsely attributing to another his or her own unacceptable feelings, impulses, or thoughts.

projective identification As in projection, the individual deals with emotional conflict or internal or external stressors by falsely attributing to another his or her own unacceptable feelings, impulses, or thoughts. Unlike simple projection, the individual does not fully disavow what is projected. Instead, the individual remains aware of his or her own affects or impulses but misattributes them as justifiable reactions to the other person. Not infrequently, the individual induces the very feelings in others that were first mistakenly believed to be there, making it difficult to clarify who did what to whom first.

Table 33–2. Glossary of specific defense mechanisms and coping styles *(continued)*

rationalization   The individual deals with emotional conflict or internal or external stressors by concealing the true motivations for his or her own thoughts, actions, or feelings through the elaboration of reassuring or self-serving but incorrect explanations.

reaction formation   The individual deals with emotional conflict or internal or external stressors by substituting behavior, thoughts, or feelings that are diametrically opposed to his or her own unacceptable thoughts or feelings (this usually occurs in conjunction with their repression).

repression   The individual deals with emotional conflict or internal or external stressors by expelling disturbing wishes, thoughts, or experiences from conscious awareness. The feeling component may remain conscious, detached from its associated ideas.

self-assertion   The individual deals with emotional conflict or stressors by expressing his or her feelings and thoughts directly in a way that is not coercive or manipulative.

self-observation   The individual deals with emotional conflict or stressors by reflecting on his or her own thoughts, feelings, motivation, and behavior, and responding appropriately.

splitting   The individual deals with emotional conflict or internal or external stressors by compartmentalizing opposite affect states and failing to integrate the positive and negative qualities of the self or others into cohesive images. Because ambivalent affects cannot be experienced simultaneously, more balanced views and expectations of self or others are excluded from emotional awareness. Self and object images tend to alternate between polar opposites: exclusively loving, powerful, worthy, nurturant, and kind—or exclusively bad, hateful, angry, destructive, rejecting, or worthless.

sublimation   The individual deals with emotional conflict or internal or external stressors by channeling potentially maladaptive feelings or impulses into socially acceptable behavior (e.g., contact sports to channel angry impulses).

suppression   The individual deals with emotional conflict or internal or external stressors by intentionally avoiding thinking about disturbing problems, wishes, feelings, or experiences.

undoing   The individual deals with emotional conflict or internal or external stressors by words or behavior designed to negate or to make amends symbolically for unacceptable thoughts, feelings, or actions.

Source. Reprinted from American Psychiatric Association: *Diagnostic and Statistical Manual of Mental Disorders,* 4th Edition, Text Revision. Washington, DC, American Psychiatric Association, 2000, pp. 811–813. Used with permission. Copyright © 2000 American Psychiatric Association.

BPD) upon entering long-term psychotherapy showed only a small effect size (0.16) at 1 year (Perry 2001). However, one case was followed until termination after 4 years of psychotherapy (180 sessions), with a follow-up at 10 years. Although termination occurred for external reasons, the patient improved 0.45 on overall defensive functioning, about a full effect size, thus attaining the threshold between personality disorder and neurotic defensive functioning. The patient was making progress toward a career, and by 10-year follow-up, the patient had continued to improve substantially (Global Assessment of Functioning score 80), attaining healthy-neurotic functioning (overall defensive functioning score 5.80), which suggested that therapy was also successful in producing delayed treatment effects. In addition, the patient's changes were largely in line with the hierarchy of defenses: decreases in low-level and increases in high adaptive level defenses. Although it is clear that defensive functioning does change with psychotherapy, more research is needed on how much of which types of psychotherapy will yield sufficient degrees of improvement in defensive functioning to enable patients to function at healthy levels.

Hersoug et al. (2002) found support for the phase model of change in brief psychotherapy (mean, 38 sessions). Symptomatic improvement began early in treatment, whereas change in defensive functioning did not begin until the midphase of treatment.

In a naturalistic study of long-term psychotherapy, Bond and Perry (2004) examined change on the Defense Style Questionnaire over a mean of 4.4 years of follow-up, including a mean of 3.0 years of psychotherapy. Seventy-five percent of the sample had a personality disorder. Those with high initial scores on the maladaptive and self-sacrificing defense styles 1 and 3 decreased significantly, with effect sizes of 0.80 and 0.67, whereas the overall defensive functioning score increased significantly (effect size 0.43).

CLINICAL WORK WITH DEFENSES IN PERSONALITY DISORDERS

In this clinical section, we describe three aims in working with defenses and end with several excerpts of

Table 33–3. Change in overall defensive functioning with psychotherapy

	Perry and Hoglend 1998		Perry 2001		Hersoug et al. 2002		Drapeau et al. 2003	
Sample size, N	37		15		39		61	
Months in therapy	6		12		9		1	
Subjects with a personality disorder, %	62		80		65		38	
GAF	52		56		55			
GSI	1.38				1.38		0.90	
Overall defensive functioning score								
mean (SD)	4.68	SD=1.05	4.27	SD=0.45	4.40	SD=0.51	4.37	SD=0.57
1-month[a]	4.94	ES =0.25			4.41	ES=0.02	4.65[b]	ES=0.49
6-month[a]	5.11	ES=0.41			4.82	ES=0.82		
12-month[a]			4.34	ES=0.16				

Note. Mean for healthy-neurotic functioning is overall defensive functioning=5.67.
ES=effect size; GAF=Global Assessment of Functioning; GSI=General Severity Index; SD=standard deviation.
[a]Mean and within-condition effect size.
[b]Improvement over four sessions.

transcripts of psychotherapy sessions with personality-disordered patients with the therapist's interventions categorized according to the Psychodynamic Intervention Rating Scale (PIRS; Cooper and Bond 1992; Milbrath et al. 1999). The PIRS intervention categories and explanations are shown in Table 33–4. The therapies were conducted as part of a naturalistic, long-term, follow-along study and all sessions were audiotaped (Bond and Perry 2004).

Principles of Working With Defenses

Identifying defenses aids psychotherapy. Each defense is a signal of distress, and reading it correctly allows the therapist to estimate how much distress the patient is feeling, how the patient is trying to protect him- or herself, what motives or conflicts may underlie the defensive activity, and whether the therapist should respond more supportively or interpretively. Because each patient uses an average of 40–60 defenses in 50 minutes (Perry and Henry 2004), defenses offer a lot of useful information for the therapist to consider. Spotting manifestations of DSM Axis II criteria does not offer the same degree of useful information.

There are three sets of aims in working with defenses: first, identifying defenses and avoiding countertransference problems; second, managing and supporting defenses; and third, exploring and interpreting defenses and developing insight. Identifying defenses and avoiding countertransference overreactions are

necessary to allow the other two aims to develop. In turn, supporting and managing defenses allows the exploratory and interpretive aims to develop.

Identifying Defenses and Avoiding Countertransference Problems

In general, use of the lower-level defenses corresponds to a state of mind in which the patient feels attacked or threatened. Even if the threat is internal, such as a conflicting wish to express oneself and fear of retaliation, the patient with personality disorder tends to externalize it and see others as the cause of the problem. Whenever the patient experiences the therapist as the source of the problem, action and major image-distorting defenses may predominate, which often evoke intense countertransference reactions from the therapist. Table 33–5 displays the five most troublesome defenses and problems that the therapist may have in dealing with the countertransference reactions. Despite the difficulty, it is valuable for the therapist to realize that his or her reaction is a clue to the patient's experience. The negative role that the therapist is tempted to step into would be a reenactment of some earlier interaction pattern, representing a role that the patient expects the therapist to play as significant others have done in the past. If the therapist successfully identifies the defense and his or her own reaction, and thus avoids reenacting the expected negative role, he or she can then consider other ways to manage, explore, and interpret the interchange.

Table 33–4. Psychodynamic Intervention Rating Scale

Interpretive interventions

Defense interpretations: Therapist remarks that try to point out, refer to, or explain the motives for processes that mitigate or diminish affect or processes that reflect shifts in the content of topics or representations of persons. These interventions may address any aspect of a dynamic conflict.

Transference interpretations: Therapist remarks that point out, refer to, wonder about, or explain the patient's experience of the therapeutic relationship.

Noninterpretive interventions

Acknowledgments: Therapist remarks intended to convey that the patient's communication has been received.

Clarification: Therapist remarks that summarize what the patient has said without interpretation and with the intent of ensuring that the therapist has understood properly the patient's communication.

Questions: Therapist inquiries about affects or details of the patient's life, relationships, or significant others. These are not considered interpretive.

Associations: Therapist remarks that reflect on something the patient has said at another point, but without making an interpretation, or that involve therapist self-disclosures or general statements of fact or opinion. These may include answers to questions or explanations.

Reflections: Therapist remarks in which the intent is to briefly express the patient's experience; usually this involves the assertion of an affect.

Work-enhancing strategies: Therapist remarks that explain the value and rationale of therapy and encourage the patient to say whatever comes to mind, no matter how seemingly unimportant or obscure.

Support strategies: Therapist remarks that make suggestions, reinforce, or question patient's solutions to various problems.

Contractual arrangements: Therapist remarks that relate to the "when's," "for how long's," and "how much's" of treatment.

Managing and Supporting Defenses

Managing and supporting defenses is appropriate whenever the patient appears to be functioning poorly with distress. At such times, there may be a rapid shift from one defense to another. The patient may feel attacked (neglected, blamed, criticized, shamed, dominated) by external sources and actively ignore internal issues. Relying on lower-level defenses at such times protects the individual from awareness of internal conflicts (e.g., fear of asserting oneself) by externalizing problems, artificially upregulating self-esteem, and counterattacking to minimize immediate distress in interactions with others. In this state of mind, individuals find psychological exploration threatening, and they mistrust others. The therapist must respect the patient's limitations in this state of mind and try to mange or diffuse it.

In extreme situations, the therapist may use *limit-setting techniques* that aim to inhibit loss of control. These limit the damage that might otherwise occur if the patient continues. A common example of acting-out might be yelling at the therapist or threatening to leave and hurt oneself. The therapist may use a *work-enhancing strategy* in such situations. These have some overlap with what are sometimes called *confrontations*. In the example of the loud patient, the therapist might say forcefully:

> "Stop yelling, I can't listen to you! [Brief pause as the patient looks at the therapist.] I can't really think how to help if you raise your voice so much."

Sometimes a defense interpretation may also be required to accomplish the limit setting. In an example in which the patient threatens to leave and hurt him or herself, the therapist may say something like:

> "I think you're putting the therapy in the same bind that you feel yourself in: life or death. [D3 Defense interpretation, including motive (described later)] Why don't you stay here and talk about the bind you're in instead of threatening to kill the therapy?" (Work-enhancing strategy)

An example of *projection* might occur in the patient who, facing a setback, questions whether the therapist is part of a vague conspiracy to harm the patient's interests in some way. In this example, the therapist might say something that has an element of transference interpretation in it but essentially suggests a limit in the service of improving the therapy:

> "It will be better if you try to resist lumping me in with the others who you're concerned about. I'll be better able to help if you keep me neutral." (Work-enhancing strategy)

The above examples manage rather than explore the negative transference underlying the defense. A more exploratory response at the same juncture would generally invite mistrust, stimulate anxiety or other negative affect, and further damage the therapeutic alliance. The more limit-setting approach tries to establish some control or limit on the defenses that are damaging the therapeutic alliance and thus reset back to a more collaborative stance.

Table 33–5.   Defense and countertransference problems in personality disorders

Defense	Countertransference problem
Splitting:	
The subject sees him- or herself as all negative or sees another person, such as the therapist, as all bad.	The therapist feels the patient is failing to see both sides of the picture and tries to argue the other side. This countertransference reaction leads to lecturing the patient, forcing the therapist's own perspective on the patient, and paradoxically entrenching the patient. When a negative self-image is activated, the patient will regress and become even more self-hating and potentially suicidal. Splitting is reinforced, making it harder for the subject to integrate positive and negative experiences.
Projective identification:	
The subject feels angry but sees this as a response to the therapist, who is perceived as angry first.	The therapist feels unjustly accused and after first trying to be rational with the patient, finally gets frustrated or feels abused and then begins to see the patient as out of control. This countertransference reaction leads to covert wishes to control the patient and to an enactment in which the therapist inadvertently becomes controlling and abusive from the patient's perspective. This enactment reinforces the subject's belief that the therapist has the very feelings imputed to him or her.
Help-rejecting complaining:	
The patient makes a series of complaints and feels increasingly angry that the therapist is not helping.	The therapist initially tries to respond to the complaints or requests with directive responses or suggestions. When help is rejected, the therapist may use reaction formation and try harder until very frustrated, at which time he or she may feel like abandoning the patient. This countertransference reaction reinforces the subject's belief that no one cares enough to help.
Acting-out:	
The subject expresses something in impulsive action that he or she feels is neither permissible nor possible to talk about.	The therapist feels that the patient is misbehaving and reacts to control and punish the patient. The patient feels blamed and abused, and the belief that there is something bad about the original wish is reinforced.
Passive aggression:	
The patient is angry but expresses it through noncooperation: lateness, missing sessions, not bringing up feelings toward the therapist.	The therapist resents the patient's lack of engagement and responds in kind: not focusing on the indirectly expressed anger. The patient then feels even more that the therapist does not care. Or the therapist confronts the patient in a scolding, blaming way; the patient feels humiliated and the belief that anger cannot be dealt with is reinforced.

Supportive Interventions

These techniques are often associated with the so-called nonspecific aspects of psychotherapy. They aim to allow the patient to return to his or her best level of functioning. They include most noninterpretive interventions. *Acknowledgements* convey that the therapist is actively listening. *Questions* help focus the patient in a new direction or better relate the details of a vignette, especially when inability to focus heightens the patient's distress. The therapist's *associations* can provide comforting examples or thoughts that help the patient feel less alone or stigmatized and more understood. *Reflections* help the patient see his or her own stated feelings as a focus of concern. *Clarifications* help untangle confusing or missing aspects of a story. *Support strategies* such as offering praise or making direct suggestions can give helpful

feedback or offer new alternatives for thinking or acting whenever the patient is receptive. Together these techniques allow the patient to reveal what is on his or her mind in a nonthreatening way. Successful supportive interventions allow emotional elaboration and set the stage for deeper exploratory work aimed at improving defensive functioning and producing insight.

If the therapist considers each session in phases, supportive interventions are most used in the beginning and middle phases to allow the patient to bring in whatever material is salient and to defuse some of the accompanying distress. Exploratory and interpretive interventions may be used gingerly in the middle phase—mostly to increase exploration of affectively meaningful material—and then more extensively and deeply in the last phase. These phases also replicate across the duration of the therapy, so that during the early and middle phases of treatment support predominates over exploration and interpretation. Later, as the patient improves, more time is spent in the middle and late phases, with a concomitant increase in exploration and interpretation.

For example, in brief therapy (mean 38 sessions) using the PIRS, Hersoug et al. (2003) found that interpretive interventions increased significantly toward the middle of the therapy, whereas supportive interventions decreased somewhat.

Exploring, Interpreting, and Developing Insight

Whereas support is designed to help the patient return to his or her usual best level of functioning, exploration and interpretation aim at developing insight and improving overall defensive functioning. This process may occur at successively deeper levels, called D1 through D5, that combine elements including affect, defensive operation, motive for the defense, objects affected, and how the defense was learned in formative relationships. In particular, defense interpretation aims to help the patient become aware of material that is outside of awareness. The successively more complex levels are as follows:

D1: Identifying a feeling of which the patient is completely or partly unaware.

D2: Pointing out the defensive activity itself and the self-deception that it provides.

D3: Deeper defense interpretations point up the more complex motives that a defense may protect against, inhibit, or gratify, such as the wish to dominate in acting-out or the gratification of a sense of victimization in passive aggression.

D4: Higher-level defense interpretations aim at providing awareness of the patterns of usage involving important objects in the patient's life.

D5: A D4 interpretation may deepen further when it includes genetic material from formative relationships and experiences related to present patterns of defenses.

Overall, defense interpretations aim to promote awareness of one's mental life, decrease anxiety, increase comfort and acceptance of one's feelings and motives, and improve the ability to reflect on and then choose to alter the choice of defenses in stressful and conflictual situations. Together, these help the patient optimize defensive functioning toward the highest-level defense possible for a given situation. More succinctly, better defenses accompany more freedom of choice.

Hersoug et al. (2003) found that more experienced therapists use more defense interpretations in short-term therapy than do less experienced therapists. In a study of brief psychotherapy for individuals dealing with grief, defense interpretations were correlated with positive reduction in symptoms after therapy (Milbrath et al. 1999). Within sessions, patients' emotional elaborations were followed by therapists' defense interpretations, which in turn led to more emotional elaboration. Noninterpretive interventions were followed by patient disclosure of facts, not emotions.

Exploration and insight are not limited to one's defenses, and thus some of the most important interpretations involve transference. Much of the content of transference interpretations involves the patient's defenses, although the focus includes the therapist. These interpretations too are offered at successively deeper levels over time. However, this discussion is beyond the scope of the present chapter.

Optimizing the Mix of Supportive and Exploratory-Interpretive Interventions

Some research suggests that supportive interventions alone are not enough, even in the earliest of sessions. In a four-session dynamic intake, Despland et al. (2001) found that whenever the alliance starts out poorly, adjusting the level of exploration to the patient's overall defensive functioning leads to improving alliances. Thus exploratory-interpretive work was necessary, but it was effective only if adjusted to one's defensive level.

Whenever the therapist relies on exploratory techniques too soon, the patient may feel threatened and respond with a flurry of defensive activity and a downward shift in his or her defense repertoire. This regression is often perceived colloquially as acting "more defensive." Managing defenses can occur in any phase in which a rupture of the alliance occurs and the patient suddenly shifts to a predominance of action, image-distorting, or disavowal defenses. Generally, if this problem arises in the third and final phase of the session, it signals a serious problem across the whole session, in which the patient's defenses have not been supported enough. The use of deep defense or transference interpretations at the end of a turbulent session, so-called "Hail Mary" interpretations, usually exacerbates rather than repairs such ruptures in the alliance.

Piper and colleagues (1991) demonstrated that the quality of object relations may influence the level of therapeutic alliance and outcome. In particular, patients with low quality of object relations—likely associated with lower defensive functioning—may not do as well in highly interpretive compared with supportive forms of short-term therapy (Piper et al. 1998).

The therapeutic alliance may be an important indicator of problems with the mix of interventions. The pattern of change in early alliance appears to be predictive of outcome. In a sample of subjects in which the majority had a personality disorder, Piper et al. (1995) found that among patients with low quality of object relations, the change pattern (slope) of the alliance was a more significant predictor than the overall level of the alliance, although both made unique contributions to change; whereas in patients with high quality of object relations there was no significant variation in slopes, so the overall level of alliance was a better predictor. This finding suggests that in the early phase of therapy with personality disorders, therapists should monitor changes in the alliance carefully, addressing concerns about the alliance when it deteriorates or fails to improve.

Defenses may play a special role in alliance formation. Bond and Perry (2004) found that high levels of maladaptive, image-distorting, and self-sacrificing defense styles were associated with poorer alliance, whereas adaptive style was associated with a good alliance. Foreman and Marmar (1985) described a series of patients with initially poor alliances that improved and led to good outcomes when the therapists addressed the patients' defenses and resistance. Gaston et al. (1988) found that higher degrees of defensiveness contributed to lower working alliance in behavioral, cognitive, and brief dynamic therapies for depression. In a study of the therapeutic process in a personality disorder sample, Winston et al. (1994) found that addressing defenses was highly correlated with improvement in target complaints. The evidence suggests, then, that the careful use of interpretation of defense and resistance can help improve the alliance and outcome of therapy, whereas aggressive use of interpretative techniques will overwhelm or threaten those patients with a lower level of defensive functioning.

Specific Examples of Working With Defenses in Psychotherapy

Parts of some transcript material have been reported in previous papers (Banon et al. 2001; Bond et al. 1998).

Case Example

In this therapy, the therapist's intellectualizing style calms down the patient so that he is open to later interpretation, and the therapist returns to the noninterpre-

tive work when the patient's anxiety seems too high. This patient's tendency to use acting-out defenses (e.g., alcohol consumption, having affairs, leaving situations such as marriage, and inconsistent attendance in therapy) indicates a high risk for disruption of therapeutic alliance and guides the therapist to be very careful with defense interpretation.

Mr. JJ had a mixed narcissistic and obsessive personality disorder and presented with a major depressive episode and comorbid substance abuse. By self-report questionnaires, his early alliance was good. Following interpretive work, he began in session four to manifest intense anxiety and mild disorganization. Responding to his anxiety over the unstructured frame, his male therapist adopted a reassuring style with intellectual explanations and support.

> Patient (Repression): I just have a bunch of rambling thoughts right now… total series of disconnected rambling thoughts that, uh—sort of nothing to do with anything.
> Therapist: But it's exactly those that we would be interested in. It's unstructured and that's how it works best. [Work-enhancing strategy] But, that has made you uncomfortable to…but, that has made you uncomfortable to start with because you're not—well, it's a new experience for you. (Reflection)

This approach appeared to settle the patient, who then continued in a calmer and more intellectual vein:

> Patient (Intellectualization): You've probably noticed also that I tend to try to structure my thoughts, and I try to sort of have one thing follow from A to B to C to D rather than just bounce around.

Early session material for this obsessional patient is consistent with a fear of emotional intensity and a fear of losing control. Later in the same session, the patient's anxiety was again apparent:

> Patient (Undoing): I know—I have the strong feeling that in time it will be that, the nonrejection of either one or the other. The acceptation of both these things is going to ultimately be very fruitful for me and will be very positive. But right now they are a source of a big problem. And sometimes I get frightened and I say well, maybe I am making a mistake. Maybe it's just one or the other.

Despite the intellectual language, the therapist responds to a build-up of emotion reflected in the patient's allusion to "strong feeling," "big problem," and "frightened" and adopts a reassuring intellectual stance:

Therapist: Okay, again I don't have an idea yet about what this is all about because I don't know you well enough. But as I have said before, I'm impressed with how exigent you are with yourself. You're quite self-critical and there's—quite self-critical in the sense of being severe and harsh with yourself. I agree that a certain self-observation, a certain self-criticism is necessary for everyone, but not in a sense that I think that I'm hearing from you in terms of the harshness and severity of your criticisms of yourself. You see, there is a parallel between this process of psychotherapy and the kind of work you do. [Defense interpretation]…there is creativity there in a certain way you have to let your mind go in whatever direction and then something forms. Well, it's similar here. The way this process works best is that if you try your best to tell me everything that you are aware of that's rushing by. (Work-enhancing strategy)

The therapist offered a defense interpretation couched in intellectual and emotionally distancing terms, followed by a return to a noninterpretive intervention—a work-enhancing strategy. This approach appeared to calm the patient without threatening his self-esteem and preserved the alliance as seen by the patient's response, in which he reported on his internal state in a nonobsessional way:

Patient (Self-observation): Well, that makes me feel good, hearing that, because I was wanting to try to be more structured and more coherent.

Later in session five, the patient discussed his extramarital affair with emotional intensity expressed in fractured and disorganized discourse. The therapist sensed that Mr. JJ tolerated this depressive affect poorly and distracted him away from these painful feelings with a task—in essence, an invitation to intellectualization:

Patient (Undoing): And of course also had I had…to suffer through a long period of loneliness of whatever, which hasn't happened…So when I say the other day…I think I do feel guilty about, uh, because it's happened, uh, I'm not giving a chance to our marriage…but at the same time I'm not—I don't feel capable whatsoever to, uh, try again.
Therapist: It might help if you told me more about your own personal set of morals and values that you have as a result of your own life experiences and how that fits in with this. (Question)

This again settled the patient, who continued:

Patient (Intellectualization): I'm a great believer in justice and equality…

In this male–male dyad, the therapist managed the alliance when intense affect emerged early in therapy through distraction and intellectualization and by normalizing his patient's feelings. The alliance remained favorable.

Case Example

Ms. KK had BPD. Her initial alliance was close to the mean for the study sample of dynamic psychotherapy in which she participated (Bond and Perry 2004) but increased steadily over the next 10 sessions. The following example occurred almost at the end of an early session. She had been exploring the point that she can never express anger directly but can only act it out. For instance, in this session she talked about having problems with expressing anger to her husband and sister. Instead of talking, she acted out by having an affair, which simultaneously got back at her husband and expressed her rivalry toward her sister.

Patient (Repression): I just can't say no. Why can't I say no?
Therapist: Exactly. (Acknowledgement)
Patient: I can't say what I want.
Therapist: I think that's the problem—that you're resorting or you have to resort to acting, doing. (Defense interpretation)
Patient: Instead of talking.
Therapist: Instead of talking. And as long as you can't talk you're stuck with having to act out all the time. (Defense interpretation)
Patient (Intellectualization): So that's why I lose the weight, that's why I act my actions?
Therapist: Yes. And that's why you have affairs and that's why you do all sorts of things. So what we have to look at is how come you can't put this into work. (Defense interpretation)
Patient: I can't.
Therapist: After all, you can do it with me quite easily. (Transference interpretation)
Patient: Yes, I can, you see.
Therapist: Uh-huh. (Acknowledgement)
Patient: But then again, not that you're a stranger, but you're—you—you won't judge me, do you understand? You won't get mad at me and walk off and start saying "da da da." You won't do that.
Therapist: I won't attack you. (Transference interpretation)
Patient: That's right. My sister will attack me. My husband will definitely attack me…But I can't talk, and I have to learn how to talk.

This excerpt illustrates well the mutual interaction of therapist and patient in a collaborative process indicative of a strong alliance. The defense interpretations helped open awareness that led the patient to face her feelings toward the therapist without the danger of her defensive structure crumbling like a dam, flooding her with overwhelming feelings. This process enabled the patient and therapist to explore the transference relationship, integrate their findings, and generalize to other areas of the patient's life.

CONCLUSIONS

The clinical-theoretical and research literatures concur that personality disorders are associated with certain defenses that are lower on the hierarchy of adaptation, and as a result the overall defensive functioning of patients with personality disorder is lower than that of neurotic or healthy-neurotic individuals. Nevertheless, personality disorders use a larger repertoire that includes a high proportion of neurotic and a low proportion of high adaptive level defenses. Certain defenses are empirically associated with certain disorders, such as BPD with the major image-distorting defenses of splitting and projective identification. These defenses, along with the action defenses such as acting-out or passive aggression, often stimulate countertransference reactions, potentially leading to reenactments of early maladaptive relationship patterns. Correct identification of defenses and attention to one's own response may help the therapist avoid such countertransference reactions.

Attending to the defenses in the interview allows the therapist to respond at the right level by managing or limit setting, supporting, or interpreting and exploring. The alliance, especially early in treatment, may serve as an indicator of how well the therapist is adjusting the mix of support and exploration to fit the patient's level of defensive functioning and ability to tolerate distress.

Psychotherapy studies of patients with personality disorders indicate that defenses change slowly. There may be some improvement early in treatment due to state changes, such as diminishing anxiety and depression, but this improvement probably represents the return to the usual level of functioning. Later in therapy, after symptoms have begun to diminish, defensive functioning may begin to improve. In the short time frame of most studies—1 year or less (Leichsenring and Leibing 2003; Perry et al. 1999)—the patient's improvement is modest and fails to attain healthy functioning. Longer-term treatments may be required for most individuals with personality disorders to attain healthy levels of defensive functioning. Treatment should continue at least until the patient develops the ability to continue the work and improve on his or her own. Further research on all these issues should have immediate clinical implications.

REFERENCES

American Psychiatric Association: Diagnostic and Statistical Manual of Mental Disorders, 3rd Edition, Revised. Washington, DC, American Psychiatric Association, 1987

American Psychiatric Association: Diagnostic and Statistical Manual of Mental Disorders, 4th Edition. Washington, DC, American Psychiatric Association, 1994

American Psychiatric Association: Diagnostic and Statistical Manual of Mental Disorders, 4th Edition, Text Revision. Washington, DC, American Psychiatric Association, 2000

Bader M, Perry JC: Defense mechanisms and relationship episodes among two brief mother–infant psychotherapies). Psychothérapies 21:123–131, 2001

Banon E, Evan-Grenier M, Bond M: Early transference interventions with male patients in psychotherapy. J Psychother Pract Res 10:79–91, 2001

Blais MA, Conboy CA, Wilcox N, et al: An empirical study of the DSM-IV Defensive Functioning Scale in personality disordered patients. Compr Psychiatry 37:435–440, 1996

Bond M, Perry JC: Long-term changes in defense styles with psychodynamic psychotherapy for depressive, anxiety and personality disorders. Am J Psychiatry 161:1665–1671, 2004

Bond M, Wesley S: Manual for the Defense Style Questionnaire. Montreal, Quebec, McGill University, 1996

Bond MP, Gardner S, Christian J, et al: Empirical study of self-rated defense styles. Arch Gen Psychiatry 40:333–338, 1983

Bond M, Paris J, Zweig-Frank H: Defense styles and borderline personality disorder. J Personal Disord 8:28–31, 1994

Bond M, Banon E, Grenier M: Differential effects of interventions on the therapeutic alliance with patients with personality disorders. J Psychother Pract Res 7:301–318, 1998

Cooper SH, Bond M: The Psychodynamic Intervention Ratings Scales (PIRS). Manual published by the authors. Montreal, Canada, 1992. Available from the authors at the Institute of Community and Family Psychiatry, 4333 Chemid de la Cote Ste-Catherine, Montreal, Quebec H3T 1E4, Canada

Dahl AA: Ego function assessment of hospitalized adult psychiatric patients with special reference to borderline patients, in The Broad Scope of Ego Function Assessment. Edited by Bellak L, Goldsmith LA. New York, Wiley, 1984, pp 167–176

Despland J-N, Despars J, de Roten Y, et al: Contribution of patient defense mechanisms and therapist interventions to the development of early therapeutic alliance in a brief psychodynamic investigation. J Psychother Pract Res 10: 155–164, 2001

Devens M, Erikson MT: The relationship between defense styles and personality disorders. J Pers Disord 12:86–93, 1998

Drapeau M, de Roten Y, Perry JC, et al: A study of stability and change in defense mechanisms during a brief psychodynamic investigation. J Nerv Ment Dis 191:496–502, 2003

Foreman SA, Marmar CR: Therapist actions that address initially poor therapeutic alliances in psychotherapy. Am J Psychiatry 142:922–926, 1985

Freud S: Inhibitions, symptoms and anxiety (1926), in The Standard Edition of the Complete Psychological Works of Sigmund Freud, Vol 20. Translated and edited by Strachey J. London, Hogarth Press, 1959, pp 77–175

Gaston L, Marmar CR, Thompson LW, et al: Relation of patient pre-treatment characteristics to the therapeutic alliance in diverse psychotherapies. J Consult Clin Psychol 56:483–489, 1988

Genden SH: A study of the relationship between developmental maturity, ego defenses and personality disorders. Dissertation Abstracts International, Section B: The Sciences and Engineering 56:2B, 1995

Goldsmith LA, Charles E, Feiner K: The use of EFA in the assessment of borderline pathology, in The Broad Scope of Ego Function Assessment. Edited by Bellak L, Goldsmith LA. New York, Wiley, 1984, pp 340–361

Hersoug AG, Sexton HC, Høglend PA: Contribution of defensive functioning to the quality of working alliance and psychotherapy outcome. Am J Psychother 56:539–554, 2002

Hersoug AG, Bøgwald KP, Høglend PA: Are patient and therapist characteristics associated with the use of defense interpretation in brief psychodynamic psychotherapy? Clin Psychol Psychother 10:209–219, 2003

Hilsenroth MJ, Callahan KL, Eudell EM: Further reliability, convergent and discriminant validity of overall defensive functioning. J Nerv Ment Dis 191:730–737, 2003

Johnson JG, Bornstein RF, Krukonis AB: Defense styles as predictors of personality disorder symptomatology. J Personal Disord 6:408–416, 1992

Kernberg OF: Borderline Conditions and Pathological Narcissism. New York, Jason Aronson, 1975

Leichsenring F, Leibing E: The effectiveness of psychodynamic therapy and cognitive behavior therapy in the treatment of personality disorders: a meta-analysis. Am J Psychiatry 160:1223–1232, 2003

Lingiardi V, Lonati C, DeLucchi F, et al: Defense mechanisms and personality disorders. J Nerv Ment Dis 187:224-228, 1999

Lyoo IK, Gunderson JG, Phillips KA: Personality dimensions associated with depressive personality disorder. J Personal Disord 12:46–55, 1998

Milbrath C, Bond M, Cooper S, et al: Sequential consequences of therapists' interventions. J Psychother Pract Res 8:40–54, 1999

Mulder RT, Joyce PR, Sullivan PF, et al: The relationship among three models of personality psychopathology: DSM-III-R personality disorder, TCI scores and DSQ defenses. Psychol Med 29:943–951, 1999

Perry JC: A prospective study of life stress, defenses, psychotic symptoms and depression in borderline and antisocial personality disorders and bipolar type II affective disorder. J Personal Disord 2:49–59, 1988

Perry JC: Defense Mechanism Rating Scales (DMRS), 5th Edition. Cambridge, MA, published by the author, May 1990a

Perry JC: Psychological defense mechanisms in the study of affective and anxiety disorders, in Comorbidity in Anxiety and Mood Disorders. Edited by Maser J, Cloninger CR. Washington, DC, American Psychiatric Press, 1990b, pp 545–562

Perry JC: The study of defense mechanisms and their effects, in Psychodynamic Treatment Research: A Handbook for Clinical Practice. Edited by Miller N, Luborsky L, Barber J, et al. New York, Basic Books, 1993, pp 276–308

Perry JC: Scala di valutazione dei meccanismi di difesa, in I Meccanismi di Defesa: Teoria Clinica e Ricerca Empirica. Edited by Lingiardi V, Madeddu F. Milano, Italy, Raffaello Cortina Editore, 1994, pp 117–198

Perry JC: Defense mechanisms in impulsive versus obsessive-compulsive disorders, in Impulsive Versus Obsessive-Compulsive Disorders. Edited by Oldham J, Skodol AE. Washington, DC, American Psychiatric Press, 1996, pp 195–230

Perry JC: A pilot study of defenses in adults with personality disorders entering psychotherapy. J Nerv Ment Dis 189:651–660, 2001

Perry JC: Defence Mechanism Rating Scales, femte udgave, Instrument til klinisk vurdering af d psykiske forsvarsmekanismer [book translated in Danish by Morton Kjolbye and Per Sorensen]. Aarhus, Denmark, Psykoterapeutisk Forlag, 2002

Perry JC: Echelles D'Evaluation des Mécanismes de Défense. Paris, Masson, 2004

Perry JC, Cooper SH: A preliminary report on defenses and conflicts associated with borderline personality disorder. J Am Psychoanal Assoc 34:865–895, 1986

Perry JC, Cooper SH: An empirical study of defense mechanisms, I: clinical interview and life vignette ratings. Arch Gen Psychiatry 46:444–452, 1989

Perry JC, Henry M: Studying defense mechanisms in psychotherapy using the Defense Mechanism Rating Scales, in Defense Mechanisms: Theoretical, Research and Clinical Perspectives. Edited by Hentschel U, Smith G, Draguns J, et al. Amsterdam, The Netherlands, Elsevier, 2004, pp 165–192

Perry JC, Hoglend P: Convergent and discriminant validity of overall defensive functioning. J Nerv Ment Dis 186:529–535, 1998

Perry JC, Ianni F: Observer-rated measures of defense mechanisms. J Pers 66:993–1024, 1998

Perry JD, Perry JC: Conflicts, defenses and the stability of narcissistic personality features. Psychiatry: Interpersonal and Biological Processes 67:310–330, 2004

Perry JC, Banon L, Ianni F: The effectiveness of psychotherapy for personality disorders. Am J Psychiatry 156:1312–1321, 1999

Piper WE, Azim HFA, Joyce AS, et al: Quality of object relations versus interpersonal functioning as predictors of therapeutic alliance and psychotherapy outcome. J Nerv Ment Dis 179:432–438, 1991

Piper WE, Boroto DR, Joyce AS, et al: Pattern of alliance and outcome in short-term individual psychotherapy. Psychotherapy 32:639–647, 1995

Piper WE, Joyce AS, McCallum M, et al: Interpretive and supportive forms of psychotherapy and patient personality variables. J Consult Clin Psychol 66:558–567, 1998

Roston D, Lee KA, Vaillant GE: A Q-sort approach to identifying defenses, in Ego Mechanisms of Defense: A Guide for Clinicians and Researchers. Edited by Vaillant GE. Washington, DC, American Psychiatric Press, 1992, pp 217–232

Sammallahti P, Aalberg V, Pentinsaari JP: Does defense style vary with severity of mental disorder? an empirical assessment. Acta Psychiatr Scand 90:290–294, 1994

Sinha BD, Watson DC: Predicting personality disorder traits with the Defense Style Questionnaire in a normal sample. J Personal Disord 13:281–286, 1999

Skodol A, Perry JC: Should an axis for defense mechanisms be included in DSM-IV? Compr Psychiatry 34:108–119, 1993

Sun L: Relationship between personality, defense style and mental health in high school students. Chinese Journal of Clinical Psychology 8:231–232, 2000

Vaillant GE: Natural history of male psychological health: the relation of choice of ego mechanisms of defense to adult adjustment. Arch Gen Psychiatry 33:535–545, 1976

Vaillant GE: The Wisdom of the Ego. Cambridge, MA, Harvard University Press, 1993

Vaillant GE, Drake RE: Maturity of ego defenses in relation to DSM-III Axis II personality disorder. Arch Gen Psychiatry 42:597–601, 1985

Winston B, Winston A, Samstag LW, et al: Patient defense/therapist interventions. Psychotherapy 31:478–491, 1994

34

Gender

Leslie C. Morey, Ph.D.
Gerianne M. Alexander, Ph.D.
Christina Boggs, M.S.

The topic of gender in personality disorders has been an issue of considerable discussion since the 1970s. These discussions, while at times fairly heated, have catalyzed a considerable amount of research aimed at understanding how gender contributes to personality disorder. The following sections provide an overview of three topics central to an understanding of the role of gender in personality disorder. First, the literature on gender differences in prevalence of personality disorders is reviewed. Next, the issue of gender bias, and research relevant to this issue, is discussed. Finally, the role of biological factors, and their interplay with social factors as influences on personality disorder, are described.

GENDER DISTRIBUTION OF PERSONALITY DISORDER

Since the first introduction of diagnostic criteria for personality disorders in DSM-III (American Psychiatric Association 1980), the gender distribution of these disorders has been a focus of interest and controversy (e.g., Kaplan 1983). In response to these controversies, some researchers concluded that, across all personality disorders, the prevalence of these disorders in men and women were roughly equivalent, with men more likely to manifest some disorders and women more likely to present with others (Kass et al. 1983; Williams and Spitzer 1983). Given these controversies, the process of developing DSM-IV (American Psychiatric Association 1994) criteria appeared to pay particular attention to gender distribution issues, and in the DSM-IV text it was suggested that 6 of the 10 official personality disorders (paranoid, antisocial, schizoid, schizotypal, narcissistic, obsessive-compulsive) are more prevalent in men, with only 1 (borderline) indicated as being more prevalent in women. However, Corbitt and Widiger (1995) noted that the statements in DSM-IV regarding gender prevalence are not always consistent with available data, and they suggested that DSM-IV may have understated the likelihood of the existence of gender differences in some disorders. In part, this is because the data on gender prevalence are difficult to interpret due to findings from different studies being fraught with problems (Corbitt and Widiger 1995). For example, although some (but not all) studies of personality disorder will publish sample gender distributions, it is typically unclear how these estimates compare to the general gender distribution for the setting in question. As Corbitt and Widiger noted, even these data can be misleading, because certain settings (e.g., eating disorder clinics, substance abuse treatment) may naturally include a disproportionate number of women or men, meaning that a correction for the setting base rate may obscure nonrandom differences.

In addition to the nature of the setting, other methodological aspects of studies also appear to influence estimates of gender distribution for personality disorders. In one study of all Axis II disorders among depressed outpatients, Golomb et al. (1995) found significant differences only for antisocial, narcissistic, and obsessive-compulsive personality disorders, all more prevalent in men when using the Personality Diagnostic Questionnaire–Revised (PDQ-R; Hyler et al. 1987) for assessment. Using a different instrument, the Structured Clinical Interview for DSM-IV Axis II Personality Disorders, the differences were limited to narcissistic and obsessive-compulsive personality disorders. However, when they attempted to control for Axis I comorbidity by examining a subset of their sample without comorbid Axis I disorders, there were no significant gender differences on any personality disorder.

Different conclusions can even be drawn when examining the same instrument in a different way; in a study using combined samples of volunteers and psychiatric patients, Ekselius et al. (1996) found that when data were analyzed by categorical diagnosis, men were more likely to have schizoid or obsessive-compulsive personality disorder, whereas women were more likely to have borderline personality. However, when the data were analyzed dimensionally by criterion count (an approach that would be expected to have greater statistical power), only the borderline difference remained significant.

In recent years, there have been some studies of the distribution of personality disorders in nonclinical settings that address some of the potential artifacts that may result from sampling in clinical settings. For the most part, these studies have supported the conclusion that the overall rate of personality disorders is comparable for men and women. Torgersen et al. (2001) reported no significant gender differences in overall prevalence of personality disorder in a Norwegian sample, with an unweighted prevalence of 12.6% for women and 13.7% for men. In an Australian study,

Jackson and Burgess (2000) also found no differences, with a 6.8% prevalence reported for men and a 6.5% prevalence for women. Using a self-reported dimensional assessment of each DSM-IV-TR (American Psychiatric Association 2000) personality disorder criterion in a college student sample, Morey et al. (2002) found that the mean criterion self-rating for men did not significantly differ from that of women across all 79 criteria. Furthermore, participants in the Morey et al. study were also asked to indicate whether the behaviors would be more problematic for men or for women, and the results indicated that the criterion set was nearly perfectly balanced in this regard, with high agreement among men and women on these ratings.

It should be noted that most studies of gender distributions for personality disorder as a whole have focused on those disorders for which specific diagnostic criteria are presented in DSM. Little is known about the group known in DSM-IV-TR as personality disorder not otherwise specified (PDNOS), which is used to describe individuals who appear to have significant personality problems but do not appear to meet criteria for any of the 10 official DSM diagnoses. In an analysis of 65 patients who would be considered as having PDNOS under DSM-III-R criteria (American Psychiatric Association 1987; Morey 1988), we found a nearly even gender distribution (49.2% women, chi-square [$df=1$] = 1.41, not significant). Within DSM-IV-TR, criteria are provided for two personality disorders (passive-aggressive and depressive) subsumed under the PDNOS category. A number of older studies of the gender distribution of passive-aggressive personality disorder have yielded equivocal results; although the genesis of the concept lies in the largely male military population, gender distribution estimates have ranged from 3:1 male (Spitzer et al. 1989) to 3:1 female (Maier et al. 1992). Relatively few studies have directly applied the DSM-IV-TR criteria for depressive personality disorder; in one large study of 198 patients meeting criteria for this disorder, McDermut et al. (2003) found that 68% of these patients were women, and the proportion of women in this group was significantly larger than the proportion of women in this setting who did not receive this diagnosis. DSM-III-R also included two other PDNOS "provisional" diagnoses, self-defeating personality disorder and sadistic personality disorder, that were quite controversial with respect to their gender implications (e.g., Caplan 1987). DSM-III-R reported that self-defeating personality disorder was more common in women; sadistic personality disorder was described as "far more common" in men and appears to have perhaps the most asymmetrical gender distribution of any specific personality disorder, with some studies reporting prevalence of males in the sample as high as 98% (Spitzer et al. 1991) to 100% (Freiman K, Widiger TA: "Co-Occurrence and Diagnostic Efficiency Statistics," unpublished raw data, Lexington, KY, University of Kentucky, 1989). Neither of these disorders was included in DSM-IV or DSM-IV-TR, and there has been limited further examination of them. Interestingly, one more recent, detailed study of gender issues in self-defeating personality disorder (Cruz et al. 2000) found neither a gender difference nor a bias in terms of the incremental validity of these criteria across gender.

There tend to be more data reported for gender distributions of the 10 standard DSM-IV-TR personality disorders, because studies of the individual disorders typically report the gender ratio in their sample. However, as noted earlier, studies of individual disorders can be misleading because they can mask distributions that are representative of the population being sampled rather than of the specific disorder (Corbitt and Widiger 1995). The following sections describe some of the most important findings across the different specific clusters of personality disorders.

Cluster A Personality Disorders

According to DSM-IV-TR, all three of the Cluster A personality disorders—paranoid, schizoid, and schizotypal—are diagnosed more commonly in men than in women. Of the three, gender differences in schizoid personality tend to be most pronounced, with many studies demonstrating a minimum 2:1 male-to-female gender ratio (Corbitt and Widiger 1995) and some studies suggesting that few if any women meet criteria for this disorder (Ekselius et al. 1996; Maier et al. 1992). However, such ratios tend to be based on very small sample sizes because of the overall low prevalence of schizoid personality disorders, and often the gender differences obtained do not reach statistical significance (Jackson and Burgess 2000; Torgersen et al. 2001). At the level of individual criteria, there have been some consistent findings to suggest that "indifference to praise or criticism" represents a schizoid feature found to be particularly prevalent in males (Ekselius et al. 1996; Morey et al. 2002).

DSM also describes schizotypal personality disorder as more commonly observed among men, although the data are somewhat inconsistent. Whereas some studies support the contention of greater prevalence among men (Dahl 1986; Maier et al. 1992; Zim-merman and Coryell 1989), others obtain no gender differences (Golomb et al. 1995; Reich 1987; Torgersen et al. 2001). Because schizotypal personality disorder is thought to reflect a schizophrenia spectrum condition, the finding that schizophrenia (which may be slightly more prevalent in men) tends to express itself differently as a function of gender (Bardenstein and McGlashan 1990) may be instructive. There appear to be suggestions that a similar pattern exists for schizotypal personality, with men tending to score higher on "negative symptom" features such as social isolation, anhedonia, and constricted affect, whereas women are more likely to demonstrate positive symptom features such as magical thinking, ideas of reference, and social anxiety (Raine 1992; Roth and Baribeau 1997).

Although DSM describes paranoid personality disorder as more common among men in clinical samples, data in support of this conclusion are mixed. For example, in two separate studies of outpatients using the same diagnostic instrument (the Structured Interview for DSM Personality Disorders), one found that 73% of paranoid personality disorder samples were male (Reich 1987), whereas the other found that only 47% were male (Alnaes and Torgersen 1988). In nonpatient samples, many studies find no gender differences (Ekselius et al. 1996; Jackson and Burgess 2000; Maier et al. 1992; Torgersen et al. 2001), suggesting that sampling issues may be influencing findings of gender differences in clinical settings. In a clinical sample of depressed outpatients, Carter et al. (1999) reported that although more men than women met criteria for paranoid personality disorder, there was no gender difference with respect to the number of paranoid personality disorder criteria met, suggesting that the diagnostic difference may be partially an artifact of the diagnostic threshold selected in DSM. It has been suggested that such a result may often be obtained when a categorical threshold is applied to the extreme of a personality dimension that displays relatively minor gender differences (Corbitt and Widiger 1995).

Cluster B Personality Disorders

The Cluster B personality disorders are perhaps the most widely discussed of these disorders with respect to their gender implications. Antisocial personality disorder (ASPD) has long been assumed to be more prevalent in males, and DSM-IV-TR indicates that it is "much more common" among men. These conclusions are borne out by consistent findings across community samples (Blazer et al. 1985) as well as clinical samples (Kass et al. 1983) and across structured interview (Jackson et al. 1991) as well as self-report (Millon 1987) instruments. Similar gender differences are also found in alternative representations of this construct, such as psychopathy (Salekin et al. 1997), although the factor structure may differ between men and women. It is important to note that greater frequency of antisocial item endorsement among males was also noted in both community and clinical normative samples of the Personality Assessment Inventory (PAI; Morey 1991), a self-report instrument that used differential item functioning analyses to eliminate items that were potentially gender-biased. The greater prevalence of antisocial features among men relative to women is perhaps the most well-replicated finding in personality disorder research.

In contrast, DSM-IV-TR indicates that borderline personality disorder (BPD) is diagnosed predominantly in women, and it provides a prevalence estimate for women of 75%. This estimate derives from a meta-analysis from Widiger and Trull (1993), who summarized the results of 75 studies that provided unbiased estimates of the sex ratio of a diagnosis of BPD. Across these studies, the average proportion of women was 76% (±3%), a number comparable with that reported by Akhtar et al. (1986) in a meta-analysis of 23 studies. Widiger and Trull (1993) noted that studies using a semi-structured interview yielded higher proportions of women (80% on average) than studies where diagnosis was based on unstructured interviews (73%). However, it is important to note that most of these prevalence estimates have been based on clinical samples in particular settings rather than on nonclinical or epidemiological community studies.

A number of studies of nonclinical samples reveal no significant gender differences in BPD and its features, including data from both community (Bernstein et al. 1993; Jackson and Burgess 2000; Morey 1991; Torgersen et al. 2001; Zimmerman and Coryell 1989) and college student (Morey et al. 2002) samples. One well-known study of college students (Henry and Cohen 1983) indicated that borderline features were more common among males in their sample; in fact, this is not an isolated finding but has also been obtained in clinical samples as well, including samples of panic disordered patients (Barzega et al. 2001) as well as depressed outpatients (Carter et al. 1999). The causes of the variability of these findings, particularly the discrepancy between clinical and nonclinical distributions, are unclear. Hartung and Widiger (1998) explored a number of potential artifacts that can distort the results of samples obtained in clinical settings, such as the methodology for assigning diagnosis, type of sample

selected, and base rate of disorder within that sample. Skodol and Bender (2003) suggested that perhaps the prevalence differences in community and clinical samples simply reflect a sampling bias.

Although research on narcissistic personality disorder is at a more preliminary stage than that for the two disorders just described, available research reports disagree on its gender distribution. Some studies support the idea that narcissistic personality disorder is more common in males than in females (Golomb et al. 1995; Ronningstam and Gunderson 1990), whereas others indicate that narcissistic personality disorder is equally prevalent in both sexes. DSM-IV-TR claims that 50%–75% of those diagnosed with narcissistic personality disorder are male, but the results are fairly variable, with one study of inpatients finding that 67% of narcissistic patients were women (Dahl 1986). As with many other disorders, gender differences among nonpatients are less frequently found, with most studies reporting no significant differences (Bernstein et al. 1993; Ekselius et al. 1996; Morey et al. 2002; Torgersen et al. 2001). Although this lack of significant findings may be in part a result of the apparently low prevalence of the disorder, the pattern is consistent even in samples with relatively high occurrence rates (Ekselius et al. 1996) and also when scores are dimensionalized by criterion count to include the entire sample under study (Ekselius et al. 1996; Morey et al. 2002). Again, sampling differences may be accounting for the different findings in clinical versus nonclinical settings; for example, 95% of patients diagnosed as narcissistic (with traits or personality disorder) in a military sample were male (Bourgeois et al. 1993), a setting that includes many more men than women.

Histrionic personality disorder has had a long history of controversy with respect to gender issues. One of Freud's earliest presentations in psychiatry involved the thesis that hysteria was underrecognized in men, and an early review by Chodoff and Lyons (1958) expressed the concern that the diagnosis focused primarily on personality traits of women rather than men. DSM-IV-TR notes that this diagnosis is more frequently assigned to women but that the gender distribution is often not significantly different from the base rate gender distribution in the clinical setting in question. DSM-IV-TR also suggests that studies using structured interviews do not find a gender difference, although in fact a number of studies using such interviews in clinical settings have found a preponderance of women receiving the diagnosis (Alnaes and Torgersen 1988; Jackson et al. 1991; Reich 1987). It does appear that diagnostic instrumentation can have a substantial effect on the conclusions drawn for this disorder. For example, Wierzbicki and Goldade (1993) found that the Millon Clinical Multiaxial Inventory (MCMI; Millon 1980) histrionic scale score was more commonly elevated in men than women; these authors suggested that Millon's construct of this disorder may differ from that which is portrayed in the DSM-III criteria. Hynan (2004) pointed out that the most recent version of this instrument, the MCMI-III, has substantially different interpretations for men and women based on the same raw score on the Histrionic scale, a difference that he identified as unsupported by the research literature. Sinha and Watson (2001) administered the MCMI-II, the Minnesota Multiphasic Personality Inventory (MMPI) personality disorder scales (Morey et al. 1985), and the Coolidge Axis II Inventory (Coolidge and Merwin 1992) to a group of 293 college students and found that only the Coolidge Axis II Inventory demonstrated a significant gender difference for the histrionic scale. Finally, as with BPD, the nature of the sampling strategy appears to have a major impact on estimated gender distribution, with a number of community studies finding no difference in prevalence between men and women outside of clinical settings (Jackson and Burgess 2000; Nestadt et al. 1990; Torgersen et al. 2001; Zimmerman and Coryell 1989).

Cluster C Disorders

Dependent personality disorder has been a frequent source of controversy with respect to gender and personality disorder (Kaplan 1983; Kass et al. 1983, Widiger 1998). Bornstein (1993) conducted a meta-analysis of 18 studies that used structured interviews to assign dependent personality disorder diagnoses, with samples gathered from inpatient, outpatient, and community settings; he found a pooled prevalence rate of 11% for women and 8% for men, a significant difference. Corbitt and Widiger (1995) similarly summarized results for a number of studies of this disorder, finding that nearly every study identified more women than men as having the diagnosis. Recent studies of nonclinical samples also tend to indicate greater prevalence of dependent features among women, although the magnitude of the differences tends to be modest (Morey et al. 2002; Torgersen et al. 2001). Bornstein (1996) suggested that the magnitude of gender differences in dependent personality disorder tends to vary as a function of the nature of the diagnostic instrument; indicators that are more transparent and clearly related to dependency are more likely to show a gender difference than those that are less face valid, such

as Rorschach indicators. He hypothesized that these findings may indicate that many observed sex differences in dependent personality disorder may reflect a difference in willingness to publicly acknowledge dependency needs, rather than a true difference in the prevalence of marked manifestations of these needs. However, it is still an open question as to whether possibly differential validity of face-valid versus subtle indicators might contribute to the pattern of findings that Bornstein noted.

DSM-IV-TR describes avoidant personality disorder as equally prevalent among men and women. Most studies report no significant gender prevalence differences, despite the disorder being fairly prevalent in the community (e.g., Torgersen et al. 2001). It is worthy to note that gender distributions in nonclinical samples have demonstrated a wide range, from 75% male (Bernstein et al. 1993) to 80% female (Zimmerman and Coryell 1989), but a preponderance of studies seem to suggest no difference. Studies of the gender distribution of individual avoidant criteria do not yield consistent differences across the criteria. Ekselius et al. (1996) reported finding that women far outnumbered men who endorsed that they are "easily hurt by criticism or disapproval," but this criterion was eliminated in DSM-IV. A somewhat similar criterion, "reluctance to take risks for fear of embarrassment," was endorsed by women more frequently than by men in a study by Morey et al. (2002).

Obsessive-compulsive personality disorder is described by DSM-IV-TR as occurring twice as often in men as in women. This conclusion is supported by some studies (Maier et al. 1992; Torgersen et al. 2001; Zimmerman and Coryell 1989), but others suggest less dramatic gender differences (Alnaes and Torgersen 1988; Ekselius et al. 1996; Gunderson et al. 2000; Morey et al. 2002). In an analysis of individual DSM-III-R criteria, Ekselius et al. (1996) found that only one criterion, "lack of generosity in giving," displayed gender differences, demonstrating the stated 2:1 male-to-female ratio. Interestingly, this criterion underwent considerable revision in the transition to DSM-IV ("adopts a miserly spending style"), and this revised criterion did not display a gender difference in a more recent study (Morey et al. 2002), suggesting that gender differences for this disorder may be smaller under DSM-IV criteria.

ISSUES OF GENDER BIAS

The concern that some psychiatric concepts may be problematically employed as a function of gender has a lengthy history. Broverman et al. (1970) brought the issue of gender bias in the diagnosis of mental disorders to the forefront, a report that continues to be cited as leading evidence of gender-biased judgments of psychopathology. This seminal study found that clinicians were significantly more likely to characterize males with traits of healthy adults than they were to attribute such terms to females. Gender bias has been a controversial topic, spanning several versions of DSM and surrounding several clinical diagnoses, such as depression (Sprock and Yoder 1997), somatization disorders (Hartung and Widiger 1998), and particularly the personality disorders (Kaplan 1983; Kass et al. 1983, Widiger 1998). For example, Kaplan (1983) suggested that the DSM-III task force that created the first sets of diagnostic criteria for personality disorders largely consisted of white males who may have subsequently perpetuated a masculine bias in the personality disorder criteria, a bias that led to stereotypically feminine behavior being labeled as pathological. Labeling processes have been implicated specifically in the overdiagnosis of women with BPD; in other words, the same traits may be seen as more tolerable in men but less tolerated in women (Henry and Cohen 1983). It also has been suggested that the personality disorders involve sex role stereotypes that are as applicable to men as to women. For example, Landrine (1989) asked undergraduates to describe the gender, marital status, and social status of individuals likely to receive specific personality disorder diagnoses. The study found that students perceived the histrionic, dependent, and self-defeating personality disorder cases as women and the antisocial, sadistic, and obsessive-compulsive personality disorder cases as men; no differences were noted in the assignment of the BPD case.

According to Garb (1997), "bias occurs when the accuracy of judgments varies as a function of client race, social class, or gender" (p. 99). Methodologically, gender bias has been a difficult topic in personality disorders research due to the lack of a clear operational definition of the term *bias* and the lack of a universally accepted gold standard against which to evaluate the presence or absence of bias. The gender bias controversy largely originated with claims based solely on differential sex prevalence rates (Kaplan 1983; Kass et al. 1983). However, discrepant prevalence rates do not provide sufficient evidence of gender bias, although they may indicate that a particular disorder is gender-typed, either correctly or incorrectly. Gender-neutral variants of mental disorders are not necessarily desirable, because the etiologies of certain disorders may be indicative of a valid sex difference (Widiger 1998). For exam-

ple, anorexia nervosa diagnoses are made up of 90% women, which may simply indicate a largely gender-typed manifestation of body dissatisfaction. An emphasis on equating gender prevalence may lead to elimination of valid criteria, in which case salient manifestations of the construct in one gender remain undetected and subsequently underdiagnosed.

Two primary types of diagnostic bias have been distinguished: criterion bias and assessment bias (Bornstein 1996; Widiger and Spitzer 1991). *Criterion sex bias* refers to bias inherent within the diagnostic criteria for each mental disorder as set forth by a diagnostic system, such as categories of personality disorder provided in DSM or ICD. In contrast, *assessment sex bias* involves a bias in the process by which individuals are assigned to these categories. The following sections review some of the findings in each of these areas.

Criterion Bias

Criterion bias can be said to exist when the sets of diagnostic criteria that define particular disorders are not equally valid across gender groups. Criterion bias within DSM has been evaluated using a variety of different methodologies (Anderson et al. 2001; Kass et al. 1983; Morey et al. 2002). Morey et al. (2002) suggested a number of strategies for exploring the possibility of bias within the defining criteria for a diagnosis, including the approaches described in the following sections.

Pathologizing Normative/Common Behaviors

Kaplan (1983) suggested that "male centered assumptions—the sunglasses through which we view each other—are causing clinicians to see normal females as abnormal" (p. 787). To support this argument, Kaplan discussed the Broverman et al. (1970) study, which found that clinicians are more likely to attribute traits depicting a healthy adult to a male rather than a female. This study has often been cited as evidence that stereotypically masculine behaviors are viewed as healthier than stereotypically feminine behaviors (Kaplan 1983; Widiger and Settle 1987). However, Widiger and Settle (1987) demonstrated that the Broverman finding is an artifact of an imbalanced ratio of "male-valued" to "female-valued" items in the dependent measure that was used to demonstrate the gender bias. Once Widiger and Settle balanced the number of stereotypic items to include an equal number of items valued by men and women, the behaviors or items were viewed as equally healthy across gender.

Morey et al. (2002) examined this issue empirically, building on Morey and Glutting's (1994) proposal that abnormal personality traits should have a marked positive skew in community samples, whereas normal traits should have a roughly normal (Gaussian) distribution in such samples. Morey et al. (2002) found that all 79 of the DSM-IV-TR criteria demonstrated positive skew in dimensional self-ratings in a nonclinical college student sample and that for 74 (men) to 76 (women) subjects the skew was markedly positive, suggesting that these personality features could not be considered normal personality characteristics for either gender.

Perceived Implications of Criteria Being Different for Men and Women

Some writers (e.g., Lerman 1996; Widiger 1998) have suggested that because the personality disorder workgroups have been predominantly male, the males in the workgroup may have tended to pathologize feminine traits to a greater extent than masculine ones (Widiger 1998). There have been studies that have examined differences in the way that personality disorder–related behaviors are viewed by males and females. Sprock (1996) asked students to rate each personality disorder criterion for abnormality, with three groups receiving different instructions: abnormality for women, abnormality for men, and abnormality without a request to consider gender. Sprock found undergraduates perceived 27 symptoms as more abnormal when they received the female instruction condition compared with the group that received the male instruction condition. This finding may suggest that the threshold for an abnormality rating of certain criteria may be lower when a woman's behavior is being evaluated. Sprock (1996) also examined the effect of participant gender on the abnormality ratings. For most criteria, there did not appear to be a difference between men and women in their perceptions of the implications of these criteria (antisocial criteria tended to be a noteworthy exception).

Anderson et al. (2001) examined the perceptions of clinicians of the maladaptiveness of the behaviors represented by the DSM-IV-TR personality disorders criteria. Although clinicians did describe certain criteria as being more typical of one gender, the criteria were found to be equally maladaptive for males and females. Morey et al. (2002) examined the degree to which the DSM-IV-TR criteria were perceived as having greater implications for one gender than another and found that across all criteria the implications appeared to be equally balanced as rated by either men or women; the undergraduates rating these implications also demonstrated a high degree of reliability (intraclass correlation=0.958) in rating the implications of these criteria.

Gender Differences in Relationship of Diagnostic Criteria to Functioning or to Other Indicators of the Same Disorder

One empirical way in which bias has been examined in the psychometric literature is through a comparison of relationships between indicators and validity criteria in different demographic subgroups (e.g., Cleary et al. 1975). In this approach, linear or logistic regression is typically used to describe indicator/criteria relationships, and differences in the parameters of these regression lines are used as evidence of bias. In an examination of indicator-diagnosis relationships, Morey et al. (2002) found few gender differences, although the schizoid criteria did seem to intercorrelate more highly for men (coefficient $\alpha=0.71$) than for women (coefficient $\alpha=0.41$). This finding may suggest that the schizoid personality disorder criteria may not be useful indicators of the disorder for women. In a more comprehensive examination using this approach, Boggs (2003) used a multimethod external assessment of functional impairment as a benchmark against which to evaluate the differential validity of the DSM criteria for avoidant, borderline, obsessive-compulsive, and schizotypal personality disorders. No consistent gender differences were found, although many of the BPD criteria seem to have different global functional implications for women than for men.

Assessment Bias

Assessment bias refers to the biased application of the diagnostic criteria by both clinicians and assessment inventories (Widiger and Spitzer 1991). Methodologically speaking, this type of bias has been more straightforward to investigate experimentally. The typical delineation of bias in this research involves an examination of potentially different rates of false-positive diagnoses (for example, the overdiagnosis of women with histrionic personality disorder) and false-negative diagnoses (the underdiagnosis of men with histrionic personality disorder; e.g., Widiger and Spitzer 1991).

One means of investigating assessment bias involves examining the role of gender in how DSM diagnostic criteria are applied by clinicians. The problem of clinicians straying from the diagnostic criteria set forth in DSM was investigated by Morey and Ochoa (1989), who found a low rate of correspondence between clinician-assigned clinical diagnoses and an algorithmic diagnosis calculated from a checklist of DSM criteria completed by these same clinicians. The results suggested that the presence of specific features or criteria did lead to an overdiagnosis or underdiagnosis of a particular disorder, but importantly, the gender of the patient was typically not one of these features. For example, in predicting the overdiagnosis of BPD, the gender of the patient was not a significant factor, but the gender of the clinician was (women clinicians were more likely to overdiagnose the disorder). These results were replicated by Blashfield and Herkov (1996), who also found that clinicians tended not to adhere to the DSM criteria when making diagnoses.

Perhaps the most common method of studying assessment bias has been having clinicians make diagnoses based on case vignettes to examine whether manipulating the stated gender of the client influences the diagnosis. An early study by Warner (1978) is typical of such studies; varying the gender of an otherwise identical case vignette led clinicians to assign a diagnosis of ASPD when the gender of the case was male—but to assign a diagnosis of histrionic personality disorder when the case was identified as female. A follow-up investigation by Hamilton et al. (1986) found that histrionic personality disorder was significantly more likely to be applied to females than males who exhibit identical symptoms; small differences were found for ASPD such that the diagnosis was applied to men more often than women, but these differences were not significant. Hamilton et al. (1986) suggested that the behavioral nature of the DSM-III ASPD diagnostic criteria (which were not in use at the time the Warner 1978 study was conducted) allowed for the diagnosis to be more accurately applied without the interference of gender stereotypes and personal biases. However, Belitsky et al. (1996) conducted a similar vignette study and found the opposite result: male patients were more likely to be diagnosed as antisocial, whereas there was no gender difference in the assignment of the histrionic diagnosis. With respect to Hamilton et al.'s hypothesis about the influence of diagnostic criteria on biased diagnosis, Ford and Widiger (1989) did find that clinicians overdiagnosed histrionic personality disorder in women who present some histrionic symptoms, but when asked to systematically use DSM diagnostic criteria, clinicians accurately diagnosed case histories for males and females.

Although most vignette studies have focused on the antisocial/histrionic contrast (Garb 1997), recent attention has turned to the study of BPD. In a study evaluating clinician gender bias in the diagnosis of BPD, Becker and Lamb (1994) analyzed clinician's ratings of the applicability of various Axis I and Axis II disorders to a written case vignette presented as either male or female. Each vignette presented a case that displayed an equal number of BPD and posttraumatic stress disorder

symptoms, although there was not sufficient evidence for a clear-cut diagnosis of either disorder. Clinicians displayed a significant tendency to rate the borderline criteria as more applicable to the female case than the male case, suggesting a possible influence of gender bias upon diagnosis. Crosby and Sprock (2004) administered male and female case vignettes containing antisocial features to a national sample of clinicians; the number of BPD diagnoses assigned to the female case far exceeded the number assigned to the male case. Although there was no significant difference in antisocial personality disorder diagnoses assigned to male and female cases, clinicians did rate themselves as feeling more confident when applying the diagnosis to the male case than the female case.

It is important to note that the biases demonstrated in such vignette studies are invariably in the direction of the stated prevalence rates of the disorders, such that clinicians are more likely to diagnose males with disorders that are thought to be more prevalent in males. It has been suggested that clinicians make decisions by taking into account base rates of disorders as a method of determining diagnoses (Koehler 1996), which may be an appropriate strategy from a Bayesian probability perspective. However, this type of behavior in and of itself may influence the differential sex prevalence rates that have been identified.

To investigate how base rate information might influence clinicians, Flanagan and Blashfield (2003) gave undergraduates descriptive information about the Cluster B personality disorders, using letters to represent the official names of the disorders in an effort to avoid any preconceived biases. Students were then taught three types of base rate information (none, stereotype-consistent, and stereotype-inconsistent) about each personality disorder. Three different student groups then rated five case vignettes, designating each as gender consistent, gender inconsistent, or ambiguous. The study concluded that when students were given no gender association, the ratings did not differ based on gender. However, when stereotype-consistent associations were taught, students tended to rate the specific gender as more representative of each disorder. When the stereotype-inconsistent associations were taught, students had difficulty learning the inconsistent associations, and gender association only appeared to influence ratings for histrionic personality disorder, which was rated as more common in men, and narcissistic personality disorder, which was rated as more common in women. This study concluded that individuals do use base rate information, but only when the information is stereotype consistent.

In addition to clinician application of the diagnostic criteria, assessment bias may be evident in particular assessment inventories that systematically overdiagnose or underdiagnose one sex. Wierzbicki and Goldade (1993) found that 10 of the 11 Millon Clinical Multiaxial Inventory personality disorder scales were significantly more associated with one sex than the other. Avoidant, dependent, passive-aggressive, schizotypal, borderline, and compulsive were found to be more related to women, whereas histrionic, narcissistic, antisocial, and paranoid were found to be more associated with men. Hynan (2004) pointed out that a number of gender differences on the most recent version of this measure, the Millon Clinical Multiaxial Inventory–III, are not supported by the literature; in particular, women receive a more pathological interpretation of the same raw score than for the histrionic, narcissistic, and compulsive scales of this instrument. Lindsay et al. (2000) evaluated the MCMI–III (Millon et al. 1994) as well as the MMPI–2 (Butcher et al. 1989) and the PDQ-4 (Hyler 1994) for gender-biased items. The authors used the sum of scale scores of the PAI (Morey 1991) as a criterion indicator of dysfunction, because the PAI is one of the few instruments that sought to eliminate gender-biased items in its construction. In addition, another measure was administered as an indicator of masculinity and femininity. Items that failed to correlate with dysfunction yet correlated positively with socially desirable gender characteristics were identified as potentially gender biased. Twenty-nine potentially biased items were found on the narcissistic scales of the MCMI-III and the MMPI-2 as well as five histrionic, one antisocial, and one dependent ($P<0.05$). When the level of statistical significance was more restricted ($P<0.001$), all problematic items were on the narcissistic scales of each inventory. No biased items were identified on the PDQ-4, potentially due to more questions pertaining to dysfunction. Lindsay et al. raised the concern that the MMPI-2 and the MCMI-III may pathologize normal levels of self-confidence and self-esteem.

Summary

Although the potential of gender bias in personality disorder diagnoses has been discussed extensively, there is little unequivocal evidence of the operation of diagnostic biases. Perhaps the most common finding is that clinicians are more likely to diagnose histrionic personality disorder in women than men and more likely to diagnose antisocial personality disorder in men than women, even when the symptoms are identical (Garb 1997). A number of procedures have been recommended that can further reduce the likelihood of bias, particularly assessment bias. Based on their results, Ford and Widiger (1989) recommended that training programs emphasize the systematic use of and adherence to the DSM criteria. In a discussion of issues related to the assessment of women, Robinson and Worell (2002) suggested that clinicians frequently reference current research on gender bias to understand issues related to the assessment of women as well as to become aware of and dispute their own attitudes and expectations of the behavior of women. McLaughlin (2002) offered a more in-depth discussion of methods for reducing and avoiding diagnostic sampling bias, diagnostic assessment bias, and diagnostic criterion bias, as well as implications for training programs.

GENDER-RELATED BIOSOCIAL INFLUENCES ON PERSONALITY DISORDER

Overview of Gender and Personality

It is unlikely that all obtained gender differences in personality disorder are a function of sampling or diagnostic biases. Gender differences exist in personality traits and related behaviors. In research on the five-factor model of personality, men score higher on dimensions of "extraversion," whereas women score higher on dimensions of "agreeableness" and "neuroticism," the latter of which includes depression and anxiety measures (Corbitt and Widiger 1995). Consistent with these findings, human males compared with human females are more active (Cambell and Eaton 1999), more physically aggressive (Archer 1991), report higher levels of sexual desire (Baldwin and Baldwin 1997), prefer rough active play (DiPietro 1981), and typically report feeling more assertive and less dependent on others (Feingold 1994). Gender differences also exist in cognitive abilities. Males tend to excel at spatial tasks, such as mental rotation or spatial navigation (Linn and Petersen 1974; Voyer et al. 1995). Females excel at verbal tasks (Hyde and Linn 1988) and spatial memory (Alexander et al. 2002b; Silverman and Eals 1992) and show an advantage in processing facial expressions (McClure 2000). For the most part, these human sex differences are consistent with cultural stereotypes (e.g., Bem 1974) that derive from the prescribed social roles for men and women as provider-protectors and nurturers, respectively. Therefore, although considerable overlap exists in the distribution of most gender-linked traits in men and women (Collaer and Hines 1995), individuals displaying high levels of cross-sex personality traits are typically categorized as "feminine" men or "masculine" women.

A large body of empirical research has demonstrated powerful social and cognitive influences on the development of gender-linked characteristics or gender role behavior (Ruble and Martin 1998). A gender label at birth activates a lifelong process of gender socialization that extends far beyond the gender-specific toys or colors selected for a child's physical environment (Pomerleau et al. 1990). Gender labels activate social perceptions and modeling and reinforcement of "gender-appropriate" behavior (Bussey and Bandura 1999). A baby with no obvious gender cues, for example, is described as more fearful when labeled as a girl than when labeled as a boy (Condry and Condry 1976). In later development, females report higher levels of anxiety than do males (Pigott 1999). The apparent internalization of social norms for gender-linked traits is thought to occur with the formation of a gender identity. From this self-identification as "male" or "female" in early childhood emerge internal elaborations of gender-behavior associations called *gender schemas* that guide behavior by filtering the encoding and retrieval of social information so to be gender consistent (Bradbard et al. 1986; Martin and Halverson 1983). As a consequence, gender-typical behavior in later childhood resists modification—even when consistent reinforcement of cross-gender behavior is applied (Martin 1994). Gender identification is also recognition of belonging to a gender group (Maccoby 1988). A far-reaching implication of gender group identification is the subsequent development of gender subcultures in childhood that, through their gender-specific play and relational styles, appear to promote sex differences in adult cognitive and emotional processing (Maccoby 1998). Not surprisingly, these cognitive-social processes are thought sufficient to explain sex-specific personality development and to influence abilities to process cognitive-emotional stimuli that might precipitate gender-linked psychological disorders.

Gender labels, the primary activators of the gender socialization processes just described, are initiated by the dichotomous categorization of the external genitalia. From this perspective, the ultimate origin of gender-linked traits and behaviors is the permanent masculinization and defeminization of the genitalia, one endpoint in a cascade of hormonal processes during prenatal life termed *organizational effects* (Breedlove et al. 1999; Phoenix et al. 1959). Also important is the maturation of the reproductive system at puberty, a developmental process that reflects the nonpermanent actions of critical amounts of sex steroids, termed *acti-*

vational effects (Arnold and Breedlove 1985). There is likely general agreement among contemporary theorists that, by initiating a process of gender socialization (and by increasing identification with adult gender groups at puberty), prenatal and postnatal gonadal hormones contribute indirectly to gender differences in personality. For example, implicit motives or unconscious preferences for incentives such as power or affiliation (McClelland 1987) are hypothesized to develop from very early socialization experiences. If so, then the postnatal onset of gender socialization should logically result in sex differences in the development of these behavioral response systems. Increasingly, however, animal and human research indicates that sex steroids may also have more direct effects on gender role development by influencing the organization and activation of the central nervous system, including brain regions integral to mood and behavioral regulation (e.g., the amygdala and hypothalamus).

Overview of Hormonal Effects on Gender Role Behavior

In many mammalian species, including nonhuman primates, hormones play a major role in directing the development of brain systems that subserve sex-typed behaviors (Arnold and Breedlove 1985; Breedlove et al. 1999). Testicular androgens aromatized to estrogens in the brain produce sex-specific changes in the central nervous system (MacLusky et al. 1997), including increased volumes of nuclei in the hypothalamus, amygdala, and hippocampus (Arnold and Gorski 1984; MacLusky and Naftolin 1981). Higher levels of testosterone also appear to produce a masculine pattern of brain asymmetry, such that the cortex of the right hemisphere is thicker than that of the left (Diamond 1991). Hormone actions in the brain during prenatal life also direct the development of sex-specific behavioral phenotypes by influencing the frequencies or expression of reproductive behavior (Gorski 1979), play (Meaney 1988), and spatial memory (Williams and Meck 1991). For example, female animals exposed to high levels of androgens during critical periods of prenatal development will show an increased potential for male-typical behavior, such as higher frequencies of rough-and-tumble play (Meaney and McEwen 1986). The expression of most other sex-typed behavior also requires critical amounts of hormones in postnatal life. Adult male sexual and aggressive behavior, for instance, is abolished by castration in male animals and reinstated following androgen administration. Thus, sexual differentiation of behavioral systems, like the sexual differentiation of the reproductive system, appears to depend on the combined influences of hormone levels during prenatal and postnatal development.

In humans, support for organizational influences of hormones on gender role behavior comes from research on both typical and atypical reproductive development. In studies of women and men with typical reproductive development, sex differences in brain development include findings that females have smaller brain weights and a higher percentage of grey matter (Gur et al. 1999). Some research also indicates males and females differ in the size and shape of interhemispheric commissures (Allen et al. 1991; de Lacoste-Utamsing and Holloway 1982) and the size of some subcortical structures (Allen and Gorski 1990) and neocortical regions (Frederiskse et al. 1999; Rademacher et al. 2001). The functional significance of differences in brain areas influencing reproductive and nonreproductive function is not established. However, sex-specific brain systems may be associated with a sex-specific response to stimuli that explains, in part, gender-linked personality traits. For example, sex-specific brain systems contributing to greater anxiety and depression in women compared with men is suggested by structural and functional brain research showing that the amygdala is larger in women than in men and larger in individuals with chronic dysphoria (Tebartz van Elst et al. 2000) and that sex-specific patterns of activation occur in the amygdala following exposure to emotional stimuli (Cahill et al. 2001; Canli et al. 2002; Killgore and Yurgelun-Todd 2001).

Although mechanisms explaining sex differences in brain development likely include both genetic and social factors, human research measuring gender-linked behavior in individuals who have atypical prenatal development (because of endocrine disorders or maternal ingestion of synthetic steroids during pregnancy) supports the hypothesis that hormonal effects on brain development influence gender role behavior. Girls with congenital adrenal hyperplasia, for example, are exposed to androgen levels more typical of the prenatal hormonal environment in normal males (Carson et al. 1982). In postnatal life these girls tend to show more aggression (Berenbaum and Resnick 1997), enhanced (i.e., more masculine) visuospatial abilities (Hampson et al. 1998; Resnick et al. 1986), more masculine occupational preferences (Berenbaum 1999), and increased bisexual or homosexual sexual preferences in fantasy or behavior (Zucker et al. 1996).

Some adult gender role behaviors also appear activated by the onset of adult levels of sex steroids at puberty. Sexual interest and sexual desire increase in boys and girls coincident with increases in androgens (McClintock and Herdt 1996). Sex differences in aggression and spatial abilities also increase following puberty (Archer 1991). Similarly, motivational sexual behaviors are enhanced following androgen administration to men with androgen deficiencies (Everitt and Bancroft 1991) and surgically menopausal women (Sherwin et al. 1985). Still other evidence suggests that individual differences in adult gender-linked traits and behavior are associated with individual differences in hormone levels. In men, for instance, testosterone levels predict social dominance (Dabbs 1998; Mazur and Booth 1998). In women, menstrual cycle phase effects have been reported on sexual desire (Alexander and Sherwin 1991), cognitive abilities (Hampson 1990), and measures of brain functional asymmetry (Alexander et al. 2002a). One suggestion is that higher testosterone levels in postnatal life indicate higher testosterone levels in prenatal life and so activate more masculine behaviors even within women. Consistent with this hypothesis, higher testosterone levels appear to enhance spatial abilities in women (Kimura and Hampson 1994) and characterize "butch" lesbians relative both to their more stereotypically feminine counterparts and to heterosexual women (Singh et al. 1999).

Activational influences on mood and sexual motivation in men with hormone deficiencies are well-established (Everitt and Bancroft 1991). However, despite positive results (such as those described earlier), postnatal hormone effects on other gender-linked behaviors are equivocal. Menstrual cycle effects on gender-linked cognitive abilities, for example, are elusive (Epting and Overman 1998; Gordon and Lee 1993; Phillips and Sherwin 1992). More critically, gender-linked behavior (i.e., aggression and spatial abilities) appears unaltered by treatment resulting in marked elevations in hormone levels (Alexander et al. 1998; Liben et al. 2002). One obvious implication of the failure of hormone administration to influence gender-linked behavior is that increased sex steroid levels at puberty or across the menstrual cycle are an insufficient explanation for any observed hormone-behavior association at these times. Notably, hormone administration does not replicate events at the level of the brain that trigger increased levels of gonadal hormones and any resulting activation of behavior. Because experiential factors clearly impact brain processes, it seems reasonable to propose that variables such as the central processing of social cues or social context may contribute to the inconsistent results in research on hormone activation of human behavior.

Dynamic Biosocial Interface

Sex steroids in postnatal life appear to influence sensitivity to stimuli associated with gender-linked traits or motives. For example, in women using oral contraceptives, higher levels of free testosterone predicted greater sensitivity to descriptions of romantic interactions in a dichotic listening task (Alexander and Sherwin 1993). Increased levels of sex steroids are also associated with increased behavioral responsiveness to achievement expectations (Josephs et al. 2003), mate characteristics associated with reproductive success (Penton-Voak et al. 1999), and threatening facial expressions (van Honk et al. 1999). A direct test of the hypothesis that implicit motives are sensitive to gonadal steroid levels in adults found that higher testosterone levels are associated with higher levels of power motivation in men, as measured by men's response to the Picture Story Exercise (Schultheiss and Rohde 2002). In women, a similar measure of affiliation motive increased at midcycle of the menstrual cycle, a time of increased ovarian steroid production and greater reproductive potential (Schultheiss et al. 2003). The association between hormones and social cues also appears bidirectional. Social cues or social interactions appear to activate hormone secretion (Harding 1981; LaFerla et al. 1978; Turner et al. 1999), consistent with the proposal of both social (Eagly and Wood 1999; Wood and Eagly 2002) and evolutionary theorists (Geary 1999) that gonadal hormones assist an individual in fulfilling a gender role—presumably by activating an appropriate behavioral response.

It should not be too surprising, then, that socialization of males and females typically appears to elaborate on hormonally determined behavioral tendencies for masculine or feminine behavior (Alexander 2003; Cambell and Eaton 1999; Geary 1999). Consider, for example, gender-typical play preferences that are clearly shaped by social processes, such as modeling and reinforcement (Bussey and Bandura 1999). Visual preferences in infants for gender-linked toys (dolls, vehicles) exist earlier in development than predicted by cognitive-social theories of gender role development (Campbell et al. 2000; O'Brien and Huston 1985; Serbin et al. 2001). Masculine play preferences are also increased in girls exposed prenatally to levels of androgens more typical of male development compared with their unaffected relatives (Berenbaum and Hines 1992; Hines and Kaufman 1994; Hines et al. 2003). Biological influences on play are further indicated by findings that vervet monkeys show sex differences in toy preferences (defined as toy contact time) similar to those documented in children (Alexander and Hines 2003). Together, these results suggest that prenatal androgen levels may direct visual preferences for "masculine" and "feminine" objects and thus provide a fertile ground for the growth of sex-specific brain and behavior systems in postnatal life (Alexander 2003).

Application and Findings for Personality Disorder

Personality traits such as assertiveness and independence (i.e., instrumental traits) and others such as emotionality and compassion (i.e., expressive traits) are associated with masculine and feminine gender roles, respectively. Gender differences in instrumental and expressive traits are thought to contribute to the general finding that girls compared with boys are twice as likely to report "internalizing" symptoms (e.g., depression, anxiety), whereas boys compared with girls are twice as likely to report "externalizing" symptoms (e.g., delinquency, aggression) (for review, see Hoffmann et al. 2004). Indeed, findings that the direction and degree of gender role identification between and within the sexes contributes to the expression of externalizing and internalizing symptoms (Huselid and Cooper 1994) have been replicated recently in a large sample of adolescents (Hoffmann et al. 2004). In that research, stronger female-typical traits in both sexes predicted less externalizing symptoms, whereas stronger male-typical traits were associated with increased competence and fewer internalizing symptoms. Masculine personality traits were also associated with increased externalizing behavior, perhaps because "dominance, assertiveness, and independence may become exaggerated in individuals who identify strongly with the instrumental gender role and thus lead to more externalizing behaviors such as arguing, aggression, and treating others poorly" (p. 807). This explanation for sex differences in internalizing/externalizing symptom expression is consistent with the earlier proposal that personality disorders showing large gender differences, such as ASPD and BPD, may represent extremes of normal gender-specific traits such as aggression or dependency (Skodol 2000).

If gender roles contribute to the expression of internalizing and externalizing symptoms and the development of gender-linked personality disorders, then their biosocial determinants may also warrant closer inspection in studies of personality disorders (Alexander and Peterson 2001). Research indicating that hormones influence gender-specific traits suggests that the extreme sexual differentiation of the brain and behavior in prenatal life may contribute to the extreme and maladaptive expression of behaviors associated with gender-linked personality disorders. This possibility is consistent with the proposal that varying degrees of exposure of the brain to sex steroid hormones promotes phenotypic differences between and within the sexes (i.e., the gradient model of hormone effects; Collaer and Hines 1995). Indeed, researchers studying male-typical psychopathology in the broader construct of gender-linked behavior have noted that core phenotypic features of autism (impaired socialization and language) and Tourette's syndrome (disinhibition of sexual or aggressive impulses), disorders showing strong male-to-female sex ratio (Peterson et al. 2001; Rutter and Garmezy 1983), appear "hypermasculine" or as very high levels of characteristics typically associated with the masculine gender role (Baron-Cohen and Hammer 1997; Peterson et al. 1992). Consistent with a role for prenatal androgens in their development, one physical marker of prenatal androgen levels—the ratio of the lengths of the second and fourth digits—is masculinized (i.e., smaller) in autism (Manning et al. 2001). Thresholds for disorders may be increased in one gender over another because specific traits are viewed by society as compatible with one's gender label (Al-Issa 1982). Therefore, it is particularly noteworthy that girls with a male-typical disorder (Tourette's syndrome) also report greater gender dysphoria, stronger preferences for masculine play styles, and a more masculinized pattern of cognitive abilities (Alexander and Peterson in press). No evidence of an altered process of gender socialization exists in female infants who later develop tics in childhood. Therefore, the similarity of these findings with those for girls exposed to higher prenatal androgen levels because they have an endocrine disorder suggests that increased masculinization of the brain in prenatal development may contribute to the development of Tourette's syndrome, at least in girls. It may be useful to examine whether females with male-typical personality disorder (i.e., ASPD) or males with a female-typical personality disorder (i.e., BPD) also report greater gender dysphoria and a cross-sex pattern of play, cognitive abilities, and digit ratio consistent with the hypothesized shift in the sexual differentiation of brain and behavior.

Because masculinization and feminization are independent hormonal processes (Collaer and Hines 1995), different mechanisms may be required to account for "hyperfeminization" or very high levels of "feminine" traits, such as excessive dependency. Therefore, it may be pertinent that prenatal stress in rats demasculinizes and feminizes sexually dimorphic brain structures and

behavior such as sexual behavior and social play (Ward and Reed 1985; Ward and Stehm 1991). In humans, prenatal stress produces attentional deficits, excess anxiety, dysregulation of the adrenal axis, and a subsequent impaired stress response (Koehl et al. 1999; Weinstock 1997). Significantly, these effects are greater in females compared with males (McCormick et al. 1995). Prenatal stress has also been implicated in the pathogenesis of some gender-linked disorders such as depression (Weinstock 2000). In a recent investigation of the behavioral effects of prenatal stress, female rats compared with male rats were found to display greater "depressive" behavior (defined as longer periods of immobility in a forced swim test) that was reduced by administration of androgens (Frye and Wawrzycki 2003). Although evidence that prenatal stress affects a range of human gender-linked behavior is equivocal (Hines 2002), the animal research showing that prenatal stress alters sex-linked behavior, including analogs of depression, suggests a mechanism whereby high levels of prenatal stress may predispose males to female-typical personality traits or female-typical personality disorders.

Research on human hormone–behavior relations has also shown that sensitivity to sex steroids in postnatal life is a general characteristic of behaviors that are influenced by prenatal hormones. Therefore, a role for steroids in pathogenesis of disorders that show sex differences predicts that symptoms will vary across normative reproductive development (e.g., at puberty or across the menstrual cycle). Periods of increased adrenal and gonadal steroid production, for example, coincide with the onset or expression of motor and vocal tics (Peterson et al. 1992). In boys, lower testosterone levels and smaller diurnal changes in testosterone are positively associated with internalizing symptoms (Granger et al. 2003). Normative changes in sex steroids in women (i.e., premenstrual period, postpartum, menopause) are also associated with increased depression (Seeman 1997; Weissman and Klerman 1977). Therefore, it is particularly interesting that the expression of borderline symptoms in young women was found increased during the late follicular phase of the menstrual cycle (i.e., a period of increasing estrogen levels) and following administration of synthetic estrogens in oral contraceptive form (DeSoto et al. 2003). These changes in symptom severity may reflect the modulatory effects of hormones on neurotransmitter systems implicated in the etiology of psychological disorders (Epperson et al. 1999). However, whether sex-specific hormonal effects on brain functional asymmetry or response to emotional stimuli contribute to these findings may be an informative area for future investigations on gender differences in personality disorders.

Finally, human hormone–behavior research also indicates that extreme sensitivity to changing levels of sex steroids may exist in some individuals. For example, cognitive impairment has been reported to occur in a small percentage of women following a sudden decrease in estrogen levels at postpartum period (Hamilton 1989) or following ovarian suppression (Varney et al. 1993). Similarly, a small number of men experience mania and aggressiveness following hormone administration, resulting in supraphysiological levels of testosterone (Pope and Katz 1988). Characteristics of individuals highly responsive to hormone variations are not well established. Animal research suggests that individual differences in hormone responsiveness may be associated with variables such as individual differences in tissue sensitivity, prenatal stress, and prior exposure to the social context (Hull et al. 2002). Research identifying factors associated with a transient adverse response to acute changes in hormone levels may provide information relevant to understanding the development of the more stable behavioral characteristics associated with gender-linked personality disorders.

CONCLUSIONS

Gender differences in typical and atypical personality development have been explained primarily in terms of the differential socialization and life experiences of males and females. However, it appears that socialization in many instances elaborates on innate behavioral tendencies. For example, feminine traits of communality appear evident in neonatal girls who, unlike neonatal boys, show visual preferences for faces with natural movement over objects with mechanical motion (Connellan et al. 2000). Significantly, in a recent long-term study of wild baboons, females displaying greater social integration (defined as grooming and proximity to other adults) were more likely than other females to rear infants successfully (Silk et al. 2003). These data suggest that complementary forces of nature and nurture on the development of personality likely exist because gender-linked personality traits have adaptive significance. They also suggest that gender-linked personality disorders may occur in part because these traits are highly sensitive to variables that alter the sexual differentiation of the brain (e.g., prenatal stress) or desynchronize the typical pattern of hormone–behavior relations in postnatal development (e.g., because of

atypical pubertal development or atypical social development, such as extreme prepubertal exposure to aggressive or sexual stimuli).

REFERENCES

Akhtar S, Byrne J, Doghramhi K: The demographic profile of borderline personality disorder. J Clin Psychiatry 47:196–198, 1986

Alexander GM: An evolutionary perspective of sex-typed toy preferences: pink, blue and the brain. Arch Sex Behav 32:7–14, 2003

Alexander GM, Hines M: Sex differences in responses to children's toys in a non-human primate (Cercopithecus aethiops sabaeus). Evol Hum Behav 23:467–479, 2003

Alexander GM, Peterson BS: Sex steroids and human behavior: implications for developmental psychopathology. CNS Spectr 6:75–88, 2001

Alexander GM, Peterson BS: Testing the prenatal hormone hypothesis of tic-related disorders: gender identity and gender role behavior. Dev Psychopathol 16:407–420, 2004

Alexander GM, Sherwin BB: The association between testosterone, sexual arousal, and selective attention for erotic stimuli in men. Horm Behav 25:367–381, 1991

Alexander GM, Sherwin BB: Sex steroids, sexual behavior, and selection attention for erotic stimuli in women using oral contraceptives. Psychoneuroendocrinology 18:91–102, 1993

Alexander GM, Swerdloff RS, Wang C, et al: Androgen-behavior correlations in hypogonadal men and eugonadal men, II: cognitive abilities. Horm Behav 33:85–94, 1998

Alexander GM, Altemus M, Peterson BS, et al: Replication of a premenstrual decrease in right-ear advantage on a language-related dichotic listening test of cerebral laterality. Neuropsychologia 40:1293–1299, 2002a

Alexander GM, Packard MG, Peterson BS: Sex and spatial position effects on object location memory following intentional learning of object identities. Neuropsychologia 40:1516–1522, 2002b

Al-Issa I: Gender and psychopathology in perspective, in Gender and Psychopathology. Edited by Al-Issa I. New York, Academic Press, 1982, pp 3–30

Allen LS, Gorski RA: Sex difference in the bed nucleus of the stria terminalis of the human brain. J Comp Neurol 302:697–706, 1990

Allen LS, Richey MF, Chai YM, et al: Sex differences in the corpus callosum of the living human being. J Neurosci 11:933–942, 1991

Alnaes R, Torgersen S: DSM-III symptom disorders (Axis I) and personality disorders (Axis II) in an outpatient population. Acta Psychiatr Scand 78:348–355, 1988

American Psychiatric Association: Diagnostic and Statistical Manual of Mental Disorders, 3rd Edition. Washington, DC, American Psychiatric Association, 1980

American Psychiatric Association: Diagnostic and Statistical Manual of Mental Disorders, 3rd Edition, Revised. Washington, DC, American Psychiatric Association, 1987

American Psychiatric Association: Diagnostic and Statistical Manual of Mental Disorders, 4th Edition. Washington, DC, American Psychiatric Association, 1994

American Psychiatric Association: Diagnostic and Statistical Manual of Mental Disorders, 4th Edition, Text Revision. Washington, DC, American Psychiatric Association, 2000

Anderson KG, Sankis LM, Widiger TA: Pathology versus statistical infrequency: potential sources of gender bias in personality disorder criteria. J Nerv Ment Dis 189:661–668, 2001

Archer J: The influence of testosterone on human aggression. Br J Psychol 82:1–28, 1991

Arnold AP, Breedlove SM: Organizational and activational effects of sex steroids on brain and behavior: a reanalysis. Horm Behav 19:469–498, 1985

Arnold AP, Gorski RA: Gonadal steroid induction of structural sex differences in the central nervous system. Annu Rev Neurosci 7:413–442, 1984

Baldwin JD, Baldwin JI: Gender differences in sexual interest. Arch Sex Behav 26:181–210, 1997

Bardenstein KK, McGlashan TH: Gender differences in affective, schizoaffective and schizophrenic disorders: a review. Schizophr Res 3:159–172, 1990

Baron-Cohen S, Hammer J: Is autism an extreme form of the male brain? Advances in Infancy Research 11:193–217, 1997

Barzega G, Maina G, Venturello S, et al: Gender-related distribution of personality disorders in a sample of patients with panic disorder. Eur Psychiatry 16:173–179, 2001

Becker D, Lamb S: Sex bias in the diagnosis of borderline personality disorder and posttraumatic stress disorder. Prof Psychol Res Pr 25:55–61, 1994

Belitsky CA, Toner BB, Ali A, et al: Sex-role attitudes and clinical appraisal in psychiatry residents. Can J Psychiatry 41:503–508, 1996

Bem SL: The measurement of psychological androgyny. J Consult Clin Psychol 42:155–162, 1974

Berenbaum SA: Effects of early androgens on sex-typed activities and interests in adolescents with congenital adrenal hyperplasia. Horm Behav 35:102–110, 1999

Berenbaum SA, Hines M: Early androgens are related to childhood sex-typed toy preferences. Psychol Sci 3:203–206, 1992

Berenbaum SA, Resnick SM: Early androgen effects on aggression in children and adults with congenital adrenal hyperplasia. Psychoneuroendocrinology 22:505–515, 1997

Bernstein DP, Cohen P, Velez CN, et al: Prevalence and stability of the DSM-III-R personality disorders in a community-based survey of adolescents. Am J Psychiatry 150:1237–1243, 1993

Blashfield RK, Herkov MJ: Investigating clinician adherence to diagnosis by criteria: a replication of Morey and Ochoa (1989). J Personal Disord 10:219–228, 1996

Blazer D, George LK, Landerman R, et al: Psychiatric disorders: a rural/urban comparison. Arch Gen Psychiatry 42:651–654, 1985

Boggs C: Gender bias in four personality disorders. Masters Thesis, Department of Psychology, Texas A&M University, College Station, TX, 2003

Bornstein RF: The Dependent Personality. New York, Guilford, 1993

Bornstein RF: Sex differences in dependent personality disorder prevalence rates. Clin Psychol Sci Pract 3:1–12, 1996

Bourgeois JJ, Hall MJ, Crosby RM, et al: An examination of narcissistic personality traits as seen in a military population. Mil Med 158:170–174, 1993

Bradbard MR, Martin CL, Endsley RC, et al: Influence of sex stereotypes on children's exploration and memory: a competence versus performance distinction. Dev Psychol 22:481–486, 1986

Breedlove SM, Cooke BM, Jordan CL: The orthodox view of brain sexual differentiation. Brain Behav Evol 54:8–14, 1999

Broverman IK, Broverman D, Clarkson FE, et al: Sex role stereotypes and clinical judgments of mental health. J Consult Clin Psychol 34:1–7, 1970

Bussey K, Bandura A: Social-cognitive theory of gender development and differentiation. Psychol Rev 106:676–713, 1999

Butcher JN, Dahlstrom WG, Graham JR, et al: Minnesota Multiphasic Personality Inventory-2: Manual for Administration and Scoring. Minneapolis, MN, University of Minnesota Press, 1989

Cahill L, Haier RJ, White NS, et al: Sex-related difference in amygdala activity during emotionally influenced memory storage. Neurobiol Learn Mem 75:1–9, 2001

Cambell DW, Eaton WO: Sex differences in the activity level of infants. Infant and Child Development 8:1–17, 1999

Campbell A, Shirley L, Heywood C: Infants' visual preference for sex-congruent babies, children, toys and activities: a longitudinal study. British Journal of Developmental Psychology 18:479–498, 2000

Canli T, Desmond JE, Zhao Z, et al: Sex differences in the neural basis of emotional memories. Proc Natl Acad Sci 99:10789–10794, 2002

Caplan P: The psychiatric association's failure to meet its own standards: the dangers of self-defeating personality disorder as a category. J Personal Disord 1:178–182, 1987

Carson DJ, Okuno A, Lee PA, et al: Amniotic fluid steroid levels: fetuses with adrenal hyperplasia, 46, XXY fetuses, and normal fetuses. Am J Dis Child 136:218–222, 1982

Carter JD, Joyce PR, Mulder RT, et al: Gender differences in the frequency of personality disorders in depressed outpatients. J Personal Disord 13:67–74, 1999

Chodoff P, Lyons H: Hysteria, the hysterical personality, and hysterical conversion. Am J Psychiatry 114:734–740, 1958

Cleary T, Humphreys L, Kendrick S, et al: Educational uses of tests with disadvantaged students. Am Psychol 30:15–41, 1975

Collaer ML, Hines M: Human behavioral sex differences: a role for gonadal hormones during early development? Psychol Bull 118:55–107, 1995

Condry J, Condry S: Sex differences: a study of the eye of the beholder. Child Dev 47:812–819, 1976

Connellan J, Baron-Cohen S, Wheelwright S, et al: Sex differences in human neonatal social perception. Infant Behavior and Development 23:113–118, 2000

Coolidge FL, Merwin MM: Reliability and validity of the Coolidge Axis II Inventory: a new inventory for the assessment of personality disorders. J Pers Assess 59:223–238, 1992

Corbitt EM, Widiger TA: Sex differences among the personality disorders: an exploration of the data. Clin Psychol Sci Pract 2:225–248, 1995

Crosby JP, Sprock J: Effect of patient sex, clinician sex, and sex role on the diagnosis of antisocial personality disorder: models of underpathologizing and overpathologizing biases. J Clin Psychol 60:583–604, 2004

Cruz J, Joiner TE Jr, Johnson JG, et al: Self-defeating personality disorder reconsidered. J Personal Disord 14:64–71, 2000

Dabbs JM Jr: Testosterone and the concept of dominance. Behav Brain Sci 21:370–371, 1998

Dahl AA: Some aspects of the DSM-III personality disorders illustrated by a consecutive sample of hospitalized patients. Acta Psychiatr Scand 228:61–67, 1986

de Lacoste-Utamsing C, Holloway RL: Sexual dimorphism in the human corpus callosum. Science 216:1431–1432, 1982

DeSoto MC, Geary DC, Hoard MK, et al: Estrogen fluctuations, oral contraceptives, and borderline personality. Psychoneuroendocrinology 28:751–766, 2003

Diamond MC: Hormonal effects on the development of cerebral lateralization. Psychoneuroendocrinology 16:121–129, 1991

DiPietro JA: Rough and tumble play: a function of gender. Dev Psychol 17:50–58, 1981

Eagly AH, Wood W: The origins of sex differences in human behavior: evolved dispositions versus social roles. Am Psychol 54:408–423, 1999

Ekselius L, Bodlund O, von Knorring L, et al: Sex differences in DSM-III-R, Axis II personality disorders. Pers Individ Diff 20:457–461, 1996

Epperson CN, Wisner KL, Yamamoto B: Gonadal steroids in the treatment of mood disorders. Psychosom Med 61:676–697, 1999

Epting LK, Overman WH: Sex-sensitive tasks in men and women: a search for performance fluctuations across the menstrual cycle. Behav Neurosci 112:1304–1317, 1998

Everitt BJ, Bancroft J: Of rats and men: the comparative approach to male sexuality. Annu Rev Sex Res 2:77–117, 1991

Feingold A: Gender differences in personality: a meta-analysis. Psychol Bull 116:429–456, 1994

Flanagan EH, Blashfield RK: Gender bias in the diagnosis of personality disorders: the role of base rates and social stereotypes. J Personal Disord 17:431–446, 2003

Ford M, Widiger TA: Sex bias in the diagnosis of histrionic and antisocial personality disorders. J Consult Clin Psychol 57:301–305, 1989

Frederiskse ME, Lu A, Aylward E, et al: Sex differences in the inferior parietal lobule. Cereb Cortex 9:896–901, 1999

Frye CA, Wawrzycki J: Effect of prenatal stress and gonadal hormone condition on depressive behaviors of female and male rats. Horm Behav 44:319–326, 2003

Garb HN: Race bias, social class bias and gender bias in clinical judgment. Clin Psychol Sci Pract 4:99–120, 1997

Geary DC: Male, Female: The Evolution of Human Sex Differences. Washington, DC, American Psychological Association, 1999

Golomb M, Fava M, Abraham M, et al: Gender differences in personality disorders. Am J Psychiatry 152:579–582, 1995

Gordon HW, Lee PA: No difference in cognitive performance between phases of the menstrual cycle. Psychoneuroendocrinology 18:521–531, 1993

Gorski RA: The neuroendocrinology or reproduction: an overview. Biol Reprod 20:111–127, 1979

Granger DA, Shirtcliff EA, Zahn-Waxler C, et al: Salivary testosterone diurnal variation and psychopathology in adolescent males and females: individual differences and developmental effects. Dev Psychopathol 15:431–449, 2003

Gunderson JG, Shea MT, Skodol AE, et al: The Collaborative Longitudinal Personality Disorders Study, I: development, aims, design, and sample characteristics. J Personal Disord 14:300–315, 2000

Gur RC, Turetsky BI, Matsui M, et al: Sex differences in brain gray and white matter in healthy young adults. J Neurosci 19:4065–4072, 1999

Hamilton JA: Postpartum psychiatric syndromes. Psychiatr Clin North Am 12:89–103, 1989

Hamilton S, Rothbart M, Dawes RM: Sex bias, diagnosis and DSM-III. Sex Roles 15:269–274, 1986

Hampson E: Variations in sex-related cognitive abilities across the menstrual cycle. Brain Cogn 14:26–43, 1990

Hampson E, Rovet JF, Altmann D: Spatial reasoning in children with congenital adrenal hyperplasia due to 21-hydroxylase deficiency. Dev Neuropsychol 14:299–320, 1998

Harding CF: Social modulation of circulating hormone levels in the male. American Zoology 21:223–231, 1981

Hartung CM, Widiger TA: Gender differences in the diagnosis of mental disorders: conclusions and controversies of the DSM-IV-TR. Psychol Bull 123:260–278, 1998

Henry KA, Cohen CI: The role of labeling process in diagnosing borderline personality disorder. Am J Psychiatry 140:1527–1529, 1983

Hines M: Sexual differentiation of the human brain and behavior, in Hormones, Brain and Behavior, Vol 4. Edited by Pfaff DW, Arnold AP, Etgen AM, et al. San Diego, CA, Academic Press, 2002, pp 425–462

Hines M, Kaufman FR: Androgen and the development of human sex-typical behavior: rough-and-tumble play and sex of preferred playmates in children with congenital adrenal hyperplasia (CAH). Child Dev 65:1042–1053, 1994

Hines M, Fane BA, Pasterski VL, et al: Spatial abilities following prenatal androgen abnormality: targeting and mental rotations performance in individuals with congenital adrenal hyperplasia. Psychoneuroendocrinology 28:1010–1026, 2003

Hoffmann ML, Powlishta KK, White KJ: An examination of gender differences in adolescent adjustment: the effect of competence on gender role differences in symptoms of psychopathology. Sex Roles 50:795–810, 2004

Hull EM, Meisel RL, Sachs BD: Male sexual behavior, in Hormones, Brain and Behavior, Vol 1. Edited by Pfaff DW, Arnold AP, Etgen AM, et al. San Diego, CA, Academic Press, 2002, pp 1–138

Huselid RF, Cooper ML: Gender roles as mediators of sex differences in expressions of pathology. J Abnorm Psychol 103:595–603, 1994

Hyde JS, Linn MC: Gender differences in verbal ability: a meta-analysis. Psychol Bull 104:53–69, 1988

Hyler SE: Personality Diagnostic Questionnaire—4+. New York, New York State Psychiatric Institute, 1994

Hyler SE, Rieder RO, Williams JB, et al: Personality Diagnostic Questionnaire–Revised (PDQ-R). New York, New York State Psychiatric Institute, 1987

Hynan DJ: Unsupported gender differences on some personality disorder scales of the Millon Clinical Multiaxial Inventory-III. Prof Psychol Res Pr 35:105–110, 2004

Jackson HJ, Burgess PM: Personality disorders in the community: a report from the Australian National Survey of Mental Health and Well-Being. Soc Psychiatry Psychiatr Epidemiol 35:531–538, 2000

Jackson HJ, Whiteside HL, Bates GW, et al: Diagnosing personality disorders in psychiatric inpatients. Acta Psychiatr Scand 83:206–213, 1991

Josephs RA, Newman ML, Brown RP, et al: Status, testosterone, and human intellectual performance: stereotype threat as status concern. Psychol Sci 14:158–163, 2003

Kaplan M: A woman's view of the DSM-III. Am Psychol 38:786–792, 1983

Kass F, Spitzer R, Williams J: An empirical study of the issue of sex bias in the diagnostic criteria of DSM-III Axis II personality disorders. Am Psychol 38:799–801, 1983

Killgore WDS, Yurgelun-Todd DA: Sex differences in amygdala activation during the perception of facial affect. Neuroreport 12:2543–2547, 2001

Kimura D, Hampson E: Cognitive pattern in men and women is influenced by fluctuations in sex hormones. Current Directions in Psychological Science 3:57–61, 1994

Koehl M, Carnaudery M, Dulluc J, et al: Prenatal stress alters circadian activity of hypothalamo-pituitary-adrenal axis and hippocampal corticosteroid receptors in adult rats of both gender. J Neurobiol 40:302–315, 1999

Koehler JJ: The base-rate fallacy reconsidered: descriptive, normative, and methodological challenges. Behav Brain Sci 19:1–53, 1996

LaFerla JJ, Anderson DL, Schalch DS: Psychoendocrine response to sexual arousal in human males. Psychosom Med 40:166–172, 1978

Landrine H: The politics of personality disorder. Psychol Women Q 13:325–339, 1989

Lerman H: Pigeonholing Women's Misery: A History and Critical Analysis of the Psychodiagnosis of Women in the Twentieth Century. New York, Basic Books, 1996

Liben LS, Susman EJ, Finkelstein JW, et al: The effects of sex steroids on spatial performance: a review and an experimental clinical investigation. Dev Psychol 38:236–263, 2002

Lindsay KA, Sankis LM, Widiger TA: Gender bias in self-report personality disorder inventories. J Personal Disord 14:218–232, 2000

Linn MC, Petersen AC: Emergence and characterization of sex differences in spatial ability: a meta-analysis. Child Dev 56:1479–1498, 1974

Maccoby EE: Gender as a social category. Dev Psychol 24:755–765, 1988

Maccoby EE: The Two Sexes: Growing Up Apart, Coming Together. Cambridge, MA, Belknap Press/Harvard University Press, 1998

MacLusky NJ, Naftolin F: Sexual differentiation of the central nervous system. Science 211:1294–1302, 1981

MacLusky NJ, Bowlby DA, Brown TJ, et al: Sex and the developing brain: suppression of neuronal estrogen sensitivity by developmental androgen exposure. Neurochem Res 22:1395–1414, 1997

Maier W, Lichtermann D, Klinger T, et al: Prevalences of personality disorders (DSM-III-R) in the community. J Personal Disord 6:187–196, 1992

Manning JT, Baron-Cohen S, Wheelwright S, et al: The 2nd to 4th digit ratio and autism. Dev Med Child Neurol 43:160–164, 2001

Martin CL: Cognitive influences on the development and maintenance of gender segregation, in Childhood Gender Segregation: Causes and Consequences (New Directions for Child Development, No. 65). Edited by Leaper C. San Francisco, CA, Jossey-Bass, 1994, pp 35–51

Martin CL, Halverson CF: The effects of sex-typing schemas on young children's memory. Child Dev 54:563–574, 1983

Mazur A, Booth A: Testosterone and dominance in men. Behav Brain Sci 21:353–363, 1998

McClelland DC: Human Motivation. New York, Cambridge University Press, 1987

McClintock MK, Herdt G: Rethinking puberty: the development of sexual attraction. Current Directions in Psychological Science 5:178–183, 1996

McClure EB: A meta-analytic review of sex differences in facial expression processing and their development in infants, children, and adolescents. Psychol Bull 126:424–453, 2000

McCormick MC, Smythe JW, Sharma S, et al: Sex-specific effects of prenatal stress on hypothalamic-pituitary-adrenal responses to stress and brain glucocorticoid receptor density in adult rats. Dev Brain Res 84:55–61, 1995

McDermut W, Zimmerman M, Chelminski I: The construct validity of depressive personality disorder. J Abnorm Psychol 112:49–60, 2003

McLaughlin JE: Reducing diagnostic bias. Journal of Mental Health Counseling 24:256–269, 2002

Meaney MJ: The sexual differentiation of social play. Trends Neurosci 11:54–58, 1988

Meaney MJ, McEwen BS: Testosterone implants into the amygdala during the neonatal period masculinize the social play of juvenile female rats. Brain Res 398:324–328, 1986

Millon T: Manual for the MCMI. Minneapolis, MN, National Computer Systems, 1980

Millon T: Manual for the MCMI-II, 2nd Edition. Minneapolis, MN, National Computer Systems, 1987

Millon T, Millon C, Davis R: MCMI-III Manual. Minneapolis, MN, National Computer Systems, 1994

Morey LC: Personality disorders under DSM-III and DSM-III-R: an examination of convergence, coverage, and internal consistency. Am J Psychiatry 145:573–577, 1988

Morey LC: The Personality Assessment Inventory Professional Manual. Odessa, FL, Psychological Assessment Resources, 1991

Morey LC, Glutting JH: The Personality Assessment Inventory: correlates with normal and abnormal personality, in Differentiating Normal and Abnormal Personality. Edited by Strack S, Lorr M. New York, Springer, 1994, pp 402–420

Morey LC, Ochoa ES: An investigation of clinical adherence to diagnostic criteria: clinical diagnosis of DSM-III personality disorders. J Personal Disord 3:180–192, 1989

Morey LC, Waugh MH, Blashfield RK: MMPI scales for DSM-III personality disorders: their derivation and correlates. J Pers Assess 49:245–251, 1985

Morey LC, Warner MB, Boggs CD: Gender bias in the personality disorders criteria: an investigation of five bias indicators. Journal of Psychopathology and Behavioral Assessment 24:55–65, 2002

Nestadt G, Romanoski AJ, Chalel R, et al: An epidemiological study of histrionic personality disorder. Psychol Med 20:413–422, 1990

O'Brien M, Huston AC: Activity level and sex stereotyped toy choice in toddler boys and girls. J Genet Psychol 146:527–534, 1985

Penton-Voak IS, Perrett DI, Castles DL, et al: Menstrual cycle alters face perception. Nature 399:741–742, 1999

Peterson BS, Leckman JF, Scahill L, et al: Steroid hormones and CNS sexual dimorphisms modulate symptom expression in Tourette's syndrome. Psychoneuroendocrinology 17:553–563, 1992

Peterson BS, Pine DS, Cohen P, et al: A prospective, longitudinal study of tic, obsessive-compulsive, and attention deficit-hyperactivity disorders in an epidemiological sample. J Am Acad Child Adolesc Psychiatry 40:685–694, 2001

Phillips SM, Sherwin BB: Variations in memory function and sex steroid hormones across the menstrual cycle. Psychoneuroendocrinology 17:497–506, 1992

Phoenix CH, Goy RW, Gerall AA, et al: Organizing action of prenatally administered testosterone propionate on the tissues mediating mating behavior in the female guinea pig. Endocrinology 65:163–196, 1959

Pigott TA: Gender differences in the epidemiology and treatment of anxiety disorders. J Clin Psychiatry 60:4–15, 1999

Pomerleau A, Bolduc D, Malcuit G, et al: Pink or blue: environmental gender stereotypes in the first two years of life. Sex Roles 22:359–367, 1990

Pope HG, Katz DL: Psychiatric and medical effects of anabolic-androgenic steroid use. Arch Gen Psychiatry 51:375–382, 1988

Rademacher J, Morosan P, Schleicher A, et al: Human primary auditory cortex in women and men. Neuroreport 12:1561–1565, 2001

Raine A: Sex differences in schizotypal personality in a nonclinical population. J Abnorm Psychol 101:361–364, 1992

Reich J: Sex distribution of DSM-III personality disorders in psychiatric outpatients. Am J Psychiatry 144:485–488, 1987

Resnick SM, Berenbaum SA, Gottesman II, et al: Early hormonal influences on cognitive functioning in congenital adrenal hyperplasia. Dev Psychol 22:191–198, 1986

Robinson DA, Worell J: Issues in clinical assessment with women, in Clinical Personality Assessment: Practical Approaches, 2nd Edition. New York, Oxford University Press, 2002, pp 190–207

Ronningstam E, Gunderson J: Identifying criteria for narcissistic personality disorder. Am J Psychiatry 147:918–922, 1990

Roth RM, Baribeau J: Gender and schizotypal personality features. Pers Individ Dif 22:411–416, 1997

Ruble DN, Martin CL: Gender development, in Handbook of Child Psychology, Vol 3, 5th Edition. Edited by Eisenberg N. New York, Wiley, 1998, pp 933–1016

Rutter M, Garmezy N: Developmental psychopathology, in Socialization, Personality and Social Development, Vol 4. Edited by Hetherington EM. New York, Wiley, 1983, pp 775–911

Salekin RT, Rogers R, Sewell KW: Construct validity of psychopathy in a female offender sample: a multitrait-multimethod evaluation. J Abnorm Psychol 106:576–585, 1997

Schultheiss OC, Rohde W: Implicit power motivation predicts men's testosterone changes and implicit learning in a contest situation. Horm Behav 41:195–202, 2002

Schultheiss OC, Dargel A, Rohde W: Implicit motives and gonadal steroid hormones: effects of menstrual cycle phase, oral contraceptive use, and relationship status. Horm Behav 43:293–301, 2003

Seeman MV: Psychopathology in women and men: focus on female hormones. Am J Psychiatry 154:1641–1647, 1997

Serbin LA, Poulin-Dubois D, Colburne KA, et al: Gender stereotyping in infant: visual preferences for and knowledge of gender-stereotyped toys in the second year of life. Int J Behav Dev 25:7–15, 2001

Sherwin BB, Gelfand MM, Brender W: Androgen enhances sexual motivation in females: a prospective, cross-over study of sex steroid administration in the surgical menopause. Psychosom Med 47:339–351, 1985

Silk JB, Alberts SC, Altmann J: Social bonds of female baboons enhance infant survival. Science 302:1231–1233, 2003

Silverman I, Eals M: Sex differences in spatial abilities: evolutionary theory and data, in The Adapted Mind. Edited by Barkow JH, Cosmides L, Tooby J. New York, Oxford, 1992, pp 533–549

Singh D, Vidaurri M, Sambarano RJ, et al: Behavioral, morphological, and hormonal correlates of erotic role identification among lesbian women. J Pers Soc Psychol 76:1035–1049, 1999

Sinha BK, Watson DC: Personality disorder in university students: a multitrait-multimethod matrix study. J Personal Disord 15:235–244, 2001

Skodol AE: Gender-specific etiologies for antisocial and borderline personality disorders? in Gender and Its Effects on Psychopathology. Edited by Frank E. Washington, DC, American Psychiatric Press, 2000, pp 37–60

Skodol A, Bender D: Why are women diagnosed borderline more than men? Psychiatr Q 74:349–360, 2003

Spitzer RL, Williams JBW, Kass F, et al: National field trial of the DSM-III-R diagnostic criteria for self-defeating personality disorder. Am J Psychiatry 146:1561–1567, 1989

Spitzer RL, Feister S, Gay M, et al: Results of a survey of forensic psychiatrists on the validity of the sadistic personality disorder diagnosis. Am J Psychiatry 148:875–879, 1991

Sprock J: Abnormality ratings of the DSM-III-R personality disorder criteria for males vs. females. J Nerv Ment Dis 184:314–316, 1996

Sprock J, Yoder CY: Women and depression: an update on the report of the APA Task Force. Sex Roles 36:269–303, 1997

Tebartz van Elst L, Woerman L, Lemieux L, et al: Increased amygdala volumes in female and depressed humans: a quantitative magnetic resonance imaging study. Neurosci Lett 281:103–106, 2000

Torgersen S, Kringlen E, Cramer V: The prevalence of personality disorders in a community sample. Arch Gen Psychiatry 58:590–596, 2001

Turner RA, Altemus M, Enos T, et al: Preliminary research on plasma oxytocin in normal cycling women: investigating emotion and interpersonal distress. Psychiatry 62:97–113, 1999

van Honk J, Tuiten A, Verbaten R, et al: Correlations among salivary testosterone, mood, and selective attention to threat in humans. Horm Behav 36:17–24, 1999

Varney NR, Syrop C, Kubu CS, et al: Neuropsychologic dysfunction in women following leuprolide acetate induction of hypoestrogenism. J Assist Reprod Genet 10:53–57, 1993

Voyer D, Voyer S, Bryden MP: Magnitude of sex differences in spatial abilities: a meta-analysis and consideration of critical variables. Psychol Bull 117:250–270, 1995

Ward IL, Reed J: Prenatal stress and prepubertal social rearing conditions interact to determine sexual behavior in male rats. Behav Neurosci 99:301–309, 1985

Ward IL, Stehm KE: Prenatal stress feminizes juvenile play patterns in male rats. Physiol Behav 50:601–605, 1991

Warner R: The diagnosis of antisocial and hysterical personality disorders. J Nerv Ment Dis 166:839–845, 1978

Weinstock M: Does prenatal stress impair coping and regulation of hypothalamic-pituitary-adrenal axis? Neurosci Biobehav Rev 21:1–10, 1997

Weinstock M: Behavioral and neurohormonal sequelae of prenatal stress: a suggested model of depression, in Contemporary Issues in Modeling Psychopathology. Edited by Myslobodsky M, Weiner I. Dordrecht, Holland, Kluwer, 2000, pp 45–54

Weissman MM, Klerman GL: Sex differences and the epidemiology of depression. Arch Gen Psychiatry 34:98–111, 1977

Widiger TA: Invited essay: sex biases in the diagnosis of personality disorders. J Personal Disord 12:95–118, 1998

Widiger TA, Settle S: Broverman et al. revisited: an artifactual sex bias. J Pers Soc Psychol 53:463–469, 1987

Widiger TA, Spitzer RL: Sex bias in the diagnosis of personality disorders: conceptual and methodological issues. Clin Psychol Rev 11:1–22, 1991

Widiger TA, Trull TJ: Borderline and narcissistic personality disorders, in Comprehensive Handbook of Psychopathology, 2nd Edition. Edited by Sutker PB, Adams HE. New York, Plenum, 1993, pp 371–394

Wierzbicki M, Goldade P: Sex-typing of the Millon Clinical Multiaxial Inventory. Psychol Rep 72:1115–1121, 1993

Williams CL, Meck WH: The organizational effects of gonadal steroids on sexually dimorphic spatial ability. Psychoneuroendocrinology 16:155–176, 1991

Williams JB, Spitzer RL: The issue of sex bias in DSM-III: a critique of "A Woman's View of DSM-III." Am Psychol 38:793–798, 1983

Wood W, Eagly AH: A cross-cultural analysis of the behavior of women and men: implications for the origins of sex differences. Psychol Bull 128:699–727, 2002

Zimmerman M, Coryell W: DSM-III personality disorder diagnoses in a nonpatient sample. Arch Gen Psychiatry 46:682–689, 1989

Zucker KJ, Bradley SJ, Oliver G, et al: Psychosexual development of women with congenital adrenal hyperplasia. Horm Behav 30:300–318, 1996

35

Cross-Cultural Issues

Renato D. Alarcón, M.D., M.P.H.

Culture is defined as the set of norms or behavioral patterns, meanings, lifestyles, and values shared and utilized by members of a determined human group. It includes variables such as social relationships, language, religion, ethical principles, traditions, technology, legal norms, and even financial philosophies (Group for the Advancement of Psychiatry 2002). In ancient periods, material elements (e.g., tools, housing, diet) constituted the core of the concept of culture, but centuries of instrumental and conceptual evolution forged the "nonmaterial culture"—the beliefs, deeds, and legacies of generations that have shaped social organizations of singular complexity. Culture may also modify its parameters as a result of social changes that are sometimes unpredictable.

Two other notions are often discussed vis-à-vis the definition of culture. *Race* is a term that fundamentally groups individuals on the basis of physiognomic characteristics (e.g., height, skin color, facial features). Although its scientific validity is controversial, its emotional impact has been crucial. This concept has generated in good measure the existence of "minorities" from demographic and social perspectives and the subproduct of racism in intergroup transactions. *Ethnicity*, on the other hand, entails differentiation, distinction, and identification of groups on the basis of

a common historical and/or geographic origin; it reflects the sense of belongingness, self-image, and intrapsychic life, and it forms the basis of identity through its impact on personality development.

Accumulated experience and systematic knowledge make clear that culture is an integral part of psychiatric theory and practice. Cultural psychiatry attempts to systematize all these interactions. It deals with the definition, description, evaluation, and management of all psychiatric conditions as they reflect the influence of cultural factors within a biopsychosocial context. Cultural psychiatry uses concepts and instruments of both social and biological sciences to advance the global understanding and treatment of psychopathological entities. It promotes culturally relevant clinical care of every patient and the elaboration of ideas and hypotheses aimed at a universally valid management of emotional suffering. Unquestionably, cultural psychiatry has contributed to the depathologization of culturally determined behaviors, the clarification of the role of culture in the etiopathogenesis and pathoplasty of psychiatric syndromes, the diagnosis and treatment of those syndromes, and the acceptance of demographic diversity, help-seeking patterns, and cultural competence in all aspects of professional work (Alarcón et al. 1999).

Clinical perspectives on personality disorders may vary among different countries or different regions of the world (Tyrer et al. 1984). For a number of years after the advent of the concept of borderline personality in the U.S. psychiatric literature, the concept was not accepted in many parts of Western Europe, where, on the contrary, it was severely questioned and criticized. Swedish psychiatrists emphasize the subjective aspects of their borderline patients as opposed to the lability and socially disruptive behavior prominent in American patients with the same diagnosis (Burns 1986). It is possible that in other countries, similar personality disorders can be described or labeled differently—an example is the use of the term *anankastic* in Europe to describe what U.S. psychiatrists know as obsessive-compulsive personality disorder (Berrios 2000). Also, a distinction should be made about the use of the antisocial personality label in the United States versus the use of antisocial behavior as a survival mechanism in societies where poverty, violence, or social unrest are prominent features of everyday life (Reid 1985).

CULTURE AND THE ETIOPATHOGENESIS OF PERSONALITY DISORDERS

Whereas personality traits cover a normal range of behaviors, personality disorders are characterized by enduring maladaptive patterns related to a variety of social, psychological, neurocognitive, and genetic mechanisms (Karterud 1988; Nash 1998; Paris 1998; Robbins 1989; Samuelian et al. 1994). Culture plays an etiopathogenic role, in close interaction with biological factors, influencing cognitive/perceptual structures, regulation of impulsivity, aggressiveness, and affective stability—all areas that, when altered or in disarray, lead to the behavioral and emotional manifestations of personality disorders.

Pathogenic Processes

A variety of situations and culture-based pathogenic sources throughout the developmental cycle contribute to the gradual articulation of personality disorders.

Child-Rearing Practices

Childhood experiences continue operating in later phases of the life cycle at both the biological and the psychological levels. Child-rearing practices are heavily

dictated by cultural norms transmitted from generation to generation. It is not mere coincidence, for example, that maternal anxiety significantly correlates with "child difficultness" (Mednick et al. 1996). The quality of the caregiving environment during the child's second year of life plays a significant role in the development of early conduct problems (Shaw et al. 2000). Historically, the Hutterites, an ethnic enclave living for over a century in the United States and Canada, and the Samoans in the South Pacific (Mead 1928) showed a remarkable absence of "undesirable" (antisocial) behaviors such as violence, crime, delinquency, neglect, and selfishness until the strong entry of so-called Western cultural features into the everyday life of these communities. Similarly, machismo (understood as exaggerated masculine behaviors such as toughness, mastery, and pride) seems to have a close relationship with punitive child-rearing practices (DeYoung and Ziegler 1994).

Family-Based Experiences

Childhood physical and sexual abuse within the family and negative relationships with parents and caretakers (and later, boyfriends or spouses) are well-known events in the past personal history of patients with borderline personality disorder (BPD), and other Cluster B and C categories (Green and Kaplan 1994). In cultures in which family life is revered and intrafamily hierarchies are well established, the risk for Cluster C (particularly passive-dependent, avoidant or obsessive-compulsive) personality disorders is higher. Wu (1992) postulated that the masochistic trends of subservience and long-suffering found in Chinese women are the result of clashing pressures from within and outside family life. Similar identity problems, emptiness, abandonment, absence of autonomy, and low anxiety threshold have been found in child and adult immigrants (Laxenaire et al. 1982; Trouve et al. 1983). In many cultures, a number of personality and behavior problems have emerged from family tensions, maladaptation, emotional disturbance, psychosomatic illnesses, addiction, severe social and network disruption, and status dislocation. The single-parent family and a cultural milieu of poverty may also contribute to the occurrence of personality disorders.

Religion

Rohr (1993) found that Evangelicals, Protestants, and Mormons focus on the ambivalence of desire and drive of their potential followers, thereby directly influencing three different aspects of identity-building processes: collective and symbiotic experiences, mother–child symbiosis, and the yet "uncivilized" corporeality and sensuality of a child. In a sample of Egyptian outpatients, Okasha et al. (1994) explored the impact of ritualistic upbringing on obsessive-compulsive symptomatology: Muslim rituals appeared to be different in quality and resulted in a higher frequency of obsessive features than Christian rituals. One-third of Christian subjects had a comorbid depressive disorder, but another 34% had paranoid, anxious, or emotionally labile personality disorder—whereas only 14% had obsessive personality disorder, half the rate of Muslim subjects. Personalities developed under the rigid Catholic rules—that, until the relatively recent past, emphasized guilt and shame as a response to perceived sins—may show characteristics that either predispose these individuals to specific personality disorders (i.e., avoidant or dependent) or are already part of a well-established diagnosis.

Finally, episodes such as the Guyana mass suicide or the group suicide of alien-expecting members of a religious cult are clinical expressions of personality disorders, extreme behaviors reflecting exaggerated beliefs. Religious experiences as well as political persuasion and recruitment processes have been called "brainwashing mechanisms" and may very well have operated in the pathogenesis of personality disorders in different historical periods (Frank and Frank 1993).

Societal Influences

Hamilton (1971) decried the lack of meaningful internalization of values in contemporary American society that then creates "unresolved dependency strivings" and subsequent individual psychopathology. On the other hand, even though so-called risk-taking behavior can arguably have a strong neurobiological basis (Siever and Davis 1991), some authors (Dake 1991) still see significant cultural biases such as hierarchy, individualism, and egalitarianism predicting distinctive rankings of dangers and preferences for risk taking at the societal level. Millon (2000) speculated about the divisive impact of rapid sociocultural changes (e.g., the diminished power of once-reparative institutions) that no longer compensate for early developmental and intrafamily deficiencies. Paris (1996) ascertained this mechanism in his biopsychosocial etiopathogenic model of antisocial personality disorder.

Members of individualistic cultures (United States and Australia) exhibit higher self-monitoring tendencies than those from collectivistic cultures (Japan, Hong Kong, and Taiwan) (Gudykunst et al. 1989). Smith

(1990) found that Asian American women have significantly lower narcissism scores than their white American counterparts; the variance is similar among Hispanic women. Grilo et al. (2002) postulated that the BPD diagnosis may represent a broader range of psychopathology in Hispanic men than Hispanic women.

Hispanics are known for strong somatizing tendencies, religiosity, strong sense of family and community, fatalism, emotionalism, preferential witchcraft practices, and pride, all against a background of machismo (Koss 1990; Padilla et al. 1987; Ramirez 1967). These are certainly pathogenic sources of some personality features and, eventually, of personality disorders such as obsessive-compulsive, avoidant, paranoid, dependent, or schizotypal.

Personality disorders are more frequent in urban than in rural settings (Cooper et al. 1972; Dohrenwend and Dohrenwend 1974), probably reflecting the effects of harsher stress in the everyday life of urban families. Relevant to these findings are Dohrenwend and Dohrenwend's (1969) suggestion that environmentally induced disjunctions between goals and the means to achieve them—and Wu's (1992) finding that discrepancies between aspirations (a culturally relevant variable of personality) and achievements—can lead to distress and pervasive personality disorder symptoms.

Life Events

Patients with personality disorders have experienced more frequent and more intense life events (cultural occurrences) such as incest, sexual assault, domestic violence, suicide attempts, and abuse of alcohol, tranquilizers, and other substances than the average population (Berenstein et al. 1993; Ward and Searle 1991). Issues of sexuality are a predominant feature among women diagnosed with BPD. Almost half of patients reporting a childhood history of abuse showed significantly higher sexual assertiveness, greater erotophilic attitudes, and higher sexual self-esteem (Noll 1993); yet despite these findings they evidenced significantly greater sexual preoccupation, sexual depression, and sexual dissatisfaction. The provision of care in psychiatric, forensic, penal, and other institutions "may degenerate into a form of unconscious abuse perpetrated against those in care" (Hinshelwood 2002, p. 28), thus perpetuating personality pathology.

The pathogenic power of the Nazi holocaust on its victims is an extraordinary example of an extreme cultural event (war) playing a pathogenic role in a number of psychopathologies, particularly personality disorders. Being outlawed and uprooted; becoming targets of discrimination and defamation; being deprived of rights; receiving constant death threats; losing individuality, language, culture, and home, with no survivors in one's family or elsewhere; and lacking appropriate burial for the dead (Peters 1989) set the pathogenic stage for behaviors such as paranoia, chronic anxiety, avoidant/phobic behavior, identity problems (borderline character), defensive narcissism, or histrionic style of interactions among Holocaust survivors. Some studies indicate that there may be a form of transmission of personality changes even to the second and third generation of Holocaust survivors (Sierles et al. 1983). Permanent personality changes as a result of traumatic events are a diagnostic category in both DSM-IV-TR (American Psychiatric Association 2000) and ICD-10.

Economic Factors

Rothman (1992) has argued that the decay of liberal capitalism is linked to a transformation of U.S. society into an adversarial culture that reinforces expressive individualism, collectivist liberalism, and ultimately alienation from both society and culture. The emphasis on materialism, narcissistic achievements, and competitiveness can lead to a breakdown of values that most cultures link to contentedness or inner peace. The resulting alienation operates as a possible premonitory factor of a variety of personality disorders.

Conversely, lingering feudal and colonial socioeconomic structures in so-called developing societies, and the chaos created by the discrimination against indigenous values and the postcolonial void, present an enormous obstacle to the development of autonomous individual personalities and effective social interactions (Montero and Sloan 1988). Dependent behavior is postulated to result from the influence of institutional structures interacting with traditional ways of life.

Acculturation

It is clear that modernization and industrialization have ruptured traditional family bonds, as family members move from rural areas to the city or to industrial areas (Boucebci and Bouchefra 1982; Laxenaire et al. 1982). Centuries of internal migration from small towns to large cities have delineated a set of "cultural illusions" that conflict with the everyday realities of citizenship in contemporary societies. The ambivalence toward a host culture doubtlessly contributes also to maladjustment, chronic bitterness, discouragement, or disillusionment that harbors further psychopathology. Rogler (1996) maintained that idioms of

aggression, assertiveness, and vindictiveness, mediated by anxiety symptoms, lead to different types of anger expression among Puerto Ricans in New York.

Pathoplastic Processes

The form and other descriptive features of personality disorder symptoms are clearly shaped by culture. The expressiveness of antisocial behaviors among Latino, African American, or Asian American patients may be different both in terms of external appearance and in severity or intensity. Robbins (1989) suggested that the absence of integration, inability of self-evaluation, and lack of adaptability (pathology of cognition and affect) in Clusters A and B personality disorders are both cause and effect of the pathological events. Accordingly, pathogenic factors also influence the symptomatological expression of each personality type—that is, dependency from inability of self-evaluation, paranoia from lack of adaptability, avoidance from absence of integration. In discussing BPD, Paris (1991) proposed that the disorder emerges when cultures change too rapidly, leaving behind those without adaptive skills. This rapid shift leads, for instance, to loss of identity expressed in the form of social protest, interpersonal instability, and poor self-image. Youth suicide and parasuicide might best be understood as the epiphenomena of contemporary social disintegration in postindustrial societies—an epidemic of personality disorders as a pathological yet understandable response against what is perceived as an oppressive, cold, distant, or unengaging society (Ishii 1985). The old notion of "cry for help" can be an ill-fated behavioral resource in a number of personality disorder types.

There are additional examples of the influence of social forces on the pathoplasty of behaviors. Investigating narcissism, social character, and communication in American culture, Goldman (1991) identified a "problematic selfhood"—fractured public culture and public actions reflecting the inner workings of personality rather than personal codes of meaning. External stimuli are both a setting and an audience for the narcissistic personality. Weatherill (1991) described culture's destabilization of the inner world and identified narcissistic pathology as correlated with and exacerbated by cultural trends that foster regression, violence, the breaking of social bonds, an illusory freedom, and an artificial sense of omnipotence.

Table 35–1 summarizes the main clinical features of personality disorders in different ethnic and cultural groups from a cultural psychiatry perspective.

Table 35–1. Clinical dimensions of cultural psychiatry as applied to personality disorders

Cultural groups	Interpretive/ Explanatory	Pathogenic/ Pathoplastic	Diagnostic/ Nosological	Therapeutic/ Protective	Services/ Management
Caucasian/White	Individualistic behaviors Arrogance	Media/Internet Television Family fragmentation Contemporary symbols	Strict use of existing classifications Cluster B	Reliance on oneself Group activities Internet	Conventional
Hispanic/Latino	Affective expressiveness Parental authority Pride, privacy	Migration/ Acculturation Barriers to host culture	Need to use cultural formulation Clusters B and C	Familism Religiosity Folk healers Role models	Cultural competence Interpreters Local staff
African American	Distrustfulness Suspiciousness Aggressive self-affirmation	Single parents Prison populations Criminalized behaviors	Need to use cultural formulation Cluster A	Political presence	Cultural competence Same ethnicity
Asian American	Passivity/Dependence Social hierarchies	Barriers to host culture Limited communication	Need to use cultural formulation Cluster C	Sociocentrism Role models Family support Group aspirations	Cultural competence Adaptable to different ethnicities
Native American/ Pacific Islanders	Melancholic Passive/Aggressive	Youth gangs Alienation Alcohol and substance abuse	Need to use cultural formulation Clusters A and B	Spirituality Folk healers Sense of community History	Cultural competence Scarcity of local staff

Note. See Alarcón et al. 1999.

CULTURE AND THE DIAGNOSIS OF PERSONALITY DISORDERS

The influence of the social and cultural environment on the psychiatric diagnostic process is undeniable. Nosology, reflecting efforts at systematizing such diagnostic knowledge, also is influenced by schools of thought, the personal training and cultural perspectives of the diagnostician, and the approachability and accessibility of patients, families, and social groups. It is pertinent to remember that the concept of disease, the science of epidemiology and the honing of the scientific method, the emphasis on empiricism, and the proving or disproving of hypotheses arose from Western culture; most aspects of the mental status examination and the labeling, diagnosis, and classification of personalities, temperaments, and personality disorders are all Western concepts. Furthermore, the continuous variation of cultural norms may result in the "normalization" of formerly described personality disorders or the addition of new ones (Mombour and Bronisch 1998). Some authors postulate that the whole category of personality disorders may be the result of a mistaken effort to medicalize some behavioral styles and is therefore an artifact of the reductionistic Western approach. Ideally, a culturally informed clinician will avoid the dual risks of stereotyping or trivializing human behavior and will be able to distinguish between personality styles and personality disorders (Alarcón and Foulks 1995a, 1995b).

The two most influential classification and diagnostic systems of this era, DSM-IV-TR and ICD-10, do have a cultural relevance greater than all of their predecessors. A pragmatic way for reducing the risk of "cultural fallacies" (Kleinman 1988) resides, for instance, in the systematic utilization of the cultural formulation included in DSM-IV-TR that allows the description of the cultural identity of the patient, his or her model of understanding and explanation of the symptoms, the nature and functioning of the psychosocial environment, and the relationship with the clinical or professional agent. Use of the cultural formulation will not only prevent mislabeling but in most instances will make possible a more appropriate contextual characterization of symptoms and behaviors of patients with personality disorder.

As a diagnostic and nosological factor in personality disorders, culture fulfills a variety of functions:

1. Helps refine clinical descriptors and diagnostic criteria and, in doing so, may also help to reveal even-

tual biases in the standard diagnostic approaches (Iwamasa et al. 2000)
2. Assists in differential diagnosis by helping to describe, explain, and/or understand different diagnostic types
3. Assists in generating treatment alternatives on the basis of a diagnostic approach that takes into account cultural factors such as child-rearing practices, societal influences, community attitudes, and other factors (Dunbar 1997)
4. Contributes to the understanding of clinical relationships or phenotypic variations between Axis I and Axis II conditions in DSM-IV-TR and other classification systems (Asaad et al. 2002)
5. Influences the diagnostician's or the nosologist's approach to data gathering, interpretation, and utilization of clinical information provided by the patient
6. Affects the structure, performance, evaluation, and usefulness of diagnostic instruments such as scales, questionnaires, and epidemiological surveys
7. Contributes to the ongoing debate about whether personality disorders should be considered true mental illnesses or variations of the so-called culture-bound syndromes (Nakamura et al. 2002)

Clinico-Cultural Diagnostic Assessment

Clinician and patient possess preexisting conceptions regarding the causes, treatment interventions, and eventual outcome of the condition under scrutiny. The interaction (sometimes, collision) of these two perspectives is crucial throughout the process and in the planning and implementation of treatment approaches.

The clinician who is culturally sensitive and competent will try to use simple, accessible language compatible with the patient's cultural background, psychological sophistication, and emotional needs. In this connection, nonverbal language is extremely important, and the clinician would do well to become familiar with the way the patient relates to his or her own relatives or to others. If a consultation is done in the outpatient environment, a preliminary observation of interactions in the waiting area may be very useful. It is important for the clinician to acknowledge the family members accompanying the patient to the visit as well as call them by their names, making a conscious effort to adapt to all the important social clues.

If necessary, the service system or care delivery organization should not hesitate to recruit an adequate number of interpreters as staff members. The use of interpreters in clinical diagnostic assessment is not without polemics, but overall, the consensus seems to be that they should be used whenever necessary. In using an interpreter, the questions to be asked should be as focused and thorough as if the patient and clinician shared a common language. The clinician should look at the patient intently and exchange words and sentences with the interpreter in a friendly, but at the same time very professional, way. The interpreter, in turn, should try to clarify the intent and sense of the question but should deliberately avoid introducing his or her own perceptions into the process. The clinician should be aware of the length of his or her own questions as well as the length of the sentences used by the interpreter and must gently question the interpreter about the clarity of his or her own words and statements.

The clinician should also pay attention to the affective component of the patient's clinical stance. The expressions of sadness, anger, frustration, fear, anxiety, and suspiciousness should be evaluated, and the depth of these thoughts and feelings, as well as their causal factors and personal impact, should be thoroughly recognized. In this context and in other aspects of the diagnostic process, a key approach for the clinician is not to question or refute the cultural beliefs that transpire during the interview. The clinician must remember that these statements reflect beliefs and values that the patient may or may not be accustomed to share and may thereby expose him- or herself to questioning, criticism, or misunderstanding. Interfering with or objecting to them may vitiate not only an accurate clinico-cultural diagnosis but also any treatment plans that may emerge.

In putting together the information about cultural background, cultural variables, explanatory models of illness and idioms of distress, and cultural beliefs in etiology, pathogenesis, therapy, and outcomes, the clinician's opinions should avoid sounding paternalistic, extremely technical, distant, or devoid of emotion and spontaneity. The same applies to the presentation of therapeutic recommendations. While using the official terminology and nomenclatures, the most important part of this phase of the assessment for the clinician is trying to find cultural equivalents to the patient's symptoms or syndromes, showing also thorough willingness to answer questions, no matter how simplified, off-topic, or inadequate they may sound.

Use of Diagnostic Instruments

Only a small number of personality disorder scales and similar instruments have been made available to individuals from different cultures. Once again, the tendency to "Westernize" comparative approaches, as well as the manualization and interpretation of test results, may be significant obstacles affecting the validity and reliability of such instruments. The need to cross-culturally validate them is essential in gathering meaningful data that may ultimately guide clinical work, delivery of services, and formulation of mental health policies (Cheung et al. 2003; Zheng et al. 2002).

A variety of personality measurement instruments have been used in different cultural groups. The Minnesota Multiphasic Personality Inventory (MMPI) is the most frequently utilized personality test. Nevertheless, its cultural value remains debatable because, among other reasons, it often confuses "cultural" factors with "socioeconomic" factors (McCreary and Padilla 1977). Choca et al. (1990) found that 45 of the 175 items of the Millon Clinical Multiaxial Inventory were answered in significantly different manners by white and African American patients, which suggests possible deficiencies regarding the cultural fairness of the test. African American subjects scored higher than white subjects in 9 of the 20 scales (histrionic, narcissistic, antisocial, paraphrenia, hypomania, dysthymia, alcohol abuse, drug abuse, and psychotic delusion). Sugihara and Warner (1999) found that Mexican American male batterers scored higher than nonbatterers on the avoidant and passive-aggressive scales, whereas nonbatterers frequently scored higher on the histrionic scale. The possibility that the instruments may be measuring different aspects of a disordered personality structure makes the need for cultural clarity in the instruments even more pervasive.

A number of other scales and instruments have been only partially used in intercultural comparative studies or, better yet, have been assessed with a cultural perspective in mind. Such is the case of the Eysenck Personality Questionnaire, several scales influenced by Cattell's work, the Hotzman Ink Blot Technique, and the Rorschach test (Goldsmith et al. 1989; Hyler et al. 1990; Inch and Crossley 1993; Jacobsson and Johansson 1985; Shattopadhyaya et al. 1990).

Several questionnaires or scales address the criteria set by classification systems such as DSM-IV-TR in the United States. The Personality Disorder Examination (Loranger et al. 1987) was adopted by the World Health Organization as an instrument for multinational studies on personality disorders, first in Europe and later in other continents, with acceptable interrater reliability and temporal stability (Loranger et al. 1994). The Structured Clinical Interview for DSM-IV Axis II Personality Disorders has been translated into several languages (Gomez-Beneyto et al. 1994). Grilo et al. (2003) found pervasive overlap of Cluster A personality disorders with other personality disorder criteria sets in the Spanish version of the Diagnostic Interview for DSM-IV Personality Disorders (S-DIPD-IV). The Personality Assessment Inventory has also been used for comparing monolingual and bilingual Hispanic individuals residing in Mexican American communities (Roberts 1980). The clinical scales have had moderate to good correspondence from English to Spanish versions, generally good stability for the Spanish version, and modest to good internal consistency for Hispanic subjects. Much more variation, however, was observed for the validity scales and the treatment/interpersonal scales. The cross-cultural value of other instruments such as the NEO Personality Inventory (Costa and McCrae 1992; Egger et al. 2003), the Wisconsin Personality Inventory (Klein et al. 1994), or the Differential Personality Questionnaire (Tellegen et al. 1988) remains to be fully established.

In summary, the diagnostic concepts imbedded in most personality disorder instruments do not seem to be sufficiently relevant to non-Western societies, cultures, and ethnic groups. The improvement in reliability of assessment devices, processes, and outcomes for the intercultural and multicultural use of these instruments is mandatory both in the present state of research development in this area and in responding to the clinical demands of social and demographic realities across the globe (Lucio et al. 1999). This goal requires a careful adaptation process that goes beyond mere language translation. The preservation of cultural fairness in epidemiologic and clinical instruments requires steps such as bilingual expert committees, conscientious back translation, systematic instrument testing in large samples, and cogent international correlational comparisons (Massoubre et al. 2002).

CULTURE AND THE TREATMENT OF PERSONALITY DISORDERS

As in other psychopathological conditions, the management of personality disorders from a cultural perspective entails the use of both psychotherapy and pharmacotherapy.

Psychotherapy

The recognition of a dual cultural context in the psychotherapeutic encounter is essential for the success of this intervention. Contextualization also applies to the setting in which the therapeutic experience takes place: a better social adjustment may be achieved by providing treatment within the patient's natural social habitat (Mauri et al. 1991). It is important to reformulate the concept and construct of empathy to more clearly address cultural and historical factors in the personal experience of the patient. Two other ingredients should be added: adaptability or flexibility and a clear measurability of the therapeutic work. Gaw (2001) listed the cultural factors that every psychotherapist or counselor has to take into account to attain successful results. They include culture-bound processes in transference and countertransference and microsocial and macrosocial issues that influence both the process and the structural elements of the clinician–patient relationship.

General Principles

Several authors (Gunderson and Gabbard 2000; Sanislow and McGlashan 1998; Target 1998) have agreed that, in general, the effects of psychotherapy on personality disorders are two to four times greater than in control conditions. However, the range of positive results oscillates between 5% and 52%. The cultural dimension, strictly speaking, has not been appropriately measured and validated in most studies. Measurement of trust, acceptance of authority, compliance, and active participation are seen more often among Asian American and Hispanic patients, whereas challenging positions, limit-testing behaviors, tendency to drop out, and—at the same time—more perseverance when the therapeutic alliance has been solidly established appear to be more evident among African American patients.

Frank and Frank (1993) hypothesized that demoralization plays a significant role in the patient's help-seeking patterns. Demoralization reflects a pathogenic way in which the individual responds to social challenges within the context of his or her own culture, how the patient has dealt with rules of social transactions, how he or she handles success and failure, and to what extent the patient has support from or is neglected by peers. In general, three steps must be taken into account when using a culturally relevant therapeutic approach to patients with personality disorders:

1. The recognition of the role of culture in personality development and social intercourse (Clauss 1998; Comas-Diaz and Greene 1994) entails the ongoing evaluation of factors such as the degree of individualism, socialization, family relationships, religious factors, and modalities of facing adverse situations. Knowing these factors allows the counselor or therapist to show flexibility in helping the patient with

vocational assistance efforts, language acquisition, and the unique sense of self in the appropriate context, all means of personal self-validation deeply affected in personality disorders.

2. The identification of these factors also ensures the establishment of effective therapeutic alliances. This feature is essential in the development of what Pellicier (1985) called the "psychic economy" in Western culture. Environmental factors disturb the "individual ergosphere" leading to losses, frustration, conflict, or changes. The concept of cognitive dissonance (or the discordances between personal estimations of individual performance and external assessments of the same) helps also to accurately formulate the cultural components of personality disturbances.

3. Appropriate and specific treatment techniques must be adopted. There is agreement that the treatment of personality disorders is complex, usually intensive, highly individualized, and perhaps has less-favorable outcomes than some other conditions. Every therapeutic modality ought to encompass a change in interconnectivity and the emergence of cooperative competition as the primary tools. Stone (1993) described the treatment of personality disorders as a series of steps from ecological selection to social integration and cultural transmission, followed by introspective reflection and "linguistical intentional sharing." Ultimately, the purpose of treatment is to change or enhance the "social intelligence" of individuals and communities.

Therapeutic Alliance

An essential notion of every psychotherapy, including those based on cultural precepts, is the establishment and strengthening of a good therapeutic alliance. The elements of curiosity, empathy, motivation, and subsequent outcomes are based on the fact that a cultural encounter is aimed at changing both patient and therapist. In the case of personality disorders, examples provided by folk stories, identification with heroes and heroines, problem resolution, social support, tolerance, and adaptability are essential therapeutic ingredients.

Moreover, different cultures offer the possibility of dealing with personality disorders in different ways. For instance, Asian Americans emphasize more the possibility of "self-effacement" to deal with either too-hostile or extremely avoidant types of personalities. African American healers emphasize assertiveness and idealization of historical figures as ways to vindi-cate or extricate the patient out of a convoluted set of interpersonal conflicts.

In general, the debate in psychotherapeutic circles about how supportive versus how exploratory the psychotherapy of personality disorders should be acquires even more relevance in dealing with patients with a unique cultural background. There is agreement that supportive and interpretive interventions can be mixed, sometimes without the therapist's awareness, and can lead to desirable changes in personality structure and personality functioning. Transferential interpretations—the essence of psychodynamic approaches—are, however, a more controversial topic. A number of authors dismiss the use of psychodynamic approaches in a number of personality disorders, and even studies considered to be very solid in the 1980s and 1990s have been questioned in recent years. Nevertheless, in Cluster C personality disorders, short-term dynamic psychotherapy may be useful, particularly if it pays attention to an interpersonal or cultural context in which memories, ideas, or reports of current emotional states are appropriately interpreted. This approach implies a good knowledge of social relationships, family interactions, coping styles, and explanatory models of the psychological conflict. It also entails an assessment of the patient's defenses or coping mechanisms: higher degrees of defensiveness weaken the therapeutic alliance, and whether the therapist should address that depends very much on the patient's articulateness, psychological sophistication, and tolerance threshold.

Settings

Several characteristics of the human and the physical setting in which therapy occurs have cultural implications. The more a physical setting resembles the patient's cultural environment, the better the outcome may be. In practical terms, such a setting may not be at all possible, even though the therapist and the service organization should always aim at making the patient feel more comfortable, cooperative, and forthcoming.

A clear description of the roles during the therapeutic process; who does what in the encounter; early measurement of assertiveness or dependence, detachment or active co-working; objective hierarchization of the therapist–patient relationship and roles; and assessment of the levels of intimidation versus collaboration are important steps in paving the way toward a successful therapeutic outcome. The use of forms or pencil-and-paper instruments may have an important cultural resonance. The multidisciplinary treatment team approach alleviates role conflicts by furthering flexibility. In some cases, having one person as a depository of the individual's trust and the group's general knowledge and confidence can be most helpful.

The therapist's credibility (Sue and Zane 1987)—that is, the patient's perception of the therapist as an effective and trustworthy helper—is even more relevant in a culturally charged context. Such credibility can be accomplished if the therapist conceptualizes the patient's problem in a manner that is congruent with the patient's belief systems; at the same time, the therapist can provide culturally appropriate means for problem resolution and for defining goals that are compatible with the patient's cultural background. A point of debate is whether therapist and patient should be of the same cultural background; those who object to this viewpoint argue that it may lead to "fusion," a real enmeshment of the therapeutic dyad that then becomes unproductive, oversimplistic in its approach, role confusing, and ultimately damaging (Comas-Diaz and Greene 1994).

Face-saving approaches on the part of Asian American patients, and the acceptance of pride as an element of privacy, hiding, and even denial of symptoms among Hispanic patients are frequently cited; the same applies to the detachment, hypercautiousness, and guardedness among African American patients in the initial phases of psychotherapy. Recognizing different ways to approach the elderly, children, and adolescents is also culturally important. Avoiding the use of adjectives that can be misinterpreted in their meaning and context would overcome some obstacles in the process.

Cultural Competence

Cultural competence plays a significant role in the psychotherapy of personality disorders. A culturally competent system of care 1) respects the unique, culturally defined needs of various populations; 2) acknowledges culture as a predominant force in shaping behaviors, values, and institutions; 3) views natural systems (e.g., family, community, church, healers) as primary mechanisms of support; 4) starts with the individual and family, as defined by each culture, as the primary and preferred points of intervention; 5) maintains that diversity within cultures is as important as diversity between cultures; 6) acknowledges that awareness of the dignity of the person is not guaranteed unless the dignity of his/her people is preserved; 7) accepts that cultural differences exist and treats all patients in their cultural context; and 8) respects cultural preferences that may value process rather than product and the harmony or balance within one's life rather than achievements (Cross et al. 1988).

Therapists of all origins and backgrounds must gain culturally competent skills based on cognitive changes through didactic models centered on case studies. This goal has an even more practical implication because it is clearly impossible to have "same-ethnicity" therapists available to respond to the demands of patients from all ethnic and cultural groups in the country. Parson (1985) advanced the notion of "ethnotherapeutic empathy." Koss-Chioino and Vargas (1999) advocated trainees being exposed, immersed, and shared into a process that allows them to better understand their own world and self-views as well as those of the people they are trying to help. This process is particularly important for personality disorders and includes study of conflict, conflict resolution, anger, and irritability as well as despondency and hopelessness.

The role of the provider stems from his or her professional identity, previous socialization, interpersonal transactions, and personal experiences. The patient's role has to do with internal fears, self-perceptions, and the possibility of misinterpretations regarding specific actions (Landrine 1992). Both the issue of confidentiality and the related concept of privacy have different cultural overtones, with some groups defending these issues more zealously than others.

The therapist's attitude of inquiry, a genuine curiosity about the people encountered as patients, should not be prurient but motivated by a desire to know and to feel what is most important to the subject of inquiry. Kleinman and Smilkstein (1980) had a type of case conference called "biopsychosocial grand rounds" in which each domain of a particular case was represented by at least one specialist who discussed the patient according to his or her perspective. The use of technological aids such as videotaping, PowerPoint presentations, telepsychiatry, and open forums or round table discussions can be very effective in developing this type of training in cultural competence (Alarcón 2004).

Techniques

Assuming that the patient accepts coming to treatment on a voluntary basis, Acosta et al.'s (1982) approach includes a process of "presocialization." A description of the clinic setting, including cultural trappings for the comfort of ethnic populations, is essential. A psychoeducational intervention that is, for instance, adaptive to the situation of differential acculturation can be used in the context of the "bicultural effectiveness approach" developed by Szaposnik et al. (1986).

Patients with a personality disorder should also be able to recognize the linkage between personal experience, social relations, and cultural meanings. This awareness would help the therapist not to appear as an intimidating or establishment-driven agent. The healer or therapist is "authorized" by the system to deliver a treatment that has cultural meaning. It is crucial for the patient to accept this redefinition of the problem in order to adapt his or her communication style to such requirements. The transformation of such meaning covers most of the therapeutic process throughout time. This "restoration of meaningfulness" (Gaw 2001) implies a renewed sense of connectedness with the culturally sanctioned value system.

Cultural Implications of Specific Psychotherapeutic Schools

The literature on proving the effectiveness of psychotherapy in personality disorders is relatively scarce. Each school poses a set of problems, resulting in uneven reports. Nevertheless, the consensus is that even minor results should not be underestimated. The same applies to improving techniques and outcomes on the basis of a better manualization of procedures or familiarity of the therapists with different techniques.

Psychodynamic psychotherapy. The goal of psychodynamic psychotherapy is to allow the patient to develop a relationship that ultimately becomes a healing, corrective, and genuine interpersonal experience that will lead him or her to new ways of thinking, feeling, and reacting in crucial interpersonal situations (Gunderson and Gabbard 2000). From the cultural vantage point, patients with personality disorder can see therapy as an opportunity to exercise their own distorted feelings of self-esteem or self-affirmation. This situation becomes even more complicated because the therapist's attitude in the traditional psychodynamic setting invites limit-testing behaviors, excessive identification with the "authority figure," or an increased suspiciousness on the side of the patient. If the therapist puts concepts such as splitting, regression in the service of the ego, triangulation, and acting-out in an appropriate cultural perspective, acting-out can be mastered, self-doubt can be erased or alleviated, boundary recognition can be better ascertained, and elusive interpersonal transactions can be significantly reduced.

Cognitive-behavioral therapies. The cultural implications of the cognitive-behavioral approach (Beck and Freeman 1990) are obvious. In cognitive-behavioral therapy (CBT) and similar techniques, the therapist acts as a participant observer. This approach refines the therapist's cultural view of some maladaptive cognitions and behaviors and eventually helps in the adaptation of cognitive-behavioral techniques (and the changes they induce) to such cultural perspectives.

Brief supportive psychotherapies. Focusing on current problems, brief and supportive psychotherapies should be solution oriented and limited in their scope. If the primary focus is a major maladaptive pattern, brief psychotherapy can be intensive while still respecting the time-limited context (Pollack et al. 1990). The treatment techniques should exhibit a sufficient degree of flexibility on cultural background and familiarity with the patient's interpersonal, culturally based resources. Ten to 12 sessions over a 6 to 12 month period can be appropriate (and acceptable for patients from different cultural backgrounds), with the understanding that the goals are limited and pragmatically dictated. The here-and-now problems of daily life, whether in the context of interpersonal or work relations, social adjustment, anger management, or others, allow for supportive psychotherapy to strengthen healthy psychological coping mechanisms, problem solving, and handling of environmental issues (Winston et al. 1991).

Group therapies. In group therapy the risk of pathological transference is more diffuse, and the patient experiences affiliation with other group members as well as with principles such as altruism, empathy, modeling, and solidarity. Because the group conveys to the individual patient a "cultural message" (Alarcón et al. 1998), group therapy adds a dimension that individual work cannot achieve. From self psychology modalities to techniques such as body awareness (Friis et al. 1989), group therapy works with what is preserved of the patient's "permeability" in order to secure a better adaptation to interpersonal and external realities (Dolan et al. 1992).

Religious/Spiritual approaches. Criticized and dismissed in the past as weak or irrelevant approaches to the management of personality disorders, religious and spiritual approaches are currently regaining popularity. The enhancement of empathy, understanding, and concepts such as forgiveness, "starting again" approaches, and a strong supportive basis for the explanation and understanding of symptoms are giving renewed strength to these approaches. Features such as unconditional empathy and cognitive changes cannot be dismissed as part of the therapeutic outcome with religious and spiritual approaches. The therapist joins in the patient's explanatory model and healing beliefs, generating a new understanding of the latter's shattered interpersonal relationships (Daie et al. 1992; Lukoff et al. 1992).

The spiritual component deals with previously ignored elements. Personality disorders are conceived, at a generic level, as a sort of spiritual emptiness. It only makes sense that well-trained therapists could address this need not by providing rhetoric, prayers, or invocations for divine help but rather by addressing notions such as a sense of belongingness, the need to transcend, and the possibility of personal redemption inherent in the religious and spiritual approaches.

"Cultural" therapeutic approaches. Most of the culturally specific therapies are based on popular or folk ethnomedical beliefs and practices (Tseng 2001). Erickson and Schultz (1982) and Pedersen (1983) have led efforts related to potential innovative modalities of existing techniques. The aim is to facilitate what these and other authors call "cultural responsiveness." For instance, one approach uses a trainee and a coach, with the team including a "client" and an "anticounselor." The latter makes explicit cultural assumptions expressed by the trainee and formulates critical comments about the trainee's approach to the client. Four skills are enhanced through the use of this model: the capacity to articulate the client's problems, the ability to recognize resistance, the opportunity for the therapist to deal with his or her own feelings of defensiveness when confronted by the "anticounselor," and the implementation of self-correcting approaches whenever necessary.

Comparative studies have been conducted mostly among children and adolescents (Constantino et al. 1994; Rogler et al. 1987). The so-called *dichos* (sayings) therapy is popular among Hispanic patients. This, and another technique called *cuento* (storytelling) therapy, allows culturally patterned topics to be "personalized" in the relationship with the patient, thus achieving greater effectiveness than modalities used in mainstream populations. A number of publications, manuals, and procedural norms with Mexican American adolescents have been published (Baca and Koss-Chioino 1997). These techniques emphasize issues dealing with ethnic identity, culturally specific patterns of family and peer interactions, creation of aspirational catalogues, encouragement and interpersonal stimulation or emulation, and other valid accomplishments. Most authors agree that the techniques as well as the outcomes vary in relationship to the generational status and length of stay in the country.

Culture and Psychotherapeutic Approaches to Specific Personality Disorders

BPD is the personality disorder most exhaustively studied by psychotherapy practitioners and researchers. In their classical work on this disorder, Kernberg et al. (1972) advocated the use of warmth and neutrality as well as specific expressions of respect for the patient's suffering. Clarification, confrontation, and interpretation can be used, but authors such as Kohut (1977) and Park et al. (1992) advocated more of a "holding environment" that can improve the prognosis of these patients.

Dialectical behavior therapy (DBT) emphasizes social skills training, new learning, self-soothing exercises, and group dynamics for patients with BPD (Linehan et al. 1993). The modeling approaches and the use of Zen Buddhist principles of acceptance, meditation, and mindfulness are heavily incorporated into this technique, making DBT a truly multicultural therapy that mixes elements of Eastern philosophy with methods and techniques of Western empiricism (Alarcón et al. 1998).

Duration of treatment is important in the management of borderline patients. It should not be forgotten that the time dimension is also heavily culturally influenced: Latino patients and European Mediterranean patients handle time differently than Far Eastern patients or African patients. If one wants to be more or less homogeneous in the application of some techniques, the patient should receive intermittent continuous therapy because the expectation of a definite termination can induce frustration, hopelessness, and ultimately noncompliance.

Among patients with narcissistic personality disorder, the results of this cognitive approach seem to be less dramatic, an outcome subsequently confirmed among ethnic group patients. The same applies to antisocial personality disorder, although as indicated earlier, antisocial behaviors could be considered essentially cultural survival devices. Cloninger (2004) has developed an approach he calls "coherence therapy" for antisocial personality patients; interestingly enough, it combines well-known therapeutic precepts (e.g., the establishment of a solid "therapeutic alliance" and respect for the human dignity of the patient) with heavily interculturally colored modalities such as meditation, music therapy, and "consciousness self-awareness."

Finally, the anxious personality disorders such as avoidant and obsessive-compulsive may respond to CBT if the underlying cognitive distortions are addressed and corrected on the basis of a relationship that recognizes the patient's social and cultural background (Andrews 1991). Cultural tools may contribute to alleviate extreme behaviors of patients with paranoid, schizotypal, and schizoid personality disorder who often present for treatment in the midst of a crisis and often see crisis resolution as the only objective of therapy.

Other issues in the culturally oriented therapeutic management of personality disorders have to do with comorbidity, for example, patients infected with HIV, personality disorders associated with drug abuse or mood disturbance, and/or greater use of denial and helplessness as coping strategies, plus an overall greater social conflict. When the comorbidity occurs between eating and personality disorders, Nozoe et al. (1995) made clear that all techniques, whether they are didactic, interpretive, cognitive, or existential, should pay attention to cultural elements such as dietetic habits, nutritional status, and body image.

Ethnopsychopharmacology

An emerging subfield in psychopharmacology is, undoubtedly, the approach to both cultural and biological singularities of ethnic groups different from the white population. Since the 1980s, vigorous research has described differences not only in clinical responses and the presence or absence of greater or lesser side effects—but also in specific distinctions in metabolic patterns—and ultimately in the genetic bases of these processes (Lin et al. 1993). Parameters such as plasma levels (peak and stabilized), half-life, rate of clearance, and others vary from group to group. Unfortunately, there is a dearth in the study of ethnopsychopharmacological interventions among personality disorder patients. Only since the 1990s have clinicians started the systematic evaluation of the impact of pharmacotherapy on these conditions. Prior to this time, the consensus was that medications had not been shown to be effective in the management of personality disorders.

In this context, different ethnic groups possessing probably different genetic make-ups can both metabolize medications in different ways and show variations in terms of time of initial response, quality of response, side effects, therapeutic levels of the different psychotropic agents, and other pharmacokinetic and pharmacodynamic patterns (Smith and Mendoza 1996). Different polymorphisms result in different patterns of enzymatic activities. Liver cytochrome P450 (CYP) enzymes catalyze oxidative reactions and therefore play a major role in the metabolism of both endogenous and exogenous compounds. Individuals can be classified according to the evaluation of cytochrome P450 enzyme expression as poor, intermediate, extensive, rapid, and ultrarapid metabolizers (Kirchheiner et al. 2001).

Poor metabolizers vary in terms of percentage among white, Asian American, African American, and Hispanic patients. Among Asian patients, only 1% lack the enzyme CYP 2D6 compared with 19% among the Suns bushmen, a tribe in the Australian forest, and 10%

among whites. Metabolic levels related to CYP 2C19 (another P450 enzyme) are relatively low among whites (about 3%), and substantially high among Asians and African Americans (18%–22%). Polymorphisms of alcohol and aldehyde dehydrogenase are more common among patients of Asian origin than among whites or African Americans. These result in the fast response of peripheral vasodilation (facial flashes) observed in Asian individuals after a small alcohol intake.

Among the tricyclic antidepressants, desipramine and nortriptyline clearances are significantly lower in Asians than in whites. African American patients treated with either nortriptyline or amitriptyline had a 50% higher plasma level of the former than did whites; however, no significant increase was observed with amitriptyline. The percentages of poor metabolizers of, for instance, risperidone (oxidized by CYP 2D6) is 5%–10% among whites and only 1%–2% among Asian Americans and African Americans. There are also significant differences in the metabolization by the same enzyme of fluoxetine, sertraline, venlafaxine, and nefazodone, with more poor metabolizers among whites than in the rest of the ethnic groups. In contrast, bupropion shows only 15% of poor metabolizers among whites versus 70% among Asian Americans; diazepam, metabolized by CYP 2C19, showed 20% of poor metabolizers among Asian Americans versus 2%–6% among whites. Among Hispanics, Mexican Americans are more intermediate and extensive metabolizers than Caribbean Americans.

The case of lithium is also intriguing: among African Americans, lithium has a longer half-life and a significantly higher ratio of red blood cells to plasma. Red blood cell lithium levels are believed to correlate with neuronal levels, which suggests that lithium dosage requirements may need to be lowered for African Americans.

Other factors contributing to the metabolization of pharmacological agents should be taken into account, among them culturally determined behaviors such as diet, tobacco consumption, and use of coffee, alcohol, herbs, and other agents. The adoption of new dietetic habits on the part of immigrants has resulted in well-demonstrated changes in the enzymatic repertoire of these individuals, thus changing transport and binding interactions at the pharmacogenomic level.

CASE EXAMPLE

Ms. LL was a 24-year-old Hispanic woman, the second of four children of an immigrant family, born in the United States. She came to a community mental health center seeking help for "depression and confusion." She grew up in a family led by an authoritarian, proud father who had to have itinerant jobs in different states to provide for his wife and five children. As a result, throughout the patient's childhood, her father was continuously out of the house, returning only for brief periods. Her mother was a quiet, very religious and resilient woman. Nevertheless, the patient perceived at times that her mother was overwhelmed by the demands on her time and energies. When her husband came back home, the patient remembers initial shows of joy and happiness soon followed by some bitter, shouting discussions. Nevertheless, each time the father was about to leave again, it seemed like both he and his wife had reconciled genuinely, father promising to return with "gifts" that only rarely materialized.

The patient had some difficulties with her English at the beginning of her school years. She attributed this to the fact that the family spoke only Spanish at home. Although she was born in the United States, she was still somewhat ridiculed by her peers because of her accent. She also had difficulties "understanding" some teachers and classes and was sent to the school counselors on two occasions; at one point, they administered psychological testing and told her that she had a "borderline IQ." During her adolescent years, her father apparently left the family for an extended period of time; her mother became significantly depressed and talked about her father having become "a drunkard." It was not until about 4 years later that the father reappeared in the patient's life.

Ms. LL's present illness had started about 1 year before the initial clinical contact. She started noticing herself as very nervous, irritable, and impulsive. She had several boyfriends who left her "because they got bored and even scared with my moodiness." At times, she was "the most charming girl," at other times she became angry, cold, hypercritical, and dismissive. She found herself without friends. The situation became complicated when a boyfriend whom she had been dating for a few months became "mean and violent." She resorted to drugs "to alleviate my emotional pain" and later decided to start cutting herself "to experience physical pain more than emotional pain." She entered college and was majoring in education, with aspirations of becoming a teacher. She did very well in most of her courses in spite of her emotional difficulties. She had not entertained suicidal thoughts. She found it difficult to talk with her mother "because she may be even more depressed than I am."

During the initial interview, the patient was at times very talkative and provided what sounded like useful information; at other times, she became "silly," giggling, somewhat seductive, and refusing to provide more information. When the clinician questioned her about these quick mood changes, she became defensive. She denied auditory or visual hallucinations. Her speech was a mix of English and Spanish, and when she did not want to provide information she either said that she did not under-

stand the question or that her English was "very poor," which was certainly not the case.

The initial tentative diagnostic impression included dysthymia and borderline personality features, with dysphoria and moodiness, plus ruling out cyclothymic disorder. The clinician referred her for psychological testing. The MMPI showed significant histrionic and "psychotic" features. Her IQ was 95, but the psychologist ascertained that the patient appeared to be "smarter than the IQ shows."

Ms. LL was referred to a counselor for weekly sessions on a regular basis. She politely requested a woman therapist who could speak Spanish. When this was granted, she seemed to be very happy and said she was willing to work hard on her case. In fact, a good therapeutic alliance was established with a therapist who was about 8 years older than the patient. The therapist used at first supportive approaches, then decided to start CBT to ascertain goals, help the patient learn some habits, and favor more open contact with the outside world. The patient learned quickly the nuances of CBT and after about 8 months in therapy said that she had recently met a number of "gringo" girls and had found it easier to establish friendly contacts. The therapist referred her to group therapy oriented toward anger management and further socialization. The patient liked particularly the use of short stories with Latino women as heroines and identified with those who "prevailed against all odds." On several occasions by the end of her therapy she brought in her mother, practically referring her for evaluation and treatment, which the mother accepted.

Six months after her last visit, the patient came to see her therapist and told her that she was about to graduate from college and was planning to get into a master's program. She was dating occasionally, still living with her mother, and also hoping that her father would get a more stable job in the city and return fully to the family's midst.

CONCLUSIONS

From this review, it is evident that culture contributes to the appearance and symptomatology of personality disorders. At the same time, culture can validate or eliminate some diagnostic labels in clinical practice. It is also clear that culture can be a preventive tool in the occurrence of these disorders because it can protect individuals and families from environmental factors that may trigger this type of psychopathology in vulnerable, predisposed individuals. The use of culture in the treatment of personality disorders has been widely shown to be a valid approach.

Overall, the clinical variations among personality disorders may be due not in small part to environmental or cultural factors. The clinician should be aware, therefore, not only of the patient's geographic place of origin but also of the ethnocultural background of the patient. The recognition of variability among seemingly homogeneous ethnic groups (including the white population in the United States) dictates clear differences in the history taking, diagnostic elucidation, therapeutic management, follow-up strategies, and ultimate outcomes. The judicious use of these variables will only have positive repercussions in the quality of life and on the fate of these patients and their families.

The clinical vignette presented at the end of the chapter illustrates, among others, features related to the influence of culture in child-rearing practices, the development of behavioral resources aimed at dealing with issues of abandonment and neglect in the household, and hostility and discrimination in the outside environment. The vignette also shows the depressogenic and anxiogenic impact of such factors and the deployment of interpersonal styles resembling a well-known personality disorder. Although this disorder was not the ultimate diagnosis, cognitively and behaviorally based individual and group therapies (strengthened by cultural features such as gender and language similarities with the therapist, both powerful factors in the Hispanic culture) enhanced healthy inner resources in the patient—and eventually led to a favorable outcome.

REFERENCES

Acosta FX, Yamamoto J, Evans LA (eds): Effective Psychotherapy for Low-Income and Minority Patients. New York, Plenum, 1982

Alarcón RD: La revolución didáctica en psiquiatria: retos y posibilidades en América Latina. Salud Mental 27:1–10, 2004

Alarcón RD, Foulks EF: Personality disorders and culture: contemporary clinical views, part A. Cult Divers Ment Health 1:3–17, 1995a

Alarcón RD, Foulks EF: Personality disorders and culture: contemporary clinical views, part B. Cult Divers Ment Health 1:79–91, 1995b

Alarcón RD, Foulks EF, Vakkur N: Personality Disorders and Culture: Clinical and Conceptual Interactions. New York, Wiley, 1998

Alarcón RD, Westermeyer J, Foulks EF, et al: Clinical dimensions of contemporary cultural Psychiatry. J Nerv Ment Dis 187:465–471, 1999

American Psychiatric Association: Diagnostic and Statistical Manual of Mental Disorders, 4th Edition, Text Revision. Washington, DC, American Psychiatric Association, 2000

Andrews G: The evaluation of psychotherapy. Curr Opin Psychiatry 4:379–383, 1991

Asaad T, Okasha T, Okasha A: Sleep EEG findings in ICD-10 borderline personality disorder in Egypt. J Affect Disord 71:11–18, 2002

Baca LM, Koss-Chiono JD: Development of a culturally responsive group therapy model. J Multicult Couns Devel 25:130–141, 1997

Beck AT, Freeman A: Cognitive Therapy of Personality Disorders. New York, Guilford, 1990

Berenstein VP, Cohen P, Velez CN, et al: Prevalence and stability of the DSM-III-R personality disorders in a community-based survey of adolescents. Am J Psychiatry 150:1237–1243, 1993

Berrios GE: History of Psychiatric Symptoms. Oxford, England, Oxford University Press, 2000

Boucebci M, Bouchefra A: Migration et psychopathologie familiale en milieu algerien. Ann Med Psychol (Paris) 140:638–644, 1982

Burns T: Use of the term "borderline patient" by Swedish psychiatrists. Int J Soc Psychiatry 32:32–39, 1986

Cheung FM, Kwong JY, Zhang J: Clinical validation of the Chinese Personality Assessment Inventory. Psychol Assess 15:89–100, 2003

Choca JP, Shanley LA, Peterson CA, et al: Racial bias and the MCMI. J Pers Assess 54:479–490, 1990

Clauss CS: Cultural intersections and system levels in counseling. Cult Divers Ment Health 4:127–134, 1998

Cloninger RC: Designs of Well-Being. London, Oxford University Press, 2004

Comas-Diaz L, Greene B (eds): Women of Color: Integrating Ethnic and Gender Identity in Psychotherapy. New York, Guilford, 1994

Constantino G, Malgady RG, Rogler LH: Storytelling through pictures: culturally sensitive psychotherapy for Hispanic children and adolescents. J Clin Child Psychol 23:13–20, 1994

Cooper JE, Kendell RE, Gurland BJ, et al: Psychiatric Diagnoses in New York and London. London, Oxford University Press, 1972

Costa PT, McCrae RR: The five-factor model of personality and its relevance to personality disorders. J Personal Disord 6:343–359, 1992

Cross T, Bazron B, Dennis K, et al: Towards a culturally competent system of care. Washington, DC, Georgetown University Child Development Center, 1988

Daie N, Witztum C, Mark M, et al: The belief in the transmigration of souls: psychotherapy of a Druze patient with severe anxiety reaction. Br J Med Psychol 65:119–130, 1992

Dake K: Orienting dispositions in the perception of risk: an analysis of contemporary world views and cultural biases. J Cross Cult Psychol 22:61–82, 1991

DeYoung Y, Ziegler EF: Machismo in two cultures: relation to punitive child-rearing practices. Am J Orthopsychiatry 64:386–395, 1994

Dohrenwend BP, Dohrenwend BS: Social Status and Psychological Disorder: A Causal Inquiry. New York, Wiley, 1969

Dohrenwend BP, Dohrenwend BS: Social and cultural influences in psychopathology. Ann Rev Psychol 25:417–452, 1974

Dolan B, Evans C, Wilson J: Therapeutic community treatment for personality disordered adults: changes in neurotic symptomatology on follow-up. Int J Soc Psychiatry 38:243–250, 1992

Dunbar E: The relationship of DSM diagnostic criteria and Gough's Prejudice Scale: exploring the clinical manifestations of the prejudiced personality. Cult Divers Ment Health 3:247–257, 1997

Egger JI, De Mey HR, Deksen JJ, et al: Cross-cultural replication of the five-factor model and comparison of the NEO-PI-R and MMPI-2 PSY-5 scales in a Dutch psychiatric sample. Psychol Assess 15:81–88, 2003

Erickson F, Schultz J: The Counselor as Gatekeeper. New York, Academic Press, 1982

Frank JD, Frank J: Persuasion and Healing, 3rd Edition. Baltimore, MD, Johns Hopkins University Press, 1993

Friis S, Skatteboe UB, Hope MK, et al: Body awareness group therapy for patients with personality disorders. Psychother Psychosom 51:18–24, 1989

Gaw A: Concise Guide to Cross-Cultural Psychiatry. Washington, DC, American Psychiatric Publishing, 2001

Goldman I: Narcissism, social character and communication: a Q-methodological perspective. Psychol Rec 41:343–360, 1991

Goldsmith SJ, Jacobsberg LB, Bell R: Personality disorder assessment. Psychiatr Ann 19:139–142, 1989

Gomez-Beneyto M, Dillarm, Renovell M, et al: The diagnosis of personality disorder with a modified version of the SCID-II in a Spanish clinical sample. J Personal Disord 8:104–110, 1994

Green AH, Kaplan MS: Psychiatric impairment and childhood victimization experiences in female child molesters. J Am Acad Child Adolesc Psychiatry 33:954–961, 1994

Grilo CM, Anez ML, McGlashan TH: DSM-IV Axis II comorbidity with borderline personality disorder in monolingual Hispanic psychiatric outpatients. J Nerv Ment Dis 190:324–330, 2002

Grilo CM, Anez LM, McGlashan TH: The Spanish-language version of the diagnostic interview for DSM-IV personality disorders: development and initial psychometric evaluation of diagnoses and criteria. Compr Psychiatry 44:154–161, 2003

Group for the Advancement of Psychiatry: Cultural Assessment in Clinical Psychiatry. Washington, DC, American Psychiatric Publishing, 2002

Gudykunst WB, Gao G, Nishida T, et al: A cross-cultural comparison of self-monitoring. Communication Research Report 6:7–12, 1989

Gunderson JG, Gabbard GO (eds): Psychotherapy for Personality Disorders (Review of Psychiatry Series, Vol 19; Oldham JM and Riba MB, series eds). Washington, DC, American Psychiatric Press, 2000

Hamilton JW: Some cultural determinants of intrapsychic structure and psychopathology. Psychoanal Rev 58:279–294, 1971

Hinshelwood L: Abusive help—helping abuse: the psychodynamic impact of severe personality disorder on caring institutions. Crim Behav Ment Health 12:S20–S30, 2002

Hyler SE, Skodol AE, Kellman HD, et al: Validity of the Personality Diagnostic Questionnaire–Revised: comparison with two structured interviews. Am J Psychiatry 147:1043–1048, 1990

Inch R, Crossley M: Diagnostic utility of the MCMI-I and MCMI-II with psychiatric outpatients. J Clin Psychol 49:358–366, 1993

Ishii K: Backgrounds of higher suicide rates among "name university" students: a retrospective study of the past 25 years. Suicide Life Threat Behav 15:56–68, 1985

Iwamasa GY, Larrabee AL, Merritt RD: Are personality disorder criteria ethnically biased? A card-sort analysis. Cultur Divers Ethnic Minor Psychol 6:284–296, 2000

Jacobsson L, Johansson S: Aspects of personality structure in Ethiopian and Swedish adolescents: a transcultural study with the Holzman Ink Blot technique. Acta Psychiatr Scand 72:291–295, 1985

Karterud S: The valence theory of Bion and the significance of DSM-III diagnoses for inpatient group behavior. Acta Psychiatr Scand 78:462–470, 1988

Kernberg OF, Burstein T, Coyne L, et al: Psychoanalysis and psychotherapy: trial report of the Menninger Foundation Psychotherapy Research Project. Bull Menninger Clin 36:1–275, 1972

Kirchheiner J, Brosen, K, Dahl ML, et al: CYP2D6 and CYP2C19 genotype-based dose recommendations for antidepressants: a first step towards subpopulation-specific dosages. Acta Psychiatr Scand 104:173–192, 2001

Klein RH, Quimette PC, Kelly HS, et al: Test-retest reliability of team consensus: best estimate diagnosis of Axis I and II disorders in a family study. Am J Psychiatry 151:1043–1047, 1994

Kleinman A: Rethinking Psychiatry. New York, Free Press, 1988

Kleinman A, Smilkstein G: Psychosocial issues in primary care, in Behavioral Science in Family Practice. Edited by Rosen G. New York, Appleton Century Crofts, 1980, pp 185–193

Kohut H: The Restoration of Self. New York, International University Press, 1977

Koss JD: Somatization and somatic complaint syndromes among Hispanics: overview and ethnopsychological prospective. Transcultural Psychiatric Research and Review 27:5–29, 1990

Koss-Chiono JD, Vargas LA: Working With Latino Youth: Culture, Development and Context. San Francisco, CA, Jossey-Bass, 1999

Landrine H: Clinical implications of cultural differences: the referential vs. the indexical self, in The Culture and Psychology Reader. Edited by Goldberger NR, Veroff JV. New York, New York University Press, 1992, pp 235–241

Laxenaire M, Ganne-Devonec MO, Streiff O: Les problemes d'identite chez les enfants des migrants. Ann Med Psychol (Paris) 140:602–605, 1982

Lin KM, Poland RE, Nakasaki G: Psychopharmacology and Psychobiology of Ethnicity. Washington, DC, American Psychiatric Press, 1993

Linehan M, Heard HL, Armstrong HE: Naturalistic follow-up of a behavioral treatment of chronically parasuicidal patients. Arch Gen Psychiatry 50:971–974, 1993

Loranger AW, Susman VL, Oldham JM, et al: The Personality Disorder Examination: a preliminary report. J Personal Disord 1:1–13, 1987

Loranger AW, Sartorius N, Andreoli A, et al: The International Personality Disorder Examination: the World Health Organization/Alcohol, Drug Abuse, and Mental Health Administration international pilot study of personality disorders. Arch Gen Psychiatry 51:215–224, 1994

Lucio E, Palacios H, Duran C, et al: MMPI-2 with Mexican psychiatric inpatients: basic and content scales. J Clin Psychol 55:1541–1552, 1999

Lukoff D, Turner R, Lu F: Transpersonal psychology research review. Journal of Transpersonal Psychology 24:41–45, 1992

Massoubre C, Lang F, Jaeger B, et al: The translation of questionnaires and of tests: techniques and problems. Can J Psychiatry 47:61–67, 2002

Mauri M, Sarno N, Armani A, et al: Differential social adjustment correlates of Axis I and Axis II psychopathology, I: anxiety and depressive disorders. Eur Psychiatry 6:127–130, 1991

McCreary C, Padilla E: MMPI differences among Blacks, Mexican American and white male offenders. J Clin Psychol 33:171–177, 1977

Mead M: Coming of Age in Samoa. New York, Blue Ribbon Press, 1928

Mednick BR, Hocevar D, Baker RL, et al: Personality and demographic characteristics of mothers and their ratings of child difficultness. Int J Behav Dev 19:121–140, 1996

Millon T: Sociocultural conceptions of the borderline personality. Psychiatr Clin North Am 23:123–136, 2000

Mombour W, Bronisch T: The modern assessment of personality disorders. Part 1: definition and typology of personality disorders. Psychopathology 31:274–280, 1998

Montero M, Sloan PS: Understanding behavior in conditions of economic and cultural dependency. Int J Psychiatry 23:597–617, 1988

Nakamura K, Kitanishi K, Miyake Y, et al: The neurotic vs. delusional subtypes of taijin-kyofu-sho: their DSM diagnoses. Psychiatry Clin Neurosci 56:595–601, 2002

Nash WP: Information gating: an evolutionary model of personality function and dysfunction. Psychiatry 61:46–60, 1998

Noll R: Multiple personality and the complex theory: a correction and a rejection of C. J. Jung's complex theory. J Anal Psychol 38:321–323, 1993

Nozoe SI, Soegima Y, Yoshioka M, et al: Clinical features of patients with anorexia nervosa: assessment of factors influencing the duration of inpatient treatment. J Psychosom Res 39:271–281, 1995

Okasha A, Saad A, Khalil AH, et al: Phenomenology of obsessive-compulsive disorder: a transcultural study. Compr Psychiatry 35:191–197, 1994

Padilla AM, Salgado-Snyder N, Cervantes RC: Self-regulation and risk-taking behavior: a Hispanic perspective. Spanish-Speaking Mental Health Research Center Bulletin Summer:1–5, 1987

Paris J: Personality disorders, parasuicide, and culture. Transcultural Psychiatric Research Review 28:25–39, 1991

Paris J: Social Factors in the Personality Disorders: A Biopsychosocial Approach to Etiology and Treatment. Cambridge, UK, Cambridge University Press, 1996

Paris J: Anxious traits, anxious attachment, and anxious-cluster personality disorders. Harv Rev Psychiatry 6:142–148, 1998

Park LC, Imboden JD, Park CJ, et al: Giftedness and psychological abuse in borderline personality disorder: the relevance to genesis and treatment. J Personal Disord 6:226–240, 1992

Parson ER: Ethnotherapeutic empathy, part II: techniques in interpersonal cognition and vicarious experiencing across cultures. Journal of Contemporary Psychotherapy 23:171–182, 1985

Pedersen PB: Intercultural training of mental health providers, in Handbook of Intercultural Training, Vol 2. Edited by Landis D, Brislin R. New York, Pergamon, 1983, pp 316–325

Pellicier Y: Diversities of work, diversities of unemployment. Psicopatologia 5:231–234, 1985

Peters UH: The psychological sequelae of persecution: the survivor's syndrome. Fortschr Neurol Psychiatrie 57:169–191, 1989

Pollack J, Winston A, McCullough L, et al: Efficacy of brief adaptational psychotherapy. J Personal Disord 4:244–250, 1990

Ramirez M: Identification with Mexican family values and authoritarianism in Mexican Americans. J Soc Psychol 73:3–11, 1967

Reid WH: The antisocial personality: a review. Hosp Community Psychiatry 36:831–837, 1985

Robbins M: Primitive personality organization as an interpersonally adaptive modification of cognition and affect. Int J Psychoanal 70:443–459, 1989

Roberts RE: Prevalence of psychological distress among Mexican Americans. J Health Soc Behav 21:134–145, 1980

Rogler LH: Framing research on culture in psychiatric diagnosis: the case of the DSM-IV. Psychiatry 59:145–155, 1996

Rogler LH, Malgady RG, Constantino G: What do culturally sensitive mental health services mean? Am Psychol 49:565–570, 1987

Rohr E: In the church: ethnopsychoanalytic research in Ecuador. Group analysis and anthropology, II: using group analysis in social and cultural anthropology and related sciences. Group Analysis 26:295–306, 1993

Rothman S: Liberalism and the decay of the American political economy. Journal of Sociology and Economics 21:277–301, 1992

Samuelian JC, Charlot V, Derynck F, et al: Adjustment disorders: an epidemiological study. Encephale 20:755–765, 1994

Sanislow CA, McGlashan TH: Treatment outcome of personality disorders. Can J Psychiatry 43:237–250, 1998

Shattopadhyaya TK, Biswas TK, Bhattacharyya AK, et al: The Eysenck Personality Questionnaire (EPQ): psychoticism, neuroticism, and extroversion in educated Bengalee adults. Manas 37:41–44, 1990

Shaw DS, Bell RQ, Gilliom M: A truly early starter model of antisocial behavior revisited. Clin Child Fam Psychol Rev 3:155–172, 2000

Sierles FS, McFarland RE, Chen JJ, et al: Posttraumatic stress disorder and concurrent psychiatric illness: a preliminary report. Am J Psychiatry 140:1177–1179, 1983

Siever L, Davis K: A psychobiological perspective on the personality disorders. Am J Psychiatry 148:1647–1658, 1991

Smith BM: The measurement of narcissism in Asian, Caucasian and Hispanic American women. Psychol Rep 67:779–785, 1990

Smith MW, Mendoza RP: Ethnicity and pharmacogenetics. Mt Sinai J Med 63:285–290, 1996

Stone MH: Long-term outcome in personality disorders. Br J Psychiatry 162:299–313, 1993

Sue S, Zane N: The role of culture and cultural techniques in psychotherapy: a critique and reformulation. Am Psychol 42:37–45, 1987

Sugihara Y, Warner JA: Mexican-American male batterers on the MCMI-III. Psychol Rep 85:163–169, 1999

Szaposnik J, Rio A, Perez-Vidal A, et al: Family Effectiveness Training (FET) for Hispanic families, in Cross-Cultural Training for Mental Health Professionals. Edited by Lefley HP, Pedersen PB. Springfield, IL, Charles C. Thomas, 1986, pp 245–261

Target M: Outcome research on the psychosocial treatment of personality disorders. Bull Menninger Clin 62:215–230, 1998

Tellegen A, Lykken DT, Bouchard TJ, et al: Personality similarity in twins reared apart and together. J Pers Soc Psychol 54:1031–1039, 1988

Trouve JN, Lianger JP, Colvet P, et al: Sociological aspects of identity problems in immigration pathology. Ann Med Psychol (Paris) 141:1041–1062, 1983

Tseng WW: Textbook of Cultural Psychiatry. San Diego, CA, Academic Press, 2001

Tyrer P, Sicchetti V, Casey PR, et al: Crossnational reliability study of schedule for assessing personality disorders. J Nerv Ment Dis 172:718–721, 1984

Ward C, Searle W: The impact of value discrepancies and cultural identity on psychological and sociocultural adjustment of sojourners. International Journal of Intercultural Relations 15:209–225, 1991

Weatherhill R: The psychical realities of modern culture. Br J Psychother 7:268–277, 1991

Winston A, Pollack J, McCullough L, et al: Brief Psychotherapy of personality disorders. J Nerv Ment Dis 179:188–193, 1991

Wu J: Masochism and fear of success in Asian women: psychoanalytic mechanisms and problems in therapy. Am J Psychoanal 52:1–12, 1992

Zheng W, Wang W, Huang Z, et al: The structure of traits delineating personality disorder in a Chinese sample. J Personal Disord 16:477–486, 2002

36

Correctional Populations: Criminal Careers and Recidivism

Jeremy Coid, M.D.

Approximately 9 million people are imprisoned worldwide, mostly as pretrial detainees or after having been convicted and sentenced. In some countries, these populations continue to show a steady increase in numbers. A significant proportion of prisoners have serious mental disorders such as psychosis, major depression, and antisocial personality disorder (ASPD). However, the provision of health care services in correctional systems is highly challenging for clinical, administrative, and structural reasons. Furthermore, mental health care is inadequate in some secure settings and in others perceived as an alternative to inadequate mental health care facilities in the community. In most prison surveys, the prevalence of "any" personality disorder is higher than that of other psychiatric conditions, and yet imprisonment is rarely perceived as an opportunity for therapeutic intervention, largely because of therapeutic pessimism but also because few correctional professionals use constructs such as "personality disorder" in their everyday working lives. Indeed, few recognize prisoners as necessarily "disordered" in a psychiatric sense.

This chapter reviews the relationship between criminal behavior leading to imprisonment and personality disorder; the implications of the high prevalence of personality disorder among prisoners, including the burden of care imposed by these conditions; and the special problems that inmates with personality disorder pose for correctional services; the chapter concludes with a review of the risks for further reoffending.

CRIMINAL CAREERS, CAREER CRIMINALS, AND ANTISOCIAL PERSONALITY DISORDER

Before examining the prevalence of personality disorder among prisoners, it is important to consider key issues in the relationship between criminal behavior leading to imprisonment and personality disorder. Imprisonment is just one of a range of sanctions within the criminal justice system, although it would appear to be applied more to individuals with a diagnosis of personality disorder than to the rest of the population. Many Westernized countries have reported an increase in crime in recent years and a substantial minority of males can expect to receive a conviction at some time in their lives. However, first convictions are predominantly recorded in the early and mid-teenage years in most Westernized countries, with the peak age for all convictions between 18 and 20 years among males and approximately 15 years among females (Coid 2003). Taking the population as a whole, criminal convictions demonstrate that the number of persons who are convicted will progressively decline with age and is almost negligible in older age groups. Although most offenders desist from crime in their late teenage and early adult years, persistence is observed in a subgroup associated with an additional range of indicators of poor social adjustment. Similar associated factors have been adopted, together with criminal and violent behavior, as the criteria for ASPD (American Psychiatric Association 2000) and as a continuous measure of psychopathy (Hare 1991). Both demonstrate considerable overlap between criminological and psychiatric constructs. It is therefore unsurprising that the prevalence of individuals meeting these criteria is high in prison populations.

Criminological research has also demonstrated that a large proportion of serious crime is committed by a small segment of the criminal population (Blumstein and Cohen 1979; Petersilia et al. 1978; Peterson and Braiker 1980; Wolfgang et al. 1972), with 5%–6% of offenders accounting for 50%–60% of crimes (Farrington et al. 1986; Wolfgang et al. 1972). This subgroup typically demonstrates characteristics such as having other family members with criminal histories, drug abuse, and social disruption (such as abandonment of families and illegitimate children), together with unemployment despite work being readily available (Langan and Greenfeld 1983). These individuals begin their criminal careers earlier and continue them longer. The financial cost to society as a result of police and court involvement, failed rehabilitation, and the direct consequences of the offending behaviors are considerable, as are the emotional and interpersonal burdens these individuals present for those around them. Some spend much of their adult lives in correctional facilities, a further subgroup demonstrating progressively shorter periods in the community between prison sentences. Overall, these persistent "high density" offenders make up the core population of correctional settings in most countries, they place the heaviest burden of care on correctional institutions, and their characteristic features match those of ASPD.

Delinquent careers can develop along several trajectories (Smith et al. 1984), but there is surprisingly little research on the correlations between personality disorder and subgroups of delinquents who have been identified using these age-related patterns of offending. This paucity exists in spite of other important correlates having been observed in criminological study and with increasing evidence about the etiology of criminality that can be derived from these subgroups (Loeber 1988; Moffitt 1993, 1994; Patterson et al. 1991). For example, studies in several countries have identified four distinct groups of offenders (Di-Lalla and Gottesman 1989; Farrington 1983; Kratzer and Hodgins 1999; Nagin and Land 1993) that could be examined according to their Axis II personality disorder profiles. These include 1) those displaying a stable pattern of antisocial behavior from early childhood through adulthood (stable early starters); 2) those who commit crimes only as adolescents (adolescence limited); 3) those who commit crimes irregularly at different times in their lives (discontinuous offenders); and 4) those who begin offending as adults (adult starters).

Most investigations have estimated that approximately 5%–7% of boys and 0%–2% of girls can be classified as early starters. However, early starters are not a homogenous group (Christian et al. 1997; Hodgins et al. 1998; Lynam 1996; Rutter 1996). Further research is required into the relationship between psychiatric morbidity, including personality disorder, and those who are placed within this category. Nevertheless, it is reasonable to assume considerable overlap between early-start offenders and ASPD. Persistence through four successive stages can be observed for career criminals who fit the pattern of the stable early starter: 1) precriminal (10–18 years), 2) early criminal (18–mid/late 20s), 3) advanced (late 20s–early 40s), and 4) criminal burnout/maturity stage (early 40s onward) (Walters 1990). In the precriminal stage, most arrests of adolescents and children are for nuisances and misdemeanors (Petersilia et al. 1978). Criminal behavior is rarely specialized (Hindelang 1971; Wolfgang et al. 1972), but larceny, burglary, and car theft are the most common offenses (LeBlanc and Frechette 1989). These offenses are frequently committed in the company of other adolescents, and thrill seeking is an important motive. A significant proportion of these juveniles do not carry their criminality into adulthood, as demonstrated in Table 36–1. During the second stage, early criminal, the overall number of individuals committing offenses progressively declines (Blumstein and Cohen 1987). However, a subgroup of individuals begin to move toward career criminality as they find themselves in contact with new criminal asso-

Table 36–1. Four stages of criminal careers

Precriminal (10–18 years of age)	Mostly nuisances and misdemeanors Rarely specialized Larceny, burglary, car theft Usually with other adolescents Thrill seeking Majority desist from crime
Early criminal (18–mid/late 20s)	Progressive decline in number of individuals who offend Subgroup moves toward career criminality Crimes decrease in number but increase in seriousness; appearance of violent offenses Money for drugs, material goods Criminal associations, incarceration, status in criminal world
Advanced (late 20s–early 40s)	Lowest proportion of dropouts during this phase Criminal lifestyle shows escalation
Criminal burnout/maturity (early 40s onward)	Further proportion drop out from crime Changes in values, motivations Many still on fringes of crime and irresponsible Maturity or burnout?

ciates, often met during periods in correctional settings; learn new criminal techniques; and acquire status in the criminal world (Gibbs and Shelley 1982). Their overall number of crimes may decrease, but the seriousness of their crimes increases in both the value of the property they steal (Langan and Farrington 1983) and the appearance of violent offenses (Petersilia et al. 1978; West and Farrington 1977). Their motives also change from thrill seeking and obtaining peer status to a desire to obtain money for drugs and nonessential material goods.

Voluntarily dropping out of criminal activity appears lowest during the advanced stage. These individuals are described as having committed themselves to a criminal lifestyle with an associated cognitive style (Walters 1990). Their antisocial behavior appears more driven and out of control, and they compensate by becoming increasingly concerned with gaining a sense of power and control over others. In the early 40s, a further stage is reached, corresponding with midlife transition, at which termination from a criminal lifestyle occurs at a higher rate (Hirschi and Gottfredson 1983). Choosing to end a criminal lifestyle corresponds to the improvement noted in a subgroup of individuals with ASPD (Robins 1966, 1978). At this stage, some individuals begin to exhibit greater maturity associated with a change in their thinking, values, and motivation accompanying their decline in physical and mental energy. However, Walters (1990) argued that maturity is not necessarily part of the process of desisting from criminal behavior. Many individuals remain on the fringes of crime, behaving in an irresponsible and self-indulgent manner but being less intrusive in their criminal behavior.

Criminological research into criminal careers and career criminals has, until recently, proceeded independently from psychiatric research into ASPD. The concept of a psychiatric "syndrome" of persistent antisocial behavior in adulthood is embodied in the diagnostic construct of ASPD. This syndrome is defined by a series of behaviors that must be present before the age of 15 and continue in adulthood. This construct has been identified by Farrington (1995) as equivalent to delinquency that persists into adulthood and the associated features demonstrated by individuals with this pattern of criminal development over the lifespan. However, ASPD is a much wider diagnostic construct because it embodies the notion that not only criminal behaviors should be included as criteria but also a wide range of behavioral disorders. Robins (1966) initially developed the criteria for the construct *sociopathic personality disorder*, from which the DSM diagnostic category *antisocial personality disorder* was derived, from a follow-up of children with conduct disorder who were referred to a child guidance clinic. This study was later replicated using additional cohorts growing up in different eras and living in different parts of the United States (Robins 1978). These studies indicated that all types of antisocial behavior in childhood could predict a high level of antisocial behavior in adulthood and that each kind of adult antisocial behavior was predicted by the overall number of factors of antisocial behavior. Robins thought her findings indicated that adult and childhood antisocial behavior constituted two syndromes and that these two syndromes were closely connected. However, most children with conduct disorder would not become adults with sociopathy or ASPD. Variety of antisocial behavior in childhood was a better predictor of subsequent adult antisocial behavior than any particular individual form of behavior. Loeber (1982) determined four factors predictive of chronic delinquency following childhood conduct disorder from a review of the literature: 1) frequency of antisocial behaviors, 2) their variety, 3) age of onset, and 4) the presence of antisocial behavior in more than one setting. These factors predispose not only to adult ASPD (Robins and Regier 1991) but also to substance abuse (Hesselbrock 1986), major mental disorder in a subgroup (Robins and Price 1991), and a higher rate of violent death (Rydelius 1988). Up to 40% of children diagnosed with conduct disorder can be expected to have serious psychosocial disturbance of one form or another in adulthood (Farrington 1995; Robins 1970; Rutter and Giller 1983; Rutter et al. 1998).

Community surveys of ASPD demonstrate several key epidemiological findings that should be considered in relation to surveys of correctional populations: the lifetime prevalence for males is significantly higher than for females (usually between four and six times), highest in the 25–44 age groups, no higher in blacks than whites, most common in those who have dropped out of high school, and most commonly found in inner-city populations (Robins 1985). ASPD appears to be strongly associated with poverty and other indices of social failure. For example, Koegel et al. (1988) found five times more ASPD among homeless persons in Los Angeles, California, than in the general population. Poor school success and poor work history predispose to low-status jobs and unemployment. The important finding of an association between ASPD and inner-city residence also corresponds to the criminological tradition of linking urbanization with increasing rates of crime (Baldwin and Bottoms 1976; Bottoms and Wiles 1997; Herbert 1979; Shaw and McKay 1942). Each of these epidemiological findings relates to an increased risk for imprisonment independent of ASPD, except for ethnicity, for which blacks in both the United States and United Kingdom are at disproportionate risk (see the following discussion).

PREVALENCE STUDIES

Of approximately 9 million people held in penal institutions throughout the world, about half are in the United States (1.96 million), Russia (920,000), and China (1.43 million, plus pretrial detainees and prisoners in "administrative detention"). At the beginning of the twenty-first century, the United States had the highest prison population rate in the world at 686 per 10,000 of the national population, following by the Cayman Is-

lands (664), Russia (638), Belarus (554), Kazakhstan (552), Turkmenistan (486), Belize (459), and The Bahamas (447). Prison population rates vary between different regions of the world and between different parts of some continents. For example, the median rate for Western and Central African countries is 50, whereas for Southern Africa it is 362. The United Kingdom rate of 139 per 10,000 persons is above the central point of the worldwide list, and it is now the highest in Europe (Walmsley 2003). Prison populations also show fluctuations in different countries, which means that the measured prevalence of personality disorder may become inaccurate within a relatively short time of any survey. It is unclear, however, whether an increase in a national prison population is necessarily accompanied by a corresponding increase in the number of prisoners with personality disorder. Increasing punitiveness (in terms of numbers in a population who are sentenced to imprisonment for crimes that were previously otherwise dealt with) could result in more persons without psychiatric morbidity being incarcerated, thereby leading to a drop in the prevalence of personality disorder. However, currently no evidence confirms this possibility one way or the other.

Surprisingly limited evidence confirms the assumption that personality disorder independently increases the risks of imprisonment, other than the observation that prevalence studies show high proportions of prisoners with these conditions. Most general-population surveys of personality disorder do not examine whether imprisonment and criminality are independently related to these conditions. However, an unpublished survey of adults ages 16–74 years in private households in England, Scotland, and Wales, carried out in 2000, did demonstrate that Cluster B personality disorders (antisocial and borderline) were associated with increased risks of self-reported previous criminal convictions (OR 10.60, 95% CI 2.72–41.30) and previous imprisonment (OR 7.57, 95% CI 1.01–56.6). These associations were independent of demographic factors, comorbid Axis I disorder (including substance misuse and dependence), and other Axis II clusters. Cluster A and Cluster C disorders did not show independent associations with imprisonment (Coid et al. in press).

PREVALENCE OF PERSONALITY DISORDER IN EARLY PRISON SURVEYS

Moran (1999) pointed out that accurate determination of the prevalence rate of mental disorder in prison settings is difficult because several factors affect the estimations, making comparisons difficult. These include location of the study (European and American courts operate differently), the type of prison (sentenced and remanded prisoners may be in different institutions), the type of prisoner studied (gender, offense type, type of sentence, or stage of sentence), and other factors determining the number of mentally disordered offenders entering the criminal justice system at any one point in time. These include the prevalence of mental disorder, including personality disorder, in the community; police practices of diverting mentally disordered persons to the hospital; and the operation of court diversion schemes. However, many of the latter factors are more likely to influence prevalences of Axis I disorder than personality disorder, because few countries have developed hospital services specifically for individuals with personality disorders.

Table 36–2. Sentenced population studies up until 1983

Author	Location	Sample	Procedure	Findings
Gluek 1918	Sing Sing Prison, Ossining, NY	600 consecutive male receptions	Clinical interview	Psychopathy, 18.0%
Roper 1950, 1951	Wakefield Prison, United Kingdom	1,100 males, consecutive mixed sentences	Clinical interview, Raven's Progressive Matrices	Psychopathy, 8%
Bluglass 1966	Perth Prison, Scotland	300 males, every fourth reception	Clinical interview	Personality disorder, 13%
Faulk 1976	Winchester Prison, United Kingdom	72 males, consecutive releases, mixed sentence	Clinical interview	Alcoholism and personality disorder, 75%
Jones 1976	Tennessee State Penitentiary, Nashville, TN	1,040 males, entire population	Screened for illness; case notes, DSM-II diagnosis	Personality disorder, 5.5%
Guze 1976	Missouri Probation Board	223 male parolees and flat-timers[a]; 66 females	Clinical interview, Feighner's criteria	Sociopathy in males, 78%; in females, 68%
Gunn et al. 1978	South East Prisons, Surrey, United Kingdom	106 males, random sample, three security grades	Clinical interview, ICD-9 diagnoses	Personality disorder, 22%
James et al. 1980	Oklahoma prisons	174 males, stratified sample	Clinical interview, self-report score	Personality disorder, 35%

Note. [a]Those who have completed their sentences.
Source. Adapted from Coid 1984.

A review of earlier studies in the twentieth century included those that had attempted to obtain random or otherwise representative samples of the overall prison population and excluded retrospective and nonrandom sampling procedures (Coid 1984). Only 11 met criteria for inclusion, 5 from the United States and 5 from the United Kingdom, with 8 estimating the prevalence of psychopathy or personality disorder, as shown in Table 36–2. Most were carried out in single prisons that were not representative of the entire prison estate. Furthermore, there was variation in sampling and only three studies in Table 36–2 made use of standardized diagnoses. It is therefore not possible to draw firm conclusions about the distribution of personality disorder from these earlier studies because the definitions vary widely.

PRISON SURVEYS OF ANTISOCIAL AND BORDERLINE PERSONALITY DISORDER

Since the publication of the DSM-III classification (American Psychiatric Association 1980), a growing number of community surveys have provided data on the prevalence of personality disorder. More information is available on ASPD than for other categories because it was included as a single personality disorder diagnosis in a number of epidemiological studies of major mental disorder. The most useful data have been provided in large-scale studies using the Diagnostic Interview Schedule (Robins et al. 1981) and more recently, the Composite International Diagnostic Interview (Wittchen et al. 1991). These instruments have subsequently been used in correctional settings. More recently, the Structured Clinical Interview for DSM-IV Axis II Personality Disorders (SCID-II; First et al. 1997) has also been used in prisons.

Fazel and Danesh (2002) carried out the most extensive systematic review of studies of the prevalence of antisocial, borderline, and "any" personality disorder in general prison populations of Western countries, published between January 1966 and January 2001. Information was collected through computer-based searches, scanning of relevant reference lists, searches of forensic psychiatry and other relevant journals by hand, and discussion and correspondence with authors. Non-English articles were translated. Surveys that sampled prisoners referred for psychiatric assessment were excluded, but those that related diagnoses of personality disorder to lifelong behavior and included diagnoses made by clinical examination

or interviewers using diagnostic instruments were included. Studies using self-report instruments were ineligible. To reduce variability in the diagnosis of personality disorders, only those studies that used validated instruments were included. Prisoners were separated into detainees (remand prisoners) and sentenced inmates. Studies that did not provide separate results for detainees and sentenced prisoners were combined in these analyses and referred to as "mixed" studies. Prevalence rates were combined from different studies by direct summation of numerators and denominators (providing weighted averages), subdivided by sex and by prisoners' status.

Table 36–3 shows the prevalence of ASPD in the 28 prison surveys identified by these authors, which included a total of 13,844 prisoners. Overall, 47% (5,113 of 10,797) of male prisoners were diagnosed with ASPD. In a subsidiary analysis of the four studies in which the investigators reported on any personality disorder in men, 65% (989 of 1,529) of male prisoners were diagnosed with some category of personality disorder (including ASPD). Overall, 21% (631 of 3,047) of female prisoners were diagnosed with ASPD. In the subsidiary analysis of the seven studies in which the investigators reported on any personality disorder in women, 42% (532 of 1,281) of female prisoners were diagnosed with some category of personality disorder (including ASPD). In the five studies in which borderline personality disorder (BPD) was reported, this diagnosis was made in 25% (307 of 1,208) female prisoners.

There was substantial heterogeneity among these studies, much of which was accounted for by differences between the larger and smaller studies and between studies done before and after 1990. There were also differences between studies done in the United States and those done elsewhere and between studies in which interviews were done by psychiatrists and other professionals and those in which interviews were done by lay persons. However, the authors concluded that approximately 1 in 2 male prisoners and approximately 1 in 5 female prisoners have ASPD. These ratios meant that, compared with the general United States and British populations, there was at least a tenfold excess of ASPD in these countries' prison populations.

These surveys confirm the high probability that individuals with ASPD will spend time in correctional facilities at some time in their lives. However, it is important to consider the limitations of imprisonment as a means to reducing the numbers of individuals with ASPD in the general population by removing them from the community. Lifetime prevalences of ASPD in

Table 36–3. Prevalence of antisocial personality disorder in 28 prison surveys

References	Location	Prevalence
Men detainees		
Roesch 1995	Canada	508/790 (64%)
Teplin 1994	United States	344/728 (47%)
Powell et al. 1997	United States	206/500 (41%)
Simpson et al. 1999	New Zealand	181/405 (45%)
Five smaller studies (Andersen et al. 1996; Brinded et al. 1999; Gingell 1991; Schoemaker and Van Zessen 1997; Singleton et al. 1998)	Denmark, New Zealand, Holland, Canada, United Kingdom	279/690 (40%)
One mixed study[a] (Robins and Regier 1991)	United States	191/604 (32%)
Subtotal		**1,709/3,717 (46%)**
Sentenced men		
Motiuk and Porporino 1992	Canada	1,095/1,925 (57%)
Collins et al. 1988	United States	325/1,149 (28%)
Neighbors et al. 1987	United States	533/1,035 (51%)
Powell et al. 1997	United States	388/750 (52%)
Simpson et al. 1999	New Zealand	243/592 (41%)
Twelve smaller studies (Bland et al. 1990; Brinded et al. 1999; Bulten 1998; Chiles et al. 1990; Darke et al. 1998; Fabregat and Sanchez 1994; Gibson et al. 1999; Schoemaker and Van Zessen 1997; Singleton et al. 1998; Walters and Chlumsky 1993; Widiger et al. 1996)	New Zealand, Holland, United States, Canada, United Kingdom, Australia, Spain, Norway	820/1,629 (50%)
Subtotal		**3,404/7,080 (48%)**
Total men		**5,113/10,797 (47%)**
Women detainees		
Teplin et al. 1996	United States	174/1,272 (14%)
Four smaller studies (Andersen et al. 1996; Hurley and Dunne 1991; Robertson et al. 1987; Salekin et al. 1997)	Denmark, Australia, United States, Canada	123/239 (51%)
Three mixed studies[a] (Robins and Regier 1991; Singleton et al. 1998; Vine 1994)	United States, United Kingdom, Australia	51/202 (25%)
Subtotal		**348/1,713 (20%)**
Sentenced women		
Jordan et al. 1996	United States	96/805 (12%)
Six smaller studies (Hurley and Dunne 1991; Robertson et al. 1987; Robins and Regier 1991; Salekin et al. 1997; Singleton et al. 1998; Vine 1994)	Australia, United States, United Kingdom, Canada	187/529 (35%)
Subtotal		**283/1,334 (21%)**
Total women		**631/3,047 (21%)**

Note. [a]Mixed studies=surveys that did not report results separately for detainees and sentenced inmates.
Source. Adapted from Fazel and Danesh 2002.

community surveys in Westernized countries tend to range from 0.6% to 3.7%. Although the prevalence of ASPD is considerably higher in prisons than in the general population, if the size of the general population is considered in relation to the size of a country's correctional population, then the overwhelming majority of individuals with ASPD at any one time are in the general population.

PREVALENCE OF OTHER PERSONALITY DISORDERS AMONG PRISONERS

Few studies have measured a full range of personality disorders in a representative sample. However, a two-stage survey was carried out in all prisons in England and Wales by the Office of National Statistics (Singleton et al. 1998), sampling a representative number from each institution and in all locations of different prisons. More than 3,000 prisoners were interviewed in the first phase by lay interviewers, who administered a screening version of the SCID-II interview using laptop computers. A one-in-six sample was then randomly selected for re-interview by trained clinicians using the SCID-II. Table 36–4 shows the prevalence of personality disorder by prisoner type. As expected, ASPD demonstrated the highest prevalence of any category. However, paranoid personality disorder was the second most prevalent condition in men and the third most prevalent in women. BPD was the second most common in women. Table 36–4 also indicates that most individual categories of personality disorder were somewhat more prevalent in remanded than sentenced male prisoners (this finding was not examined in female prisoners because both categories were combined due to the smaller sample sizes in the second phase).

These figures can be compared with those from a community sample of adults in households in England and Wales who were surveyed by the same company using the same instruments in 2000. The sampling method was different, however, in that this was a true two-phase survey (Shrout and Newman 1989) with selection for SCID-II interview in the second phase determined by scores on responses to the SCID-II screen administered in the first phase. These data are weighted to take account of the selection procedure and nonresponse. Table 36–4 shows that the prevalence of any personality disorder among male remanded prisoners is 14 times, and among sentenced prisoners is 11 times, that found in the male household population; and that the prevalence among female prisoners is 21 times that

of the female household population. Personality disorder was more prevalent among men than among women in general households, similar to the pattern observed in prisoners. However, obsessive-compulsive personality disorder was the most prevalent Axis II disorder in men and avoidant personality disorder was most prevalent in women.

ETHNIC DIFFERENCES IN PERSONALITY DISORDER IN PRISONERS

Concerns over the differential representation of ethnic groups in the criminal justice process have been highlighted, particularly in the United States, where one in three black men between the ages of 20 and 29 were under some form of criminal justice supervision (prison, probation, or parole) in 1994. Overall, black men were estimated to be imprisoned at a rate six times that of white men (Donziger 1996). However, standardized imprisonment ratios in England and Wales in 1997 had demonstrated that black men were 5.26 times more likely to be imprisoned than white men and black women 8.1 times more likely than white women (Coid et al. 2002a). Black men were also more likely to be imprisoned for robbery and firearm offenses than were white men in England and Wales but were less likely to be imprisoned for burglary and theft. Similarly, black women were less likely to be imprisoned for theft but more likely to be imprisoned for drugs offenses than were white women.

The processes leading to disproportionate numbers of black persons in prison settings in parts of Europe and North America are complex. A criminological review has concluded that "although some bias against black people has been demonstrated at several stages of the process, and although some decision-making criteria clearly work to the disadvantage of black people, in large part the difference in rates of arrest and imprisonment between black and white people arises from a difference in the rate of offending" (Smith 1997, p. 703). In the United Kingdom, it has also been pointed out that persons of Indian, Pakistani, and Bangladeshi origin are not overrepresented among offenders. For example, white women are three times more likely to be imprisoned than women of South Asian origin in England and Wales (Coid et al. 2002a).

These findings suggest the possibility of differences in the profile of personality disorders, primarily ASPD, among different ethnic groups. However, Robins and Regier (1991) found no differences in rates of ASPD in the Epidemiologic Catchment Area (ECA)

Table 36–4. Prevalence of personality disorders using SCID-II clinical interviews in prisoners and persons (ages 16–64 years) in households in England and Wales

Personality disorder	Males remanded (n=181), %	Males sentenced (n=120), %	Males in households[a] (n=251), %	Female prisoners (n=105), %	Females in households[a] (n=250), %
Antisocial	63	49	1.2	31	0.4
Paranoid	29	20	1.6	16	0.4
Borderline	23	14	1.2	20	0.4
Avoidant	14	7	1.2	11	0.8
Obsessive-compulsive	7	11	2.4	11	0.4
Narcissistic	8	7	—	6	—
Schizoid	8	6	0.8	4	0.4
Dependent	4	1	0.4	5	0.0
Schizotypal	2	2	—	4	—
Histrionic	1	2	—	4	—
Any	78	64	5.6	50	2.4

Note. SCID-II=Structured Clinical Interview for DSM-IV Axis II Personality Disorders.
[a]Weighted data.

study among blacks, whites, and Hispanics. Questioning whether the apparent ethnic equality was an artifact (in view of minority groups being overrepresented in arrested and incarcerated populations), Robins and Regier (1991) excluded the possibility that this was due to questions in the survey or that the low rate for blacks was accounted for by many with ASPD having been sent to prison, leaving the black community residents with low rates of ASPD. The ECA sample included prisoners, and as expected, their prisoner sample showed the expected high proportion of blacks overall. They also discounted the possibility that the phenomenon was caused by missing young black males from the U.S. census and differential reporting. In the case of the latter, more black than white men reported having been convicted of a felony, confirming the excess of convictions among blacks. The authors concluded that blacks truly appeared to have more convictions than whites but without a correspondingly higher rate of ASPD.

There was evidence that blacks in the community may be arrested and convicted more readily than whites who committed the same acts, although it was also possible that blacks had committed more frequent or more serious offenses than whites. Robins et al. 1991 found that fewer black than white users of weapons qualified as having antisocial personalities (21% versus 35% of whites). They also found that the use of weapons by blacks was less often preceded by the multiplicity of childhood behaviors that predicted adult antisocial behavior. This finding suggested that there is a greater acceptance of weapon use in the black than in the white community and that weapon use put blacks without a serious predisposition to antisocial behavior at greater risk of imprisonment. The authors also found, as expected, that black arrestees less often met criteria for ASPD than did white arrestees. Similarly, blacks with felony convictions met all criteria for ASPD in only 35% of cases, whereas half of white felons did so. The authors concluded that arrested blacks, including those convicted of a felony, were more "normal" than whites with the same arrest history.

Disadvantage in the criminal justice system was also suggested by the findings of Coid et al. (2002a) who demonstrated that both male and female black prisoners were significantly less likely to have previous convictions than white prisoners (although this finding characterized a subgroup), suggesting that black defendants may have been treated more harshly in the courts. In this survey in England and Wales, differences also were found in the profiles of individual personality disorders between black and white male prisoners but with no difference in their overall rate. For example, black male prisoners were less likely to have ASPD and BPD but more likely to have narcissistic personality disorders. In contrast, black women prisoners appeared to have a higher overall prevalence than white women of any personality disorder and were more likely to have paranoid, schizoid, and narcissistic personality disorders.

These findings contrasted with a previous survey of inmates in secure psychiatric hospitals in which it was demonstrated that black patients were considerably less likely than their white counterparts to have a primary diagnosis of personality disorder (Coid et al. 1999). Based on the prevalences of personality disorders in the prison population, it might have been expected that black women with personality disorder would be found more frequently in secure hospitals. One explanation for the discrepancy may have been that black prisoners do not have an excess of BPD and ASPD, the conditions most commonly observed in secure hospital services (Coid et al. 1999). However, the effect of ethnic group on treatment-seeking behaviors of prisoners and the gatekeeping process governing access to treatment are likely to have been of considerably greater importance. Further examination of the prison survey data revealed that if black prisoners presented with the same personality disorder as whites, they were less likely to have previously been treated in a psychiatric hospital or to have received psychiatric treatment in prison. This finding was particularly the case for black women prisoners. For example, 44% of all white women with BPD had previously been psychiatric inpatients compared with less than 6% of black women with the same condition (Coid et al. 2002b). BPD is typically characterized by seeking help from psychiatric services (Reich and de Girolamo 1997), and these findings suggest that this behavior may differ between different ethnic groups.

PSYCHOPATHY IN PRISONERS

Psychopathy has a significant impact on prisons and prisoners, and it can be argued that the study of psychopathy has had considerably more impact on policy and the management of prisoners than the study of Axis II personality disorders. In the context of the criminal career research described earlier, Hart and Hare (1997) emphasized the distinction between psychopathy and criminal conduct, even though the association between the two is strong. *Psychopathy* is a personality disorder—a formal, chronic mental disorder associated with a specific set of symptoms impairing psychosocial functioning in a relatively small number of people in society. One important aspect of psychopathy is the persistent, frequent, and varied asocial and antisocial behavior, which starts at an early age. The clinical construct was first described by Cleckley (1941) in The Mask of Sanity and was later developed into a rating scale, the most recent version being the Psychopathy Checklist–Revised (PCL-R; Hare 2003), which is designed for use in adult male forensic populations.

Psychopaths are described interpersonally as grandiose, arrogant, callous, superficial, and manipulative; affectively they are short-tempered, unable to form strong emotional bonds with others, and lacking in empathy, guilt, or remorse; and behaviorally they are irresponsible, impulsive, and prone to violent social and legal norms and expectations. Using 20 items derived from these features, the PCL-R can be scored on each item as 0 (item does not apply), 1 (item applies somewhat), or 2 (item definitely applies). Total scores can range from 0 to 40 and reflect the extent to which an individual matches the "prototypical" psychopath. Scores of 30 or higher are considered diagnostic of psychopathy. Individuals can be rated according to a total score or according to two factors derived from factor analysis: Factor 1 reflects the interpersonal and affective features of psychopathy (callous and remorseless use of others), and Factor 2 reflects antisocial behavior (chronically unstable and antisocial lifestyle) (Hare 2003). More recently, Cooke and Michie (2001) suggested a three-factor model. Furthermore, Cooke and Michie (1999) argued that a lower cutoff of 25 may be more appropriate in European offender populations. In a study of Scottish male offenders, it was argued that this score reflected the same level of the latent construct of psychopathy as a score of 30 in North American male offenders, although Hare (2003) disagreed with this conclusion.

Prevalence of Psychopathy Among Prisoners

Hare (2003) provided mean and standard deviations of PCL-R total scores for 15 samples of male offenders. Of this pooled sample of 5,408 male offenders, the mean PCL-R score was 22.1 (SD 7.9). For a pooled sample of 1,218 female offenders derived from six samples, the mean score was 19.0 (SD 7.5). However, these samples were taken from different institutions in North America and largely consisted of volunteers to participate in experiments. These samples were not

obtained for the purpose of determining prevalences and were not representative of an entire prison population. Only two European studies have measured prevalence using an appropriate sampling frame. These suggested that the prevalence of psychopathy in prisoners was much lower than expected. Cooke (1994) found that only 3% of male prisoners in a Scottish survey were psychopaths, using a cutoff score of 30 and above on the PCL-R. A somewhat higher prevalence was found in the survey of prisoners in England and Wales by Coid et al. 2002a, described earlier. Using the same cutoff with prisoners interviewed using the PCL-R in the second phase of this survey (n=497), prevalences were 9% among male remand prisoners, 6% among male sentenced prisoners, and 2% among female prisoners.

These findings should be compared with the considerably higher prevalences described earlier for ASPD. The PCL-R and ASPD are highly correlated in most studies of forensic populations. However, this association has been described as "asymmetric" (Hare 2003). A PCL-R diagnosis of psychopathy is more predictive of ASPD than an ASPD diagnosis is of psychopathy. Most criminal psychopaths meet the criteria for ASPD, whereas most offenders with ASPD do not meet the PCL-R criteria for psychopathy. For example, Hart et al. (1991) found in a sample of 119 prisoners that whereas 79% of psychopaths were diagnosed with ASPD, only 30% with ASPD received diagnoses of psychopathy. The base rate for PCL-R–defined psychopathy in correctional populations is much lower than the base rate for ASPD. Furthermore, the PCL-R predicts ASPD well because most criminal psychopaths engage in some sort of antisocial behavior and therefore have high scores on Factor 2. Most prisoners with ASPD do not show evidence of the personality characteristics defined by Factor 1 in the PCL-R. In contrast, the first factor (interpersonal and affective symptoms) correlates positively with narcissistic and histrionic personality disorder and negatively with avoidant and dependent personality disorder; the second factor correlates positively with ASPD and BPD (Hart and Hare 1989).

Criminal Careers of Psychopaths

Psychopaths typically begin their criminal careers at a younger age than other offenders, as reflected in formal contact with the criminal justice system. There is evidence that their criminal activities are also more extensive and more varied than that of other offenders, even controlling for time "at risk" of committing further offenses while in the community. Psychopaths are therefore described as "high density, versatile" offenders. In terms of their violent behavior, there is evidence that it is qualitatively different from that of other offenders, being more likely to be predatory in nature, motivated by readily identifiable goals, and carried out in a callous, calculated manner without the emotional context that usually characterizes the violence of other offenders. Although psychopathy tends to be strongly associated with general and violent criminality, a series of studies has indicated that it is only weakly or inconsistently related to the number of convictions or charges for sexual offenses. Psychopathy is considerably lower among child molesters than among rapists or "mixed" sex offenders who both molest and rape. The relatively high proportion of rapists with high PCL-R scores is consistent with research that demonstrates an association between psychopathy and instrumental violence. The PCL-R score is not consistently related to measures of deviant sexual arousal. However, sex offenders with a combination of a high PCL-R score and evidence of deviant sexual arousal are believed to be at particularly high risk for reoffending (discussed later) (Hare 2003; Hart and Hare 1997).

COMORBIDITY OF AXIS II DISORDERS AMONG PRISONERS

The importance of comorbidity between personality disorders and other mental disorders is increasingly recognized. When assessing mentally disordered offenders, comorbidity between conditions in the different axes may indicate unmet service needs and can determine pathways into psychiatric care (Coid et al. 1999). However, there is no universally accepted definition of comorbidity, and it currently has no comprehensive and coherent theoretical framework (Wittchen 1996). It is generally taken to imply co-occurrence of independent psychiatric disorders in an individual patient. Studies in clinical samples demonstrate that at least 50% of subjects will have two or more coexisting personality disorders (Loranger et al. 1987; Oldham et al. 1992; Pfohl et al. 1986). Although the prevalence of both Axis II and clinical syndromes is high among prisoners, this does not necessarily mean that there will be a higher level of comorbidity between these conditions in studies carried out in correctional settings when compared with clinical community samples. A study of dangerous offenders in high-security hospitals and

special units for high-risk prisoners demonstrated a lower level of Axis II/Axis II comorbidity than in previous studies in clinical samples, especially for BPD. However, comorbidity between Axis II disorders and Axis I disorders appeared high (Coid et al. 2003b).

In a study of the comorbidity of personality disorder and clinical syndromes in prisoners in England and Wales (Coid et al. in press), the patterns observed were generally similar to those found in previous clinical samples (Becker et al. 2000; Dahl 1986; Grilo et al. 2002; Hyler and Lyons 1988; McGlashan et al. 2000; Moldin et al. 1994; Oldham et al. 1992; Pfohl et al. 1991; Stuart et al. 1998; Widiger et al. 1991; Zanarini et al. 1998a, 1998b; Zimmerman and Coryell 1989). ASPD was comorbid with BPD and paranoid personality disorder and with alcohol and drug misuse. In contrast to the study of offender patients (Coid et al. 2003b), BPD showed more extensive comorbidity than the other Axis II disorders, co-occurring with schizotypal, avoidant, dependent, paranoid, and histrionic personality disorders as well as Axis I depressive disorder, schizophrenia, and alcohol misuse. Narcissistic personality disorder was comorbid with histrionic, paranoid, and obsessive-compulsive personality disorder; and paranoid personality disorder was comorbid with Axis I schizophrenia and depressive disorder. Schizoid personality disorder was comorbid with schizotypal, and dependent personality disorder with avoidant, as observed in previous clinical studies.

These findings ultimately raise the question of whether certain Axis II disorders represent a true predisposition for developing certain Axis I disorders, but this cannot be answered from cross-sectional studies, either in correctional or community settings. For example, residual or subclinical symptoms or an Axis I disorder could be misdiagnosed as Axis II disorder, especially in cases such as schizophrenia and schizotypal personality disorder and delusional disorder and paranoid personality disorder. This question would require prospective study of these diagnostic associations.

Caron and Rutter (1991) proposed four potential processes that can lead to true comorbidity: 1) shared risk factors, 2) overlap between risk factors, 3) the comorbid pattern constituting a meaningful syndrome, and 4) one disorder creating an increased risk for the other. They also emphasized that patterns of comorbidity observed within clinic and selected samples, such as those in correctional settings, must be confirmed by investigations carried out in epidemiologically representative community samples. Nevertheless, despite higher prevalences of Axis II disorders, the patterns observed in correctional samples do appear similar to those carried out in psychiatric clinics.

EXPLANATIONS OF THE ASSOCIATIONS BETWEEN PERSONALITY DISORDER AND OFFENDING BEHAVIOR

This chapter examines the associations between criminal careers research and ASPD. However, there are surprisingly few studies on the specific associations between personality disorder and offending behaviors leading to imprisonment. From a theoretical standpoint, these associations can be divided into three main areas: criterion overlap, the secondary effects of personality disorder, and a cognitive model in which the offending behavior is the direct result of motivations that are a consequence of the personality disorder.

Criterion Overlap

Many clinicians assume that the relationship between personality disorder and offending is a direct one. This notion is encouraged by the inclusion of criteria in the Axis II disorder ASPD that overlap with both acquisitive and violent offending behavior. Essential features of ASPD are described in DSM-IV-TR as a "pervasive pattern of disregard for, and violation of, the rights of others that begins in childhood or early adolescence and continues into adulthood" (American Psychiatric Association 2000, p. 701). Although DSM-IV-TR and ICD-10 have moved to become more similar and to use trait-based systems, ASPD still comprises behaviors originally observed in the empirical study of conduct disordered children with persistence of antisocial behavior into adulthood. Although it is emphasized that these behaviors are not necessarily criminal, observation of the 15 conduct disorder items with an onset before age 15 shows that 11 of these (initiating physical fights, using a weapon, being physically cruel to people, physical cruelty to animals, stealing while confronting a victim, forcing sexual activity on another, fire setting, destroying property, breaking into a house or building, lying to obtain goods, stealing items without confronting a victim) could all result in criminal charges. Similarly, four of the seven items occurring since age 15 could also result in criminal convictions and imprisonment (failure to conform to social norms with respect to lawful behaviors as indicated by repeatedly perform-

ing acts that are grounds for arrest, use of aliases or conning others for personal profit or pleasure, irritability and aggressiveness as indicated by repeated physical fights or assault, and reckless disregard for safety of self or others).

Violent behavior is a defining feature of two of the personality disorders included in DSM-IV-TR: BPD and ASPD. Antagonistic, hostile traits are also evident in seven of the personality disorders (paranoid, antisocial, borderline, histrionic, narcissistic, schizotypal, and obsessive-compulsive). Widiger and Trull (1994) pointed out that complementary traits of agreeableness are prominent in only one—dependent personality disorder. However, they also pointed out that neither a diagnosis of BPD nor of ASPD, in the absence of a history of violent or aggressive behavior, is likely in itself to indicate a risk with substantial clinical or social significance. Violent behavior should be perceived as the result of a complex interaction among a variety of social, clinical, personality, and environmental factors whose relative importance varies across situations and time. The complexity of this interaction should raise the issue of the extent to which one should conceive violent behavior as resulting from a personality disorder rather than a situational, environmental, or other factor. For example, the effects of substance misuse can be seen within a complex interaction in which it may be difficult to determine whether the violent act is due to the effects of substance use or the personality disorder. Even if violent behavior occurs only when under the influence of a substance, the substance use may itself be a manifestation or an effect of the personality disorder. Alternatively, the substance may be acting simply as a disinhibitor of premorbid aggressive tendencies. On the other hand, a substance use disorder can contribute to the development, maintenance, and escalation of antisocial behaviors.

Widiger and Trull (1994) argued that the trend in measuring personality to understand and predict violent behavior has moved toward the development of interactive, multifactorial models and that the current personality disorder taxonomy is inadequate within these models for three reasons: 1) the Axis II categorization is a dichotomous model imposing arbitrary categorical distinctions between the presence and absence of a disorder that may have little relationship to the predictability of violent behavior; 2) these diagnostic categories are substantially heterogeneous with respect to the personality variables that are most likely to be predictive of violent behavior; and 3) the Axis II categorization does not provide a comprehensive model of personality dysfunction.

Secondary Effects of Personality Disorder

A second hypothesis is that personality disorder is not central to the criminal behavior, does not constitute a "drive," and merely shapes certain aspects of the offense. In this context, personality disorder would be seen as secondary to another factor. For example, a man with dependent personality disorder takes part in a serious group assault on another man as a result of his need for support from other group members and to belong to the group. These factors lead him to participate in causing injuries to a man toward whom he feels no personal animosity. Another example is a serial child murderer whose offenses are driven primarily by pedophilia and sexual sadism but whose obsessive-compulsive personality results in careful attention to the crime scene, such as folding the child's clothing. Other examples include the removal of trophy items from a victim for subsequent grandiose enhancement of self-esteem as a result of narcissistic personality disorder or a rapist whose sexual assault is driven by other dynamic factors, such as displaced anger, but whose robbery of the woman after the rape is better understood in the context of his ASPD.

In these situations, personality disorder may shape the modus operandi of the individual, reflecting specific personality characteristics but not directly triggering the criminal behavior. The personality disorder may in certain circumstances constitute a deficit in criminal skills, and in other situations it may enhance them.

Personality Disorder and Criminal Motivation

An alternative approach, and one that fits within the complex multifactorial model proposed by Widiger and Trull (1994), is that personality disorder leads to motivations and dispositional factors in potential offenders. Criminal behavior can be broken down into characteristics that describe the act itself; characteristics of the offender and victim; motives or motivating factors that induced the offender to act in a certain way; and additional shaping factors such as the disinhibiting influences of intoxication, incitement, or encouragement from others. Dynamic relationships can act among several of these factors within a single criminal act. Furthermore, the time frame for each of these interactions, and the addition of external circumstances, may result in further complexities. Within this model, certain offending behaviors and Axis II psychopathology would have a direct link; for example, repetitive impulsive behaviors, the orchestration of circumstances that lead to interpersonal conflict, and the tendency to experience intense affects or paranoid ideation when under stress.

A body of literature has attempted to investigate the psychology of the violent offender by examining the links between personality and violence. An early model was proposed by Megargee (1966), in which violence was hypothesized to occur when the instigation to violence, mediated by anger, would exceed the individual's level of control of aggressive feelings or impulses. An "undercontrolled" person would have very low inhibition and would therefore frequently act in a violent manner to any provocation perceived. On the other hand, an "overcontrolled" person would have extremely strong inhibitions, and violence would only occur if the provocation had been intense or endured over a long period of time. Megargee predicted that an overcontrolled personality would be found in those who had committed acts of extreme violence but not in those with histories of frequent minor assault. Blackburn (1968) confirmed these predictions in a group of violent offenders, although Crawford (1977) failed to replicate the findings. Nevertheless, subsequent work by Quinsey et al. (1983) and Henderson (1983) confirmed that there are deficiencies in the assertive behavior of overcontrolled offenders and that individuals with low psychometric measures of control report difficulty in controlling their temper and in avoiding fights.

Blackburn (1989) later argued that it is important to distinguish between the occurrence of a violent act and the tendency to repeat such an act, because the act of violence in itself does not necessarily imply an aggressive personality. More emphasis has subsequently been placed on situational approaches that have largely been developed in studies of sexual offending. These have led to a series of descriptive analyses of offense characteristics (see review by Hollin 1989). In the case of rape, a range of approaches has been used in categorization, including specific aspects of the offense, characteristics of the victim, and psychiatric and legal subgroupings. An alternative approach has been to classify the act according to the motives of the rapists (Box 1983; Prentsky et al. 1985). For example, Groth (1979) described three types of rape according to varying degrees of hostility and control associated with the rape. For example, "anger" rape typically follows arguments, sexual jealousies, and social rejection. The offender typically reports experiencing anger and rage together with feelings of being wrongly treated prior to the act. During the assault, the rapist uses more force than necessary to inflict physical injury, and the rape is an additional way of inflicting pain. In "power" rape, sexual conquest is the goal and physical aggression is used as necessary to force compliance. "Sadistic" rape combines sexuality and aggression. The victim is often bound and helpless, is humiliated, and may be tortured, which also provides a source of sexual excitement for the rapist.

Ressler et al. (1988) proposed a motivational model to explain sexual homicide. This model comprised a more complex and detailed framework than that used by previous authors, demonstrating parallels with the biosocial interaction hypothesis (Raine 2002) of abnormal personality development. The model incorporates interacting components, including the murderer's social environment, child and adolescent formative events, patterns of responses to these events, resulting actions toward others, and reaction via a mental "feedback" filtered to his murderous acts. Within this model, the authors proposed a series of processes that were closely interwoven with the offender's personality, had developed over the lifespan, led up to the homicide, and had origins in several components within the offender's childhood environments. In some cases, it is probable that constitutional abnormalities, including neurodevelopmental abnormality and genetic factors, had made substantial contributions to the development of the offending behavior by interacting with environmental factors over the lifespan.

The association between motivational and dispositional factors, Axis II disorders, and serious offending was examined in a study by Coid (1998a). Motivational factors described by the participants as operating immediately before, and the situational factors during, the commission of the criminal act were examined in relation to subjects' psychopathology, measured using Axis II and lifetime Axis I categories. In what was a highly selected group of offenders with a history of very serious offenses, significant associations were found between narcissistic personality disorder and homicide; paranoid personality disorder and other serious violent offenses such as attempted murder and wounding; BPD and arson; schizoid personality and kidnapping and abduction; and ASPD and robbery, firearm offenses, and thefts and burglary. Associations between narcissistic personality disorder and incarceration for a violent crime were observed in female prisoners by Warren et al. (2002). However, associations were also observed with Cluster A diagnoses in this sample, with both prostitution and violent reoffending.

Serious violent offending in the case of narcissistic personality disorder in the United Kingdom sample of serious offenders (Coid 1998a) appeared to be motivated by blows to self-esteem and the need to exert power, domination, and control over victims, which is entirely consistent with the psychodynamic literature on narcissistic personality organization. Subjects with paranoid personality disorder appeared to have offended in states of undercontrolled aggression and for motives of revenge, corresponding to the paranoid, sensitive, and vengeful traits of many of these individuals. Schizoid subjects appeared to demonstrate expressive aggression, where the primary motive for the offense had been anger, not sexual gratification, for the purpose of or accompanied by excitement and/or exhilaration. Subjects with BPD, although most strongly associated with offenses of arson, also committed serious violent and sexual offenses. These subjects demonstrated multiple motivations for their crimes, including relief of tension and dysphoria after carrying out the act; subjects behaved violently in a state of extreme hyperirritability, demonstrated revenge, displaced aggression onto other persons or objects (particularly in the case of arson), committed offenses in a state of excitement or exhilaration, offended to deliberately resolve their problems such as homelessness; and demonstrated pyromania in a small number of cases. ASPD was associated with offenses carried out in gangs or within groups for the purpose of financial gain and with violence when in a state of hyperirritability.

A cognitive model was subsequently proposed to explain the relationship between personality disorder, motivation, and behavioral disorder (Coid 2002). It was hypothesized that individuals with personality disorder demonstrated predispositions, operating in the form of preexisting Axis II disorder, that led to the development of cognitive schemas that integrate and attach meaning to events and the environment. It was proposed that these schemas lead to attributions and motivation that in turn result in action in the form of violence or deliberate disruptive behavior. In personality disorders, schemas are considered to operate on a continuous basis, processing information; regulating cognition, affect, motivation, and tendency to action; inhibiting behavior; and directing the individual's actions. Certain schemas are concerned with evaluation of others and self (Beck and Freeman 1990). It was proposed that future developments using such a model might include a more complex longitudinal approach similar to that described by Ressler et al. (1988) as applied to sexual homicide. However, further research would ultimately be needed to resolve the difficulties in predicting which situational factors are most important in precipitating examples of criminal behavior in the presence of Axis II personality disorder.

PERSONALITY DISORDER AND PROBLEMS OF CONTROL IN PRISONS

Most prisoners serve their sentences uneventfully, conform to prison discipline, and make no attempt to escape. However, the risk of behavioral problems, especially violence, is greatly increased within correctional settings among prisoners with personality disorder. This has been demonstrated by surveys of prisoners who have committed disciplinary infractions resulting in additional punishments and in surveys of individuals placed in special settings with increased levels of security as a result of their dangerous and disruptive behavior.

Within the context of the prison environment, management's responsibility is to maintain good order and discipline in the day-to-day running of the institution. All penal systems have a series of punitive sanctions that can be applied in response to behavioral problems. In Westernized countries, these sanctions usually range from the withdrawal of privileges to segregation, which involves placement in solitary confinement for varying periods. In some countries, including the United States, prisoners may be placed in physical restraints for periods of time. Despite the punitive approach usually taken with problems of disorder, containment and management of the most disruptive, psychopathic prisoners can still be highly stressful for prison staff. It may also pose ethical questions as to what level of retribution is acceptable. A small subgroup of determined and often psychopathic prisoners can continue to remain unresponsive to all therapeutic attempts at treatment and rehabilitation, recalcitrant in the face of all punishment, and still be able to exert a malign and destructive influence even from within the most highly secure and segregated environments (see Coid 1998b).

It has been argued that an emphasis on situational and environmental manipulation, rather than on direct interactions with individuals, is often more productive with difficult prisoners (Cooke 1991). In the simplest form, this approach may merely involve transfer of a highly disruptive inmate to another penal institution where the behavioral disorder may show a dramatic improvement because staff members are more skilled in handling the individual in the new location. Megargee (1977) observed that characteristics of the milieu in which a violent incident takes place are often more important than characteristics of the individual. It may be possible to change a prisoner's behavior to a greater extent by modifying the environment than by attempting to modify psychological functioning. Cooke (1991) emphasized the importance of the characteristics of staff members who deliver the regimen to prisoners, identifying key elements in this area as including staff–inmate communication and staff training, experience, and morale. Quality of relationships between prisoners and outside visitors can be especially important for some inmates and the implementation of incentives for good behavior (Ditchfield 1990). The location of the prison itself can have important implications for behavior; some inmates behave badly if they think it will result in transfer to a more accessible prison that would allow visits from friends and relatives.

The relationship between prison population density leading to overcrowding and inmate discipline has been the subject of considerable research, but it is still difficult to draw firm conclusions regarding the effects of personality disorder (see Coid 1998b). It is widely assumed that prisoner programs and activities promote control in prison. For example, Hare (1970) suggested that psychopathic prisoners may employ manipulational violence to "liven up" their institution in search for stimulation. Ditchfield (1990) observed that poor work opportunities and curtailment of certain facilities contributed to subsequent mass disturbances in certain United Kingdom prisons. However, research suggests that relative levels of facilities and privileges are what primarily concern inmates rather than absolute levels. Inmates feel more threatened by a perceived deterioration in their standard of living than by a poor standard of living overall.

Administrative changes and uncertainty also influence the level of violence. Ellis (1984) noted that when there is a high turnover of prisoners, the rate of violence tends to be higher. Ward (1987) observed that chaotic administration contributed to an escalation of violence in Folsom Prison in California. Paradoxically, increasing security levels may sometimes increase the probability of violence, because prisoners resort to violence as a means of saving face by resisting the regimen (Cooke 1991).

The mix of prisoners may be of prime importance. In some cases, it is necessary for prisoners to be identified and separated into groups to prevent predatory behavior by one group against another. This segregation is frequently carried out by prison staff without recourse to the diagnostic approaches used by psychiatrists and psychologists. Prison classification systems have been developed for prison officers' observations of prisoners' behaviors that are intended to identify those who are frequently aggressive and should be assigned to a particular wing or cell block or, alternatively, to identify weaker individuals, more prone to victimization, who should be housed elsewhere for protective purposes. The intention of this approach is to reduce problematic behavior by identifying and separating particular groups of prisoners.

For example, Quay (1984) developed a classification system dividing prisoners into one of five types. Group 1 prisoners include those who display hostile, aggressive, and violent behavior; are resentful of rules and regulations; crave excitement; and become bored easily. They have little concern for the feelings or welfare of others and present serious disciplinary problems in institutions. They are most likely to be involved in fighting, assaults, threats of bodily harm, extortion, destruction of property, and possession of weapons. This group has features of psychopathy. Inmates in Group 2 do not have the same degree of outward aggression but are hostile toward authority and tend to deal with others through cunning or manipulative behavior. They may organize inmate gangs or illicit enterprises within the institution. They are generally seen by staff as untrustworthy and unreliable. Group 3 inmates are neither excessively aggressive nor dependent, although the experience of being in prison may demoralize them. They do not have extensive criminal histories and have a low frequency of disciplinary problems. They are often the type of prisoners upon whom the staff can rely, and they tend to maintain prison activities and industries. Prisoners in Group 4 are withdrawn, sluggish, unhappy, and passive. They are easily victimized by those in Groups 1 and 2 because they are often friendless and perceived as weak, indecisive, and submissive. Group 5 consists of prisoners who constantly display anxiety; are easily upset and unhappy; appear sad, depressed, or tense; and are unable to relate to prison officers. They are also easily preyed upon by others. They do not have a high rate of disciplinary infractions in the institution, but when they are involved in misconduct it is often of a serious nature, because they tend to explode when unable to handle stress.

Quay (1984) argued that after prisoners are separated into these groups, they should be placed in different types of regimens. For example, regimens for the first two groups should be staffed by officers who treat them in a "no-nonsense" and "by the rules" manner. Those in Group 3 should be treated in a "hands off" manner. Those in Groups 4 and 5 should be treated in a supportive and highly verbal manner. The rates of inmate–staff and inmate–inmate assaults dropped significantly in a large maximum security

penitentiary during a 4-year period in which inmates were separated according to this classification.

Solitary Confinement

Most Westernized countries have a formal system of prison rules whereby adjudications are held following prisoner misbehavior, and the misbehavior is dealt with by loss of privileges or (for more severe examples) by loss of remission of sentence. The most serious behavior may result in further police investigation, formal charges, and a further sentence following a conviction in an outside court. However, placement in solitary confinement for varying periods of time, and with varying levels of privileges and facilities while confined, is the primary disincentive in most correctional systems.

Ditchfield (1990) observed that certain individual characteristics were associated with disciplinary infraction rates in prison. The most important was age, with most (but not all) studies demonstrating that involvement in disciplinary offenses was greater for younger inmates than older prisoners. Offenders serving sentences for robbery, aggravated burglary, attempted murder, or assault had above-average involvement in prison violence in the United Kingdom, whereas those serving sentences for homicide or sexual and drug offenses were below average. In general, those serving longer sentences tended to have lower infraction rates than did short-term inmates. However, Toch and Adams (1989) in the United States and Coid (1998b) in the United Kingdom observed a subgroup of exceptionally difficult prisons who deviated from these general findings in that they were somewhat older, a proportion was serving sentences for homicide offenses, and some had extensive histories of psychiatric treatment.

In the survey of prisoners in England and Wales, characteristics of those who had been placed in disciplinary segregation were examined in over 3,000 subjects interviewed using self-report data (Coid et al. 2003a). There was no evidence that prisoners with severe mental illness were more likely to experience disciplinary segregation than other prisoners. Those who reported this experience corresponded to previous studies, tending to be younger, with criminal histories characterized by offenses of robbery and violence, but they differed in that more were sentenced or charged after homicide offenses. The overall impression of segregated prisoners was that they tended to be "career criminals" with personality disorder, together with additional features of emotional instability and impulsivity and drug misuse, especially crack cocaine. Both men and women were significantly more likely to have a diagnosis of ASPD and had higher scores of psychopathy on the PCL-R. Men who had been segregated were more likely to have additional diagnoses of paranoid and narcissistic personality disorder, and women were more likely to have paranoid and borderline personality disorders. Prisoners who had been segregated were more likely to have demonstrated conduct disorder during childhood, corresponding to their increased likelihood of placements in local authority care and special schools for disruptive children as well as juvenile correctional facilities (for men), and to have reported experiences of sexual abuse (for women). Women who had histories of institutional violence were also likely to have a diagnosis of ASPD in a sample of incarcerated women in the United States (Warren et al. 2002).

A further subgroup of prisoners had been placed in special cells (also known as "strip cells") in which prisoners can be placed after the removal of belongings and clothing. The application of this regimen may be specific to the United Kingdom but is meant to be differentiated from the standard use of segregation. A special cell may be used for the "temporary confinement of a violent or refractory prisoner" but must be authorized by the senior management of the prison and used only if necessary to prevent the prisoner carrying out self-injury, injuring another prisoner or staff, damaging property, or causing a disturbance. The use of special cells is not officially for punishment, and use is expected to continue only as long as the initial justification remains. In contrast to disciplinary segregation, survey respondents who had been placed in special "strip" cell conditions were more likely to have severe mental illness, suicidal tendencies, and a history of deliberate self-injury. The personality disorder profile of these patients contrasted with those who had been placed in segregation, with men demonstrating more Cluster A (paranoid, schizotypal, schizoid) and Cluster C (avoidant, dependent) traits. They did not exhibit Cluster B disorders except for BPD. Women were characterized by borderline, paranoid, and avoidant traits. There were also fewer associations with substance misuse in this subgroup, and they had significantly lower PCL-R scores. Instead of the associations with impulsive offenses such as robbery, violence, and burglary observed in segregated prisoners, those placed in special cells were more likely to have histories of arson, sexual offending, and abduction/kidnapping. Violent offending was, however, more characteristic of the women in this subgroup, but they were also more likely to have previous

convictions for arson. This group appeared to have many of the characteristics of Groups 4 and 5 described by Quay (1984), who require protection from the more aggressive and predatory groups (many of whom show characteristics typically associated with placement in disciplinary segregation) and from whom it is preferable to keep them separate due to their vulnerability.

Special Facilities for Difficult and Disruptive Prisoners

Although disruptive prisoners can be sent for periods to a segregation unit, isolated from the main part of the prison, it is still possible in some institutions for a prisoner in segregation to continue to exert a powerful influence on other prisoners. Some countries operate a system of repeated transfers between establishments for the most disruptive inmates. However, for the most extreme problems (e.g., those who have killed other prisoners or prison staff or who present a real and continued threat of homicide) some penal systems have developed special high-security cells or even supermaximum-security prisons (Boin 2001; Clare et al. 2001; Coid 2002; King 1999). There has been little study of individuals within these institutions, however, largely due to difficulty in gaining access.

In a small sample of 81 prisoners admitted to special units for difficult and dangerous prisoners in England, offenses clustered among the most serious forms of violence against the person: robbery and aggravated burglary (48%), murder and manslaughter (47%), attempted murder and grievous bodily harm (36%), assault (16%), and serious sexual offenses (12%). Violence in the prison setting was the most common type of behavior, including violence toward other inmates (68%), violence toward staff (68%), and weapon making (52%). Most of the subjects received DSM-III Axis II diagnoses of ASPD (84%) and 73% were designated as psychopaths using a cutoff score of 30 on the PCL-R. ASPD was highly comorbid with additional Axis II disorders including paranoid, narcissistic, borderline, and passive-aggressive personality disorders (Coid 1998a).

Personality Disorder and Motivation for Prison Disorder

Associations were examined among DSM-III Axis II disorders, disruptive behavior, and motivation for the behavior (Coid 2002). Specific associations supported a cognitive model explaining the functional association between personality disorder and the antisocial behavior. It was hypothesized that personality disorders acted as predisposing factors influencing the development of motivations and subsequently facilitating the enactment of disordered behavior in a linear progression, as described earlier in the example of criminal behavior. In this sample, ASPD was highly prevalent and did not discriminate well between the different motivational variables. However, psychopathy characterized prisoners with low frustration tolerance and threshold for aggression, together with reported episodes of hyperirritability leading to violence against other inmates, but with an additional predatory tendency to make and conceal weapons (see also Hart and Hare 1997).

Subjects with narcissistic personality disorder demonstrated general intolerance of rules and regulations as well as the belief that violence was the only solution to their interpersonal difficulties, corresponding to the DSM construct of a pervasive pattern of grandiosity, lack of empathy, and hypersensitivity to evaluation by others combined with the overinflated self-image considered the source of the narcissistic personality style (Beck and Freeman 1990). Narcissistic subjects in these special prison units were particularly likely to have exhibited violence against both inmates and staff and to have been involved in incidents of cell barricading. Major discrepancies were observed between their expectations of how they should be managed and the reality of prison discipline, and this led to multiple serious behavioral problems (Coid 2002).

Paranoid personality disorder was highly prevalent and strongly comorbid with ASPD. The paranoid, sensitive, and vengeful traits of these subjects added an additional dimension of potential risk to their preexisting criminal disposition, operating through their ASPD. This personality disorder exacerbated their tendency to become involved in fights after minimal provocation. In some incidents, violence toward other inmates and making weapons to carry out their attacks were additionally motivated by revenge for real or imagined slights that had resulted in a blow to their fragile self-esteem. Chronic vigilance for signs of malicious intent by others and the view that others cannot be trusted resulted in any slights or mistreatments being perceived as intentional and malicious and therefore deserving of retaliation. Protests that the slights were unintentional or accidental were seen by these men as further evidence of deception (Coid 2002).

Features of overdramatic, reactive, and intensely expressed behavior, with characteristic disturbances in interpersonal relationships due to shallowness, egocentricity, vanity, and demanding behavior in histrionic subjects appeared closely related to their need to adver-

tise their toughness within the prison environment and their minimal ability to tolerate stress (Coid 2002). These individuals had additional histories of escaping from custody. In contrast, however, BPD was a less significant factor in overt violence toward others in this group of men than had been expected. BPD was associated with a history of hostage-taking incidents and a subgroup described compulsive urges to kill others. Behavioral disorder associated with relief of tension and dysphoria corresponded to a previous study of female subjects detained in maximum-security hospitals who had demonstrated a range of behaviors, including fire-setting, self-mutilation, binge eating, property damage, assaults, and compulsive homicidal urges during mood swings (Coid 1993). These subjects reported relief and reduction of the intensity of these symptoms as a result of these behaviors, many of which were carried out deliberately for this purpose, and in these cases one behavior could be substituted for another. This model, linking BPD and dangerous behaviors through a disorder of mood, contrasted with the conventional view that associates abnormal behaviors with individual personality traits embodied within the DSM construct. In this context, behavioral disorder would be perceived as the outcome of instability in interpersonal relationships, self-image, and affects accompanied by impulsivity in the subject.

Schizoid personality disorder among this group of prisoners corresponded to the syndrome described by Wolff and Chick (1980), based on the developmental observation of a group of emotionally withdrawn and socially detached children. Behavioral disorder in this subgroup of men was not motivated by obvious external precipitants and sometimes involved acting out homicidal fantasies rehearsed in their imagination over a prolonged period. Serious assaults on other prisoners had usually been unprovoked and therefore unexpected. Schizoid individuals had better control over their behavior and were therefore highly unlikely to have carried out violence against prison staff. Associations with pleasure and excitement in enacting violence were observed in certain subjects with schizotypal personality disorder, which may have related to their pervasive pattern of detachment from social relations, restricted range of expression of emotions in interpersonal settings, associated cognitive and perceptual distortions, and eccentricities of behavior. For these men, taking pleasure and deriving excitement from violence may have reflected a distortion of their affective functioning and a tendency to retreat into magical thinking. A small subgroup with avoidant personality disorder, comorbid with the more prevalent conditions such as antisocial and paranoid personality disorder, added an additional dimension. These individuals described profound anxiety and intolerance of association with other prisoners to the extent that they were willing to act with extreme violence to ensure their isolation. Being placed in segregation did not act as a punishment for these men and was their preferred option (Coid 2002).

Although carried out in a small sample that was not representative of the general prison population, the study did demonstrate the importance of the assessment of Axis II personality disorders when evaluating the behavior of dangerous and disruptive prisoners. Although the major challenge for future research is to predict which situational factors are most important in precipitating examples of behavioral disorder in the presence of an Axis II personality disorder, the study suggested that situational factors were not always the essential precipitants to behavioral disorder. Sometimes situational factors acted in a cumulative manner over time, or the situation in which the problem behavior occurred had been engineered by the subjects themselves. These findings suggested indications for the management of these highly disturbed individuals and the creation of more suitable prison environments in which to contain them. For example, prisoners with highly avoidant personalities comorbid with psychopathic personality disorder who are prepared to stop at nothing to obtain solitude and respite from the normal regime will perceive little deterrence from being placed in solitary confinement. Men with comorbid narcissistic and antisocial personalities can be highly predatory in a conventional prison setting. Their behavioral problems may be reduced when they are placed in conditions containing similar individuals and kept apart from inadequate prisoners and those with mental health problems whom they tend to victimize (Quay 1984). It might be possible in the future to develop treatment interventions to modify some of the distorted beliefs of these men by taking a cognitive behavioral approach (Beck and Freeman 1990), but for some prisoners it may still be necessary to reduce the intensity of their extreme affective states and their distortions in reality testing by using psychotropic medication before such treatments can be safely undertaken.

PREDICTING REOFFENDING AND INSTITUTIONAL BEHAVIOR

In many countries, mental health and criminal justice personnel are increasingly required to make predic-

tions regarding future criminal and violent conduct. In certain U.S. states, measures of psychopathy have influenced death penalty decisions, and in the United Kingdom, risk assessments and risk management have been key components of the government's proposal to detain and treat persons with severe personality disorder who challenge public safety. More recent proposals have been made for new legislation to extend prison sentences on the basis of future risk of reoffending. Research in this field has progressed from previous skepticism regarding clinicians' ability to make accurate predictions of dangerousness (Cocozza and Steadman 1976; Ennis and Litwack 1974; Megargee 1989; Menzies et al. 1994; Monahan 1981; Webster et al. 1985) to the increasing recognition of the accuracy and importance of risk assessment. This recognition has led to a "rejuvenation" of risk assessment research (Monahan and Steadman 1994; Monahan et al. 2001) and the development of improved risk assessment instruments. However, accuracy in the process of assessment increasingly will be expected from professionals by both policy makers and the public in the future. It should be anticipated that criteria for detention will be challenged by legal representatives on an increasingly frequent basis if decisions are made or influenced by scores on these instruments.

Predictive Ability of Axis II Disorders

Risk factors for future violent behaviors have been divided into either static or dynamic categories. *Static risk factors* include those that remain the same when measured, including age, sex, and psychopathy ratings, and would, according to the DSM-IV-TR definition implying stability over time, include the presence or absence of Axis II disorder. *Dynamic risk factors* are those that may change and therefore may be more amenable to interventions, such as employment, housing, substance misuse, and so on.

The ability of the Axis II personality disorders to predict criminal recidivism has been a relatively underresearched area. However, the presence of an Axis II disorder is included as an item of risk in certain instruments, such as the Historical, Clinical, and Risk Management Scales (HCR-20; Webster et al. 1997). Although the high prevalence of personality disorder in the cross-sectional surveys described earlier would suggest increased risk of offending, meta-analyses of longitudinal research also suggest that antisocial and impulsive personality features are substantial risk factors for criminal recidivism among adult offenders in the criminal justice system (Gendreau et al. 1996) and among former forensic psychiatric patients (Bonta et al. 1998). Prospective studies of clinical and forensic samples have found that personality disorders predict violent reoffending (Gandhi et al. 2001; Hernandez-Avila et al. 2000; Tardiff et al. 1997). The presence of Cluster B personality disorders independently increased the likelihood of violent acts by adolescents in the general population of upstate New York who were followed up several years later. Yet despite the recommendation that DSM-IV-TR Axis II disorders should be included in the assessment of risk of violent behavior (e.g., Tardiff 2001), little research has been carried out using this diagnostic system in correctional samples.

Nevertheless, a study in Sweden of subjects who had received court-mandated, pre-sentence forensic psychiatric evaluations (some of whom were subsequently sentenced to compulsory forensic psychiatric treatment, and others to imprisonment, as well as sanctions that did not include detention [$n=168$]) revealed age-adjusted odds ratios of 4.8 times higher risk for any recidivism and 3.7 higher risk for violent recidivism among subjects whose self-report diagnoses suggested a categorical diagnosis of ASPD (Hiscoke et al. 2003). The remaining nine categorical DSM-IV-TR personality disorder diagnoses were not significantly related to recidivism. The subjects had been followed for an average of 36 months after release from prison, discharge from a forensic psychiatric hospital, or onset of nondetaining sentences. Using dimensional analyses, each additional antisocial and schizoid personality disorder symptom endorsed by participants at baseline increased the risk for violent reoffending. Results suggested a relationship between self-reported behavior instability and interpersonal dysfunction captured primarily by the DSM-IV-TR antisocial and schizoid personality disorder constructs.

Predictive Ability of Ratings of Psychopathy

The predictive ability of psychopathy, measured using the PCL, PCL-R and PCL:SV, has been studied more extensively than that of Axis II, although these instruments were not originally designed to predict criminal behavior or to assess risk for violence. In a review of studies examining the evidence for convergent validity of the PCL-R with instruments specifically designed to predict recidivism and violence, Hare (2003) demonstrated the PCL-R's consistent relationship with actuarial instruments that have been designed to predict general criminal recidivism. These included the Violence Risk Appraisal Guide (Harris et al. 1993; Quinsey et al. 1998), four sex offender risk

scales, the Level of Service Inventory–Revised (Andrews and Bonta 1995), the HCR-20 (Webster et al. 1997), and the Spousal Assault Risk Assessment Guide (Kropp et al. 1999). Statistical associations between these instruments remained when removing items from the PCL:SV of PCL-R, as measures of psychopathy are included in most of these scales. Because most measures contain items that reflect or predict criminal behaviors, it was not surprising that Factor 2 of the PCL-R showed the strongest associations. Exceptions were the HCR-20 and Spousal Assault Risk Assessment Guide, each of which contained items requiring clinical judgment, and each of which was found to be quite strongly related to both Factor 1 and Factor 2.

Three recent meta-analyses (Hemphill et al. 1998; Salekin et al. 1996; Walters 2003) provided quantitative evaluations of the predictive validity of the PCL, PCL-R, and PCL:SV expressed in several ways, including correlation coefficients, relative risk, odds ratios, receiver operating characteristic analyses, and effect size estimates. Salekin et al. (1996) reported a meta-analysis of 18 studies that investigated the relationship between the PCL/PCL-R and violent and nonviolent recidivism. The average effect size across all predictive studies was 0.68. To examine how the instruments performed in three areas of prediction, including violent recidivism and institutional violence (combined), general recidivism, and sexual sadism and deviant sexual arousal, studies were divided to examine these three groups. The effect sizes when violence was used as a primary outcome ranged from 0.42 to 1.92, with a mean effect size of 0.79. When general recidivism was the outcome, substantially lower effect sizes were obtained. In this case, effect sizes ranged from 0.24 to 2.3, with a mean effect size of 0.55. In the three studies that addressed deviant sexual arousal and sexual sadism, effect sizes ranged from 0.47 to 0.77, with a mean of 0.61.

The studies were examined according to their positive and negative predictive values. Of the 13 studies that measured subsequent violent behavior, the mean positive predictive value was 0.72 and the mean negative predictive value 0.59. Salekin and colleagues (1996) concluded that these classification rates were unprecedented in their predictions of dangerousness (Webster et al. 1994), but that optimism should be tempered for several reasons. First, the mean negative predictive value was relatively low, in that 41% of nonviolent offenders were incorrectly classified as violent. Second, clinicians might have difficulty in selecting the optimum cutoff score for their correctional settings.

Third, the generalized ability of the research instruments to apply to other clinical populations had yet to be determined. These studies related overwhelmingly to white male offenders. In studies of general criminal recidivism, a mean positive predictive value of 0.70 and mean negative predictive value of 0.58 were obtained, indicating that whereas 30% of recidivists were missed with high PCL scores, 42% of the low scorers who had not reoffended were misclassified as recidivists. Overall, results from this meta-analysis also indicated that Factor 2 was a stronger predictor of both violence and general recidivism than Factor 1.

Hemphill et al. (1998) confirmed the effectiveness of psychopathy ratings in measuring recidivism, but in a subanalysis, these authors recommended the use of criminal careers profiles rather than survival techniques analysis. Survival analysis appeared less sensitive than criminal career profiles when subjects were separated by low, medium, and high scorers according to the PCL. The criminal careers profile methodology incorporated the time interval between criminal behaviors, allowed for varying follow-up length between groups, and provided a statistical comparison of criminal behaviors simultaneously across a range of time periods and between groups.

Walters (2003) explored the validity of PCL/PCL-R factor scores in predicting institutional adjustment and recidivism in forensic clinical samples and prison inmates. Forty-two studies in which institutional adjustment, release outcome (recidivism), or both were assessed prospectively when using these instruments resulted in 50 effect size estimates between factor scores and measures of institutional adjustment/recidivism. The meta-analysis indicated that Factor 2 (antisocial/unstable lifestyle) correlated moderately well with institutional adjustments in recidivism, whereas Factor 1 (affective/interpersonal traits) was less robustly associated with these outcomes. Direct comparisons of the mean effect sizes obtained by Factors 1 and 2 revealed that Factor 2 was significantly more predictive of total outcomes, general recidivism, violent recidivism, and outcomes from the 12 most methodologically sound studies compared with Factor 1. There was less differentiation between Factors 1 and 2 on measures of institutional adjustment. The mean weighted effect sizes for Factor 1 scores as predictors of general recidivism were 0.15, violent recidivism 0.18, and sexual recidivism 0.05. The mean weighted effect sizes for Factor 2 scores as predictors of general recidivism were 0.32, violent recidivism 0.26, and sexual recidivism 0.08. There was less differentiation in the predictive efficacy for Factor 1 and

Factor 2 among females and in juvenile samples, possibly due to low statistical power in some of these studies.

CONCLUSIONS

Prison populations vary in size between different countries and explain more about their criminal justice systems and societal attitudes toward what is acceptable punishment for criminal behavior than about levels of psychiatric morbidity in different correctional populations. However, research into the prevalence and correlates of personality disorder in correctional populations must be considered in relation to the epidemiology of personality disorder in the general population. In most countries, the core prison population consists of individuals, mainly men, whose criminal careers started at an early age and have persisted into adulthood despite attempts from professionals to intervene. In many cases, persisting criminality has remained intractable in the face of repetitive punishments, including imprisonment. This pattern of criminal behavior is associated with a range of social problems and noncriminal behavioral disorders corresponding to a diagnosis of ASPD, the most prevalent Axis II category in correctional settings.

ASPD is frequently comorbid with other Axis II disorders, and future research should examine patterns of comorbidity in relation to criminal behavior and behavioral problems subsequently demonstrated within the correctional setting. At the present time, few theoretical models explain the functional links between personality disorder and violent and criminal behaviors. These models have largely been restricted to observed associations between the specific traits that are considered to directly predispose to behavioral disorder and a more recent model that proposed that persons with certain forms of Axis II psychopathology are predisposed to dispositions and motivations that in turn lead to criminal and violent behavior. In the future, the challenge for this area of research is to demonstrate the key situational variables that increase the risks of behavioral disorder in the presence of Axis II disorders.

Criminal justice personnel and mental health professionals working in correctional settings are increasingly being called on to assess the risk of reoffending and of institutional misbehavior. Risk assessment has traditionally been carried out with a view to the day-to-day management of prisoners in the correctional setting, including the separation of vulnerable individuals from other, more predatory prisoners. However, certain jurisdictions require advice to courts on sentencing as well as more accurate information for those who must make decisions on parole. In some countries, increasing consideration is being given to the question of new interventions in correctional settings with a view to reducing future risk, together with extension of periods of mandatory surveillance in the community following release. These will be determined by formal risk assessments and will include clinical assessment for the diagnosis of personality disorder.

REFERENCES

American Psychiatric Association: Diagnostic and Statistical Manual of Mental Disorders, 3rd Edition. Washington, DC, American Psychiatric Association, 1980

American Psychiatric Association: Diagnostic and Statistical Manual of Mental Disorders, 4th Edition, Text Revision. Washington, DC, American Psychiatric Association, 2000

Andersen J, Sestoft D, Lilleback T, et al: Prevalence of ICD-10 psychiatric morbidity in random samples of prisoners on remand. Int J Law Psychiatry 19:61–74, 1996

Andrews DA, Bonta J: The Level of Service Inventory–Revised. Toronto, ON, Multi-Health Systems, 1995

Baldwin J, Bottoms AE: The Urban Criminal. London, England, Tavistock, 1976

Beck AT, Freeman A: Cognitive Therapy of Personality Disorders. New York, Guilford, 1990

Becker DF, Grilo CM, Edell WS, et al: Comorbidity of borderline personality disorder with other personality disorders in hospitalized adolescents and adults. Am J Psychiatry 157:2011–2016, 2000

Blackburn R: Personality in relation to extreme aggression in psychiatric offenders. Br J Psychiatry 114:821–828, 1968

Blackburn R: Psychopathology and Personality Disorder in Relation to Violence, in Clinical Approaches to Violence. Edited by Howells K, Hollin CR. Chichester, England, Wiley, 1989, pp 61–87

Bland R, Newman S, Dyck R, et al: Prevalence of psychiatric disorders and suicide attempts in a prison population. Can J Psychiatry 35:407–413, 1990

Bluglass R: A Psychiatric Study of Scottish Convicted Prisoners. M.D. thesis, University of St. Andrews, Scotland, 1966

Blumstein A, Cohen J: Estimation of individual crime rates from arrest records. Journal of Criminal Law and Criminology 70:561–585, 1979

Blumstein A, Cohen J: Characterising criminal careers. Science 237:985–991, 1987

Boin A: Securing safety in the Dutch prison system: pros and cons of a supermax. The Howard Journal of Criminal Justice 40:335–346, 2001

Bonta J, Law M, Hanson K: The prediction of criminal and violent recidivism among mentally disordered offenders: a meta-analysis. Psychol Bull 123:123–142, 1998

Bottoms AE, Wiles P: Environmental criminology, in The Oxford Handbook of Criminology, 2nd Edition. Edited by Maguire M, Morgan M, Reiner R. Oxford, England, Clarendon, 1997, pp 305–360

Box S: Power, Crime, and Mystification. London, England, Tavistock, 1983

Brinded P, Mulder R, Stevens J, et al: The Christchurch prisons psychiatric epidemiology study: personality disorders assessment in a prison population. Crim Behav Mental Health 9:144–155, 1999

Bulten B: Gevangen tussen straf en zorg. Deventer, The Netherlands, Kluwer, 1998

Caron C, Rutter M: Comorbidity in child psychopathology: concepts, issues and research strategies. J Child Psychol Psychiatry 32:1063–1080, 1991

Chiles J, von Cleve E, Jemelka R, et al: Substance abuse and psychiatric disorders in prison inmates. Hosp Community Psychiatry 41:1132–1134, 1990

Christian RE, Frick PJ, Hill NL, et al: Psychopathy and conduct problems in children, II: implications for subtyping children with conduct problems. J Am Acad Child Adolesc Psychiatry 36:233–241, 1997

Clare E, Bottomley K, Grounds A, et al: Evaluation of Close Supervision Centres. Home Office Research Study, No 219. London, Stationery Office, 2001

Cleckley H: The Mask of Sanity. St Louis, MO, Mosby, 1941

Cocozza JJ, Steadman HJ: The failure of psychiatric predictions of dangerousness: clear and convincing evidence. Rutgers Law Review 29:1084–1101, 1976

Coid J[W]: How many psychiatric patients in prison? Br J Psychiatry 145:78–86, 1984

Coid JW: An affective syndrome in psychopaths with borderline personality disorder? Br J Psychiatry 162:641–650, 1993

Coid JW: Axis II disorders and motivation for serious criminal behavior, in Psychopathology and Violent Crime. Edited by Skodol AE. Washington, DC, American Psychiatric Press, 1998a, pp 53–98

Coid JW: The management of dangerous psychopathy in prison, in Psychopathy: Antisocial, Criminal, and Violent Behavior. Edited by Millon T, Simonsen E, Birket-Smith M, et al. New York, Guilford, 1998b, pp 431–457

Coid JW: Personality disorders in prisoners and their motivation for dangerous and disruptive behavior. Crim Behav Ment Health 12:209–226, 2002

Coid JW: Formulating strategies for the primary prevention of adult antisocial behavior: "high risk" or "population" strategies? in Early Prevention of Adult Antisocial Behaviour. Edited by Farrington DP, Coid JW. Cambridge, UK, Cambridge University Press, 2003, pp 32–78

Coid J[W], Kahtan N, Gault S, et al: Patients with personality disorder admitted to secure forensic psychiatric services. Br J Psychiatry 175:528–536, 1999

Coid J[W], Petruckevitch A, Bebbington P, et al: Ethnic differences in prisoners, 1: criminality and psychiatric morbidity. Br J Psychiatry 181:473–480, 2002a

Coid J[W], Petruckevitch A, Bebbington P, et al: Ethnic differences in prisoners, 2: risk factors and psychiatric service use. Br J Psychiatry 181:481–487, 2002b

Coid J[W], Petruckevitch A, Bebbington P, et al: Psychiatric morbidity in prisoners and solitary cellular confinement, I: disciplinary segregation. Journal of Forensic Psychiatry and Psychology 14:298–319, 2003a

Coid J[W], Petruckevitch A, Bebbington P, et al: Psychiatric morbidity in prisoners and solitary cellular confinement, II: special ("strip") cells. Journal of Forensic Psychiatry and Psychology 14:320–340, 2003b

Coid J[W], Moran P, Bebbington P, et al: The co-morbidity of personality disorder and clinical syndromes in prisoners. Crim Behav Ment Health (in press)

Collins J, Schlenger W, Jordan B: Antisocial personality and substance abuse disorders. Bull Am Acad Psychiatry Law 16:187–198, 1988

Cooke DJ: Violence in prisons: the influence of regime factors. The Howard Journal of Criminal Justice 30:95–109, 1991

Cooke DJ: Psychological Disturbance in the Scottish Prison System: Prevalence, Precipitants, and Policy. Edinburgh, Scotland, Scottish Home and Health Department, 1994

Cooke DJ, Michie C: Psychopathy across cultures: Scotland and North America compared. J Abnorm Psychol 108:58–68, 1999

Cooke DJ, Michie C: Refining the construct of psychopathy: towards a hierarchical model. Psychol Assess 13:171–188, 2001

Crawford DA: The HDHQ results of long-term prisoners: relationships with criminal and institutional behavior. Br J Clin Soc Psychol 16:391–394, 1977

Dahl A: Some aspects of the DSM-III personality disorders illustrated by a consecutive sample of hospitalized patients. Acta Psychiatr Scand 73:62–66, 1986

Darke S, Kaye S, Finlay-Jones R: Antisocial personality disorder, psychopathy and injecting heroin use. Drug Alcohol Depend 52:63–69, 1998

DiLalla LF, Gottesman II: Heterogeneity of causes for delinquency and criminality: lifespan perspectives. Dev Psychopathol 1:339–349, 1989

Ditchfield J: Control in Prisons: A Review of the Literature. Home Office Research Study No 118. London, The Stationery Office, 1990

Donziger SR: The Real War on Crime: The Report of the National Criminal Justice Commission. New York, Harper Perennial, 1996

Ellis D: Crowding and prison violence: integration of research and theory. Crim Justice Behav 11:277–308, 1984

Ennis BJ, Litwack TR: Psychiatry and the presumption of expertise: flipping coins in the courtroom. California Law Review 62:693–752, 1974

Fabregat AA, Sanchez JP: Medida del trastorno antisocial de la personalidad del DSM-III mediante la escala de desviacion psicipatica del MMPI. Psiquis 15:41–52, 1994

Farrington DP: Offending from 10 to 25 years of age, in Prospective Studies of Crime and Delinquency. Edited by Van Dusen KT, Mednick SA. The Hague, Kluwer-Nijhoff, 1983

Farrington DP: The development of offending and antisocial behavior from childhood: key findings from the Cambridge Study in Delinquent Development. J Child Psychol Psychiatry 360:929–964, 1995

Farrington DP, Ohlin LE, Wilson JQ: Understanding and Controlling Crime. New York, Springer-Verlag, 1986, pp 17–37

Faulk M: A psychiatric study of men serving a sentence in Winchester Prison. Med Sci Law 16:244–251, 1976

Fazel S, Danesh J: Serious mental disorder in 23,000 prisoners: a systematic review of 62 surveys. Lancet 359:545–550, 2002

First MB, Gibbon M, Spitzer RL, et al: Structured Clinical Interviews for DSM-IV Axis-II Personality Disorders. Washington, DC, American Psychiatric Press, 1997

Gandhi N, Tyrer P, Evans K, et al: A randomised controlled trial of community-oriented and hospital-oriented care for discharged psychiatric patients: influence of personality disorder on police contacts. J Personal Disord 15:94–102, 2001

Gendreau P, Goggin C, Paparozzi MA: Principles of effective assessment for community corrections. Fed Probat 60:64–70, 1996

Gibbs JJ, Shelly PL: Life in the fast lane: a retrospective view of commercial thieves. Journal of Research in Crime and Delinquency 19:299–330, 1982

Gibson L, Holt J, Fondacaro K, et al: An examination of antecedent traumas and psychiatric comorbidity among male inmates with PTSD. J Trauma Stress 12:473–484, 1999

Gingell R: The criminalization of the mentally ill: an examination of the hypothesis. PhD thesis, Simon Fraser University, 1991

Gluek B: A study of 608 admissions to Sing Sing prison. Ment Hyg 2:85–151, 1918

Grilo CM, Sanislow CA, McGlashan TH: Co-occurrence of DSM-IV personality disorders with borderline personality disorder. J Nerv Ment Dis 190:552–554, 2002

Groth AN, Birnbaum HJ: Men Who Rape: The Psychology of the Offender. New York, Plenum, 1979

Gunn J, Robertson G, Dell S, et al: Psychiatric Aspects of Imprisonment. London, England, Academic Press, 1978

Guze SB: Criminality and Psychiatric Disorders. New York, Oxford University Press, 1976

Hare RD: Psychopathy: Theory and Research. New York, Wiley, 1970

Hare RD: The Hare Psychopathy Checklist–Revised. Toronto, ON, Multi-Health Systems, 1991

Hare RD: Hare Psychopathy Checklist–Revised (PCL-R), 2nd Edition. Toronto, ON, Multi-Health Systems, 2003

Harris GT, Rice ME, Quinsey VL: Violent recidivism of mentally disordered offenders: the development of a statistical prediction instrument. Crim Justice Behav 20:315–335, 1993

Hart SD, Hare RD: Discriminant validity of the Psychopathy Checklist in a forensic psychiatric population. J Consult Clin Psychol 1:211–218, 1989

Hart SD, Hare RD: Psychopathy: assessment and association with criminal conduct, in Handbook of Antisocial Behavior. Edited by Stoff DM, Breiling J, Maser J. New York, Wiley, 1997, pp 22–35

Hart SD, Forth AE, Hare RD: The MCMI-II as a measure of psychopathy. J Personal Disord 5:318–327, 1991

Hemphill JF, Templeman R, Wong S, et al: Psychopathy and crime: recidivism and criminal careers, in Psychopathy: Theory, Research, and Implications for Society. Edited by Cooke DJ, Forth AE, Hare RD. Dordrecht, The Netherlands, Kluwer Academic, 1998, pp 375–399

Henderson M: Self-reported assertion and aggression among violent offenders with high or low levels of overcontrolled hostility. Pers Individ Dif 4:113–115, 1983

Herbert DT: Urban crime: a geographical perspective, in Social Problems and the City: Geographical Perspectives. Edited by Herbert DT, Smith DM. New York, Oxford University Press, 1979

Hernandez-Avila CA, Burleson JA, Poling J, et al: Personality and substance use disorders as predictors of criminality. Compr Psychiatry 41:276–283, 2000

Hesselbrock MN: Childhood behavior problems and adult antisocial personality disorder in alcoholism, in Psychopathology and Addictive Disorders. Edited by Myer RE. New York, Guilford, 1986, pp 78–94

Hindelang MJ: The social versus solitary nature of delinquent involvements. Br J Criminol 11:167–175, 1971

Hirschi T, Gottfredson M: Age and the explanation of crime. Am J Sociol 89:552–584, 1983

Hiscoke UL, Langstrom N, Ottosson H, et al: Self-reported personality traits and disorders (DSM-IV) and risk of criminal recidivism: a prospective study. J Personal Disord 17:293–305, 2003

Hodgins S, Cote G, Toupin J: Major mental disorders and crime: an aetiological hypothesis, in Psychopathy: Theory, Research, and Implications for Society. Edited by Cooke D, Forth A, Hare RD. Dordrecht, The Netherlands, Kluwer Academic, 1998, pp 231–256

Hollin CR: Psychology and Crime. London, England, Routledge, 1989

Hurley W, Dunne M: Psychological distress and psychiatric morbidity in women prisoners. Aust N Z J Psychiatry 25:461–470, 1991

Hyler S, Lyons M: Factor analysis of the DSM-III personality disorder clusters: a replication. Compr Psychiatry 29:304–308, 1988

James JF, Gregory D, Jones RK, et al: Psychiatric morbidity in prisons. Hosp Community Psychiatry 31:674–677, 1980

Jones DA: The Health Risks of Imprisonment. Lexington, MA, Lexington Books, 1976

Jordan BK, Schlenger WE, Fairbank JA, et al: Prevalence of psychiatric disorders among incarcerated women, II: convicted felons entering prison. Arch Gen Psychiatry 53:513–519, 1996

King RD: The rise and rise of supermax: an American solution in search of a problem? International Journal of Penology 1:163–186, 1999

Koegel P, Burman A, Farr RK: The prevalence of specific psychiatric disorders among homeless individuals in the inner city of Los Angeles. Arch Gen Psychiatry 45:1085–1092, 1988

Kratzer L, Hodgins S: A typology of offenders: a test of Moffitt's theory among males and females from childhood to age 30. Crim Behav Ment Health 9:57–73, 1999

Kropp PR, Hart SD, Webster CD, et al: Spousal Assault Risk Assessment Guide (SARA). Toronto, ON, Multi-Health Systems, 1999

Langan PA, Farrington DP: Two-track or one-track justice? Some evidence from an English longitudinal survey. Journal of Criminal Law and Criminology 74:519–546, 1983

Langan PA, Greenfeld LA: Career Patterns in Crime: Bureau of Criminal Statistic Special Report NCJ-88672. Washington, DC, Bureau of Justice Statistics, 1983

LeBlanc M, Frechette M: Male Criminal Activity from Childhood Through Youth: Multilevel and Developmental Perspectives. New York, Springer-Verlag, 1989

Loeber R: The stability of antisocial and delinquent child behavior: a review. Child Dev 53:1431–1446, 1982

Loeber R: Natural histories of conduct problems, delinquency and associated substance use: evidence for developmental progressions, in Advances in Clinical Child Psychology, Vol 11. Edited by Lahey BB, Kazdin AE. New York, Plenum, 1988

Loranger A, Susman VL, Oldham JM, et al: The Personality Disorder Examination: a preliminary report. J Personal Disord 1:1–13, 1987

Lynam DR: Early identification of chronic offenders: who is the fledgling psychopath? Psychol Bull 120:209–234, 1996

McGlashan TH, Grilo CM, Skodol AE, et al: The Collaborative Longitudinal Personality Disorders Study: baseline Axis I/II and II/II diagnostic co-occurrence. Acta Psychiatr Scand 102:256–264, 2000

Megargee EI: Undercontrolled and overcontrolled personality types in extreme antisocial aggression. Psychol Monogr 80:1–29, 1966

Megargee EI: The association of population density, reduced space and uncomfortable temperatures with misconduct in a prison community. Am J Community Psychol 5:289–298, 1977

Megargee EI: Putting the criminal back into criminology [review of life style and criminality]. Contemporary Psychology 34:562–564, 1989

Menzies R, Webster CD, McMain S, et al: The dimensions of dangerousness revisited: assessing forensic predictions about violence. Law Hum Behav 18:1–28, 1994

Moffitt TE: Adolescence-limited and life-course-persistent antisocial behavior: a developmental taxonomy. Psychol Rev 100:674–701, 1993

Moffitt TE: Natural histories of delinquency, in Cross-national Longitudinal Research on Human Development and Criminal Behavior. Edited by Weitekamp EGM, Kerner H-J. The Netherlands, Kluwer Academic, 1994, pp 3–61

Moldin SO, Rice JP, Erlenmeyer-Kimling L, et al: Latest structure of DSM-III-R Axis II psychopathology in a normal sample. J Abnorm Psychol 103:259–266, 1994

Monahan J: Predicting Violent Behavior: An Assessment of Clinical Techniques. Beverly Hills, CA, Sage, 1981

Monahan J, Steadman HJ: Towards a rejuvenation of risk assessment research, in Violence and Mental Disorder: Developments and Risk Assessment. Edited by Monahan J, Steadman HJ. Chicago, IL, University of Chicago Press, 1994, pp 1–17

Monahan J, Steadman HJ, Silver E, et al: Rethinking Risk Assessment. The MacArthur Study of Mental Disorder and Violence. Oxford, England, Oxford University Press, 2001

Moran P: Antisocial Personality Disorder: An Epidemiological Perspective. London, Gaskell, 1999

Motiuk L, Porporino F: The prevalence, nature, and severity of mental health problems among federal male inmates in Canadian pententiaries. Ottawa, Canada, Research and Statistical Branch, Correctional Service, 1992

Nagin DS, Land KC: Age, criminal careers, and population heterogeneity: specification and estimation of a nonparametric, mixed poisson model. Criminology 31:327–362, 1993

Neighbors H, Williams D, Gunnings T, et al: The prevalence of mental disorder in Michigan prisons. Detroit, Michigan Department of Corrections, 1987

Oldham JM, Skodol AE, Kellman HD, et al: Diagnosis of DSM-III-R personality disorders by two structured interviews: patterns of comorbidity. Am J Psychiatry 149:213–220, 1992

Patterson GR, Capaldi D, Bank C: An early starter model for predicting delinquency, in The Development and Treatment of Childhood Aggression. Edited by Pepler DJ, Rubin KH. Hillsdale, NJ, Lawrence Erlbaum, 1991

Petersilia J, Greenwood PW, Lavin M: Criminal Careers of Habitual Felons. Washington, DC, U.S. Government Printing Office, 1978

Peterson MA, Braiker HB: Doing Crime: A Survey of California Prison Inmates. Santa Monica, CA, RAND, 1980

Pfohl B, Coryell W, Zimmerman M, et al: DSM-III personality disorders: diagnostic overlap and internal consistency of individual DSM-III criteria. Compr Psychiatry 27:21–34, 1986

Pfohl B, Black DW, Noyes R, et al: Axis I and Axis II comorbidity findings: implications for validity, in Personality Disorders: New Perspectives on Diagnostic Validity. Edited by Oldham J. Washington, DC, American Psychiatric Press, 1991, pp 145–161

Powell TA, Holt JC, Fondacaro KM: The prevalence of mental illness among inmates in a rural state. Law Hum Behav 21:427–438, 1997

Prentsky R, Cohen M, Seghorn T: Development of a rational taxonomy for the classification of rapists: the Massachusetts treatment center system. Bull Am Acad Psychiatry Law 13:39–70, 1985

Quay HC: Managing Adult Inmates: Classification for Housing and Program Assignments. College Park, MD, American Correctional Association, 1984

Quinsey VL, Maguire A, Varney GW: Assertion and overcontrolled hostility among mentally disordered murderers. J Consult Clin Psychol 51:550–556, 1983

Quinsey VL, Harris GT, Rice ME, et al: Violent Offenders: Appraising and Managing Risk. Washington, DC, American Psychological Association, 1998

Raine A: Biosocial studies of antisocial and violent behavior in children and adults: a review. J Abnorm Child Psychol 30:311–326, 2002

Reich JH, de Girolamo G: Epidemiology of DSM-III personality disorders in the community and in clinical populations, in Assessment and Diagnosis of Personality Disorders. Edited by Loranger AW, Janca A, Sartorius N. Cambridge, England, Cambridge University Press, 1997

Ressler RK, Burgess AW, Douglas JE: Sexual Homicide: Patterns and Motives. New York, Lexington Books, 1988

Robertson RG: The female offender: a Canadian study. Can J Psychiatry 32:749–755, 1987

Robins LN: Deviant Children Grown Up: A Sociological and Psychiatric Study of Sociopathic Personality. Baltimore, MD, Williams and Wilkins, 1966

Robins LN: Follow-up studies of childhood conduct disorder, in Psychiatric Epidemiology. Edited by Hare EH, Wing JK. London, Oxford University Press, 1970, pp 29–89

Robins LN: Sturdy childhood predictors of adult antisocial behavior: replications from longitudinal studies. Psychol Med 8:611–622, 1978

Robins LN: Epidemiology of antisocial personality, in Psychiatry, Vol 3. Edited by Cavenar JO. Philadelphia, PA, Lippincott, 1985, pp 1–14

Robins LN, Price RK: Adult disorders predicted by childhood conduct problems: results from the NIMH Epidemiologic Catchment Area project. Psychiatry 54:116–132, 1991

Robins LN, Helzer JE, Croughan J, et al: National Institute of Mental Health Diagnostic Interview Schedule: its history, characteristics and validity. Arch Gen Psychiatry 39:381–389, 1981

Robins LN, Tipp J, Przybeck T: Antisocial personality, in Psychiatric Disorder in America. Edited by Robbins LN, Regier DA. New York, The Free Press, 1991, pp 258–290

Robins R, Regier D: Psychiatric Disorders in America: The Epidemiologic Catchment Area Study. New York, The Free Press, 1991

Roesch R: Mental health interventions in pretrial jails, in Psychology, Law and Criminal Justice. Edited by Davies G, Lloyd-Bostock S. Berlin, Germany, De Greuter, 1995, pp 520–531

Roper WF: A comparative study of the Wakefield Prison population in 1948, part I. British Journal of Delinquency 1:15–28, 1950

Roper WF: A comparative study of the Wakefield Prison population in 1948 and 1949, part II. British Journal of Delinquency 1:243–270, 1951

Rutter M: Concepts of antisocial behavior, of cause, and of genetic influences, in Genetics of Criminal and Antisocial Behavior. Edited by Bock GR, Goode JA. New York, Wiley, 1996, pp 1–15

Rutter M, Giller H: Juvenile Delinquency: Trends and Perspectives. Harmondsworth, UK, Penguin, 1983

Rutter M, Giller H, Hagell A: Antisocial Behavior by Young People. Cambridge, England, Cambridge University Press, 1998

Rydelius PA: The development of antisocial behavioral and sudden violent death. Acta Psychiatr Scand 77:398–403, 1988

Salekin R, Rogers R, Sewell K: A review and meta-analysis of the Psychopathy Checklist and Psychopathy Checklist–Revised: predictive validity of dangerousness. Clin Psychol Sci Pract 3:203–215, 1996

Salekin R, Rogers R, Sewell K: Construct validity of psychopathy in a female offender sample: a multitrait-multimethod evaluation. J Abnorm Psychol 106:576–585, 1997

Schoemaker C, Van Zessen G: Psychische stoornissen bij gedetineerden. Utrecht, The Netherlands, Trimbos-Instituut, 1997

Shaw CR, McKay HD: Juvenile Delinquency and Urban Areas. Chicago, IL, Chicago University Press, 1942

Shrout PE, Newman SC: Design of two-phase prevalence surveys of rare disorders. Biometrics 45:549–555, 1989

Simpson A, Brinded P, Laidlaw T, et al: The national study of psychiatric morbidity in New Zealand prisons. Auckland, New Zealand, Department of Corrections, 1999

Singleton N, Meltzer H, Gatward R, et al: Psychiatric Morbidity Among Prisons in England and Wales. London, England, The Stationery Office, 1998

Smith DJ: Ethnic origins, crime and criminal justice, in The Oxford Textbook of Criminology, 2nd Edition. Edited by Maguire M, Morgan R, Reiner R. Oxford, England, Clarendon, 1997, pp 703–759

Smith DR, Smith W, Noma E: Delinquent career-lines: a conceptual link between theory and juvenile offences. Sociol Q 25:155–172, 1984

Stattin M, Magnusson D: Stability and change in criminal behavior up to age 30: findings from a prospective, longitudinal study in Sweden. Br J Criminol 31:327–346, 1991

Stuart S, Pfohl B, Battaglia M, et al: The co-occurrence of DSM-III-R personality disorders. J Personal Disord 12:302–315, 1998

Tardiff K: Axis II disorders and dangerousness, in Clinical Assessment of Dangerousness: Empirical Contributions. Edited by Pinard G-F, Paganini L. New York, Cambridge University Press, 2001, pp 103–120

Tardiff K, Marzuk PM, Leon AC, et al: A prospective study of violence by psychiatric patients after hospital discharge. Psychiatr Serv 48:678–681, 1997

Teplin LA: Psychiatric and substance abuse disorders among male urban jail detainees. Am J Public Health 84:290–293, 1994

Teplin LA, Abram KM, McClelland G: Prevalence of psychiatric disorders among incarcerated women, I: practical jail detainees. Arch Gen Psychiatry 53:505–512, 1996

Toch H, Adams K: Coping: Maladaptation in Prisons. New Brunswick, NJ, Transaction Publishers, 1989

Vine R: Benzodiazepine use in women prisoners: association with personality disorder and behavioral dyscontrol. Psychiatry Psychol Law 1:53–58, 1994

Walmsley R: World prison population list (4th edition). London, Home Office Research, Development and Statistics Directorate, Findings 188, 2003. Available at: http://www.homeoffice.gov.uk/rds/pdfs2/r188.pdf. Accessed December 6, 2004.

Walters GD: The Criminal Lifestyle: Patterns of Serious Criminal Conduct. Newbury Park, CA, Sage, 1990

Walters GD: Predicting institutional adjustment and recidivism with the Psychopathy Checklist factor scores: a meta-analysis. Law Hum Behav 27:541–558, 2003

Walters G, Chlumsky M: The lifestyle criminality screening form and antisocial personality disorder. Behav Sci Law 11:111–115, 1993

Ward DA: Control strategies for problem prisoners in American penal systems, in Problems of Long-Term Imprisonment. Edited by Bottoms AE, Light R. Aldershot, England, Gower, 1987

Warren JI, Burnette M, South SC, et al: Personality disorders and violence among female prison inmates. J Am Acad Psychiatry Law 30:502–509, 2002

Webster CD, Dickens B, Addario S: Constructing Dangerousness: Scientific, Legal and Policy Implications (Research Report). Toronto, ON, Centre for Criminology, University of Toronto, 1985

Webster CD, Harris GT, Rice ME, et al: The Violence Prediction Scheme: Assessing Dangerousness in High Risk Men. Toronto, ON, Centre for Criminology, University of Toronto, 1994

Webster CD, Douglas KS, Eaves D, et al: HCR-20: Assessing the Risk for Violence (Version 2). Vancouver, BC, Mental Health, Law, and Policy Institute, Simon Fraser University, 1997

West D, Farrington DP: The Delinquent Way of Life: Third Report of the Cambridge Study in Delinquent Development. London, England, Heinemann, 1977

Widiger TA, Trull TJ: Personality disorders and violence, in Violence and Mental Disorder: Developments in Risk Assessment. Edited by Monahan J, Steadman HJ. Chicago, IL, University of Chicago Press, 1994, pp 203–226

Widiger TA, Frances AJ, Harris MJ, et al: Comorbidity among Axis II disorders, in Personality Disorders: New Perspectives on Diagnostic Validity. Edited by Oldham J. Washington, DC, American Psychiatric Press, 1991, pp 163–194

Widiger T, Hare R, Rutherford M: DSM-IV antisocial personality disorder field trial. J Abnorm Psychol 105:3–16, 1996

Wittchen H-V: Critical issues in the evaluation of comorbidity of psychiatric disorders. Br J Psychiatry 168 (suppl 30):9–16, 1996

Wittchen H-V, Robins LN, Cottler LB, et al., participants in the multicentre WHO/ADAMHA field trials: Cross-cultural feasibility, reliability and sources of variance of the Composite International Diagnostic Interview (CIDI). Br J Psychiatry, 159:645–653, 1991

Wolff S, Chick J: Schizoid personality in childhood: a controlled follow-up study. Psychol Med 10:85–100, 1980

Wolfgang M, Figli RF, Sellin T: Delinquency in a Birth Cohort. Chicago, IL, University of Chicago Press, 1972

Zanarini MC, Frankenburg FR, Dubo ED, et al: Axis I comorbidity of borderline personality disorder. Am J Psychiatry 155:1733–1739, 1998a

Zanarini MC, Frankenburg FR, Dubo ED, et al: Axis II comorbidity of borderline personality disorder. Compr Psychiatry 39:296–302, 1998b

Zimmerman M, Coryell W: DSM-III personality disorder diagnoses in a nonpatient sample: demographic correlates and comorbidity. Arch Gen Psychiatry 46:682–689, 1989

37

Medical Settings

Peter Tyrer, M.D.

The data presented in Chapter 8, "Epidemiology," illustrate the wide variation in the prevalence of personality disorders in different settings. In many of these settings, the figures are remarkably high, but many clinicians working in these environments are unaware that so many of their patients have personality disorders. Creating better awareness will be one of the major objectives over the next few years, because comorbid personality disorder in patients seen in these settings seems to have important implications for the service.

There are four major settings in which we know personality disorders have an important impact: primary care, general hospitals (all medical disciplines), emergency medical settings, and specialized psychiatric settings in which personality disorder is often ignored.

PRIMARY CARE

There is considerable international variation in the extent to which primary care forms the cornerstone of medical services. In some countries, paradoxically including the most developed (including the United States) and least developed countries, primary care is often bypassed in favor of a direct route to secondary care (Goldberg and Huxley 1992). In other countries, illness of any type is almost always seen first in primary care, and the primary care physician (PCP) acts as a gatekeeper for other services. It is the latter group that has normally been studied with regard to personality pathology and its implications.

The most accurate estimate suggests that between 1 in 3 and 1 in 5 of all patients visiting their PCPs have a comorbid personality disorder using current criteria of diagnosis (which may be too lax) (Casey et al. 1984; Moran et al. 2000). Only a small proportion of these patients are recognized as such by the PCP (Gross et al. 2002), and many who are thought by the PCP to have a personality disorder turn out to have no personality disorder after formal testing (Moran 2002). Therefore, a major deficiency in the identification and recognition of personality disorders must be overcome if any useful form of intervention, or modification of interventions for treatment of other conditions, is to be undertaken in the primary care setting.

I thank Drs. Paul Moran, Giovanni di Girolamo, and Helen Seivewright for the valuable information they contributed to the research for this chapter.

The distribution of personality disorders in primary care since 1960, split by decades, is shown in Tables 37–1 through 37–4. The prevalences of personality disorder increased greatly after the introduction of DSM-III in 1980 (American Psychiatric Association 1980). The groups of personality disorders presenting in primary care have been Cluster B (notably borderline personality disorder) and Cluster C; this prevalence might be expected in view of these disorders' strong association with anxiety and depression, which constitute the greater proportion of primary care psychiatric consultations (Goldberg and Huxley 1992).

There is some debate, reflected elsewhere in this book, about the validity of epidemiological data on personality disorder in the presence of other psychiatric morbidity; the general consensus is that the prevalence may be inflated, although a possible alternative explanation is that treatment of comorbid disorders (particularly with antidepressants) may also improve the personality disorder (Fava et al. 2002; Tyrer et al. 1993). It is also possible that the characteristics related to affective personality traits (more marked in Cluster C) are less stable than others and are directly influenced by changes in state affect (Clark et al. 2003; Vaidya et al. 2002). The reader should nevertheless retain a certain skepticism about the higher levels of prevalence in Tables 37–2 through 37–4, but even if we discount the possibility that a proportion of these patients are incorrectly diagnosed, the fact remains that personality disturbance is surprisingly common.

Impact of Personality Disorder in Primary Care

Taking personality disorders as a whole, their presence in primary care is associated with 1) more frequent attendance at the surgery; 2) more frequent referral to psychiatric services (more marked in urban areas than rural ones) (Casey et al. 1984); 3) a greater drop out from care (possibly associated with greater mobility); 4) greater vulnerability and more presentations with these conditions; and 5) somewhat greater costs of care, although the results are somewhat equivocal (Table 37–5). The prevalence of personality disorder in primary care populations is (unsurprisingly) higher than in the general community, but great variation among studies is really of too high a magnitude to be explained by local factors alone.

Various terms, most of which are emotive, have been used to describe primary care patients who are difficult to care for: "problem patients" (Emerson et al. 1994), "hateful patients" (Groves 1978), and "heartsink patients" (O'Dowd 1988). Although these labels refer to patients with a variety of different physical, psychological, and social problems, these patients share the characteristic of evoking strongly negative emotional reactions in their doctors—a characteristic that may have important prognostic significance (Groves 1978).

In primary care, the prevalence of "difficult patients" has been estimated to be between 15% and 30% (Hahn et al. 1996; Lin et al. 1991). Physiological and functional health outcomes have been reported to be worse for this group of patients. Hahn et al. (1996) found that compared with a control group, "difficult patients" in primary care make more frequent medical visits, have poorer social function scores, receive more prescriptions, undergo more laboratory investigations, and receive more referrals.

Some evidence indicates that although the overall prevalence of personality disorder is similar in urban and rural settings, the distribution of personality abnormality is different. There is a greater proportion of Cluster C personality disorders in those who present in rural communities, particularly obsessive-compulsive personality disorder (Scott et al. 1982), and there is a greater tendency for those in primary care in a rural setting to have their psychiatric services provided from primary rather than secondary care services (a form of medical offset) (Seivewright et al. 1991).

In all studies in which assessment by the PCP is also included in the process, there is a distressing absence of agreement between PCP and external (research) assessment, indicating that at least one, or possibly both, are invalid. For example, in one study of 195 patients in the United Kingdom who visited their PCP and were rated for personality disorder by both their PCP and a trained researcher using a standardized assessment, the level of agreement was extremely low ($\kappa = 0.03$) (Moran et al. 2001). One explanation for why PCPs diagnose personality disorder when it may not exist is because those who present repeatedly for assessment or who argue or have some difference of opinion with the PCP are viewed as having a personality disorder. PCP ratings of personality disorder seem to be strongly associated with the perception of difficult consulting behavior, and although such behavior may sometimes be associated with personality disorder, there is a risk of the label being misapplied to a proportion of non-personality-disordered but difficult patients. There is a well-established prejudice that doctors diagnose people they do not like as having personality disorders (Lewis and Appleby 1988), and unfortunately this prejudice is still extant.

Table 37–1. Studies of personality disorder carried out in primary care (1960–1981)

Study	Location	Sample	Study design	Procedure	Findings
Kessel 1960	1 suburban general practice in the United Kingdom	911 randomly selected patients	Cross-sectional survey	Clinical interview	5% described as having an "abnormal personality"
Cooper 1965	10 general practices in the United Kingdom	100 selected patients with "chronic psychiatric disorder"	Cross-sectional survey	Clinical interview	8% identified by psychiatrist as having a personality disorder
Cooper 1972	8 general practices in the United Kingdom	115 selected patients with psychiatric disorder	Cross-sectional survey	Clinical interview using ICD-8 criteria	6% diagnosed with personality disorder
Hoeper et al. 1979	Family practice clinic in Wisconsin, United States	247 family practice patients	Cross-sectional survey	SADS-L	3.7% diagnosed as labile personality; 2% diagnosed as cyclothymic personality
Mann et al. 1981b	2 general practices in the United Kingdom	87 patients with nonpsychotic disorder identified by primary care physician	Cross-sectional survey with 1-year follow-up	SAP	35.6% had abnormal personalities; consumption of psychotropic agents at 1 year associated with personality abnormality

Note.   SADS-L=Schedule for Affective Disorders and Schizophrenia (Lifetime Version); SAP=Standardized Assessment of Personality.

Table 37–2. Studies of personality disorder carried out in primary care (1984–1989)

Author	Location	Sample	Study design	Procedure	Findings
Casey et al. 1984	Inner-city general practice in the United Kingdom	171 primary care patients with conspicuous psychiatric morbidity	Cross-sectional survey	PAS	33.9% point prevalence for unspecified personality disorder; explosive personality disorder most frequent Personality disorder rarely diagnosed as primary problem by primary care physician
Kessler et al. 1985	Primary care clinic in Wisconsin, United States	192 randomly selected patients	Cross-sectional survey with 1-year follow-up	SADS-L	Of continuing cases of psychiatric disorder, 33.3% had labile personality disorder and 20.4% had other personality disorder
Regier et al. 1985	Primary care clinic in Wisconsin, United States	247 consecutive attenders (sampled from 1,072 recruited and screened over 3 months)	Cross-sectional survey	SADS-L	Prevalence of personality and prolonged disorders, 7.4%; this group of disorders contributed the highest proportion of the total population with severe disability
Dilling et al. 1989	18 general practices in upper Bavaria, Germany	Representative sample of 1,274 attenders consulted doctors during a 14-day period	Cross-sectional survey	CIS and ICD-8 criteria	Prevalence of personality disorder, 9.4%

Note. CIS=Clinical Interview Schedule; PAS=Personality Assessment Schedule; SADS-L=Schedule for Affective Disorders and Schizophrenia (Lifetime Version).

Table 37–3. Studies of personality disorder carried out in primary care (1990–1996)

Author	Location	Sample	Study design	Procedure	Findings
Casey and Tyrer 1990	2 general practices in the United Kingdom; 1 urban, 1 rural	358 patients with conspicuous psychiatric morbidity	Cross-sectional survey	PAS	Prevalence of any personality disorder, 28%; more urban than rural
Seivewright et al. 1991	2 general practices in the United Kingdom; 1 urban, 1 rural	301 patients with conspicuous psychiatric morbidity (24% with a personality disorder)	Prospective cohort	Previously assessed with PAS; case records examined at 3 years	At 3 years, patients with personality disorder received more psychotropic drugs and had more contact with psychiatric services
Ceroni et al. 1992	11 general practices in northern Italy	66 consecutive attenders	Cross-sectional survey	Clinical Interview for DSM-III disorders	Prevalence of DSM-III personality disorder, 12.1%
Patience et al. 1995	14 general practices in Scotland	113 patients with DSM-III major depression	Clinical trial	PAS; treatment study with PAS administered after improvement	Personality disorder prevalence, 26%; presence of personality pathology delayed recovery from depression
Schramm et al. 1995	General practice clinic in Germany	105 attenders with chronic insomnia	Cross-sectional survey	SCID-II	14% had at least one Axis II diagnosis
Hueston et al. 1996	Family medical center in Wisconsin	93 registered patients	Cross-sectional survey	SCID-II screening questionnaire	70% of patients judged to be at high risk for personality disorder

Note. PAS=Personality Assessment Schedule; SCID-II=Structured Clinical Interview for DSM-III-R Personality Disorders.

Table 37–4. Studies of personality disorder carried out in primary care (1996–2002)

Author	Location	Sample	Study design	Procedure	Findings
Sansone et al. 1996	Family health care facility in Indiana	194 consecutive nonemergency attenders seen by a family physician	Cross-sectional survey	Borderline personality disorder scale of the PDQ-R	20% reported symptoms suggestive of BPD; BPD subjects used significantly more health resources
Barry et al. 1997	Offices of 64 primary care physicians in Wisconsin	Sample of all attenders to offices of 64 primary care physicians ($n=1,898$)	Cross-sectional survey	DIS-R	Prevalence of ASPD, among men 8%, among women 3.1%; ASPD significantly associated with male gender, being unmarried, younger age, lifetime depression, and alcohol and drug problems
Sansone et al. 1998	Offices of primary care physicians in Ohio	39 primary care patients being treated for depression	Cross-sectional survey	MCMI-III	33% had clinically significant levels of personality pathology
Hueston et al. 1999	13 family practices in Wisconsin	250 practice attenders	Cross-sectional study	SCID-II screening questionnaire	32% judged to be at high risk for personality disorder; high-risk group made more visits to hospital and had significantly lower health functional status scores
El-Rufaie et al. 2002	Primary care patients in Al Ain, United Arab Emirates	Schizoid and anankastic (obsessive-compulsive) personality disorders most common in this Arabian sample	Cross-sectional study	Administration of IPDE (ICD-10 version)	12.7% had definite personality disorder, higher rates in females (15.8F: 9.8M). Schizoid (5%), anankastic (4%), and BPD (4%) most common.
Gross et al. 2002	Urban primary care practice	218 patients from a systematic sample	Cross-sectional survey	Structured interview for Borderline Personality Disorder (Lifetime Prevalence)	6.4% (BPD only)

Note. ASPD=antisocial personality disorder; BPD=borderline personality disorder; DIS-R=Diagnostic Interview Schedule–Revised; IPDE=International Personality Disorder Examination; MCMI-III=Millon Clinical Multiaxial Inventory–III; PDQ-R=Personality Diagnostic Questionnaire–Revised; SCID-II= Structured Clinical Interview for DSM-III-R Personality Disorders.

Table 37–5. Impact of personality disorders on primary care services

Authors	Reported influence of personality disorder	Comments
Mann et al. 1981a	Greater consumption of psychotropic drugs in those with personality disorder	
Kessler et al. 1985	One in three of all patients with continuing care after 1 year had personality disturbance	No formal assessment of personality disorder
Seivewright et al. 1991	Greater number of prescriptions for benzodiazepines (and disulfiram) but not other drugs in those with personality disorder; more loss to follow-up in those with personality disorder	Difference in benzodiazepine prescription accounted for mainly by anxiolytic member of group
Patience et al. 1995	Patients with DSM diagnosis of major depressive episode and personality disorder in primary care had greater pathology at outset and took longer to recover than those with no personality disorder, but at 18 months the groups were equivalent	26% of patients identified with personality disorder; likely that a large proportion of these would be regarded as having treatment-resistant depression after 6 months to 1 year of treatment
Seivewright et al. 1998, 2004b; Tyrer et al. 2003b	More psychiatric symptomatology and worse social function in those with personality disorder after 5 and 12 years	Largest effects in those with severe personality disorder (Tyrer and Johnson 1996)
Moran et al. 2000, 2001	More psychiatric morbidity in those with Cluster B personality disorder; those with research diagnosis of personality disorder significantly more likely to be frequent attenders (more than eight consultations per year); those with primary care diagnosis of personality disorder more likely to receive psychotropic drugs	Cluster B associated with greater psychiatric morbidity but overall no increase in referral to secondary care
Rendu et al. 2002	Personality disorder significantly associated with higher mean total costs, but in univariate and multivariate analysis this difference was no longer sustained	Interaction found between personality disorders and psychiatric morbidity: excess costs only associated with personality disorder in presence of additional psychiatric morbidity

What is apparent from the clear disparity in the results of assessment (Casey et al. 1984; Gross et al. 2002; Moran et al. 2001) is that standard diagnostic procedures for assessing personality disorder in ordinary practice are inadequate. Many of those with personality disorder who present in primary care seem likely to have their diagnosis missed, and the training of PCPs to improve recognition of personality disorder is likely to become a priority in the near future. However, we should be careful not to assume that the poor level of agreement between PCP ratings and those of structured interviews indicates differential validity. The finding that PCPs tend to give the diagnosis of personality disorder to those from whom they derive negative connotations may indicate a prejudiced and unfair view. On the other hand, it may identify a core component of personality disorder that the structured interview (in this case the Standardized Assessment of Personality; Mann et al. 1981a) has failed to detect. Until we can be more confident about the validity of our assessment procedures, both hypotheses have to stay in the frame.

Course of Patients Presenting With Personality Disorders in Primary Care

In the short term, patients with personality disorder tend to consult PCPs more frequently if they have Cluster B disorders, but this trend is not so marked with other groups (Moran et al. 2000) (Table 37–2). It is also important to note that those who have a mental illness and comorbid personality disorder tend to have greater pathology than those who have a mental illness alone (Gross et al. 2002; Tyrer et al. 1990). They will therefore appear to make greater demands on services, but this may not be a direct effect of the personality disorder.

We have limited long-term (i.e., more than 5 years) evidence of the impact of personality disorders in primary care. The main study that has been carried out in this area is the Nottingham Study of Neurotic Disorder. However, although this study deals with the most common mental disorders—anxiety and depression—the results only refer to general practice psychiatric clinics. These clinics are somewhat unusual (particularly to those in the United States) and followed a movement into primary care that was initiated in the United Kingdom in the late 1960s but reduced toward the end of the 1980s. This movement involved greater liaison between secondary and primary care but was initiated primarily by psychiatrists, who took a personal initiative to go and consult with general practitioners about their patients in the primary care setting. This practice initially was highly praised and copied (Mitchell 1985; Tyrer

1984; Tyrer et al. 1984; Williams and Clare 1981) but was later criticized (Horder 1988), and direct contact with patients was replaced to some extent by increased liaison between primary and secondary care (Creed and Marks 1989; Emmanuel et al. 2002).

In personal work, we have seen most patients in general practice psychiatric clinics. These are halfway between conventional primary and secondary mental health care, with patients having more severe pathology than those seen in primary care alone but less severe pathology than those seen in psychiatric outpatient clinics, and the results have to be taken in this context. However, the findings are in keeping with other studies. They show that those with personality disorder have higher rates of consultation but also higher rates of dropout; more diagnostic changes between anxiety, depression, and other common mental disorders (Seivewright et al. 2000); a poorer outcome after 5 years and 12 years (Seivewright et al. 1998; Tyrer et al. 2004a); and a better response to drug treatment than psychotherapeutic approaches in the medium term (Tyrer et al. 1993).

The main implication of these findings is that those who have personality disorder would benefit greatly from being identified early in care. The general negative impact of personality disorder has to be tempered with the knowledge that those who have comorbid personality disorder and mental illness usually have greater psychiatric morbidity at the beginning of treatment and therefore might not be expected to improve as much as those without personality disorder. However, when this is taken into account using appropriate regression techniques, those with personality disorder have a significantly worse outcome than those who do not (Seivewright et al. 1998; Tyrer et al. 2003b), although this greater morbidity is usually only manifest strongly in the longer term. In short-term studies those with personality disorder often do as well as those without (Mulder 2002).

The data on the long-term implications of a comorbid personality disorder in primary care remain limited, but it is reasonable to conclude that the importance of the comorbidity increases over time. The long-term outcome of disorders in primary care tends to be more of academic than clinical interest, but the level of increased costs that usually accompanies personality disorder is a matter of great concern to PCPs (although the only study in primary care [Rendu et al. 2002] throws some doubt on this increased cost), and further work needs to be done in this area. Thus, for example, urban practices, which have a greater excess of Cluster B personality disorders than rural practices, are likely to cost more, although some of this cost will be offset by care transferred to psychiatric services (Seivewright et al. 1991).

There are two good reasons why it would be helpful for PCPs to be able to identify personality disorder in clinical practice. First, it would help to predict the course of most mental illnesses more accurately, and second, it would give a broader picture of a person's problems. The "broader picture" is sometimes lost in this era, in which the psychiatrist is taught to identify key features of mental illness and intervene with a treatment appropriate for the label that he or she has just attached. This broader picture assessment of personality gives a longitudinal perspective and helps to place current problems in better perspective. As treatments for personality disorder become better established in psychiatry, then these treatments could also be considered in addition to treatments for specific mental disorders and should, if successful, improve the general outcome.

Case Example

Mr. MM, a young man of 24 years, was referred by his PCP to a psychiatric clinic because of recurrent depression that had failed to respond to vigorous treatment with antidepressants. Assessment of the patient showed features of both borderline and antisocial personality, amounting to a disorder in the Cluster B category. The patient was not keen on being labeled as mentally ill and wanted most of his care to be given by his PCP. It was therefore arranged that the contacts with the psychiatrist would be infrequent, but that the PCP would be kept in touch with the psychiatrist's thinking on the problem. The psychiatrist felt that antidepressant medication was not of particular value because the depressive disturbance was usually precipitated by arguments with the patient's girlfriend and because impulsive self-harming with antidepressants could easily lead to (an unintentional) death.

The PCP still felt it better to continue with antidepressants and gave these in relatively low dosage and in small supplies—concentrating on drugs with low toxicity in overdose (mainly lofepramine and sertraline)—and continued to see the patient regularly. Problems persisted, but after 18 months there was a sudden improvement. The psychiatrist related this significant change to the patient's relationship with a new girlfriend with whom he was now living; the PCP felt it was related to the prescription of a new antidepressant, citalopram. There were no major upsets in the next year, and the patient decided to stop taking the antidepressant halfway through this time. There were no ill effects immediately after stopping, but 3 months later the patient again became depressed and suicidal after his girlfriend started seeing another man. The PCP and psychiatrist met socially shortly afterward. The PCP commented, "I think our experience with Mr. MM has taught me that your jabbering on about personality disorder is relevant to me after all. I now realize that Mr. MM has a 'personality-induced' depression; it is certainly not like the ordinary ones I treat." The psychiatrist replied, "Yes, but your interest in his depression kept him in touch with you and was probably a great help; if you had just thought of him having a personality disorder he might have been treated, and responded, very differently."

PERSONALITY DISORDER IN OTHER MEDICAL SETTINGS

It is rare for personality disorder to be given much prominence in other medical settings, although it is likely to be a significant influence in the presentation and course of many disorders. We nonetheless have clues about its presence from a number of sources.

General Medicine and Psychiatry

Factitious disorder, formerly called Münchausen's syndrome after the celebrated paper published by Richard Asher (1951), is characterized by the deliberate feigning of physical or psychological illness for emotional—rather than financial—gains, including the induction of illnesses or the manipulation or distortion of existing medical conditions in order to receive emotional reinforcement such as attention, support, and care from health care professionals, friends, and coworkers. It classically covers the presentation of somatic symptomatology, expressed clearly in Asher's original paper, and psychiatric symptoms such as dissociation but may also stretch to simulated (instrumental) psychosis, where it has been called the Good Soldier Svejk syndrome after the famous fictional Czech antihero of the same name (Tyrer et al. 2001). It also overlaps with malingering, the conscious contrived simulation of illness, and some blurred medical conditions in which the pathology is uncertain but is likely to include a strong psychiatric component. These include hysteroepilepsy, factitious dermatitis, and associated conditions such as trichotillomania and dermatotillomania and some chronic pain disorders. Excoriating skin disease is commonly associated with personality disorder, and a case has been made for including "psychogenic excoriation" in DSM-V (Arnold et al. 2001), in which both compulsive and impulsive personality features would be measured. There is also the alarming introduction of another diagnosis, rather unfortunately and inappropriately called Münchausen's syndrome by proxy

(Bools 1996), in which the patient makes a person under his or her care ill by giving poisonous substances or inappropriate treatment, not through ignorance but deliberately as part of a pathological syndrome.

There have been relatively few formal studies of the prevalence of personality disorder in factitious disorders; Bauer and Boegner (1996) found that all patients with classic Münchausen's syndrome seen at a neurology clinic also satisfied the criteria for personality disorder, and Rechlin et al. (1997) found that of 15 patients with hysterical pseudoseizures, 10 had borderline personality disorder, 2 had antisocial personality disorder, and 3 had histrionic personality disorder. In this context, it is also important for clinicians to be aware of a change in personality as a consequence of traumatic or other forms of brain injury. Personality change occurring after brain damage is a separate diagnosis in ICD-10 (World Health Organization 1992), and "organic personality disorders," seemingly indistinguishable from their natural counterparts occurring earlier in life, are well represented in neurology clinics (Franulic et al. 2000).

Genitourinary Medicine

Genitourinary medicine and sexual health clinics are difficult for the epidemiologist to evaluate because of the need to maintain strict confidentiality and anonymity. However, personality disorder has been evaluated in one small study of those attending such clinics (n=118). In this group, 38% of homosexually active and 28% of heterosexually active men were found to have personality disorder, and sexual risk-taking behavior was most marked in those with antisocial personality disorder (Ellis et al. 1995). Similar risky behavior leads to hepatitis B and C infections, and a significant proportion of those with these conditions also have personality disorder, particularly antisocial personality disorder (Martinez-Raga et al. 2001).

It is likely that at least one in four of all patients attending these and other medical clinics are likely to meet the formal criteria for the diagnosis of personality disorder. The extent to which this ratio is likely to be significant is impossible to say in our present state of knowledge, and our recommendations would be stronger and carry more weight if we had greater confidence in our diagnostic evaluation of the condition.

Emergency Medical Settings

The most common example of patients with personality disorder presenting in emergency settings is self-harm, and this constitutes a major public health problem. A majority of those with recurrent self-harm also have personality disorder or significant personality disturbance (Dirks 1998; Tyrer et al. 2003a; Yen et al. 2003), with borderline personality disorder showing the greatest frequency of presentation. The management of such personality disorders is described elsewhere in this book; here I discuss only the implications and management in the accident and emergency departments where most of the cases of self-harm present.

Most staff in these settings are antipathetic to those who present with self-harm; such patients are perceived as wasting valuable time and diverting resources from others who are more worthy. As a result, many patients who have self-harmed get short shrift and little therapeutic input. This staff response is particularly likely if the patient has a personality disorder. However, there are suggestive indicators that a more positive attitude and possibly some intervention in those with personality disorder might pay dividends. Crawford and Wessely (1998) found that those who did not attend appointments after being seen in an accident and emergency clinic following self-harm were more likely to repeat the self-harm, and the authors recommended that further training be given in the immediate management of such patients in accident and emergency settings.

Personality disorder is normally diagnosed only in early adulthood or later (American Psychiatric Association 2000). Nevertheless, some studies have reported that a minority of children and adolescents who self-harm also have many of the characteristics associated with personality disorder, although personality traits are usually not measured formally (Deykin and Buka 1994). The nature and impact of personality disorder in the pediatric population is rather less marked than those in older people (Fritsch et al. 2000), and although guidelines take personality factors into account in some respects (Shaffer et al. 2001), they do not give the same emphasis as with borderline personality disorder in adulthood and in late adolescence.

IMPLICATIONS OF EVIDENCE TO DATE

The findings from all these studies can be summarized in one short sentence: Patients with personality disorders in medical settings are more morbid and go to these settings more frequently than patients without personality disorders. Other chapters in this book reinforce this conclusion and also show that what happens in medical settings is only a reflection of what happens in general psychiatric practice. As Bender et al. (2001) recently found in a cross-collaborative study, those with personality disorder have greater contacts and more extensive histories of psychiatric outpatient, inpatient, and drug treatment than patients with major depressive disorder, and this tendency is true for those with borderline personality disorder more than any other group. Thus, we should not be surprised that this pattern is replicated across medicine.

Even if we knew nothing about the management of personality disorder, the message that personality disorder carries greater morbidity would need to be known to practitioners wherever they happen to be. Purely from an economic viewpoint, those with personality disorder need to be recognized, because, when everything is taken into consideration, care for these patients carries a greater economic cost. For example, a recent large-scale study of 480 patients involved in a comparison of treatments for recurrent self-harm showed that personality disorder was the best cost predictor, with those having a personality disorder of any type incurring 16% more costs over 1 year compared with those without personality disorder, a total difference of $550,000 dollars in this single study (Tyrer et al. 2004b).

FURTHER DEVELOPMENTS

Our ignorance of personality disorders in general medical settings remains profound, and it is likely that our detection and management of these conditions are so primitive at present that they handicap our knowledge development as much as they help it. Nevertheless, personality disorders in general medical settings is a subject that cannot be ignored. It is likely to come into greater prominence over the next few years as health economics becomes a driving force in making the best use of valuable resources. Not to dismiss their problems as unimportant, but those who present to medical clinics with personality disorders and related conditions are cost-inefficient; they use up a large amount of valuable health resources expensively and inappropriately (Powell and Boast 1993; Seivewright et al. 2004a). If we are to tackle these issues squarely and fairly, we need to have alternative ways of detecting and managing patients within the whole range of psychological disturbance, and according to present evidence, personality disorders are vying for the top spot in importance.

Case Example

Ms. NN, a woman of 45 years of age, presented at a genitourinary medicine clinic after being referred by her new general practitioner (GP). Her former GP had crossed her off his list because she had, in his view, consulted him inappropriately so many times (in the United Kingdom everyone has access to free health care, but GPs have the power to remove patients from their lists). She was found to have marked health anxiety (hypochondriasis) on assessment; she was convinced that past impulsive sexual behavior had infected her whole body and influenced her stomach, liver, brain, heart, and other organs. Ms. NN spent up to 6 hours each day ruminating about her symptoms and deciding whom to consult about them. Each time she was seen by a GP or specialist she initially felt reassured, but improvement seldom lasted for more than a few hours. Examination of her records showed that she had made over 40 consultations with different doctors in the previous 6 months. At assessment she also revealed a history of serious sexual abuse as an adolescent and qualified for the diagnoses of borderline and dependent personality disorders. At the clinic she was treated with an adapted form of cognitive-behavioral therapy for hypochondriasis and made slow improvement. For short periods she was also treated with antidepressants and atypical antipsychotic drugs when her hypochondriacal worries became delusional in their intensity. After 18 months she had made significant improvement but was by no means well. However, the time she spent ruminating about her symptoms had fallen to less than 2 hours each day, and she had obtained a part-time job.

REFERENCES

American Psychiatric Association: Diagnostic and Statistical Manual of Mental Disorders, 3rd Edition. Washington, DC, American Psychiatric Association, 1980

American Psychiatric Association: Diagnostic and Statistical Manual of Mental Disorders, 4th Edition, Text Revision. Washington, DC, American Psychiatric Association, 2000

Arnold LM, Auchenbach MB, McElroy SL: Psychogenic excoriation: clinical features, proposed diagnostic criteria, epidemiology and approaches to treatment. CNS Drugs 15:351–359, 2001

Asher R: Münchausen's syndrome. Lancet i:339–341, 1951

Barry LK, Fleming MF, Manwell LB, et al: Conduct disorder and antisocial personality disorder in adult primary care patients. J Fam Pract 45:151–158, 1997

Bauer M, Boegner F: Neurological syndromes in factitious disorder. J Nerv Ment Dis 184:281–288, 1996

Bender DS, Dolan RT, Skodol AE, et al: Treatment utilization by patients with personality disorders. Am J Psychiatry 158:295–302, 2001

Bools C: Factitious illness by proxy: Münchausen syndrome by proxy. Br J Psychiatry 169:268–275, 1996

Casey P, Tyrer P: Personality disorder and psychiatric illness in general practice. Br J Psychiatry 156:261–265, 1990

Casey PR, Dillon S, Tyrer PJ: The diagnostic status of patients with conspicuous psychiatric morbidity in primary care. Psychol Med 14:673–681, 1984

Ceroni GB, Ceroni FB, Bivi R, et al: DDM-III mental-disorders in general medical sector: a follow-up and incidence study over a 2-year period. Soc Psychiatry Psychiatr Epidemiol 27:234–241, 1992

Clark LA, Vittengl J, Kraft D, et al: Separate personality traits from the states to predict depression. J Personal Disord 17:152–172, 2003

Cooper B: A study of one hundred chronic psychiatric patients identified in general practice. Br J Psychiatry 111:595–605, 1965

Cooper B: Clinical and social aspects of chronic neurosis. Proc R Soc Med 65:509–512, 1972

Crawford MJ, Wessely S: Does initial management affect the rate of repetition of deliberate self harm? A cohort study. BMJ 317:985, 1998

Creed F, Marks B: Liaison psychiatry in general practice: a comparison of the liaison-attachment scheme and shifted out-patient models. J R Coll Gen Pract 39:514–517, 1989

Deykin EY, Buka SL: Suicidal ideation and attempts among chemically dependent adolescents. Am J Public Health 84:634–639, 1994

Dilling H, Weyerer S, Fichter M: The upper Bavarian studies. Acta Psychiatr Scand Suppl 348:113–139, 1989

Dirks BL: Repetition of parasuicide: ICD-10 personality disorders and adversity. Acta Psychiatr Scand 98:208–213, 1998

El-Rufaie OEF, Al-Sabosy M, Abuzeid MSO, et al: Personality profile among primary care patients: experimenting with the Arabic IPDE ICD-10. Acta Psychiatr Scand 105:38–41, 2002

Ellis D, Collis I, King M: Personality disorder and sexual risk-taking among homosexually active and heterosexually active men attending a genitourinary medicine clinic. J Psychosom Res 39:901–910, 1995

Emerson J, Pankratz L, Joos S, et al: Personality disorders in problematic medical patients. Psychosomatics 35:469–473, 1994

Emmanuel JS, McGee A, Ukouminne OC, et al: A randomised controlled trial of enhanced key-worker liaison psychiatry in general practice. Soc Psychiatry Psychiatr Epidemiol 37:261–266, 2002

Franulic A, Horta E, Maturana R, et al: Organic personality disorder after traumatic brain injury: cognitive, anatomic and psychosocial factors. A 6 month follow-up. Brain Inj 14:431–439, 2000

Fava M, Farabaugh AH, Sickinger AH, et al: Personality disorders and depression. Psychol Med 32:1049–1057, 2002

Fritsch S, Donaldson D, Spirito A, et al: Personality characteristics of adolescent suicide attempters. Child Psychiatry Hum Dev 30:219–235, 2000

Goldberg D, Huxley P: Common Mental Disorders: A Biosocial Model. London, England, Tavistock/Routledge, 1992

Gross R, Olfson M, Gameroff M, et al: Borderline personality disorder in primary care. Arch Intern Med 162:53–60, 2002

Groves JE: Taking care of the hateful patient. N Engl J Med 298:883–887, 1978

Hahn SR, Kroenke K, Spitzer RL: The difficult patient: prevalence, psychopathology, and functional impairment. J Gen Intern Med 11:1–8, 1996

Hoeper EW, Nyez GR, Cleary PD, et al: Estimated prevalence of RDC mental disorder in primary medical care. Int J Ment Health 8:6–15, 1979

Horder J: Working with general practitioners. Br J Psychiatry 153:513–520, 1988

Hueston WJ, Mainous AG, Schilling R: Patients with personality disorders: functional status, health care utilization, and satisfaction with care. J Fam Pract 42:54–60, 1996

Hueston WJ, Werth J, Mainous AG: Personality disorder traits: prevalence and effects on health status in primary care patients. Int J Psychiatry Med 29:63–74, 1999

Kessel N: Psychiatric morbidity in a London general practice. Br J Prev Soc Med 14:16–22, 1960

Kessler LG, Cleary PD, Burke JD: Psychiatric disorders in primary care: results of a follow-up study. Arch Gen Psychiatry 42:583–587, 1985

Lewis G, Appleby L: Personality disorder: the patients psychiatrists dislike. Br J Psychiatry 153:44–49, 1988

Lin EH, Katon W, Von Korff M: Frustrating patients: physician and patient perspectives among distressed high users of medical services. J Gen Intern Med 6:241–246, 1991

Mann AH, Jenkins R, Cutting JC, et al: The development and use of a standardized assessment of abnormal personality. Psychol Med 11:839–847, 1981a

Mann AH, Jenkins R, Belsey E: The twelve-month outcome of patients with neurotic illness in general practice. Psychol Med 11:535–550, 1981b

Martinez-Raga J, Marshall EJ, Keaney F, et al: Hepatitis B and C in alcohol-dependent patients admitted to a UK alcohol inpatient treatment unit. Addict Biol 6:363–372, 2001

Mitchell AR: Psychiatrists in primary health care settings. Br J Psychiatry 147:371–379, 1985

Moran P: Personality disorder in general practice. MD Thesis: University of London, 2002

Moran P, Jenkins R, Tylee A, et al: The prevalence of personality disorder among UK primary care attenders. Acta Psychiatr Scand 102:52–57, 2000

Moran P, Rendu A, Jenkins R, et al: The impact of personality disorder in UK primary care: a 1-year follow-up of attenders. Psychol Med 31:1447–1454, 2001

Mulder RT: Personality pathology and treatment outcome in major depression: a review. Am J Psychiatry 159:359–371, 2002

O'Dowd TC: Five years of heartsink patients in general practice. BMJ 297:528–530, 1988

Patience DA, McGuire RJ, Scott AI, et al: The Edinburgh Primary Care Depression Study: personality disorder and outcome. Br J Psychiatry 167:324–330, 1995

Powell R, Boast N: The million dollar man: resource implications for chronic Münchausen's syndrome. Br J Psychiatry 162:253–256, 1993

Rechlin T, Loew TH, Joraschky P: Pseudoseizure "status." J Psychosom Res 42:495–498, 1997

Regier DA, Burke JDJ, Manderscheid RW, et al: The chronically mentally ill in primary care. Psychol Med 15:265–273, 1985

Rendu A, Moran P, Patel A, et al: Economic impact of personality disorders in UK primary care attenders. Br J Psychiatry 181:62–66, 2002

Sansone RA, Sansone LA, Wiederman MW: Borderline personality disorder and health care utilization in a primary care setting. South Med J 89:1162–1165, 1996

Sansone RA, Wiederman MW, Sansone LA, et al: Early onset dysthymia and personality disturbance among patients in a primary care setting. J Nerv Ment Dis 186:57–58, 1998

Schramm E, Hohagen F, Kappler C, et al: Mental comorbidity of chronic insomnia in general-practice attenders using DSM-III-R. Acta Psychiatr Scand 91:10–17, 1995

Scott A, Kelleher MJ, Smith A, et al: Regional differences in obsessionality and obsessional neurosis. Psychol Med 12:131–134, 1982

Seivewright H, Tyrer P, Casey P, et al: A three-year follow-up of psychiatric morbidity in urban and rural primary care. Psychol Med 21: 495–503, 1991

Seivewright H, Tyrer P, Johnson T: Prediction of outcome in neurotic disorder: a five year prospective study. Psychol Med 28:1149–1157, 1998

Seivewright N, Tyrer P, Ferguson B, et al: Longitudinal study of the influence of life events and personality status on diagnostic change in three neurotic disorders. Depress Anxiety 11:105–113, 2000

Seivewright H, Salkovskis P, Green J, et al: Prevalence and service implications of health anxiety in genitourinary medicine clinics. Int J STD AIDS 15:519–522, 2004a

Seivewright H, Tyrer P, Johnson T: Persistent social dysfunction in anxious and depressed patients with personality disorder. Acta Psychiatr Scand 109:104–109, 2004b

Shaffer D, Pfeffer CR, Bernet W, et al: Practice parameter for the assessment and treatment of children and adolescents with suicidal behavior. J Am Acad Child Adolesc Psychiatry 40 (suppl):24S–51S, 2001

Tyrer P: Psychiatric clinics in General Practice: an extension of community care. Br J Psychiatry 145: 9-14, 1984

Tyrer P, Johnson T: Establishing the severity of personality disorder. Am J Psychiatry 153:1593–1597, 1996

Tyrer P, Seivewright, N, Wollerton S: General practice psychiatric clinics: impact on psychiatric services. Br J Psychiatry 145:15–19, 1984

Tyrer P, Seivewright N, Ferguson B et al: The Nottingham Study of Neurotic Disorder: relationship between personality status and symptoms. Psychol Med 20:423–431, 1990

Tyrer P, Seivewright N, Ferguson B, et al: The Nottingham Study of Neurotic Disorder: effect of personality status on response to drug treatment, cognitive therapy and self-help over two years. Br J Psychiatry 162:219–226, 1993

Tyrer P, Emmanuel J, Babidge N, et al: Instrumental psychosis: the syndrome of the Good Soldier Svejk. J R Soc Med 94:22–25, 2001

Tyrer P, Jones V, Thompson S, et al, for the POPMACT Group: Service variation in baseline variables and prediction of risk in a randomised controlled trial of psychological treatment in repeated parasuicide: the POPMACT study. Int J Soc Psychiatry 49:58–69, 2003a

Tyrer P, Seivewright H, Johnson T: The core elements of neurosis: mixed anxiety-depression (cothymia) and personality disorder. J Personal Disord 17:109–118, 2003b

Tyrer P, Seivewright H, Johnson T: The Nottingham Study of Neurotic Disorder: predictors of 12 year outcome of dysthymic, panic and generalised anxiety disorder. Psychol Med 34:1385–1394, 2004a

Tyrer P, Tom B, Byford S, et al: Differential effects of manual assisted cognitive behavior therapy in the treatment of recurrent deliberate self-harm and personality disturbance: the POPMACT study. J Personal Disord 18:82–96, 2004b

Vaidya J, Gray E, Haigh J, et al: On the temporal stability of personality: evidence for differential stability and the role of life experiences. J Pers Soc Psychol 83:1469–1484, 2002

Williams P, Clare A: Changing patterns of psychiatric care. BMJ 282:375–377, 1981

World Health Organization: International Statistical Classification of Diseases and Related Health Problems, 10th Revision. Geneva, Switzerland, World Health Organization, 1992

Yen S, Shea MT, Pagano M, et al: Axis I and Axis II disorders as predictors of prospective suicide attempts: findings from the collaborative longitudinal personality disorders study. J Abnorm Psychol 112:375–381, 2003

Part VI

New Developments and Future Directions

38

Brain Imaging

Ziad Nahas, M.D.
Chris Molnar, Ph.D.
Mark S. George, M.D.

Findings about neurobiological substrates of normal and abnormal personality in humans allow researchers to constrain theory so that it results both in improved understanding of disorders and in development of treatment interventions that are tailored to the needs of individuals. Consider findings, for example, that extremes of arousal will functionally decerebrate an individual, thereby making it harder for him or her to benefit from the inhibitory functions of the prefrontal cortex. In light of such findings, both the limitations of people with personality disorders and the need to tailor treatments to address these limitations are appreciated. Although our understanding of disorders and their treatments has improved with research about brain structure and function, researchers attempting to make inferences about the neurobiological correlates of personality still face several challenges. These challenges are due to technical limitations of brain imaging tools, some of which are described here; methodological features of studies; and the failure of researchers to adequately define constructs and to design studies within shared theoretical frameworks. In this chapter, we describe the imaging methods used to study structural and functional correlates of personality disorders and review some of the technical and methodological challenges. Following this review, we summarize limitations of current personality disorder constructs as defined in DSM-IV-TR (American Psychiatric Association 2000) and describe a recently proposed theoretical framework that researchers of the neurobiology of personality disorders can use. Next, we summarize research findings about imaging correlates of personality dimensions in healthy individuals because of these findings' applicability to improving understanding of disorders. We then describe findings about the neurobiology of personality disorders and present a clinical vignette. We use the vignette to highlight the potential of research about functional neuronal circuitry to improve treatment of often disabling and underdetected Axis II diagnoses.

Acknowledgment: The chapter authors would like to thank Ashley Leinbach for her assistance in preparing this chapter.

IMAGING MODALITIES

One of the most important distinctions in imaging is whether one is looking at brain structure or brain function. As the British neurologist John Hughlings Jackson (1874/1958) noted in the 1870s, brain structure does not equal function and vice versa. That is, structural brain damage, such as a tumor, can obliterate the function normally subserved by that portion, can heighten the function of that portion of the brain, or can have no measurable functional consequences due to plastic, distributed, or compensatory processes. Additionally, one can have normal brain structure (at least as measurable using current technology) and have markedly abnormal function. In contrast to computed tomography (CT) and traditional magnetic resonance imaging (MRI), which images the structure of the brain, several technologies have been developed recently with the power to look at brain function. Radiotracer-based techniques such as positron emission tomography (PET) and single-photon emission computed tomography (SPECT) provide an image of brain activity or function as do special MRI imaging sequences that do not involve any exposure to radiation (Lauterbur 1973; Mansfield 1977). Brain regions that are more active consume more glucose for energy consumption and receive more blood flow in order to provide oxygen and carry off waste. Thus areas that are more active will provide a larger signal if one injects a radiotracer that is coupled to blood flow (oxygen-15 PET) or glucose (fluoro-2-deoxy-D-glucose [FDG] PET). Under most conditions, blood flow and metabolism are coupled. Using more sophisticated tracers, one can label specific neurotransmitter receptors and transporters, providing information about regional pharmacological activity. In schizotypal personality disorder, for example, abnormalities in glucose metabolism and dopamine receptors have been found in frontal lobes, cingulate, striatum, and temporal lobes (Buchsbaum et al. 2002).

TECHNICAL AND METHODOLOGICAL CHALLENGES

Investigators encounter several technical and methodological challenges when they attempt to link findings about brain structure and function to the cognitive, behavioral, and physiological indices of personality disorders. As technology has improved, researchers have been able to image structure with greater resolution

and precision, yet significant challenges in imaging remain. For example, image resolution is improved with more powerful magnets yet the problem of movement artifact is increased. We are still unable to link functional processes in real time to dependent variables because there is a time delay between response and its measurement using functional MRI (fMRI). Images obtained across sessions are marked by low reliability (McGonigle et al. 2000). The technical features of fMRI constrain the nature of questions that can be asked about patient groups. For example, to obtain the most robust responses to emotional stimuli, such stimuli must be repeated across several blocks and interspersed with comparator stimuli. Unfortunately, turning emotions on and off across blocks is difficult for healthy participants, let alone individuals diagnosed with personality disorders. Challenges in interpretation also exist and are tightly linked to method of investigation used. For example, increased activity may be causally linked to a behavior or disease, may reflect a compensatory process, or may merely be an artifact related to the method of investigation (Phan et al. 2002) or the choice of comparator condition (Gusnard et al. 2001). Finally, more sophisticated analytic techniques (McIntosh et al. 1996) and nonlinear models of brain function are essential if researchers are to understand the dynamic and recursive processes they seek to study.

CONSTRUCTS AND THEORETICAL FRAMEWORKS

The particular challenges associated with the construct of personality disorders as operationalized in the DSM categorical diagnostic system are delineated in Chapter 3, "Categorical and Dimensional Models of Personality Disorders," and include comorbidity, heterogeneity within groups of individuals who meet diagnostic criteria for a particular disorder, arbitrary boundaries between normal and abnormal levels of functioning, and incomplete coverage of the personality dysfunction often found in individuals with a personality disorder diagnosis. An alternative dimensional conceptualization of personality can overcome these problems. Moreover, recent empirical evidence suggests that many disorders once thought of as categorical in nature are actually more accurately thought of as dimensional in nature (e.g., Ruscio and Ruscio 2000). Fortunately, several dimensional models of personality have been proposed, yet all are parsimoniously captured by four broad dimensions of personality functioning that include 1) emotional dysregulation versus emotional stability, 2) extraversion versus introversion, 3) agreeableness versus antagonism, and 4) constraint versus impulsivity (Chapter 3, "Categorical and Dimensional Models"). Some models also suggest a fifth domain captured by the five-factor model's (FFM's) broad dimension of openness. Unlike the first four dimensions, however, openness is not empirically related to the broad construct of trait emotionality (Watson 2000). The reader is referred to Chapter 3 of this volume, Table 3–1, for the relationships among several personality theories of relevance to personality disorders. The unique, and empirically supported, dimensional profiles of DSM personality disorders are described in Chapter 3. Next we summarize findings about neurobiological correlates of personality dimensions in primarily nonclinical samples, because research that examines central nervous system (CNS) correlates of the broadly accepted personality dimensions has the benefit of not losing personality-related variance as occurs when personality is dichotomized. Moreover, findings from research conducted using a dimensional model can be applied to diagnostic personality conceptualizations and, for the clinician, allow for refined and tailored case conceptualization.

Personality is fundamentally emotional in nature and several theoretical frameworks exist to capture the construct of emotion (Miller and Kozak 1993). Moreover, the use of imaging tools to integrate existing theoretical frameworks for emotion holds potential to elucidate the neurobiology of personality disorders. One group of researchers recently used just such a strategy of integrating existing theory with imaging findings to facilitate interpretation of a morass of brain imaging findings. In particular, Phillips and colleagues (2003a, 2003b) recently published a set of articles about the neurobiology of emotion, neurobiological perception of emotion, and neurobiological implications of emotion for understanding neuropsychiatric disorders. Phillips and colleagues' approach to inference is also especially useful for approaching investigation of neurobiological correlates of Axis II conditions. In Phillips' reviews, the authors explicitly state the theory of emotion processing by which they are guided (i.e., appraisalist theory) and identify three processes of theoretical importance to brain imaging researchers who investigate emotion and its disorders within this framework. In particular, first is the process of appraising the emotional significance of a stimulus. As is described in Chapter 18, "Schema Therapy," personality disorders are marked by serious cognitive biases and distortions that result in inaccurate appraisals of stimuli. The second process de-

lineated is the production of CNS-initiated efferent activity that follows the appraisal and automatic attempts to regulate emotional responses. Inaccurate appraisals of stimuli by individuals with personality disorders result in extreme and maladaptive emotional responses and associated automatic but maladaptive behaviors aimed at regulating those responses. The third process is the effortful regulation of emotional reactions produced in response to stimuli. As is described repeatedly when correlates of personality disorders are reviewed, often the prefrontal regions are "offline" in personality disorders, and thus effortful and controlled regulation of emotional responses is not possible until arousal intensity diminishes. Using this three-process account, Phillips et al. (2003b) go on to apply their framework to the understanding of some Axis I disorders and suggest that "distinct patterns of structural and functional abnormalities in neural systems important for emotion processing are associated with specific symptoms of particular Axis I disorders" (p. 515). Phillips and colleagues organize what is otherwise a morass of findings by positing that a ventral cortical system is linked to appraisal, efferent activity, and automatic regulatory processes, whereas a dorsal system is linked to the controlled regulation of emotional responses. Particular hypotheses about neurobiological correlates of the symptoms of not just Axis I, but also Axis II disorders, can be generated using this framework. Moreover, dimensional measurement of personality should be combined with this framework to uniquely capture both Axis I and II disorders because both "types" of disorders are actually disorders of emotion, and emotion is a construct that is parsimoniously described using personality theory. Thus, findings about the neurobiology of personality dimensions are described next. The reader is referred to Table 38–1 for further information about brain regions of interest described in the following section that play an important role in the neurobiology of personality and its disorders.

STRUCTURAL FINDINGS

Few structural studies have been conducted on the relationship between a dimensional personality construct and brain structure. Knutson et al. 2001 found a significant negative association between neuroticism, an index of emotion dysregulation (Costa and McCrae 1992) and the ratio of brain matter volume to the entire intracranial volume. In particular, the specific neuroticism facets of anxiety and self-consciousness were negatively associated with the ratio, suggesting that

Table 38–1.   Abbreviations of brain regions of interest and their functions

Frontal regions

dF	Dorsal frontal	Executive functions
mFr	Medial prefrontal	Extinction of conditioned responding, experiential emotion, object recognition, self, thought, cognition, movement, planning
pFr	Prefrontal	Executive functions, thought, working memory
pm	Premotor	Planning of movements

Limbic and paralimbic regions

amyg	Amygdala	Appraisal of hedonic value and novelty of stimuli, control of physiological response to stimuli
aCg	Anterior cingulate	Cognitive-related inhibition of automatic emotional responding
Hc	Hippocampus	Explicit memory, learning
Hth	Hypothalamus	Modulates autonomic nervous system and endocrine activity
pCg	Posterior cingulate	Cognitive-related inhibition of automatic emotional responding
rCg	Rostral cingulate	Appraisal of hedonic value of stimuli, emotions, learning, memory
mOF	Medial orbital frontal	Part of limbic association cortex, reward, thought, cognition, movement, planning

Other regions

bstem	Brain stem	Primitive regulatory functions
	Cerebellum	Coordinated movement
DR	Dorsal raphe	Source of serotonin that projects widely to telencephalic and diencephelic regions
ins	Insular cortex	Sensory representation including taste and pain; balance
LC	Locus coeruleus	Reward, principle source of noradrenaline
Par	Parietal	Heteromodal association, perception, vision, reading, speech
	Striatum	Gating, comprises the caudate nucleus, putamen, and nucleus accumbens
Temp	Temporal	Learning, memory, perception
Thal	Thalamus	Gating, part of diencephalons, major site of relay nuclei that transmit sensory information to cerebral cortex
VTA	Ventral tegmental area	Reward

Note.   Numbers refer to Brodmann areas.

neuronal atrophy was associated with each. A study by Matsui et al. 2002 revealed that lack of self-control, a trait linked to both high neuroticism and low conscientiousness (conscientiousness being an index of constraint [Costa and McCrae 1992]) was associated with reduced volume of the supplementary motor cortex, a prefrontal region involved in behavior planning. Reduced prefrontal regions have also been linked to the presence of schizotypal personality traits (Raine et al. 1992). Finally, a positive relationship between the size of the anterior cingulate gyrus and alexithymia in men and harm avoidance in women has been reported (Gundel et al. 2004).

FUNCTIONAL IMAGING

Several researchers have investigated functional correlates of constructs conceptually and empirically linked to the broad dimension of emotional dysregulation versus stability. Some constructs related to emotion dysregulation include harm avoidance (Cloninger et al. 1993), neuroticism (Costa and McCrae 1992; Eysenck 1967), and trait negative affect (Watson 2000). Trait negative affect was directly related to activity in both anterior and posterior ventromedial prefrontal cortex (VMPFC) regions (Zald et al. 2002). In this study, no relationship between positive affect at the core of extraversion and VMPFC activity was found, thus ruling out the alternative explanation that intensity of affect alone was associated with VMPFC activity. A positive relationship between neuroticism and activity in left frontal and limbic regions in response to negative pictures and an inverse relationship between neuroticism and right frontal activity was reported in another study (Canli et al. 2001). An inverse relationship between harm avoidance and activity in frontal regions was also reported in two other studies (Moresco et al. 2002; Sugiura et al. 2000). An inverse relationship between neuroticism and serotonin activity in frontal, paralimbic, parietal, and occipital regions has also been reported (Tauscher et al. 2001). Findings from another study revealed links between brain activity and measures of self-control that are conceptually linked to emotion dysregulation (Horn et al. 2003). The ability to inhibit a behavioral response is associated with low neuroticism and high conscientiousness and was associated with activation in several frontal regions, cingulate, superior temporal gyrus, and parietal regions. Significant inverse correlations were found between activations in some of these regions and scores on a dimensional measure of impulsivity. Notably, however, an index of intelligence accounted for a large portion of variance in self-control difficulties.

A trait that can be thought of as related to low reported levels of neuroticism is the personality trait alexithymia. *Alexithymia* literally means "without words to describe mood" and is marked by difficulties in identifying and communicating both positive and negative emotions and an associated decrease in the experience of such emotions. Interestingly, stimuli designed to evoke negative emotions were linked to deactivation in medial prefrontal cortex, whereas positive emotional stimuli were associated with activation in anterior cingulate cortex (ACC), medial prefrontal cortex, and middle frontal gyrus (Berthoz et al. 2002). These results suggest that more attention is paid to positive than to negative stimuli in individuals high on the alexithymia personality dimension. If replicated, these results may call for a revision of the construct of alexithymia as associated with biased attention toward stimuli that evoke positive emotions.

Finally, several laboratories reported no relationship between trait anxiety and regional cerebral blood flow (rCBF; Canli et al. 2001; Ebmeier et al. 1994; Fischer et al. 1997; Simpson et al. 2001).

Several studies have investigated brain activity correlates of the second broad personality dimension, extraversion, that is measured by numerous scales (Cloninger et al. 1993; Costa and McCrae 1992; Eysenck 1967). Stenberg and colleagues (1990, 1993) were the first to report that extraversion was related inversely to rCBF in temporal lobe regions. These results were replicated and extended by Ebmeier et al. (1994), who also reported an inverse relationship between activity in the cingulate regions and extraversion. Low levels of extraversion (i.e., introversion) were linked to increases in activity during a resting state in the caudate nucleus, putamen, and secondary visual cortex in one study that used a categorical approach to analysis by splitting extraversion at the median and comparing activity between the resultant groups (Fischer et al. 1997). In another study, higher levels of extraversion were linked to activity in the amygdala in response to happy faces relative to neutral faces (Canli et al. 2002). In a separate study by this group of investigators, brain activity resulting from the contrast of positive relative to negative, rather than neutral, pictures revealed that extraversion was directly related to activity in the amygdala, caudate, putamen, and the middle frontal gyrus (Canli et al. 2001). An inverse relationship between extraversion and activity in frontal regions, hippocampus, Broca's area, putamen, thalamus, and cingulate has also been reported (Johnson et al. 1999). Extraversion also was positively related to activity in different thalamic and cingulate regions, amygdala, and temporal lobe regions. Finally, no relationship between serotonin receptor-related activity and extraversion was found by another laboratory (Tauscher et al. 2001).

Brain activity correlates of the broad dimension of agreeableness (Costa and McCrae 1992) versus antagonism can be inferred from investigations into the dimension of reward dependence (Cloninger et al. 1993) as well as other constructs. No relationship was found between agreeableness and rCBF (Tauscher et al. 2001). Detachment, a dimension negatively related to agreeableness, was inversely related to the density of dopamine receptors (Farde et al. 1997) in another study. Finally, reward dependence was inversely related to activity in frontal, hippocampal, cingulate, insula, and precuneus regions (Sugiura et al. 2000).

Brain activity correlates of the broad dimension of constraint versus impulsivity can be inferred not just from studies of neuroticism-related constructs, which are negatively related to impulsivity, but also from investigation of facets of the broad personality domain of constraint (Costa and McCrae 1992) and associated constructs such as persistence and novelty seeking (Cloninger et al. 1993). Persistence was positively related to activity in lateral orbital and medial prefrontal cortex as well as ventral striatum regions (Gray and Braver 2002; Gusnard et al. 2003). Two laboratories reported that no significant relationship between conscientiousness and rCBF was found (Gusnard et al. 2003; Tauscher et al. 2001). Finally, two studies have suggested that several traits reflecting high levels of constraint (and thus low reward dependence) including rigidity, stoicism, persistence, and orderliness are associated with low levels of dopamine function in Parkinson's disease (Menza et al. 1993a, 1993b). Such findings suggest that brain regions implicated in Parkinson's disease will also be implicated in the personality dimension of constraint.

To date only one study is available about the personality dimension of openness (Costa and McCrae 1992), indicating no relationship between openness and brain function (Tauscher et al. 2001).

In general, findings suggest that frontal regions associated with the ability to inhibit emotional responding are less active when extremes of personality dimensions are present, whereas the medial prefrontal cortex, which is associated with the experience of emotions, is more active in the presence of such extremes of experience. In addition, regions of interest associated with attention are differentially active at times when stimuli relevant to a particular personality dimension are present or when those high in neuroticism attend to stimuli that evoke negative emotions. Another generalization worth mention is that limbic regions associated with the experience of intense emotion and with efferent activity are also associated with extreme levels of personality dimensions. Findings from these studies can guide hypotheses about personality disorders that are validly conceptualized as extreme levels of various unique combinations of these dimensions (Costa and Widiger 2002; Chapter 3, "Categorical and Dimensional Models of Personality Disorders"). For example, although not one study exists about imaging correlates of any Cluster C disorder, predictions about these disorders can be guided from findings about personality dimensions in healthy individuals. Obsessive-compulsive personality disorder (OCPD) is marked by an extremely high level of constraint and low level of agreeableness, thus it is hypothesized that regional activation patterns in OCPD will resemble those found in healthy participants who exhibit extremes of these dimensions.

CLUSTER A

Almost all the Cluster A studies focus on schizotypal personality disorder. This is due in part to the disorder's close genetic, phenomenologic, and biologic relationship with schizophrenia. Many of these studies have also been modeled to a large extent on schizophrenia neuroimaging research. Thus, brain regions under investigation in schizotypal personality disorder are primarily regions that have been hypothesized to be dysfunctional in schizophrenia. These brain regions include the prefrontal lobes, superior temporal gyrus, and amygdala, each of which plays a role, respectively, in executive functions, assessment of the relevance of external events to the self, and appraisal of hedonic value or novelty. Regions associated with dopaminergic function, which is known to be dysfunctional in schizophrenia, have also been investigated in schizotypal personality disorder. Researchers focusing on schizotypal personality disorder have attempted to look for a "protective" biological marker or compensatory process that precludes the development of fully manifested psychosis.

Schizotypal Personality Disorder

Schizotypal personality disorder is characterized by difficulties with social interactions and language along with odd behavior and magical thinking. The most notable difference from schizophrenia is the lack of psychosis. There are two hypotheses regarding schizotypal personality disorder's relationship to schizophrenia. Some researchers have argued that schizotypal personality is a less severe form of schizophrenia and lies on a continuum of psychotic spectrum disorders (Siever and Davis 2004), whereas other theorists have advocated for schizotypal personality disorder as a separate category of illness. It is difficult to draw any final conclusions from the host of studies reviewed. It is clear, however, that individuals with schizotypal personality disorder present with abnormalities in the superior temporal gyrus, the thalamus, the corpus callosum, and asymmetry of the hippocampus. Individuals with schizotypal personality disorders also exhibit a host of functional abnormalities in response to cognitive or affective probes.

Structural Imaging

More than 20 studies have investigated structural abnormalities in schizotypal personality disorder. Some of the earlier investigations were confounded by comorbidities and marked by the use of less sensitive imaging modalities (e.g., CT scan). Despite its similarity with schizophrenia, schizotypal personality disorder has not shown volumetric decrease in frontal volumes (Buchsbaum et al. 2002; Dickey et al. 2000). There does appear to be, however, an inverse correlation between the size of the frontal lobe and executive functions in schizotypal personality disorder (Raine et al. 1992). Most recently, Dickey et al. (2003) have shown no gray matter volume differences in the left or right superior temporal gyrus between a group of 21 females with schizotypal personality disorder and 29 healthy control subjects; however, patients demonstrated a negative correlation between left superior temporal gyrus volume and odd speech. These results are different from an earlier study by the same group in schizotypal personality disorder male patients that had shown decreased gray matter volume in the left superior temporal gyrus (Dickey et al. 2003).

Downhill et al. (2001) found similar results with the addition of normal white matter connectivity that potentially could explain the difference between behavioral manifestations of schizotypal personality disorder as compared with schizophrenia, where white matter disconnections are present on top of temporal lobe abnormalities (Dickey et al. 1999; Downhill et al. 2001). The thalamus is another structure that has been linked to the pathophysiology of schizophrenia and has been also found to be abnormal in schizotypal personality disorder. The thalamus encompasses a number of distinct nuclei that play key intermediate roles in processing external and internal information. High resolution MRI scan and advanced image processing have allowed measurement of the pulvinar and the medial dorsal nucleus (Byne et al. 2001). Unlike the medial dorsal nucleus with its primary connections to the frontal lobes, the pulvinar volume is equally reduced in schizotypal and schizophrenic patients compared with control subjects. Along with smaller volumes of the splenium of the corpus callosum, which connects inferior temporal and part of superior temporal regions (Downhill et al. 2000), the pulvinar abnormality highlights again the abnormalities in superior temporal gyrus in schizotypal personality disorder pathophysiology (Siever and Davis 2004). The basal ganglia have also been shown to be abnormal in individuals with schizotypal personality disorder. In the striatum, the putamen is significantly smaller in subjects with schizotypal personality disorder than in control subjects, whereas in schizophrenia patients, it is larger than in control subjects, presumably due to exposure to neuroleptics (Shihabuddin et al. 2001). Although Shihabuddin et al. (2001) reported no differences in caudate volumes among their three groups, Levitt et al. (2004) showed an "edgy" shaped head of the caudate that was different from control subjects and correlated with neuropsychological deficits. Finally, the greater prevalence of cavum septum pellucidum, which may reflect neurodevelopmental abnormalities in surrounding limbic and corpus callosum structures, in 27% of those with schizotypal personality disorder compared with 13% of control subjects (George et al. 1989; Kwon et al. 1998) suggests that this structure may play a role in the pathophysiology of this disorder.

Functional Imaging

Resting Studies.   Functional imaging studies have also been modeled on schizophrenia research and primarily have used cognitive probes, with fewer studies examining emotional processing in schizotypal personality disorder. These studies have shown in general a similar topography to what is found in schizophrenia but generally less severe (Siever and Davis 2004). The brain regions most often indicated in schizotypal personality disorder are the frontal and temporal lobes. Schizotypal patients show intermediate activity in lateral temporal regions compared with normal volunteers and schizophrenic patients. Schizotypal patients also show higher than normal metabolic rates in both medial frontal and medial temporal areas. Metabolic rates in Brodmann area 10 were distinctly higher in patients with schizotypal personality disorder than in either normal volunteers or schizophrenic patients (Buchsbaum et al. 2002). The ventral putamen has also shown a significantly higher glucose metabolic rate in 16 schizotypal personality disorder patients compared with 42 schizophrenia patients and 47 control subjects (Shihabuddin et al. 2001). This finding, in addition to the structural results cited earlier, may help explain why patients with schizotypal personality disorder did not develop psychotic symptoms.

Cognitive Functions.   Research suggests that the frontal lobe of patients with schizotypal personality disorder may be engaged in a compensatory activity and a utilization of a different circuit to accomplish similar executive cognitive tasks than psychotic patients.

Buchsbaum et al. (1997) measured rCBF in normal control subjects and in patients with schizophrenia and with schizotypal personality disorder during administration of the Wisconsin Card Sorting Test (WCST). The Symbol-Matching Test (SMT), which does not require abstract reasoning, was administered as a control task. The direction of the change in schizotypal subjects was opposite to that of control subjects in the prefrontal cortex and medial temporal regions. During the WCST, the control subjects showed the greatest activation in the precentral gyrus, whereas schizotypal subjects showed the greatest activation in the middle frontal gyrus. In control subjects, cerebral blood flow was higher in the left medial temporal lobe during the WCST versus the SMT; the opposite effect was seen in the schizotypal personality disorder group. In an analysis of the entire cortical surface, temporal activity was diminished in the schizotypal personality disorder group during the WCST. Underactivity of the temporal gyrus along with altered prefrontal cortex activity during a word list learning task, the California Verbal Learning Test, has also been reported in schizotypal personality disorder (Buchsbaum et al. 2002). A marked difference in hemispheric activation has been observed, suggesting altered lateralization. Finally, thalamus activity can be dysregulated (Buchsbaum et al. 2002). Hazlett et al. (1999) had used earlier a similar probe (California Verbal Learning Test) and did not show any decreases in mediodorsal nucleus of the thalamus activity in patients with schizotypal personality disorder compared with control subjects. During this task, however, Shihabuddin et al. (2001) reported that patients with schizotypal personality disorder demonstrated an increased activity in ventral putamen, which the authors attributed to a decreased dopaminergic inhibitory activity in the thalamic nucleus. This dysregulated dopaminergic activity, with a reduction in dopamine release, has also been shown in the striatum using SPECT, which measures binding of iodine-methoxybenzamide and its displacement following amphetamine administration (Siever et al. 2002).

In summary, these findings provide support for the hypothesis that schizotypal personality disorder falls on a spectrum of psychotic disorders as evidenced by structural and metabolic abnormalities of dopaminergic transmission. Patients with schizotypal personality disorder present with a distinctive activity in medial prefrontal cortex (Brodmann area 10) that may be protective.

CLUSTER B

Similar to Cluster A, many researchers have investigated the biological underpinnings of Cluster B personality disorders, driven in part by the high health and socioeconomic burden associated with these disorders. A limited number of structural and functional imaging studies have been described, utilizing different techniques, in which the recruited populations are heterogeneous. These studies are nevertheless a necessary first step in identifying the underlying neurobiological basis for Cluster B disorders. They predominantly focus on borderline and antisocial personality disorders. No studies have been published to date about neurobiological substrates of narcissistic or histrionic personality disorder. It is noteworthy that unlike studies in Cluster A, which have predominantly focused on cognitive processing, studies in Cluster B deal with emotional processing, impulsivity, and social relatedness. The brain regions involved are likely homologous to the ones identified in mood and anxiety disorders. By drawing on previous network models in mood disorder research, many of the studies reviewed here focus on identifying key subset regions involved in mood and impulse dysregulation. Not surprisingly, the implicated regions are similar to ones invoked by mood and anxiety disorders. These regions are associated with both decreased activity in dorsal neocortical regions and relative increased activity in ventral limbic and paralimbic areas (Drevets et al. 2002). Increased rCBF and metabolism have been shown (but not always [Abercrombie et al. 1998]) in the amygdala, orbitofrontal cortex, and medial thalamus—and decreases in rCBF and metabolism were found in the dorsomedial/dorsal anterolateral prefrontal cortex, subgenual ACC, and dorsal ACC in mood and anxiety disorder subjects relative to healthy control subjects. Dysfunction of these subset regions is hypothesized to explain the combination of clinical symptoms seen in depressed and anxious patients. Similarly, these regions may be differentially affected in subtypes of personality disorders in which the core symptoms studied are emotion dysregulation (Koenigsberg et al. 1999). Other important regions that are likely implicated in Cluster B include the hippocampus, insula, ventral striatum, putamen, and midbrain monoamine nuclei (Figure 38–1).

Borderline Personality Disorder

Borderline personality disorder (BPD) is marked by high levels of the dimensions of emotion dysregulation and extraversion and low levels of agreeableness and constraint (Chapter 3, "Categorical and Dimensional Models of Personality Disorders"). During extreme states of arousal, transient, stress-induced paranoid ideation or severe dissociative symptoms can also be exhibited (Skodol et al. 2002a, 2002b).

Structural Imaging

Earlier volumetric studies using CT scan revealed no volumetric or asymmetric abnormalities in BPD patients (Lucas et al. 1989; Schulz et al. 1983; Snyder et al. 1983). MRI studies have shown a 6.2% frontal lobe vol-

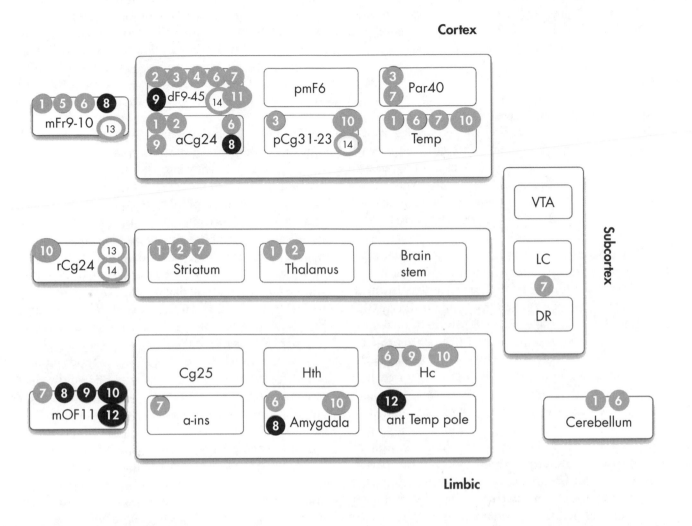

Figure 38–1. Brain regions of interest implicated in Cluster B personality disorders.

Open circles represent mixed or antisocial personality disorder; *filled circles* represent borderline personality disorder. *Dark circles* signify increased brain activity; *light circles* signify decreased brain activity. *Numbers* indicate studies: 1=Leyton et al. 2001; 2, 4, 5=De La Fuente et al. 1997; 3=Goyer et al. 1994; 6=Schmahl et al. 2003a; 7=Soloff et al. 2000; 8=Herpertz et al. 2001; 9=Juengling et al. 2003; 10=Kiehl et al. 2001; 11=Tebartz van Elst et al. 2003; 12=Driessen et al. 2004; 13=Siever et al. 1999; 14=New et al. 2002.

a-ins=anterior insular cortex; ant Temp pole=anterior temporal pole; Cg25=cingulate cortex. See Table 38–1 for additional abbreviations.
Source. Simplified diagram modeled after Mayberg et al. 2000.

ume reduction in 25 BPD patients compared with control subjects (Lyoo et al. 1998). Efforts to replicate this finding have been negative so far (Rusch et al. 2003). Rusch et al. 2003 attempted to control for highly prevalent comorbid Axis I and II diagnoses and failed to control for total brain volume. Teicher et al. (2002) have undertaken a comprehensive summary of the neurobiological consequences of developmentally early stress, highly predominant in this cluster, and the deleterious effect of stress hormones on hippocampal size. They also noted an association between a history of sexual abuse in girls and neglect in boys and

diminished corpus callosum size. Driessen at al. (2000) also showed a decrease of 16% in hippocampal volume in 21 BPD patients with a history of sexual or physical abuse compared with control subjects and a smaller difference in amygdala volume (8%). They did not control for comorbid depression and failed to differentiate their results based on a concurrent posttraumatic stress disorder (PTSD) diagnosis. Rusch et al. (2003) found gray matter volume loss in the left amygdala, which supports the hypothesis that temporolimbic abnormalities play a role in the pathophysiology of BPD (Rusch et al. 2003). Similarly, Tebartz van Elst et al. (2003) found a significant reduction of hippocampal and amygdala volumes in eight patients with BPD along with 24% reduction of the left orbitofrontal and a 26% reduction of the right ACC.

Functional Imaging

Emotional Lability.   Affective instability and disturbed interpersonal relations are key characteristics of BPD (American Psychiatric Association 2000). People with BPD have difficulty processing and responding to emotional information and characteristically exhibit emotional overreaction and mood lability. Functional imaging studies have begun linking this dysregulation to specific regions.

The prefrontal cortex is instrumental in planning, thinking, executing responses, and regulating mood. Abnormal functioning of this brain region is implicated in the emotional instability experienced by BPD patients. De La Fuente et al. (1997) studied the resting brain activity of 10 unmedicated BPD patients with FDG PET and found relative hypometabolism in the prefrontal cortex in addition to the premotor cortical areas, ACC, and the thalamic, caudate, and lenticular nuclei. However, these results are inconsistent with those of Juengling et al. (2003), who used a similar methodology and found increased activity of superior frontal gyrus bilaterally and the right inferior frontal gyrus. In addition, these authors found increased activity in the ACC and decreased activity in the left hippocampus. These presumably opposite results in small but well-screened BPD patients may be due in part to the differences in control groups or could reflect a more heterogeneous sample of patients.

Using fMRI, Herpertz et al. (2001) found BPD women to show increased activity in the amygdala, fusiform gyrus, orbital prefrontal region, and anterior cingulate region when seeing aversive scenes. It is hypothesized that the increased activation of the limbic and visual associative areas may reflect an intense perceptual style especially in line with BPD patients' self-report on the State-Trait Anxiety Inventory (Spielberger et al. 1970) and the State-Trait Anger Expression Scale (Schocken et al. 1987), reflecting a pervasive readiness to react with intense emotions. This increased activity may also be explained by slow habituation as opposed to increased response and hypervigilance. It is unclear whether or not increased orbitofrontal activity is a self-monitoring and top-down control of the amygdala. Knowing that BPD is associated with early abuse, Driessen et al. (2004) recently published an fMRI study where BPD patients with and without comorbid PTSD, recalled autobio-

graphical memory. All subjects showed activation of the orbitofrontal cortex, anterior temporal lobes, and occipital areas. The group with PTSD showed marked orbitofrontal activation with lateralization weighted to the right hemisphere. This study may help researchers understand the pathophysiology of different BPD subgroups and perhaps begin separating them based on their neurobiological signatures (Driessen et al. 2004). During autobiographical memories of abandonment, the BPD group showed significantly greater activation than did control subjects with comparable trauma histories in bilateral superior frontal gyrus, right middle frontal gyrus, right inferior temporal gyrus, cerebellum, cuneus, and right middle occipital gyrus. BPD patients showed significantly greater deactivation than control subjects during memories of abandonment in different cerebellum regions, left superior temporal gyrus, left middle temporal gyrus, right medial frontal gyrus, right inferior frontal gyrus, right anterior cingulate, right hippocampus/amygdala, and left visual association cortex (Schmahl et al. 2003a, 2003b).

The frontal lobes are seen as major modulators of impulsive behavior, and thus several PET studies have found abnormal frontal activity in impulsive subjects versus normal control subjects (Juengling et al. 2003; Oquendo and Mann 2000; Siever et al. 1999; Soloff et al. 2000). One of the earlier studies (Goyer et al. 1994) used PET in 17 patients with DSM-III-R (American Psychiatric Association 1987) diagnoses of different personality disorders (including six with BPD and six with antisocial personality disorder). Overall, there was a significant inverse correlation between a life history of aggressive impulse difficulties and regional activity in the frontal cortex. In addition, dysfunction of the central serotonergic system has been postulated to play a role in suicidal and/or impulsive aggressive behavior (Coccaro et al. 1989). Siever et al. (1999) hypothesized that BPD would show diminished serotonin availability. They studied six impulsive-aggressive patients and five healthy volunteers in a placebo-controlled fenfluramine challenge. BPD patients showed significantly blunted metabolic responses and a reduced serotonergic modulation in orbital frontal, ventral medial, and cingulate cortex (Siever et al. 1999).

Soloff et al. (2000) replicated these findings in five BPD subjects and eight control subjects using a similar paradigm and reported a diminished response to serotonergic stimulation in areas of prefrontal cortex in BPD patients, adding support to the regulatory role played by this region in modulating impulsive behavior (Soloff et al. 2000). Various functional imaging techniques have documented aberrant functioning in the cingulate cortex associated with impulsivity (De La Fuente 1997; Gurvits 2000; Herpertz et al. 2001; Leyton et al. 2001; Oquendo and Mann 2000; Siever et al. 1999; Sugiura et al. 2000; Young 1999). The hippocampus also plays an active role in behavior inhibition. It receives serotonin from the raphe nuclei, which facilitates inhibition of inappropriate emotional and behavioral responses. A PET study by Juengling et al. (2003) found the hippocampus of BPD subjects to be hypoactive at rest compared with control subjects. Juengling suggested that this malfunction may explain some of the clinical symptoms observed in these patients, because it would also be seen in many other disorders marked by extremes of negative emotions like major depressive disorder (Sheline et al. 1999).

Norepinephrine is a neurotransmitter also associated with regulation of aggression. Abnormally high levels of this neurotransmitter contribute to the aggressive nature of the impulsive behaviors observed in patients with BPD (Oquendo and Mann 2000). Increased norepinephrine levels can also result in hyperactivity of the sympathetic nervous system, producing symptoms of increased arousal. This heightened arousal has been self-treated with alcohol and other substances that lower norepinephrine levels and may contribute to the alcoholism and substance abuse among patients with BPD. Dopamine and γ-aminobutyric acid (GABA) neurotransmitters have been linked to aggressive impulsive behaviors in animal studies. Further studies are required for these neurotransmitters to be implicated in human behavior (Oquendo and Mann 2000).

Antisocial Personality Disorder

Many researchers and clinicians tend to consider antisocial personality disorder (ASPD) and psychopathy synonymous; whereas in fact the latter is defined based on the Psychopathy Checklist (Hare et al. 1991). This distinction becomes more relevant when discussing functional imaging results. Although deficits in frontal executive function may increase the likelihood of future aggression, no study has reliably demonstrated a characteristic pattern of frontal network dysfunction predictive of violent crime. ASPD and antisocial or criminal behaviors have been linked to structural and functional frontal lobe dysfunction ever since Phineas Gage's mining accident (Damasio et al. 1994). Brower and Price (2001) conducted a comprehensive review of the literature for both functional and structural imaging studies and found supportive evidence associating frontal lobe dysfunction and increased impulsive aggressive and antisocial behavior.

For example, patients with temporal lobe epilepsy and aggressive episodes were found to have decreased left frontal gray matter (Woermann et al. 2000). Injury to the focal orbitofrontal or ACC are specifically associated with increased aggression (Anderson et al. 1999; Heinrichs 1989). As studies accumulate, there is more imaging support (Volkow and Tancredi 1987) for the theories of frontotemporal deficits that initially originated from neuropsychological testing in aggressive and antisocial individuals (Brower and Price 2001). Despite the importance of studies in ASPD and violent offenders, these studies are the most controversial of all personality disorder neuroimaging research, given the legal ramifications that could follow the claims that these individuals may not be responsible for their crimes (Canli and Amin 2002).

Structural Imaging

Early structural studies in ASPD were nonconclusive, due in part to poor control of comorbid conditions and low imaging resolution. More recently, Raine et al. (2000) studied 21 antisocial patients and found an 11% reduction in orbitofrontal gray matter compared with 34 control subjects and a 13% reduction compared with 26 substance abusers. They also showed differences in more violent crimes and greater psychopathic traits. This relationship did not hold true in a study by Laakso et al. (2002), in which observed volume deficits of dorsolateral, orbitofrontal, and medial frontal cortex in 24 antisocial subjects were related more to comorbid alcoholism or differences in education compared with control subjects—rather than to the diagnosis of ASPD. Moreover, no significant correlations between any of the volumes and the degree of psychopathy were found. The same authors applied a similar method to study the hippocampal volume of 18 male violent offenders. Experimental lesions of the dorsal hippocampus in animals impair the acquisition of conditioned fear, which in turn may relate to the pathophysiology of psychopathy. The authors found posterior hippocampi volumes to correlate with the subjects' degree of psychopathy (Laakso et al. 2001). A complement to these prefrontal and hippocampal findings is a study by Dolan et al. (2002) in which 18 psychopaths showed lower mean right temporal volumes compared with 19 control subjects and with an inverse correlation to the belligerence factor on the Antisocial Personality Questionnaire. They also found smaller dorsomedial prefrontal cortex in their personality disorder sample (Dolan et al. 2002). A complementary line of structural investigations is to focus on white matter interhemispheric connectivity by measuring the corpus callosum.

Psychopathic patients with ASPD show a 22.6% increase in volume but a 15.3% reduction in thickness compared with control subjects. These larger callosum volumes correlated with affective and interpersonal deficits and low autonomic stress reactivity, and they may reflect an arrest in early axonal pruning or increased white matter myelination (Raine et al. 2003).

Functional Imaging

Aggression. There are several studies that have attempted to explore aggression and impulsivity by crossing the boundaries of DSM-IV-TR classification and including several subgroups of personality disorders. This approach is due in part to a preference for a dimensional construct rather than a categorical one (Blackburn 1998), limiting our ability to link findings to current nomenclature. Some of these studies were described earlier in the chapter (Goyer et al. 1994), as were the important modulatory functions of serotonin and norepinephrine in aggressive behavior.

PET studies have shown abnormalities in the prefrontal and anterior cingulate in violent offenders (Bassarath 2001). Raine et al. (1994) reported on 22 murderers who showed lower medial and lateral prefrontal cortex metabolic activity compared with control subjects. This finding was evident in the affective murderers as opposed to predatory murderers. Although groups were matched, a limitation of this study was the inclusion of schizophrenia and head injury patients (Raine et al. 1994). Soderstrom et al. (2002) used SPECT imaging and correlated brain activity with the Psychopathy Checklist–Revised (PCL-R), which rates three aspects of psychopathy: disturbed interpersonal attitudes, affective unresponsiveness, and impulsive antisocial behavior. Significant negative correlations were found between interpersonal features of psychopathy and the medial and lateral frontal and temporal perfusion. The two most clearly associated regions of interest were the head of the caudate nuclei and the hippocampi. Out of 23 incarcerated violent offenders, high scores on impulsivity correlated with less perfusion in lateral prefrontal cortex (Soderstrom et al. 2002).

New et al. (2002) assessed brain activity of impulsive aggressive patients and normal control subjects after administration of *meta*-chlorophenylpiperazine (m-CPP), a serotonergic probe. These 13 patients met criteria for one or more personality disorders (including BPD), but all met criteria for intermittent explosive disorder. m-CPP or placebo was administered on two separate visits, and image analyses focused on prefrontal cortex (medial and lateral cortex) and anterior, middle, and posterior cingulate cortex. They showed

a decreased activation of inhibitory regions (left anteromedial orbital cortex and ACC) in patients compared with control subjects that may explain why these patients have a hard time modulating their aggressive impulses. Interestingly, there was no difference in bilateral prefrontal cortex activity, and the posterior cingulate was more responsive to m-CPP in patients than in control subjects. It is postulated that the inhibitory chain of command in these patients may begin in the posterior cingulate and ineffectively modulate the orbitofrontal cortex (New et al. 2002).

Affect Processing. Normally, anger-induction models in men show increased brain activity in the left orbitofrontal cortex and right ACC, presumably in an effort to inhibit an aggressive response (Dougherty et al. 1999). Findings of abnormal control of reactions in aggressive patients have already been described. It may also be possible that patients with ASPD process affect differently than do control subjects. Intrator et al. (1997) found greater activation in temporofrontal cortex using single-slice SPECT in psychopaths processing affective compared with neutral information. Kiehl et al. (2001) looked at activation during emotional processing in nonpsychopathic criminals, psychopathic criminals, and control subjects and found criminal psychopaths to show less affect-related activity in inferior frontal gyrus, rostral and caudal ACC, right amygdala, and ventral medial prefrontal cortex during negative affective encoding and rehearsal than during neutral phrases. Other areas showed increases, such as the left anterior superior temporal gyrus/inferior frontal gyrus and right inferior frontal gyrus.

In summary, both structural and functional imaging abnormalities have been associated with Cluster B disorders. A history of stress or trauma may lead to smaller hippocampi, whereas emotional lability and aggression are associated with a dysregulation of prefrontal-limbic networks that could also be seen in other Axis I disorders characterized by excessive emotional reactivity or poor executive control.

CLUSTER C AND PERSONALITY DIMENSIONS

To date, only one imaging study of brain function (Laasonen-Balk et al. 2001) and no study of brain structure have been published about individuals diagnosed with Cluster C personality disorders. Cluster C disorders include avoidant personality disorder, marked by a pervasive pattern of social inhibition, feelings of inade-

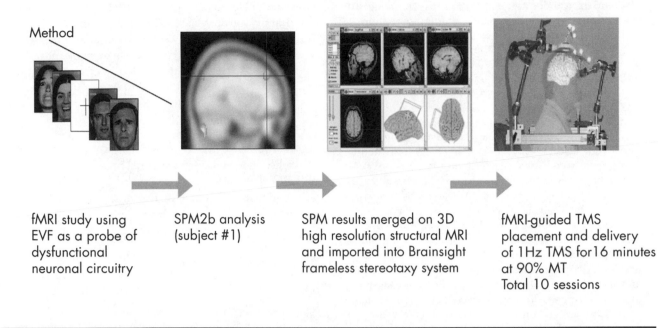

Method

fMRI study using EVF as a probe of dysfunctional neuronal circuitry

SPM2b analysis (subject #1)

SPM results merged on 3D high resolution structural MRI and imported into Brainsight frameless stereotaxy system

fMRI-guided TMS placement and delivery of 1 Hz TMS for 16 minutes at 90% MT Total 10 sessions

Figure 38–2. Illustration of functional imaging used to identify, target, and modulate via transcranial magnetic stimulation the functional circuitry used by a patient with borderline personality disorder who is viewing emotional faces.

EVF=Eckman emotion-evoking faces; fMRI=functional magnetic resonance imaging; MRI=magnetic resonance imaging; MT=motor threshold; SPM=statistical parametric mapping; 3D=three-dimensional; TMS=transcranial magnetic stimulation.

quacy, and hypersensitivity to negative evaluation; dependent personality disorder, marked by a pervasive pattern of submissive and clinging behavior related to a need to be taken care of; and OCPD, marked by a pervasive pattern of preoccupation with orderliness, perfectionism, and control (American Psychiatric Association 2000). In the one study of brain function in Cluster C personality disorders, dopamine transporter density in the basal ganglia was examined in two groups of individuals with major depression with and without Cluster C personality disorders (Laasonen-Balk et al. 2001). No differences were found in dopamine transporter density in the basal ganglia between the two depressed groups. This study was quite limited in its focus and thus aids only minimally in hypothesis generation about the neurobiology of Cluster C disorders. As has been said earlier, hypotheses regarding neurobiological substrates of these disorders can be derived from findings about the dimensions that uniquely capture not only Axis II but also Axis I disorders.

FUTURE INTEGRATION WITH BRAIN STIMULATION

As previously discussed, BPD likely encompasses several abnormal dimensions of cognition and behavior

with associated neurobiologic substrates. It remains unclear whether targeted noninvasive modulation of the circuits implicated in BPD can be modulated using transcranial magnetic stimulation (TMS) to treat BPD symptoms (Figure 38–2). One method to study this question utilizes fMRI and an Eckman emotion-evoking faces block design to guide TMS placement. The emotion recognition/regulation circuitry activated during this paradigm is targeted with TMS in an effort to modulate its activity. The following case report illustrates this avenue of clinical investigation.

Case Example

Functional neuroimaging-based targeted repetitive TMS (rTMS) in a patient with emotional lability diagnosed BPD.

Ms. OO, a 35-year-old married female, had a long history of emotional lability and a poorly organized sense of self. She had been through numerous pharmacological trials and a number of relatively unsuccessful courses of psychotherapy, including dialectical behavioral therapy. Her main concerns were her outbursts of anger, her lack of attachment to her 10-year-old daughter, and her inability to emotionally appreciate the support that her husband had given her over the years. Ironically, the threat of losing her husband and child would invariably lead to clinical decompensation and at times micropsychotic episodes. She struggled constantly with impulses to hurt herself and had several failed suicide attempts.

Ms. OO moved in with her parents for a while, away from her husband and daughter. She was enrolled in a 2-week double-blind, placebo-controlled clinical trial using fMRI-guided rTMS. Before TMS, Ms. OO underwent a functional imaging study to probe what has now been demonstrated as an overactive prefrontal/limbic circuit in BPD subjects when processing Eckman emotion-evoking faces compared with healthy control subjects. TMS placement over her right prefrontal cortex was based on the results of her individualized image analysis and was accomplished using Brainsight (a frameless stereotactic system). Over the course of the first 2 weeks, and with placebo stimulation, Ms. OO reported very limited changes in her symptoms. Her baseline scores on interviews designed for assessment of depression and borderline personality symptoms remained essentially unchanged. She later received compassionate open-label TMS treatment for an additional 2 weeks.

Interestingly, during her time away from her nuclear family, her symptoms worsened; she reported more paranoid distortions and extreme anguish from graphically violent self-destructive fantasies. The repetitive stimulation appeared to have reduced her anxiety and impulsivity, and to some extent she subjectively reported less distress from her daytime fantasies. Although by the end of the treatment her scores were still markedly elevated, both she and her father were convinced of the overall calming effect TMS had had on her, and thus her improvement was much more noticeable on her subjective ratings than on objective scales.

This vignette illustrates an approach by which a dysfunctional neuronal basis underlying a personality disorder dimension can be identified and studied utilizing TMS neuromodulation, with the goal of identifying new effective clinical interventions.

REFERENCES

Abercrombie HC, Schaefer SM, Larson CL, et al: Metabolic rate in the right amygdala predicts negative affect in depressed patients. Neuroreport 9:3301–3307, 1998

American Psychiatric Association: Diagnostic and Statistical Manual of Mental Disorders, 3rd Edition, Revised. Washington, DC, American Psychiatric Association, 1987

American Psychiatric Association: Diagnostic and Statistical Manual of Mental Disorders, 4th Edition, Text Revision. Washington, DC, American Psychiatric Association, 2000

Anderson SW, Bechara A, Damasio H, et al: Impairment of social and moral behavior related to early damage in human prefrontal cortex. Nat Neurosci 2:1032–1037, 1999

Bassarath L: Neuroimaging studies of antisocial behaviour. Can J Psychiatry 46:728–732, 2001

Berthoz S, Artiges E, Van De Moortele, et al: Effect of impaired recognition and expression of emotions on frontocingulate cortices: an fMRI study of men with alexithymia. Am J Psychiatry 159:961–967, 2002

Blackburn R: Relationship of personality disorders to observer ratings of interpersonal style in forensic psychiatric patients. J Personal Disord 12:77–85, 1998

Brower MC, Price BH: Neuropsychiatry of frontal lobe dysfunction in violent and criminal behaviour: a critical review. J Neurol Neurosurg Psychiatry 71:720–726, 2001

Buchsbaum MS, Trestman RL, Hazlett E, et al: Regional cerebral blood flow during the Wisconsin Card Sort Test in schizotypal personality disorder. Schizophr Res 27:21–28, 1997

Buchsbaum MS, Nenadic I, Hazlett EA, et al: Differential metabolic rates in prefrontal and temporal Brodmann areas in schizophrenia and schizotypal personality disorder. Schizophr Res 54:141–150, 2002

Byne W, Buchsbaum MS, Kemether E, et al: Magnetic resonance imaging of the thalamic mediodorsal nucleus and pulvinar in schizophrenia and schizotypal personality disorder. Arch Gen Psychiatry 58:133–140, 2001

Canli T, Amin Z: Neuroimaging of emotion and personality: scientific evidence and ethical considerations. Brain Cogn 50:414–431, 2002

Canli T, Zhao Z, Desmond JE, et al: An fMRI study of personality influences on brain reactivity to emotional stimuli. Behav Neurosci 115:33–42, 2001

Canli T, Sivers H, Whitfield SL, et al: Amygdala response to happy faces as a function of extraversion. Science 296:2191, 2002

Cloninger CR, Svrakic DM, Przybeck TR: A psychobiological model of temperament and character. Arch Gen Psychiatry 50:975–990, 1993

Coccaro EF, Siever LJ, Klar HM, et al: Serotonergic studies in patients with affective and personality disorders: correlates with suicidal and impulsive aggressive behavior. Arch Gen Psychiatry 46:587–599, 1989

Costa PT, McCrae RR: NEO PI-R Professional Manual: Revised NEO Personality Inventory (NEO PI-R) and NEO Five-Factor Inventory (NEO-FFI). Odessa, FL, Psychological Assessment Resources, 1992

Costa PT, Widiger TA: Personality Disorders and the Five-Factor Model of Personality, 2nd Edition. Washington, DC, American Psychological Association, 2002

Damasio H, Grabowski T, Frank R, et al: The return of Phineas Gage: clues about the brain from the skull of a famous patient. Science 264:1102–1105, 1994

De La Fuente JM, Goldman S, Stanus E, et al: Brain glucose metabolism in borderline personality disorder. J Psychiatr Res 31:531–541, 1997

Dickey CC, McCarley RW, Voglmaier MM, et al: Schizotypal personality disorder and MRI abnormalities of temporal lobe gray matter. Biol Psychiatry 45:1393–1402, 1999

Dickey CC, Shenton ME, Hirayasu Y, et al: Large CSF volume not attributable to ventricular volume in schizotypal personality disorder. Am J Psychiatry 157:48–54, 2000

Dickey CC, McCarley RW, Voglmaier MM, et al: An MRI study of superior temporal gyrus volume in women with schizotypal personality disorder. Am J Psychiatry 160:2198–2201, 2003

Dolan M, Millington J, Park I: Personality and neuropsychological function in violent, sexual and arson offenders. Med Sci Law 42:34–43, 2002

Dougherty DD, Shin LM, Alpert NM, et al: Anger in healthy men: a PET study using script-driven imagery. Biol Psychiatry 46:466–472, 1999

Downhill JE Jr, Buchsbaum MS, Wei T, et al: Shape and size of the corpus callosum in schizophrenia and schizotypal personality disorder. Schizophr Res 42:193–208, 2000

Downhill JE Jr, Buchsbaum MS, Hazlett EA, et al: Temporal lobe volume determined by magnetic resonance imaging in schizotypal personality disorder and schizophrenia. Schizophr Res 48:187–199, 2001

Drevets WC, Bogers W, Raichle ME: Functional anatomical correlates of antidepressant drug treatment assessed using PET measures of regional glucose metabolism. Eur Neuropsychopharmacol 12:527–544, 2002

Driessen M, Herrmann J, Stahl K, et al: Magnetic resonance imaging volumes of the hippocampus and the amygdala in women with borderline personality disorder and early traumatization. Arch Gen Psychiatry 57:1115-1122, 2000

Driessen M, Beblo T, Mertens M, et al: Posttraumatic stress disorder and fMRI activation patterns of traumatic memory in patients with borderline personality disorder. Biol Psychiatry 55:603–611, 2004

Ebmeier KP, Deary IJ, O'Carroll RE, et al: Personality associations with the uptake of the cerebral blood flow marker ^{99m}Tc-Exametazime estimated with single photon emission tomography. Pers Individ Dif 17:587–595, 1994

Eysenck HJ: The Biological Bases of Personality. Baltimore, MD, University Park Press, 1967

Farde L, Gustavson P, Jonsson E: D2 dopamine receptors and personality traits. Nature 385:590, 1997

Fischer H, Wik G, Fredrikson M: Extraversion, neuroticism, and brain function: a PET study of personality. Pers Individ Dif 23:345–352, 1997

George MS, Scott T, Kellner CH, et al: Abnormalities of the septum pellucidum in schizophrenia: two case reports and a discussion. J Neuropsychiatry Clin Neurosci 1:3 85–390, 1989

Goyer PF, Andreason PJ, Semple WE, et al: Positron-emission tomography and personality disorders. Neuropsychopharmacology 10:21–28, 1994

Gray JR, Braver TS: Personality predicts working-memory-related activation in the caudal anterior cingulate cortex. Cogn Affect Behav Neurosci 2:64–75, 2002

Gundel H, Lopez-Sala A, Ceballos-Baumann AO, et al: Alexithymia correlates with the size of the right anterior cingulate. Psychosom Med 66:132–140, 2004

Gusnard DA, Raichle ME, Raichle ME: Searching for a baseline: functional imaging and the resting human brain. Nat Rev Neurosci 2:685–694, 2001

Gusnard DA, Ollinger JM, Shulman GL, et al: Persistence and brain circuitry. Proc Natl Acad Sci U S A 100:3479–3484, 2003

Hare RD, Hart SD, Harpur TJ: Psychopathy and the DSM-IV criteria for antisocial personality disorder. J Abnorm Psychol 100:391–398, 1991

Hazlett EA, Buchsbaum MS, Byne W, et al: Three-dimensional analysis with MRI and PET of the size, shape, and function of the thalamus in the schizophrenia spectrum. Am J Psychiatry 156:1190–1199, 1999

Heinrichs RW: Frontal cerebral lesions and violent incidents in chronic neuropsychiatric patients. Biol Psychiatry 25:174–178, 1989

Herpertz SC, Dietrich TM, Wenning B, et al: Evidence of abnormal amygdala functioning in borderline personality disorder: a functional MRI study. Biol Psychiatry 50:292–298, 2001

Horn NR, Dolan M, Elliott R, et al: Response inhibition and impulsivity: an fMRI study. Neuropsychologia 41:1959–1966, 2003

Intrator J, Hare R, Stritzke P, et al: A brain imaging (single photon emission computerized tomography) study of semantic and affective processing in psychopaths. Biol Psychiatry 42:96–103, 1997

Jackson JH (1874): On the nature of the duality of the brain, in Medical Press and Circular 1, 19, 41, 63: Selected Writings of John Hughlings Jackson. Edited by Taylor J. New York, Basic Books, 1958

Johnson DL, Wiebe JS, Gold SM, et al: Cerebral blood flow and personality: a positron emission tomography study. Am J Psychiatry 156:252–257, 1999

Juengling FD, Schmahl C, Hesslinger B, et al: Positron emission tomography in female patients with borderline personality disorder. J Psychiatr Res 37:109–115, 2003

Kiehl KA, Smith AM, Hare RD, et al: Limbic abnormalities in affective processing by criminal psychopaths as revealed by functional magnetic resonance imaging. Biol Psychiatry 50:677–684, 2001

Knutson B, Momenan R, Rawlings RR, et al: Negative association of neuroticism with brain volume ratio in healthy humans. Biol Psychiatry 50:685–690, 2001

Koenigsberg HW, Anwunah I, New AS, et al: Relationship between depression and borderline personality disorder. Depress Anxiety 10:158–167, 1999

Kwon JS, Shenton ME, Hirayasu Y, et al: MRI study of cavum septi pellucidi in schizophrenia, affective disorder, and schizotypal personality disorder. Am J Psychiatry 155:509–515, 1998

Laakso MP, Vaurio O, Koivisto E, et al: Psychopathy and the posterior hippocampus. Behav Brain Res 118:187–193, 2001

Laakso MP, Gunning-Dixon F, Vaurio O, et al: Prefrontal volumes in habitually violent subjects with antisocial personality disorder and type 2 alcoholism. Psychiatry Res 114:95–102, 2002

Laasonen-Balk T, Viinamaki H, Kuikka J, et al: Cluster C personality disorder has no independent effect on striatal dopamine transporter densities in major depression. Psychopharmacology (Berl) 155:113–114, 2001

Lauterbur PC: Image formation by induced local interactions: examples employing nuclear magnetic resonance. Nature 242:190–191, 1973

Levitt JJ, Westin CF, Nestor PG, et al: Shape of caudate nucleus and its cognitive correlates in neuroleptic-naive schizotypal personality disorder. Biol Psychiatry 55:177–184, 2004

Leyton M, Okazawa H, Diksic M, et al: Brain regional alpha-[11C]methyl-L-tryptophan trapping in impulsive subjects with borderline personality disorder. Am J Psychiatry 158:775–782, 2001

Lucas PB, Gardner DL, Cowdry RW, et al: Cerebral structure in borderline personality disorder. Psychiatry Res 27:111–115, 1989

Lyoo IK, Han MH, Cho DY: A brain MRI study in subjects with borderline personality disorder. J Affect Disord 50:235–243, 1998

Mansfield P: Multi-planar image formation using NMR spin-echoes. Journal of Physics C: Solid State Physics 10:L55–L58, 1977

Mayberg HS, Brannan SK, Tekell JL, et al: Regional metabolic effects of fluoxetine in major depression: serial changes and relationship to clinical response. Biol Psychiatry 48:830–843, 2000

Matsui M, Yoneyama E, Sumiyoshi T, et al: Lack of self-control as assessed by a personality inventory is related to reduced volume of supplementary motor area. Psychiatry Res 116:53–61, 2002

McGonigle DJ, Howseman AM, Athwal BS, et al: Variability in fMRI: an examination of intersession differences. Neuroimage 11:708–734, 2000

McIntosh AR, Bookstein FL, Haxby JV, et al: Spatial pattern analysis of functional brain images using partial least squares. Neuroimage 3:143–157, 1996

Menza MA, Golbe LI, Cody RA, et al: Dopamine-related personality traits in Parkinson's disease. Neurology 43:505–508, 1993a

Menza MA, Forman NE, Sage JI, et al: Parkinson's disease and smoking: the relationship to personality. Neuropsychiatry Neuropsychol Behav Neurol 6:214–218, 1993b

Miller GA, Kozak MJ: Three systems assessment and the construct of emotion, in The Structure of Emotion. Edited by Ohman A, Birbaumer N. Toronto, ON, Hogrefe and Huber, 1993, pp 31–47

Moresco FM, Dieci M, Vita A, et al: In vivo serotonin 5HT(2A) receptor binding and personality traits in healthy subjects: a positron emission tomography study. Neuroimage 17:1470–1478, 2002

New AS, Hazlett EA, Buchsbaum MS, et al: Blunted prefrontal cortical 18fluorodeoxyglucose positron emission tomography response to meta-chlorophenylpiperazine in impulsive aggression. Arch Gen Psychiatry 59:621–629, 2002

Oquendo MA, Mann JJ: The biology of impulsivity and suicidality. Psychiatr Clin North Am 23:11–25, 2000

Phan KL, Wager T, Taylor SF, et al: Functional neuroanatomy of emotion: a meta-analysis of emotion activation studies in PET and fMRI. Neuroimage 16:331–348, 2002

Phillips ML, Drevets WC, Rauch SL, et al. Neurobiology of emotion perception, I: the neural basis of normal emotion perception. Biol Psychiatry 54:504–514, 2003a

Phillips ML, Drevets WC, Rauch SL, et al: Neurobiology of emotion perception, II: implications for major psychiatric disorders. Biol Psychiatry 54:515–528, 2003b

Raine A, Sheard C, Reynolds GP, et al: Pre-frontal structural and functional deficits associated with individual differences in schizotypal personality. Schizophr Res 7:237–247, 1992

Raine A, Buchsbaum MS, Stanley J, et al: Selective reductions in prefrontal glucose metabolism in murderers. Biol Psychiatry 36:365–373, 1994

Raine A, Lencz T, Bihrle S, et al: Reduced prefrontal gray matter volume and reduced autonomic activity in antisocial personality disorder. Arch Gen Psychiatry 57:119–129, 2000

Raine A, Lencz T, Taylor K, et al: Corpus callosum abnormalities in psychopathic antisocial individuals. Arch Gen Psychiatry 60:1134–1142, 2003

Rusch N, van Elst LT, Ludaescher P, et al: A voxel-based morphometric MRI study in female patients with borderline personality disorder. Neuroimage 20:385–392, 2003

Ruscio J, Ruscio AM: Informing the continuity controversy: a taxometric analysis of depression. J Abnorm Psychol 109:473–487, 2000

Schmahl CG, Vermetten E, Elzinga BM, et al: Magnetic resonance imaging of hippocampal and amygdala volume in women with childhood abuse and borderline personality disorder. Psychiatry Res 122:193–198, 2003a

Schmahl CG, Elzinga BM, Vermetten E, et al: Neural correlates of memories of abandonment in women with and without borderline personality disorder. Biol Psychiatry 54:142–151, 2003b

Schocken DD, Greene AF, Worden TJ, et al: Effects of age and gender on the relationship between anxiety and coronary artery disease. Psychosom Med 49:118–126, 1987

Schulz SC, Koller MM, Kishore PR, et al: Ventricular enlargement in teenage patients with schizophrenia spectrum disorder. Am J Psychiatry 140:1592–1595, 1983

Sheline Y, Sanghavi M, Mintun M, et al: Depression duration but not age predicts hippocampal volume loss in women with recurrent major depression. J Neurosci 19:5034–5043, 1999

Shihabuddin L, Buchsbaum MS, Hazlett EA, et al: Striatal size and relative glucose metabolic rate in schizotypal personality disorder and schizophrenia. Arch Gen Psychiatry 58:877–884, 2001

Siever LJ, Davis KL: The pathophysiology of schizophrenia disorders: perspectives from the spectrum. Am J Psychiatry 161:398–413, 2004

Siever LJ, Buchsbaum MS, New AS, et al: d,l-Fenfluramine response in impulsive personality disorder assessed with [18F]fluorodeoxyglucose positron emission tomography. Neuropsychopharmacology 20:413–423, 1999

Siever LJ, Koenigsberg HW, Harvey P, et al: Cognitive and brain function in schizotypal personality disorder. Schizophr Res 54:157–167, 2002

Simpson JR Jr, Drevets WC, Snyder AZ, et al: Emotion-induced changes in human medial prefrontal cortex, II: during anticipatory anxiety. Proc Natl Acad Sci U S A 98:688–693, 2001

Skodol AE, Gunderson JG, Pfohl B, et al: The borderline diagnosis, I: psychopathology, comorbidity, and personality structure. Biol Psychiatry 51:936–950, 2002a

Skodol AE, Siever LJ, Livesley WJ, et al: The borderline diagnosis, II: biology, genetics, and clinical course. Biol Psychiatry 51:951–963, 2002b

Snyder S, Pitts WM Jr, Gustin Q, et al: CT scans of patients with borderline personality disorder. Am J Psychiatry 140:272, 1983

Soderstrom H, Hultin L, Tullberg M, et al: Reduced frontotemporal perfusion in psychopathic personality. Psychiatry Res 114:81–94, 2002

Soloff PH, Meltzer CC, Greer PJ, et al: A fenfluramine-activated FDG-PET study of borderline personality disorder. Biol Psychiatry 47:540–547, 2000

Spielberger CD, Gorsuch RL, Lushene RD: Manual for the State-Trait Anxiety Inventory. Palo Alto, CA, Consulting Psychologists Press, 1970

Stenberg G, Risberg J, Warkentin S, et al: Regional patterns of cortical blood flow distinguish extraverts from introverts. Pers Individ Dif 11:663–673, 1990

Stenberg G, Wendt PE, Risberg J: Regional cerebral blood flow and extraversion. Pers Individ Dif 15:547–554, 1993

Sugiura M, Kawashima R, Nakagawa M, et al: Correlation between human personality and neural activity in cerebral cortex. Neuroimage 11:541–546, 2000

Tauscher J, Bagby RM, Javanmard M, et al: Inverse relationship between serotonin 5-HT(1A) receptor binding and anxiety: a [(11)C]WAY-100635 PET investigation in healthy volunteers. Am J Psychiatry 158:1326–1328, 2001

Teicher MH, Andersen SL, Polcari A, et al: Developmental neurobiology of childhood stress and trauma. Psychiatr Clin North Am 25:397–426, 2002

Tebartz van Elst L, Hesslinger B, Thiel T, et al: Frontolimbic brain abnormalities in patients with borderline personality disorder: a volumetric magnetic resonance imaging study. Biol Psychiatry 54:163–171, 2003

Volkow ND, Tancredi L: Neural substrates of violent behaviour. A preliminary study with positron emission tomography. Br J Psychiatry 151:668–673, 1987

Watson D: Mood and Temperament. New York, Guilford, 2000, pp 174–203

Woermann FG, van Elst LT, Koepp MJ, et al: Reduction of frontal neocortical grey matter associated with affective aggression in patients with temporal lobe epilepsy: an objective voxel by voxel analysis of automatically segmented MRI. J Neurol Neurosurg Psychiatry 68:162–169, 2000

Young SN, Leyton M, Benkelfat C: Pet studies of serotonin synthesis in the human brain. Adv Exp Med Biol 467:11–18, 1999

Zald DH, Mattson DL, Pardo JV: Brain activity in ventromedial prefrontal cortex correlates with individual differences in negative affect. Proc Natl Acad Sci U S A 99:2450–2454, 2002

39

Translational Research

Martin Bohus, M.D.

Christian Schmahl, M.D.

The large field encompassed by brain science is currently undergoing an era of unpredicted developments. This advancement applies not only to basic sciences, such as molecular and quantitative genetics, neurochemistry, or neurophysiology, but also to the fields of neuroimaging and experimental neuropsychology. With the fascinating progress in these research areas, the opportunity emerges to develop psychopathological concepts based on translations of knowledge from basic science rather than on pure clinical observation or hypothetical constructs. In most other specialties of medicine, clinical and laboratory scientists cooperate to solve overriding problems and make headway toward understanding and treating somatic disorders. However, in the field of neurobehavioral science, translational approaches are only beginning.

In this chapter, we first sketch the prerequisites and basic strategies of translational processes in research on personality disorders. Afterward, an example of this process is explained more concretely for the phenomenon of dissociation.

PRAGMATIC METHODOLOGICAL CONSIDERATIONS

The categorical classification schema in psychiatry is currently based on clusters of behaviors and symptoms that are not based on measures of the underlying genetic or biological pathophysiology of the disorders. Against the backdrop of dramatic research progress within these areas, this initially useful syndromal approach to classification is losing some of its value, particularly in the area of the personality disorders. DSM-based categorical diagnoses are conceived and grouped as complex clusters of response patterns to environmental stimuli. It is more than evident that the complexity of personological phenomena makes it difficult or impossible to establish clear-cut relationships among such divergent phenomena as cognition, impulse control, interpersonal behavior, and emotion regulation. Meanwhile, there is a common sense that categorical diagnostic systems are certainly reliable but of dubious validity.

Translational research holds promise for contributing important delineations applicable to the refinement of a diagnostic model for personality disorders. The following critical steps will leverage the benefits of translational research toward the revision and validation of the diagnostic schema.

1. **Identify and differentiate clinically relevant phenotypes, independent of categorical diagnoses.** Impulsivity, for example, plays an important role within a subgroup of patients with borderline personality disorder (BPD) as well as in patients with antisocial, histrionic, and paranoid personality disorders. If we attempt to study the role of serotonergic dysfunctions in BPD, we cannot expect to obtain valid results when comparing a group of patients with BPD with a mixed group of patients with other personality disorders if we do not control for concomitant impulsivity within the latter group. In addition, the construct of impulsivity comprises a heterogeneous cluster of lower-order traits. Depue and Lenzenweger (2001) postulated at least five different neurobehavioral systems that might underlie this trait complex: positive incentive motivation, lack of fear of physical harm, affective aggression, instrumental aggression, and disinhibition of impulse control. Thus, there is growing evidence that impulsivity emerges from the interaction of at least four to five independent neurobehavioral subsystems that should be carefully classified.

2. **Break down the clinically based phenotypes into lower-order traits that can be studied on an experimental level.** Most behaviors are both dimensional and multifactorial. In this sense, individual differences and variations are considered normal, and personality disorders are thought to be the quantitative extreme of the normal distribution. This conceptualization has some far-reaching implications for research designs: rather than creating differences between experimental and control groups through manipulation, the individual difference perspective focuses on naturally occurring differences between individuals.

3. **Focus on quantitative aspects rather than qualitative differences of the lower-order traits.** As mentioned previously, most behaviors have multifactorial and polygenic origins. Thus, even when the quantitative differentiation of the clinically defined phenotypes might be successful, studies of the neurobiological underpinnings are hampered by the etiological heterogeneity of psychopathologically defined phenotypes of personality disorders. A phenotype always represents observable characteristics that are the joint product of both genotypic and environmental influences, and the phenotypic output of brain—that is, behavior—is more than the sum of its parts. It stands to reason that reduction of degrees of complexity should be a prerequisite to study underlying neurobiological and genetic mechanisms. To reduce complexity and bridge the gap between "the gene and the elusive disease," Gottesman and Gould (2003) suggested the term *endophenotype* or *internal phenotype*, discoverable by biochemical tests or microscopic examination. Endophenotypes should provide a means for identifying the "downstream" traits or facets of clinical phenotypes as well as the "upstream" consequences of genes and, in principle, could assist in the identification of aberrant genes in the hypothesized polygenetic systems conferring vulnerability to disorders. As such, endophenotypes could mark the path between the genotype and the behavior of interest (Gottesman and Gould 2003). As for methods available for endophenotype analysis, Gottesman and Gould 2003 mention "neurophysiological, biochemical, endocrinological, neuroanatomical, cognitive, and neuropsychological" measures (p. 636). To discriminate the term *endophenotype* from synonyms like *intermediate phenotype*, *biological marker*, or *vulnerability marker*, which may not necessarily reflect genetic underpinnings but rather reflect associated findings, the endophenotype should fulfill the following criteria:

   a. The endophenotype is associated with the disorder in the population.
   b. The endophenotype is heritable.
   c. The endophenotype is primarily state-independent.
   d. Within families, endophenotypes and disorders co-segregate.
   e. The endophenotype found in affected family members is found in nonaffected family members at a higher rate than in the general population.

4. **Decompose observable behavioral patterns and search for multiple endophenotypes.** If animal models are based on endophenotypes rather than on clinical observations (like pseudodepressive behavior in the learned helplessness paradigm), these models should represent evolutionarily selected and quantifiable traits.

5. **Define methodological issues to describe the transformation of data and degrees of validity during translational processes.**

THEORETICAL METHODOLOGICAL CONSIDERATIONS

Translational processes basically have to consider the degree of complexity of our findings. *Degree of complexity* can be defined as a measure of the number of interacting subcomponents involved in a process. With that, a clear duality results: the parts of a system are distinguished from each other and are simultaneously bound together. It can thus be assumed that a system is more complex in proportion to the distinctiveness of its parts (functional specialization) and the interconnectivity of its parts (functional integration) (Heylighten 1990). In addition, a distinction should be drawn between structural and dynamic complexity (Strogatz 2001): *structural complexity* represents the architectonics of relationships, whereas *dynamic complexity* describes the processes of change. Electroencephalographic research (e.g., Nunez 2000) distinguishes *local processes* (in which functional segregations are dominant) from *global processes* (in which functional integration is dominant); however distinct, both processes are found in permanent interaction.

As long as we thought in traditional, linear, and closed models that were hierarchically organized, it should have been theoretically—that is, logically—possible to organize a finite number of subcomponents into a finite number of partial aspects, examine them for their conformity to law, and finally develop inferences from the manner in which the complex system operated. This process, however, presupposes that the manner of operation of a subcomponent in the isolated (i.e., experimental) system is identical with its manner of operation in the complex context. In the field of biology, this level of conformity to law is abandoned. The transmission of stimuli of an isolated neuron under experimental conditions does not unconditionally underlie the same conformities to law as they become noticeable within a complex neuronal network. On the contrary, the neuron becomes subordinate in the entire system of feedback processes, which decisively influence the electrical as well as the chemical components of the transmission of stimuli. In other words, the complex network influences the manner of functioning of its subcomponents, and thus the fundamental axioms of the inductive method are overturned. This phenomenon applies to the major part of complex biological systems. For example, protein synthesis is not a unidirectional process but is subordinated to interactions between the synthesized protein products and the RNA expression.

In the analysis of subcomponents within complex systems, it must be considered that the influence of the subsystems on the entire network, as well as the feedback influence of the network on its subsystems, is differentially manifested. Thus, many rudimentary (i.e., phylogenetically old) processes, such as the production of energy in the citric acid cycle, appear to be guided relatively consistently—that is, only by extremely tight feedback loops. It would be highly disadvantageous if cognitive or emotional processes, such as the news of a person's death, had an effect on the intracellular production of energy. Conversely, the subcomponents of cellular production of energy influence to the highest degree the functionality of all other subcomponents of the entire network. The respective subcomponents can be categorized first, therefore, relative to their degree of interlinkage and second, relative to their modulative (deterministic) valence. Four categories may be distinguished:

Type I: Relatively "autonomous" subcomponents with limited interlinkage, weakly active and passive modulation competence (e.g., hair growth)

Type II: Subcomponents with prominent interlinkage and preponderantly active modulation competence (e.g., conveyance of oxygen through membranes)

Type III: Subcomponents with relatively stronger interlinkage and preponderantly passive modulation competence (e.g., basal emotions like fear)

Type IV: Subcomponents with relatively weak interlinkage and comparably prominent active and passive modulation competence (e.g., breathing)

The clarification of these connections is in its infancy but is a fundamental element of translational research. It may thus be assumed that operationalizable patterns of behavior are controlled, such as impulse control or operative cognitive processes (e.g., the focusing of attention and sealing off of stimuli), and that in these processes dopaminergic bunches of neurons in the prefrontal area play an essential role. A translational process occurs that defines the connections between dopaminergic neurotransmitters and observable behavior. The validity of this statement now depends on the degree of complexity of the respective subcomponents. The higher the degree of interlinkage of impulse controls—and thus the stronger this pattern of behavior is influenced by different subcomponents operating independently of the dopaminergic system (e.g., the serotonergic system, motivational aspects, and so on)—the less valid the statement becomes. The opposite also applies: the stronger the active modulation interlinkage, for example the prefrontal dopaminergic system in which no alterations are found, the less valid is a causal connection between the disorders of the dopaminergic system and disorders of impulse control.

In essence, the following applies: the smaller the degree of interlinkage of a research process, the more valid are statements pertaining to the determinability through alterations of interlinked subcomponents. To express it another way: the statement that the disturbance of a process influenced by 100 variables, of which one proves to be the disturbing agent, is conditioned precisely by this single variable, has a smaller degree of validity than if the same statement is made about a process determined solely by 10 variables. As long as experimental procedures cannot be followed, such as evoking the process of disturbance by inducing a disturbance of subcomponents, a presentation of evidence requires the exclusion of participation of all other subcomponents in the origination of disturbance.

Therefore, the first strategies in top-down analysis would be

1. The complex patterns of disturbance in cases of comparative analysis are broken down as much as possible to hold the number of determining variables as small as possible. If a process proves to be disturbed, then this should influence all further active modulation components. Expressed more simply, if a process is disturbed that is interlinked with 20 other components and influences their processing, then it would be required that not only two or three of these subcomponents demonstrate disturbances but all of them, insofar as they are not again compensated by the activity of other components. If, for example, a disturbance of function of the amygdala is postulated in cases of anxiety disorders, then not only the startle reaction but also the distribution of electrodermal activity should manifest itself.

2. It should be explored under experimental conditions which partial components of a disturbance would be affected by the postulated subcomponent, in order to analyze these postulated disturbances in light of further comparative analyses. Even if this influence occurs, it is still uncertain whether a further subcomponent is inducing a newly discovered disturbance. As a result, the statement is valid only until further disturbances are uncovered that are not classifiable as the consequences of a disturbance of the aforementioned subcomponent.

In a nutshell, translational research in the domain of personality disorders deals with complex, nonlinear, organized, open systems. The manner of functioning of these systems should be understood as an interactive process of subcomponents. The results are to be carefully interpreted as candid shots that alter the validity of recent findings and create the condition for further questions. To illustrate these theoretical considerations, we now attempt to describe a translational approach to the phenomenon of dissociation.

DISSOCIATION

Dissociation is currently defined as a disruption in the usually integrated functions of consciousness, memory, identity, or perceptions, leading to a fragmentation of the self (American Psychiatric Association 2000). It took quite a long time to achieve the first step in a translational research process: the definition of a distinct, highly consistent, and measurable phenomenon. The term *dissociation* was developed concurrently with the emergence of the concept of hysteria at the turn of the nineteenth century (see Nemiah 1998). Pierre Janet (1907) described dissociation as an inability of the personal self to bind together the various mental components into an integrated whole under its control. These components consist of somatic (e.g., pain perception) as well as psychological (e.g., amnesia) components. In contrast, Freud (1895/1977) considered dissociative phenomena a result of active repression (e.g., repression of traumatic memories) and introduced the concept of *defense hysteria*.

There are currently two models of nosological classification of dissociation: 1) dimensional models describe a continuum that ranges from mild symptoms (e.g., nonreflective driving) that are relatively normative—to more severe forms of dissociation, such as amnesia; 2) categorical models divide the population into subjects displaying high or low dissociation. Categorical models also underlie the current DSM-IV (American Psychiatric Association 1994) conceptualization of dissociative disorders, although this spectrum ranges from less severe conditions (depersonalization disorder) to the most extreme form of pathological dissociation as represented by dissociative identity disorder. On closer inspection, evidence for both dimensional and categorical models can be found with nonpathological dissociation (e.g., absorption) distributed dimensionally and pathological dissociation (e.g., identity alterations) distributed categorically (Waller et al. 1996). A further nosological dichotomy concerns the temporal structure of dissociation and distinguishes between dissociative traits (e.g., in depersonalization disorder) and dissociative states, which are of shorter duration (minutes to days). These dissociative states are a central feature of BPD. Patients with BPD frequently engage in self-destructive behavior, which may function to terminate dissociative states. This disorder occurs in the general population with a relatively high prevalence of 1.3% (Torgersen et al. 2001) and is associated with high health care utilization (Bender et al. 2001). Dissociative states correlate with the chronicity and resistance to therapy of BPD, thus playing an important economic role in our general health systems. This influence may be due to the interference of dissociative states with cognitive-behavioral and exposure-based treatment approaches in traumatized individuals. Dissociative disorders occur at a prevalence of about 1%–2% (Freyberger and Stieglitz 1999; Simeon 2004).

Meanwhile, several instruments assess the DSM-IV dissociative disorders (dissociative amnesia, dissociative fugue, dissociative identity disorder, depersonalization disorder) and dissociative symptoms. Well-validated measures of DSM-IV dissociative disorders include the Dissociative Disorders Interview Schedule (Ross et al. 1989) and the Structured Clinical Interview for DSM-IV Dissociative Disorders (Steinberg 1994). The most commonly used self-rating questionnaire for the long-term assessment of dissociative symptoms is the Dissociative Experiences Scale (DES; Bernstein and Putnam 1986). DES scores range from 8.3 in healthy individuals to 13.2 in affective disorders, 21.6 in BPD, and as high as 31.5 in posttraumatic stress disorder (PTSD) and 44.6 in dissociative identity disorder (Putnam et al. 1996). The German Fragebogen zu Dissoziativen Symptomen (Freyberger et al. 1999) is an adaptation of the DES but also assesses somatoform dissociative symptoms as defined in ICD-10.

Acute dissociative states can be assessed with the Clinician-Administered Dissociative States Scale (Bremner et al. 1998a), a reliable and valid 27-item scale for the measurement of current dissociative states, including several observer-based items. In Germany, dissociative states can be assessed with a self-rating questionnaire, the Dissoziations-Spannungs-Skala akut (Dissociation-Tension-Scale acute; Stiglmayr et al. 2003). Homogeneity of this instrument was demonstrated, and a reliability analysis resulted in Cronbach's α between 0.88 and 0.94. Thus, the prerequisite to make use of translational processes (the operationalization of a homogenous phenomenon) has been achieved. This fact opens the focus to physiological pathways underlying dissociative features.

There are different possible approaches. First, one can investigate potential physiological correlates of dissociative states, such as the visceral nervous system, the endocrine system, respiration, movement coordination, electrodermal activity, and so on. This approach makes sense because, on an observer-based behavioral level, severe dissociative states seem to be correlated with tonic immobility, often in combination with aphonia, bradycardia, and hypoventilation.

Methods that enable us to induce dissociative states under experimental conditions will facilitate these investigations. Otherwise, we would have to depend on pure coincidence. For example, our group found a significant influence of dissociation on physiological reactivity measured by the startle response. Patients with self-reported low dissociative experiences during the experiment revealed enhanced startle responses, whereas patients with high dissociative experiences during the experiment showed reduced responses (Ebner-Priemer et al. 2004). Even if these data could be interpreted to suggest that dissociation is correlated with dampening amygdala reactivity, the fact that this finding can also be interpreted as an unspecific group effect renders this evidence problematic.

Thus, the development of methods to induce dissociative states has top priority. At least three different categories of induction can be defined: 1) pharmacological induction, 2) electric stimulation, 3) psychological induction.

Pharmacological Induction Methods

Several neurotransmitter systems have been implicated in dissociative symptoms. Evidence, however, is scant and in some cases indirect. Tentatively, four classes of neurochemicals were suggested to be involved in the generation of dissociative states, including N-methyl-D-aspartate (NMDA) antagonists, serotonergic hallucinogens, opioid agonists, and neurochemicals of the hypothalamic-pituitary-adrenal (HPA) axis.

NMDA Antagonists

Noncompetitive NMDA antagonists such as phencyclidine and ketamine, also known as the "dissociative anesthetic" and as the street drug "Special K," produce a derealized and depersonalized state characterized by marked perceptual alterations at subanesthetic doses (Domino et al. 1965; Krystal et al. 1994). NMDA receptors are distributed widely in the cortex, as well as in the hippocampus and the amygdala, and are thought to mediate associative functioning and long-term potentiation of memory processes. Thus, it is plausible that diminished NMDA neurotransmission may be related to dissociative states. The dissociative effects of cannabinoids such as marijuana, which consistently have been shown to induce depersonalization, might be mediated by their antagonistic action at NMDA receptors (Feigenbaum et al. 1989). Brain imaging studies stress the importance of the medial prefrontal cortex in the generation of dissociative symptoms. In healthy subjects, severity of tetrahydrocannabinol-induced depersonalization was correlated with blood flow increase in the right frontal cortex and the anterior cingulate cortex (ACC) (Mathew et al. 1999).

Serotonergic Hallucinogens

Serotonergic hallucinogens such as lysergic acid diethylamide (better known as LSD), mescaline, psilocybin, and dimethyltryptamine also produce dissociative symptoms (Freedman 1968; Klee 1963; Simeon 2004). These substances stimulate 5-HT_{2A} and 5-HT_{2C} receptors (Rasmussen et al. 1986; Titeler et al. 1988). Neurochemical challenge studies with the 5-HT_{2C} receptor agonist *meta*-chlorophenylpiperazine demonstrated the induction of significantly more depersonalization than placebo (Simeon et al. 1995) as well as the induction of flashbacks and dissociative symptoms in patients with PTSD (Southwick et al. 1991). Vollenweider and colleagues (1998) found increased fluorodeoxyglucose positron emission tomography (PET) metabolism in ACC, striatum, and thalamus after amphetamine-induced depersonalization.

Opioid Agonists

The endogenous opioid system involves three classes of substances: endorphins, enkephalins, and dynorphins. In addition, a recently discovered neuropeptide, Orphanin FQ, has antiopioid activity (Griebel et al. 1999). The endogenous opioid system mediates stress-induced analgesia (Madden et al. 1997), and analgesia in response to combat stimuli in PTSD can be at least partially blocked by the opioid antagonist naloxone (Pitman et al. 1990). Surgical stress in humans is accompanied by β-endorphin release (Cohen et al. 1981; Dubois et al. 1981), and an increase of dynorphin A release was found with hypoxia stress, thus suggesting that not only β-endorphin is involved in the stress response (Chen 1998). Cerebrospinal fluid β-endorphin was found to be low in dissociative patients with eating disorders (Demitrack et al. 1993), and blood levels of noradrenaline, dopamine, and β-endorphin were elevated during trance states (Kawai et al. 2001). Several

conflicting reports show alterations of endogenous opioid levels in disorders associated with elevated levels of stress, such as PTSD and BPD. Plasma β-endorphin immunoreactivity was low in patients with non-major depression, many of whom met criteria for BPD (Cohen et al. 1984). Also in patients with BPD, Coid and colleagues (1983) reported raised plasma met-enkephalin levels, whereas Pickar and colleagues (1982) reported low levels of opioid activity in cerebrospinal fluid. Low plasma levels of opioid activity have also been reported for patients with PTSD (Hoffman et al. 1989; Wolf et al. 1991), and one study reported a negative correlation between β-endorphin activity and intrusive and avoidant symptoms in PTSD (Baker et al. 1997).

The kappa opioid receptor agonists ketocyclazocine, MR-2033, and enadoline can induce depersonalization, derealization, and perceptual alterations (Kumor et al. 1986; Pfeiffer et al. 1986; Walsh et al. 2001). Along these lines, opioid receptor antagonists have been reported to reduce dissociation, such as naltrexone in BPD (Bohus et al. 1999) and intravenous naloxone in chronic depersonalization (Nuller et al. 2001). The role of the recently discovered antiopioid neuropeptide orphanin FQ in dissociation is unclear, although this substance has demonstrated anxiolytic as well as stress-reducing effects (Griebel et al. 1999; Jenck et al. 1997).

Neurochemicals of the Hypothalamic-Pituitary-Adrenal Axis

The HPA axis is known to play a central role in the stress response. Exposure to stressful events is associated with a marked increase in cortisol release from the adrenal gland as well as an increase in dissociative symptoms, especially in stress-related disorders such as PTSD and BPD. However, the role of the HPA axis in mediating dissociation is still unclear. For instance, two studies on depersonalization disorder have revealed rather conflicting results. One study (Stanton et al. 2001) reported nonsignificantly lower basal salivary cortisol in patients with depersonalization disorder compared with control subjects. In contrast, another study demonstrated a tendency toward elevated basal urinary and plasma cortisol as well as a resistance to low-dose dexamethasone suppression in these patients as compared with control subjects (Simeon et al. 2001).

Electric and Mechanic Stimulation

Penfield and Perot (1963) elicited dreamlike states, memories, and complex experiential phenomena by direct electrical stimulation of structures in the temporal lobe, temporoparietal association areas, hippocampus, and amygdala. However, even if depersonalization is also common in temporal lobe epilepsy with left-sided foci (Devinsky et al. 1989; Sedman and Kenna 1963), the reported symptoms are quite vague, and there is little more than a hint that these areas may be even marginally involved.

Psychological Induction Paradigms

In analogy to the field of research on stress induction paradigms, one should distinguish between "objective" induction paradigms and "subjective, biographically relevant" induction paradigms. Because dissociation usually is triggered by biographically relevant aversive stimuli, the latter normally will be the first choice. Because subjective stimuli are very difficult to compare or assess and dissociation is not an on/off but rather a dimensional phenomenon, a method independent of subjective appraisal of the participant would be required to assess the level of dissociation under experimental conditions. Evoked potentials might be a possible approach. Patients report analgesia, numbness, and increased auditory thresholds during dissociative states, thus evoked sensory potentials might reveal electroencephalographic alterations correlated with the grade of dissociative states.

One of the major fields of translational research compares these three different induction paradigms. Given that the dependent variable—the "dissociative state"—is a consistent entity, all three methods should lead to the same results. Psychological induction is clinically the most relevant, and thus it should be used as a "positive control variable" when searching for adequate pharmacological or electric induction mechanisms.

Because currently standardized psychological inductive methods are not available, one must examine spontaneous dissociative states in patients with a high probability of experiencing dissociative features under experimental conditions. This widespread approach has several intrinsic problems. Most important, and usually underestimated, is the simple clinical observation that psychiatric disorders are never monosymptomatic but generally are organized as a bundle of interlacing symptoms with anxiety, stress, anger, and shame (the basic emotions) playing important roles either as primary or as secondary symptoms. Thus, any neurobiological finding within a specific group of patients can mean anything as long as it is not proven to be specific for a single symptomatic entity. As simple as this observation sounds, it is the most repeated fault in biological psychiatric research and covers the whole spectrum of research from study of the HPA axis to evoked potentials and most recently the fashionable amygdala hyperreactivity and volume loss of hippocampal or prefrontal areas.

Thus, with regard to experiments based on comparisons between patients and healthy control subjects, translational research aims to clarify the specificity of the findings, requiring inclusion of thorough controls not only between different patient groups but also among patients with the same diagnosis (e.g., BPD) and differentiation of subtypes (with and without dissociative experience).

Concerning neuroanatomy, the elucidation of the brain circuit underlying dissociation is a first step, and several regions were identified that appear to be involved in the generation of dissociative symptoms. Studies in patients with PTSD found a correlation between hippocampal atrophy and the extent of dissociative symptoms; thus, the hippocampus was implicated in dissociative processes (Bremner, personal communication, January 20, 2004; Stein et al. 1997). In addition, given the important role of the hippocampus in declarative memory, a putative role of this brain region involves amnestic symptoms as well as the generation of intrusive memories (Bremner 1998; Bremner et al. 1998b).

Lanius and colleagues (2002) studied women with PTSD secondary to childhood sexual abuse using functional magnetic resonance imaging with script-driven imagery. Among the 30% of patients who dissociated in response to the scripts, the authors found increased activation in the medial prefrontal cortex, inferior frontal gyrus, ACC, superior and middle temporal gyrus, and parietal and occipital lobes compared with PTSD patients without dissociation and control subjects. Furthermore, dissociating patients revealed no concomitant increase in heart rate as compared with patients without dissociative response. In addition, another study found heightened activation in the ventral prefrontal cortex as well as a failure of activation in the insula among patients with depersonalization disorder with high levels of state dissociation (Phillips et al. 2001). In a PET study of patients with depersonalization disorder, Simeon and colleagues (2000) found higher activity in somatosensory association areas compared with control subjects, and dissociation scores were strongly correlated with this activity.

The prefrontal cortex, including the ACC, also appears to play a role in states of dissociative sensory loss (nondermatomal somatosensory deficits). Mailis-

Gagnon and colleagues (2003) found a failure of activation in Brodmann area 10 and posterior ACC with unperceived stimuli in contrast to perceived stimuli at the contralateral limb. In contrast, unperceived stimuli resulted in activation in anterior ACC, a pattern that was not seen with perceived stimuli.

Animal Research

To bridge the gap between human and animal research concerning dissociative features, one should be sure that the methodological domains are not confused. This distinction means that behavioral levels in humans should be compared with behavioral levels in animals, intrapsychic observation or appraisals cannot be compared at all, physiological levels in animals should be compared with those in human beings, and so on. Models that switch between different levels (e.g., the learned helplessness paradigm for depression, which compares intrapsychic experience in humans to observable behavior in animals) are usually not valid and should be carefully discussed.

Concerning dissociation, the construct has been derived from clinical experience as well as from research in humans. There is to date no animal model for dissociation; hence, animal research must rely on analogues of this phenomenon. Animal research in this domain has two decisive advantages. First, only in animals are real experimental designs possible, in which only one independent variable in an experimental setting can be selectively changed, for example, by using genetically altered ("knockout") animals. Second, intraspecies correlation analyses can be conducted on a more sophisticated level. On a neurobiological level, there are several decisive advantages of animal research. One is the higher spatial resolution in neuroanatomy (e.g., in the differentiation of amygdala subnuclei or periaqueductal grey substructures). A second significant advantage is the possibility of specific and experimental pharmacological interventions that should throw light on the neurochemical pathways involved in dissociative features. Thus, the animal model is the primary prerequisite for developing pharmacological interventions within human subjects.

One possible analogue of dissociation in animals can be derived from behavioral research using fear-conditioning paradigms. The behavior systems approach views an animal as having a set of several genetically determined, prepackaged behaviors that it uses to solve particular functional problems. If the problem has to be solved immediately, the animal's behavioral repertoire becomes restricted to those genetically hard-wired behaviors. This approach was outlined by Bolles (1970) in his species-specific defense reaction theory. When an animal is confronted by a natural environmental threat (e.g., a predator) or an artificial one (e.g., an electrical shock), its behavioral repertoire becomes restricted to its species-specific defense reaction. Freezing, fight, and flight are examples of these reactions. The so-called defensive behavior system (Fanselow 1994) is organized by the imminence of a predator and can be divided into three stages—preencounter, postencounter, and circa-strike. *Preencounter* defensive behaviors comprise reorganization of meal patterns and protective nest maintenance if an animal has to leave a safe nesting area. When the level of fear increases (e.g., because of actual detection of a predator), *postencounter* defensive behavior mode becomes active. This mode includes several dimensions (Bohus et al. 1996; Cleroux et al. 1985; Fanselow 1994; Mayer and Fanselow 2003; Nijsen et al. 1998; Overton 1993): a motor component (freezing), a sensory component (opiate analgesia), an autonomic component, an endocrinological component (HPA axis), and an emotional component (anxiety). In the case of physical contact, for example, by the notion of pain, the animal engages in more active defenses such as biting and jumping. The latter is an example of *circa-strike* behavior.

Translational research has to develop research designs to study these components in parallel with animals and human beings. Because the hypothesis is based on the assumption that dissociation is activated as part of a phylogenetically conservative pattern, there should be mechanisms common to all mammals.

Critical anatomical structures for postencounter defensive behavior are the amygdala, the ventral periaqueductal grey, and the hypothalamus. The amygdala has a central relay function for mediation of postencounter defensive behavior with important glutamatergic input from the thalamus to the lateral amygdala (Fanselow 1994). Furthermore, the central amygdala mediates transfer of information about the threat level to the ventral periaqueductal grey, which in turn appears to mediate analgesia and freezing by opioidergic neurotransmission (Fanselow and Gale 2003; LeDoux 1992). Autonomic and endocrinological responses are mediated by connections of the amygdala with the hypothalamus (LeDoux et al. 1988). The exact localization of the emotional component is unclear but can be assumed to rely on amygdala-prefrontal cortex pathways (LeDoux 2002). Circa-strike behavior is mediated by the superior colliculus and the dorsolateral periaqueductal grey, which receives nociceptive input from the spinal cord and the trigeminal nucleus (Blomqvist and Craig 1991). In phylogenetically more recent species such as humans, these systems can be assumed to be usually controlled by higher cortical regions and to be activated under high levels of stress. It could be hypothesized that dissociation is the representation of the postencounter defense mode in humans, comprising the same dimensions as described in animals extended by an emotional-psychological component (depersonalization, derealization, and emotional numbness). In this model, self-destructive behavior, which can be observed frequently during dissociative states (e.g., in patients with BPD), may represent an analogue of the pain-induced switch of behavioral modes from postencounter to circa-strike in a human being faced with high levels of aversive stress.

The development of this dissociative model exemplifies both the advantages and disadvantages of an animal model for mental disturbances. On the one hand, animal models enable the analysis and elucidation of components currently involved on physiological and neuroanatomical levels under experimental conditions. On the other hand, the relevance of these animal models to the human species is always one of analogy insofar as the experience of depersonalization or derealization cannot be simply made parallel. The validity of this analogy, however, can be strengthened on the human level through experimental transfer, as gained, for example, through pharmacological interventions in the animal model.

SUMMARY

In a nutshell, translational research processes can be summarized as a circumplex procedure.

In the first place, the most precise and concise possible operationalizability of clinical symptoms is achieved on the phenomenological level. This achievement enables the parallel analysis of coincident physiological and neuroanatomical variables, in which one fundamentally strives on this level to arrive at experimentally inductive methods as derived from parallel analysis (patient and healthy control subjects). This procedure again enables the development of animal models. On this level, experimental pharmacological and molecular-genetic operations can again be conducted. The transfer back ensues through application of the methods of intervention acquired in the animal model and examination into whether the above-mentioned clinical phenomena have been influenced by it.

REFERENCES

American Psychiatric Association: Diagnostic and Statistical Manual of Mental Disorders, 4th Edition. Washington, DC, American Psychiatric Association, 1994

American Psychiatric Association: Diagnostic and Statistical Manual of Mental Disorders, 4th Edition, Text Revision. Washington, DC, American Psychiatric Association, 2000

Baker DG, West SA, Orth DN, et al: Cerebrospinal fluid and plasma β-endorphin in combat veterans with posttraumatic stress disorder. Psychoneuroendocrinology 22: 517–529, 1997

Bender DS, Dolan RT, Skodol AE, et al: Treatment utilization by patients with personality disorders. Am J Psychiatry 158:295–302, 2001

Bernstein E, Putnam FW: Development, reliability and validity of a dissociation rating scale. J Nerv Ment Dis 174:727–735, 1986

Blomqvist A, Craig AD: Organization of spinal and trigeminal input to the PAG, in The Midbrain Periaqueductal Grey Matter: Functional, Anatomical and Immunohistochemical Organization. NATO ASI Series A, Vol 213. Edited by Depaulis A, Bandler R. New York, Plenum, 1991, pp 345–363

Bohus B, Koolhaas JM, Korte SM, et al: Forebrain pathways and their behavioural interactions with neuroendocrine and cardiovascular function in the rat. Clin Exp Pharmacol Physiol 23:177–182, 1996

Bohus MJ, Landwehrmeyer GB, Stiglmayr CE, et al: Naltrexone in the treatment of dissociative symptoms in patients with borderline personality disorder: an open-label trial. J Clin Psychiatry 60:598–603, 1999

Bolles RC: Species-specific defense reactions and avoidance learning. Psychol Rev 77:32–48, 1970

Bremner JD: Traumatic memories lost and found: can lost memories of abuse be found in the brain? In Trauma and Memory. Edited by Williams LM, Banyard VL. New Delhi, Sage, 1998

Bremner JD, Krystal JH, Putnam F, et al: Measurement of dissociative states with the Clinician-Administered Dissociative States Scale (CADSS). J Trauma Stress 11:125–136, 1998a

Bremner JD, Vermetten E, Southwick SM, et al: Trauma, memory, and dissociation: an integrative formulation, in Trauma, Memory, and Dissociation. Edited by Bremner JD, Marmar CR. Washington, DC, American Psychiatric Press, 1998b, pp 365–402

Chen D: Changes of plasma level of neurotensin, somatostatin, and dynorphin A in pilots under acute hypoxia. Mil Med 163:120–121, 1998

Cleroux J, Peronnet F, De Champlain J: Sympathetic indices during psychological and physical stimuli before and after training. Physiol Behav 35:271–275, 1985

Cohen M, Pickar D, Dubois M, et al: Surgical stress and endorphins. Lancet 1:213–214, 1981

Cohen MR, Pickar D, Extein I, et al: Plasma cortisol and β-endorphin immunoreactivity in nonmajor and major depression. Am J Psychiatry 141:628–632, 1984

Coid J, Allolio B, Rees LH: Raised plasma metenkephalin in patients who habitually mutilate themselves. Lancet 2:545–546, 1983

Demitrack MA, Putnam FW, Rubinow DR, et al: Relation of dissociative phenomena to levels of cerebrospinal fluid monoamine metabolites and beta-endorphin in patients with eating disorders: a pilot study. Psychiatry Res 49:1–10, 1993

Depue RA, Lenzenweger MF: A neurobehavioral dimensional model, in Handbook of Personality Disorder. Edited by Livesley WJ. New York, Guilford, 2001, pp 136–177

Devinsky O, Putnam F, Grafman J, et al: Dissociative states and epilepsy. Neurology 39:835–840, 1989

Domino EF, Chodoff P, Corssen G: Pharmacologic effects of CI-581, a new dissociative anesthetic in man. Clin Pharmacol Ther 6:279–291, 1965

Dubois M, Pickar D, Cohen MR, et al: Surgical stress in humans is accompanied by an increase in plasma beta-endorphin immunoreactivity. Life Sci 29:1249–1254, 1981

Ebner-Priemer UW, Badeck S, Beckmann C, et al: Affective dysregulation and dissociative experience in female patients with borderline personality disorder: a startle response study. J Psychiatr Res 39:85–92, 2005

Fanselow MS: Neural organization of the defensive behavior system responsible for fear. Psychol Bull Rev 1:429–438, 1994

Fanselow MS, Gale GD: The amygdala, fear, and memory. Ann N Y Acad Sci 985:125–134, 2003

Feigenbaum JJ, Bergamnn F, Richmond SA, et al: Nonpsychotropic cannabinoid acts as a functional N-methyl-D-aspartate receptor blocker. Proc Natl Acad Sci U S A 86:9584–9587, 1989

Freedman DX: On the use and abuse of LSD. Arch Gen Psychiatry 18:330–347, 1968

Freud S, Breuer J: Studien über Hysterie (1895), in Gesammelte Werke, Vol 1. Frankfurt, Germany, Fischer, 1977, pp 75–312

Freyberger HJ, Stieglitz RD: Dissoziative Störungen (Dissociative Disorders), in Psychiatrie und Psychotherapie. Edited by Berger M. München, Germany, Urban und Schwarzenberg, 1999

Freyberger HJ, Spitzer C, Stieglitz RD: Fragebogen zu Dissoziativen Symptomen (FDS). Bern, Germany, Verlag Hans Huber, 1999

Gottesman IL, Gould TD: The endophenotype concept in psychiatry: etymology and strategic intentions. Am J Psychiatry 160: 636–645, 2003

Griebel G, Perrault G, Sanger DJ: Orphanin FQ, a novel neuropeptide with anti-stress-like activity. Brain Res 836:221–224, 1999

Heylighten F: Relational closure: a mathematical concept for distinction making and complexity analysis, in Cybernetics and Systems '90. Edited by Trappl R. Singapore, World Scientific, 1990, pp 335–342

Hoffman L, Burges Watson P, Wilson G, et al: Low plasma beta-endorphin in posttraumatic stress disorder. Aust N Z J Psychiatry 23:268–273, 1989

Janet P: The Major Symptoms of Hysteria. New York, Macmillan, 1907

Jenck F, Moreau JL, Martin JR, et al: Orphanin FQ acts as an anxiolytic to attenuate behavioral responses to stress. Proc Natl Acad Sci U S A 94:14854–14858, 1997

Kawai N, Honda M, Nakamura S, et al: Catecholamines and opioid peptides increase in plasma in humans during possession states. Neuroreport 12:3419–3423, 2001

Klee GD: Lysergic acid diethylamide (LSD-25) and ego functions. Arch Gen Psychiatry 8:57–70, 1963

Krystal JH, Karper LP, Seibyl JP, et al: Subanesthetic effects of the NMDA antagonist, ketamine, in humans: psychotomimetic, perceptual, cognitive, and neuroendocrine effects. Arch Gen Psychiatry 51:199–214, 1994

Kumor KM, Haertzen CA, Johnson RE, et al: Human psychopharmacology of ketocyclazocine as compared with cyclazocine, morphine and placebo. J Pharmacol Exp Ther 238:960–968, 1986

Lanius RTA, Williamson PC, Boksman K, et al: Brain activation during script-driven imagery induced dissociative responses in PTSD: a functional magnetic resonance imaging investigation. Biol Psychiatry 52:305–311, 2002

LeDoux JE: Emotion and the amygdala, in The Amygdala: Neurobiological Aspects of Emotion, Memory, and Mental Dysfunction. Edited by Aggleton JP. New York, Wiley-Liss, 1992, pp 339–351

LeDoux JE: Synaptic Self: How Our Brains Become Who We Are. New York, Viking, 2002

LeDoux JE, Cicchetti P, Xagoraris A, et al: Different projections of the central amygdaloid nucleus mediate autonomic and behavioral correlates of conditioned fear. J Neurosci 8:2517–2529, 1988

Madden J, Akil H, Patrick RL, et al: Stress-induced parallel changes in central opioid levels and pain responsiveness in the rat. Nature 265:358–360, 1997

Mailis-Gagnon A, Giannoylis I, Downar J, et al: Altered central somatosensory processing in chronic pain patients with "hysterical" anesthesia. Neurology 60:1501–1507, 2003

Mathew RJ, Wilson WH, Chiu NY, et al: Regional cerebral blood flow and depersonalization after tetrahydrocannabinol administration. Acta Psychiatr Scand 100:67–75, 1999

Mayer EA, Fanselow MS: Dissecting the components of the central response to stress. Nat Neurosci 6:1011–1012, 2003

Nemiah JC: Early concepts of trauma, dissociation, and the unconscious: their history and current implications, in Trauma, Memory, and Dissociation. Edited by Bremner JD, Marmar CR. Washington, DC, American Psychiatric Press, 1998, pp 1–26

Nijsen MJMA, Croiset G, Diamant M, et al: Conditioned fear-induced tachycardia in the rat: vagal involvement. Eur J Pharmacol 350:211–222, 1998

Nuller YL, Morozova MG, Kushnir ON, et al: Effect of naloxone therapy on depersonalization. J Psychopharmacol 15:93–95, 2001

Nunez PL: Toward a quantitative description of larger-scale neocortical dynamic function and EEG. Behav Brain Sci 23:371–437, 2000

Overton JM: Influence of autonomic blockade on cardiovascular responses to exercise in rats. J Appl Physiol 75:155–161, 1993

Penfield W, Perot P: The brain's record of auditory and visual experience: a final summary and discussion. Brain 86:595–696, 1963

Pfeiffer A, Brantl V, Herz A, et al: Psychotomimesis mediated by κ opiate receptors. Science 233:774–776, 1986

Phillips ML, Medford N, Senior C, et al: Depersonalization disorder: thinking without feeling. Psychiatry Research: Neuroimaging 108:145–160, 2001

Pickar D, Cohen MR, Naber D, et al: Clinical studies of the endogenous opioid system. Biol Psychiatry 17:1243–1276, 1982

Pitman RK, van der Kolk BA, Orr SP: Naloxone-reversible analgesic response to combat-related stimuli in posttraumatic stress disorder. Arch Gen Psychiatry 54:749–758, 1990

Putnam FW, Carlson EB, Ross CA, et al: Patterns of dissociation in clinical and nonclinical samples. J Nerv Ment Dis 184:673–679, 1996

Rasmussen K, Glennon RA, Aghajanian GK: Phenethylamine hallucinogens in the locus coeruleus: potency of action correlates with rank order of 5-HT2 binding affinity. Eur J Pharmacol 32:79–82, 1986

Ross CA, Heber S, Norton GR, et al: The Dissociative Disorders Interview Schedule: a structured interview. Dissociation: Progress in the Dissociative Disorders 2:169–189, 1989

Sedman G, Kenna JC: Depersonalization and mood changes in schizophrenia. Br J Psychiatry 109:669–673, 1963

Simeon D: Depersonalization disorder: A contemporary overview. CNS Drugs 18:343–354, 2004

Simeon D, Hollander E, Stein DJ: Induction of depersonalization by the serotonin agonist *meta*-chlorophenylpiperazine. Psychiatry Res 58:161–164, 1995

Simeon D, Guralnik O, Hazlett Spiegel-Cohen J, et al: Feeling unreal: a PET study of depersonalization disorder. Am J Psychiatry 157:1782–1788, 2000

Simeon D, Guralnik O, Knutelska M, et al: Hypothalamic-pituitary-adrenal axis dysregulation in depersonalization disorder. Neuropsychopharmacology 25:793–795, 2001

Southwick SM, Krystal JH, Bremner JD, et al: Noradrenergic and serotonergic function in posttraumatic stress disorder. Arch Gen Psychiatry 54:749–758, 1991

Stanton BR, David AS, Cleare AJ, et al: Basal activity of the hypothalamic-pituitary-adrenal axis in patients with depersonalization disorder. Psychiatry Res 104:85–89, 2001

Stein MB, Koverola C, Hanna C, et al: Hippocampal volume in women victimized by childhood sexual abuse. Psychol Med 27:951–959, 1997

Steinberg M: Interviewer's Guide to the Structured Clinical Interview for DSM-IV Dissociative Disorders. Washington, DC, American Psychiatric Press, 1994

Stiglmayr C, Braakmann D, Haaf B, et al: Development and characteristics of Dissociation-Tension Scale acute (DSS-Akute). Psychother Psychosom Med Psychol 53:287–294, 2003

Strogatz SH: Exploring complex networks. Nature 410:268–276, 2001

Titeler M, Lyon RA, Glennon RA: Radioligand binding evidence implicates the brain 5-HT2 receptor as a site of action for LSD and phenylisopropylamine hallucinogens. Psychopharmacology 94:213–216, 1988

Torgersen S, Kringlen E, Cramer V: The prevalence of personality disorders in a community sample. Arch Gen Psychiatry 58:590–596, 2001

Vollenweider FX, Maguire RP, Leenders KL, et al: Effects high amphetamine dose on mood and cerebral glucose metabolism in normal volunteers using positron emission tomography (PET). Psychiatry Research: Neuroimaging 83:149–162, 1998

Waller NG, Putnam FW, Carlson EB: Types of dissociation and dissociative types: a taxometric analysis of dissociative experiences. Psychol Methods 1:300–321, 1996

Walsh SL, Geter-Douglas B, Strain EC, et al: Enadoline and butorphanol: evaluation of κ-agonists on cocaine pharmacodynamics and cocaine self-administration in humans. J Pharmacol Exp Ther 299:147–158, 2001

Wolf ME, Mosnaim AD, Puente J, et al: Plasma methionine enkephalin in PTSD. Biol Psychiatry 29:305–307, 1991

40

Development of Animal Models in Neuroscience and Molecular Biology

Michael J. Meaney, Ph.D.

Discussions of animal models in psychiatry are often frustrating. There is understandable skepticism about the expression of psychiatric symptoms in nonhuman subjects. Is there really a depressed rat? Do monkeys obsess? Do ruminants, well, ruminate? How can one hope to meaningfully depict clinical psychiatric syndromes in nonhuman species? Actually, there is frustration on both sides of the table. How, for example, do researchers interested in uncovering the neurobiology of depression model a disorder that shows such wide variation among patients? Indeed, it is probably unrealistic to believe that we can develop a satisfying animal model of anything so complex as psychiatric illnesses or syndromes, the definition of which remains a moving target. Faced with these concerns, researchers often work with models that offer far more modest promise, such as behavioral assays that help predict drug efficacy in human populations. Moreover, with

the advent of human neuroimaging, animal models are no longer the only tool in the shed when defining underlying neural mechanisms. Techniques such as functional magnetic resonance imaging (fMRI), along with advances in bioinformatics, will describe activated neural circuits in the human brain. Some might argue that such advances render animal models substantially less necessary in the study of brain and behavior. I think the opposite is true. With the popularization of human neuroimaging, there is now a crucial bridge linking psychology and the biological sciences. Neuroimaging with human populations reveals that information previously obtained from neurobehavioral models with nonhuman species was indeed accurate in describing relevant neural circuits in the human brain and provides a wonderfully improved platform for the development of a generation of far more ambitious research with nonhuman populations.

OVERVIEW

It has always been reasonable to expect useful animal models of specific features of psychiatric disorders (e.g., anhedonia), and there is a history of success on this front. Much of the controversy that surrounds the topic of animal models derives from confusion concerning the intent: what is the intended purpose of the model? Many models were not intended to model anything human in form but simply to provide a fast and reliable way of predicting specific drug effects. The use of the Prosolt swim test to predict antidepressant actions is a case in point. Such tests provide little information on the mechanism for drug effects on behavior. Other tests are clearly more ambitious, but the point here is that models should be judged in terms of their intended purpose. Shekhar et al. (2001) and Nestler et al. (2002) provided extensive and critical surveys of many of the existing animal models of psychiatric illnesses and in the process defined the various strengths and weaknesses of several approaches. I do not attempt to repeat this effort. Instead, I focus on reasons for optimism in the development of more ambitious animal models of human misbehavior. I believe that over the next decade we will be able to develop substantially more powerful animal models of psychiatric symptoms. I will focus on the rationale underlying such optimism and the challenges that we face in realizing the potential afforded us with technological and conceptual advances in neuroscience and molecular biology. I believe that these considerations are important for all areas of psychiatry but especially for the study of personality disorders.

With advances in genomics and proteomics, the potential for understanding the mechanisms of mental illness has expanded considerably. However, ultimately research will have gone beyond simple linkage of genotype with phenotypes by analyzing the intermediate levels of function that characterize states of vulnerability and/or resistance. Developments in neuroimaging are of obvious importance; however, many of the findings remain correlational as, for that matter, do findings from gene linkage or association studies. Animal models remain a powerful approach in the quest of establishing causal relations between genomic and environmental factors and the risk for illness. Animal models are also invaluable in our efforts to conceptually understand the importance of findings from genetics research. What exactly is the importance of specific genetic polymorphisms in the development of individual differences in neural and psychological function? How can we best understand gene–environment interactions? In many areas, the conceptual approach to these issues is unchanged over the past 50 years. Animal models of relevant gene–environment interactions are invaluable not only in the specific information they provide but also in the way they influence our understanding of phenotypic development.

Another approach to the development of animal models is to focus on "exposures" that are known to increase the risk of illness in human populations. Animal models that focus on such risk factors have the potential to define causal relations between genomic variations or environmental events and illness. Such models focus not on symptoms but on vulnerability. The more we learn from epidemiological studies about the possible etiology of specific diseases, the better able we are to create models that focus on more specific and relevant classes of risk factors. Taken together with a dimensional rather than categorical approach to psychiatric illness, there is reason for considerable optimism that models of psychiatric illness based on nonhuman species can be very meaningful. The dimensional approach is of course essential in the study of personality disorders. The focus on operationally defined intermediate states of function, or endophenotypes, provides an empirical link between studies with human and nonhuman models.

Neuroimaging technology provides another reason for optimism. The problems that confront the development of animal models of psychiatric illness cannot be separated from those associated with diagnosis. The latter basically defines the former. Until recently, psychiatry was severely handicapped because the primary organ responsible for the relevant forms of illness lay largely outside the domain of scientific investigation. Studies of the neurobiological basis of psychiatric illness in human subjects were largely confined either to postmortem analysis or to research using nonneuronal cells such as platelets or lymphocytes. In truth, despite obvious constraints, such studies probably yielded more information than is often assumed to have been the case. Nevertheless the limitations are certainly important. Advances in neuroimaging are changing the landscape dramatically. It is now entirely reasonable to define many psychiatric symptoms in terms of neuroanatomical variations as well as changes in patterns of neural and neurochemical activity. The base from which we develop animal models of psychiatric symptoms is now substantially stronger. The confluence of human and nonhuman models can now be defined on the basis of structure as well as function. Animal models work best when they are integrated into experimental programs that involve studies with human populations. Neuroimaging provides the necessary link for this level of integration.

A final reason for optimism for the development of future animal models is that, to be honest, we have not really tried all that hard in the past. Although there are notable exceptions, animal models have been constructed in the absence of the relevant genetic or environmental conditions known to influence risk for mental illness. It is perhaps surprising that any useful models have emerged from the study of genetically low-risk animals housed in standard laboratory conditions, free from viral pathogens, hunger, social strife, and bill collectors. The potential to examine relevant genetically engineered animals living in more complex and challenging environments has yet to be fully explored. We must become more creative and adventuresome in our efforts to model the risks of the real world.

DIMENSIONAL APPROACHES IN PSYCHIATRY

It is obviously not the intent of this chapter to argue the merits of a categorical versus a dimensional approach for clinical psychiatry (see Chapter 3, "Categorical and Dimensional Models of Personality Disorders"). However, from the standpoint of a basic scientist, the dimensional approach offers advantages that are especially important for the study of personality disorders. For example, borderline personality disorder (BPD) appears to be composed of key psychobiological domains that include impulsive aggression associated with reduced serotonergic activity in the brain and affective instability (Siever and Davis 1991). BPD has been linked to personality traits such as neuroticism, impulsivity, anxiousness, affect lability, and insecure attachment. Specific features of BPD or its underlying traits can be studied in nonhuman populations, where they are represented on a continuum. Stable individual differences in nonhuman species can be defined for impulsivity, fearfulness, aggressivity, and so on (Suomi 1997; Westergaard et al. 2003). Although the measurement of personality in nonhuman species is not without some concern, it is substantially less arduous than attempting to bring to bear the definition of depression or anxiety. Individual features of personality can be operationally defined in nonhuman species, and such definitions can then be empirically compared in studies with humans.

As those concerned with the measurement of psychopathology will readily attest, categorical descriptions of mental illness are inferential even in humans. Whereas specific features of mood disorders, such as anhedonia or irritability, can be successfully measured in nonhuman species, models of entire disease syndromes will likely remain elusive. We are more successful when we examine specific features of a syndrome. Thus discussions of the relevant dimensions of psychopathology provide a far more productive conversation between behavioral neuroscientists and clinicians.

The advantages extend beyond such rather obvious considerations. There are no genes for mental health syndromes. Genes encode for proteins, not illnesses. Nor are there neural circuits for mental disorders. Pathology is inferred on the basis of the cognitive, emotional, and behavioral functions of the individual. Function, but not diagnosis, has a neural basis. Neural systems produce dysfunctional outcomes within specific domains, for example, impulse regulation and attention. The identification of the relevant domains for any particular illness is critical. Thus, the identification of relevant dimensions for psychopathology permits neuroscientists to examine the activity of specific neural pathways in relation to clinically relevant functions as opposed to more vague and heterogeneous categories. This focus is important not only for the development of animal models but also for the discovery of relevant variations in genotype. The dimensional approach permits researchers to focus on specific aspects of function and define relevant endophenotypes. These studies identify intermediate, high-risk phenotypes (New and Siever 2003). Taken together with advances in neuroimaging, a dimensional approach to psychopathology allows behavioral neuroscientists and molecular biologists to develop models that are based on precise measures of functions as well as on information concerning relevant neural and pharmacological substrates. Endophenotypes may be more precisely measured and may be more easily translated from animal to human (Nestler et al. 2002). It is reasonable to assume that the better the specification of the endophenotypes, the more realistic are the chances of defining the relevant genomic and neurobiological mechanisms.

Finally, dimensional approaches provide continuous measures that are correlated with clinical outcomes. Hence the relevance of animal studies becomes more obvious as the range of measures extends along a continuum of normal to abnormal function, rather than in cases where categories of pathology exist as independent entities. It is far more realistic to model variations in impulsivity in nonhuman species, which is nevertheless closely associated with antisocial and borderline personality, than to mimic the more extreme conditions of pathology. Moreover, the existing literature on the neuropharmacological mechanisms of many forms of emotional/cognitive function is formidable and provides a substantial base for the development of more sophisticated models with the advent of molecular technology (discussed later). These considerations also argue for greater communication between researchers examining personality in human populations and behavioral neuroscientists studying the issue of measurement.

NEUROIMAGING

Advances since the mid-1990s in imaging of the human brain provide a remarkable opportunity for the coordination of human and nonhuman models of behavior, emotion, and cognition. First, it is now possible to respond to the question often posed by clinicians of what studies with nonhuman species really tell us about the function of the human brain. In truth, such skepticism always rested on a rather tenuous understanding of biology and evolution. It would be difficult to understand how activity of the human brain in the service of emotional and cognitive processes that are common to mammalian species would differ greatly across species. Nevertheless, it is a source of comfort that neuroimaging studies of human populations have largely validated neural models derived from studies with primates and rodents. However, the real power of neuroimaging with human populations lies not simply in the discovery of brain structure–function relations. Often such studies largely recapitulate what is known from research with nonhuman species or neuropsychological assessments of various patient populations, such as lesion studies. The greater value of such approaches is the ability to understand how dynamic variations in neural activity and function relate to emotional and cognitive states and to behavior. For those interested in understanding the neural basis of behavior, the issue now is how best to coordinate studies of neural function with human and nonhuman models. A few examples reveal the potential for such an approach.

Neural Basis of Addiction

Animal models that focus on specific behavioral symptoms have been substantially more successful than attempts to model complex syndromes. One of the most useful models for the study of mood disorders has been that of anhedonia. The reward systems of the brain have been a major focus of research in behavioral neuroscience since the pioneering work of Olds and Milner (1954; also Olds 1955). These systems are known targets for all drugs of abuse, and the resulting activation of ascending catecholaminergic systems is considered a major substrate for addiction (Stewart 2003; Wise 2000). Such systems have also emerged as regulators of responses to natural reinforcers such as food or sex as well as nonpharmacologically based addictions such as gambling (Breiter et al. 2001; Everitt et al. 2001). The major focus of such studies has been the mesocorticolimbic dopamine system, which arises from the ventral tegmental region. Most notable are projections from the ventral tegmental area to the amygdala and nucleus accumbens as well as to the medial prefrontal cortex. This system is responsive to all major drugs of abuse and in rodent models is considered essential for the acquisition and maintenance of drug self-administration. Importantly, studies with rats established that all major drugs of abuse activate this pathway and that drug-seeking behavior is dependent on the dopamine release at the terminal regions of this projection. This topic is of particular relevance for the study of personality disorders, considering the common comorbidity between personality disorders, especially those marked by impulsivity and/or novelty-seeking, and substance abuse (see Chapter 30, "Substance Abuse").

Studies with human subjects, including addicts, reveal a remarkably similar neural circuit. Studies with addicts show that opioid-, cocaine-, and nicotine-related compounds activate the prefrontal cortex, largely anterior cingulated and orbitofrontal cortex, basal ganglia, and ventral tegmental area in humans (Breiter et al. 1997; see Daglish and Nutt 2003 for a review). Breiter et al. (1997) demonstrated a rapid "rush" following cocaine administration that was associated with activity of the ventral tegmental area and the basal forebrain. As in animal models, the hedonic value of the drug was associated with activity in structures along the mesocorticolimbic dopamine pathway. Moreover, the subjective experience of craving is associated with activity in the nucleus accumbens and amygdala. In rodents, exposure to cues previously associated with rewarding drugs comes to elicit activity in those same brain regions that respond to direct administration of the drug (Stewart 2003). Likewise, in human subjects, cues associated with psychostimulants activate the medial prefrontal cortex, nucleus accumbens, amygdala, and ventral tegmental area (see Daglish and Nutt 2003 for a review). As in the rat, the magnitude of drug effect, for example methylphenidate, is proportional to the increase in intrasynaptic dopamine as measured using positron emission tomography (PET) with the dopamine-2 receptor ligand, raclopride (Volkow et al. 1999).

These findings have greatly advanced our understanding of the neural basis of addiction in humans. Note, however, that such research was drawn directly from preclinical studies with rodents. Our ability to define neural systems that mediate behavior in nonhuman species forms scaffolding for studies with relevant human populations, but the utility of animal models is certainly not unique to the description of relevant neural systems. Indeed, the use of animal models is perhaps even more important for the definition of the various psychological components of complex behavioral and cognitive functions. Berridge and Robinson (2003) provided a wonderfully useful example with respect to the study of reward and drug-seeking behavior. As they described, drug-seeking behavior results as a function of at least two psychological processes: 1) *Learning:* what the individual knows about the drug or drug-related stimuli will direct behavior; such knowledge can emerge as a function of declarative- (conscious) or procedural- (habit) based forms of learning. 2) *Emotions:* Emotional and motivational processes influence goal-directed approach or avoidance; recent advances, much through the studies of Berridge and Robinson (2003), have provided compelling evidence for the distinction between "wanting" (motivational processes) and "liking" (emotional processes). The latter is commonly associated with hedonic reactions and "reward." Interestingly, dopamine, the neurotransmitter commonly associated with feelings of pleasure, is not necessary for "liking." Instead, the increased activity in the mesocorticolimbic dopamine system is more closely associated with the motivational state (wanting). Such findings are consistent with the studies using in vivo voltammetry to examine dynamic variations in dopamine signals in areas such as the nucleus accumbens over intervals as short as 1–2 seconds. The results of such studies reveal that increased dopamine release occurs prior to (i.e., in anticipation of) the delivery of the rewarding stimulus, and this response is true for food, sex, or drugs of abuse (Gratton and Wise 1994). Hence in studies with rats, "wanting" and "liking" can be dissociated on the basis of the relevant neural substrates.

Such findings prompted similar studies with humans. Thus Leyton et al. (2002) found that in human subjects dopamine activity in the accumbens-striatal system is better correlated with subjective feelings of craving or wanting than with sensations of pleasure.

In addition to the nucleus accumbens, other brain regions involved in the motivational circuit include the amygdala and the prefrontal cortex (Everitt and Wolf 2002). Interestingly, this same circuit is responsive to aversive stimuli, which was always a source of concern for those describing this system as a pleasure circuit. Stress activates dopamine release in the nucleus accumbens, amygdala, and medial prefrontal cortex in the rat (Stewart 2003) as well as in humans (Pruessner et al. 2004). Indeed, there is evidence for cross-sensitization of the corticolimbic dopamine system between stressors and, for example, psychostimulant drugs (Shaham et al. 2003). These findings underscore the importance of this system as a motivational network not solely dedicated to pleasurable events.

Humans, of course, process an enormous amount of information concerning hedonically relevant stimuli, and this process is reflected in the findings of increased activation of the cingulate cortex and orbitofrontal cortex by stimuli previously associated with a commonly self-administered drug. Feelings of "reward" are an emergent property of multiple psychological processes, any one of which can serve as the basis for individual differences in vulnerability for drug dependence. Similar processes can be modeled in the rat and provide evidence for cognitive representations of stimuli that produce "expectations" of outcomes based on learned contingencies (Balleine and Dickson 2000; Berridge and Robinson 2003). In the rat, such processes depend on activity in the medial prefrontal cortex.

These studies provide strong evidence for the importance of animal models. Clearly drug addiction is maintained by activity in multiple brain regions and occurs as an emergent property of multiple, diverse psychological processes. The virtue of animal models is not simply to define relevant neural systems but to be better able to parse the relevant psychological processes that underlie drug-seeking behavior. Understanding the individual components of such processes is critical for the development of effective treatments for addiction—especially true for psychologically as well as pharmacologically based interventions. The implications are certainly not unique to the study of drug addiction. Animals might, for example, demonstrate excessive, maladaptive levels of fear comparable to that of a patient with a generalized anxiety disorder, but for reasons that are completely different. The psychological process underlying the fear behavior of the rat may or may not be the same as that of the patient. Such information is critical in determining the utility of that particular model for examining the neurobiological basis of generalized anxiety disorder. Of course the origin of the anxiety disorder in these patients will vary, reflecting the importance of diagnosis and the definition of relevant subpopulations (see earlier discussion of the dimensional approach). Hence the development of effective research approaches in biological psychiatry requires a constant exchange of information between clinicians and neuroscientists (including researchers examining both human and nonhuman populations). This is precisely the level of interaction that is common at recent meetings such as that of the American College of Neuropsychopharmacology.

Fear/Anxiety

One of the most exciting areas of research in biological psychiatry since the mid-1990s has been in the study of fear and anxiety. This topic is of obvious importance for the study of the Cluster C personality disorders, the so-called anxious/fearful cluster. Two lines of research fuel such advances (Davidson et al. 1999). First is the description of the neural circuitry that mediates the expression of fear in rodents. Second is the emergence of neuroimaging studies of fear in human subjects. Again, what is particularly noteworthy is the degree to which advances in one area have served to direct the research in the other. This practice continues and forms the basis for the emerging discipline of affective neuroscience.

Studies of rodents provide a model for understanding how stimuli associated with aversive events are processed and stored in the brain (Cahill and McGaugh 1998; Davis and Whalen 2001; Davis et al. 1997; LeDoux 2000). These studies focus on the role of the amygdala and its anatomical extensions, notably the bed nucleus of the stria terminalis. The lateral and basolateral segments of the amygdala are essential in processing the relevant sensory input and for the establishment of "emotional memories." A crucial extension of this model has emerged from the studies of Davis and colleagues (Davis and Whalen 2001; Davis et al. 1997), revealing the differences in the function of the amygdala and the bed nucleus of the stria terminalis in states of "fear" versus "anxiety." Interestingly, so-called stress hormones, the glucocorticoids and norepinephrine, serve to facilitate the recall of information associated with aversive events (Cahill and McGaugh 1998). These effects contrast with the inhibitory effects of glucocorticoids on hippocampal function and declarative memory formation in both human and nonhuman species (Lupien and Meaney 1998).

The basic elements of this model have been replicated in studies with human populations. Emotionally adverse stimuli activate the human amygdala. Indeed, the degree of amygdaloid activation is highly correlated ($r = 0.93$) with recall of emotionally disturbing, but not neutral, material. Using fMRI, LaBar et al. (1995) found increased amygdala activity during the acquisition phase of fear conditioning, and patients with amygdala damage show profound deficits in fear conditioning (Bechara et al. 1995; LaBar et al. 1998). Interestingly, individual differences in the degree of amygdaloid activation occurring during fear conditioning were highly correlated with the strength of a conditioned autonomic fear response (Furmark et al. 1997). Moreover, stress hormones also facilitate the establishment of emotional memories in humans as well as rodents, and the critical site of action lies in the amygdala (Cahill and McGaugh 1998).

Studies of blood flow and metabolism as well as fMRI reveal a common pattern of decreased activation of the prefrontal cortex–cingulate gyrus and increased amygdala activity in patients with mood disorders (Davidson et al. 1999). Amygdaloid dysfunction is associated with both anxiety and depression (Drevets et al. 1997), and amygdaloid activity in PET scans, particularly in the right amygdala, is strongly correlated with negative affect (Abercrombie et al. 1998). PET studies indicate that right amygdala blood flow is increased in patients with posttraumatic stress disorder (Rauch et al. 1996; Shin et al. 1997). Importantly, the reciprocal dysfunction in the prefrontal cortex–amygdala is normalized with successful treatment of the mood disorder (Mayberg et al. 1997). Such findings serve as the basis for a renewed interest among neuroscientists in the circuitry that connects regions commonly thought to be involved in mood disorders, notably the hippocampus, amygdala, and medial prefrontal cortex.

Advances in the understanding of the pharmacological bases of mental illness are more challenging due to the obstacles associated with ligand development for PET studies. Nevertheless, important findings here have served as the platform for some of the most exciting research in molecular neuroscience. For example, studies with humans support the idea that alterations in the $GABA_A$/benzodiazepine receptor complex might form the basis for individual differences in vulnerability for anxiety disorders. Unmedicated patients with a history of panic disorder show a significant decrease in labeling of the benzodiazepine receptor antagonist [11C]flumazenil in the orbitoprefrontal cortex and amygdala/hippocampal region in PET studies (Malizia et al. 1998). The findings are consistent with those of pharmacological measures of benzodiazepine receptor sensitivity. Subjects high on measures of neuroticism, a trait that is common among patients with personality disorders, show reduced sensitivity to the benzodiazepine receptor agonist midazolam (Glue et al. 1995). Roy-Byrne et al. (1990, 1996) found reduced sensitivity to diazepam in patients with panic disorders and proposed that the reduced benzodiazepine receptor sensitivity was related to anxiety. Patients with panic attacks or high levels of general anxiety show decreased sensitivity to benzodiazepine-induced amnesia, sedation, and dampening of noradrenergic function compared with control subjects (Melo de Paula 1977; Oblowitz and Robins 1983). These findings are at least consistent with the idea that decreased benzodiazepine binding levels in critical sites, such as the amygdala, are related to increased vulnerability to anxiety disorders (Gorman et al. 2000).

These findings, together with the well-defined anxiolytic effects of benzodiazepine agonists, have inspired studies on the molecular basis of $GABA_A$/benzodiazepine receptor function in rodents (McKernan and Whiting 1997). Predictably, behavioral responses to stress are inhibited by benzodiazepines, which exert their potent anxiolytic effect by enhancing GABA-mediated Cl currents through $GABA_A$ receptors (McKernan and Whiting 1997; Mehta and Ticku 1999). Benzodiazepine receptor agonists exert anxiolytic effects via their actions at a number of limbic areas depending on the test conditions. However, to date the evidence is perhaps strongest for effects at the level of the basolateral complex of the amygdala, comprising the lateral, basal, and anterior basal nuclei (Pitkanen et al. 1997) and the central nucleus of the amygdala. Direct administration of benzodiazepines into the basolateral or central regions of the amygdala yields an anxiolytic effect.

The $GABA_A$ receptor complex in the rat brain, which often includes a benzodiazepine binding site, is most commonly arranged in a pentameric structure—essentially five proteins clustered together to form a single, functional membrane receptor that binds GABA and regulates Cl permeability across the cell membrane. The $GABA_A$ receptor is thus composed of α, β, and γ subunits in the form of two α, two β, and one γ subunit or of two α, one β, and two γ subunits (McKernan and Whiting 1997; Mehta and Ticku 1999). The α subunit forms the GABA binding site, and the interface between the α and γ subunits appears to form the benzodiazepine receptor site. $GABA_A$ receptor activity is allosterically regulated by compounds acting at benzodiazepine receptor sites. Interestingly, dynamic variations in $GABA_A$ receptor function often

occur as a result of such allosteric modulation of the $GABA_A$ receptor, including, of course, actions at the benzodiazepine site. These findings have led to a focus on the α and γ subunits that form the benzodiazepine receptor. Point mutations in either subunit are sufficient to eliminate benzodiazepine receptor binding, and animals bearing a null mutation of the γ_2 subunit show approximately an 85% loss of $[^3H]$flunitrazepam binding (Gunther et al. 1995). Perhaps some of the strongest evidence linking differences in the expression of the $GABA_A$ receptor subunits and those in fear conditioning comes from studies of animals bearing a null mutation of the γ_2 subunit ($\gamma_2-/-$). Predictably, these animals show very significantly reduced benzodiazepine receptor binding and increased fear-conditioned freezing as well as conditioned inhibitory avoidance (Crestani et al. 1999). What makes these animals so interesting is the remarkable phenotype of the heterozygotes ($\gamma_2+/-$). By comparison with the wild-type ($\gamma_2+/+$) mouse, the $\gamma_2+/-$ animals also show significantly decreased $[^3H]$flunitrazepam binding and increased fearfulness under conditions of novelty as well as enhanced fear conditioning. The results with the heterozygotes are intermediate between those of the wild type and homozygous ($-/-$) animals, suggesting a gene–dosage effect. These animals represent a model of genetic vulnerability (i.e., the γ_2- allele) for high trait anxiety.

One approach to the development of preclinical models with human or nonhuman populations is to focus on factors that are involved in the etiology of human psychiatric disorders. The quality of early family life influences the risk for anxiety disorders. Individuals experiencing parental loss or divorce before the age of 10 as well as victims of abuse are at a seven-times greater risk for anxiety disorders in adulthood. Indeed, the maternal care score on the Parental Bonding Index is significantly correlated with state anxiety in young adults (Pruessner et al. 2004). Evidence from clinical studies is at least consistent with the idea that variation in the $GABA_A$/benzodiazepine receptor system in the amygdala predisposes individuals to anxiety disorders (Gorman et al. 2000). Recent studies with rodents suggest that variations in parental care over the first week of life permanently alter the expression of genes that encode for various $GABA_A$/benzodiazepine receptor subunits and thus alter $GABA_A$/benzodiazepine receptor function. The adult offspring of mothers that exhibit increased pup licking show enhanced expression of the α_1 and γ of the GABAA/benzodiazepine receptor compared with those reared by low-licking mothers; these differences are reversed with cross-fostering

(Caldji et al. 2003). The $\alpha_1\gamma_2$ confer increased sensitivity to benzodiazepine agonists, and thus these effects could serve as the basis for an environmentally determined individual difference in $GABA_A$/benzodiazepine receptor function.

Individual Differences

The issue of development of such individual differences in neural function and personality is seminal for the study of personality. Two points are worth noting in the present context. First, individual differences in personality can be meaningfully studied in relation to neural substrates. In an exhaustive study, Pujol et al. (2002) correlated variations in anterior cingulate gyrus morphometry to scores on the Temperament and Character Inventory. Anatomical asymmetry was prevalent, confirming earlier electroencephalographic studies (Davidson et al. 1999), and it was demonstrable in 83% of the subjects. Surface area of the right anterior cingulate gyrus accounted for 24% of the variance in the harm avoidance measure. Men and women with larger right anterior cingulated gyrus or with increased right prefrontal electroencephalogram results tend to describe themselves as worriers, more fearful, shy, and easily fatigued (Davidson et al. 1999; Pujol et al. 2002). Larger surface area of the left anterior cingulated or greater electroencephalographic results is associated with extraversion and sociability. Likewise, individual differences in stress reactivity and perhaps even their developmental origins can be examined with neuroimaging technology. Pruessner et al. (2004) found that dopamine responses to stress in the nucleus accumbens, as well as cortisol release, were strongly correlated ($r>0.6$) with ratings on questionnaire measures of maternal care.

Kalin et al. (1998) provided compelling evidence for similar relations between prefrontal structure/activity and individual differences in personality in the rhesus monkey. There are stable individual differences in asymmetries in prefrontal electroencephalogram in the rhesus monkey. As in humans, macaques with increased prefrontal electroencephalographic activity in the right hemisphere exhibit increased fearfulness (Kalin et al. 1998). In humans and macaques, increased activity in the right prefrontal cortex is associated with elevated cortisol levels suggestive of increased hypothalamic-pituitary-adrenal (HPA) activity. Consistent with this finding, monkeys with right-biased prefrontal electroencephalographic activity show increased cerebrospinal fluid levels of corticotropin-releasing factor (CRF).

Stable individual differences in behavior and neuroendocrine function are well established in the rat. The extensive studies by Piazza and LeMoal (1996) revealed stable individual differences in behavior that predict function outcomes. Perhaps the most successful rodent model of individual differences is based on stable differences in locomotor activity in a novel environment. The model addresses a crucially important feature of individual differences in vulnerability for drug abuse: Whereas many individuals experiment with drugs, only a few develop true addictions. Such individual differences are also apparent in populations of experimental animals, such as the rat (Piazza and LeMoal 1996). Animals that exhibit spontaneous hyperactivity in novel test environments show greater amphetamine-induced increases in nucleus accumbens dopamine release, and this characteristic is glucocorticoid dependent. This finding laid the foundation for studies focusing on such behavioral responses to novelty to define high-responsive and low-responsive animals. The inhibition of glucocorticoid secretion eliminates the difference in nucleus accumbens dopamine release in low- and high-responsive animals (Piazza and LeMoal 1996; Piazza et al. 1996). Finally, under normal conditions, spontaneously hyperactive high-responsive animals show increased adrenal glucocorticoid responses to acute or chronic stress (Piazza et al. 1991). Stimulant self-administration is attenuated following destruction of ascending dopamine pathways or treatment with dopamine receptor antagonists. Moreover, group differences in dopamine responses to stimulants or stressors are associated with differences in the degree to which animals develop stimulant dependence (Piazza and LeMoal 1996). It is important to note the degree to which the fundamental elements of the Piazza model have been replicated in neuroimaging studies of human addiction.

These findings support the idea that stable individual differences in selected traits can be meaningful models in nonhuman species. The information to be gleaned from such efforts increases markedly when the functional model maps onto established individual differences in humans. Tests such as HPA activity, fear-potentiated startle, attentional tests, and prepulse inhibition are some of the obvious candidates for exploitation. There will be no single, simple model of human traits and vulnerability. Simpler tests, such as the Prosolt swim test, that are amenable to high-throughput analysis bear an important limitation: we have little or no idea what psychological processes are actually studied in such tests! More informative models derive from basic research in behavioral neuroscience and neuroendocrinology. Such models examine fundamental elements of behavior and biology that are common across multiple mammalian species (e.g., attentional processes, fear conditioning). Studies on the neural basis of such functions as well as on the origins and significance of individual differences will prove invaluable in defining the direction of studies with human populations and in defining casual relations, an issue of particular importance for studies that attempt to define the developmental origins of individual differences in personality and health.

MODELS OF VULNERABILITY BASED ON GENE–ENVIRONMENT INTERACTIONS

A journalist once asked Donald Hebb (1904–1985) what, in his view, was more important for the development of personality: nature or nurture? Hebb responded that to ask which factor lent more to development was akin to asking what contributes more to the area of a rectangle, the length or the width? The nature–nurture debate is essentially an argument about the relative contribution of genetics versus environment. Molecular biology illustrates the futility of any perspective that treats gene and environment as independent entities. Rather, phenotype emerges from a lifelong developmental process that is, at all times, the product of continuous gene–environment interactions. The genome is a dynamic entity, the structure and activity of which is continuously subject to environmental regulation. Recent developments in molecular genetics reveal that DNA operates within a highly dynamic chromatin environment that actively determines the process of gene expression. The nature of chromatin structure is, in turn, shaped by environmental influences. Indeed, the highly modifiable histone proteins that furnish the bulk of the chromatin milieu may be considered a crucial interface between the fixed genome and the dynamic environment. At the same time, genomic variations influence the individual's response to environmental events through variations in the function of cells that process sensory information, as well as through an influence on temperament and other traits. Gene and environment are biologically inseparable.

Vulnerability for psychiatric illness, like any form of chronic illness, emerges as the result of continuous gene–environment interactions through development and into adulthood. Epidemiological studies reveal specific environmental events or genetic variations that increase the statistical probability of specific forms of illness. Yet it is clear that the net result is a probability that falls well short of certainty. Even where genomic inheritance is clearly influential, the variation in predicted outcomes is considerable. Individuals with a schizophrenic identical twin are still only about 40%–45% likely to develop the illness. The figure is less still for depression and substance abuse, and lower yet for anxiety disorders. Yet obviously such risks are well above those in the normal population. So where does this leave us? From the perspective of the individual, what does it mean to carry a 30% risk for depression? What are the factors that determine health outcomes under conditions of inherited risk? How does genetic variation interact with environmental conditions to influence the development and health of the individual? How do macrovariables, such as socioeconomic factors, so potently influence the risk for chronic illness, and why are some individuals so much more affected by environmental adversity than others? What is actually meant by gene–environment interactions, how do they occur, and what do they imply in terms of clinical interventions? The challenge is to identify the pathways by which specific risk factors lead to illness.

Advances in genomics are critical. Analyses of single nucleotide polymorphisms (SNPs) permit the association of specific genomic variants with health outcomes. Such studies also provide viable genomic targets for studies of gene expression: How might environmental factors regulate the expression of the genes implicated through SNP analysis? We can work from the other direction. Epidemiological studies serve to identify relevant environmental risk factors. Neuroimaging studies provide structural correlates of disease states. The question then becomes whether the environmental events might alter gene expression within the relevant neural structures and whether such effects are more apparent in one genotype than another: might a specific polymorphism render the gene more or less vulnerable to environmental regulation? Gene expression arrays that examine the activity of literally thousands of targets, although still in need of optimization, are designed to address such issues. The results provide an obvious target for studies on the mechanism of specific and relevant forms of gene–environment interactions.

The gene–environment approach may appear to some as the ideal or as only one approach. I would argue that to pursue animal models of chronic illness in the absence of a gene–environment approach is naïve in the extreme. Indeed, I think that the dismay that is often expressed by those examining either genomic *or* environmental determinants of health is due not to the impotence of individual factors but to our failure to examine these factors in the relevant context. The effects of genomic variation on phenotype are, in most cases, contextually dependent. Some might argue that the identification of the polymorphism in the serotonin transporter, as an example, accounts for only about 3%–5% of the variance in predicting the probability of depression in the general population. Yet the general population does not live under circumstances that constantly promote the development of depression. Those who do are inevitably the victims of circumstances that extend beyond the presence of a single polymorphism. It may well be that the influence of the genomic variation is fully appreciated only under specific environmental conditions: the effects of certain polymorphisms may be unique to individuals living under conditions of severe adversity. Indeed, the scientific evidence from studies of serotonin transporter mutations with human or nonhuman populations support this contention.

In humans, a length variation (long vs. short) in the promoter region of the serotonin transporter (5-HTT) is associated with anxiety, depression, and aggressivity (Lesch et al. 1996). Such variation is associated with a common 44-base pair insertion/deletion polymorphism in the promoter region of the serotonin transporter (5-HTTPR) resulting in short (*S) and long (*L) variants. The 5-HTTPR polymorphism is associated with effects on 5-HTT mRNA expression in brain, 5-HTT binding, and serotonin (5-HT) reuptake (Holmes et al. 2003). The 5-HTTPR polymorphism has also been associated with individual differences in personality, such as neuroticism and harm avoidance, and an increased risk for alcoholism as well as mood and anxiety disorders.

Earlier studies (see Owens and Nemeroff 1998 for a review) provided a link between mood disorders and 5-HTT binding in platelets and brain. Hariri et al. (2002) found that the 5-HTTPR polymorphism was associated with differences in the magnitude of limbic activation in response to emotional provocation. Individuals bearing one or two copies of the *5-HTTPR*S* allele exhibit greater amygdala neuronal activation in responses to fearful stimuli than individuals homozygous for the *5-HTTPR*L* allele. These findings suggest that a genomically based alteration in 5-HTT gene expression might underlie an increased vulnerability for specific forms of psychopathology. However, such studies are inherently correlational. To better define the relation between 5-HTT gene expression and be-

havioral phenotype, researchers developed a 5-HTT knockout mouse model (a knockout model is a genetically engineered strain in which a specific genomic target has been rendered dysfunctional through targeted mutation). Importantly, subsequent studies with the null mutant (*5-HTT*–/–) reveal abnormalities in fear behavior, sleep, activity, and hormonal stress responses that are strikingly similar to the clinical features of mood and anxiety disorders (see Holmes et al. 2003). The results of the knockout studies would seem to suggest a causal relation between the 5-HTT genomic variant and mood and anxiety states.

However, as is commonly the case, failures to replicate the original results of the 5-HTT gene linkage studies (see Furlong et al. 1998 and Veenstra-Vander-Weele et al. 2000 for reviews) suggest a more modest overall effect of the 5-HTT genotype. Such findings are common and perhaps expected in dealing with complex, non-Mendelian disorders. The common conclusion is that specific polymorphisms add "small effects" to such complex syndromes. Yet this somewhat peculiarly additive approach is likely a misleading assessment of the importance of the 5-HTTPR variant. A remarkably relevant animal model has proved invaluable in providing clarity.

A comparable 5-HTTPR variant is found in rhesus monkeys, and as in humans, transcriptional activity associated with the longer variant of the promoter is greater than that driven by the shorter variant (Bennett et al. 2002). In humans, the shorter variant is also associated with decreased 5-HT uptake into lymphocytes and decreased 5-HT mRNA in brain (Little et al. 1998). In the rhesus monkey the 5-HTTPR variants are associated with differences in 5-HT synthesis and metabolism as indicated by 5-hydroxyindoleacetic acid (5-HIAA) measures in cerebrospinal fluid samples. However, the effect is dependent on the rearing environment (Bennett et al. 2002). Regardless of 5-HTTPR genotype, monkeys reared with their mothers do not differ in cerebrospinal fluid levels of 5-HIAA. Monkeys reared in nurseries show very significant impairments in serotonin metabolism. A similar pattern of results emerged in studies of infant temperament (Champoux et al. 2002). These findings reveal environmentally dependent effects of genotype in the rhesus monkey.

Caspi et al. (2003) provided evidence for a comparable gene–environment interaction in humans. A prospective study of the Dunedin Multidisciplinary Health and Development Study cohort revealed that the 5-HTTPR polymorphism mediated the influence of stressful life events on the probability of depression.

Among the cohort as a whole, the number of stressful life events increased the probability of self-reported or confirmed depressive episodes. However, this effect was almost entirely accounted for by individuals bearing one or two copies of the *5-HTTPR*S* allele. Among subjects homozygous for the *5-HTTPR*L* allele, there was little or no effect of stressful life events on the probability of depression. Likewise, the effect of maltreatment in childhood was apparent only in those with the *5-HTTPT*S/*S* or *S/*L* genotype; there was no effect of childhood adversity on individuals with the *5-HTTPR *L/*L* genotype.

These findings reflect the gene–environment interactions previously described in the primate model. Of course, similar comments could be made concerning the potential for gene–gene interactions (see Chapter 9, "Genetics"). The alterations in phenotype associated with the 5-HTT knockout in the mouse depend on the genomic background. Mice strains differ in genotype, by definition, as well as phenotype. Interestingly, there are considerable strain differences in fearfulness, and such differences predict the effect associated with genomic disruption of the 5-HTT gene. The 5-HTT knockout produced against a C57BL/6J background produces significant effects on fear behavior that is not apparent when the same construct is employed using a 129S6 strain (Holmes et al. 2003). There is no effect of the 5-HTT knockout on anxiety-like behavior in the 129S6 strain. There are differences in fear behavior in the C57 and 129S6 strains that might mask or otherwise influence the effects of the 5-HTT null mutation; under normal conditions, C57 mice are markedly less fearful than are 129S6 animals. Alternatively, the genomic background might provide a basis for different forms of gene–gene interactions that altered the phenotype associated with the 5-HTT mutation. Gene–gene interactions appear to moderate the effects of specific polymorphisms in human populations. Ebstein et al. (1998) found a highly significant effect of the dopamine receptor 4 (*DRD4*) repeat variant on infant temperament, with 2-month-olds bearing *DRD4* short variants showing more negative emotion than those bearing a longer number of repeats. Interestingly, this association was *only* apparent among children bearing the short variant of the 5-HTTPR gene (Arbelle et al. 2003; Auerbach et al. 1999). Among children with the longer version of the 5-HTTPR gene, the variants on the *DRD4* gene were inconsequential with respect to temperament. Interestingly, variants in the *DRD4* gene are also associated with attachment behavior in the Stranger Situation Test at 1 year of age (Lakatos et al. 2000). Such effects are apparent even in a nonclinical, low-risk population and

speak to the potential importance of gene–gene interactions. Certainly direct interactions between central dopamine and serotonin systems are well known, and it is not difficult to imagine that variation in the respective gene products might alter both dopaminergic and serotonergic systems. However, it is also important to note that embedded with such interactions are gene–environment effects. Certainly infants with more negative emotion or those who differ in attachment elicit differential parenting. The early appearance of the functional correlates of these genetic variants underscores the potential gene–environment interactions. Such differences in infant temperament might well be associated with variations in parental care such that an apparent gene–gene interaction is actually a gene–gene–environment interaction. An example of such interactions emerges from nonhuman primate studies (Bennett et al. 2002; Suomi 1997). Rhesus monkeys show the same 5-HTTP polymorphism, with strong linkage to temperament and stress reactivity, as well as evidence for effects of central 5-HT activity. However, animals bearing the short variant of the 5-HTTP gene but reared by highly nurturing mothers do not differ from animals with the long 5-HTTP variant on measures of temperament, stress reactivity, or 5-HT function. It can get complicated.

Such findings might serve as a profound source of discouragement. How might we ever clearly define the relevant gene–environment events that mediate vulnerability to psychopathology? Here, of course, is the importance of animal models. Yet to be relevant, such models must begin to incorporate the level of sophistication revealed in the previous discussion. The wonderful studies of Suomi (1997) and Higley et al. (1991) with the rhesus monkey demonstrated one of the rare examples of an animal model that respects the importance of gene–environment interactions. Woefully, despite the remarkable appeal of gene–environment interactions, we are generally in a poor position to study such events even with rodent models—and not for lack of molecular tools. The primary molecular focus for gene–environment studies lies in the area of gene expression. The logical targets for such studies are the regulatory DNA regions (promoters, enhancers, suppressors) that direct the expression of the coding genes. The cloning of even longer regulatory sequences is remarkably simple by comparison with the state of affairs as recent as 10 years ago. Chromatin immunoprecipitation assays permit researchers to describe protein–DNA interactions under physiologically and behaviorally relevant conditions. Protein biochemistry has advanced to the point where very specific alterations in single amino acids can define the essential conditions for protein–DNA and protein–protein interactions.

Perhaps one of the most important advances for neuroscience is the emergence of gene expression arrays that permit researchers to evaluate changes in mRNA levels across a wide range of genes. Sensitivity remains an issue at this point in the development of array technology, and this situation is particularly troubling for neuroscientists who wish to examine somewhat more subtle changes in discrete brain regions. However, these problems will be resolved with increased sensitivity and better methods to amplify signals from smaller tissue samples. Moreover, the development of behavioral tests has improved greatly over the past decade, especially in rat models. The comparative approach advocated earlier has resulted in a number of models in which testing procedures and, presumably, relevant neural circuits are examined in much the same way across rodents and humans. Examples involve attentional tests (Robbins 2001), spatial learning and memory, sensory-gating with prepulse inhibition (Swerdlow et al. 2001), fear conditioning (LeDoux 2000), and fear-potentiated startle (Davis and Whalen 2001). Certainly tests unique to rodents can be of considerable value, but in the hunt for relevant gene products it is comforting to have the face validity offered by testing procedures that can be used across multiple species.

Indeed, the major obstacle to vastly improved animal models lies not in biochemistry or test procedures but in simple animal husbandry. The embarrassing truth is that we examine gene–environment interactions in a complex, social species like the rat that is housed for its entire life in an 18 cm × 30 cm plastic cage. Some environment! If indeed we buy into the idea that behavior emerges as a function of genotype and prevailing environmental conditions, then it is difficult to understand how we are to truly advance our understanding of gene–environment interactions under housing conditions as uniformly insipid as those in use in modern animal research facilities. Even reasonably modest attempts at replicating some of the relevant conditions of normal social life for rats reveal a remarkable range of behavior and health outcomes. This point has long been championed by Blanchard and Blanchard (2003), who have developed a "visual burrow system" that measures only 1 m × 1 m but permits wonderfully intricate social interactions and the emergence of easily defined dominance hierarchies. The impact of housing under such conditions for periods as short as 14 days can completely alter neuroendocrine function, leading to a loss of the HPA response to stress in certain subordinates. Such phenotypes are never apparent among animals housed in pairs in small "shoebox" cages. One can only imagine the richness of a gene–environment model that examines changes in gene expression over time in the visual burrow system in relation to such fundamental modifications in phenotype. The reemerging interest in environmental enrichment and the molecular mechanisms underlying enrichment-induced synaptic outgrowth (Kempermann et al. 1997) further argue for more creative animal housing conditions. Considering the remarkably rich behavioral repertoire of the highly social rat (Calhoun 1962), the potential for gene–environment studies with this species has barely been realized (ask those who own these animals as pets).

ANIMAL MODELS OF MACROVARIABLES

Advances in epidemiology reveal the potent influence of social and economic factors on health. Health is socially and economically defined. The incidence of many forms of chronic illness, including arthritis, diabetes, heart disease, and depression, is several-fold higher in economically disadvantaged populations, and the trend is apparent throughout the Western world. Such findings are often hastily translated into major policy initiatives. Unfortunately, only in rare cases are such policy decisions based on a clear understanding of the mechanisms that link such social and environmental factors with health outcomes. The risk is that of developing expensive interventions that fail to target critical processes or appropriate populations. Indeed, the issues here are comparable with those that emerge from the Human Genome Project, because the genetic and the epidemiological approaches bear the same limitation; both are inherently correlational. The challenge is to functionally link high-risk socioeconomic conditions to health and thus understand the pathways by which relevant gene–environment interactions lead to disease. This approach is fundamental to understanding individual differences in vulnerability and resistance to disease.

Nowhere is the interplay between genes and environment more evident than in the relationships that exist between family environment and vulnerability or resistance to chronic illness. The quality of family life influences health over the lifespan and is itself a product of social and economic forces. Thus, low socioeconomic status and poor mental health of the parents both predict patterns of parent–child interactions that promote vulnerability to illness. As adults, victims of childhood abuse, emotional neglect, family conflict, and conditions of harsh, inconsistent discipline are at significantly greater risk for mental illness including personality disorders as well as for obesity, diabetes, and heart disease. These conditions also compromise intellectual development such that the cost to society and the individual is reflected in diminished human potential.

Recent studies on the topics of "environmental programming" of gene expression provide an understanding of the mechanisms by which parental care can directly influence function. In rodents, maternal care directly activates the expression of genes that encode for neurotrophic factors, increasing synaptic development in the neocortex and permanently altering the capacity for learning and memory (Bredy et al. 2003; Liu et al. 2000). The expression of genes that regulate fat and glucose metabolism in the offspring is permanently influenced by maternal conditions such as nutritional deprivation and stress during fetal life, thus affecting the likelihood of diabetes and hypertension (Seckl 2004). In rodent and primate models, environmental adversity compromises mother–infant interactions that, in turn, result in sustained changes in the expression of genes that regulate endocrine, behavioral, and autonomic responses to stress. Moreover, because mother–infant interactions influence the development of individual differences in the female offspring, the effects of environmental adversity can be transmitted from parent to child through nongenomic mechanisms (Francis et al. 1999; Meaney 2001). Obviously, the poor mental health of the parents can reflect the influence of genetic factors that predispose for depression, drug abuse, and anxiety. The transmission of the high-risk condition from parent to offspring occurs at multiple and converging levels. This bidirectionality defies any simple solution and begs for studies of mechanism. How does stress affect parental behavior? How do variations in parent–child interactions promote changes in organ function? Are such changes linked to altered patterns of gene expression, and if so, how are changes in gene expression sustained throughout life? Why are some individuals more affected by environmental adversity than others? Do such interactions reflect the importance of the genome in determining sensitivity to environmental events? If so, what do such gene–environment interactions imply for current methods employed in genetic epidemiology? The answers to such questions will define the relevant gene–environment interactions that underlie vulnerability and resistance for chronic ill-

ness and identify critical targets for intervention programs. These are issues that must be addressed in the next generation of animal models, and such models should then serve to guide the direction and design of human studies. The issue of variation among individuals in response to environmental events as a function of genotype (see Caspi et al. 2003 for a recent and compelling example) can be addressed using genetically engineered animals housed in complex and varied environmental conditions. Yet few, if any, such studies have been undertaken. Moreover, if we are to establish meaningful animal models, the level of environmental manipulations must become more sophisticated and better reflect the social and economic reality of life.

Perhaps the most compelling evidence for this process emerges from the studies of Rosenblum, Coplan, and colleagues (Coplan et al. 1996, 1998; Rosenblum and Andrews 1994). Bonnet macaque mother–infant dyads were maintained under one of three foraging conditions: low foraging demand, where food was readily available; high foraging demand, where ample food was available but required long periods of searching; and variable foraging demand, a mixture of the two conditions on a schedule that did not allow for predictability. At the time that these conditions were imposed, there were no differences in the nature of mother–infant interactions. However, after a number of months of these conditions there were highly significant differences in mother–infant interactions. The variable condition was clearly the most disruptive (Rosenblum and Andrews 1994): mother–infant conflict increased, and infants of mothers housed under these conditions were significantly more timid and fearful. They showed signs of depression commonly observed in maternally separated macaque infants, even while in contact with their mothers. As adolescents, the infants reared in the variable conditions were more fearful and submissive and showed less social play behavior.

More recent studies have demonstrated the effects of these conditions on the development of neural systems that mediate behavioral and endocrine response to stress. As adults, monkeys reared under variable foraging demand conditions showed increased cerebrospinal fluid levels of CRF (Coplan et al. 1996, 1998). Increased central CRF drive would suggest altered noradrenergic and serotonergic responses to stress, and this stress response is exactly what was seen in adolescent variable foraging demand–reared animals.

These remarkable studies reveal a direct effect of experimental manipulations that vary the availability of economic resources on parent–infant interactions and their consequences for development. Indeed, the literature in behavioral ecology is replete with examples of the effects of "economic" factors on the biology and social organization of a wide range of species (Krebs and Davies 1991). Such factors can be modeled in the laboratory setting but will require the cooperation of veterinary medicine and a willingness to abandon easy and convenient methods of animal husbandry. The study of animals housed under conditions of environmental enrichment reveals the potent effects of environmental complexity on gene expression and behavior (Kempermann et al. 1997) and suggests that if we can indeed become more creative in such matters, the scientific information to be gleaned will allow us to begin to address the complex issues outlined above.

CONCLUSIONS

With recent advances in genetics and molecular biology, the level of research questions has become substantially more sophisticated and complex. If animal models are to become more relevant to the study of mental health, they will need to become more creative, and testing paradigms will need to better map onto human psychological function. Since the 1990s, there has been considerable improvement with respect to the latter. Neuroimaging studies provide an understanding of the neural systems mediating social, cognitive, and emotional function in humans and thus a broader basis for translational research across species. Experimental models of attention processes and fear, to name but a few, have improved, and in many cases the same testing procedures are used in human and nonhuman species. These advances have emerged from a closer working relationship between clinical psychiatrists and behavioral neuroscientists, with neuroimaging techniques often forming the common ground. However, where we continue to lag is in the area of gene–environment studies. Here the challenges are daunting. However, molecular biology has provided the tools by which such research might be pursued. We can now clearly define and manipulate specific genomic targets with the use of conditional knockouts in which genomic targets are disrupted in certain regions of the central nervous system at specific stages in development. Personality and thus personality-based disorders emerge as a function of complex gene–environment interactions. The challenge for those working with animal models is to understand how such interactions produce these stable individual differences in psychological function. If animal models are to remain relevant, this challenge cannot be ignored. As the examples cited above should indicate, this problem will not be amendable to quick, high-throughput solutions.

REFERENCES

Abercrombie HC, Schaefer SM, Larson CL, et al: Metabolic rate in the right amygdala predicts negative affect in depressed patients. Neuroreport 9:3301–3307, 1998

Arbelle S, Benjamin J, Golin M, et al: Relation of shyness in grade school children to the genotype for the long form of the serotonin transporter promoter region polymorphism. Am J Psychiatry 160:671–676, 2003

Auerbach J, Geller V, Lezer S, et al: Dopamine D4 receptor (D4DR) and serotonin transporter promoter (5-HTTLPR) polymorphisms in the determination of temperament in 2-month-old infants. Mol Psychiatry 4:369–373, 1999

Balleine BW, Dickson A: The effects of lesions of the insular cortex on instrumental conditioning: evidence for a role in incentive memory. J Neurosci 20:8954–8964, 2000

Bechara A, Tranel D, Damasio H, et al: Double dissociation of conditioning and declarative knowledge relative to the amygdala and hippocampus in humans. Science 269:1115–1118, 1995

Bennett AJ, Lesch KP, Heils A, et al: Early experience and serotonin transporter gene variation interact to influence primate CNS function. Mol Psychiatry 7:118–122, 2002

Berridge KC, Robinson TE: Parsing reward. Trends Neurosci 26:507–513, 2003

Blanchard RJ, Blanchard DC: Bringing natural behaviors into the laboratory: a tribute to Paul MacLean. Physiol Behav 79:515–524, 2003

Bredy TW, Diorio J, Grant R, et al: Maternal care influences hippocampal neuron survival in the rat. Eur J Neurosci 18:2903–2909, 2003

Breiter HC, Gollub RL, Weisskoff RM, et al: Acute effects of cocaine on human brain activity and emotion. Neuron 19:591–611, 1997

Breiter HC, Aharon I, Kahneman D, et al: Functional imaging of neural responses to expectancy and experience of monetary gains and losses. Neuron 30:619–639, 2001

Cahill L, McGaugh JL: Mechanisms of emotional arousal and lasting declarative memory. Trends Neurosci 21:294–299, 1998

Caldji C, Diorio J, Meaney MJ: Variations in maternal care alter $GABA_A$ receptor subunit expression in brain regions associated with fear. Neuropsychopharmacology 28:150–159, 2003

Calhoun JB: The Ecology and Sociology of the Norway Rat. Bethesda, MD, H.E.W. Public Health Service, 1962

Caspi A, Sugden K, Moffitt TE, et al: Influence of life stress on depression: moderation by a polymorphism in the 5-HTT gene. Science 301:386–390, 2003

Champoux M, Bennett A, Shannon C, et al: Serotonin transporter gene polymorphism, differential early rearing, and behavior in rhesus monkey neonates. Mol Psychiatry 7:1058–1063, 2002

Coplan JD, Andrews MW, Rosenblum LA, et al: Persistent elevations of cerebrospinal fluid concentrations of corticotropin-releasing factor in adult nonhuman primates exposed to early life stressors: implications for the pathophysiology of mood and anxiety disorders. Proc Natl Acad Sci U S A 93:1619–1623, 1996

Coplan JD, Trost RC, Owens MJ, et al: Cerebrospinal fluid concentrations of somatostatin and biogenic amines in grown primates reared by mothers exposed to manipulated foraging conditions. Arch Gen Psychiatry 55:473–477, 1998

Crestani F, Lorez M, Baer K, et al: Decreased GABAA-receptor clustering results in enhanced anxiety and a bias for threat cues. Nat Neurosci 2:833–839, 1999

Daglish MRC, Nutt DJ: Brain imaging studies in human addicts. Eur Neuropsychopharmacol 13:453–458, 2003

Davidson RJ, Abercrombie H, Nitschke JB, et al: Regional brain function, emotion and disorders of emotion. Curr Opin Neurobiol 9:228–234, 1999

Davis M, Whalen PJ: The amygdala: vigilance and emotion. Mol Psychiatry 6:13–34, 2001

Davis M, Walker DL, Lee Y: Amygdala and bed nucleus of the stria terminalis: different roles in fear and anxiety measured with the acoustic startle reflex. Philos Trans R Soc Lond B Biol Sci 352:1675–1687, 1997

Drevets W, Price JL, Simpson JR, et al: Subgenual prefrontal cortex abnormalities in mood disorders. Nature 386:824–827, 1997

Ebstein RP, Levine J, Geller V, et al: Dopamine DR receptor and serotonin receptor promoter in the determination of neonatal temperament. Mol Psychiatry 3:238–246, 1998

Everitt BJ, Wolf ME: Psychomotor stimulant addiction: a neural systems perspective. J Neurosci 22:3312–3320, 2002

Everitt BJ, Dickinson A, Robbins TW: The neuropsychological basis of addictive behaviour. Brain Res Brain Res Rev 36:129–138, 2001

Francis DD, Diorio J, Liu D, et al: Nongenomic transmission across generations in maternal behavior and stress responses in the rat. Science 286:1155–1158, 1999

Furlong RA, Ho L, Walsh C, et al: Analysis and meta-analysis of two serotonin transporter gene polymorphisms in bipolar and unipolar affective disorders. Am J Med Genet 81:58–63, 1998

Furmark T, Fischer H, Wik G, et al: The amygdala and individual differences in human fear conditioning. Neuroreport 8:3957–3960, 1997

Glue P, Wilson S, Coupland N, et al: The relationship between benzodiazepine receptor sensitivity and neuroticism. J Anxiety Disord 9:33–45, 1995

Gorman JM, Kent JM, Sullivan GM, et al: Neuroanatomical hypothesis of panic disorder, revised. Am J Psychiatry 157:493–505, 2000

Gratton A, Wise RA: Drug- and behavior-associated changes in dopamine-related electrochemical signals during intravenous cocaine self-administration in rats. J Neurosci 14:4130–4146, 1994

Gunther U, Benson J, Benke D, et al: Benzodiazepine-insensitive mice generated by targeted disruption of the gamma 2 subunit gene of gamma-aminobutyric acid type A receptors. Proc Natl Acad Sci U S A 92:7749–7753, 1995

Hariri A, Mattay V, Tessitore A, et al: Serotonin transporter genetic variation and the response of the human amygdala. Science 297:400–403, 2002

Higley JD, Hasert MF, Suomi SJ, et al: Nonhuman primate model of alcohol abuse: effects of early experience, personality, and stress on alcohol consumption. Proc Natl Acad Sci U S A 88:7261–7265, 1991

Holmes A, Yang R, Lesch K-P, et al: Mice lacking the serotonin transporter exhibit 5-HT(1A) receptor-mediated abnormalities in tests for anxiety-like behavior. Neuropsychopharmacology 28:2077–2088, 2003

Kalin N, Larson C, Shelton SE, et al: Asymmetric frontal brain activity, cortisol and behavior associated with fearful temperaments in rhesus monkeys. Behav Neurosci 112:1–7, 1998

Kempermann G, Kuhn HG, Gage FH: More hippocampal neurons in adult mice living in an enriched environment. Nature 386:493–495, 1997

Krebs JR, Davies NB: Behavioral Ecology: An Evolutionary Approach. Blackwell Scientific, Cambridge, MA, 1991

LaBar KS, LeDoux JE, Spencer DD, et al: Impaired fear conditioning following unilateral temporal lobectomy in humans. J Neurosci 15:6846–6855, 1995

LaBar KS, Gatenby JC, Gore JC, et al: Human amygdala activation during conditioned fear acquisition and extinction: a mixed-trial fMRI study. Neuron 20:937–945, 1998

Lakatos K, Toth I, Nemoda Z, et al: Dopamine D4 receptor (DRD4) gene polymorphism is associated with attachment disorganization in infants. Molec Psychiatry 5:633–637, 2000

LeDoux JE: Emotion circuits in the brain. Ann Rev Neurosci 23:155–184, 2000

Lesch KP, Bengel D, Heils A, et al: Association of anxiety-related traits with a polymorphism in the serotonin transporter gene regulatory region. Science 274:1527–1531, 1996

Leyton M, Boileau I, Benkelfat C, et al: Amphetamine-induced increases in extracellular dopamine, drug wanting, and novelty seeking: a PET/[11C]raclopride study in healthy men. Neuropsychopharmacology 27:1027–1035, 2002

Little KY, McLaughlin DP, Zhang L, et al: Cocaine, ethanol, and genotype effects on human midbrain serotonin transporter binding sites and mRNA levels. Am J Psychiatry 155:207–213, 1998

Liu D, Diorio J, Day JC, et al: Maternal care, hippocampal synaptogenesis and cognitive development in the rat. Nat Neurosci 3:799–806, 2000

Lupien S, Meaney MJ: Stress, glucocorticoids, and hippocampus aging in rat and human, in Handbook of Human Aging. Edited by Wang E, Snyder S. New York, Academic Press, 1998, pp 19–50

Malizia AL, Cunningham VJ, Bell CJ, et al: Decreased brain GABA(A)-benzodiazepine receptor binding in panic disorder: preliminary results from a quantitative PET study. Arch Gen Psychiatry 55:715–720, 1998

Mayberg HS, Brannan SK, Mahurin RK, et al: Cingulate function in depression: a potential predictor of treatment response. Neuroreport 8:1057–1061, 1997

McKernan RM, Whiting PJ: Which GABAA-receptor subtypes really occur in the brain? Trends Neurosci 19:139–143, 1997

Meaney MJ: The development of individual differences in behavioral and endocrine responses to stress. Ann Rev Neurosci 24:1161–1192, 2001

Mehta AK, Ticku MJ: An update on GABAA receptors. Brain Res Brain Res Rev 29:196–217, 1999

Melo de Paula AJ: A comparative study of lormetazepam and flurazepam in the treatment of insomnia. Clin Ther 64:500–508, 1977

Nestler EJ, Gould E, Manji H, et al: Preclinical models: status of basic research in depression. Biol Psychiatry 52:503–528, 2002

New AS, Siever LJ: Biochemical endophenotypes in personality disorders. Methods Mol Med 77:199–213, 2003

Oblowitz H, Robins AH: The effect of clobazam and lorazepam on the psychomotor performance of anxious patients. Br J Clin Pharmacol 16:95–99, 1983

Olds J: "Reward" from brain stimulation in the rat. Science 122:878, 1955

Olds J, Milner P: Positive reinforcement produced by electrical stimulation of septal area and other regions of rat brain. J Comp Physiol Psychol 47:419–427, 1954

Owens MJ, Nemeroff CB: The serotonin transporter and depression. Depress Anxiety 8 (suppl)1:5–12, 1998

Piazza PV, LeMoal M: Pathophysiological basis of vulnerability to drug abuse: interaction between stress, glucocorticoids and dopaminergic neurons. Ann Rev Pharmacol Toxicol 36:359–378, 1996

Piazza PV, Maccari S, Deminière J-M, et al: Corticosterone levels determine individual vulnerability to amphetamine self-administration. Proc Natl Acad Sci U S A 88:2088–2092, 1991

Piazza PV, Barrot M, Rougé-Pont F, et al: Suppression of glucocorticoid secretion and antipsychotic drugs have similar effects on the mesolimbic dopaminergic transmission. Proc Natl Acad Sci U S A 93:15445–15450, 1996

Pitkanen A, Savander V, LeDoux JE: Organization of intra-amygdaloid circuitries in the rat: an emerging framework for understanding functions of the amygdala. Trends Neurosci 20:517–523, 1997

Pruessner JL, Champagne FA, Meaney MJ, et al: Parental care and neuroendocrine and dopamine responses to stress in humans: a PET imaging study. J Neurosci 24:2825–2831, 2004

Pujol A, Lopez A, Deus J, et al: Anatomical variability of the anterior cingulate gyrus and basic dimensions of human personality. Neuroimage 15:847–855, 2002

Rauch SL, van der Kolk BA, Fisler RA, et al: A symptom provocation study of posttraumatic stress disorder using positron emission tomography and script-driven imagery. Arch Gen Psychiatry 53:380–386, 1996

Robbins TW: The 5-choice serial reaction time task: behavioural pharmacology and functional neurochemistry. Psychopharmacology 163:362–380, 2001

Rosenblum LA, Andrews MW: Influences of environmental demand on maternal behavior and infant development. Acta Paediatr Suppl 397:57–63, 1994

Roy-Byrne P, Cowley DS, Greenblatt DJ, et al: Reduced benzodiazepine sensitivity in panic disorder. Arch Gen Psychiatry 47:534–538, 1990

Roy-Byrne P, Wingerson DK, Radant A, et al: Reduced benzodiazepine sensitivity in patients with panic disorder: comparison with patients with obsessive-compulsive disorder and normal subjects. Am J Psychiatry 153:1444–1449, 1996

Seckl JR: Prenatal glucocorticoids and long-term programming. Eur J Endocrinol 151 (suppl 3):U49–U62, 2004

Shaham Y, Shalev U, Lu L, et al: The reinstatement model of drug relapse: history, methodology and major findings. Psychopharmacology 168:3–20, 2003

Shekhar A, McCann UD, Meaney MJ, et al: Summary of a National Institute of Mental Health workshop: developing animal models of anxiety disorders. Psychopharmacology (Berl) 157:327–339, 2001

Shin LM, Kosslyn SM, McNally RJ, et al: Visual imagery and perception in post-traumatic stress disorder. Arch Gen Psychiatry 54:233–241, 1997

Siever LJ, Davis KL: A psychobiological perspective on the personality disorders. Am J Psychiatry 148:1647–1658, 1991

Stewart J: Stress and relapse to drug seeking: studies in laboratory animals shed light on mechanisms and sources of long-term vulnerability. Am J Addict 12:1–17, 2003

Suomi SJ: Early determinants of behaviour: evidence from primate studies. Br Med Bull 53:170–184, 1997

Swerdlow NR, Geyer MA, Braff DL: Neural circuit regulation of prepulse inhibition of startle in the rat: current knowledge and future challenges. Psychopharmacology (Berl) 156:194–215, 2001

Veenstra-VanderWeele J, Anderson GM, Cook EH: Pharmacogenetics and the serotonin system: initial studies and future directions. Eur J Pharmacol 410:165–181, 2000

Volkow ND, Wang G-J, Fowler JS, et al: Prediction of reinforcing responses to psychostimulants in humans by brain dopamine D2 receptor levels. Am J Psychiatry 156:1440–1443, 1999

Westergaard GC, Suomi SJ, Chavanne TJ, et al: Physiological correlates of aggression and impulsivity in free-ranging female primates. Neuropsychopharmacol 28:1045–1055, 2003

Wise RA: Interactions between medial prefrontal cortex and meso-limbic components of brain reward circuitry. Prog Brain Res 126:255–262, 2000

41

Biology in the Service of Psychotherapy

Amit Etkin, M.Phil.
Christopher J. Pittenger, M.D., Ph.D.
Eric R. Kandel, M.D.

Neuroscience has developed a number of useful methods for analyzing cognitive function. As a result, our understanding of normal and abnormal mental function has grown substantially. These insights have improved the ability to intervene pharmacotherapeutically in the treatment of patients with mental illness. Can this new understanding also inform and improve psychotherapeutic interventions?

Psychotherapy remains one of the cornerstones of treatment for many psychopathologies, including various personality disorders. There also is evidence that the combined use of psychotherapy and medications can lead to better treatment outcome (Newton-Howes and Tyrer 2003; Zanarini and Frankenburg 2001). Despite the extensive use of psychotherapy for a number of mental disorders, we lack a biological perspective on how psychotherapy works. Investigation of the biological underpinnings of psychotherapy is important for two reasons. First, an understanding of psychotherapy is important in psychiatry's attempt to link specific mental functions with specific brain mecha-

nisms and may aid in the analysis of how the environment affects the brain. Psychotherapy is a controlled form of learning that occurs in the context of a therapeutic relationship—and from this perspective, the biology of psychotherapy can be understood as a special case in the biology of learning (Kandel 1979). Second, insight into the biological mechanisms of psychotherapeutic action would revolutionize psychiatry by enhancing our understanding of premorbid vulnerabilities, selection of the optimal course of therapy, and evaluation of treatment outcome.

Because the neurobiological study of psychotherapy is in its infancy, any attempt to address the biology of psychotherapy at this early point will be incomplete. Nonetheless, the initial research into the biological underpinnings of psychotherapy has already provided several new insights. In this chapter, we outline where we are and how future refinements might advance the field further. Our discussion centers primarily on depression, obsessive-compulsive disorder (OCD), and anxiety, where neuroimaging work is most advanced. By contrast, little is known about the neurobiology of personality disorders. In considering these illnesses, we focus in particular on the use of neuroimaging for diagnosing and understanding psychopathology and for predicting the outcome of treatment and following its course.

Basal Brain Imaging: Detecting Changes Associated With Psychotherapy

Most early neuroimaging studies of psychotherapy focused on depression and OCD and examined basal brain metabolism or basal cerebral blood flow (Baxter et al. 1992; Brody et al. 1998, 2001; Martin et al. 2001; Schwartz et al. 1996). These studies have consistently demonstrated changes in brain activity in patients with these disorders when compared with healthy control subjects. Successful treatment frequently restored the brain to a state that superficially resembled the brain state of control subjects. Particularly interesting is the finding that some of the changes accompanying successful psychotherapy resembled those seen with pharmacotherapy, suggesting that, at least in some cases, both psychotherapy and drugs may act on a common set of brain targets.

Early neuroimaging studies of OCD used fluorodeoxyglucose–positron emission tomography (FDG-PET). A typical scan involves continuous acquisition for 30–40 minutes while patients are at rest and is therefore not sensitive to moment-to-moment changes in neuronal activity, as might happen during performance of a cognitive task.

In the first such study, Baxter et al. (1992) found an increase in basal glucose metabolism in the caudate nucleus of OCD patients. Treatment with either the selective serotonin reuptake inhibitor (SSRI) fluoxetine or exposure psychotherapy reversed the metabolic abnormality caused by this disorder. A subsequent study found that patients who responded to psychotherapy showed greater decreases in right caudate metabolism than patients who did not respond (Schwartz et al. 1996). Although both lacked important controls, the two studies demonstrated for the first time that psychotherapy can produce a detectable change in brain activity.

Subsequent FDG-PET studies of psychotherapy have focused primarily on depression. The most common finding in depression is a decrease in the basal activity of the dorsolateral prefrontal cortex (PFC). Less consistently reported is increased activity in the ventrolateral PFC (Drevets 1998; Kennedy et al. 1997; Mayberg 1997;

Mayberg et al. 1999). Both SSRIs and electroconvulsive therapy reversed these abnormalities (Drevets 1998).

To relate these findings to psychotherapy, two studies compared interpersonal psychotherapy (IPT) with either the SSRI paroxetine or the serotonin-norepinephrine reuptake inhibitor venlafaxine in the treatment of depression (Brody et al. 2001; Martin et al. 2001). Again, psychotherapy reversed pretreatment abnormalities, including those in the PFC, similar to the effects of pharmacotherapy.

The conclusion from these two sets of studies that psychotherapy is similar to pharmacotherapy in normalizing functional abnormalities in brain circuits that give rise to symptoms is, however, potentially simplistic. With further research it should be possible to distinguish common from distinct changes among therapies. This may allow one to distinguish between brain regions that contribute to symptom improvement per se and those that contribute to the mechanisms of a particular therapy. For example, Goldapple et al. (2004) found that depressed patients treated with cognitive-behavioral therapy (CBT) show some common and some different brain changes when compared with patients treated with paroxetine. Thus, the initial idea in the literature that psychotherapy and pharmacotherapy produce similar changes is not likely to prove generally true. Indeed, firm conclusions should not yet be drawn from any of these early studies, because they are hampered by lack of or incomplete randomization for treatment types, as well as by missing controls.

Beyond Basal Brain Function: Stimulus-Responsive Imaging and Psychotherapy

Recent studies have sought to go beyond the measurement of basal metabolism by examining the effect of psychotherapy on context-specific neural responses in disease-relevant tasks (Furmark et al. 2002; Paquette et al. 2003). In one such study, Furmark et al. (2002) examined patients with social phobia treated with either citalopram or CBT, using PET measures of changes in regional blood flow secondary to neuronal activation. They had previously found that when patients with social phobia gave a prepared speech in the scanner while in the presence of others (as compared with giving the speech alone), they showed a larger increase in regional blood flow in the amygdala and hippocampus, compared with control subjects (Tillfors et al. 2001). Improvement in symptoms with treatment was accom-

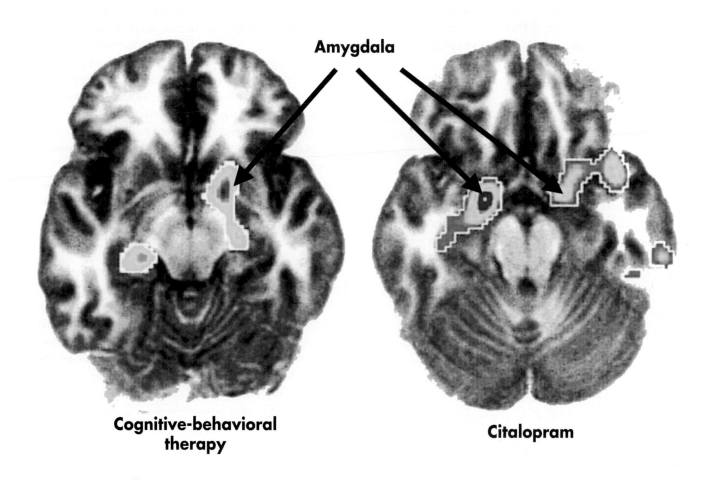

Amygdala

Cognitive-behavioral therapy

Citalopram

Figure 41–1. Effects of cognitive-behavioral therapy (CBT) or citalopram treatment on brain activity in patients with social phobia while carrying out a public speaking task.

CBT **(left)** and citalopram **(right)** treatment are both associated with decreased activation of the amygdala during performance of an anxiogenic public speaking task after therapy, compared with before therapy. Depicted are regions showing a significant post- versus pretreatment decrease in activity.

Source. Reprinted from Furmark T, Tillfors M, Marteinsdottir I, et al.: "Common Changes in Cerebral Blood Flow in Patients With Social Phobia Treated with Citalopram or Cognitive-Behavioral Therapy." *Archives of General Psychiatry* 59:425–433, 2002. Copyright 2002, American Medical Association. Used with permission.

panied by decreased activity in the amygdala and the medial temporal lobe in the stressful public speaking condition (Figure 41–1). No such changes were seen in waiting-list control subjects. Comparing treatment groups with a control group of waiting-list patients who received no treatment allowed the authors to rule out changes related only to subject rescanning or simply to the passage of time. Decreases in the activity of the amygdala were seen in both the CBT and the citalopram groups. The two treatment groups, however, differed with respect to neural changes outside the amygdala. Interestingly, the degree to which amygdala activity decreased as a result of therapy predicted patients' reduction in symptoms 1 year later. Unfortunately, because of

small sample sizes, the study was not able to distinguish between responders and nonresponders for each modality, which might have dissociated the symptom-improving effects of the treatment from the consequences of having received the treatment per se.

Despite their limitations, both the basal metabolism and stimulus-responsive imaging investigations have demonstrated that psychotherapy produces changes in the brain, some of which may be shared with those induced by pharmacotherapy, whereas others are modality-specific. As the neurobiological substrates of psychotherapeutic change are better defined, more directed animal studies can also be focused on those brain regions and the functional networks in which they participate.

FURTHER CLINICAL APPLICATIONS OF NEUROIMAGING TO PSYCHOTHERAPY

Neuroimaging can be a highly sensitive mode of investigation. Instead of looking at a single dependent measure (e.g., reaction times), neuroimaging simultaneously assesses the activity of every part of the brain. This flexibility can be enhanced by use of a variety of stimuli and tasks, as well as data analytic techniques that can separately probe the data for activations, connectivity, network-level interactions, and so forth.

This sensitivity has several implications. Neuroimaging may give an independent way of grouping patients based on biological variables closer to the pathogenesis of the disease. Personality disorders, for example, are even more likely than other psychiatric disorders to have distinct etiologies, yet these distinct etiologies (and mechanisms) may lead to clinically indistinguishable presentations. Subgrouping patients may reveal why some patients improve with particular therapies, and others do not, and this may better inform therapeutic decisions.

The power of novel data analysis techniques for objectively subgrouping subjects on the basis of biological criteria was illustrated by Meyer-Lindenberg et al. (2001). They found, using a multivariate analysis approach, that the expression of a brainwide pattern of activity in an individual can almost perfectly separate a group of schizophrenic patients from a control group (like a diagnostic marker). In this way they were able to separate out two independent cohorts with 94% accuracy, using only resting brain scans. Most neuroimaging studies use univariate analysis methods and examine the activity of single brain regions at a time rather than groups of areas across the whole brain. This can result in a great degree of overlap between regional activation in a disease group and in a control group—a distinction that may otherwise be easily made by multivariate analysis methods.

Alternatively, predictions of whether a particular therapy will work for a given patient may depend more on the functional characteristics of that individual's brain and less on what diagnostic group the patient is put in. In other words, understanding how that individual's brain processes particular stimuli may provide critical information for predicting treatment outcome. Neuroimaging-based quantification of regional brain function during disease-relevant and irrelevant tasks in a standardized way across patients may bring out many subtle differences. These differences may predict how a patient will process and respond to stimuli in the

context of particular forms of psychotherapy, or after pharmacological treatment. Such an approach can be thought of as a "cognitive and emotional stress test" much as a cardiologist may use an exercise stress test to bring out subtle differences in cardiovascular function that will predict disease progression and possibly the medications the patient should take to achieve the optimal outcome. This approach may predict which of several treatment courses is most suitable, or may allow the progress of treatment to be monitored, and thus provide early markers of the likelihood of success long before changes in behavior can be seen. Prediction of outcome may be successful even without a full understanding of why a particular pattern of brain activation predicts better outcome.

Our arguments are based on the assumption that biological variables are causal to the behavioral manifestations of psychiatric disorders and can be more sensitive indices of cognitive function. Importantly, neuroimaging measures are equally sensitive to processes at the conscious and unconscious levels, as they must both be reflected by underlying processes in the brain. Thus, neuroimaging approaches can be equally well used, no matter how the psychopathology or psychotherapy is conceptualized.

PREDICTING OUTCOME WITH NEUROIMAGING: PRELIMINARY EVIDENCE FROM DEPRESSION AND OBSESSIVE-COMPULSIVE DISORDER

The most convincing outcome predictions come from neuroimaging studies of depression. While these studies relate to the pharmacotherapy of depression, they can be at least conceptually extended to psychotherapy.

A landmark FDG-PET study of the pharmacological treatment of unipolar depression found that activity in the rostral anterior cingulate cortex (ACC) uniquely differentiated treatment responders from nonresponders (Mayberg et al. 1997). Responders were hypermetabolic prior to treatment with respect to controls, while nonresponders were hypometabolic (see Figure 41–2A). The predictive value of pretreatment activity in the rostral cingulate in depression has been confirmed by subsequent studies. Rostral cingulate activity predicted better response to paroxetine treatment (Saxena et al. 2003) as well as to partial sleep deprivation therapy (see Figure 41–2B) (Volk et al. 1997; Wu et al. 1999). More recently, Pizzagalli et al. (2001) recorded scalp EEG activity in nortriptyline-treated

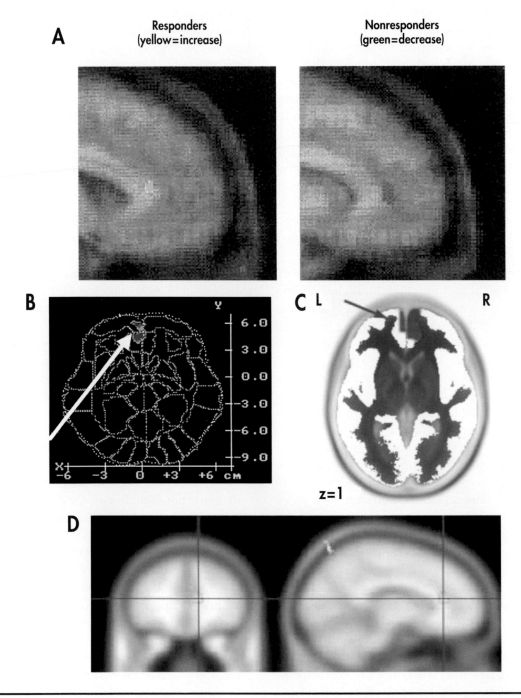

A Responders
(yellow=increase)

Nonresponders
(green=decrease)

Figure 41–2. Prediction of better outcome in depression by higher pretreatment levels of rostral anterior cingulate cortex metabolism or activity.

In **(A)**, responders to antidepressants were found to be *hyper*metabolic in the rostral cingulate, whereas nonresponders were *hypo*metabolic (Mayberg et al. 1997). Basal brain metabolism (Wu et al. 1999) and theta frequency EEG signal (Pizzagalli et al. 2001) in the rostral cingulate predicted better outcome to sleep deprivation therapy **(B)** or antidepressants **(C)**, respectively. **(D)** Greater functional recruitment of the rostral cingulate in an emotional activation task prior to antidepressant treatment also predicted better outcome (Davidson et al. 2003).

Source. **A:** Reprinted from Mayberg HS, Brannan SK, Mahurin RK, et al.: "Cingulate Function in Depression: A Potential Predictor of Treatment Response." *Neuroreport* 8 (4):1057–1061, 1997. **B:** Wu J, Buchsbaum MS, Gillin JC, et al.: "Prediction of Antidepressant Effects of Sleep Deprivation by Metabolic Rates in the Ventral Anterior Cingulate and Medial Prefrontal Cortex." *American Journal of Psychiatry* 156:1149–1158, 1999. Copyright 1999, American Psychiatric Association. Used with permission. **C:** Pizzagalli D, Pascual-Marqui RD, Nitschke JB, et al.: "Anterior Cingulate Activity as a Predictor of Degree of Treatment Response in Major Depression: Evidence From Brain Electrical Tomography Analysis." *American Journal of Psychiatry* 158:405–415, 2001. Copyright 2001, American Psychiatric Association. Used with permission. **D:** Davidson RJ, Irwin W, Anderle MJ, et al.: "The Neural Substrates of Affective Processing in Depressed Patients Treated With Venlafaxine." *American Journal of Psychiatry* 160:64–75, 2003. Copyright 2003, American Psychiatric Association. Used with permission.

depressed patients, focusing on one EEG frequency band thought to be generated by the anterior cingulate. Here again patients showing electrical hyperactivity in the rostral cingulate before treatment showed better response 4–6 months after treatment, an effect that was not related to pretreatment depression severity (see Figure 41–2C). In the first study to examine functional recruitment of the rostral cingulate, rather than its baseline activity or metabolism, Davidson et al. (2003) examined functional magnetic resonance imaging (fMRI) activation in response to viewing negatively valenced visual stimuli, compared with neutral stimuli. They likewise found that higher pretreatment activation of the rostral cingulate predicted a lower depression symptom scale score 8 weeks after treatment (see Figure 41–2D).

The anterior cingulate can be divided into three divisions by anatomical and functional imaging criteria (Bush et al. 2000; Devinsky et al. 1995). Changes in both the dorsal and ventral regions of the cingulate have been seen in depression (Davidson et al. 2002; Drevets 2001; Mayberg 1997). The dorsal ("cognitive") division of the ACC is often activated by nonemotional tasks that produce conflicts between potential responses (i.e., a color-word Stroop task in which the font color of the word to be identified is incongruent with the word itself—"red" in green ink). The ventral ("affective") division of the ACC can be recruited by mood induction protocols (Bush et al. 2000; Mayberg et al. 1999).

The rostral cingulate, located between these other two subdivisions and implicated in the studies of depression summarized above, receives input from both of the other divisions of the ACC and is thought to integrate them (Devinsky et al. 1995). Thus, the rostral cingulate may be important for detecting conflict in the emotional domain and recruiting cognitive-attentional processes to resolve the conflict. In support of this view, the rostral cingulate becomes more active when subjects are asked to ignore emotional words in a word counting task than when they are instructed to ignore neutral words (Whalen et al. 1998). In this task, ignoring emotional content would be expected to increase conflict in the emotional domain.

Conflict resolution and cognitive control by the rostral cingulate may be analogous to the functions of the dorsal cingulate under conflict conditions. Kerns et al. (2004) found that the dorsal division of the ACC was activated by conflict in a color-word Stroop task. Dorsal ACC activation by this conflict predicted greater recruitment of the dorsolateral PFC on the subsequent trial. This increase in cognitive control decreased the incongruency effect, thereby leading to shorter reaction times for incongruent trials that were preceded by an incongruent trial than for incongruent trials that were preceded by a congruent trial. The dorsal ACC appeared to both resolve cognitive conflict and prime cognitive systems to better reduce conflict on the subsequent trial.

By analogy, the rostral cingulate may be recruited to resolve conflict between emotional stimuli or between conflicting mental content. In major depression, cognitive control may be important for regulating the effects of negative mood over perception, thoughts, and behavior. Patients with higher levels of activity in the rostral cingulate before therapy may thereby be in a better position for recovery.

Preliminary imaging studies of OCD implicate a different area of the PFC, the orbitofrontal cortex (OFC), in predicting treatment response. The OFC is highly activated during symptom provocation in OCD patients (McGuire et al. 1994; Rauch et al. 1994). One FDG-PET study of OCD found that lower pretreatment levels of activity predicted better response to drug therapy (Figure 41–3A) (Saxena et al. 1999). More intriguing was the finding that lower pretreatment metabolism of the OFC predicted better response to drugs than to psychotherapy, whereas higher OFC metabolism predicted the opposite (see Figure 41–3B). As in many of the other studies cited earlier, several major caveats must be considered. Subjects were not randomized, blinded, or compared with a placebo group.

Why lower OFC metabolism predicts treatment outcome is not clear. It may, for example, be related to the recruitment of this region in behavioral control and inhibition (Horn et al. 2003; Lubman et al. 2004). OFC metabolism may reflect the degree of control that patients feel they must exert on their behavior in order to satisfy their compulsions. Why OFC metabolism may predict opposite results for psychotherapy and pharmacotherapy is also unclear. Finally, because none of the outcome prediction studies in depression contrasted psychotherapy and pharmacotherapy, it is unknown whether the rostral cingulate in depression may differentially predict outcome depending on the treatment type as the OFC may in OCD.

ROLE OF AWARENESS: IMPLICATIONS OF CONSCIOUS AND UNCONSCIOUS FOR PSYCHOPATHOLOGY AND PSYCHOTHERAPY

Most theories of psychopathology, both psychodynamic and cognitive, emphasize the importance of unconscious processes and differentiate them from con-

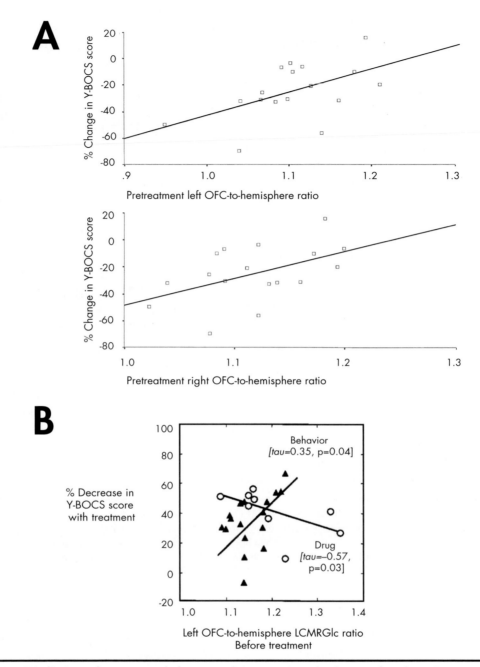

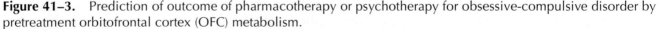

Figure 41–3. Prediction of outcome of pharmacotherapy or psychotherapy for obsessive-compulsive disorder by pretreatment orbitofrontal cortex (OFC) metabolism.

(A) Lower pretreatment metabolism in the OFC predicted better response to antidepressants (Saxena et al. 1999), reflected by a greater decrease in Y-BOCS scores, a measure of OCD symptoms. **(B)** The relationship between pretreatment OFC metabolism and outcome of behavioral psychotherapy (Brody et al. 1998) may be opposite that between pretreatment OFC metabolism and outcome of drug therapy. LCMRGlc=local cerebral metabolic rates for glucose.

Source. **A:** Reprinted from Saxena S, Brody AL, Maidment KM, et al.: "Localized Orbitofrontal and Subcortical Metabolic Changes and Predictors of Response to Paroxetine Treatment in Obsessive-Compulsive Disorder." *Neuropsychopharmacology* 21:683–693, 1999. Used with permission. **B:** Reprinted from Brody AL, Saxena S, Schwartz JM, et al.: "FDG-PET Predictors of Response to Behavioral Therapy and Pharmacotherapy in Obsessive-Compulsive Disorder." *Psychiatry Research* 84:1–6, 1998. Copyright 1998, with permission from Elsevier.

scious processes (Beck and Clark 1997; Gabbard 2005; Wong 1999). This is particularly clear in anxiety disorders. For all of their differences, these theories generally agree that an anxiety-related unconscious 1) should differ between individuals with different anxiety levels and 2) is probably the sum of a family of processes occurring outside of subjective awareness. A recent fMRI study from our laboratory (Etkin et al. 2004) has investigated these features of unconscious processing in anxiety. The results shed light on the conscious and uncon-

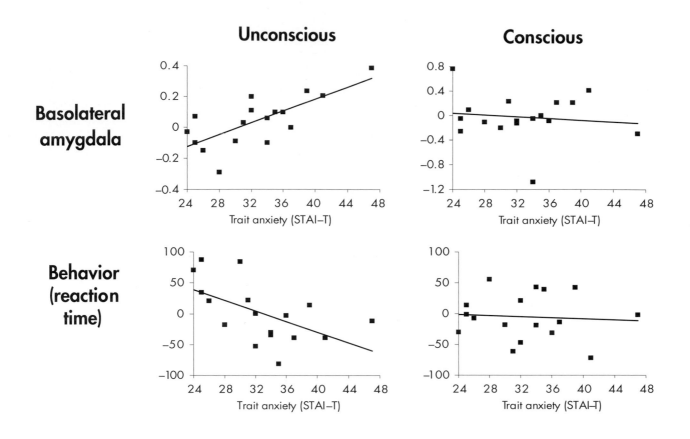

Figure 41–4. Prediction of basolateral subregion amygdalar activity by differences in baseline (trait) anxiety within a normal population during unconscious, but not conscious, processing of fearful faces.

Individual differences in baseline (trait) anxiety predicted activity in the basolateral subregion of the amygdala during unconscious, but not conscious, processing of fearful faces. Similarly, differences in trait anxiety predicted behavior (color identification reaction times) specifically during unconscious processing. STAI-T=Spielberger State-Trait Anxiety Inventory—Trait Anxiety.

Source.   Adapted from Etkin A, Klemenhagen KC, Dudman JT, et al.: "Individual Differences in Trait Anxiety Predict the Response of the Basolateral Amygdala to Unconsciously Processed Fearful Faces." *Neuron* 44:1043–1055, 2004. Copyright 2004, with permission from Elsevier.

scious components of anxiety and delineate new ways of evaluating the mechanisms whereby anxious subjects respond to treatment.

Etkin et al. (2004) examined a group of normal volunteers and exposed them to fearful faces. While none of these participants had anxiety disorders, they represented the range of baseline (trait) anxiety present in the normal population. Fearful facial expressions are culturally conserved signals of threat that have been shown to stimulate activity in the amygdala (Aggleton 2000; Ekman et al. 1969). These faces were presented for conscious or unconscious processing; the latter was achieved through backward masking, which entails presenting a fearful face very rapidly and immediately followed by a neutral face. This procedure renders stimuli consciously nonreportable. While viewing these faces, subjects were engaged in a color identifica-

tion task not related to the emotion expressed on the face. Reaction times in this task could show the effects of emotion if processing the emotional content affected the attentional resources available for the color identification task.

Etkin et al. (2004) found that individual differences in trait anxiety predicted activity in the amygdala, as well as reaction times and activity in cortical regions important in attention (see Figures 41–4 and 41–5). However, the relationships of brain activity or behavior to trait anxiety were seen only when stimuli were processed unconsciously. Etkin et al. therefore identified a network of brain regions important in the unconscious emotional vigilance commonly described behaviorally for nonclinically anxious individuals and patients with anxiety disorder (see Figure 41–5) (Mogg and Bradley 1998). This network involved the amygdala in emo-

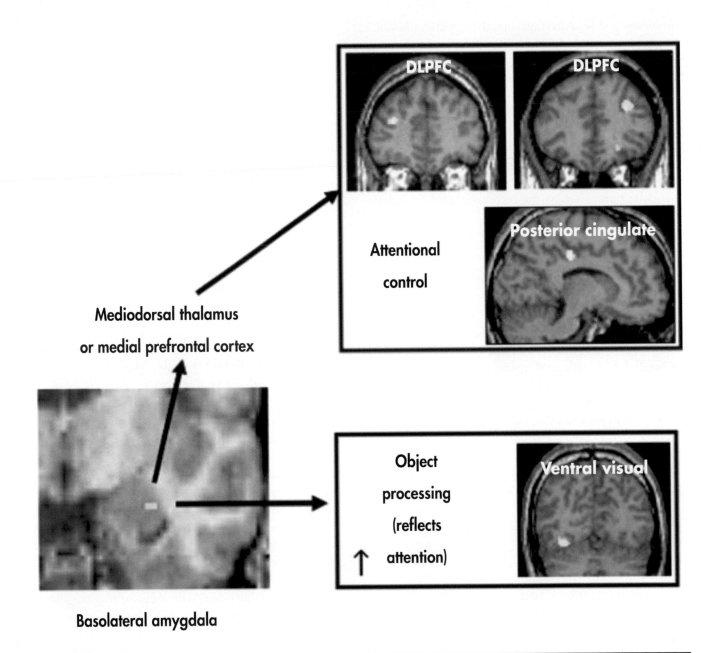

Figure 41–5. Identification of an unconscious emotional vigilance network in anxiety (Etkin et al. 2004).

Unconscious trait anxiety–correlated activations are seen in the basolateral amygdala, dorsolateral prefrontal cortex (DLPFC), posterior cingulate, and a number of ventral visual areas. These regions may thus form an unconscious emotional vigilance network that directs attention for enhanced processing of unconscious threat (DLPFC and posterior cingulate), which was reflected in enhanced activation of object processing areas in the ventral visual stream.

Source. Adapted from Etkin A, Klemenhagen KC, Dudman JT, et al.: "Individual Differences in Trait Anxiety Predict the Response of the Basolateral Amygdala to Unconsciously Processed Fearful Faces." *Neuron* 44:1043–1055, 2004. Copyright 2004, with permission from Elsevier.

tional evaluation and the dorsolateral PFC and the posterior cingulate cortex in directing attention for better processing of the unconscious threat. The network also contained a number of ventral visual regions important in the processing of objects, particularly faces. Enhanced activity in these visual regions is thought to reflect the effects of enhanced attention. Emotional arousal led to faster color identification reaction times, but, again, only when emotion was processed unconsciously.

The fact that brain activations and reaction times were not correlated with anxiety during consciously processed fear illustrates another important point: conscious processes may secondarily regulate unconscious biases. Distinguishing between conscious and unconscious processes may be essential for understanding both psychopathology and psychotherapy. For example, certain therapies (or drugs) may alter the capacity for secondary regulation of unconscious biases, but not the biases per se. Alternatively, the effectiveness of a therapy may relate to its ability to normalize unconscious biases. One can imagine two simple ways in which biases may be corrected. Excessive unconscious amygdala activation brought about by anxiety may be normalized through changes occurring primarily in the amygdala or by recruitment of additional areas, perhaps top-down inhibitory areas in the frontal cortex. Thus, neuroimaging can help distinguish conscious from unconscious brain changes and identify which particular brain changes are responsible for the behavioral improvement.

FUNCTIONAL CORRELATES OF PERSONALITY DISORDERS

Relatively few studies have examined the neural basis of personality disorders. Of these, most have focused on borderline personality disorder (BPD) or antisocial personality disorder, and in particular on patients' impulsivity. Despite limited data, results from these studies generally point to abnormalities in the ventromedial PFC and OFC. These areas have been implicated in the inhibition of inappropriate behavior (Horn et al. 2003; Lubman et al. 2004) and appropriate decision making within the emotional or personal domains (Bechara et al. 1997; A.R. Damasio et al. 1990; H. Damasio et al. 1994). Deficits in impulse control are important elements of several personality disorders (American Psychiatric Association 2000).

Several studies have found, using FDG-PET, broad decreases in prefrontal metabolism in BPD patients (De La Fuente et al. 1997; Soloff et al. 2000, 2003). De la Fuente et al. (1997) found decreased activity in the medial and lateral PFC, including in the ACC in BPD patients. Soloff et al. (2000, 2003) found decreased metabolism in the medial OFC of BPD patients (see Figure 41–6A and B), with the degree of orbitofrontal hypometabolism related to self-report and interviewer-assessed measures of impulsivity (Soloff et al. 2003). Schmahl et al. (2003) compared neural activation during script-guided imagination of abandonment situations with activation during imagination of neutral situations in BPD patients and control subjects. The BPD patients showed decreased activation, relative to controls, in the ACC and amygdala/hippocampus, and increased activation in the dorsolateral PFC.

Other studies point to serotonergic dysfunction in the ventromedial PFC in BPD. Fenfluramine is a compound with serotonergic activity. Challenge with fenfluramine leads to increased metabolism in the PFC.

This increase was blunted in the medial and orbitofrontal regions of the PFC of patients with BPD, as well as in several regions outside of the frontal lobe (see Figure 41–6A) (Schmahl et al. 2002; Soloff et al. 2000). To more directly probe the serotonergic system, one can inject subjects with a radioactively labeled compound that binds proteins important for serotonin function, and image the degree of binding throughout the brain with the PET camera. Leyton et al. (2001) found decreased binding of a serotonin precursor in the medial PFC and ACC in BPD patients (see Figure 41–6C). This deficit was more severe in patients with higher impulsivity scores. Finally, two studies of impulsive aggressive patients with a variety of personality disorders found baseline and fenfluramine-induced deficits in the ventromedial PFC, similar to those described above for BPD patients (Goyer et al. 1994; Siever et al. 1999).

FUNCTIONS OF REDUCED ACTIVITY IN THE VENTRAL FRONTAL CORTEX

What are the consequences of reduced activity in ventromedial and orbitofrontal circuitry in individuals with BPD or antisocial personality disorder? Some insight into this question comes from studies of damage to these areas. Antonio Damasio and colleagues characterized subjects with lesions in the ventromedial PFC and found that they displayed problems in decision making, particularly in the interpersonal and emotional domains (Bechara et al. 1997; A.R. Damasio et al. 1990; H. Damasio et al. 1994). When asked to carry out tasks that require the development of a strategy for long-term benefit, subjects with ventromedial PFC lesions developed neither a discriminative skin conductance response indicating the correct choice nor a successful long-term strategy (Bechara et al. 1997). Lesions of the medial OFC in experimental animals result in reduced behavioral inhibition, and the "orbitofrontal syndrome" in humans consists of disinhibited, socially inappropriate behaviors; impulsivity and aggression; and emotional lability (Blair 2001; A.R. Damasio et al. 1990; H. Damasio et al. 1994; Goldman-Rakic 1987; Malloy et al. 1993). These personality changes can even result in sociopathic behavior.

Taken together, these findings suggest that the abnormalities in the ventromedial and orbitofrontal cortex found in BPD and antisocial personality disorder may reflect the deficits in behavioral inhibition that are common across several personality disorders. Other than impulse control, however, our understanding of the neurobiology of personality disorders is rudimentary.

A

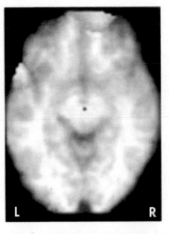
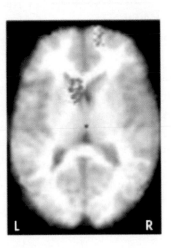

Baseline   Fenfluramine

B

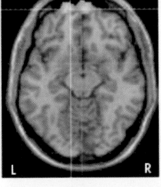

Baseline

C

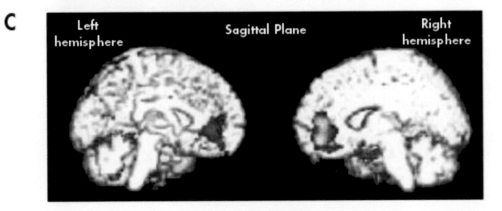

Figure 41–6. Deficits in basal brain metabolism and serotonergic function in patients with borderline personality disorder (BPD).

(A and B) The medial orbitofrontal cortex (OFC) showed less basal brain metabolism in BPD patients (indicated by the blue clusters in **(A)** and the orange cluster in **(B)** (Soloff et al. 2000, 2003). Challenge with fenfluramine, a compound with serotonergic properties, also revealed less recruitment of orbital regions in BPD patients than in control subjects (Soloff et al. 2000). **(C)** The binding of a serotonin precursor was decreased in the anterior cingulate and ventromedial prefrontal cortices of BPD patients (Leyton et al. 2001).

Source. **A and B:** Reprinted from Soloff PH, Meltzer CC, Greer PJ, et al.: "Fenfluramine-Activated FDG-PET Study of Borderline Personality Disorder." *Biological Psychiatry* 47:540–547, Copyright 2000, with permission from Society of Biological Psychiatry; Soloff PH, Meltzer CC, Becker C, et al.: "Impulsivity and Prefrontal Hypometabolism in Borderline Personality Disorder." *Psychiatry Research* 123:153–163, Copyright 2003, with permission from Elsevier. **C:** Leyton M, Okazawa H, Diksic M, et al.: "Brain Regional Alpha-[11C]Methyl-L-Tryptophan Trapping in Impulsive Subjects With Borderline Personality Disorder. *American Journal of Psychiatry* 158:775–782, 2001. Used with permission.

OUTCOME PREDICTION IN PATIENTS WITH PERSONALITY DISORDERS

How might the findings summarized above—on the role of the rostral cingulate and OFC in prediction of treatment response in patients with depression and OCD—apply to patients with personality disorders? The mutually exclusive relationship between rostral cingulate and depression versus OFC and OCD suggests that there may be disease-specificity to brain areas with prognostic value, even in diseases that can be treated with the same treatment modality or drug. Personality disorders are a highly varied category of mental illnesses and are often comorbid with mood and anxiety disorders. As such, prediction of treatment outcome may be less readily accomplished than with depression and OCD. Outcome prediction for each dimension of a personality disorder may need to be examined separately, which would necessitate use of more stimulus-responsive imaging modalities.

The conflict detection and resolution function of the rostral cingulate and the behavioral inhibition function of the OFC may both turn out to be very relevant for the capacity of patients with personality disorders to recover. Psychotherapies call on patients to understand the beliefs underlying their actions and exert control over those beliefs and over their own behavior. One can imagine that conflicts would be frequently created between patients' hardened (likely unconscious) beliefs and their attempts to understand their behavior and correct these maladaptive beliefs. The ability to respond to and resolve these conflicts may involve recruitment of rostral cingulate–based neural circuitry. Those patients who can better recruit the rostral cingulate may be those who better resolve these conflicts and better respond to therapy. Similarly, patterns of thought or action in personality disorders may be so characteristic as to become compulsive, and a role for the OFC in regulating these patterns, as in OCD, may also relate to the capacity of patients to correct their thoughts and actions.

CONCLUSION

The biological study of psychotherapy is in its infancy, but several lines of evidence point to an important future role for neuroimaging in evaluating the mechanisms and outcome of psychotherapy. Imaging can contribute to an analysis of the mechanisms of pathogenesis of a mental disorder and it may provide meaningful predictions of treatment outcome. Although only a handful of neu-

roimaging studies have probed the biological deficits in personality disorders, they have been useful in identifying an important role for the ventral prefrontal cortices in impulse control among patients with BPD or antisocial personality disorder. A clearer direction for how neuroimaging will contribute to the psychotherapeutic treatment of patients with personality disorders will come when the biology of psychotherapy and personality disorders is more fully examined. We propose several points that may guide this process.

First, it is now clear that psychotherapy can induce robust changes in brain function that are detectable with neuroimaging. These findings must now be systematically explored. For example, the anxiety results described above suggest important mechanistic differences between processes operating at conscious and unconscious levels.

Second, prior to psychopharmacological treatment, the function of certain brain regions can predict the degree of patient improvement at follow-up, and there may be some degree of disease-specificity with respect to which region is most predictive of outcome. The anterior cingulate and orbitofrontal cortices, regions identified for the drug treatment of depression and OCD, may also be prognostic regions for psychotherapy outcome, as they are involved in conflict detection and resolution and in behavioral inhibition—functions that may be central targets of psychotherapy. Further investigation will show whether regions with prognostic value are specific to the type of disease or the form of treatment, and whether differential response to drug or psychotherapy can be predicted before treatment. In addition, understanding the brain regions and cognitive functions that best predict treatment response may allow the development of pharmacological agents that specifically enhance these cognitive processes and activity within prognostic regions. Combining novel pharmacological agents with psychotherapy may therefore lead to improved outcome (Ressler et al. 2004).

Third, deficits in impulse control in certain personality disorders have been associated with abnormalities in the ventromedial prefrontal and orbitofrontal cortices. Identification of deficits in these regions may point to the type of tasks and stimuli that will best probe the role of ventral prefrontal regions in behavioral inhibition, which may be very relevant for the ability of a patient to recover through psychotherapeutic treatment.

There is no longer doubt that psychotherapy can result in detectable changes in the brain. We now need to focus on the best neuroimaging approaches that will assist clinically relevant decisions relating to psychopathology and psychotherapy.

REFERENCES

Aggleton JP: The Amygdala: A Functional Analysis. New York, Oxford University Press, 2000

American Psychiatric Association: Diagnostic and Statistical Manual of Mental Disorders, 4th Edition, Text Revision. Arlington, VA, American Psychiatric Association, 2000

Baxter LR Jr, Schwartz JM, Bergman KS, et al: Caudate glucose metabolic rate changes with both drug and behavior therapy for obsessive-compulsive disorder. Arch Gen Psychiatry 49:681–689, 1992

Bechara A, Damasio H, Tranel D, et al: Deciding advantageously before knowing the advantageous strategy. Science 275:1293–1295, 1997

Beck AT, Clark DA: An information processing model of anxiety: automatic and strategic processes. Behav Res Ther 35:49–58, 1997

Blair RJ: Neurocognitive models of aggression, the antisocial personality disorders, and psychopathy. J Neurol Neurosurg Psychiatry 71:727–731, 2001

Brody AL, Saxena S, Schwartz JM, et al: FDG-PET predictors of response to behavioral therapy and pharmacotherapy in obsessive compulsive disorder. Psychiatry Res 84:1–6, 1998

Brody AL, Saxena S, Stoessel P, et al: Regional brain metabolic changes in patients with major depression treated with either paroxetine or interpersonal therapy: preliminary findings. Arch Gen Psychiatry 58:631–640, 2001

Bush G, Luu P, Posner MI: Cognitive and emotional influences in anterior cingulate cortex. Trends Cogn Sci 4: 215–222, 2000

Damasio AR, Tranel D, Damasio H: Individuals with sociopathic behavior caused by frontal damage fail to respond autonomically to social stimuli. Behav Brain Res 41:81–94, 1990

Damasio H, Grabowski T, Frank R, et al: The return of Phineas Gage: clues about the brain from the skull of a famous patient. Science 264:1102–1105, 1994

Davidson RJ, Pizzagalli D, Nitschke JB, et al: Depression: perspectives from affective neuroscience. Annu Rev Psychol 53:545–574, 2002

Davidson RJ, Irwin W, Anderle MJ, et al: The neural substrates of affective processing in depressed patients treated with venlafaxine. Am J Psychiatry 160:64–75, 2003

De la Fuente JM, Goldman S, Stanus E, et al: Brain glucose metabolism in borderline personality disorder. J Psychiatr Res 31:531–541, 1997

Devinsky O, Morrell MJ, Vogt BA: Contributions of anterior cingulate cortex to behaviour. Brain 118 (pt 1):279–306, 1995

Drevets WC: Functional neuroimaging studies of depression: the anatomy of melancholia. Annu Rev Med 49: 341–361, 1998

Drevets WC: Neuroimaging and neuropathological studies of depression: implications for the cognitive-emotional features of mood disorders. Curr Opin Neurobiol 11: 240–249, 2001

Ekman P, Sorenson ER, Friesen WV: Pan-cultural elements in facial displays of emotion. Science 164:86–88, 1969

Etkin A, Klemenhagen KC, Dudman JT, et al: Individual differences in trait anxiety predict the response of the basolateral amygdala to unconsciously processed fearful faces. Neuron 44:1043–1055, 2004

Furmark T, Tillfors M, Marteinsdottir I, et al: Common changes in cerebral blood flow in patients with social phobia treated with citalopram or cognitive-behavioral therapy. Arch Gen Psychiatry 59:425–433, 2002

Gabbard GO: Psychodynamic Psychiatry in Clinical Practice, 4th Edition. Washington, DC, American Psychiatric Publishing, 2005

Goldapple K, Segal Z, Garson C, et al: Modulation of cortical-limbic pathways in major depression: treatment-specific effects of cognitive behavior therapy. Arch Gen Psychiatry 61:34–41, 2004

Goldman-Rakic PC: Circuitry of the Primate Prefrontal Cortex and Regulation of Behavior by Representational Knowledge. Bethesda, MD, American Physiological Society, 1987

Goyer PF, Andreason PJ, Semple WE, et al: Positron-emission tomography and personality disorders. Neuropsychopharmacology 10:21–28, 1994

Horn NR, Dolan M, Elliott R, et al: Response inhibition and impulsivity: an fMRI study. Neuropsychologia 41:1959–1966, 2003

Kandel ER: Psychotherapy and the single synapse: the impact of psychiatric thought on neurobiologic research. N Engl J Med 301:1028–1037, 1979

Kennedy SH, Javanmard M, Vaccarino FJ: A review of functional neuroimaging in mood disorders: positron emission tomography and depression. Can J Psychiatry 42:467–475, 1997

Kerns JG, Cohen JD, MacDonald AW 3rd, et al: Anterior cingulate conflict monitoring and adjustments in control. Science 303:1023–1026, 2004

Leyton M, Okazawa H, Diksic M, et al: Brain regional alpha-[^{11}C]methyl-L-tryptophan trapping in impulsive subjects with borderline personality disorder. Am J Psychiatry 158:775–782, 2001

Lubman DI, Yucel M, Pantelis C: Addiction, a condition of compulsive behaviour? Neuroimaging and neuropsychological evidence of inhibitory dysregulation. Addiction 99:1491–1502, 2004

Malloy P, Bihrle A, Duffy J, et al: The orbitomedial frontal syndrome. Arch Clin Neuropsychol 8:185–201, 1993

Martin SD, Martin E, Rai SS, et al: Brain blood flow changes in depressed patients treated with interpersonal psychotherapy or venlafaxine hydrochloride: preliminary findings. Arch Gen Psychiatry 58:641–648, 2001

Mayberg HS: Limbic-cortical dysregulation: a proposed model of depression. J Neuropsychiatry Clin Neurosci 9:471–481, 1997

Mayberg HS, Brannan SK, Mahurin RK, et al: Cingulate function in depression: a potential predictor of treatment response. Neuroreport 8:1057–1061, 1997

Mayberg HS, Liotti M, Brannan SK, et al: Reciprocal limbic-cortical function and negative mood: converging PET findings in depression and normal sadness. Am J Psychiatry 156:675–682, 1999

McGuire PK, Bench CJ, Frith CD, et al: Functional anatomy of obsessive-compulsive phenomena. Br J Psychiatry 164:459–468, 1994

Meyer-Lindenberg A, Poline JB, Kohn PD, et al: Evidence for abnormal cortical functional connectivity during working memory in schizophrenia. Am J Psychiatry 158:1809–1817, 2001

Mogg K, Bradley BP: A cognitive-motivational analysis of anxiety. Behav Res Ther 36:809–848, 1998

Newton-Howes G, Tyrer P: Pharmacotherapy for personality disorders. Expert Opin Pharmacother 4:1643–1649, 2003

Paquette V, Levesque J, Mensour B, et al: Change the mind and you change the brain: effects of cognitive-behavioral therapy on the neural correlates of spider phobia. Neuroimage 18:401–409, 2003

Pizzagalli D, Pascual-Marqui RD, Nitschke JB, et al: Anterior cingulate activity as a predictor of degree of treatment response in major depression: evidence from brain electrical tomography analysis. Am J Psychiatry 158:405–415, 2001

Rauch SL, Jenike MA, Alpert NM, et al: Regional cerebral blood flow measured during symptom provocation in obsessive-compulsive disorder using oxygen-15–labeled carbon dioxide and positron emission tomography. Arch Gen Psychiatry 51:62–70, 1994

Ressler KJ, Rothbaum BO, Tannenbaum L, et al: Cognitive enhancers as adjuncts to psychotherapy: use of D-cycloserine in phobic individuals to facilitate extinction of fear. Arch Gen Psychiatry 61:1136–1144, 2004

Saxena S, Brody AL, Maidment KM, et al: Localized orbitofrontal and subcortical metabolic changes and predictors of response to paroxetine treatment in obsessive-compulsive disorder. Neuropsychopharmacology 21:683–693, 1999

Saxena S, Brody AL, Ho ML, et al: Differential brain metabolic predictors of response to paroxetine in obsessive-compulsive disorder versus major depression. Am J Psychiatry 160:522–532, 2003

Schmahl CG, McGlashan TH, Bremner JD: Neurobiological correlates of borderline personality disorder. Psychopharmacol Bull 36:69–87, 2002

Schmahl CG, Elzinga BM, Vermetten E, et al: Neural correlates of memories of abandonment in women with and without borderline personality disorder. Biol Psychiatry 54:142–151, 2003

Schwartz JM, Stoessel PW, Baxter LR Jr, et al: Systematic changes in cerebral glucose metabolic rate after successful behavior modification treatment of obsessive-compulsive disorder. Arch Gen Psychiatry 53:109–113, 1996

Siever LJ, Buchsbaum MS, New AS, et al: d,l-Fenfluramine response in impulsive personality disorder assessed with [^{18}F]fluorodeoxyglucose positron emission tomography. Neuropsychopharmacology 20:413–423, 1999

Soloff PH, Meltzer CC, Greer PJ, et al: A fenfluramine-activated FDG-PET study of borderline personality disorder. Biol Psychiatry 47:540–547, 2000

Soloff PH, Meltzer CC, Becker C, et al: Impulsivity and prefrontal hypometabolism in borderline personality disorder. Psychiatry Res 123:153–163, 2003

Tillfors M, Furmark T, Marteinsdottir I, et al: Cerebral blood flow in subjects with social phobia during stressful speaking tasks: a PET study. Am J Psychiatry 158:1220–1226, 2001

Volk SA, Kaendler SH, Hertel A, et al: Can response to partial sleep deprivation in depressed patients be predicted by regional changes of cerebral blood flow? Psychiatry Res 75:67–74, 1997

Whalen PJ, Bush G, McNally RJ, et al: The emotional counting Stroop paradigm: a functional magnetic resonance imaging probe of the anterior cingulate affective division. Biol Psychiatry 44:1219–1228, 1998

Wong PS: Anxiety, signal anxiety, and unconscious anticipation: neuroscientific evidence for an unconscious signal function in humans. J Am Psychoanal Assoc 47:817–841, 1999

Wu J, Buchsbaum MS, Gillin JC, et al: Prediction of antidepressant effects of sleep deprivation by metabolic rates in the ventral anterior cingulate and medial prefrontal cortex. Am J Psychiatry 156:1149–1158, 1999

Zanarini MC, Frankenburg FR: Olanzapine treatment of female borderline personality disorder patients: a double-blind, placebo-controlled pilot study. J Clin Psychiatry 62:849–854, 2001

Appendix

DSM-IV-TR Diagnostic Criteria for Personality Disorders

General diagnostic criteria for a personality disorder

A. An enduring pattern of inner experience and behavior that deviates markedly from the expectations of the individual's culture. This pattern is manifested in two (or more) of the following areas:
   (1) cognition (i.e., ways of perceiving and interpreting self, other people, and events)
   (2) affectivity (i.e., the range, intensity, lability, and appropriateness of emotional response)
   (3) interpersonal functioning
   (4) impulse control
B. The enduring pattern is inflexible and pervasive across a broad range of personal and social situations.
C. The enduring pattern leads to clinically significant distress or impairment in social, occupational, or other important areas of functioning.
D. The pattern is stable and of long duration, and its onset can be traced back at least to adolescence or early adulthood.
E. The enduring pattern is not better accounted for as a manifestation or consequence of another mental disorder.
F. The enduring pattern is not due to the direct physiological effects of a substance (e.g., a drug of abuse, a medication) or a general medical condition (e.g., head trauma).

Personality disorder not otherwise specified

This category is for disorders of personality functioning (refer to the general diagnostic criteria for a personality disorder) that do not meet criteria for any specific personality disorder. An example is the presence of features of more than one specific personality disorder that do not meet the full criteria for any one personality disorder ("mixed personality"), but that together cause clinically significant distress or impairment in one or more important areas of functioning (e.g., social or occupational). This category can also be used when the clinician judges that a specific personality disorder that is not included in the classification is appropriate. Examples include depressive personality disorder and passive-aggressive personality disorder.

CLUSTER A

Diagnostic criteria for paranoid personality disorder

A. A pervasive distrust and suspiciousness of others such that their motives are interpreted as malevolent, beginning by early adulthood and present in a variety of contexts, as indicated by four (or more) of the following:

   (1) suspects, without sufficient basis, that others are exploiting, harming, or deceiving him or her

   (2) is preoccupied with unjustified doubts about the loyalty or trustworthiness of friends or associates

   (3) is reluctant to confide in others because of unwarranted fear that the information will be used maliciously against him or her

   (4) reads hidden demeaning or threatening meanings into benign remarks or events

   (5) persistently bears grudges, i.e., is unforgiving of insults, injuries, or slights

   (6) perceives attacks on his or her character or reputation that are not apparent to others and is quick to react angrily or to counterattack

   (7) has recurrent suspicions, without justification, regarding fidelity of spouse or sexual partner

B. Does not occur exclusively during the course of schizophrenia, a mood disorder with psychotic features, or another psychotic disorder and is not due to the direct physiological effects of a general medical condition.

Diagnostic criteria for schizoid personality disorder

A. A pervasive pattern of detachment from social relationships and a restricted range of expression of emotions in interpersonal settings, beginning by early adulthood and present in a variety of contexts, as indicated by four (or more) of the following:

   (1) neither desires nor enjoys close relationships, including being part of a family

   (2) almost always chooses solitary activities

   (3) has little, if any, interest in having sexual experiences with another person

   (4) takes pleasure in few, if any, activities

   (5) lacks close friends or confidants other than first-degree relatives

   (6) appears indifferent to the praise or criticism of others

   (7) shows emotional coldness, detachment, or flattened affectivity

B. Does not occur exclusively during the course of schizophrenia, a mood disorder with psychotic features, another psychotic disorder, or a pervasive developmental disorder and is not due to the direct physiological effects of a general medical condition.

CLUSTER A *(CONTINUED)*

Diagnostic criteria for schizotypal personality disorder

A. A pervasive pattern of social and interpersonal deficits marked by acute discomfort with, and reduced capacity for, close relationships as well as by cognitive or perceptual distortions and eccentricities of behavior, beginning by early adulthood and present in a variety of contexts, as indicated by five (or more) of the following:

(1) ideas of reference (excluding delusions of reference)

(2) odd beliefs or magical thinking that influences behavior and is inconsistent with subcultural norms (e.g., superstitiousness, belief in clairvoyance, telepathy, or "sixth sense"; in children and adolescents, bizarre fantasies or preoccupations)

(3) unusual perceptual experiences, including bodily illusions

(4) odd thinking and speech (e.g., vague, circumstantial, metaphorical, overelaborate, or stereotyped)

(5) suspiciousness or paranoid ideation

(6) inappropriate or constricted affect

(7) behavior or appearance that is odd, eccentric, or peculiar

(8) lack of close friends or confidants other than first-degree relatives

(9) excessive social anxiety that does not diminish with familiarity and tends to be associated with paranoid fears rather than negative judgments about self

B. Does not occur exclusively during the course of schizophrenia, a mood disorder with psychotic features, another psychotic disorder, or a pervasive developmental disorder.

CLUSTER B

Diagnostic criteria for antisocial personality disorder

A. There is a pervasive pattern of disregard for and violation of the rights of others occurring since age 15 years, as indicated by three (or more) of the following:
   (1) failure to conform to social norms with respect to lawful behaviors as indicated by repeatedly performing acts that are grounds for arrest
   (2) deceitfulness, as indicated by repeated lying, use of aliases, or conning others for personal profit or pleasure
   (3) impulsivity or failure to plan ahead
   (4) irritability and aggressiveness, as indicated by repeated physical fights or assaults
   (5) reckless disregard for safety of self or others
   (6) consistent irresponsibility, as indicated by repeated failure to sustain consistent work behavior or honor financial obligations
   (7) lack of remorse, as indicated by being indifferent to or rationalizing having hurt, mistreated, or stolen from another
B. The individual is at least age 18 years.
C. There is evidence of conduct disorder with onset before age 15 years.
D. The occurrence of antisocial behavior is not exclusively during the course of schizophrenia or a manic episode.

Diagnostic criteria for borderline personality disorder

A pervasive pattern of instability of interpersonal relationships, self-image, and affects, and marked impulsivity beginning by early adulthood and present in a variety of contexts, as indicated by five (or more) of the following:
   (1) frantic efforts to avoid real or imagined abandonment
   Note: Do not include suicidal or self-mutilating behavior covered in Criterion 5.
   (2) a pattern of unstable and intense interpersonal relationships characterized by alternating between extremes of idealization and devaluation
   (3) identity disturbance: markedly and persistently unstable self-image or sense of self
   (4) impulsivity in at least two areas that are potentially self-damaging (e.g., spending, sex, substance abuse, reckless driving, binge eating)   **Note:** Do not include suicidal or self-mutilating behavior covered in Criterion 5.
   (5) recurrent suicidal behavior, gestures, or threats, or self-mutilating behavior
   (6) affective instability due to a marked reactivity of mood (e.g., intense episodic dysphoria, irritability, or anxiety usually lasting a few hours and only rarely more than a few days)
   (7) chronic feelings of emptiness
   (8) inappropriate, intense anger or difficulty controlling anger (e.g., frequent displays of temper, constant anger, recurrent physical fights)
   (9) transient, stress-related paranoid ideation or severe dissociative symptoms

Diagnostic criteria for histrionic personality disorder

A pervasive pattern of excessive emotionality and attention seeking, beginning by early adulthood and present in a variety of contexts, as indicated by five (or more) of the following:
   (1) is uncomfortable in situations in which he or she is not the center of attention
   (2) interaction with others is often characterized by inappropriate sexually seductive or provocative behavior
   (3) displays rapidly shifting and shallow expression of emotions
   (4) consistently uses physical appearance to draw attention to self
   (5) has a style of speech that is excessively impressionistic and lacking in detail
   (6) shows self-dramatization, theatricality, and exaggerated expression of emotion
   (7) is suggestible, i.e., easily influenced by others or circumstances
   (8) considers relationships to be more intimate than they actually are

CLUSTER B *(CONTINUED)*

Diagnostic criteria for narcissistic personality disorder

A pervasive pattern of grandiosity (in fantasy or behavior), need for admiration, and lack of empathy, beginning by early adulthood and present in a variety of contexts, as indicated by five (or more) of the following:

(1) has a grandiose sense of self-importance (e.g., exaggerates achievements and talents, expects to be recognized as superior without commensurate achievements)

(2) is preoccupied with fantasies of unlimited success, power, brilliance, beauty, or ideal love

(3) believes that he or she is "special" and unique and can only be understood by, or should associate with, other special or high-status people (or institutions)

(4) requires excessive admiration

(5) has a sense of entitlement, i.e., unreasonable expectations of especially favorable treatment or automatic compliance with his or her expectations

(6) is interpersonally exploitative, i.e., takes advantage of others to achieve his or her own ends

(7) lacks empathy: is unwilling to recognize or identify with the feelings and needs of others

(8) is often envious of others or believes that others are envious of him or her

(9) shows arrogant, haughty behaviors or attitudes

Cluster C

Diagnostic criteria for avoidant personality disorder

A pervasive pattern of social inhibition, feelings of inadequacy, and hypersensitivity to negative evaluation, beginning by early adulthood and present in a variety of contexts, as indicated by four (or more) of the following:

  (1) avoids occupational activities that involve significant interpersonal contact, because of fears of criticism, disapproval, or rejection
  (2) is unwilling to get involved with people unless certain of being liked
  (3) shows restraint within intimate relationships because of the fear of being shamed or ridiculed
  (4) is preoccupied with being criticized or rejected in social situations
  (5) is inhibited in new interpersonal situations because of feelings of inadequacy
  (6) views self as socially inept, personally unappealing, or inferior to others
  (7) is unusually reluctant to take personal risks or to engage in any new activities because they may prove embarrassing

Diagnostic criteria for dependent personality disorder

A pervasive and excessive need to be taken care of that leads to submissive and clinging behavior and fears of separation, beginning by early adulthood and present in a variety of contexts, as indicated by five (or more) of the following:

  (1) has difficulty making everyday decisions without an excessive amount of advice and reassurance from others
  (2) needs others to assume responsibility for most major areas of his or her life
  (3) has difficulty expressing disagreement with others because of fear of loss of support or approval
      Note: Do not include realistic fears of retribution.
  (4) has difficulty initiating projects or doing things on his or her own (because of a lack of self-confidence in judgment or abilities rather than a lack of motivation or energy)
  (5) goes to excessive lengths to obtain nurturance and support from others, to the point of volunteering to do things that are unpleasant
  (6) feels uncomfortable or helpless when alone because of exaggerated fears of being unable to care for himself or herself
  (7) urgently seeks another relationship as a source of care and support when a close relationship ends
  (8) is unrealistically preoccupied with fears of being left to take care of himself or herself

Diagnostic criteria for obsessive-compulsive personality disorder

A pervasive pattern of preoccupation with orderliness, perfectionism, and mental and interpersonal control, at the expense of flexibility, openness, and efficiency, beginning by early adulthood and present in a variety of contexts, as indicated by four (or more) of the following:

  (1) is preoccupied with details, rules, lists, order, organization, or schedules to the extent that the major point of the activity is lost
  (2) shows perfectionism that interferes with task completion (e.g., is unable to complete a project because his or her own overly strict standards are not met)
  (3) is excessively devoted to work and productivity to the exclusion of leisure activities and friendships (not accounted for by obvious economic necessity)
  (4) is overconscientious, scrupulous, and inflexible about matters of morality, ethics, or values (not accounted for by cultural or religious identification)
  (5) is unable to discard worn-out or worthless objects even when they have no sentimental value
  (6) is reluctant to delegate tasks or to work with others unless they submit to exactly his or her way of doing things
  (7) adopts a miserly spending style toward both self and others; money is viewed as something to be hoarded for future catastrophes
  (8) shows rigidity and stubbornness

Index

Page numbers printed in *boldface* type refer to tables or figures.